OPTUM360°®

ICD-10-PCS

The complete official code set

Codes valid from October 1, 2021, through September 30, 2022

2022 **optum360coding.com**

Notice

ICD-10-PCS: The Complete Official Code Set is designed to be an accurate and authoritative source regarding coding and every reasonable effort has been made to ensure accuracy and completeness of the content. However, Optum360 makes no guarantee, warranty, or representation that this publication is accurate, complete, or without errors. It is understood that Optum360 is not rendering any legal or other professional services or advice in this publication and that Optum360 bears no liability for any results or consequences that may arise from the use of this book. Please address all correspondence to:

Optum360
2525 Lake Park Blvd
Salt Lake City, UT 84120

Our Commitment to Accuracy

Optum360 is committed to producing accurate and reliable materials. To report corrections, please visit www.optum360coding.com/accuracy or email accuracy@optum.com. You can also reach customer service by calling 1.800.464.3649, option 1.

Copyright

Made in the USA
ISBN 978-1-62254-776-0 (Spiral)
ISBN 978-1-62254-777-7 (Softbound)

Acknowledgments

Marianne Randall, CPC, *Product Manager*

Anita Schmidt, BS, RHIA, AHIMA-approved ICD-10-CM/PCS Trainer, *Subject Matter Expert*

Karen Krawzik, RHIT, CCS, AHIMA-approved ICD-10-CM/PCS Trainer, *Subject Matter Expert*

LaJuana Green, RHIA, CCS, *Subject Matter Expert*

Stacy Perry, *Manager, Desktop Publishing*

Tracy Betzler, *Senior Desktop Publishing Specialist*

Hope M. Dunn, *Senior Desktop Publishing Specialist*

Katie Russell, *Desktop Publishing Specialist*

Kate Holden, *Editor*

Anita Schmidt, BS, RHIA, AHIMA-approved ICD-10-CM/PCS Trainer

Ms. Schmidt has expertise in ICD-10-CM/PCS, DRG, and CPT with more than 15 years' experience in coding in multiple settings, including inpatient, observation, and same-day surgery. Her experience includes analysis of medical record documentation, assignment of ICD-10-CM and PCS codes, and DRG validation. She has conducted training for ICD-10-CM/PCS and electronic health record. She has also collaborated with clinical documentation specialists to identify documentation needs and potential areas for physician education. Most recently she has been developing content for resource and educational products related to ICD-10-CM, ICD-10-PCS, DRG, and CPT. Ms. Schmidt is an AHIMA-approved ICD-10-CM/PCS trainer and is an active member of the American Health Information Management Association (AHIMA) and the Minnesota Health Information Management Association (MHIMA).

Karen Krawzik, RHIT, CCS, AHIMA-approved ICD-10-CM/PCS Trainer

Ms. Krawzik has expertise in ICD-10-CM, ICD-9-CM, CPT/HCPCS, DRG, and data quality and analytics, with more than 30 years' experience coding in multiple settings, including inpatient, observation, ambulatory surgery, ancillary, and emergency room. She has served as a DRG analyst and auditor of commercial and government payer claims, as a contract administrator, and worked on a team providing enterprise-wide conversion of the ICD-9-CM code set to ICD-10. More recently, she has been developing print and electronic content related to ICD-10-CM and ICD-10-PCS coding systems, MS-DRGs, and HCCs. Ms. Krawzik is credentialed by the American Health Information Management Association (AHIMA) as a Registered Health Information Technician (RHIT) and a Certified Coding Specialist (CCS) and is an AHIMA-approved ICD-10-CM/PCS trainer. She is an active member of AHIMA and the Missouri Health Information Management Association.

Product Updates

Significant updates to this manual will also be provided on our product updates page at Optum360coding.com, which can be accessed at the following:

https://www.optum360coding.com/ProductUpdates/
Password: PCS22UPD

Contents

What's New for 2022 iii

Introduction 1
- Number of Codes in ICD-10-PCS 1
- ICD-10-PCS Manual 1
- Medical and Surgical Section (Ø) 4
- Obstetrics Section (1) 7
- Placement Section (2) 8
- Administration Section (3) 9
- Measurement and Monitoring Section (4) 9
- Extracorporeal or Systemic Assistance and Performance Section (5) 10
- Extracorporeal or Systemic Therapies Section (6) 10
- Osteopathic Section (7) 11
- Other Procedures Section (8) 11
- Chiropractic Section (9) 12
- Imaging Section (B) 12
- Nuclear Medicine Section (C) 13
- Radiation Therapy Section (D) 13
- Physical Rehabilitation and Diagnostic Audiology Section (F) 14
- Mental Health Section (G) 15
- Substance Abuse Treatment Section (H) 15
- New Technology Section (X) 16

ICD-10-PCS Index and Tabular Format 19
- Index 19
- Code Tables 19

ICD-10-PCS Additional Features 21
- Use of Official Sources 21
- Table Notations 21
- Appendixes 22

ICD-10-PCS Official Guidelines for Coding and Reporting 2022 25
- Conventions 25
- Medical and Surgical Section Guidelines (section Ø) 26
- Obstetric Section Guidelines (section 1) 30
- Radiation Therapy Section Guidelines (section D) 31
- New Technology Section Guidelines (section X) 31

ICD-10-PCS Index 33

ICD-10-PCS Tables 131
- Central Nervous System and Cranial Nerves 131
- Peripheral Nervous System 153
- Heart and Great Vessels 171
- Upper Arteries 193
- Lower Arteries 219
- Upper Veins 243
- Lower Veins 263
- Lymphatic and Hemic Systems 283
- Eye 301
- Ear, Nose, Sinus 319
- Respiratory System 339
- Mouth and Throat 355
- Gastrointestinal System 373
- Hepatobiliary System and Pancreas 401
- Endocrine System 415
- Skin and Breast 425
- Subcutaneous Tissue and Fascia 443
- Muscles 463
- Tendons 485
- Bursae and Ligaments 499
- Head and Facial Bones 521
- Upper Bones 541
- Lower Bones 561
- Upper Joints 579
- Lower Joints 599
- Urinary System 621
- Female Reproductive System 637
- Male Reproductive System 657
- Anatomical Regions, General 673
- Anatomical Regions, Upper Extremities 685
- Anatomical Regions, Lower Extremities 695
- Obstetrics 705
- Placement 709
- Administration 715
- Measurement and Monitoring 727
- Extracorporeal or Systemic Assistance and Performance 731
- Extracorporeal or Systemic Therapies 733
- Osteopathic 735
- Other Procedures 737
- Chiropractic 739
- Imaging 741
- Nuclear Medicine 771
- Radiation Therapy 781
- Physical Rehabilitation and Diagnostic Audiology 799
- Mental Health 811
- Substance Abuse Treatment 813
- New Technology 815

Appendixes 825
- Appendix A: Components of the Medical and Surgical Approach Definitions 825
- Appendix B: Root Operation Definitions 828
- Appendix C: Comparison of Medical and Surgical Root Operations 833
- Appendix D: Body Part Key 835
- Appendix E: Body Part Definitions 851
- Appendix F: Device Classification 863
- Appendix G: Device Key and Aggregation Table 865
- Appendix H: Device Definitions 874
- Appendix I: Substance Key/Substance Definitions 880
- Appendix J: Sections B–H Character Definitions 885
- Appendix K: Hospital Acquired Conditions 894
- Appendix L: Procedure Combination Tables 913
- Appendix M: Coding Exercises and Answers 932

What's New for 2022

The Centers for Medicare and Medicaid Services is the agency charged with maintaining and updating ICD-10-PCS. CMS released the most current revisions, a summary of which may be found on the CMS website at https://www.cms.gov/medicare/icd-10/2022-icd-10-pcs.

Due to the unique structure of ICD-10-PCS, a change in a character value may affect individual codes and several code tables.

Change Summary Table

2021 Total	New Codes	Revised Titles	Deleted Codes	2022 Total
78,136	191	62	107	78,220

ICD-10-PCS Code FY 2022 Totals, By Section

Medical and Surgical	67,754
Obstetrics	304
Placement	861
Administration	1,253
Measurement and Monitoring	422
Extracorporeal or Systemic Assistance and Performance	52
Extracorporeal or Systemic Therapies	46
Osteopathic	100
Other Procedures	78
Chiropractic	90
Imaging	2,977
Nuclear Medicine	463
Radiation Therapy	2,087
Physical Rehabilitation and Diagnostic Audiology	1,380
Mental Health	30
Substance Abuse Treatment	59
New Technology	264
Total	78,220

ICD-10-PCS Table Changes Highlights

- New rows added to root operation table Extraction in the Central Nervous System and Cranial Nerves body system, capturing body part values Brain and Cerebral Hemisphere
- New qualifier Orbital Atherectomy Technique added to root operation table Extirpation in the Heart and Great Vessels body system, Percutaneous approach, for body parts Coronary Artery, One; Coronary Artery, Two; Coronary Artery, Three Arteries; and Coronary Artery, Four or More Arteries
- New row added to root operation table Fragmentation in the Heart and Great Vessels body system, capturing body parts Coronary Artery, One; Coronary Artery, Two; Coronary Artery, Three Arteries; and Coronary Artery, Four or More Arteries
- New rows added to root operation table Replacement in the Heart and Great Vessels body system, adding body part Heart, Open approach, with Devices Biologic with Synthetic Substitute, Autoregulated Electrohydraulic and Synthetic Substitute, Pneumatic, and new rows added to body part Pulmonary Valve, device Zooplastic Tissue, to capture new Device qualifiers In Existing Conduit and Native Site
- New body part value Ventricle, Left, added to root operation table Restriction in the Heart and Great Vessels body system
- Approach value Percutaneous added to body parts Brachial Artery, Left, and Brachial Artery, Right, in the root operation table Bypass in the Upper Arteries body system
- New body part value Intracranial Artery added to root operation table Fragmentation in the Upper Arteries body system
- New approach values Via Natural or Artificial Opening and Via Natural or Artificial Opening Endoscopic added to root operation table Occlusion in the Lower Veins body system, body part Lower Vein
- New body part value Bone Marrow added to root operation table Extraction in the Lymphatic and Hemic Systems body system
- New body part values Liver; Liver, Right Lobe; and Liver, Left Lobe, added to root operation table Division in the Hepatobiliary System and Pancreas body system
- New row added specific to body part Tongue, Palate, Pharynx Muscle, to root operation table Division in the Muscles body system with two new approach values, Via Natural and Artificial Opening and Via Natural and Artificial Opening Endoscopic
- New device value added to body part Skull in the root operation table Insertion in the Head and Facial Bones body system to capture Infusion Device
- New device value for Spinal Stabilization Device, Vertebral Body Tether, added to root operation table Reposition in the Upper Bones body system for body part Thoracic Vertebra and root operation table Reposition in the Lower Bones body system for body part Lumbar Vertebra
- New rows added to root operation table Excision in the Lower Bones body system, specific to body parts Metatarsal, Right, and Metatarsal, Left, adding new qualifier value Sesamoid Bone(s) 1st Toe
- New rows added specific to body parts Shoulder Joint, Right, and Shoulder Joint, Left, adding new qualifier values Humeral Surface and Glenoid Surface to root operation tables Removal and Revision in the Upper Joints body system
- New substance Pathogen Reduced Cryoprecipitated Fibrinogen Complex, with qualifier Nonautologous, added to root operation table Transfusion, Circulatory, in the Administration section
- New approach Percutaneous Endoscopic added to root operation table Irrigation, Physiological Systems and Anatomical Regions, in the Administration section, for body part Peritoneal Cavity
- New row added to root operation table Measurement, Physiological Devices, in the Measurement and Monitory section for body system Central Nervous with Function/Device value Cerebrospinal Fluid Shunt and qualifier Wireless Sensor
- New qualifier Automated added to root operation table Performance, Physiological Systems, for body system Cardiac, Duration Continuous, Function Output
- New rows added for body part Liver to root operation table Fluoroscopy, Hepatobiliary System and Pancreas, in the Imaging section
- New row added to New Technology root operation table Extirpation, Cardiovascular System New Technology Group 7, and deleted rows for New Technology Group 1

- New body part Thoracic Aorta, Arch, added to New Technology root operation table Replacement, Cardiovascular System, with device Branched Synthetic Substitute with Intraluminal Device, New Technology Group 7
- New row added to New Technology root operation table Replacement, Skin, Subcutaneous Tissue, Fascia and Breast, to capture Device/Substance/Technology Bioengineered Allogeneic Construct, New Technology Group 7
- New device value Posterior (Dynamic) Distraction Device added to New Technology root operation table Reposition, Bones, New Technology Group 7
- New device value Interbody Fusion Device, Customizable, added to New Technology root operation table Fusion, Joints, New Technology Group 7
- Multiple Device/Substance/Technology values added to New Technology root operation table Introduction, Anatomical Regions
- New Device/Substance/Technology values Hyperimmune Globulin and High-Dose Intravenous Immune Globulin added to New Technology root operation table Transfusion, Anatomical Regions
- New row added in New Technology root operation table Measurement, Physiological Systems, for body part Central Nervous, Device/Substance/Technology Computer-aided Triage and Notification, New Technology Group 7, and body part Arterial, Device/Substance/Technology Pulmonary Artery Flow, Computer-Aided Triage and Notification, and body part Nose, Device/Substance/Technology Infection, Nasopharyngeal Fluid SARS-CoV-2 Polymerase Chain Reaction
- New row added to New Technology root operation table Introduction, Extracorporeal, for body part Extracorporeal, Device/Substance/Technology Nafamostat Anticoagulant, New Technology Group 7
- Seven new tables in New Technology section:
  - — X2J Cardiovascular System, Inspection
  - — X2K Cardiovascular System, Bypass
  - — X2V Cardiovascular System, Restriction
  - — XD2 Gastrointestinal System, Monitoring
  - — XDP Gastrointestinal System, Irrigation
  - — XFJ Hepatobiliary System and Pancreas, Inspection
  - — XWH Anatomical Regions, Insertion
- Two deleted tables in the New Technology Section:
  - — XR2 Joints, Monitoring
  - — XW2 Anatomical Regions, Transfusion

New Definitions Addenda

Section 0 — Medical and Surgical Body Part Definitions

ICD-10-PCS Value	Definition
Cervical Spinal Cord	Add Dorsal root ganglion
Lumbar Spinal Cord	Add Dorsal root ganglion
Metatarsal, Left	Add Fibular sesamoid Add Tibial sesamoid
Metatarsal, Right	Add Fibular sesamoid Add Tibial sesamoid
Neck	Add Parapharyngeal space Add Retropharyngeal space
Spinal Cord	Add Dorsal root ganglion
Thoracic Spinal Cord	Add Dorsal root ganglion

Section 0 — Medical and Surgical Device Definitions

ICD-10-PCS Value	Definition
Add Biologic with Synthetic Substitute, Autoregulated Electrohydraulic for Replacement in Heart and Great Vessels	Add Carmat total artificial heart (TAH)
Add Other Device	Add Alfapump® system
Stimulator Generator, Multiple Array for Insertion in Subcutaneous Tissue and Fascia	Add PERCEPT™ PC neurostimulator
Stimulator Generator, Single Array for Insertion in Subcutaneous Tissue and Fascia	Delete InterStim® Therapy neurostimulator Add InterStim™ II Therapy neurostimulator
Stimulator Generator, Single Array Rechargeable for Insertion in Subcutaneous Tissue and Fascia	Add InterStim™ Micro Therapy neurostimulator
Synthetic Substitute, Pneumatic for Replacement in Heart and Great Vessels	Add SynCardia (temporary) total artificial heart (TAH)

Section 0 — Medical and Surgical Device Aggregation Table

Specific Device	for Operation	in Body System	General Device
Add Spinal Stabilization Device, Vertebral Body Tether	Add Reposition	Add Lower Bones Add Upper Bones	Add 4 Internal Fixation Device

Section 3 - Administration Substance Definitions

ICD-10-PCS Value	Definition
Add Globulin	Add Gammaglobulin Add Hyperimmune globulin Add Immunoglobulin Add Polyclonal hyperimmune globulin
Hematopoietic Stem/Progenitor Cells, Genetically Modified	Add OTL-101 Add OTL-103 Add OTL-200
Add Other Anti-infective	Add AVYCAZ® (ceftazidime-avibactam) Add Ceftazidime-avibactam Add CRESEMBA® (isavuconazonium sulfate) Add Isavuconazole (isavuconazonium sulfate)
Add Other Antineoplastic	Add Blinatumomab Add BLINCYTO® (blinatumomab)
Add Other Therapeutic Substance	Add Idarucizumab, Pradaxa®(dabigatran) reversal agent Add Praxbind® (idarucizumab), Pradaxa®(dabigatran) reversal agent
Add Pathogen Reduced Cryoprecipitated Fibrinogen Complex	Add INTERCEPT Blood System for Plasma Pathogen Reduced Cryoprecipitated Fibrinogen Complex Add INTERCEPT Fibrinogen Complex

Section X — New Technology Root Operation Definitions

ICD-10-PCS Value	Definition
Add Bypass	Add Definition: Altering the route of passage of the contents of a tubular body part.
Add Insertion	Add Definition: Putting in a nonbiological appliance that monitors, assists, performs, or prevents a physiological function but does not physically take the place of a body part.
Add Inspection	Add Definition: Visually and/or manually exploring a body part.
Add Irrigation	Add Definition: Putting in or on a cleansing substance
Add Restriction	Add Definition: Partially closing an orifice or the lumen of a tubular body part.

Section X — New Technology Device/Substance/Technology Definitions

ICD-10-PCS Value	Definition
Add Antibiotic-eluting Bone Void Filler	Add CERAMENT® G
Add Axicabtagene Ciloleucel Immunotherapy	Add Axicabtagene Ciloleucel Add Yescarta®
Add Bioengineered Allogeneic Construct	Add StrataGraft®
Add Branched Synthetic Substitute with Intraluminal Device in New Technology	Add Thoraflex™ Hybrid device
Brexucabtagene Autoleucel Immunotherapy	Add Tecartus™
Delete Engineered Autologous Chimeric Antigen Receptor T-cell Immunotherapy	Delete Axicabtagene Ciloeucel Delete KYMRIAH Delete Tisagenlecleucel
Add Bromelain-enriched Proteolytic Enzyme	Add NexoBrid™
Add Ciltacabtagene Autoleucel	Add cilta-cel
Add High-Dose Intravenous Immune Globulin	Add GAMUNEX-C, for COVID-19 treatment Add hdIVIG (high-dose intravenous immunoglobulin), for COVID-19 treatment Add High-dose intravenous immunoglobulin (hdIVIG), for COVID-19 treatment Add Octagam 10%, for COVID-19 treatment
Add Hyperimmune Globulin	Add Anti-SARS-CoV-2 hyperimmune globulin Add HIG (hyperimmune globulin), for COVID-19 treatment Add hIVIG (hyperimmune intravenous immunoglobulin), for COVID-19 treatment Add Hyperimmune intravenous immunoglobulin (hIVIG), for COVID-19 treatment Add IGIV-C, for COVID-19 treatment
Add Idecabtagene Vicleucel Immunotherapy	Add ABECMA® Add Ide-cel Add Idecabtagene Vicleucel
Add Interbody Fusion Device, Customizable in New Technology	Add aprevo™
Add Lifileucel Immunotherapy	Add Lifileucel
Add Lurbinectedin	Add ZEPZELCA™
Add Nafamostat Anticoagulant	Add LTX Regional Anticoagulant Add Niyad™
Add Posterior (Dynamic) Distraction Device in New Technology	Add ApiFix® Minimally Invasive Deformity Correction (MID-C) System
Add Reduction Device in New Technology	Add Neovasc Reducer™ Add Reducer™ System
Add REGN-COV2 Monoclonal Antibody	Add Casirivimab (REGN10933) and Imdevimab (REGN10987) Add Imdevimab (REGN10987) and Casirivimab (REGN10933)
Add Satralizumab-mwge	Add ENSPRYNG™
Add Terlipressin	Add TERLIVAZ®
Add Tisagenlecleucel Immunotherapy	Add KYMRIAH® Add Tisagenlecleucel
Add Trilaciclib	Add COSELA™

List of Updated Files

2022 Official ICD-10-PCS Coding Guidelines

- Guidelines B3.7, B4.1c, B4.8, E.1a, and E.1b revised in response to public comment and internal review
- Downloadable PDF

2022 ICD-10-PCS Code Tables and Index (Zip file)

- Code tables for use beginning October 1, 2021
- Downloadable PDF, file name is pcs_2022.pdf
- Downloadable xml files for developers, file names are icd10pcs_tables_2022.xml, icd10pcs_index_2022.xml, icd10pcs_definitions_2022.xml
- Accompanying schema for developers, file names are icd10pcs_tables.xsd, icd10pcs_index.xsd, icd10pcs_definitions.xsd

2022 ICD-10-PCS Codes File (Zip file)

- ICD-10-PCS codes file is a simple format for nontechnical uses, containing the valid FY 2022 ICD-10-PCS codes and their long titles
- File is in text file format: file name is icd10pcs_codes_2022.txt
- Accompanying documentation for codes file: file name is icd10pcsCodesFile.pdf
- Codes file addenda in text format: file name is codes_addenda_2022.txt

2022 ICD-10-PCS Order File (Long and Abbreviated Titles) (Zip file)

- ICD-10-PCS order file is for developers, provides a unique five-digit "order number" for each ICD-10-PCS table and code, as well as a long and abbreviated code title.
- ICD-10-PCS order file name is icd10pcs_order_2022.txt
- Accompanying documentation for tabular order file: file name is icd10pcsOrderFile.pdf
- Tabular order file addenda in text format: file name is order_addenda_2022.txt

2022 ICD-10-PCS Final Addenda (Zip file)

- Addenda files in downloadable PDF: file names are tables_addenda_2022.pdf, index_addenda_2022.pdf, definitions_addenda_2022.pdf
- Addenda files also in machine readable text format for developers: file names are tables_addenda_2022.txt, index_addenda_2022.txt, definitions_addenda_2022.txt

2022 ICD-10-PCS Conversion Table (Zip file)

- ICD-10-PCS code conversion table is provided to assist users in data retrieval, in downloadable Excel spreadsheet: file name is icd10pcs_conversion_table_2022.xlsx
- Conversion table also in machine readable text format for developers: file name is icd10pcs_conversion_table_2022.txt
- Accompanying documentation for code conversion table: file name is icd10pcsConversionTable.pdf

Introduction

ICD-10-PCS: The Complete Official Code Set is your definitive coding resource for procedure coding in acute inpatient hospitals. In addition to the official ICD-10-PCS Coding System Files, revised and distributed by the Centers for Medicare and Medicaid Services (CMS), Optum360's coding experts have incorporated Medicare-related coding edits and proprietary features, such as coding tools and appendixes, into a comprehensive and easy-to-use reference.

This manual provides the most current information that was available at the time of publication. For updates to official source documents that may have occurred after this manual was published, please refer to the following:

- **CMS International Classification of Disease, 10th Revision, Procedural Coding System (ICD-10-PCS):**
  https://www.cms.gov/medicare/icd-10/2022-icd-10-pcs
- **CMS Inpatient Prospective Payment System Proposed Rule, FY2022**
  https://www.cms.gov/medicare/acute-inpatient-pps/fy-2022-ipps-proposed-rule-home-page
- **CMS Inpatient Prospective Payment System Proposed Rule, FY 2022 - Proposed, version 39, MS-DRG Grouper software, Definitions Manual files and Medicare Code Editor (MCE) files**
  https://www.cms.gov/Medicare/Medicare-Fee-for-Service-Payment/AcuteInpatientPPS/MS-DRG-Classifications-and-Software
- **American Hospital Association (AHA) Coding Clinics**
  https://www.codingclinicadvisor.com/

ICD-10-PCS Code Structure

ICD-10-PCS has a seven-character alphanumeric code structure. Each character contains up to 34 possible values. Each value represents a specific option for the general character definition. The 10 digits Ø–9 and the 24 letters A–H, J–N, and P–Z may be used in each character. The letters O and I are not used so as to avoid confusion with the digits Ø and 1. An ICD-10-PCS code is the result of a process rather than as a single fixed set of digits or alphabetic characters. The process consists of combining semi-independent values from among a selection of values, according to the rules governing the construction of codes.

	Section	Body System	Root Operation	Body Part	Approach	Device	Qualifier
Characters:	1	2	3	4	5	6	7

A code is derived by choosing a specific value for each of the seven characters. Based on details about the procedure performed, values for each character specifying the section, body system, root operation, body part, approach, device, and qualifier are assigned. Because the definition of each character is also a function of its physical position in the code, the same letter or number placed in a different position in the code has a different meaning.

The seven characters that make up a complete code have specific meanings that vary for each of the 17 sections of the manual.

Procedures are then divided into sections that identify the general type of procedure (e.g., Medical and Surgical, Obstetrics, Imaging). The first character of the procedure code always specifies the section. The second through seventh characters have the same meaning within each section, but may mean different things in other sections. In all sections, the third character specifies the general type of procedure performed (e.g., Resection, Transfusion, Fluoroscopy), while the other characters give additional information such as the body part and approach.

In ICD-10-PCS, the term *procedure* refers to the complete specification of the seven characters.

Number of Codes in ICD-10-PCS

The table structure of ICD-10-PCS permits the specification of a large number of codes on a single page. At the time of this publication, there are 78,220 codes in the 2022 ICD-10-PCS.

ICD-10-PCS Manual

Index

Codes may be found in the index based on the general type of procedure (e.g., resection, transfusion, fluoroscopy), or a more commonly used term (e.g., appendectomy). For example, the code for percutaneous intraluminal dilation of the coronary arteries with an intraluminal device can be found in the Index under *Dilation*, or a synonym of *Dilation* (e.g., angioplasty). The Index then specifies the first three or four values of the code or directs the user to see another term.

Example:

Dilation
Artery
Coronary
One Artery Ø27Ø

Based on the first three values of the code provided in the Index, the corresponding table can be located. In the example above, the first three values indicate table Ø27 is to be referenced for code completion.

The tables and characters are arranged first by number and then by letter for each character (tables for ØØ-, Ø1-, Ø2-, etc., are followed by those for ØB-, ØC-, ØD-, etc., followed by ØB1, ØB2, etc., followed by ØBB, ØBC, ØBD, etc.).

Note: The Tables section must be used to construct a complete and valid code by specifying the last three or four values.

Tables

The tables in ICD-10-PCS provide the valid combination of character values needed to build a unique procedure code. Each table is preceded by the first three characters of the code, along with their descriptions. In the Medical and Surgical section, for example, the first three characters contain the name of the section (character 1), the body system (character 2), and the root operation performed (character 3).

Listed underneath the first three characters is a table comprising four columns and one or more rows. The four columns in the table specify the last four characters needed to complete the ICD-10-PCS code. Depending on the section, the labels for each column may be different. In the Medical and Surgical section, they are labeled body part (character 4), approach (character 5), device (character 6), and qualifier (character 7). Each row in the table specifies the valid combination of values for characters 4 through 7.

Introduction

Table 1: Row from table Ø27

Ø Medical and Surgical
2 Heart and Great Vessels
7 Dilation Definition: Expanding an orifice or the lumen of a tubular body part

Explanation: The orifice can be a natural orifice or an artificially created orifice. Accomplished by stretching a tubular body part using intraluminal pressure or by cutting part of the orifice or wall of the tubular body part.

Body Part Character 4	Approach Character 5	Device Character 6	Qualifier Character 7
Ø Coronary Artery, One Artery **1 Coronary Artery, Two Arteries** **2 Coronary Artery, Three Arteries** **3 Coronary Artery, Four or More Arteries**	**Ø Open** **3 Percutaneous** **4 Percutaneous Endoscopic**	**4 Intraluminal Device, Drug-eluting** **5 Intraluminal Device, Drug-eluting, Two** **6 Intraluminal Device, Drug-eluting, Three** **7 Intraluminal Device, Drug-eluting, Four or More** **D Intraluminal Device** **E Intraluminal Device, Two** **F Intraluminal Device, Three** **G Intraluminal Device, Four or More** **T Intraluminal Device, Radioactive** **Z No Device**	**6 Bifurcation** **Z No Qualifier**

For instance, table 1 above shows the first row from table Ø27 in ICD-10-PCS. The values *Ø27* specify the section *Medical and Surgical (Ø)*, the body system *Heart and Great Vessels (2)*, and the root operation *Dilation (7)*. As shown, the root operation (Dilation) is also accompanied by its corresponding definition and explanation. Note, a definition of the root operation is provided for every table in ICD-10-PCS; however, an explanation may not always be applicable.

In total, this single row can be used to construct 240 unique procedure codes. The valid codes shown in table 2 (below) are constructed using the body part (character 4) value of Ø, Coronary artery, one artery, combined with all valid approach (character 5) values, device (character 6) values, and a qualifier (character 7) value of Z, No Qualifier.

Table 2: Code titles for dilation of one coronary artery (Ø27Ø)

Ø27ØØ4Z	Dilation of Coronary Artery, One Artery with Drug-eluting Intraluminal Device, Open Approach
Ø27ØØ5Z	Dilation of Coronary Artery, One Artery with Two Drug-eluting Intraluminal Devices, Open Approach
Ø27ØØ6Z	Dilation of Coronary Artery, One Artery with Three Drug-eluting Intraluminal Devices, Open Approach
Ø27ØØ7Z	Dilation of Coronary Artery, One Artery with Four or More Drug-eluting Intraluminal Devices, Open Approach
Ø27ØØDZ	Dilation of Coronary Artery, One Artery with Intraluminal Device, Open Approach
Ø27ØØEZ	Dilation of Coronary Artery, One Artery with Two Intraluminal Devices, Open Approach
Ø27ØØFZ	Dilation of Coronary Artery, One Artery with Three Intraluminal Devices, Open Approach
Ø27ØØGZ	Dilation of Coronary Artery, One Artery with Four or More Intraluminal Devices, Open Approach
Ø27ØØTZ	Dilation of Coronary Artery, One Artery with Radioactive Intraluminal Device, Open Approach
Ø27ØØZZ	Dilation of Coronary Artery, One Artery, Open Approach
Ø27Ø34Z	Dilation of Coronary Artery, One Artery with Drug-eluting Intraluminal Device, Percutaneous Approach
Ø27Ø35Z	Dilation of Coronary Artery, One Artery with Two Drug-eluting Intraluminal Devices, Percutaneous Approach
Ø27Ø36Z	Dilation of Coronary Artery, One Artery with Three Drug-eluting Intraluminal Devices, Percutaneous Approach
Ø27Ø37Z	Dilation of Coronary Artery, One Artery with Four or More Drug-eluting Intraluminal Devices, Percutaneous Approach
Ø27Ø3DZ	Dilation of Coronary Artery, One Artery with Intraluminal Device, Percutaneous Approach
Ø27Ø3EZ	Dilation of Coronary Artery, One Artery with Two Intraluminal Devices, Percutaneous Approach
Ø27Ø3FZ	Dilation of Coronary Artery, One Artery with Three Intraluminal Devices, Percutaneous Approach
Ø27Ø3GZ	Dilation of Coronary Artery, One Artery with Four or More Intraluminal Devices, Percutaneous Approach
Ø27Ø3TZ	Dilation of Coronary Artery, One Artery with Radioactive Intraluminal Device, Percutaneous Approach
Ø27Ø3ZZ	Dilation of Coronary Artery, One Artery, Percutaneous Approach
Ø27Ø44Z	Dilation of Coronary Artery, One Artery with Drug-eluting Intraluminal Device, Percutaneous Endoscopic Approach
Ø27Ø45Z	Dilation of Coronary Artery, One Artery with Two Drug-eluting Intraluminal Devices, Percutaneous Endoscopic Approach
Ø27Ø46Z	Dilation of Coronary Artery, One Artery with Three Drug-eluting Intraluminal Devices, Percutaneous Endoscopic Approach
Ø27Ø47Z	Dilation of Coronary Artery, One Artery with Four or More Drug-eluting Intraluminal Devices, Percutaneous Endoscopic Approach
Ø27Ø4DZ	Dilation of Coronary Artery, One Artery with Intraluminal Device, Percutaneous Endoscopic Approach
Ø27Ø4EZ	Dilation of Coronary Artery, One Artery with Two Intraluminal Devices, Percutaneous Endoscopic Approach
Ø27Ø4FZ	Dilation of Coronary Artery, One Artery with Three Intraluminal Devices, Percutaneous Endoscopic Approach
Ø27Ø4GZ	Dilation of Coronary Artery, One Artery with Four or More Intraluminal Devices, Percutaneous Endoscopic Approach
Ø27Ø4TZ	Dilation of Coronary Artery, One Artery with Radioactive Intraluminal Device, Percutaneous Endoscopic Approach
Ø27Ø4ZZ	Dilation of Coronary Artery, One Artery, Percutaneous Endoscopic Approach

Table 3: Rows from table ØØH

Ø Medical and Surgical
Ø Central Nervous System and Cranial Nerves
H Insertion Definition: Putting in a nonbiological appliance that monitors, assists, performs, or prevents a physiological function but does not physically take the place of a body part

Explanation: None

Body Part Character 4		Approach Character 5	Device Character 6	Qualifier Character 7
Ø Brain Cerebrum Corpus callosum Encephalon		**Ø Open**	**1 Radioactive Element** **2 Monitoring Device** **3 Infusion Device** **4 Radioactive Element, Cesium-131 Collagen Implant** **M Neurostimulator Lead** **Y Other Device**	**Z No Qualifier**
Ø Brain Cerebrum Corpus callosum Encephalon		**3 Percutaneous** **4 Percutaneous Endoscopic**	**1 Radioactive Element** **2 Monitoring Device** **3 Infusion Device** **M Neurostimulator Lead** **Y Other Device**	**Z No Qualifier**
6 Cerebral Ventricle Aqueduct of Sylvius Cerebral aqueduct (Sylvius) Choroid plexus Ependyma Foramen of Monro (intraventricular) Fourth ventricle Interventricular foramen (Monro) Left lateral ventricle Right lateral ventricle Third ventricle	**E Cranial Nerve** **U Spinal Canal** Epidural space, spinal Extradural space, spinal Subarachnoid space, spinal Subdural space, spinal Vertebral canal **V Spinal Cord** Dorsal root ganglion	**Ø Open** **3 Percutaneous** **4 Percutaneous Endoscopic**	**1 Radioactive Element** **2 Monitoring Device** **3 Infusion Device** **M Neurostimulator Lead** **Y Other Device**	**Z No Qualifier**

Table 3, is split into three rows; values of characters must all be selected from within the same row of the table. Rows 1 and 2 have the same body part (character 4) value of Ø Brain and the same qualifier value (character 7) of Z No Qualifier. However, the approach (character 5) values are not the same for these two rows, and there is one additional device (character 6) value in row 1 that is not included in row 2. As shown in row 1, body part value Brain (Ø) with device value Radioactive Element, Cesium-131 Collagen Implant (4) can only be used with approach value Open (Ø). In other words, code ØØHØ34Z would be invalid as the approach value 3 is only applicable to row 2 and the device value 4 is only applicable to row 1. It would be inappropriate to build a code for body part Ø if all of the values are not contained in its own row.

Note: In this manual, there are instances in which some tables due to length must be continued on the next page. Each section must be used separately and value selection must be made within the same row of the table.

Character Meanings

In each section, each character has a specific meaning, and this character meaning remains constant within that section. Character meaning tables have been provided at the beginning of each body system in the Medical and Surgical section (Ø) and the Obstetric section (1) to help the user identify the character members available within that section. These tables have purple headers, unlike the official code tables that have green headers and **SHOULD NOT** be used to build a PCS code. Following is an excerpt of a character meaning table.

Table 4: Rows from Central Nervous System and Cranial Nerves - Character Meanings Table

Operation–Character 3	Body Part–Character 4	Approach–Character 5	Device–Character 6	Qualifier–Character 7
1 Bypass	Ø Brain	Ø Open	Ø Drainage Device	Ø Nasopharynx
2 Change	1 Cerebral Meninges	3 Percutaneous	1 Radioactive Element	1 Mastoid Sinus
5 Destruction	2 Dura Mater	4 Percutaneous Endoscopic	2 Monitoring Device	2 Atrium
7 Dilation	3 Epidural Space, Intracranial	X External	3 Infusion Device	3 Blood Vessel
8 Division	4 Subdural Space, Intracranial		4 Radioactive Element, Cesium-131 Collagen Implant	4 Pleural Cavity
9 Drainage	5 Subarachnoid Space, Intracranial		7 Autologous Tissue Substitute	5 Intestine
B Excision	6 Cerebral Ventricle		J Synthetic Substitute	6 Peritoneal Cavity
C Extirpation	7 Cerebral Hemisphere		K Nonautologous Tissue Substitute	7 Urinary Tract
D Extraction	8 Basal Ganglia		M Neurostimulator Lead	8 Bone Marrow
F Fragmentation	9 Thalamus		Y Other Device	9 Fallopian Tube
H Insertion	A Hypothalamus		Z No Device	A Subgaleal space
J Inspection	B Pons			B Cerebral Cisterns

Sections

Procedures are divided into sections that identify the general type of procedure (e.g., Medical and Surgical, Obstetrics, Imaging). The first character of the procedure code always specifies the section.

The sections are listed below:

Medical and Surgical section

Ø Medical and Surgical

Medical and Surgical-related sections

1 Obstetrics

2 Placement

3 Administration

4 Measurement and Monitoring

5 Extracorporeal or Systemic Assistance and Performance

6 Extracorporeal or Systemic Therapies

7 Osteopathic

8 Other Procedures

9 Chiropractic

Ancillary Sections

B Imaging

C Nuclear Medicine

D Radiation Therapy

F Physical Rehabilitation and Diagnostic Audiology

G Mental Health

H Substance Abuse Treatment

New Technology Section

X New Technology

Medical and Surgical Section (Ø)

Character Meaning

The seven characters for Medical and Surgical procedures have the following meaning:

Character	Meaning
1	Section
2	Body System
3	Root Operation
4	Body Part
5	Approach
6	Device
7	Qualifier

The Medical and Surgical section constitutes the vast majority of procedures reported in an inpatient setting. Medical and Surgical procedure codes all have a first character value of Ø. The second character indicates the general body system (e.g., Mouth and Throat, Gastrointestinal). The third character indicates the root operation, or specific objective, of the procedure (e.g., Excision). The fourth character indicates the specific body part on which the procedure was performed (e.g., Tonsils, Duodenum). The fifth character indicates the approach used to reach the procedure site (e.g., Open). The sixth character indicates whether a device was left in place during the procedure (e.g., Synthetic Substitute). The seventh character is qualifier, which has a specific meaning for each root operation. For example, the qualifier can be used to identify the destination site of a *Bypass*. The first through fifth characters are always assigned a specific value, but the device (sixth character) and the qualifier (seventh character) are not applicable to all procedures. The value *Z* is used for the sixth and seventh characters to indicate that a specific device or qualifier does not apply to the procedure.

Section (Character 1)

Medical and Surgical procedure codes all have a first character value of Ø.

Body Systems (Character 2)

Body systems for Medical and Surgical section codes are specified in the second character.

Body Systems

Ø Central Nervous System and Cranial Nerves

1 Peripheral Nervous System

2 Heart and Great Vessels

3 Upper Arteries

4 Lower Arteries

5 Upper Veins

6 Lower Veins

7 Lymphatic and Hemic Systems

8 Eye

9 Ear, Nose, Sinus

B Respiratory System

C Mouth and Throat

D Gastrointestinal System

F Hepatobiliary System and Pancreas

G Endocrine System

H Skin and Breast

J Subcutaneous Tissue and Fascia

K Muscles

L Tendons

M Bursae and Ligaments

N Head and Facial Bones

P Upper Bones

Q Lower Bones

R Upper Joints

S Lower Joints

T Urinary System

U Female Reproductive System

V Male Reproductive System

W Anatomical Regions, General

X Anatomical Regions, Upper Extremities

Y Anatomical Regions, Lower Extremities

Root Operations (Character 3)

The root operation is specified in the third character. In the Medical and Surgical section there are 31 different root operations. The root operation identifies the objective of the procedure. Each root operation has a precise definition.

- *Alteration:* Modifying the natural anatomic structure of a body part without affecting the function of the body part
- *Bypass:* Altering the route of passage of the contents of a tubular body part
- *Change:* Taking out or off a device from a body part and putting back an identical or similar device in or on the same body part without cutting or puncturing the skin or a mucous membrane
- *Control:* Stopping, or attempting to stop, postprocedural or other acute bleeding
- *Creation:* Putting in or on biological or synthetic material to form a new body part that to the extent possible replicates the anatomic structure or function of an absent body part
- *Destruction:* Physical eradication of all or a portion of a body part by the direct use of energy, force, or a destructive agent
- *Detachment:* Cutting off all or a portion of the upper or lower extremities
- *Dilation:* Expanding an orifice or the lumen of a tubular body part
- *Division:* Cutting into a body part without draining fluids and/or gases from the body part in order to separate or transect a body part
- *Drainage:* Taking or letting out fluids and/or gases from a body part
- *Excision:* Cutting out or off, without replacement, a portion of a body part
- *Extirpation:* Taking or cutting out solid matter from a body part
- *Extraction:* Pulling or stripping out or off all or a portion of a body part by the use of force
- *Fragmentation:* Breaking solid matter in a body part into pieces
- *Fusion:* Joining together portions of an articular body part rendering the articular body part immobile
- *Insertion:* Putting in a nonbiological appliance that monitors, assists, performs, or prevents a physiological function but does not physically take the place of a body part
- *Inspection:* Visually and/or manually exploring a body part
- *Map:* Locating the route of passage of electrical impulses and/or locating functional areas in a body part
- *Occlusion:* Completely closing an orifice or lumen of a tubular body part
- *Reattachment:* Putting back in or on all or a portion of a separated body part to its normal location or other suitable location
- *Release:* Freeing a body part from an abnormal physical constraint by cutting or by use of force
- *Removal:* Taking out or off a device from a body part
- *Repair:* Restoring, to the extent possible, a body part to its normal anatomic structure and function
- *Replacement:* Putting in or on biological or synthetic material that physically takes the place and/or function of all or a portion of a body part
- *Reposition:* Moving to its normal location or other suitable location all or a portion of a body part
- *Resection:* Cutting out or off, without replacement, all of a body part
- *Restriction:* Partially closing an orifice or lumen of a tubular body part
- *Revision:* Correcting, to the extent possible, a portion of a malfunctioning device or the position of a displaced device
- *Supplement:* Putting in or on biological or synthetic material that physically reinforces and/or augments the function of a portion of a body part
- *Transfer:* Moving, without taking out, all or a portion of a body part to another location to take over the function of all or a portion of a body part
- *Transplantation:* Putting in or on all or a portion of a living body part taken from another individual or animal to physically take the place and/or function of all or a portion of a similar body part

The above definitions of root operations illustrate the precision of code values defined in the system. There is a clear distinction between each root operation.

A root operation specifies the objective of the procedure. The term *anastomosis* is not a root operation, because it is a means of joining and is always an integral part of another procedure (e.g., Bypass, Resection) with a specific objective. Similarly, *incision* is not a root operation, since it is always part of the objective of another procedure (e.g., Division, Drainage). The root operation *Repair* in the Medical and Surgical section functions as a "not elsewhere classified" option. *Repair* is used when the procedure performed is not one of the other specific root operations.

Appendix B provides additional explanation and representative examples of the Medical and Surgical root operations. Appendix C groups all root operations in the Medical and Surgical section into subcategories and provides an example of each root operation.

Body Part (Character 4)

The body part is specified in the fourth character. The body part indicates the specific anatomical site of the body system on which the procedure was performed (e.g., Duodenum). Tubular body parts are defined in ICD-10-PCS as those hollow body parts that provide a route of passage for solids, liquids, or gases. They include the cardiovascular system and body parts such as those contained in the gastrointestinal tract, genitourinary tract, biliary tract, and respiratory tract.

Approach (Character 5)

The technique used to reach the site of the procedure is specified in the fifth character. There are seven different approaches:

- *Open*: Cutting through the skin or mucous membrane and any other body layers necessary to expose the site of the procedure
- *Percutaneous*: Entry, by puncture or minor incision, of instrumentation through the skin or mucous membrane and any other body layers necessary to reach the site of the procedure
- *Percutaneous Endoscopic*: Entry, by puncture or minor incision, of instrumentation through the skin or mucous membrane and any other body layers necessary to reach and visualize the site of the procedure
- *Via Natural or Artificial Opening*: Entry of instrumentation through a natural or artificial external opening to reach the site of the procedure
- *Via Natural or Artificial Opening Endoscopic*: Entry of instrumentation through a natural or artificial external opening to reach and visualize the site of the procedure

- *Via Natural or Artificial Opening with Percutaneous Endoscopic Assistance:* Entry of instrumentation through a natural or artificial external opening and entry, by puncture or minor incision, of instrumentation through the skin or mucous membrane and any other body layers necessary to aid in the performance of the procedure
- *External*: Procedures performed directly on the skin or mucous membrane and procedures performed indirectly by the application of external force through the skin or mucous membrane

The approach comprises three components: the access location, method, and type of instrumentation.

Access location: For procedures performed on an internal body part, the access location specifies the external site through which the site of the procedure is reached. There are two general types of access locations: skin or mucous membranes, and external orifices. Every approach value except external includes one of these two access locations. The skin or mucous membrane can be cut or punctured to reach the procedure site. All open and percutaneous approach values use this access location. The site of a procedure can also be reached through an external opening. External openings can be natural (e.g., mouth) or artificial (e.g., colostomy stoma).

Method: For procedures performed on an internal body part, the method specifies how the external access location is entered. An open method specifies cutting through the skin or mucous membrane and any other intervening body layers necessary to expose the site of the procedure. An instrumentation method specifies the entry of instrumentation through the access location to the internal procedure site. Instrumentation can be introduced by puncture or minor incision, or through an external opening. The puncture or minor incision does not constitute an open approach because it does not expose the site of the procedure. An approach can define multiple methods. For example, *Via Natural or Artificial Opening with Percutaneous Endoscopic Assistance* includes both the initial entry of instrumentation to reach the site of the procedure, and the placement of additional percutaneous instrumentation into the body part to visualize and assist in the performance of the procedure.

Type of instrumentation: For procedures performed on an internal body part, instrumentation means that specialized equipment is used to perform the procedure. Instrumentation is used in all internal approaches other than the basic open approach. Instrumentation may or may not include the capacity to visualize the procedure site. For example, the instrumentation used to perform a sigmoidoscopy permits the internal site of the procedure to be visualized, while the instrumentation used to perform a needle biopsy of the liver does not. The term "endoscopic" as used in approach values refers to instrumentation that permits a site to be visualized.

Procedures performed directly on the skin or mucous membrane are identified by the external approach (e.g., skin excision). Procedures performed indirectly by the application of external force are also identified by the external approach (e.g., closed reduction of fracture).

Appendix A compares the components (access location, method, and type of instrumentation) of each approach and provides an example and illustration of each approach.

Device (Character 6)

The device is specified in the sixth character. There are four general types of devices:

- Biological or synthetic material that takes the place of all or a portion of a body part (e.g, skin graft, joint prosthesis).
- Biological or synthetic material that assists or prevents a physiological function (e.g., IUD).
- Therapeutic material that is not absorbed by, eliminated by, or incorporated into a body part (e.g., radioactive implant).
- Mechanical or electronic appliances used to assist, monitor, take the place of or prevent a physiological function (e.g., cardiac pacemaker, orthopedic pin).

Appendix F compares the general device types and provides examples of each.

While all devices can be removed, some cannot be removed without putting in another nonbiological appliance or body-part substitute.

When a specific device value is used to identify the device for a root operation, such as *Insertion* and that same device value is not an option for a more broad range root operation such as *Removal*, select the general device value. For example, in the body system Heart and Great Vessels, the specific device character for Cardiac Lead, Pacemaker in root operation *Insertion* is J. For the root operation *Removal*, the general device character M Cardiac Lead would be selected for the pacemaker lead.

ICD-10-PCS contains a PCS Device Aggregation Table (see appendix G) that crosswalks the *specific* device character values that have been created for specific root operations and specific body part character values to the *general* device character value that would be used for root operations that represent a broad range of procedures and general body part character values, such as Removal and Revision.

Instruments used to visualize the procedure site are specified in the approach, not the device, value.

If the objective of the procedure is to put in the device, then the root operation is *Insertion*. If the device is put in to meet an objective other than *Insertion*, then the root operation defining the underlying objective of the procedure is used, with the device specified in the device character. For example, if a procedure to replace the hip joint is performed, the root operation *Replacement* is coded, and the prosthetic device is specified in the device character. Materials that are incidental to a procedure such as clips, ligatures, and sutures are not specified in the device character. Because new devices can be developed, the value *Other Device* is provided as a temporary option for use until a specific device value is added to the system.

Qualifier (Character 7)

The qualifier is specified in the seventh character. The qualifier contains unique values for individual procedures. For example, the qualifier can be used to identify the destination site in a *Bypass*.

Medical and Surgical Section Principles

In developing the Medical and Surgical procedure codes, several specific principles were followed.

Composite Terms Are Not Root Operations

Composite terms such as colonoscopy, sigmoidectomy, or appendectomy do not describe root operations, but they do specify multiple components of a specific root operation. In ICD-10-PCS, the

components of a procedure are defined separately by the characters making up the complete code. The only component of a procedure specified in the root operation is the objective of the procedure. With each complete code the underlying objective of the procedure is specified by the root operation (third character), the precise part is specified by the body part (fourth character), and the method used to reach and visualize the procedure site is specified by the approach (fifth character). While colonoscopy, sigmoidectomy, and appendectomy are included in the Index, they do not constitute root operations in the Tables section. The objective of colonoscopy is the visualization of the colon and the root operation (character 3) is *Inspection*. Character 4 specifies the body part, which in this case is part of the colon. These composite terms, like colonoscopy or appendectomy, are included as cross-reference only. The index provides the correct root operation reference. Examples of other types of composite terms not representative of root operations are *partial* sigmoidectomy, *total* hysterectomy, and *partial* hip replacement. Always refer to the correct root operation in the Index and Tables section.

Root Operation Based on Objective of Procedure

The root operation is based on the objective of the procedure, such as *Resection* of transverse colon or *Dilation* of an artery. The assignment of the root operation is based on the procedure actually performed, which may or may not have been the intended procedure. If the intended procedure is modified or discontinued (e.g., excision instead of resection is performed), the root operation is determined by the procedure actually performed. If the desired result is not attained after completing the procedure (i.e., the artery does not remain expanded after the dilation procedure), the root operation is still determined by the procedure actually performed.

Examples:

- Dilating the urethra is coded as *Dilation* since the objective of the procedure is to dilate the urethra. If dilation of the urethra includes putting in an intraluminal stent, the root operation remains *Dilation* and not *Insertion* of the intraluminal device because the underlying objective of the procedure is dilation of the urethra. The stent is identified by the intraluminal device value in the sixth character of the dilation procedure code.
- If the objective is solely to put a radioactive element in the urethra, then the procedure is coded to the root operation *Insertion*, with the radioactive element identified in the sixth character of the code.
- If the objective of the procedure is to correct a malfunctioning or displaced device, then the procedure is coded to the root operation *Revision*. In the root operation *Revision*, the original device being revised is identified in the device character. *Revision* is typically performed on mechanical appliances (e.g., pacemaker) or materials used in replacement procedures (e.g., synthetic substitute). Typical revision procedures include adjustment of pacemaker position and correction of malfunctioning knee prosthesis.

Combination Procedures Are Coded Separately

If multiple procedures as defined by distinct objectives are performed during an operative episode, then multiple codes are used. For example, obtaining the vein graft used for coronary bypass surgery is coded as a separate procedure from the bypass itself.

Redo of Procedures

The complete or partial redo of the original procedure is coded to the root operation that identifies the procedure performed rather than *Revision*.

Example:

A complete redo of a hip replacement procedure that requires putting in a new prosthesis is coded to the root operation *Replacement* rather than *Revision*.

The correction of complications arising from the original procedure, other than device complications, is coded to the procedure performed. Correction of a malfunctioning or displaced device would be coded to the root operation *Revision*.

Example:

A procedure to control hemorrhage arising from the original procedure is coded to *Control* rather than *Revision*.

Examples of Procedures Coded in the Medical Surgical Section

The following are examples of procedures from the Medical and Surgical section, coded in ICD-10-PCS.

- Suture of skin laceration, left lower arm: ØHQEXZZ

  Medical and Surgical section (Ø), body system *Skin and Breast* (H), root operation *Repair* (Q), body part *Skin, Left Lower Arm* (E), *External* Approach (X) *No device* (Z), and *No qualifier* (Z).
- Laparoscopic appendectomy: ØDTJ4ZZ

  Medical and Surgical section (Ø), body system *Gastrointestinal* (D), root operation *Resection* (T), body part *Appendix* (J), *Percutaneous Endoscopic* approach (4), No Device (Z), and No qualifier (Z).
- Sigmoidoscopy with biopsy: ØDBN8ZX

  Medical and Surgical section (Ø), body system *Gastrointestinal* (D), root operation *Excision* (B), body part *Sigmoid Colon* (N), *Via Natural or Artificial Opening Endoscopic* approach (8), *No Device* (Z), and with qualifier *Diagnostic* (X).
- Tracheostomy with tracheostomy tube: ØB11ØF4

  Medical and Surgical section (Ø), body system *Respiratory* (B), root operation *Bypass* (1), body part *Trachea* (1), *Open* approach (Ø), with *Tracheostomy Device* (F), and qualifier *Cutaneous* (4).

Obstetrics Section (1)

Character Meanings

The seven characters in the Obstetrics section have the same meaning as in the Medical and Surgical section.

Character	Meaning
1	Section
2	Body System
3	Root Operation
4	Body Part
5	Approach
6	Device
7	Qualifier

The Obstetrics section includes procedures performed on the products of conception only. Procedures on the pregnant female are coded in the Medical and Surgical section (e.g., episiotomy). The term "products of conception" refers to all physical components of a pregnancy, including the fetus, amnion, umbilical cord, and placenta. There is no differentiation of the products of conception based on gestational age.

Thus, the specification of the products of conception as a zygote, embryo or fetus, or the trimester of the pregnancy is not part of the procedure code but can be found in the diagnosis code.

Section (Character 1)
Obstetrics procedure codes have a first character value of *1*.

Body System (Character 2)
The second character value for body system is *Pregnancy*.

Root Operation (Character 3)
The root operations *Change, Drainage, Extraction, Insertion, Inspection, Removal, Repair, Reposition, Resection,* and *Transplantation* are used in the obstetrics section and have the same meaning as in the Medical and Surgical section.

The Obstetrics section also includes two additional root operations, *Abortion* and *Delivery*, defined below:

- *Abortion*: Artificially terminating a pregnancy
- *Delivery*: Assisting the passage of the products of conception from the genital canal

A cesarean section is not a separate root operation because the underlying objective is *Extraction* (i.e., pulling out all or a portion of a body part).

Body Part (Character 4)
The body part values in the obstetrics section are:

- *Products of conception*
- *Products of conception, retained*
- *Products of conception, ectopic*

Approach (Character 5)
The fifth character specifies approaches as defined in the Medical and Surgical section.

Device (Character 6)
The sixth character is used for devices such as fetal monitoring electrodes.

Qualifier (Character 7)
Qualifier values are specific to the root operation and are used to capture details of the procedure, such as whether forceps or a vacuum were used during an Extraction, the type of fluid taken out during a Drainage procedure, or the products of conception body system that was repaired.

Placement Section (2)

Character Meanings
The seven characters in the Placement section have the following meaning:

Character	Meaning
1	Section
2	Body System
3	Root Operation
4	Body Region
5	Approach
6	Device
7	Qualifier

Placement section codes represent procedures for putting a device in or on a body region for the purpose of protection, immobilization, stretching, compression, or packing.

Section (Character 1)
Placement procedure codes have a first character value of *2*.

Body System (Character 2)
The second character contains two values specifying either *Anatomical Regions* or *Anatomical Orifices*.

Root Operation (Character 3)
The root operations in the Placement section include only those procedures that are performed without making an incision or a puncture. The root operations *Change* and *Removal* are in the Placement section and have the same meaning as in the Medical and Surgical section.

The Placement section also includes five additional root operations, defined as follows:

- *Compression*: Putting pressure on a body region
- *Dressing*: Putting material on a body region for protection
- *Immobilization*: Limiting or preventing motion of an external body region
- *Packing*: Putting material in a body region or orifice
- *Traction*: Exerting a pulling force on a body region in a distal direction

Body Region (Character 4)
The fourth character values are either body regions (e.g., *Upper Leg*) or natural orifices (e.g., *Ear*).

Approach (Character 5)
Since all placement procedures are performed directly on the skin or mucous membrane, or performed indirectly by applying external force through the skin or mucous membrane, the approach value is always *External*.

Device (Character 6)
The device character is always specified (except in the case of manual traction) and indicates the device placed during the procedure (e.g., cast, splint, bandage, etc.). Except for casts for fractures and dislocations, devices in the Placement section are off the shelf and do not require any extensive design, fabrication, or fitting. Placement of devices that require extensive design, fabrication, or fitting are coded in the Rehabilitation section.

Qualifier (Character 7)
The qualifier character is not specified in the Placement section; the qualifier value is always *No Qualifier*.

Administration Section (3)

Character Meanings
The seven characters in the Administration section have the following meaning:

Character	Meaning
1	Section
2	Body System
3	Root Operation
4	Body System/Region
5	Approach
6	Substance
7	Qualifier

Administration section codes represent procedures for putting in or on a therapeutic, prophylactic, protective, diagnostic, nutritional, or physiological substance. The section includes transfusions, infusions, and injections, along with other similar services such as irrigation and tattooing.

Section (Character 1)
Administration procedure codes have a first character value of *3*.

Body System (Character 2)
The body system character contains only three values: *Indwelling Device, Physiological Systems and Anatomical Regions,* or *Circulatory System*. The *Circulatory System* is used for transfusion procedures.

Root Operation (Character 3)
There are three root operations in the Administration section.

- *Introduction*: Putting in or on a therapeutic, diagnostic, nutritional, physiological, or prophylactic substance except blood or blood products
- *Irrigation*: Putting in or on a cleansing substance
- *Transfusion*: Putting in blood or blood products

Body/System Region (Character 4)
The fourth character specifies the body system/region. The fourth character identifies the site where the substance is administered, not the site where the substance administered takes effect. Sites include *Skin and Mucous Membranes, Subcutaneous Tissue,* and *Muscle*. These differentiate intradermal, subcutaneous, and intramuscular injections, respectively. Other sites include *Eye, Respiratory Tract, Peritoneal Cavity,* and *Epidural Space*.

The body systems/regions for arteries and veins are *Peripheral Artery, Central Artery, Peripheral Vein,* and *Central Vein*. The *Peripheral Artery* or *Vein* is typically used when a substance is introduced locally into an artery or vein. For example, chemotherapy is the introduction of an antineoplastic substance into a peripheral artery or vein by a percutaneous approach. In general, the substance introduced into a peripheral artery or vein has a systemic effect.

The *Central Artery* or *Vein* is typically used when the site where the substance is introduced is distant from the point of entry into the artery or vein. For example, the introduction of a substance directly at the site of a clot within an artery or vein using a catheter is coded as an introduction of a thrombolytic substance into a central artery or vein by a percutaneous approach. In general, the substance introduced into a central artery or vein has a local effect.

Approach (Character 5)
The fifth character specifies approaches as defined in the Medical and Surgical section. The approach for intradermal, subcutaneous, and intramuscular introductions (i.e., injections) is *Percutaneous*. If a catheter is placed to introduce a substance into an internal site within the circulatory system, then the approach is also *Percutaneous*. For example, if a catheter is used to introduce contrast directly into the heart for angiography, then the procedure would be coded as a percutaneous introduction of contrast into the heart.

Substance (Character 6)
The sixth character specifies the substance being introduced. Broad categories of substances are defined, such as anesthetic, contrast, dialysate, and blood products such as platelets.

Qualifier (Character 7)
The seventh character is a qualifier and is used to indicate whether the transfused substance is *Autologous, Nonautologous, or Allogeneic* (related, unrelated, unspecified), or to further specify the substance.

Measurement and Monitoring Section (4)

Character Meanings
The seven characters in the Measurement and Monitoring section have the following meaning:

Character	Meaning
1	Section
2	Body System
3	Root Operation
4	Body System
5	Approach
6	Function/Device
7	Qualifier

Measurement and Monitoring section codes represent procedures for determining the level of a physiological or physical function.

Section (Character 1)
Measurement and Monitoring procedure codes have a first character value of *4*.

Body System (Character 2)
The second character values for body system are A, *Physiological Systems* or B, *Physiological Devices*.

Root Operation (Character 3)
There are two root operations in the Measurement and Monitoring section, as defined below:

- *Measurement*: Determining the level of a physiological or physical function at a point in time
- *Monitoring*: Determining the level of a physiological or physical function repetitively over a period of time

Introduction

Body System (Character 4)

The fourth character specifies the specific body system measured or monitored.

Approach (Character 5)

The fifth character specifies approaches as defined in the Medical and Surgical section.

Function/Device (Character 6)

The sixth character specifies the physiological or physical function being measured or monitored. Examples of physiological or physical functions are *Conductivity, Metabolism, Pulse, Temperature,* and *Volume*. If a device used to perform the measurement or monitoring is inserted and left in, then insertion of the device is coded as a separate Medical and Surgical procedure.

Qualifier (Character 7)

The seventh character qualifier contains specific values as needed to further specify the body part (e.g., central, portal, pulmonary) or a variation of the procedure performed (e.g., ambulatory, stress). Examples of typical procedures coded in this section are EKG, EEG, and cardiac catheterization. An EKG is the measurement of cardiac electrical activity, while an EEG is the measurement of electrical activity of the central nervous system. A cardiac catheterization performed to measure the pressure in the heart is coded as the measurement of cardiac pressure by percutaneous approach.

Extracorporeal or Systemic Assistance and Performance Section (5)

Character Meanings

The seven characters in the Extracorporeal or Systemic Assistance and Performance section have the following meaning:

Character	Meaning
1	Section
2	Body System
3	Root Operation
4	Body System
5	Duration
6	Function
7	Qualifier

In Extracorporeal or Systemic Assistance and Performance procedures, equipment outside the body is used to assist or perform a physiological function. The section includes procedures performed in a critical care setting, such as mechanical ventilation and cardioversion; it also includes other services such as hyperbaric oxygen treatment and hemodialysis.

Section (Character 1)

Extracorporeal or Systemic Assistance and Performance procedure codes have a first character value of *5*.

Body System (Character 2)

The second character value for body system is A, *Physiological Systems*.

Root Operation (Character 3)

There are three root operations in the Extracorporeal or Systemic Assistance and Performance section, as defined below.

- *Assistance*: Taking over a portion of a physiological function by extracorporeal means
- *Performance*: Completely taking over a physiological function by extracorporeal means
- *Restoration*: Returning, or attempting to return, a physiological function to its natural state by extracorporeal means

The root operation *Restoration* contains a single procedure code that identifies extracorporeal cardioversion.

Body System (Character 4)

The fourth character specifies the body system (e.g., cardiac, respiratory) to which extracorporeal or systemic assistance or performance is applied.

Duration (Character 5)

The fifth character specifies the duration of the procedure.

Function (Character 6)

The sixth character specifies the physiological function assisted or performed (e.g., oxygenation, ventilation) during the procedure.

Qualifier (Character 7)

The seventh character qualifier specifies the type of equipment used, if any.

Extracorporeal or Systemic Therapies Section (6)

Character Meanings

The seven characters in the Extracorporeal or Systemic Therapies section have the following meaning:

Character	Meaning
1	Section
2	Body System
3	Root Operation
4	Body System
5	Duration
6	Qualifier
7	Qualifier

In extracorporeal or systemic therapy, equipment outside the body is used for a therapeutic purpose that does not involve the assistance or performance of a physiological function.

Section (Character 1)

Extracorporeal or Systemic Therapy procedure codes have a first character value of 6.

Body System (Character 2)

The second character value for body system is *Physiological Systems*.

Root Operation (Character 3)

There are 11 root operations in the Extracorporeal or Systemic Therapy section, as defined below.

- *Atmospheric Control*: Extracorporeal control of atmospheric pressure and composition
- *Decompression*: Extracorporeal elimination of undissolved gas from body fluids

  Coding note: The root operation *Decompression* involves only one type of procedure: treatment for decompression sickness (the bends) in a hyperbaric chamber.
- *Electromagnetic Therapy*: Extracorporeal treatment by electromagnetic rays
- *Hyperthermia*: Extracorporeal raising of body temperature

  Coding note: The term hyperthermia is used to describe both a temperature imbalance treatment and also as an adjunct radiation treatment for cancer. When treating the temperature imbalance, it is coded to this section; for the cancer treatment, it is coded in section *D Radiation Therapy.*
- *Hypothermia*: Extracorporeal lowering of body temperature
- *Perfusion*: Extracorporeal treatment by diffusion of therapeutic fluid
- *Pheresis*: Extracorporeal separation of blood products

  Coding note: Pheresis may be used for two main purposes: to treat diseases when too much of a blood component is produced (e.g., leukemia) and to remove a blood product such as platelets from a donor, for transfusion into another patient.
- *Phototherapy*: Extracorporeal treatment by light rays

  Coding note: Phototherapy involves using a machine that exposes the blood to light rays outside the body, recirculates it, and then returns it to the body.
- *Shock Wave Therapy*: Extracorporeal treatment by shock waves
- *Ultrasound Therapy*: Extracorporeal treatment by ultrasound
- *Ultraviolet Light Therapy*: Extracorporeal treatment by ultraviolet light

Body System (Character 4)

The fourth character specifies the body system on which the extracorporeal or systemic therapy is performed (e.g., skin, circulatory).

Duration (Character 5)

The fifth character specifies whether the procedure was performed once (single) or multiple times.

Qualifier (Character 6)

The sixth character for Extracorporeal or Systemic Therapies is *No Qualifier*, except for root operation Perfusion which has a sixth character qualifier of *Donor Organ*.

Qualifier (Character 7)

The seventh character qualifier is used in the root operation *Pheresis* to specify the blood component on which pheresis is performed and in the root operation *Ultrasound Therapy* to specify site of treatment.

Osteopathic Section (7)

Character Meanings

The seven characters in the Osteopathic section have the following meaning:

Character	Meaning
1	Section
2	Body System
3	Root Operation
4	Body Region
5	Approach
6	Method
7	Qualifier

Section (Character 1)

Osteopathic procedure codes have a first character value of *7*.

Body System (Character 2)

The body system character contains the value *Anatomical Regions*.

Root Operation (Character 3)

There is only one root operation in the Osteopathic section.

- *Treatment*: Manual treatment to eliminate or alleviate somatic dysfunction and related disorders

Body Region (Character 4)

The fourth character specifies the body region on which the osteopathic treatment is performed.

Approach (Character 5)

The approach for osteopathic treatment is always *External*.

Method (Character 6)

The sixth character specifies the method by which the treatment is accomplished.

Qualifier (Character 7)

The seventh character is not specified in the Osteopathic section and always has the value *None*.

Other Procedures Section (8)

Character Meanings

The seven characters in the Other Procedures section have the following meaning:

Character	Meaning
1	Section
2	Body System
3	Root Operation
4	Body Region
5	Approach
6	Method
7	Qualifier

The Other Procedures section includes acupuncture, suture removal, and in vitro fertilization.

Section (Character 1)

Other Procedure section codes have a first character value of *8*.

Body System (Character 2)

The second character values for body systems are *Physiological Systems and Anatomical Regions* and *Indwelling Device*.

Root Operation (Character 3)

The Other Procedures section has only one root operation, defined as follows:

- *Other Procedures*: Methodologies that attempt to remediate or cure a disorder or disease.

Body Region (Character 4)

The fourth character contains specified body-region values, and also the body-region value *None*.

Approach (Character 5)

The fifth character specifies approaches as defined in the Medical and Surgical section.

Method (Character 6)

The sixth character specifies the method (e.g., *Acupuncture, Therapeutic Massage*).

Qualifier (Character 7)

The seventh character is a qualifier and contains specific values as needed.

Chiropractic Section (9)

Character Meanings

The seven characters in the Chiropractic section have the following meaning:

Character	Meaning
1	Section
2	Body System
3	Root Operation
4	Body Region
5	Approach
6	Method
7	Qualifier

Section (Character 1)

Chiropractic section procedure codes have a first character value of *9*.

Body System (Character 2)

The second character value for body system is *Anatomical Regions*.

Root Operation (Character 3)

There is only one root operation in the *Chiropractic* section.

- *Manipulation:* Manual procedure that involves a directed thrust to move a joint past the physiological range of motion, without exceeding the anatomical limit.

Body Region (Character 4)

The fourth character specifies the body region on which the chiropractic manipulation is performed.

Approach (Character 5)

The approach for chiropractic manipulation is always *External*.

Method (Character 6)

The sixth character is the method by which the manipulation is accomplished.

Qualifier (Character 7)

The seventh character is not specified in the Chiropractic section and always has the value *None*.

Imaging Section (B)

Character Meanings

The seven characters in Imaging procedures have the following meaning:

Character	Meaning
1	Section
2	Body System
3	Type
4	Body Part
5	Contrast
6	Qualifier
7	Qualifier

Imaging procedures include plain radiography, fluoroscopy, CT, MRI, and ultrasound. Nuclear medicine procedures, including PET, uptakes, and scans, are in the nuclear medicine section. Therapeutic radiation procedure codes are in a separate radiation therapy section.

Section (Character 1)

Imaging procedure codes have a first character value of *B*.

Body System (Character 2)

In the Imaging section, the second character defines the body system, such as *Heart* or *Gastrointestinal System*.

Type (Character 3)

The third character defines the type of imaging procedure (e.g., MRI, ultrasound). The following list includes all types in the *Imaging* section with a definition of each type:

- *Computerized Tomography (CT Scan)*: Computer reformatted digital display of multiplanar images developed from the capture of multiple exposures of external ionizing radiation
- *Fluoroscopy*: Single plane or bi-plane real time display of an image developed from the capture of external ionizing radiation on a fluorescent screen. The image may also be stored by either digital or analog means
- *Magnetic Resonance Imaging (MRI)*: Computer reformatted digital display of multiplanar images developed from the capture of radiofrequency signals emitted by nuclei in a body site excited within a magnetic field
- *Other Imaging:* Other specified modality for visualizing a body part

- *Plain Radiography*: Planar display of an image developed from the capture of external ionizing radiation on photographic or photoconductive plate
- *Ultrasonography*: Real time display of images of anatomy or flow information developed from the capture of reflected and attenuated high frequency sound waves

Body Part (Character 4)

The fourth character defines the body part with different values for each body system (character 2) value.

Contrast (Character 5)

The fifth character specifies whether the contrast material used in the imaging procedure is *High Osmolar, Low Osmolar*, or *Other Contrast* when applicable.

Qualifier (Character 6)

The sixth character qualifier provides further detail regarding the nature of the substance or technologies used, such as *Unenhanced and Enhanced (contrast), Laser, or Intravascular Optical Coherence*.

Qualifier (Character 7)

The seventh character is a qualifier that may be used to specify certain procedural circumstances, the method by which the procedure was performed, or technologies utilized, such as *Intraoperative, Intravascular, or Transesophageal*.

Nuclear Medicine Section (C)

Character Meanings

The seven characters in the Nuclear Medicine section have the following meaning:

Character	Meaning
1	Section
2	Body System
3	Type
4	Body Part
5	Radionuclide
6	Qualifier
7	Qualifier

Nuclear Medicine is the introduction of radioactive material into the body to create an image, to diagnose and treat pathologic conditions, or to assess metabolic functions. The Nuclear Medicine section does not include the introduction of encapsulated radioactive material for the treatment of cancer. These procedures are included in the Radiation Therapy section.

Section (Character 1)

Nuclear Medicine procedure codes have a first character value of *C*.

Body System (Character 2)

The second character specifies the body system on which the nuclear medicine procedure is performed.

Type (Character 3)

The third character indicates the type of nuclear medicine procedure (e.g., planar imaging or nonimaging uptake). The following list includes the types of nuclear medicine procedures with a definition of each type.

- *Nonimaging Nuclear Medicine Assay:* Introduction of radioactive materials into the body for the study of body fluids and blood elements, by the detection of radioactive emissions
- *Nonimaging Nuclear Medicine Probe:* Introduction of radioactive materials into the body for the study of distribution and fate of certain substances by the detection of radioactive emissions; or alternatively, measurement of absorption of radioactive emissions from an external source
- *Nonimaging Nuclear Medicine Uptake:* Introduction of radioactive materials into the body for measurements of organ function, from the detection of radioactive emissions
- *Planar Nuclear Medicine Imaging*: Introduction of radioactive materials into the body for single-plane display of images developed from the capture of radioactive emissions
- *Positron Emission Tomography (PET) Imaging:* Introduction of radioactive materials into the body for three dimensional display of images developed from the simultaneous capture, 180 degrees apart, of radioactive emissions
- *Systemic Nuclear Medicine Therapy:* Introduction of unsealed radioactive materials into the body for treatment
- *Tomographic (Tomo) Nuclear Medicine Imaging*: Introduction of radioactive materials into the body for three dimensional display of images developed from the capture of radioactive emissions

Body Part (Character 4)

The fourth character indicates the body part or body region studied; with regional (e.g., *lower extremity veins*) and combination (e.g., *liver and spleen*) body parts commonly used.

Radionuclide (Character 5)

The fifth character specifies the radionuclide, the radiation source. The option *Other Radionuclide* is provided in the nuclear medicine section for newly approved radionuclides until they can be added to the coding system. If more than one radiopharmaceutical is given to perform the procedure, then more than one code is used.

Qualifier (Character 6 and 7)

The sixth and seventh characters are qualifiers but are not specified in the *Nuclear Medicine* section; the value is always *None.*

Radiation Therapy Section (D)

Character Meanings

The seven characters in the Radiation Therapy section have the following meaning:

Character	Meaning
1	Section
2	Body System
3	Modality
4	Treatment Site
5	Modality Qualifier
6	Isotope
7	Qualifier

Introduction

Section (Character 1)
Radiation therapy procedure codes have a first character value of *D*.

Body System (Character 2)
The second character specifies the body system (e.g., central nervous system, musculoskeletal) irradiated.

Modality (Character 3)
The third character specifies the general modality used (e.g., beam radiation).

Treatment Site (Character 4)
The fourth character specifies the body part that is the focus of the radiation therapy.

Modality Qualifier (Character 5)
The fifth character further specifies the radiation modality used (e.g., photons, electrons).

Isotope (Character 6)
The sixth character specifies the isotopes introduced into the body, if applicable.

Qualifier (Character 7)
The seventh character may specify whether the procedure was performed intraoperatively.

Physical Rehabilitation and Diagnostic Audiology Section (F)

Character Meanings
The seven characters in the Physical Rehabilitation and Diagnostic Audiology section have the following meaning:

Character	Meaning
1	Section
2	Section Qualifier
3	Type
4	Body System/Region
5	Type Qualifier
6	Equipment
7	Qualifier

Physical rehabilitation procedures include physical therapy, occupational therapy, and speech-language pathology. Osteopathic procedures and chiropractic procedures are in separate sections.

Section (Character 1)
Physical Rehabilitation and Diagnostic Audiology procedure codes have a first character value of *F*.

Section Qualifier (Character 2)
The section qualifier *Rehabilitation* or *Diagnostic Audiology* is specified in the second character.

Type (Character 3)
The third character specifies the type. There are 14 different values, which can be classified into four basic types of rehabilitation and diagnostic audiology procedures, defined as follows:

Assessment: Includes a determination of the patient's diagnosis when appropriate, need for treatment, planning for treatment, periodic assessment, and documentation related to these activities

Assessments are further classified into more than 100 different tests or methods. The majority of these focus on the faculties of hearing and speech, but others focus on various aspects of body function, and on the patient's quality of life, such as muscle performance, neuromotor development, and reintegration skills.

- *Speech Assessment*: Measurement of speech and related functions
- *Motor and/or Nerve Function Assessment*: Measurement of motor, nerve, and related functions
- *Activities of Daily Living Assessment*: Measurement of functional level for activities of daily living
- *Hearing Assessment*: Measurement of hearing and related functions
- *Hearing Aid Assessment*: Measurement of the appropriateness and/or effectiveness of a hearing device
- *Vestibular Assessment*: Measurement of the vestibular system and related functions

Caregiver Training: Educating caregiver with the skills and knowledge used to interact with and assist the patient

Caregiver Training is divided into 18 different broad subjects taught to help a caregiver provide proper patient care.

- *Caregiver Training*: Training in activities to support patient's optimal level of function

Fitting(s): Design, fabrication, modification, selection, and/or application of splint, orthosis, prosthesis, hearing aids, and/or other rehabilitation device

The fifth character used in *Device Fitting* procedures describes the device being fitted rather than the method used to fit the device. Definitions of devices, when provided, are located in the definitions portion of the ICD-10-PCS tables and index, under section F, character 5.

- *Device Fitting*: Fitting of a device designed to facilitate or support achievement of a higher level of function

Treatment: Use of specific activities or methods to develop, improve, and/or restore the performance of necessary functions, compensate for dysfunction and/or minimize debilitation

Treatment procedures include swallowing dysfunction exercises, bathing and showering techniques, wound management, gait training, and a host of activities typically associated with rehabilitation.

- *Speech Treatment*: Application of techniques to improve, augment, or compensate for speech and related functional impairment
- *Motor Treatment*: Exercise or activities to increase or facilitate motor function
- *Activities of Daily Living Treatment*: Exercise or activities to facilitate functional competence for activities of daily living
- *Hearing Treatment*: Application of techniques to improve, augment, or compensate for hearing and related functional impairment

- *Cochlear Implant Treatment*: Application of techniques to improve the communication abilities of individuals with cochlear implant
- *Vestibular Treatment*: Application of techniques to improve, augment, or compensate for vestibular and related functional impairment

The type of treatment includes training as well as activities that restore function.

Body System/Region (Character 4)

The fourth character specifies the body region and/or system on which the procedure is performed.

Type Qualifier (Character 5)

The fifth character is a type qualifier that further specifies the procedure performed. Examples include therapy to improve the range of motion and training for bathing techniques. Refer to appendix J for definitions of these types of procedures.

Equipment (Character 6)

The sixth character specifies the equipment used. Specific equipment is not defined in the equipment value. Instead, broad categories of equipment are specified (e.g., aerobic endurance and conditioning, assistive/adaptive/supportive, etc.)

Qualifier (Character 7)

The seventh character is not specified in the Physical Rehabilitation and Diagnostic Audiology section and always has the value *None*.

Mental Health Section (G)

Character Meanings

The seven characters in the Mental Health section have the following meaning:

Character	Meaning
1	Section
2	Body System
3	Type
4	Qualifier
5	Qualifier
6	Qualifier
7	Qualifier

Section (Character 1)

Mental health procedure codes have a first character value of *G*.

Body System (Character 2)

The second character is used to identify the body system elsewhere in ICD-10-PCS. In this section it always has the value *None*.

Type (Character 3)

The third character specifies the procedure type, such as crisis intervention or counseling. There are 12 types of mental health procedures.

- *Psychological Tests:* The administration and interpretation of standardized psychological tests and measurement instruments for the assessment of psychological function
- *Crisis Intervention:* Treatment of a traumatized, acutely disturbed, or distressed individual for the purpose of short-term stabilization
- *Medication Management:* Monitoring and adjusting the use of medications for the treatment of a mental health disorder
- *Individual Psychotherapy:* Treatment of an individual with a mental health disorder by behavioral, cognitive, psychoanalytic, psychodynamic, or psychophysiological means to improve functioning or well-being
- *Counseling:* The application of psychological methods to treat an individual with normal developmental issues and psychological problems in order to increase function, improve well-being, alleviate distress, maladjustment, or resolve crises
- *Family Psychotherapy:* Treatment that includes one or more family members of an individual with a mental health disorder by behavioral, cognitive, psychoanalytic, psychodynamic, or psychophysiological means to improve functioning or well-being
- *Electroconvulsive Therapy:* The application of controlled electrical voltages to treat a mental health disorder
- *Biofeedback:* Provision of information from the monitoring and regulating of physiological processes in conjunction with cognitive-behavioral techniques to improve patient functioning or well-being
- *Hypnosis:* Induction of a state of heightened suggestibility by auditory, visual, and tactile techniques to elicit an emotional or behavioral response
- *Narcosynthesis:* Administration of intravenous barbiturates in order to release suppressed or repressed thoughts
- *Group Psychotherapy:* Treatment of two or more individuals with a mental health disorder by behavioral, cognitive, psychoanalytic, psychodynamic, or psychophysiological means to improve functioning or well-being
- *Light Therapy:* Application of specialized light treatments to improve functioning or well-being

Qualifier (Character 4)

The fourth character is a qualifier to indicate that counseling was educational or vocational or to indicate type of test or method of therapy.

Qualifier (Character 5, 6 and 7)

The fifth, sixth, and seventh characters are not specified and always have the value *None*.

Substance Abuse Treatment Section (H)

Character Meanings

The seven characters in the Substance Abuse Treatment section have the following meaning:

Character	Meaning
1	Section
2	Body System
3	Type
4	Qualifier
5	Qualifier
6	Qualifier
7	Qualifier

Section (Character 1)

Substance Abuse Treatment codes have a first character value of *H*.

Body System (Character 2)

The second character is used to identify the body system elsewhere in ICD-10-PCS. In this section, it always has the value *None*.

Type (Character 3)

The third character specifies the type of procedure. There are seven values classified in this section, as listed below:

- *Detoxification Services:* Detoxification from alcohol and/or drugs
- *Individual Counseling:* The application of psychological methods to treat an individual with addictive behavior
- *Group Counseling:* The application of psychological methods to treat two or more individuals with addictive behavior
- *Individual Psychotherapy:* Treatment of an individual with addictive behavior by behavioral, cognitive, psychoanalytic, psychodynamic, or psychophysiological means
- *Family Counseling:* The application of psychological methods that includes one or more family members to treat an individual with addictive behavior
- *Medication Management:* Monitoring and adjusting the use of replacement medications for the treatment of addiction
- *Pharmacotherapy:* The use of replacement medications for the treatment of addiction

Qualifier (Character 4)

The fourth character further specifies the procedure type. These qualifier values vary dependent upon the Root Type procedure (Character 3). Root type 2, *Detoxification Services* contains only the value Z, *None* and Root type 6, *Family Counseling* contains only the value 3, *Other Family Counseling*, whereas the remainder Root Type procedures include multiple possible values.

Qualifier (Character 5, 6 and 7)

The fifth through seventh characters are designated as qualifiers but are never specified, so they always have the value *None*.

New Technology Section (X)

General Information

Section X New Technology is a section added to ICD-10-PCS beginning October 1, 2015. The new section provides a place for codes that uniquely identify procedures requested via the New Technology Application Process or that capture other new technologies not currently classified in ICD-10-PCS.

Section X does not introduce any new coding concepts or unusual guidelines for correct coding. In fact, Section X codes maintain continuity with the other sections in ICD-10-PCS by using the same root operation and body part values as their closest counterparts in other sections of ICD-10-PCS. For example, the codes for the infusion of ceftazidime-avibactam, use the same root operation (Introduction) and body part values (Central Vein and Peripheral Vein) in section X as the infusion codes in section 3 Administration, which are their closest counterparts in the other sections of ICD-10-PCS.

Character Meanings

The seven characters in the new technology section have the following meaning:

Character	Meaning
1	Section
2	Body System
3	Root Operation
4	Body Part
5	Approach
6	Device/Substance/Technology
7	Qualifier

Section (Character 1)

New technology procedure codes have a first character value of *X*.

Body System (Character 2)

The second character values for body system combine the uses of body system, body region, and physiological system as specified in other sections in ICD-10-PCS.

Root Operation (Character 3)

The third character utilizes the same root operation values as their counterparts in other sections of ICD-10-PCS.

Body Part (Character 4)

The fourth character specifies the same body part values as their closest counterparts in other sections of ICD-10-PCS.

Approach (Character 5)

The fifth character specifies approaches as defined in the Medical and Surgical section.

Device/Substance/Technology (Character 6)

The sixth character specifies the key feature of the new technology procedure. It may be specified as a new device, a new substance, or other new technology. Examples of sixth character values are *blinatumomab antineoplastic immunotherapy, orbital atherectomy technology,* and *intraoperative knee replacement sensor*.

Qualifier (Character 7)

The seventh character qualifier is used exclusively to specify the new technology group, a number or letter that changes each year that new technology codes are added to the system. For example, Section X codes added for the first year have the seventh character value 1, *New Technology Group 1*, and the next year that Section X codes are added have the seventh character value 2, *New Technology Group 2*, and so on. Changing the seventh character value to a unique letter or number every year that there are new codes in the new technology section allows the ICD-10-PCS to "recycle" the values in the third, fourth, and sixth characters as needed.

New Technology Coding Instruction

Section X codes are standalone codes. They are not supplemental codes. Section X codes fully represent the specific procedure described in the code title, and do not require any additional codes from other sections of ICD-10-PCS. When section X contains a code title which describes a specific new technology procedure, only that X code is reported for the procedure. There is no need to report a broader, non-specific code in another section of ICD-10-PCS.

For example, code XW033G5 Introduction of Sarilumab into Peripheral Vein, Percutaneous Approach, New Technology Group 5, would be reported to indicate that Sarilumab was administered via peripheral vein. A separate code from table 3EØ in the Administration section of ICD-10-PCS would not be reported in addition to this code. The X section code fully identifies the administration of the sarilumab, and no additional code is needed.

The New Technology section codes are easily found by looking in the ICD-10-PCS Index or the Tables. In the Index, the name of the new technology device, substance or technology for a section X code is included as a main term. In addition, all codes in section X are listed under the main term New Technology. The new technology code index entry for sarilumab is shown below.

Sarilumab XWØ

New Technology
    Sarilumab XWØ

ICD-10-PCS Index and Tabular Format

The *ICD-10-PCS: The Complete Official Code Set* is based on the official version of the International Classification of Diseases, 10th Revision, Procedure Classification System, issued by the U.S. Department of Health and Human Services, Centers for Medicare and Medicaid Services. This book is consistent with the content of the government's version of ICD-10-PCS and follows their official format.

Index

The Alphabetic Index can be used to locate the appropriate table containing all the information necessary to construct a procedure code, however, the PCS tables should always be consulted to find the most appropriate valid code. Users may choose a valid code directly from the tables—he or she need not consult the index before proceeding to the tables to complete the code.

Main Terms

The Alphabetic Index reflects the structure of the tables. Therefore, the index is organized as an alphabetic listing. The index:

- Is based on the value of the third character
- Contains common procedure terms
- Lists anatomic sites
- Uses device terms

The main terms in the Alphabetic Index are root operations, root procedure types, or common procedure names. In addition, anatomic sites from the Body Part Key and device terms from the Device Key have been added for ease of use.

Examples:

Resection (root operation)

Fluoroscopy (root type)

Prostatectomy (common procedure name)

Brachiocephalic artery (body part)

Bard® Dulex™ mesh (device)

The index provides at least the first three or four values of the code, and some entries may provide complete valid codes. However, the user should always consult the appropriate table to verify that the most appropriate valid code has been selected.

Root Operation and Procedure Type Main Terms

For the *Medical and Surgical* and related sections, the root operation values are used as main terms in the index. The subterms under the root operation main terms are body parts. For the Ancillary section of the tables, the main terms in the index are the general type of procedure performed.

Examples:

Biofeedback GZC9ZZZ
Destruction
  Acetabulum
    Left ØQ55
    Right ØQ54
  Adenoids ØC5Q
  Ampulla of Vater ØF5C
Planar Nuclear Medicine Imaging
  Abdomen CW1Ø

See Reference

The second type of term in the index uses common procedure names, such as "appendectomy" or "fundoplication." These common terms are listed as main terms with a "see" reference noting the PCS root operations that are possible valid code tables based on the objective of the procedure.

Examples:

Tendonectomy
  see Excision, Tendons ØLB
  see Resection, Tendons ØLT

Use Reference

The index also lists anatomic sites from the Body Part Key and device terms from the Device Key. These terms are listed with a "use" reference. The purpose of these references is to act as an additional reference to the terms located in the Appendix Keys. The term provided is the Body Part value or Device value to be selected when constructing a procedure code using the code tables. This type of index reference is not intended to direct the user to another term in the index, but to provide guidance regarding character value selection. Therefore, "use" references generally do not refer to specific valid code tables.

Examples:

CoAxia NeuroFlo catheter
  use Intraluminal Device
Epitrochlear lymph node
  use Lymphatic, Left Upper Extremity
  use Lymphatic, Right Upper Extremity
SynCardia Total Artificial Heart
  use Synthetic Substitute

Code Tables

ICD-10-PCS contains 17 sections of Code Tables organized by general type of procedure. The first three characters of a procedure code define each table. The tables consist of columns providing the possible last four characters of codes and rows providing valid values for each character. Within a PCS table, valid codes include all combinations of choices in characters 4 through 7 contained in the same row of the table. All seven characters must be specified to form a valid code.

There are three main sections of tables:

- Medical and Surgical section:
  - — *Medical and Surgical* (Ø)
- Medical and Surgical-related sections:
  - — *Obstetrics* (1)
  - — *Placement* (2)
  - — *Administration* (3)
  - — *Measurement and Monitoring* (4)
  - — *Extracorporeal or Systemic Assistance and Performance* (5)
  - — *Extracorporeal or Systemic Therapies* (6)
  - — *Osteopathic* (7)
  - — *Other Procedures* (8)
  - — *Chiropractic* (9)

- Ancillary sections:
  - *Imaging* (B)
  - *Nuclear Medicine* (C)
  - *Radiation Therapy* (D)
  - *Physical Rehabilitation and Diagnostic Audiology* (F)
  - *Mental Health* (G)
  - *Substance Abuse Treatment* (H)
- New Technology section:
  - *New Technology* (X)

The first three character values define each table. The root operation or root type designated for each table is accompanied by its official definition.

Example:

Table ØØF provides codes for procedures on the central nervous system that involve breaking up of solid matter into pieces:

Character 1, Section	Ø: Medical and Surgical
Character 2, Body System	Ø: Central Nervous System and Cranial Nerves
Character 3, Root Operation	F: Fragmentation: Breaking solid matter in a body part into pieces

Tables are arranged numerically, then alphabetically.

When reviewing tables, the user should keep in mind that:

- Some tables may cover multiple pages in the code book—to ensure maximum clarity about character choices, valid entries do not split rows between pages. For instance, the entire table of valid characters completing a code beginning with 4A1 is split between two pages, but the split is between, not within, rows. This means that all the valid sixth and seventh characters for, say, body system *Arterial* (3) and approach *External* (X) are contained on one page.
- Individual entries may be listed in several horizontal "selection" lines.
- When a table is continued onto another page, a note to this effect has been added in red.

Body Part Definitions:

An exclusive Optum360 feature in the tables is the incorporation of the body part definitions provided in appendix E into the Medical and Surgical section (Ø) tables under their appropriate body part characters in the first column (character 4). This provides the user a direct reference to all anatomical descriptions, terms, and sites that could be coded to that particular body part value.

Paired body parts typically have values for the right and left side and in some cases a value for bilateral. These paired body parts often have the same list of inclusive body part definitions. When there are paired body parts with the same body part definitions, the first listed body part (usually the right side) contains the list of body part definitions while the second listed body part (usually the left side) contains a ***See*** instruction. This ***See*** instruction references the body part value that contains the body part definitions. In the table below, body part value P – Upper Eyelid, Left is followed by a ***See*** instruction that states ***See*** *N Upper Eyelid, Right*. All body part descriptions under value N also apply to body part value P.

Example:

Ø Medical and Surgical
8 Eye
M Reattachment Definition: Putting back in or on all or a portion of a separated body part to its normal location or other suitable location
Explanation: Vascular circulation and nervous pathways may or may not be reestablished

Body Part Character 4	Approach Character 5	Device Character 6	Qualifier Character 7
N Upper Eyelid, Right Lateral canthus Levator palpebrae superioris muscle Orbicularis oculi muscle Superior tarsal plate **P Upper Eyelid, Left** *See N Upper Eyelid, Right* **Q Lower Eyelid, Right** Inferior tarsal plate Medial canthus **R Lower Eyelid, Left** *See Q Lower Eyelid, Right*	**X External**	**Z No Device**	**Z No Qualifier**

ICD-10-PCS Additional Features

Use of Official Sources

Color-coding, symbol, and other annotations in this manual that identify coding and reimbursement issues are derived from various official federal government sources, including the *Federal Register*, volume 86, number 88, May 10, 2021 ("Hospital Inpatient Prospective Payment Systems for Acute Care Hospitals and the Long Term Care Hospital Prospective Payment System and Proposed Policy Changes and Fiscal Year 2022 Rates; Proposed Rule") and the proposed, version 39, MS-DRG Grouper software, Definitions Manual files and Medicare Code Editor (MCE) files published with the fiscal 2022 IPPS proposed rule. For the most current files related to IPPS, please refer to the following:

- FY2022 IPPS Final Rule
  https://www.cms.gov/Medicare/Medicare-Fee-for-Service-Payment/AcuteInpatientPPS/IPPS-Regulations-and-Notices
- FY2022 Final Version 39, MS-DRG Grouper software
  https://www.cms.gov/Medicare/Medicare-Fee-for-Service-Payment/AcuteInpatientPPS/MS-DRG-Classifications-and-Software

Table Notations

Many tables in ICD-10-PCS contain color or symbol annotations that may aid in code selection, provide clinical or coding information, or alert the coder to reimbursement issues affected by the PCS code assignment. These annotations may be displayed on or next to a character 4, character 6, or character 7 value. Please note that some values may have more than one annotation; this is true most often with the character 4 value.

Refer to the color/symbol legend at the bottom of each page in the tables section for an abridged description of each color and symbol.

Annotation Box

An annotation box has been appended to all tables that contain color-coding or symbol annotations. The color bar or symbol attached to a character value is provided in the box, as well as a list of the valid PCS code(s) to which that edit applies. The box may also list conditional criteria that must be met to satisfy the edit.

For example, see Table ØØF. Four character 4 body part values have a gray color bar. In the annotation box below the table, the gray color bar is defined as "Non-OR," or a nonoperating room procedure edit. Following the Non-OR annotation are the PCS codes that are considered nonoperating room procedures from that row of Table ØØF.

Bracketed Code Notation

The use of bracketed codes is an efficient convention to provide all valid character value alternatives for a specific set of circumstances. The character values in the brackets correspond to the valid values for the character in the position the bracket appears.

Examples:

In the annotation box for Table ØØF the Noncovered Procedure edit (NC) applies to codes represented in the bracketed code ØØF[3,4,5,6]XZZ.

ØØF[3,4,5,6]XZZ Fragmentation in (Central Nervous System and Cranial Nerves), External Approach

The valid fourth character values (body part) that may be selected for this specific circumstance are as follows:

3 Epidural Space, Intracranial
4 Subdural Space, Intracranial
5 Subarachnoid Space, Intracranial
6 Cerebral Ventricle

The fragmentation of matter in the spinal canal, Body Part value U, is not included in the noncovered procedure code edit.

Color-Coding/Symbols

New and Revised Text

To highlight changes to the PCS tables for the current year, the new and revised text is provided in green font.

Medicare Code Edits

Medicare administrative contractors (MACs) and many payers use Medicare code edits to check the coding accuracy on claims. The coding edits provided in this manual include only those directly related to ICD-10-PCS codes used for acute care hospital inpatient admissions. These edits are based on the proposed, version 39, Medicare Code Editor (MCE) files published with the fiscal 2022 IPPS proposed rule.

The PCS related Medicare code edits are listed below:

- Invalid procedure code
- *Sex conflict
- *Questionable obstetric admission
- *Noncovered procedure
- *Limited coverage procedure

Starred edits above that are related to PCS issues are identified in this manual by symbols as described below.

Sex Edit Symbols

The sex edit symbols below are used to detect inconsistencies between the patient's sex and the procedure. The symbols below most often appear to the right of the body part (character 4) value but may also be found to the right of the qualifier (character 7) value:

♂ Male procedure only
♀ Female procedure only

QA **Questionable Obstetric Admission**

An inpatient admission is considered questionable when a vaginal or cesarean delivery code is assigned without a corresponding secondary diagnosis code describing the outcome of delivery. Both a delivery (ICD-10-PCS) code and an outcome-of-delivery (ICD-10-CM) code must be present to avoid errors in MS-DRG assignment. This symbol is found only in the Obstetrics Section, appearing to the right of the body part (character 4) value.

NC **Noncovered Procedure**

Medicare does not cover all procedures. However, some noncovered procedures, due to the presence of certain diagnoses, are reimbursed.

LC **Limited Coverage**

For certain procedures whose medical complexity and serious nature incur extraordinary associated costs, Medicare limits coverage to a portion of the cost. The limited coverage edit indicates the type of limited coverage.

ICD-10 MS-DRG Definitions Manual Edits

An MS-DRG is assigned based on specific patient attributes, such as principal diagnosis, secondary diagnoses, procedures, and discharge status. The attributes (edits) provided in this manual include only those directly related to ICD-10-PCS codes used for acute care hospital inpatient admissions. These edits are based on the proposed, version 39, MS-DRG Grouper software and Definitions Manual published with the fiscal 2022 IPPS proposed rule.

Non-Operating Room Procedures Not Affecting MS-DRG Assignment

In the Medical and Surgical section (ØØ1-ØYW) and the Obstetric section (1Ø2-1ØY) tables **only,** ICD-10-PCS procedures codes that DO NOT affect MS-DRG assignment are identified by a **gray color bar** over the body part (character 4) value and are considered non-operating room (non-OR) procedures.

NOTE: The majority of the ICD-10-PCS codes in the Medical and Surgical-Related, Ancillary and New Technology section tables are non-operating room procedures that do not typically affect MS-DRG assignment. Only the Valid Operating Room and DRG Non-Operating Room procedures are highlighted in these sections, *see* Non-Operating Room Procedures Affecting MS-DRG Assignment and Valid OR Procedure description below.

Non-Operating Room Procedures Affecting MS-DRG Assignment

Some ICD-10-PCS procedure codes, although considered non-operating room procedures, may still affect MS-DRG assignment. In all sections of the ICD-10-PCS book, these procedures are identified by a **purple color bar** over the body part (character 4) value.

Valid OR Procedure

In the Medical and Surgical-Related (2WØ-9WB), Ancillary (BØØ-HZ9) and New Technology (X2A-XYØ) section tables **only,** any codes that are considered a valid operating room procedure are identified with a **blue color bar** over the body part (character 4) value and will affect MS-DRG assignment. All codes without a color bar (blue or purple) are considered non-operating room procedures.

Hospital-Acquired Condition Related Procedures

Procedures associated with hospital-acquired conditions (HAC) are identified with the **yellow color bar** over the body part (character 4) value. Appendix K provides each specific HAC category and its associated ICD-10-CM and ICD-10-PCS codes.

Combination Only

Some ICD-10-PCS procedure codes that describe non-operating room procedures can group to a specific MS-DRG but only when used in combination with certain other ICD-10-PCS procedure codes. Such codes are designated by a **red color bar** over the body part (character 4) value.

⊞ **Combination Member**

A combination member, which can be either a valid operating room procedure or a non-operating room procedure, is an ICD-10-PCS procedure code that can influence MS-DRG assignment either on its own or in combination with other specific ICD-10-PCS procedure codes. Combination member codes are designated by a plus sign (⊞) to the right of the body part (character 4) value.

Note: In the few instances when a code is both a combination member and a non-operating room procedure affecting the MS-DRG assignment, the body part (character 4) value will have a purple color bar and the combination member icon.

See Appendix L for Procedure Combinations

Under certain circumstances, more than one procedure code is needed in order to group to a specific MS-DRG. When codes within a table have been identified as a Combination Only (**red color bar**) or Combination Member (⊞) code, there is also a footnote instructing the coder to *see Appendix L*. Appendix L contains tables that identify the other procedure codes needed in the combination and the title and number of the MS-DRG to which the combination will group.

Other Table Notations

AHA Coding Clinic:

Official citations from AHA's *Coding Clinic for ICD-10-CM/PCS* have been provided at the beginning of each section, when applicable. Each specific citation is listed below a header identifying the table to which that particular *Coding Clinic* citation applies. The citations appear in purple type with the year, quarter, and page of the reference as well as the title of the question as it appears in that *Coding Clinic's* table of contents. *Coding Clinic* citations included in this edition have been updated through second quarter 2021.

NT **New Technology Add-on Payment**

This symbol identifies procedure codes that involve new technologies or medical services that have qualified for a new technology add-on payment (NTAP). CMS provides incremental payment, in addition to the DRG payment, for technologies that have received the NTAP designation. This symbol appears to the right of the sixth character value.

Note: Only specific brand or trade named devices, substances, or technologies receive NTAP approval. The sixth character value in the PCS table provides a generalized description that may be applicable to several brand or trade names. Unless otherwise specified in the annotation box, refer to appendix H or I to determine the specific brand or trade name of the device, substance, or technology that is applicable to the new technology add-on payment. New technology add-on payments are not exclusive to the New Technology (X) section.

Appendixes

The resources described below have been included as appendixes for *ICD-10-PCS The Complete Official Code Set*. These resources further instruct the coder on the appropriate application of the ICD-10-PCS code set.

Appendix A: Components of the Medical and Surgical Approach Definitions

This resource further defines the approach characters used in the Medical and Surgical (Ø) section. Complementing the detailed definition of the approach, additional information includes whether or not instrumentation is a part of the approach, the typical access location, the method used to initiate the approach, related procedural examples, and illustrations all of which will help the user determine the appropriate approach value.

Appendix B: Root Operation Definitions

This resource is a compilation of all root operations found in the Medical and Surgical-related sections (Ø-9) of this PCS manual. It provides a definition and in some cases a more detailed explanation of the root operation, to better reflect the purpose or objective. Examples of related procedure(s) may also be provided.

Appendix C: Comparison of Medical and Surgical Root Operations

The Medical and Surgical (Ø) section root operations are divided into groups that share similar attributes. These groups, and the root operations in each group, are listed in this resource along with information identifying the target of the root operation, the action used to perform the root operation, any clarification or further explanation on the objective of the root operation, and procedure examples.

Appendix D: Body Part Key

When an anatomical term or description is provided in the documentation but does not have a specific body part character within a table, the user can reference this resource to search for the anatomical description or site noted in the documentation to determine if there is a specific PCS body part character (character 4) to which the anatomical description or site could be coded.

Appendix E: Body Part Definitions

This resource is the reverse look-up of the Body Part Key. Each table in the Medical and Surgical section (Ø) of the PCS manual contains anatomical terms linked to a body part character or value, for example, in Table ØBB the Body Part (character 4) of 1 is Trachea. The body part Trachea may have anatomical structures or descriptions that may be used in procedure documentation instead of the term trachea. The Body Part Definitions list other anatomical structures or synonyms that are included in specific ICD-10-PCS body part values. According to the body part definitions, in the example above, cricoid cartilage is included in the Trachea (character 1) body part.

Appendix F: Device Classification

This resource provides an explanation of how a device is defined in the ICD-10-PCS classification along with two tables. The first table groups devices used in the ICD-10-PCS tables into general categories, including a definition of each device type and related examples. The second table provides definitions of transplant and grafting tissue types and associated terminology that may be found in the documentation.

Appendix G: Device Key and Aggregation Table

The Device Key helps users code the appropriate PCS sixth character for device. Devices are listed alphabetically by brand name or commonly used medical terminology and are translated to the appropriate PCS language or value. The key also reflects the body system where the device is located. For example, a SAPIEN valve used for transaortic valve replacement translates to Zooplastic Tissue in Heart and Great Vessels.

The following symbol NT has been placed next to those devices that have received an NTAP (new technology add-on payment) designation. When the code for this device is applied to an inpatient encounter, CMS provides incremental payment in addition to the DRG payment.

The Aggregation Table crosswalks specific device character value definitions for specific root operations in a specific body system to the more general device character value to be used when the root operation covers a wide range of body parts and the device character represents an entire family of devices.

Appendix H: Device Definitions

This resource is a reverse look-up to the Device Key. The user may reference this resource to see all the specific devices that may be grouped to a particular device character (character 6).

Example:
The operative report states, "An internal fixation device was used to repair a fractured femur. Kirschner wire, bone screws and neutralization plate all used and left in the bone at the end of the procedure."

Although PCS requires all devices left in the body to be coded and the operative report lists three different devices, a check in the device definitions shows that all of these devices are included in the PCS value "Internal Fixation Device" and require only one code.

The following symbol NT has been placed next to those devices that have received an NTAP (new technology add-on payment) designation. When the code for this device is applied to an inpatient encounter, CMS provides incremental payment in addition to the DRG payment.

Appendix I: Substance Key/Substance Definitions

The Substance Key lists substances by trade name or synonym and relates them to a PCS character in the Administration (3) or New Technology (X) section in the Substance (sixth character) or Qualifier (seventh character) column.

The Substance Definitions table is the reverse look-up of the substance key, relating all substance categories, the sixth- or seventh character values, to all trade name or synonyms that may be classified to that particular character.

The following symbol NT has been placed next to those substances/technologies that have received an NTAP (new technology add-on payment) designation. When the code for this substance/technology is applied to an inpatient encounter, CMS provides incremental payment in addition to the DRG payment.

Appendix J: Sections B-H Character Definitions

In each ancillary section (B-H) the characters in a particular column may have different meanings depending on which section the user is working from. This resource provides the values for the characters in these sections as well as a definition of the character value.

Appendix K: Hospital Acquired Conditions

Hospital acquired conditions (HACs) are conditions that are considered reasonably preventable when occurring during the hospital admission and may prevent a case from grouping to a higher-paying MS-DRG. In certain instances the HACs are conditional, requiring a specific ICD-10-CM diagnosis code in combination with a specific ICD-10-PCS procedure code. This resource identifies these conditional HACs, listing the diagnosis and procedure codes that, in combination, may trigger a HAC edit. All codes, ICD-10-CM and ICD-10-PCS, are listed with their full descriptions.

Appendix L: Procedure Combination Tables

The procedure combination tables provided in this resource illustrate certain procedure combinations that must occur in order to assign a specific MS-DRG.

Appendix M: Coding Exercises and Answers

This resource provides the coding exercises with answers, and in some cases a brief explanation as to the reason that particular code was used.

ICD-10-PCS Official Guidelines for Coding and Reporting 2022

Narrative changes appear in **bold** text.

The Centers for Medicare and Medicaid Services (CMS) and the National Center for Health Statistics (NCHS), two departments within the U.S. Federal Government's Department of Health and Human Services (DHHS) provide the following guidelines for coding and reporting using the International Classification of Diseases, 10th Revision, Procedure Coding System (ICD-10-PCS). These guidelines should be used as a companion document to the official version of the ICD-10-PCS as published on the CMS website. The ICD-10-PCS is a procedure classification published by the United States for classifying procedures performed in hospital inpatient health care settings.

These guidelines have been approved by the four organizations that make up the Cooperating Parties for the ICD-10-PCS: the American Hospital Association (AHA), the American Health Information Management Association (AHIMA), CMS, and NCHS.

These guidelines are a set of rules that have been developed to accompany and complement the official conventions and instructions provided within the ICD-10-PCS itself. They are intended to provide direction that is applicable in most circumstances. However, there may be unique circumstances where exceptions are applied. The instructions and conventions of the classification take precedence over guidelines. These guidelines are based on the coding and sequencing instructions in the Tables, Index and Definitions of ICD-10-PCS, but provide additional instruction. Adherence to these guidelines when assigning ICD-10-PCS procedure codes is required under the Health Insurance Portability and Accountability Act (HIPAA). The procedure codes have been adopted under HIPAA for hospital inpatient healthcare settings. A joint effort between the healthcare provider and the coder is essential to achieve complete and accurate documentation, code assignment, and reporting of diagnoses and procedures. These guidelines have been developed to assist both the healthcare provider and the coder in identifying those procedures that are to be reported. The importance of consistent, complete documentation in the medical record cannot be overemphasized. Without such documentation accurate coding cannot be achieved.

Conventions

A1. ICD-10-PCS codes are composed of seven characters. Each character is an axis of classification that specifies information about the procedure performed. Within a defined code range, a character specifies the same type of information in that axis of classification.

Example:
The fifth axis of classification specifies the approach in sections Ø through 4 and 7 through 9 of the system.

A2. One of 34 possible values can be assigned to each axis of classification in the seven-character code: they are the numbers Ø through 9 and the alphabet (except I and O because they are easily confused with the numbers 1 and Ø). The number of unique values used in an axis of classification differs as needed.

Example:
Where the fifth axis of classification specifies the approach, seven different approach values are currently used to specify the approach.

A3. The valid values for an axis of classification can be added to as needed.

Example:
If a significantly distinct type of device is used in a new procedure, a new device value can be added to the system.

A4. As with words in their context, the meaning of any single value is a combination of its axis of classification and any preceding values on which it may be dependent.

Example:
The meaning of a body part value in the Medical and Surgical section is always dependent on the body system value. The body part value Ø in the Central Nervous body system specifies Brain and the body part value Ø in the Peripheral Nervous body system specifies Cervical Plexus.

A5. As the system is expanded to become increasingly detailed, over time more values will depend on preceding values for their meaning.

Example:
In the Lower Joints body system, the device value 3 in the root operation Insertion specifies Infusion Device and the device value 3 in the root operation Replacement specifies Ceramic Synthetic Substitute.

A6. The purpose of the alphabetic index is to locate the appropriate table that contains all information necessary to construct a procedure code. The PCS Tables should always be consulted to find the most appropriate valid code.

A7. It is not required to consult the index first before proceeding to the tables to complete the code. A valid code may be chosen directly from the tables.

A8. All seven characters must be specified to be a valid code. If the documentation is incomplete for coding purposes, the physician should be queried for the necessary information.

A9. Within a PCS table, valid codes include all combinations of choices in characters 4 through 7 contained in the same row of the table. In the example below, ØJHT3VZ is a valid code, and ØJHW3VZ is *not* a valid code.

Section: Ø **Medical and Surgical**
Body System: J **Subcutaneous Tissue and Fascia**
Operation: H **Insertion** Putting in a nonbiological appliance that monitors, assists, performs, or prevents a physiological function but does not physically take the place of a body part

Body Part	Approach	Device	Qualifier
S Subcutaneous Tissue and Fascia, Head and Neck **V** Subcutaneous Tissue and Fascia, Upper Extremity **W** Subcutaneous Tissue and Fascia, Lower Extremity	**Ø** Open **3** Percutaneous	**1** Radioactive Element **3** Infusion Device **Y** Other Device	**Z** No Qualifier
T Subcutaneous Tissue and Fascia, Trunk	**Ø** Open **3** Percutaneous	**1** Radioactive Element **3** Infusion Device **V** Infusion Pump **Y** Other Device	**Z** No Qualifier

A10. "And," when used in a code description, means "and/or," except when used to describe a combination of multiple body parts for which separate values exist for each body part (e.g., Skin and Subcutaneous Tissue used as a qualifier, where there are separate body part values for "Skin" and "Subcutaneous Tissue").

Example:
Lower Arm and Wrist Muscle means lower arm and/or wrist muscle.

A11. Many of the terms used to construct PCS codes are defined within the system. It is the coder's responsibility to determine what the documentation in the medical record equates to in the PCS definitions. The physician is not expected to use the terms used in PCS code descriptions, nor is the coder required to query the physician when the correlation between the documentation and the defined PCS terms is clear.

Example:
When the physician documents "partial resection" the coder can independently correlate "partial resection" to the root operation Excision without querying the physician for clarification.

Medical and Surgical Section Guidelines (section Ø)

B2. Body System

General guidelines

B2.1a. The procedure codes in Anatomical Regions, General, Anatomical Regions, Upper Extremities and Anatomical Regions, Lower Extremities can be used when the procedure is performed on an anatomical region rather than a specific body part, or on the rare occasion when no information is available to support assignment of a code to a specific body part.

Examples:
Chest tube drainage of the pleural cavity is coded to the root operation Drainage found in the body system Anatomical Regions, General.

Suture repair of the abdominal wall is coded to the root operation Repair in the body system Anatomical Regions, General.

Amputation of the foot is coded to the root operation Detachment in the body system Anatomical Regions, Lower Extremities.

B2.1b. Where the general body part values "upper" and "lower" are provided as an option in the Upper Arteries, Lower Arteries, Upper Veins, Lower Veins, Muscles and Tendons body systems, "upper" or "lower" specifies body parts located above or below the diaphragm respectively.

Example:
Vein body parts above the diaphragm are found in the Upper Veins body system; vein body parts below the diaphragm are found in the Lower Veins body system.

B3. Root Operation

General guidelines

B3.1a. In order to determine the appropriate root operation, the full definition of the root operation as contained in the PCS Tables must be applied.

B3.1b. Components of a procedure specified in the root operation definition or explanation as integral to that root operation are not coded separately. Procedural steps necessary to reach the operative site and close the operative site, including anastomosis of a tubular body part, are also not coded separately.

Examples:
Resection of a joint as part of a joint replacement procedure is included in the root operation definition of Replacement and is not coded separately.

Laparotomy performed to reach the site of an open liver biopsy is not coded separately.

In a resection of sigmoid colon with anastomosis of descending colon to rectum, the anastomosis is not coded separately.

Multiple procedures

B3.2. During the same operative episode, multiple procedures are coded if:

a. The same root operation is performed on different body parts as defined by distinct values of the body part character.
Examples:
Diagnostic excision of liver and pancreas are coded separately.
Excision of lesion in the ascending colon and excision of lesion in the transverse colon are coded separately.

b. The same root operation is repeated in multiple body parts, and those body parts are separate and distinct body parts classified to a single ICD-10-PCS body part value.
Examples:
Excision of the sartorius muscle and excision of the gracilis muscle are both included in the upper leg muscle body part value, and multiple procedures are coded.
Extraction of multiple toenails are coded separately.

c. Multiple root operations with distinct objectives are performed on the same body part.
Example:
Destruction of sigmoid lesion and bypass of sigmoid colon are coded separately.

d. The intended root operation is attempted using one approach but is converted to a different approach.
Example:
Laparoscopic cholecystectomy converted to an open cholecystectomy is coded as percutaneous endoscopic Inspection and open Resection.

Discontinued or incomplete procedures

B3.3. If the intended procedure is discontinued or otherwise not completed, code the procedure to the root operation performed. If a procedure is discontinued before any other root operation is performed, code the root operation Inspection of the body part or anatomical region inspected.

Example:
A planned aortic valve replacement procedure is discontinued after the initial thoracotomy and before any incision is made in the heart muscle, when the patient becomes hemodynamically unstable. This procedure is coded as an open Inspection of the mediastinum.

Biopsy procedures

B3.4a. Biopsy procedures are coded using the root operations Excision, Extraction, or Drainage and the qualifier Diagnostic.

Examples:
Fine needle aspiration biopsy of fluid in the lung is coded to the root operation Drainage with the qualifier Diagnostic.

Biopsy of bone marrow is coded to the root operation Extraction with the qualifier Diagnostic.

Lymph node sampling for biopsy is coded to the root operation Excision with the qualifier Diagnostic.

Biopsy followed by more definitive treatment

B3.4b. If a diagnostic Excision, Extraction, or Drainage procedure (biopsy) is followed by a more definitive procedure, such as Destruction, Excision or Resection at the same procedure site, both the biopsy and the more definitive treatment are coded.

Example:
Biopsy of breast followed by partial mastectomy at the same procedure site, both the biopsy and the partial mastectomy procedure are coded.

Overlapping body layers

B3.5. If root operations such as Excision, Extraction, Repair or Inspection are performed on overlapping layers of the musculoskeletal system, the body part specifying the deepest layer is coded.

Example:
Excisional debridement that includes skin and subcutaneous tissue and muscle is coded to the muscle body part.

Bypass procedures

B3.6a. Bypass procedures are coded by identifying the body part bypassed "from" and the body part bypassed "to." The fourth character body part specifies the body part bypassed from, and the qualifier specifies the body part bypassed to.

Example:
Bypass from stomach to jejunum, stomach is the body part and jejunum is the qualifier.

B3.6b. Coronary artery bypass procedures are coded differently than other bypass procedures as described in the previous guideline. Rather than identifying the body part bypassed from, the body part identifies the number of coronary arteries bypassed to, and the qualifier specifies the vessel bypassed from.

Example:
Aortocoronary artery bypass of the left anterior descending coronary artery and the obtuse marginal coronary artery is classified in the body part axis of classification as two coronary arteries, and the qualifier specifies the aorta as the body part bypassed from.

B3.6c. If multiple coronary arteries are bypassed, a separate procedure is coded for each coronary artery that uses a different device and/or qualifier.

Example:
Aortocoronary artery bypass and internal mammary coronary artery bypass are coded separately.

*Control vs. more **specific** root operations*

B3.7. The root operation Control is defined as, "Stopping, or attempting to stop, postprocedural or other acute bleeding." **Control is the root operation coded when the procedure performed to achieve hemostasis, beyond what would be considered integral to a procedure, utilizes techniques (e.g. cautery, application of substances or pressure, suturing or ligation or clipping of bleeding points at the site) that are not described by a more specific root operation definition, such as Bypass, Detachment, Excision, Extraction, Reposition, Replacement, or Resection. If a more specific root operation definition applies to the procedure performed, then the more specific root operation is coded instead of Control.**

Example:
Silver nitrate cautery to treat acute nasal bleeding is coded to the root operation Control.

Example:
Liquid embolization of the right internal iliac artery to treat acute hematoma by stopping blood flow is coded to the root operation Occlusion.

Example:
Suctioning of residual blood to achieve hemostasis during a transbronchial cryobiopsy is considered integral to the cryobiopsy procedure and is not coded separately.

Excision vs. Resection

B3.8. PCS contains specific body parts for anatomical subdivisions of a body part, such as lobes of the lungs or liver and regions of the intestine. Resection of the specific body part is coded whenever all of the body part is cut out or off, rather than coding Excision of a less specific body part.

Example:
Left upper lung lobectomy is coded to Resection of Upper Lung Lobe, Left rather than Excision of Lung, Left.

Excision for graft

B3.9. If an autograft is obtained from a different procedure site in order to complete the objective of the procedure, a separate procedure is coded, except when the seventh character qualifier value in the ICD-10-PCS table fully specifies the site from which the autograft was obtained.

Examples:
Coronary bypass with excision of saphenous vein graft, excision of saphenous vein is coded separately.

Replacement of breast with autologous deep inferior epigastric artery perforator (DIEP) flap, excision of the DIEP flap is not coded separately. The seventh character qualifier value Deep Inferior Epigastric Artery Perforator Flap in the Replacement table fully specifies the site of the autograft harvest.

Fusion procedures of the spine

B3.10a. The body part coded for a spinal vertebral joint(s) rendered immobile by a spinal fusion procedure is classified by the level of the spine (e.g. thoracic). There are distinct body part values for a single vertebral joint and for multiple vertebral joints at each spinal level.

Example:
Body part values specify Lumbar Vertebral Joint, Lumbar Vertebral Joints, 2 or More and Lumbosacral Vertebral Joint.

B3.10b. If multiple vertebral joints are fused, a separate procedure is coded for each vertebral joint that uses a different device and/or qualifier.

Example:
Fusion of lumbar vertebral joint, posterior approach, anterior column and fusion of lumbar vertebral joint, posterior approach, posterior column are coded separately.

B3.10c. Combinations of devices and materials are often used on a vertebral joint to render the joint immobile. When combinations of devices are used on the same vertebral joint, the device value coded for the procedure is as follows:

- If an interbody fusion device is used to render the joint immobile (containing bone graft or bone graft substitute), the procedure is coded with the device value Interbody Fusion Device
- If bone graft is the *only* device used to render the joint immobile, the procedure is coded with the device value Nonautologous Tissue Substitute or Autologous Tissue Substitute

- If a mixture of autologous and nonautologous bone graft (with or without biological or synthetic extenders or binders) is used to render the joint immobile, code the procedure with the device value Autologous Tissue Substitute

Examples:
Fusion of a vertebral joint using a cage style interbody fusion device containing morsellized bone graft is coded to the device Interbody Fusion Device.

Fusion of a vertebral joint using a bone dowel interbody fusion device made of cadaver bone and packed with a mixture of local morsellized bone and demineralized bone matrix is coded to the device Interbody Fusion Device.

Fusion of a vertebral joint using both autologous bone graft and bone bank bone graft is coded to the device Autologous Tissue Substitute.

Inspection procedures

B3.11a. Inspection of a body part(s) performed in order to achieve the objective of a procedure is not coded separately.

Example:
Fiberoptic bronchoscopy performed for irrigation of bronchus, only the irrigation procedure is coded.

B3.11b. If multiple tubular body parts are inspected, the most distal body part (the body part furthest from the starting point of the inspection) is coded. If multiple non-tubular body parts in a region are inspected, the body part that specifies the entire area inspected is coded.

Examples:
Cystoureteroscopy with inspection of bladder and ureters is coded to the ureter body part value.

Exploratory laparotomy with general inspection of abdominal contents is coded to the peritoneal cavity body part value.

B3.11c. When both an Inspection procedure and another procedure are performed on the same body part during the same episode, if the Inspection procedure is performed using a different approach than the other procedure, the Inspection procedure is coded separately.

Example:
Endoscopic Inspection of the duodenum is coded separately when open Excision of the duodenum is performed during the same procedural episode.

Occlusion vs. Restriction for vessel embolization procedures

B3.12. If the objective of an embolization procedure is to completely close a vessel, the root operation Occlusion is coded. If the objective of an embolization procedure is to narrow the lumen of a vessel, the root operation Restriction is coded.

Examples:
Tumor embolization is coded to the root operation Occlusion, because the objective of the procedure is to cut off the blood supply to the vessel.

Embolization of a cerebral aneurysm is coded to the root operation Restriction, because the objective of the procedure is not to close off the vessel entirely, but to narrow the lumen of the vessel at the site of the aneurysm where it is abnormally wide.

Release procedures

B3.13. In the root operation Release, the body part value coded is the body part being freed and not the tissue being manipulated or cut to free the body part.

Example:
Lysis of intestinal adhesions is coded to the specific intestine body part value.

Release vs. Division

B3.14. If the sole objective of the procedure is freeing a body part without cutting the body part, the root operation is Release. If the sole objective of the procedure is separating or transecting a body part, the root operation is Division.

Examples:
Freeing a nerve root from surrounding scar tissue to relieve pain is coded to the root operation Release.

Severing a nerve root to relieve pain is coded to the root operation Division.

Reposition for fracture treatment

B3.15. Reduction of a displaced fracture is coded to the root operation Reposition and the application of a cast or splint in conjunction with the Reposition procedure is not coded separately. Treatment of a nondisplaced fracture is coded to the procedure performed.

Examples:
Casting of a nondisplaced fracture is coded to the root operation Immobilization in the Placement section.

Putting a pin in a nondisplaced fracture is coded to the root operation Insertion.

Transplantation vs. Administration

B3.16. Putting in a mature and functioning living body part taken from another individual or animal is coded to the root operation Transplantation. Putting in autologous or nonautologous cells is coded to the Administration section.

Example:
Putting in autologous or nonautologous bone marrow, pancreatic islet cells or stem cells is coded to the Administration section.

Transfer procedures using multiple tissue layers

B3.17. The root operation Transfer contains qualifiers that can be used to specify when a transfer flap is composed of more than one tissue layer, such as a musculocutaneous flap. For procedures involving transfer of multiple tissue layers including skin, subcutaneous tissue, fascia or muscle, the procedure is coded to the body part value that describes the deepest tissue layer in the flap, and the qualifier can be used to describe the other tissue layer(s) in the transfer flap.

Example:
A musculocutaneous flap transfer is coded to the appropriate body part value in the body system Muscles, and the qualifier is used to describe the additional tissue layer(s) in the transfer flap.

Excision/Resection followed by replacement

B3.18. If an excision or resection of a body part is followed by a replacement procedure, code both procedures to identify each distinct objective, except when the excision or resection is considered integral and preparatory for the replacement procedure.

Examples:
Mastectomy followed by reconstruction, both resection and replacement of the breast are coded to fully capture the distinct objectives of the procedures performed.

Maxillectomy with obturator reconstruction, both excision and replacement of the maxilla are coded to fully capture the distinct objectives of the procedures performed.

Excisional debridement of tendon with skin graft, both the excision of the tendon and the replacement of the skin with a graft are coded to fully capture the distinct objectives of the procedures performed.

Esophagectomy followed by reconstruction with colonic interposition, both the resection and the transfer of the large intestine to function as the esophagus are coded to fully capture the distinct objectives of the procedures performed.

Examples:
Resection of a joint as part of a joint replacement procedure is considered integral and preparatory for the replacement of the joint and the resection is not coded separately.

Resection of a valve as part of a valve replacement procedure is considered integral and preparatory for the valve replacement and the resection is not coded separately.

B4. Body Part

General guidelines

B4.1a. If a procedure is performed on a portion of a body part that does not have a separate body part value, code the body part value corresponding to the whole body part.

Example:
A procedure performed on the alveolar process of the mandible is coded to the mandible body part.

B4.1b. If the prefix "peri" is combined with a body part to identify the site of the procedure, and the site of the procedure is not further specified, then the procedure is coded to the body part named. This guideline applies only when a more specific body part value is not available.

Examples:
A procedure site identified as perirenal is coded to the kidney body part when the site of the procedure is not further specified.

A procedure site described in the documentation as peri-urethral, and the documentation also indicates that it is the vulvar tissue and not the urethral tissue that is the site of the procedure, then the procedure is coded to the vulva body part.

A procedure site documented as involving the periosteum is coded to the corresponding bone body part.

B4.1c. If a procedure is performed on a continuous section of a tubular body part, code the body part value corresponding to the **anatomically most proximal (closest to the heart) portion of the tubular body part.**

Example:
A procedure performed on a continuous section of artery from the femoral artery to the external iliac artery with the point of entry at the femoral artery is coded to the external iliac body part.

A procedure performed on a continuous section of artery from the femoral artery to the external iliac artery with the point of entry at the external iliac artery is also coded to the external iliac artery body part.

Branches of body parts

B4.2. Where a specific branch of a body part does not have its own body part value in PCS, the body part is typically coded to the closest proximal branch that has a specific body part value. In the cardiovascular body systems, if a general body part is available in the correct root operation table, and coding to a proximal branch would require assigning a code in a different body system, the procedure is coded using the general body part value.

Examples:
A procedure performed on the mandibular branch of the trigeminal nerve is coded to the trigeminal nerve body part value.

Occlusion of the bronchial artery is coded to the body part value Upper Artery in the body system Upper Arteries, and not to the body part value Thoracic Aorta, Descending in the body system Heart and Great Vessels.

Bilateral body part values

B4.3. Bilateral body part values are available for a limited number of body parts. If the identical procedure is performed on contralateral body parts, and a bilateral body part value exists for that body part, a single procedure is coded using the bilateral body part value. If no bilateral body part value exists, each procedure is coded separately using the appropriate body part value.

Examples:
The identical procedure performed on both fallopian tubes is coded once using the body part value Fallopian Tube, Bilateral.

The identical procedure performed on both knee joints is coded twice using the body part values Knee Joint, Right and Knee Joint, Left.

Coronary arteries

B4.4. The coronary arteries are classified as a single body part that is further specified by number of arteries treated. One procedure code specifying multiple arteries is used when the same procedure is performed, including the same device and qualifier values.

Examples:
Angioplasty of two distinct coronary arteries with placement of two stents is coded as Dilation of Coronary Artery, Two Arteries with Two Intraluminal Devices.

Angioplasty of two distinct coronary arteries, one with stent placed and one without, is coded separately as Dilation of Coronary Artery, One Artery with Intraluminal Device, and Dilation of Coronary Artery, One Artery with no device.

Tendons, ligaments, bursae and fascia near a joint

B4.5. Procedures performed on tendons, ligaments, bursae and fascia supporting a joint are coded to the body part in the respective body system that is the focus of the procedure. Procedures performed on joint structures themselves are coded to the body part in the joint body systems.

Examples:
Repair of the anterior cruciate ligament of the knee is coded to the knee bursa and ligament body part in the bursae and ligaments body system.

Knee arthroscopy with shaving of articular cartilage is coded to the knee joint body part in the Lower Joints body system.

Skin, subcutaneous tissue and fascia overlying a joint

B4.6. If a procedure is performed on the skin, subcutaneous tissue or fascia overlying a joint, the procedure is coded to the following body part:

- Shoulder is coded to Upper Arm
- Elbow is coded to Lower Arm
- Wrist is coded to Lower Arm
- Hip is coded to Upper Leg
- Knee is coded to Lower Leg
- Ankle is coded to Foot

Fingers and toes

B4.7. If a body system does not contain a separate body part value for fingers, procedures performed on the fingers are coded to the body part value for the hand. If a body system does not contain a separate body part value for toes, procedures performed on the toes are coded to the body part value for the foot.

Example:
Excision of finger muscle is coded to one of the hand muscle body part values in the Muscles body system.

Upper and lower intestinal tract

B4.8. In the Gastrointestinal body system, the general body part values Upper Intestinal Tract and Lower Intestinal Tract are provided as an option for the root operations **such as** Change, **Insertion,** Inspection, Removal and Revision. Upper Intestinal Tract includes the portion of the gastrointestinal tract from the esophagus down to and including the duodenum, and Lower Intestinal Tract includes the portion of the gastrointestinal tract from the jejunum down to and including the rectum and anus.

Example:
In the root operation Change table, change of a device in the jejunum is coded using the body part Lower Intestinal Tract.

B5. Approach

Open approach with percutaneous endoscopic assistance

B5.2a. Procedures performed using the open approach with percutaneous endoscopic assistance are coded to the approach Open.

Example:
Laparoscopic-assisted sigmoidectomy is coded to the approach Open.

Percutaneous endoscopic approach with extension of incision

B5.2b. Procedures performed using the percutaneous endoscopic approach, with incision or extension of an incision to assist in the removal of all or a portion of a body part or to anastomose a tubular body part to complete the procedure, are coded to the approach value Percutaneous Endoscopic.

Examples:
Laparoscopic sigmoid colectomy with extension of stapling port for removal of specimen and direct anastomosis is coded to the approach value percutaneous endoscopic.

Laparoscopic nephrectomy with midline incision for removing the resected kidney is coded to the approach value percutaneous endoscopic.

Robotic-assisted laparoscopic prostatectomy with extension of incision for removal of the resected prostate is coded to the approach value percutaneous endoscopic.

External approach

B5.3a. Procedures performed within an orifice on structures that are visible without the aid of any instrumentation are coded to the approach External.

Example:
Resection of tonsils is coded to the approach External.

B5.3b. Procedures performed indirectly by the application of external force through the intervening body layers are coded to the approach External.

Example:
Closed reduction of fracture is coded to the approach External.

Percutaneous procedure via device

B5.4. Procedures performed percutaneously via a device placed for the procedure are coded to the approach Percutaneous.

Example:
Fragmentation of kidney stone performed via percutaneous nephrostomy is coded to the approach Percutaneous.

B6. Device

General guidelines

B6.1a. A device is coded only if a device remains after the procedure is completed. If no device remains, the device value No Device is coded. In limited root operations, the classification provides the qualifier values Temporary and Intraoperative, for specific procedures involving clinically significant devices, where the purpose of the device is to be utilized for a brief duration during the procedure or current inpatient stay. If a device that is intended to remain after the procedure is completed requires removal before the end of the operative episode in which it was inserted (for example, the device size is inadequate or a complication occurs), both the insertion and removal of the device should be coded.

B6.1b. Materials such as sutures, ligatures, radiological markers and temporary post-operative wound drains are considered integral to the performance of a procedure and are not coded as devices.

B6.1c. Procedures performed on a device only and not on a body part are specified in the root operations Change, Irrigation, Removal and Revision, and are coded to the procedure performed.

Example:
Irrigation of percutaneous nephrostomy tube is coded to the root operation Irrigation of indwelling device in the Administration section.

Drainage device

B6.2. A separate procedure to put in a drainage device is coded to the root operation Drainage with the device value Drainage Device.

Obstetric Section Guidelines (section 1)

C. Obstetrics Section

Products of conception

C1. Procedures performed on the products of conception are coded to the Obstetrics section. Procedures performed on the pregnant female other than the products of conception are coded to the appropriate root operation in the Medical and Surgical section.

Examples:
Amniocentesis is coded to the products of conception body part in the Obstetrics section.

Repair of obstetric urethral laceration is coded to the urethra body part in the Medical and Surgical section.

Procedures following delivery or abortion

C2. Procedures performed following a delivery or abortion for curettage of the endometrium or evacuation of retained products of conception are all coded in the Obstetrics section, to the root operation Extraction and the body part Products of Conception, Retained.

Diagnostic or therapeutic dilation and curettage performed during times other than the postpartum or post-abortion period are all coded in the Medical and Surgical section, to the root operation Extraction and the body part Endometrium.

Radiation Therapy Section Guidelines (section D)

D. Radiation Therapy Section

Brachytherapy

D1.a. Brachytherapy is coded to the modality Brachytherapy in the Radiation Therapy section. When a radioactive brachytherapy source is left in the body at the end of the procedure, it is coded separately to the root operation Insertion with the device value Radioactive Element.

Example:
Brachytherapy with implantation of a low dose rate brachytherapy source left in the body at the end of the procedure is coded to the applicable treatment site in section D, Radiation Therapy, with the modality Brachytherapy, the modality qualifier value Low Dose Rate, and the applicable isotope value and qualifier value. The implantation of the brachytherapy source is coded separately to the device value Radioactive Element in the appropriate Insertion table of the Medical and Surgical section. The Radiation Therapy section code identifies the specific modality and isotope of the brachytherapy, and the root operation Insertion code identifies the implantation of the brachytherapy source that remains in the body at the end of the procedure.

Exception:
Implantation of Cesium-131 brachytherapy seeds embedded in a collagen matrix to the treatment site after resection of brain tumor is coded to the root operation Insertion with the device value Radioactive Element, Cesium-131 Collagen Implant. The procedure is coded to the root operation Insertion only, because the device value identifies both the implantation of the radioactive element and a specific brachytherapy isotope that is not included in the Radiation Therapy section tables.

D1.b. A separate procedure to place a temporary applicator for delivering the brachytherapy is coded to the root operation Insertion and the device value Other Device.

Examples:
Intrauterine brachytherapy applicator placed as a separate procedure from the brachytherapy procedure is coded to Insertion of Other Device, and the brachytherapy is coded separately using the modality Brachytherapy in the Radiation Therapy section.

Intrauterine brachytherapy applicator placed concomitantly with delivery of the brachytherapy dose is coded with a single code using the modality Brachytherapy in the Radiation Therapy section.

New Technology Section Guidelines (section X)

E. New Technology Section

General guidelines

E1.a. Section X codes fully represent the specific procedure described in the code title, and do not require additional codes from other sections of ICD-10-PCS. When section X contains a code title which fully describes a specific new technology procedure, and it is the only procedure performed, only the section X code is reported for the procedure. There is no need to report an additional code in another section of ICD-10-PCS.

Example:
XW043A6 Introduction of **Cefiderocol** Anti-infective into Central Vein, Percutaneous Approach, New Technology Group **6**, can be coded to indicate that **Cefiderocol** Anti-infective was administered via a central vein. A separate code from table 3EØ in the Administration section of ICD-10-PCS is not coded in addition to this code.

E1.b. When multiple procedures are performed, New Technology section X codes are coded following the multiple procedures guideline.

Examples:
Dual filter cerebral embolic filtration used during transcatheter aortic valve replacement (TAVR), X2A5312 Cerebral Embolic Filtration, Dual Filter in Innominate Artery and Left Common Carotid Artery, Percutaneous Approach, New Technology Group 2, is coded for the cerebral embolic filtration, along with an ICD-10-PCS code for the TAVR procedure.

An extracorporeal flow reversal circuit for embolic neuroprotection placed during a transcarotid arterial revascularization procedure, a code from table X2A, Assistance of the Cardiovascular System is coded for the use of the extracorporeal flow reversal circuit, along with an ICD-10-PCS code for the transcarotid arterial revascularization procedure.

F. Selection of Principal Procedure

The following instructions should be applied in the selection of principal procedure and clarification on the importance of the relation to the principal diagnosis when more than one procedure is performed:

1. Procedure performed for definitive treatment of both principal diagnosis and secondary diagnosis
   a. Sequence procedure performed for definitive treatment most related to principal diagnosis as principal procedure.
2. Procedure performed for definitive treatment and diagnostic procedures performed for both principal diagnosis and secondary diagnosis.
   a. Sequence procedure performed for definitive treatment most related to principal diagnosis as principal procedure
3. A diagnostic procedure was performed for the principal diagnosis and a procedure is performed for definitive treatment of a secondary diagnosis.
   a. Sequence diagnostic procedure as principal procedure, since the procedure most related to the principal diagnosis takes precedence.
4. No procedures performed that are related to principal diagnosis; procedures performed for definitive treatment and diagnostic procedures were performed for secondary diagnosis
   a. Sequence procedure performed for definitive treatment of secondary diagnosis as principal procedure, since there are no procedures (definitive or nondefinitive treatment) related to principal diagnosis.

# #

3f (Aortic) Bioprosthesis valve *use* Zooplastic Tissue in Heart and Great Vessels

A

Abdominal aortic plexus *use* Abdominal Sympathetic Nerve
Abdominal esophagus *use* Esophagus, Lower
Abdominohysterectomy *see* Resection, Uterus ØUT9
Abdominoplasty
see Alteration, Abdominal Wall ØWØF
see Repair, Abdominal Wall ØWQF
see Supplement, Abdominal Wall ØWUF
Abductor hallucis muscle
use Foot Muscle, Left
use Foot Muscle, Right
ABECMA® *use* Idecabtagene Vicleucel Immunotherapy
AbioCor® Total Replacement Heart *use* Synthetic Substitute
Ablation
see Control bleeding in
see Destruction
Abortion
Abortifacient 1ØAØ7ZX
Laminaria 1ØAØ7ZW
Products of Conception 1ØAØ
Vacuum 1ØAØ7Z6
Abrasion *see* Extraction
Absolute Pro Vascular (OTW) Self-Expanding Stent System *use* Intraluminal Device
Accelerate PhenoTest™ BC XXE5XN6
Accessory cephalic vein
use Cephalic Vein, Left
use Cephalic Vein, Right
Accessory obturator nerve *use* Lumbar Plexus
Accessory phrenic nerve *use* Phrenic Nerve
Accessory spleen *use* Spleen
Acculink (RX) Carotid Stent System *use* Intraluminal Device
Acellular Hydrated Dermis *use* Nonautologous Tissue Substitute
Acetabular cup *use* Liner in Lower Joints
Acetabulectomy
see Excision, Lower Bones ØQB
see Resection, Lower Bones ØQT
Acetabulofemoral joint
use Hip Joint, Left
use Hip Joint, Right
Acetabuloplasty
see Repair, Lower Bones ØQQ
see Replacement, Lower Bones ØQR
see Supplement, Lower Bones ØQU
Achilles tendon
use Lower Leg Tendon, Left
use Lower Leg Tendon, Right
Achillorrhaphy *see* Repair, Tendons ØLQ
Achillotenotomy, achillotomy
see Division, Tendons ØL8
see Drainage, Tendons ØL9
Acoustic Pulse Thrombolysis *see* Fragmentation, Artery
Acromioclavicular ligament
use Shoulder Bursa and Ligament, Left
use Shoulder Bursa and Ligament, Right
Acromion (process)
use Scapula, Left
use Scapula, Right
Acromionectomy
see Excision, Upper Joints ØRB
see Resection, Upper Joints ØRT
Acromioplasty
see Repair, Upper Joints ØRQ
see Replacement, Upper Joints ØRR
see Supplement, Upper Joints ØRU
ACTEMRA® *use* Tocilizumab
Activa PC neurostimulator *use* Stimulator Generator, Multiple Array in ØJH
Activa RC neurostimulator *use* Stimulator Generator, Multiple Array Rechargeable in ØJH
Activa SC neurostimulator *use* Stimulator Generator, Single Array in ØJH
Activities of Daily Living Assessment FØ2
Activities of Daily Living Treatment FØ8
ACUITY™ Steerable Lead
use Cardiac Lead, Defibrillator in Ø2H
use Cardiac Lead, Pacemaker in Ø2H
Acupuncture
Breast
Anesthesia 8EØH3ØØ
No Qualifier 8EØH3ØZ
Integumentary System
Anesthesia 8EØH3ØØ
No Qualifier 8EØH3ØZ
Adductor brevis muscle
use Upper Leg Muscle, Left
use Upper Leg Muscle, Right
Adductor hallucis muscle
use Foot Muscle, Left
use Foot Muscle, Right
Adductor longus muscle
use Upper Leg Muscle, Left
use Upper Leg Muscle, Right
Adductor magnus muscle
use Upper Leg Muscle, Left
use Upper Leg Muscle, Right
Adenohypophysis *use* Pituitary Gland
Adenoidectomy
see Excision, Adenoids ØCBQ
see Resection, Adenoids ØCTQ
Adenoidotomy *see* Drainage, Adenoids ØC9Q
Adhesiolysis *see* Release
Administration
Blood products *see* Transfusion
Other substance *see* Introduction of substance in or on
Adrenalectomy
see Excision, Endocrine System ØGB
see Resection, Endocrine System ØGT
Adrenalorrhaphy *see* Repair, Endocrine System ØGQ
Adrenalotomy *see* Drainage, Endocrine System ØG9
Advancement
see Reposition
see Transfer
Advisa (MRI) *use* Pacemaker, Dual Chamber in ØJH
AFX® Endovascular AAA System *use* Intraluminal Device
Aidoc Briefcase for PE (pulmonary embolism) XXE3X27
AIGISRx Antibacterial Envelope *use* Anti-Infective Envelope
Alar ligament of axis *use* Head and Neck Bursa and Ligament
Alfapump® system *use* Other Device
Alfieri Stitch Valvuloplasty *see* Restriction, Valve, Mitral Ø2VG
Alimentation *see* Introduction of substance in or on
ALPPS (Associating liver partition and portal vein ligation)
see Division, Hepatobiliary System and Pancreas ØF8
see Resection, Hepatobiliary System and Pancreas ØFT
Alteration
Abdominal Wall ØWØF
Ankle Region
Left ØYØL
Right ØYØK
Arm
Lower
Left ØXØF
Right ØXØD
Upper
Left ØXØ9
Right ØXØ8
Axilla
Left ØXØ5
Right ØXØ4
Back
Lower ØWØL
Upper ØWØK
Breast
Bilateral ØHØV
Left ØHØU
Right ØHØT
Buttock
Left ØYØ1
Right ØYØØ
Chest Wall ØWØ8
Ear
Bilateral Ø9Ø2
Alteration — *continued*
Ear — *continued*
Left Ø9Ø1
Right Ø9ØØ
Elbow Region
Left ØXØC
Right ØXØB
Extremity
Lower
Left ØYØB
Right ØYØ9
Upper
Left ØXØ7
Right ØXØ6
Eyelid
Lower
Left Ø8ØR
Right Ø8ØQ
Upper
Left Ø8ØP
Right Ø8ØN
Face ØWØ2
Head ØWØØ
Jaw
Lower ØWØ5
Upper ØWØ4
Knee Region
Left ØYØG
Right ØYØF
Leg
Lower
Left ØYØJ
Right ØYØH
Upper
Left ØYØD
Right ØYØC
Lip
Lower ØCØ1X
Upper ØCØØX
Nasal Mucosa and Soft Tissue Ø9ØK
Neck ØWØ6
Perineum
Female ØWØN
Male ØWØM
Shoulder Region
Left ØXØ3
Right ØXØ2
Subcutaneous Tissue and Fascia
Abdomen ØJØ8
Back ØJØ7
Buttock ØJØ9
Chest ØJØ6
Face ØJØ1
Lower Arm
Left ØJØH
Right ØJØG
Lower Leg
Left ØJØP
Right ØJØN
Neck
Left ØJØ5
Right ØJØ4
Upper Arm
Left ØJØF
Right ØJØD
Upper Leg
Left ØJØM
Right ØJØL
Wrist Region
Left ØXØH
Right ØXØG
Alveolar process of mandible
use Mandible, Left
use Mandible, Right
Alveolar process of maxilla *use* Maxilla
Alveolectomy
see Excision, Head and Facial Bones ØNB
see Resection, Head and Facial Bones ØNT
Alveoloplasty
see Repair, Head and Facial Bones ØNQ
see Replacement, Head and Facial Bones ØNR
see Supplement, Head and Facial Bones ØNU
Alveolotomy
see Division, Head and Facial Bones ØN8
see Drainage, Head and Facial Bones ØN9
Ambulatory cardiac monitoring 4A12X45
Amivantamab Monoclonal Antibody XWØ

Amniocentesis *see* Drainage, Products of Conception 1Ø9Ø
Amnioinfusion *see* Introduction of substance in or on, Products of Conception 3EØE
Amnioscopy 1ØJØ8ZZ
Amniotomy *see* Drainage, Products of Conception 1Ø9Ø
AMPLATZER® Muscular VSD Occluder *use* Synthetic Substitute
Amputation *see* Detachment
AMS 8ØØ® Urinary Control System *use* Artificial Sphincter in Urinary System
Anal orifice *use* Anus
Analog radiography *see* Plain Radiography
Analog radiology *see* Plain Radiography
Anastomosis *see* Bypass
Anatomical snuffbox
use Lower Arm and Wrist Muscle, Left
use Lower Arm and Wrist Muscle, Right
Andexanet Alfa, Factor Xa Inhibitor Reversal Agent *use* Coagulation Factor Xa, Inactivated
Andexxa *use* Coagulation Factor Xa, Inactivated
AneuRx® AAA Advantage® *use* Intraluminal Device
Angiectomy
see Excision, Heart and Great Vessels Ø2B
see Excision, Lower Arteries Ø4B
see Excision, Lower Veins Ø6B
see Excision, Upper Arteries Ø3B
see Excision, Upper Veins Ø5B
Angiocardiography
Combined right and left heart *see* Fluoroscopy, Heart, Right and Left B216
Left Heart *see* Fluoroscopy, Heart, Left B215
Right Heart *see* Fluoroscopy, Heart, Right B214
SPY system intravascular fluorescence *see* Monitoring, Physiological Systems 4A1
Angiography
see Computerized Tomography (CT Scan), Artery
see Fluoroscopy, Artery
see Magnetic Resonance Imaging (MRI), Artery
see Plain Radiography, Artery
Angioplasty
see Dilation, Heart and Great Vessels Ø27
see Dilation, Lower Arteries Ø47
see Dilation, Upper Arteries Ø37
see Repair, Heart and Great Vessels Ø2Q
see Repair, Lower Arteries Ø4Q
see Repair, Upper Arteries Ø3Q
see Replacement, Heart and Great Vessels Ø2R
see Replacement, Lower Arteries Ø4R
see Replacement, Upper Arteries Ø3R
see Supplement, Heart and Great Vessels Ø2U
see Supplement, Lower Arteries Ø4U
see Supplement, Upper Arteries Ø3U
Angiorrhaphy
see Repair, Heart and Great Vessels Ø2Q
see Repair, Lower Arteries Ø4Q
see Repair, Upper Arteries Ø3Q
Angioscopy Ø2JY4ZZ, Ø3JY4ZZ, Ø4JY4ZZ
Angiotensin II *use* Synthetic Human Angiotensin II
Angiotripsy
see Occlusion, Lower Arteries Ø4L
see Occlusion, Upper Arteries Ø3L
Angular artery *use* Face Artery
Angular vein
use Face Vein, Left
use Face Vein, Right
Annular ligament
use Elbow Bursa and Ligament, Left
use Elbow Bursa and Ligament, Right
Annuloplasty
see Repair, Heart and Great Vessels Ø2Q
see Supplement, Heart and Great Vessels Ø2U
Annuloplasty ring *use* Synthetic Substitute
Anoplasty
see Repair, Anus ØDQQ
see Supplement, Anus ØDUQ
Anorectal junction *use* Rectum
Anoscopy ØDJD8ZZ
Ansa cervicalis *use* Cervical Plexus
Antabuse therapy HZ93ZZZ
Antebrachial fascia
use Subcutaneous Tissue and Fascia, Left Lower Arm
use Subcutaneous Tissue and Fascia, Right Lower Arm
Anterior cerebral artery *use* Intracranial Artery
Anterior cerebral vein *use* Intracranial Vein
Anterior choroidal artery *use* Intracranial Artery
Anterior circumflex humeral artery
use Axillary Artery, Left
use Axillary Artery, Right
Anterior communicating artery *use* Intracranial Artery
Anterior cruciate ligament (ACL)
use Knee Bursa and Ligament, Left
use Knee Bursa and Ligament, Right
Anterior crural nerve *use* Femoral Nerve
Anterior facial vein
use Face Vein, Left
use Face Vein, Right
Anterior intercostal artery
use Internal Mammary Artery, Left
use Internal Mammary Artery, Right
Anterior interosseous nerve *use* Median Nerve
Anterior lateral malleolar artery
use Anterior Tibial Artery, Left
use Anterior Tibial Artery, Right
Anterior lingual gland *use* Minor Salivary Gland
Anterior (pectoral) lymph node
use Lymphatic, Left Axillary
use Lymphatic, Right Axillary
Anterior medial malleolar artery
use Anterior Tibial Artery, Left
use Anterior Tibial Artery, Right
Anterior spinal artery
use Vertebral Artery, Left
use Vertebral Artery, Right
Anterior tibial recurrent artery
use Anterior Tibial Artery, Left
use Anterior Tibial Artery, Right
Anterior ulnar recurrent artery
use Ulnar Artery, Left
use Ulnar Artery, Right
Anterior vagal trunk *use* Vagus Nerve
Anterior vertebral muscle
use Neck Muscle, Left
use Neck Muscle, Right
Antibacterial Envelope (TYRX) (AIGISRx) *use* Anti-Infective Envelope
Antibiotic-eluting Bone Void Filler XWØVØP7
Antigen-free air conditioning *see* Atmospheric Control, Physiological Systems 6AØ
Antihelix
use External Ear, Bilateral
use External Ear, Left
use External Ear, Right
Antimicrobial envelope *use* Anti-Infective Envelope
Anti-SARS-CoV-2 hyperimmune globulin *use* Hyperimmune Globulin
Antitragus
use External Ear, Bilateral
use External Ear, Left
use External Ear, Right
Antrostomy *see* Drainage, Ear, Nose, Sinus Ø99
Antrotomy *see* Drainage, Ear, Nose, Sinus Ø99
Antrum of Highmore
use Maxillary Sinus, Left
use Maxillary Sinus, Right
Aortic annulus *use* Aortic Valve
Aortic arch *use* Thoracic Aorta, Ascending/Arch
Aortic intercostal artery *use* Upper Artery
Aortography
see Fluoroscopy, Lower Arteries B41
see Fluoroscopy, Upper Arteries B31
see Plain Radiography, Lower Arteries B4Ø
see Plain Radiography, Upper Arteries B3Ø
Aortoplasty
see Repair, Aorta, Abdominal Ø4QØ
see Repair, Aorta, Thoracic, Ascending/Arch Ø2QX
see Repair, Aorta, Thoracic, Descending Ø2QW
see Replacement, Aorta, Abdominal Ø4RØ
see Replacement, Aorta, Thoracic, Ascending/Arch Ø2RX
see Replacement, Aorta, Thoracic, Descending Ø2RW
see Supplement, Aorta, Abdominal Ø4UØ
see Supplement, Aorta, Thoracic, Ascending/Arch Ø2UX
see Supplement, Aorta, Thoracic, Descending Ø2UW
Apalutamide Antineoplastic XWØDXJ5
Apical (subclavicular) lymph node
use Lymphatic, Left Axillary
use Lymphatic, Right Axillary
ApiFix® Minimally Invasive Deformity Correction (MID-C) System *use* Posterior (Dynamic) Distraction Device in New Technology
Apneustic center *use* Pons
Appendectomy
see Excision, Appendix ØDBJ
see Resection, Appendix ØDTJ
Appendicolysis *see* Release, Appendix ØDNJ
Appendicotomy *see* Drainage, Appendix ØD9J
Application *see* Introduction of substance in or on
aprevo™ *use* Interbody Fusion Device, Customizable in New Technology
Aquablation therapy, prostate XV5Ø8A4
Aquapheresis 6A55ØZ3
Aqueduct of Sylvius *use* Cerebral Ventricle
Aqueous humour
use Anterior Chamber, Left
use Anterior Chamber, Right
Arachnoid mater, intracranial *use* Cerebral Meninges
Arachnoid mater, spinal *use* Spinal Meninges
Arcuate artery
use Foot Artery, Left
use Foot Artery, Right
Areola
use Nipple, Left
use Nipple, Right
AROM (artificial rupture of membranes) 1Ø9Ø7ZC
Arterial canal (duct) *use* Pulmonary Artery, Left
Arterial pulse tracing *see* Measurement, Arterial 4AØ3
Arteriectomy
see Excision, Heart and Great Vessels Ø2B
see Excision, Lower Arteries Ø4B
see Excision, Upper Arteries Ø3B
Arteriography
see Fluoroscopy, Heart B21
see Fluoroscopy, Lower Arteries B41
see Fluoroscopy, Upper Arteries B31
see Plain Radiography, Heart B2Ø
see Plain Radiography, Lower Arteries B4Ø
see Plain Radiography, Upper Arteries B3Ø
Arterioplasty
see Repair, Heart and Great Vessels Ø2Q
see Repair, Lower Arteries Ø4Q
see Repair, Upper Arteries Ø3Q
see Replacement, Heart and Great Vessels Ø2R
see Replacement, Lower Arteries Ø4R
see Replacement, Upper Arteries Ø3R
see Supplement, Heart and Great Vessels Ø2U
see Supplement, Lower Arteries Ø4U
see Supplement, Upper Arteries Ø3U
Arteriorrhaphy
see Repair, Heart and Great Vessels Ø2Q
see Repair, Lower Arteries Ø4Q
see Repair, Upper Arteries Ø3Q
Arterioscopy
see Inspection, Artery, Lower Ø4JY
see Inspection, Artery, Upper Ø3JY
see Inspection, Great Vessel Ø2JY
Arthrectomy
see Excision, Lower Joints ØSB
see Excision, Upper Joints ØRB
see Resection, Lower Joints ØST
see Resection, Upper Joints ØRT
Arthrocentesis
see Drainage, Lower Joints ØS9
see Drainage, Upper Joints ØR9
Arthrodesis
see Fusion, Lower Joints ØSG
see Fusion, Upper Joints ØRG
Arthrography
see Plain Radiography, Non-Axial Lower Bones BQØ
see Plain Radiography, Non-Axial Upper Bones BPØ
see Plain Radiography, Skull and Facial Bones BNØ
Arthrolysis
see Release, Lower Joints ØSN
see Release, Upper Joints ØRN
Arthropexy
see Repair, Lower Joints ØSQ
see Repair, Upper Joints ØRQ
see Reposition, Lower Joints ØSS
see Reposition, Upper Joints ØRS
Arthroplasty
see Repair, Lower Joints ØSQ

Arthroplasty — *continued*
see Repair, Upper Joints ØRQ
see Replacement, Lower Joints ØSR
see Replacement, Upper Joints ØRR
see Supplement, Lower Joints ØSU
see Supplement, Upper Joints ØRU
Arthroplasty, radial head
see Replacement, Radius, Left ØPRJ
see Replacement, Radius, Right ØPRH
Arthroscopy
see Inspection, Lower Joints ØSJ
see Inspection, Upper Joints ØRJ
Arthrotomy
see Drainage, Lower Joints ØS9
see Drainage, Upper Joints ØR9
Articulating Spacer (Antibiotic) *use* Articulating Spacer in Lower Joints
Artificial anal sphincter (AAS) *use* Artificial Sphincter in Gastrointestinal System
Artificial bowel sphincter (neosphincter) *use* Artificial Sphincter in Gastrointestinal System
Artificial Sphincter
Insertion of device in
Anus ØDHQ
Bladder ØTHB
Bladder Neck ØTHC
Urethra ØTHD
Removal of device from
Anus ØDPQ
Bladder ØTPB
Urethra ØTPD
Revision of device in
Anus ØDWQ
Bladder ØTWB
Urethra ØTWD
Artificial urinary sphincter (AUS) *use* Artificial Sphincter in Urinary System
Aryepiglottic fold *use* Larynx
Arytenoid cartilage *use* Larynx
Arytenoid muscle
use Neck Muscle, Left
use Neck Muscle, Right
Arytenoidectomy *see* Excision, Larynx ØCBS
Arytenoidopexy *see* Repair, Larynx ØCQS
Ascenda Intrathecal Catheter *use* Infusion Device
Ascending aorta *use* Thoracic Aorta, Ascending/Arch
Ascending palatine artery *use* Face Artery
Ascending pharyngeal artery
use External Carotid Artery, Left
use External Carotid Artery, Right
aScope™ Duodeno *see* New Technology, Hepatobiliary System and Pancreas XFJ
Aspiration, fine needle
Fluid or gas *see* Drainage
Tissue biopsy
see Excision
see Extraction
Assessment
Activities of daily living *see* Activities of Daily Living Assessment, Rehabilitation FØ2
Hearing *see* Hearing Assessment, Diagnostic Audiology F13
Hearing aid *see* Hearing Aid Assessment, Diagnostic Audiology F14
Intravascular perfusion, using indocyanine green (ICG) dye *see* Monitoring, Physiological Systems 4A1
Motor function *see* Motor Function Assessment, Rehabilitation FØ1
Nerve function *see* Motor Function Assessment, Rehabilitation FØ1
Speech *see* Speech Assessment, Rehabilitation FØØ
Vestibular *see* Vestibular Assessment, Diagnostic Audiology F15
Vocational *see* Activities of Daily Living Treatment, Rehabilitation FØ8
Assistance
Cardiac
Continuous
Balloon Pump 5AØ221Ø
Impeller Pump 5AØ221D
Other Pump 5AØ2216
Pulsatile Compression 5AØ2215
Intermittent
Balloon Pump 5AØ211Ø
Impeller Pump 5AØ211D
Other Pump 5AØ2116
Assistance — *continued*
Cardiac — *continued*
Intermittent — *continued*
Pulsatile Compression 5AØ2115
Circulatory
Continuous
Hyperbaric 5AØ5221
Supersaturated 5AØ522C
Intermittent
Hyperbaric 5AØ5121
Supersaturated 5AØ512C
Respiratory
24-96 Consecutive Hours
Continuous Negative Airway Pressure 5AØ9459
Continuous Positive Airway Pressure 5AØ9457
High Nasal Flow/Velocity 5AØ945A
Intermittent Negative Airway Pressure 5AØ945B
Intermittent Positive Airway Pressure 5AØ9458
No Qualifier 5AØ945Z
Continuous, Filtration 5AØ92ØZ
Greater than 96 Consecutive Hours
Continuous Negative Airway Pressure 5AØ9559
Continuous Positive Airway Pressure 5AØ9557
High Nasal Flow/Velocity 5AØ955A
Intermittent Negative Airway Pressure 5AØ955B
Intermittent Positive Airway Pressure 5AØ9558
No Qualifier 5AØ955Z
Less than 24 Consecutive Hours
Continuous Negative Airway Pressure 5AØ9359
Continuous Positive Airway Pressure 5AØ9357
High Nasal Flow/Velocity 5AØ935A
Intermittent Negative Airway Pressure 5AØ935B
Intermittent Positive Airway Pressure 5AØ9358
No Qualifier 5AØ935Z
Associating liver partition and portal vein ligation (ALPPS)
see Division, Hepatobiliary System and Pancreas ØF8
see Resection, Hepatobiliary System and Pancreas ØFT
Assurant (Cobalt) stent *use* Intraluminal Device
Atezolizumab Antineoplastic XWØ
Atherectomy
see Extirpation, Heart and Great Vessels Ø2C
see Extirpation, Lower Arteries Ø4C
see Extirpation, Upper Arteries Ø3C
Atlantoaxial joint *use* Cervical Vertebral Joint
Atmospheric Control 6AØZ
AtriClip LAA Exclusion System *use* Extraluminal Device
Atrioseptoplasty
see Repair, Heart and Great Vessels Ø2Q
see Replacement, Heart and Great Vessels Ø2R
see Supplement, Heart and Great Vessels Ø2U
Atrioventricular node *use* Conduction Mechanism
Atrium dextrum cordis *use* Atrium, Right
Atrium pulmonale *use* Atrium, Left
Attain Ability® lead Ø2H
use Cardiac Lead, Defibrillator in Ø2H
use Cardiac Lead, Pacemaker in Ø2H
Attain Starfix® (OTW) lead
use Cardiac Lead, Defibrillator in Ø2H
use Cardiac Lead, Pacemaker in Ø2H
Audiology, diagnostic
see Hearing Aid Assessment, Diagnostic Audiology F14
see Hearing Assessment, Diagnostic Audiology F13
see Vestibular Assessment, Diagnostic Audiology F15
Audiometry *see* Hearing Assessment, Diagnostic Audiology F13
Auditory tube
use Eustachian Tube, Left
use Eustachian Tube, Right
Auerbach's (myenteric) plexus *use* Abdominal Sympathetic Nerve
Auricle
use External Ear, Bilateral
use External Ear, Left
use External Ear, Right
Auricularis muscle *use* Head Muscle
Autograft *use* Autologous Tissue Substitute
Autologous artery graft
use Autologous Arterial Tissue in Heart and Great Vessels
use Autologous Arterial Tissue in Lower Arteries
use Autologous Arterial Tissue in Lower Veins
use Autologous Arterial Tissue in Upper Arteries
use Autologous Arterial Tissue in Upper Veins
Autologous vein graft
use Autologous Venous Tissue in Heart and Great Vessels
use Autologous Venous Tissue in Lower Arteries
use Autologous Venous Tissue in Lower Veins
use Autologous Venous Tissue in Upper Arteries
use Autologous Venous Tissue in Upper Veins
Automated Chest Compression (ACC) 5A1221J
AutoPulse® Resuscitation System 5A1221J
Autotransfusion *see* Transfusion
Autotransplant
Adrenal tissue *see* Reposition, Endocrine System ØGS
Kidney *see* Reposition, Urinary System ØTS
Pancreatic tissue *see* Reposition, Pancreas ØFSG
Parathyroid tissue *see* Reposition, Endocrine System ØGS
Thyroid tissue *see* Reposition, Endocrine System ØGS
Tooth *see* Reattachment, Mouth and Throat ØCM
Avulsion *see* Extraction
AVYCAZ® (ceftazidime-avibactam) *use* Other Anti-infective
Axial Lumbar Interbody Fusion System *use* Interbody Fusion Device in Lower Joints
AxiaLIF® System *use* Interbody Fusion Device in Lower Joints
Axicabtagene Ciloleucel *use* Axicabtagene Ciloleucel Immunotherapy
Axicabtagene Ciloleucel Immunotherapy XWØ
Axillary fascia
use Subcutaneous Tissue and Fascia, Left Upper Arm
use Subcutaneous Tissue and Fascia, Right Upper Arm
Axillary nerve *use* Brachial Plexus
AZEDRA® *use* Iobenguane I-131 Antineoplastic

B

BAK/C® Interbody Cervical Fusion System *use* Interbody Fusion Device in Upper Joints
BAL (bronchial alveolar lavage), diagnostic *see* Drainage, Respiratory System ØB9
Balanoplasty
see Repair, Penis ØVQS
see Supplement, Penis ØVUS
Balloon atrial septostomy (BAS) Ø2163Z7
Balloon Pump
Continuous, Output 5AØ221Ø
Intermittent, Output 5AØ211Ø
Bamlanivimab Monoclonal Antibody XWØ
Bandage, Elastic *see* Compression
Banding
see Occlusion
see Restriction
Banding, esophageal varices *see* Occlusion, Vein, Esophageal Ø6L3
Banding, laparoscopic (adjustable) gastric
Initial procedure ØDV64CZ
Surgical correction *see* Revision of device in, Stomach ØDW6
Bard® Composix® Kugel® patch *use* Synthetic Substitute
Bard® Composix® (E/X) (LP) mesh *use* Synthetic Substitute
Bard® Dulex™ mesh *use* Synthetic Substitute
Bard® Ventralex™ hernia patch *use* Synthetic Substitute
Baricitinib XWØ

Barium swallow *see* Fluoroscopy, Gastrointestinal System BD1
Baroreflex Activation Therapy® (BAT®)
use Stimulator Generator in Subcutaneous Tissue and Fascia
use Stimulator Lead in Upper Arteries
Barricaid® Annular Closure Device (ACD) *use* Synthetic Substitute
Bartholin's (greater vestibular) gland *use* Vestibular Gland
Basal (internal) cerebral vein *use* Intracranial Vein
Basal metabolic rate (BMR) *see* Measurement, Physiological Systems 4AØZ
Basal nuclei *use* Basal Ganglia
Base of Tongue *use* Pharynx
Basilar artery *use* Intracranial Artery
Basis pontis *use* Pons
Beam Radiation
Abdomen DWØ3
Intraoperative DWØ33ZØ
Adrenal Gland DGØ2
Intraoperative DGØ23ZØ
Bile Ducts DFØ2
Intraoperative DFØ23ZØ
Bladder DTØ2
Intraoperative DTØ23ZØ
Bone
Intraoperative DPØC3ZØ
Other DPØC
Bone Marrow D7ØØ
Intraoperative D7ØØ3ZØ
Brain DØØØ
Intraoperative DØØØ3ZØ
Brain Stem DØØ1
Intraoperative DØØ13ZØ
Breast
Left DMØØ
Intraoperative DMØØ3ZØ
Right DMØ1
Intraoperative DMØ13ZØ
Bronchus DBØ1
Intraoperative DBØ13ZØ
Cervix DUØ1
Intraoperative DUØ13ZØ
Chest DWØ2
Intraoperative DWØ23ZØ
Chest Wall DBØ7
Intraoperative DBØ73ZØ
Colon DDØ5
Intraoperative DDØ53ZØ
Diaphragm DBØ8
Intraoperative DBØ83ZØ
Duodenum DDØ2
Intraoperative DDØ23ZØ
Ear D9ØØ
Intraoperative D9ØØ3ZØ
Esophagus DDØØ
Intraoperative DDØØ3ZØ
Eye D8ØØ
Intraoperative D8ØØ3ZØ
Femur DPØ9
Intraoperative DPØ93ZØ
Fibula DPØB
Intraoperative DPØB3ZØ
Gallbladder DFØ1
Intraoperative DFØ13ZØ
Gland
Adrenal DGØ2
Intraoperative DGØ23ZØ
Parathyroid DGØ4
Intraoperative DGØ43ZØ
Pituitary DGØØ
Intraoperative DGØØ3ZØ
Thyroid DGØ5
Intraoperative DGØ53ZØ
Glands
Intraoperative D9Ø63ZØ
Salivary D9Ø6
Head and Neck DWØ1
Intraoperative DWØ13ZØ
Hemibody DWØ4
Intraoperative DWØ43ZØ
Humerus DPØ6
Intraoperative DPØ63ZØ
Hypopharynx D9Ø3
Intraoperative D9Ø33ZØ
Ileum DDØ4
Intraoperative DDØ43ZØ

Beam Radiation — *continued*
Jejunum DDØ3
Intraoperative DDØ33ZØ
Kidney DTØØ
Intraoperative DTØØ3ZØ
Larynx D9ØB
Intraoperative D9ØB3ZØ
Liver DFØØ
Intraoperative DFØØ3ZØ
Lung DBØ2
Intraoperative DBØ23ZØ
Lymphatics
Abdomen D7Ø6
Intraoperative D7Ø63ZØ
Axillary D7Ø4
Intraoperative D7Ø43ZØ
Inguinal D7Ø8
Intraoperative D7Ø83ZØ
Neck D7Ø3
Intraoperative D7Ø33ZØ
Pelvis D7Ø7
Intraoperative D7Ø73ZØ
Thorax D7Ø5
Intraoperative D7Ø53ZØ
Mandible DPØ3
Intraoperative DPØ33ZØ
Maxilla DPØ2
Intraoperative DPØ23ZØ
Mediastinum DBØ6
Intraoperative DBØ63ZØ
Mouth D9Ø4
Intraoperative D9Ø43ZØ
Nasopharynx D9ØD
Intraoperative D9ØD3ZØ
Neck and Head DWØ1
Intraoperative DWØ13ZØ
Nerve
Intraoperative DØØ73ZØ
Peripheral DØØ7
Nose D9Ø1
Intraoperative D9Ø13ZØ
Oropharynx D9ØF
Intraoperative D9ØF3ZØ
Ovary DUØØ
Intraoperative DUØØ3ZØ
Palate
Hard D9Ø8
Intraoperative D9Ø83ZØ
Soft D9Ø9
Intraoperative D9Ø93ZØ
Pancreas DFØ3
Intraoperative DFØ33ZØ
Parathyroid Gland DGØ4
Intraoperative DGØ43ZØ
Pelvic Bones DPØ8
Intraoperative DPØ83ZØ
Pelvic Region DWØ6
Intraoperative DWØ63ZØ
Pineal Body DGØ1
Intraoperative DGØ13ZØ
Pituitary Gland DGØØ
Intraoperative DGØØ3ZØ
Pleura DBØ5
Intraoperative DBØ53ZØ
Prostate DVØØ
Intraoperative DVØØ3ZØ
Radius DPØ7
Intraoperative DPØ73ZØ
Rectum DDØ7
Intraoperative DDØ73ZØ
Rib DPØ5
Intraoperative DPØ53ZØ
Sinuses D9Ø7
Intraoperative D9Ø73ZØ
Skin
Abdomen DHØ8
Intraoperative DHØ83ZØ
Arm DHØ4
Intraoperative DHØ43ZØ
Back DHØ7
Intraoperative DHØ73ZØ
Buttock DHØ9
Intraoperative DHØ93ZØ
Chest DHØ6
Intraoperative DHØ63ZØ
Face DHØ2
Intraoperative DHØ23ZØ
Leg DHØB
Intraoperative DHØB3ZØ

Beam Radiation — *continued*
Skin — *continued*
Neck DHØ3
Intraoperative DHØ33ZØ
Skull DPØØ
Intraoperative DPØØ3ZØ
Spinal Cord DØØ6
Intraoperative DØØ63ZØ
Spleen D7Ø2
Intraoperative D7Ø23ZØ
Sternum DPØ4
Intraoperative DPØ43ZØ
Stomach DDØ1
Intraoperative DDØ13ZØ
Testis DVØ1
Intraoperative DVØ13ZØ
Thymus D7Ø1
Intraoperative D7Ø13ZØ
Thyroid Gland DGØ5
Intraoperative DGØ53ZØ
Tibia DPØB
Intraoperative DPØB3ZØ
Tongue D9Ø5
Intraoperative D9Ø53ZØ
Trachea DBØØ
Intraoperative DBØØ3ZØ
Ulna DPØ7
Intraoperative DPØ73ZØ
Ureter DTØ1
Intraoperative DTØ13ZØ
Urethra DTØ3
Intraoperative DTØ33ZØ
Uterus DUØ2
Intraoperative DUØ23ZØ
Whole Body DWØ5
Intraoperative DWØ53ZØ
Bedside swallow FØØZJWZ
Berlin Heart Ventricular Assist Device *use* Implantable Heart Assist System in Heart and Great Vessels
Bezlotoxumab Monoclonal Antibody XWØ
Biceps brachii muscle
use Upper Arm Muscle, Left
use Upper Arm Muscle, Right
Biceps femoris muscle
use Upper Leg Muscle, Left
use Upper Leg Muscle, Right
Bicipital aponeurosis
use Subcutaneous Tissue and Fascia, Left Lower Arm
use Subcutaneous Tissue and Fascia, Right Lower Arm
Bicuspid valve *use* Mitral Valve
Bili light therapy *see* Phototherapy, Skin 6A6Ø
Bioactive embolization coil(s) *use* Intraluminal Device, Bioactive in Upper Arteries
Bioengineered Allogeneic Construct, Skin XHRPXF7
Biofeedback GZC9ZZZ
BioFire® FilmArray® Pneumonia Panel XXEBXQ6
Biopsy
see Drainage with qualifier Diagnostic
see Excision with qualifier Diagnostic
see Extraction with qualifier Diagnostic
BiPAP *see* Assistance, Respiratory 5AØ9
Bisection *see* Division
Biventricular external heart assist system *use* Short-term External Heart Assist System in Heart and Great Vessels
Blepharectomy
see Excision, Eye Ø8B
see Resection, Eye Ø8T
Blepharoplasty
see Repair, Eye Ø8Q
see Replacement, Eye Ø8R
see Reposition, Eye Ø8S
see Supplement, Eye Ø8U
Blepharorrhaphy *see* Repair, Eye Ø8Q
Blepharotomy *see* Drainage, Eye Ø89
Blinatumomab *use* Other Antineoplastic
BLINCYTO® (blinatumomab) *use* Other Antineoplastic
Block, Nerve, anesthetic injection 3EØT3BZ
Blood glucose monitoring system *use* Monitoring Device
Blood pressure *see* Measurement, Arterial 4AØ3
BMR (basal metabolic rate) *see* Measurement, Physiological Systems 4AØZ

Body of femur
use Femoral Shaft, Left
use Femoral Shaft, Right
Body of fibula
use Fibula, Left
use Fibula, Right
Bone anchored hearing device
use Hearing Device, Bone Conduction in Ø9H
use Hearing Device in Head and Facial Bones
Bone bank bone graft *use* Nonautologous Tissue Substitute
Bone Growth Stimulator
Insertion of device in
Bone
Facial ØNHW
Lower ØQHY
Nasal ØNHB
Upper ØPHY
Skull ØNHØ
Removal of device from
Bone
Facial ØNPW
Lower ØQPY
Nasal ØNPB
Upper ØPPY
Skull ØNPØ
Revision of device in
Bone
Facial ØNWW
Lower ØQWY
Nasal ØNWB
Upper ØPWY
Skull ØNWØ
Bone marrow transplant *see* Transfusion, Circulatory 3Ø2
Bone morphogenetic protein 2 (BMP 2) *use* Recombinant Bone Morphogenetic Protein
Bone screw (interlocking) (lag) (pedicle) (recessed)
use Internal Fixation Device in Head and Facial Bones
use Internal Fixation Device in Lower Bones
use Internal Fixation Device in Upper Bones
Bony labyrinth
use Inner Ear, Left
use Inner Ear, Right
Bony orbit
use Orbit, Left
use Orbit, Right
Bony vestibule
use Inner Ear, Left
use Inner Ear, Right
Botallo's duct *use* Pulmonary Artery, Left
Bovine pericardial valve *use* Zooplastic Tissue in Heart and Great Vessels
Bovine pericardium graft *use* Zooplastic Tissue in Heart and Great Vessels
BP (blood pressure) *see* Measurement, Arterial 4AØ3
Brachial (lateral) lymph node
use Lymphatic, Left Axillary
use Lymphatic, Right Axillary
Brachialis muscle
use Upper Arm Muscle, Left
use Upper Arm Muscle, Right
Brachiocephalic artery *use* Innominate Artery
Brachiocephalic trunk *use* Innominate Artery
Brachiocephalic vein
use Innominate Vein, Left
use Innominate Vein, Right
Brachioradialis muscle
use Lower Arm and Wrist Muscle, Left
use Lower Arm and Wrist Muscle, Right
Brachytherapy
Abdomen DW13
Adrenal Gland DG12
Back
Lower DW1LBB
Upper DW1KBB
Bile Ducts DF12
Bladder DT12
Bone Marrow D71Ø
Brain DØ1Ø
Brain Stem DØ11
Breast
Left DM1Ø
Right DM11
Bronchus DB11
Cervix DU11
Brachytherapy — *continued*
Chest DW12
Chest Wall DB17
Colon DD15
Cranial Cavity DW1ØBB
Diaphragm DB18
Duodenum DD12
Ear D91Ø
Esophagus DD1Ø
Extremity
Lower DW1YBB
Upper DW1XBB
Eye D81Ø
Gallbladder DF11
Gastrointestinal Tract DW1PBB
Genitourinary Tract DW1RBB
Gland
Adrenal DG12
Parathyroid DG14
Pituitary DG1Ø
Thyroid DG15
Glands, Salivary D916
Head and Neck DW11
Hypopharynx D913
Ileum DD14
Jejunum DD13
Kidney DT1Ø
Larynx D91B
Liver DF1Ø
Lung DB12
Lymphatics
Abdomen D716
Axillary D714
Inguinal D718
Neck D713
Pelvis D717
Thorax D715
Mediastinum DB16
Mouth D914
Nasopharynx D91D
Neck and Head DW11
Nerve, Peripheral DØ17
Nose D911
Oropharynx D91F
Ovary DU1Ø
Palate
Hard D918
Soft D919
Pancreas DF13
Parathyroid Gland DG14
Pelvic Region DW16
Pineal Body DG11
Pituitary Gland DG1Ø
Pleura DB15
Prostate DV1Ø
Rectum DD17
Respiratory Tract DW1QBB
Sinuses D917
Spinal Cord DØ16
Spleen D712
Stomach DD11
Testis DV11
Thymus D711
Thyroid Gland DG15
Tongue D915
Trachea DB1Ø
Ureter DT11
Urethra DT13
Uterus DU12
Brachytherapy, CivaSheet®
see Brachytherapy with qualifier Unidirectional Source
see Insertion with device Radioactive Element
Brachytherapy seeds *use* Radioactive Element
Breast procedures, skin only *use* Skin, Chest
Brexanolone XWØ
Brexucabtagene Autoleucel *use* Brexucabtagene Autoleucel Immunotherapy
Brexucabtagene Autoleucel Immunotherapy XWØ
Broad ligament *use* Uterine Supporting Structure
Bromelain-enriched Proteolytic Enzyme XWØ
Bronchial artery *use* Upper Artery
Bronchography
see Fluoroscopy, Respiratory System BB1
see Plain Radiography, Respiratory System BBØ
Bronchoplasty
see Repair, Respiratory System ØBQ
see Supplement, Respiratory System ØBU
Bronchorrhaphy *see* Repair, Respiratory System ØBQ
Bronchoscopy ØBJØ8ZZ
Bronchotomy *see* Drainage, Respiratory System ØB9
Bronchus Intermedius *use* Main Bronchus, Right
BRYAN® Cervical Disc System *use* Synthetic Substitute
Buccal gland *use* Buccal Mucosa
Buccinator lymph node *use* Lymphatic, Head
Buccinator muscle *use* Facial Muscle
Buckling, scleral with implant *see* Supplement, Eye Ø8U
Bulbospongiosus muscle *use* Perineum Muscle
Bulbourethral (Cowper's) gland *use* Urethra
Bundle of His *use* Conduction Mechanism
Bundle of Kent *use* Conduction Mechanism
Bunionectomy *see* Excision, Lower Bones ØQB
Bursectomy
see Excision, Bursae and Ligaments ØMB
see Resection, Bursae and Ligaments ØMT
Bursocentesis *see* Drainage, Bursae and Ligaments ØM9
Bursography
see Plain Radiography, Non-Axial Lower Bones BQØ
see Plain Radiography, Non-Axial Upper Bones BPØ
Bursotomy
see Division, Bursae and Ligaments ØM8
see Drainage, Bursae and Ligaments ØM9
BVS 5ØØØ Ventricular Assist Device *use* Short-term External Heart Assist System in Heart and Great Vessels
Bypass
Anterior Chamber
Left Ø8133
Right Ø8123
Aorta
Abdominal Ø41Ø
Thoracic
Ascending/Arch Ø21X
Descending Ø21W
Artery
Anterior Tibial
Left Ø41Q
Right Ø41P
Axillary
Left Ø316Ø
Right Ø315Ø
Brachial
Left Ø318
Right Ø317
Common Carotid
Left Ø31JØ
Right Ø31HØ
Common Iliac
Left Ø41D
Right Ø41C
Coronary
Four or More Arteries Ø213
One Artery Ø21Ø
Three Arteries Ø212
Two Arteries Ø211
External Carotid
Left Ø31NØ
Right Ø31MØ
External Iliac
Left Ø41J
Right Ø41H
Femoral
Left Ø41L
Right Ø41K
Foot
Left Ø41W
Right Ø41V
Hepatic Ø413
Innominate Ø312Ø
Internal Carotid
Left Ø31LØ
Right Ø31KØ
Internal Iliac
Left Ø41F
Right Ø41E
Intracranial Ø31GØ
Peroneal
Left Ø41U
Right Ø41T
Popliteal
Left Ø41N
Right Ø41M
Posterior Tibial
Left Ø41S

Bypass — *continued*
Artery — *continued*
Posterior Tibial — *continued*
Right Ø41R
Pulmonary
Left Ø21R
Right Ø21Q
Pulmonary Trunk Ø21P
Radial
Left Ø31C
Right Ø31B
Splenic Ø414
Subclavian
Left Ø314Ø
Right Ø313Ø
Temporal
Left Ø31TØ
Right Ø31SØ
Ulnar
Left Ø31A
Right Ø319
Atrium
Left Ø217
Right Ø216
Bladder ØT1B
Cavity, Cranial ØW11ØJ
Cecum ØD1H
Cerebral Ventricle ØØ16
Colon
Ascending ØD1K
Descending ØD1M
Sigmoid ØD1N
Transverse ØD1L
Duct
Common Bile ØF19
Cystic ØF18
Hepatic
Common ØF17
Left ØF16
Right ØF15
Lacrimal
Left Ø81Y
Right Ø81X
Pancreatic ØF1D
Accessory ØF1F
Duodenum ØD19
Ear
Left Ø91EØ
Right Ø91DØ
Esophagus ØD15
Lower ØD13
Middle ØD12
Upper ØD11
Fallopian Tube
Left ØU16
Right ØU15
Gallbladder ØF14
Ileum ØD1B
Intestine
Large ØD1E
Small ØD18
Jejunum ØD1A
Kidney Pelvis
Left ØT14
Right ØT13
Pancreas ØF1G
Pelvic Cavity ØW1J
Peritoneal Cavity ØW1G
Pleural Cavity
Left ØW1B
Right ØW19
Spinal Canal ØØ1U
Stomach ØD16
Trachea ØB11
Ureter
Left ØT17
Right ØT16
Ureters, Bilateral ØT18
Vas Deferens
Bilateral ØV1Q
Left ØV1P
Right ØV1N
Vein
Axillary
Left Ø518
Right Ø517
Azygos Ø51Ø
Basilic
Left Ø51C

Bypass — *continued*
Vein — *continued*
Basilic — *continued*
Right Ø51B
Brachial
Left Ø51A
Right Ø519
Cephalic
Left Ø51F
Right Ø51D
Colic Ø617
Common Iliac
Left Ø61D
Right Ø61C
Esophageal Ø613
External Iliac
Left Ø61G
Right Ø61F
External Jugular
Left Ø51Q
Right Ø51P
Face
Left Ø51V
Right Ø51T
Femoral
Left Ø61N
Right Ø61M
Foot
Left Ø61V
Right Ø61T
Gastric Ø612
Hand
Left Ø51H
Right Ø51G
Hemiazygos Ø511
Hepatic Ø614
Hypogastric
Left Ø61J
Right Ø61H
Inferior Mesenteric Ø616
Innominate
Left Ø514
Right Ø513
Internal Jugular
Left Ø51N
Right Ø51M
Intracranial Ø51L
Portal Ø618
Renal
Left Ø61B
Right Ø619
Saphenous
Left Ø61Q
Right Ø61P
Splenic Ø611
Subclavian
Left Ø516
Right Ø515
Superior Mesenteric Ø615
Vertebral
Left Ø51S
Right Ø51R
Vena Cava
Inferior Ø61Ø
Superior Ø21V
Ventricle
Left Ø21L
Right Ø21K
Bypass, cardiopulmonary 5A1221Z

C

Caesarean section *see* Extraction, Products of Conception 1ØDØ
Calcaneocuboid joint
use Tarsal Joint, Left
use Tarsal Joint, Right
Calcaneocuboid ligament
use Foot Bursa and Ligament, Left
use Foot Bursa and Ligament, Right
Calcaneofibular ligament
use Ankle Bursa and Ligament, Left
use Ankle Bursa and Ligament, Right
Calcaneus
use Tarsal, Left
use Tarsal, Right

Cannulation
see Bypass
see Dilation
see Drainage
see Irrigation
Canthorrhaphy *see* Repair, Eye Ø8Q
Canthotomy *see* Release, Eye Ø8N
Capitate bone
use Carpal, Left
use Carpal, Right
Caplacizumab XWØ
Capsulectomy, lens *see* Excision, Eye Ø8B
Capsulorrhaphy, joint
see Repair, Lower Joints ØSQ
see Repair, Upper Joints ØRQ
Caption Guidance system X2JAX47
Cardia *use* Esophagogastric Junction
Cardiac contractility modulation lead *use* Cardiac Lead in Heart and Great Vessels
Cardiac event recorder *use* Monitoring Device
Cardiac Lead
Defibrillator
Atrium
Left Ø2H7
Right Ø2H6
Pericardium Ø2HN
Vein, Coronary Ø2H4
Ventricle
Left Ø2HL
Right Ø2HK
Insertion of device in
Atrium
Left Ø2H7
Right Ø2H6
Pericardium Ø2HN
Vein, Coronary Ø2H4
Ventricle
Left Ø2HL
Right Ø2HK
Pacemaker
Atrium
Left Ø2H7
Right Ø2H6
Pericardium Ø2HN
Vein, Coronary Ø2H4
Ventricle
Left Ø2HL
Right Ø2HK
Removal of device from, Heart Ø2PA
Revision of device in, Heart Ø2WA
Cardiac plexus *use* Thoracic Sympathetic Nerve
Cardiac Resynchronization Defibrillator Pulse Generator
Abdomen ØJH8
Chest ØJH6
Cardiac Resynchronization Pacemaker Pulse Generator
Abdomen ØJH8
Chest ØJH6
Cardiac resynchronization therapy (CRT) lead
use Cardiac Lead, Defibrillator in Ø2H
use Cardiac Lead, Pacemaker in Ø2H
Cardiac Rhythm Related Device
Insertion of device in
Abdomen ØJH8
Chest ØJH6
Removal of device from, Subcutaneous Tissue and Fascia, Trunk ØJPT
Revision of device in, Subcutaneous Tissue and Fascia, Trunk ØJWT
Cardiocentesis *see* Drainage, Pericardial Cavity ØW9D
Cardioesophageal junction *use* Esophagogastric Junction
Cardiolysis *see* Release, Heart and Great Vessels Ø2N
CardioMEMS® pressure sensor *use* Monitoring Device, Pressure Sensor in Ø2H
Cardiomyotomy *see* Division, Esophagogastric Junction ØD84
Cardioplegia *see* Introduction of substance in or on, Heart 3EØ8
Cardiorrhaphy *see* Repair, Heart and Great Vessels Ø2Q
Cardioversion 5A22Ø4Z
Caregiver Training FØFZ
Carmat total artificial heart (TAH) *use* Biologic with Synthetic Substitute, Autoregulated Electrohydraulic in Ø2R

Caroticotympanic artery
use Internal Carotid Artery, Left
use Internal Carotid Artery, Right
Carotid glomus
use Carotid Bodies, Bilateral
use Carotid Body, Left
use Carotid Body, Right
Carotid sinus
use Internal Carotid Artery, Left
use Internal Carotid Artery, Right
Carotid (artery) sinus (baroreceptor) lead *use* Stimulator Lead in Upper Arteries
Carotid sinus nerve *use* Glossopharyngeal Nerve
Carotid WALLSTENT® Monorail® Endoprosthesis *use* Intraluminal Device
Carpectomy
see Excision, Upper Bones ØPB
see Resection, Upper Bones ØPT
Carpometacarpal ligament
use Hand Bursa and Ligament, Left
use Hand Bursa and Ligament, Right
Casirivimab (REGN10933) and Imdevimab (REGN10987) *use* REGN-COV2 Monoclonal Antibody
Casting *see* Immobilization
CAT scan *see* Computerized Tomography (CT Scan)
Catheterization
see Dilation
see Drainage
see Insertion of device in
see Irrigation
Heart *see* Measurement, Cardiac 4AØ2
Umbilical vein, for infusion Ø6HØ33T
Cauda equina *use* Lumbar Spinal Cord
Cauterization
see Destruction
see Repair
Cavernous plexus *use* Head and Neck Sympathetic Nerve
CBMA (Concentrated Bone Marrow Aspirate) *use* Concentrated Bone Marrow Aspirate
CBMA (Concentrated Bone Marrow Aspirate) injection, intramuscular XKØ23Ø3
CD24Fc Immunomodulator XWØ
Cecectomy
see Excision, Cecum ØDBH
see Resection, Cecum ØDTH
Cecocolostomy
see Bypass, Gastrointestinal System ØD1
see Drainage, Gastrointestinal System ØD9
Cecopexy
see Repair, Cecum ØDQH
see Reposition, Cecum ØDSH
Cecoplication *see* Restriction, Cecum ØDVH
Cecorrhaphy *see* Repair, Cecum ØDQH
Cecostomy
see Bypass, Cecum ØD1H
see Drainage, Cecum ØD9H
Cecotomy *see* Drainage, Cecum ØD9H
Cefiderocol Anti-infective XWØ
Ceftazidime-avibactam *use* Other Anti-infective
Ceftolozane/Tazobactam Anti-infective XWØ
Celiac ganglion *use* Abdominal Sympathetic Nerve
Celiac lymph node *use* Lymphatic, Aortic
Celiac (solar) plexus *use* Abdominal Sympathetic Nerve
Celiac trunk *use* Celiac Artery
Central axillary lymph node
use Lymphatic, Left Axillary
use Lymphatic, Right Axillary
Central venous pressure *see* Measurement, Venous 4AØ4
Centrimag® Blood Pump *use* Short-term External Heart Assist System in Heart and Great Vessels
Cephalogram BNØØZZZ
CERAMENT® G *use* Antibiotic-eluting Bone Void Filler
Ceramic on ceramic bearing surface *use* Synthetic Substitute, Ceramic in ØSR
Cerclage *see* Restriction
Cerebral aqueduct (Sylvius) *use* Cerebral Ventricle
Cerebral Embolic Filtration
Dual Filter X2A5312
Extracorporeal Flow Reversal Circuit X2A
Single Deflection Filter X2A6325
Cerebrum *use* Brain
Cervical esophagus *use* Esophagus, Upper
Cervical facet joint
use Cervical Vertebral Joint
use Cervical Vertebral Joint, 2 or more
Cervical ganglion *use* Head and Neck Sympathetic Nerve
Cervical interspinous ligament *use* Head and Neck Bursa and Ligament
Cervical intertransverse ligament *use* Head and Neck Bursa and Ligament
Cervical Ligamentum Flavum *use* Head and Neck Bursa and Ligament
Cervical Lymph Node
use Lymphatic, Left Neck
use Lymphatic, Right Neck
Cervicectomy
see Excision, Cervix ØUBC
see Resection, Cervix ØUTC
Cervicothoracic facet joint *use* Cervicothoracic Vertebral Joint
Cesarean section *see* Extraction, Products of Conception 1ØDØ
Cesium-131 Collagen Implant *use* Radioactive Element, Cesium-131 Collagen Implant in ØØH
Change Device in
Abdominal Wall ØW2FX
Back
Lower ØW2LX
Upper ØW2KX
Bladder ØT2BX
Bone
Facial ØN2WX
Lower ØQ2YX
Nasal ØN2BX
Upper ØP2YX
Bone Marrow Ø72TX
Brain ØØ2ØX
Breast
Left ØH2UX
Right ØH2TX
Bursa and Ligament
Lower ØM2YX
Upper ØM2XX
Cavity, Cranial ØW21X
Chest Wall ØW28X
Cisterna Chyli Ø72LX
Diaphragm ØB2TX
Duct
Hepatobiliary ØF2BX
Pancreatic ØF2DX
Ear
Left Ø92JX
Right Ø92HX
Epididymis and Spermatic Cord ØV2MX
Extremity
Lower
Left ØY2BX
Right ØY29X
Upper
Left ØX27X
Right ØX26X
Eye
Left Ø821X
Right Ø82ØX
Face ØW22X
Fallopian Tube ØU28X
Gallbladder ØF24X
Gland
Adrenal ØG25X
Endocrine ØG2SX
Pituitary ØG2ØX
Salivary ØC2AX
Head ØW2ØX
Intestinal Tract
Lower ØD2DXUZ
Upper ØD2ØXUZ
Jaw
Lower ØW25X
Upper ØW24X
Joint
Lower ØS2YX
Upper ØR2YX
Kidney ØT25X
Larynx ØC2SX
Liver ØF2ØX
Lung
Left ØB2LX
Right ØB2KX
Lymphatic Ø72NX
Change Device in — *continued*
Lymphatic — *continued*
Thoracic Duct Ø72KX
Mediastinum ØW2CX
Mesentery ØD2VX
Mouth and Throat ØC2YX
Muscle
Lower ØK2YX
Upper ØK2XX
Nasal Mucosa and Soft Tissue Ø92KX
Neck ØW26X
Nerve
Cranial ØØ2EX
Peripheral Ø12YX
Omentum ØD2UX
Ovary ØU23X
Pancreas ØF2GX
Parathyroid Gland ØG2RX
Pelvic Cavity ØW2JX
Penis ØV2SX
Pericardial Cavity ØW2DX
Perineum
Female ØW2NX
Male ØW2MX
Peritoneal Cavity ØW2GX
Peritoneum ØD2WX
Pineal Body ØG21X
Pleura ØB2QX
Pleural Cavity
Left ØW2BX
Right ØW29X
Products of Conception 1Ø2Ø7
Prostate and Seminal Vesicles ØV24X
Retroperitoneum ØW2HX
Scrotum and Tunica Vaginalis ØV28X
Sinus Ø92YX
Skin ØH2PX
Skull ØN2ØX
Spinal Canal ØØ2UX
Spleen Ø72PX
Subcutaneous Tissue and Fascia
Head and Neck ØJ2SX
Lower Extremity ØJ2WX
Trunk ØJ2TX
Upper Extremity ØJ2VX
Tendon
Lower ØL2YX
Upper ØL2XX
Testis ØV2DX
Thymus Ø72MX
Thyroid Gland ØG2KX
Trachea ØB21
Tracheobronchial Tree ØB2ØX
Ureter ØT29X
Urethra ØT2DX
Uterus and Cervix ØU2DXHZ
Vagina and Cul-de-sac ØU2HXGZ
Vas Deferens ØV2RX
Vulva ØU2MX
Change Device in or on
Abdominal Wall 2WØ3X
Anorectal 2YØ3X5Z
Arm
Lower
Left 2WØDX
Right 2WØCX
Upper
Left 2WØBX
Right 2WØAX
Back 2WØ5X
Chest Wall 2WØ4X
Ear 2YØ2X5Z
Extremity
Lower
Left 2WØMX
Right 2WØLX
Upper
Left 2WØ9X
Right 2WØ8X
Face 2WØ1X
Finger
Left 2WØKX
Right 2WØJX
Foot
Left 2WØTX
Right 2WØSX
Genital Tract, Female 2YØ4X5Z
Hand
Left 2WØFX

Index

Caroticotympanic artery — Change Device in or on

Change Device in or on — *continued*
Hand — *continued*
Right 2WØEX
Head 2WØØX
Inguinal Region
Left 2WØ7X
Right 2WØ6X
Leg
Lower
Left 2WØRX
Right 2WØQX
Upper
Left 2WØPX
Right 2WØNX
Mouth and Pharynx 2YØØX5Z
Nasal 2YØ1X5Z
Neck 2WØ2X
Thumb
Left 2WØHX
Right 2WØGX
Toe
Left 2WØVX
Right 2WØUX
Urethra 2YØ5X5Z
Chemoembolization *see* Introduction of substance in or on
Chemosurgery, Skin 3EØØXTZ
Chemothalamectomy *see* Destruction, Thalamus ØØ59
Chemotherapy, Infusion for Cancer *see* Introduction of substance in or on
Chest compression (CPR), external
Manual 5A12Ø12
Mechanical 5A1221J
Chest x-ray *see* Plain Radiography, Chest BWØ3
Chiropractic Manipulation
Abdomen 9WB9X
Cervical 9WB1X
Extremities
Lower 9WB6X
Upper 9WB7X
Head 9WBØX
Lumbar 9WB3X
Pelvis 9WB5X
Rib Cage 9WB8X
Sacrum 9WB4X
Thoracic 9WB2X
Choana *use* Nasopharynx
Cholangiogram
see Fluoroscopy, Hepatobiliary System and Pancreas BF1
see Plain Radiography, Hepatobiliary System and Pancreas BFØ
Cholecystectomy
see Excision, Gallbladder ØFB4
see Resection, Gallbladder ØFT4
Cholecystojejunostomy
see Bypass, Hepatobiliary System and Pancreas ØF1
see Drainage, Hepatobiliary System and Pancreas ØF9
Cholecystopexy
see Repair, Gallbladder ØFQ4
see Reposition, Gallbladder ØFS4
Cholecystoscopy ØFJ44ZZ
Cholecystostomy
see Bypass, Gallbladder ØF14
see Drainage, Gallbladder ØF94
Cholecystotomy *see* Drainage, Gallbladder ØF94
Choledochectomy
see Excision, Hepatobiliary System and Pancreas ØFB
see Resection, Hepatobiliary System and Pancreas ØFT
Choledocholithotomy *see* Extirpation, Duct, Common Bile ØFC9
Choledochoplasty
see Repair, Hepatobiliary System and Pancreas ØFQ
see Replacement, Hepatobiliary System and Pancreas ØFR
see Supplement, Hepatobiliary System and Pancreas ØFU
Choledochoscopy ØFJB8ZZ
Choledochotomy *see* Drainage, Hepatobiliary System and Pancreas ØF9
Cholelithotomy *see* Extirpation, Hepatobiliary System and Pancreas ØFC
Chondrectomy
see Excision, Lower Joints ØSB
Chondrectomy — *continued*
see Excision, Upper Joints ØRB
Knee *see* Excision, Lower Joints ØSB
Semilunar cartilage *see* Excision, Lower Joints ØSB
Chondroglossus muscle *use* Tongue, Palate, Pharynx Muscle
Chorda tympani *use* Facial Nerve
Chordotomy *see* Division, Central Nervous System and Cranial Nerves ØØ8
Choroid plexus *use* Cerebral Ventricle
Choroidectomy
see Excision, Eye Ø8B
see Resection, Eye Ø8T
Ciliary body
use Eye, Left
use Eye, Right
Ciliary ganglion *use* Head and Neck Sympathetic Nerve
Ciltacabtagene Autoleucel XWØ
cilta-cel *use* Ciltacabtagene Autoleucel
Circle of Willis *use* Intracranial Artery
Circumcision ØVTTXZZ
Circumflex iliac artery
use Femoral Artery, Left
use Femoral Artery, Right
CivaSheet® *use* Radioactive Element
CivaSheet® Brachytherapy
see Brachytherapy with qualifier Unidirectional Source
see Insertion with device Radioactive Element
Clamp and rod internal fixation system (CRIF)
use Internal Fixation Device in Lower Bones
use Internal Fixation Device in Upper Bones
Clamping *see* Occlusion
Claustrum *use* Basal Ganglia
Claviculectomy
see Excision, Upper Bones ØPB
see Resection, Upper Bones ØPT
Claviculotomy
see Division, Upper Bones ØP8
see Drainage, Upper Bones ØP9
Clipping, aneurysm
see Occlusion using Extraluminal Device
see Restriction using Extraluminal Device
Clitorectomy, clitoridectomy
see Excision, Clitoris ØUBJ
see Resection, Clitoris ØUTJ
Clolar *use* Clofarabine
Closure
see Occlusion
see Repair
Clysis *see* Introduction of substance in or on
Coagulation *see* Destruction
Coagulation Factor Xa, Inactivated XWØ
Coagulation Factor Xa, (Recombinant) Inactivated *use* Coagulation Factor Xa, Inactivated
COALESCE® radiolucent interbody fusion device *use* Interbody Fusion Device, Radiolucent Porous in New Technology
CoAxia NeuroFlo catheter *use* Intraluminal Device
Cobalt/chromium head and polyethylene socket *use* Synthetic Substitute, Metal on Polyethylene in ØSR
Cobalt/chromium head and socket *use* Synthetic Substitute, Metal in ØSR
Coccygeal body *use* Coccygeal Glomus
Coccygeus muscle
use Trunk Muscle, Left
use Trunk Muscle, Right
Cochlea
use Inner Ear, Left
use Inner Ear, Right
Cochlear implant (CI), multiple channel (electrode) *use* Hearing Device, Multiple Channel Cochlear Prosthesis in Ø9H
Cochlear implant (CI), single channel (electrode) *use* Hearing Device, Single Channel Cochlear Prosthesis in Ø9H
Cochlear Implant Treatment FØBZØ
Cochlear nerve *use* Acoustic Nerve
COGNIS® CRT-D *use* Cardiac Resynchronization Defibrillator Pulse Generator in ØJH
COHERE® radiolucent interbody fusion device *use* Interbody Fusion Device, Radiolucent Porous in New Technology
Colectomy
see Excision, Gastrointestinal System ØDB
Colectomy — *continued*
see Resection, Gastrointestinal System ØDT
Collapse *see* Occlusion
Collection from
Breast, Breast Milk 8EØHX62
Indwelling Device
Circulatory System
Blood 8CØ2X6K
Other Fluid 8CØ2X6L
Nervous System
Cerebrospinal Fluid 8CØ1X6J
Other Fluid 8CØ1X6L
Integumentary System, Breast Milk 8EØHX62
Reproductive System, Male, Sperm 8EØVX63
Colocentesis *see* Drainage, Gastrointestinal System ØD9
Colofixation
see Repair, Gastrointestinal System ØDQ
see Reposition, Gastrointestinal System ØDS
Colofysis *see* Release, Gastrointestinal System ØDN
Colonic Z-Stent® *use* Intraluminal Device
Colonoscopy ØDJD8ZZ
Colopexy
see Repair, Gastrointestinal System ØDQ
see Reposition, Gastrointestinal System ØDS
Coloplication *see* Restriction, Gastrointestinal System ØDV
Coloproctectomy
see Excision, Gastrointestinal System ØDB
see Resection, Gastrointestinal System ØDT
Coloproctostomy
see Bypass, Gastrointestinal System ØD1
see Drainage, Gastrointestinal System ØD9
Colopuncture *see* Drainage, Gastrointestinal System ØD9
Colorrhaphy *see* Repair, Gastrointestinal System ØDQ
Colostomy
see Bypass, Gastrointestinal System ØD1
see Drainage, Gastrointestinal System ØD9
Colpectomy
see Excision, Vagina ØUBG
see Resection, Vagina ØUTG
Colpocentesis *see* Drainage, Vagina ØU9G
Colpopexy
see Repair, Vagina ØUQG
see Reposition, Vagina ØUSG
Colpoplasty
see Repair, Vagina ØUQG
see Supplement, Vagina ØUUG
Colporrhaphy *see* Repair, Vagina ØUQG
Colposcopy ØUJH8ZZ
Columella *use* Nasal Mucosa and Soft Tissue
Common digital vein
use Foot Vein, Left
use Foot Vein, Right
Common facial vein
use Face Vein, Left
use Face Vein, Right
Common fibular nerve *use* Peroneal Nerve
Common hepatic artery *use* Hepatic Artery
Common iliac (subaortic) lymph node *use* Lymphatic, Pelvis
Common interosseous artery
use Ulnar Artery, Left
use Ulnar Artery, Right
Common peroneal nerve *use* Peroneal Nerve
Complete (SE) stent *use* Intraluminal Device
Compression
see Restriction
Abdominal Wall 2W13X
Arm
Lower
Left 2W1DX
Right 2W1CX
Upper
Left 2W1BX
Right 2W1AX
Back 2W15X
Chest Wall 2W14X
Extremity
Lower
Left 2W1MX
Right 2W1LX
Upper
Left 2W19X
Right 2W18X
Face 2W11X

Compression — *continued*
Finger
Left 2W1KX
Right 2W1JX
Foot
Left 2W1TX
Right 2W1SX
Hand
Left 2W1FX
Right 2W1EX
Head 2W1ØX
Inguinal Region
Left 2W17X
Right 2W16X
Leg
Lower
Left 2W1RX
Right 2W1QX
Upper
Left 2W1PX
Right 2W1NX
Neck 2W12X
Thumb
Left 2W1HX
Right 2W1GX
Toe
Left 2W1VX
Right 2W1UX
Computer Assisted Procedure
Extremity
Lower
No Qualifier 8EØYXBZ
With Computerized Tomography 8EØYXBG
With Fluoroscopy 8EØYXBF
With Magnetic Resonance Imaging 8EØYXBH
Upper
No Qualifier 8EØXXBZ
With Computerized Tomography 8EØXXBG
With Fluoroscopy 8EØXXBF
With Magnetic Resonance Imaging 8EØXXBH
Head and Neck Region
No Qualifier 8EØ9XBZ
With Computerized Tomography 8EØ9XBG
With Fluoroscopy 8EØ9XBF
With Magnetic Resonance Imaging 8EØ9XBH
Trunk Region
No Qualifier 8EØWXBZ
With Computerized Tomography 8EØWXBG
With Fluoroscopy 8EØWXBF
With Magnetic Resonance Imaging 8EØWXBH
Computer-aided Assessment, Intracranial Vascular Activity XXEØXØ7
Computer-aided Guidance, Transthoracic Echocardiography X2JAX47
Computer-aided Mechanical Aspiration X2C
Computer-aided Triage and Notification, Pulmonary Artery Flow XXE3X27
Computer-assisted Intermittent Aspiration *see* New Technology, Cardiovascular System X2C
Computerized Tomography (CT Scan)
Abdomen BW2Ø
Chest and Pelvis BW25
Abdomen and Chest BW24
Abdomen and Pelvis BW21
Airway, Trachea BB2F
Ankle
Left BQ2H
Right BQ2G
Aorta
Abdominal B42Ø
Intravascular Optical Coherence B42ØZ2Z
Thoracic B32Ø
Intravascular Optical Coherence B32ØZ2Z
Arm
Left BP2F
Right BP2E
Artery
Celiac B421
Intravascular Optical Coherence B421Z2Z
Common Carotid
Bilateral B325

Computerized Tomography (CT Scan) — *continued*
Artery — *continued*
Common Carotid — *continued*
Intravascular Optical Coherence B325Z2Z
Coronary
Bypass Graft
Intravascular Optical Coherence B223Z2Z
Multiple B223
Multiple B221
Intravascular Optical Coherence B221Z2Z
Internal Carotid
Bilateral B328
Intravascular Optical Coherence B328Z2Z
Intracranial B32R
Intravascular Optical Coherence B32RZ2Z
Lower Extremity
Bilateral B42H
Intravascular Optical Coherence B42HZ2Z
Left B42G
Intravascular Optical Coherence B42GZ2Z
Right B42F
Intravascular Optical Coherence B42FZ2Z
Pelvic B42C
Intravascular Optical Coherence B42CZ2Z
Pulmonary
Left B32T
Intravascular Optical Coherence B32TZ2Z
Right B32S
Intravascular Optical Coherence B32SZ2Z
Renal
Bilateral B428
Intravascular Optical Coherence B428Z2Z
Transplant B42M
Intravascular Optical Coherence B42MZ2Z
Superior Mesenteric B424
Intravascular Optical Coherence B424Z2Z
Vertebral
Bilateral B32G
Intravascular Optical Coherence B32GZ2Z
Bladder BT2Ø
Bone
Facial BN25
Temporal BN2F
Brain BØ2Ø
Calcaneus
Left BQ2K
Right BQ2J
Cerebral Ventricle BØ28
Chest, Abdomen and Pelvis BW25
Chest and Abdomen BW24
Cisterna BØ27
Clavicle
Left BP25
Right BP24
Coccyx BR2F
Colon BD24
Ear B92Ø
Elbow
Left BP2H
Right BP2G
Extremity
Lower
Left BQ2S
Right BQ2R
Upper
Bilateral BP2V
Left BP2U
Right BP2T
Eye
Bilateral B827
Left B826
Right B825
Femur
Left BQ24

Computerized Tomography (CT Scan) — *continued*
Femur — *continued*
Right BQ23
Fibula
Left BQ2C
Right BQ2B
Finger
Left BP2S
Right BP2R
Foot
Left BQ2M
Right BQ2L
Forearm
Left BP2K
Right BP2J
Gland
Adrenal, Bilateral BG22
Parathyroid BG23
Parotid, Bilateral B926
Salivary, Bilateral B92D
Submandibular, Bilateral B929
Thyroid BG24
Hand
Left BP2P
Right BP2N
Hands and Wrists, Bilateral BP2Q
Head BW28
Head and Neck BW29
Heart
Intravascular Optical Coherence B226Z2Z
Right and Left B226
Hepatobiliary System, All BF2C
Hip
Left BQ21
Right BQ2Ø
Humerus
Left BP2B
Right BP2A
Intracranial Sinus B522
Intravascular Optical Coherence B522Z2Z
Joint
Acromioclavicular, Bilateral BP23
Finger
Left BP2DZZZ
Right BP2CZZZ
Foot
Left BQ2Y
Right BQ2X
Hand
Left BP2DZZZ
Right BP2CZZZ
Sacroiliac BR2D
Sternoclavicular
Bilateral BP22
Left BP21
Right BP2Ø
Temporomandibular, Bilateral BN29
Toe
Left BQ2Y
Right BQ2X
Kidney
Bilateral BT23
Left BT22
Right BT21
Transplant BT29
Knee
Left BQ28
Right BQ27
Larynx B92J
Leg
Left BQ2F
Right BQ2D
Liver BF25
Liver and Spleen BF26
Lung, Bilateral BB24
Mandible BN26
Nasopharynx B92F
Neck BW2F
Neck and Head BW29
Orbit, Bilateral BN23
Oropharynx B92F
Pancreas BF27
Patella
Left BQ2W
Right BQ2V
Pelvic Region BW2G
Pelvis BR2C
Chest and Abdomen BW25
Pelvis and Abdomen BW21

Computerized Tomography (CT Scan) — *continued*
Pituitary Gland BØ29
Prostate BV23
Ribs
Left BP2Y
Right BP2X
Sacrum BR2F
Scapula
Left BP27
Right BP26
Sella Turcica BØ29
Shoulder
Left BP29
Right BP28
Sinus
Intracranial B522
Intravascular Optical Coherence B522Z2Z
Paranasal B922
Skull BN2Ø
Spinal Cord BØ2B
Spine
Cervical BR2Ø
Lumbar BR29
Thoracic BR27
Spleen and Liver BF26
Thorax BP2W
Tibia
Left BQ2C
Right BQ2B
Toe
Left BQ2Q
Right BQ2P
Trachea BB2F
Tracheobronchial Tree
Bilateral BB29
Left BB28
Right BB27
Vein
Pelvic (Iliac)
Left B52G
Intravascular Optical Coherence B52GZ2Z
Right B52F
Intravascular Optical Coherence B52FZ2Z
Pelvic (Iliac) Bilateral B52H
Intravascular Optical Coherence B52HZ2Z
Portal B52T
Intravascular Optical Coherence B52TZ2Z
Pulmonary
Bilateral B52S
Intravascular Optical Coherence B52SZ2Z
Left B52R
Intravascular Optical Coherence B52RZ2Z
Right B52Q
Intravascular Optical Coherence B52QZ2Z
Renal
Bilateral B52L
Intravascular Optical Coherence B52LZ2Z
Left B52K
Intravascular Optical Coherence B52KZ2Z
Right B52J
Intravascular Optical Coherence B52JZ2Z
Spanchnic B52T
Intravascular Optical Coherence B52TZ2Z
Vena Cava
Inferior B529
Intravascular Optical Coherence B529Z2Z
Superior B528
Intravascular Optical Coherence B528Z2Z
Ventricle, Cerebral BØ28
Wrist
Left BP2M
Right BP2L
Concentrated Bone Marrow Aspirate (CBMA) injection, intramuscular XKØ23Ø3
Concerto II CRT-D *use* Cardiac Resynchronization Defibrillator Pulse Generator in ØJH
Condylectomy
see Excision, Head and Facial Bones ØNB
see Excision, Lower Bones ØQB
see Excision, Upper Bones ØPB
Condyloid process
use Mandible, Left
use Mandible, Right
Condylotomy
see Division, Head and Facial Bones ØN8
see Division, Lower Bones ØQ8
see Division, Upper Bones ØP8
see Drainage, Head and Facial Bones ØN9
see Drainage, Lower Bones ØQ9
see Drainage, Upper Bones ØP9
Condylysis
see Release, Head and Facial Bones ØNN
see Release, Lower Bones ØQN
see Release, Upper Bones ØPN
Conization, cervix *see* Excision, Cervix ØUBC
Conjunctivoplasty
see Repair, Eye Ø8Q
see Replacement, Eye Ø8R
CONSERVE® PLUS Total Resurfacing Hip System *use* Resurfacing Device in Lower Joints
Construction
Auricle, ear *see* Replacement, Ear, Nose, Sinus Ø9R
Ileal conduit *see* Bypass, Urinary System ØT1
Consulta CRT-D *use* Cardiac Resynchronization Defibrillator Pulse Generator in ØJH
Consulta CRT-P *use* Cardiac Resynchronization Pacemaker Pulse Generator in ØJH
Contact Radiation
Abdomen DWY37ZZ
Adrenal Gland DGY27ZZ
Bile Ducts DFY27ZZ
Bladder DTY27ZZ
Bone, Other DPYC7ZZ
Brain DØYØ7ZZ
Brain Stem DØY17ZZ
Breast
Left DMYØ7ZZ
Right DMY17ZZ
Bronchus DBY17ZZ
Cervix DUY17ZZ
Chest DWY27ZZ
Chest Wall DBY77ZZ
Colon DDY57ZZ
Diaphragm DBY87ZZ
Duodenum DDY27ZZ
Ear D9YØ7ZZ
Esophagus DDYØ7ZZ
Eye D8YØ7ZZ
Femur DPY97ZZ
Fibula DPYB7ZZ
Gallbladder DFY17ZZ
Gland
Adrenal DGY27ZZ
Parathyroid DGY47ZZ
Pituitary DGYØ7ZZ
Thyroid DGY57ZZ
Glands, Salivary D9Y67ZZ
Head and Neck DWY17ZZ
Hemibody DWY47ZZ
Humerus DPY67ZZ
Hypopharynx D9Y37ZZ
Ileum DDY47ZZ
Jejunum DDY37ZZ
Kidney DTYØ7ZZ
Larynx D9YB7ZZ
Liver DFYØ7ZZ
Lung DBY27ZZ
Mandible DPY37ZZ
Maxilla DPY27ZZ
Mediastinum DBY67ZZ
Mouth D9Y47ZZ
Nasopharynx D9YD7ZZ
Neck and Head DWY17ZZ
Nerve, Peripheral DØY77ZZ
Nose D9Y17ZZ
Oropharynx D9YF7ZZ
Ovary DUYØ7ZZ
Palate
Hard D9Y87ZZ
Soft D9Y97ZZ
Pancreas DFY37ZZ
Parathyroid Gland DGY47ZZ
Contact Radiation — *continued*
Pelvic Bones DPY87ZZ
Pelvic Region DWY67ZZ
Pineal Body DGY17ZZ
Pituitary Gland DGYØ7ZZ
Pleura DBY57ZZ
Prostate DVYØ7ZZ
Radius DPY77ZZ
Rectum DDY77ZZ
Rib DPY57ZZ
Sinuses D9Y77ZZ
Skin
Abdomen DHY87ZZ
Arm DHY47ZZ
Back DHY77ZZ
Buttock DHY97ZZ
Chest DHY67ZZ
Face DHY27ZZ
Leg DHYB7ZZ
Neck DHY37ZZ
Skull DPYØ7ZZ
Spinal Cord DØY67ZZ
Sternum DPY47ZZ
Stomach DDY17ZZ
Testis DVY17ZZ
Thyroid Gland DGY57ZZ
Tibia DPYB7ZZ
Tongue D9Y57ZZ
Trachea DBYØ7ZZ
Ulna DPY77ZZ
Ureter DTY17ZZ
Urethra DTY37ZZ
Uterus DUY27ZZ
Whole Body DWY57ZZ
ContaCT software (Measurement of intracranial arterial flow) 4AØ3X5D
CONTAK RENEWAL® 3 RF (HE) CRT-D *use* Cardiac Resynchronization Defibrillator Pulse Generator in ØJH
Contegra Pulmonary Valved Conduit *use* Zooplastic Tissue in Heart and Great Vessels
CONTEPO™ *use* Fosfomycin Anti-Infective
Continuous Glucose Monitoring (CGM) device *use* Monitoring Device
Continuous Negative Airway Pressure
24-96 Consecutive Hours, Ventilation 5AØ9459
Greater than 96 Consecutive Hours, Ventilation 5AØ9559
Less than 24 Consecutive Hours, Ventilation 5AØ9359
Continuous Positive Airway Pressure
24-96 Consecutive Hours, Ventilation 5AØ9457
Greater than 96 Consecutive Hours, Ventilation 5AØ9557
Less than 24 Consecutive Hours, Ventilation 5AØ9357
Continuous renal replacement therapy (CRRT) 5A1D9ØZ
Contraceptive Device
Change device in, Uterus and Cervix ØU2DXHZ
Insertion of device in
Cervix ØUHC
Subcutaneous Tissue and Fascia
Abdomen ØJH8
Chest ØJH6
Lower Arm
Left ØJHH
Right ØJHG
Lower Leg
Left ØJHP
Right ØJHN
Upper Arm
Left ØJHF
Right ØJHD
Upper Leg
Left ØJHM
Right ØJHL
Uterus ØUH9
Removal of device from
Subcutaneous Tissue and Fascia
Lower Extremity ØJPW
Trunk ØJPT
Upper Extremity ØJPV
Uterus and Cervix ØUPD
Revision of device in
Subcutaneous Tissue and Fascia
Lower Extremity ØJWW
Trunk ØJWT

Contraceptive Device — *continued*
Revision of device in — *continued*
Subcutaneous Tissue and Fascia — *continued*
Upper Extremity 0JWV
Uterus and Cervix 0UWD
Contractility Modulation Device
Abdomen 0JH8
Chest 0JH6
Control bleeding in
Abdominal Wall 0W3F
Ankle Region
Left 0Y3L
Right 0Y3K
Arm
Lower
Left 0X3F
Right 0X3D
Upper
Left 0X39
Right 0X38
Axilla
Left 0X35
Right 0X34
Back
Lower 0W3L
Upper 0W3K
Buttock
Left 0Y31
Right 0Y30
Cavity, Cranial 0W31
Chest Wall 0W38
Elbow Region
Left 0X3C
Right 0X3B
Extremity
Lower
Left 0Y3B
Right 0Y39
Upper
Left 0X37
Right 0X36
Face 0W32
Femoral Region
Left 0Y38
Right 0Y37
Foot
Left 0Y3N
Right 0Y3M
Gastrointestinal Tract 0W3P
Genitourinary Tract 0W3R
Hand
Left 0X3K
Right 0X3J
Head 0W30
Inguinal Region
Left 0Y36
Right 0Y35
Jaw
Lower 0W35
Upper 0W34
Knee Region
Left 0Y3G
Right 0Y3F
Leg
Lower
Left 0Y3J
Right 0Y3H
Upper
Left 0Y3D
Right 0Y3C
Mediastinum 0W3C
Nasal Mucosa and Soft Tissue 093K
Neck 0W36
Oral Cavity and Throat 0W33
Pelvic Cavity 0W3J
Pericardial Cavity 0W3D
Perineum
Female 0W3N
Male 0W3M
Peritoneal Cavity 0W3G
Pleural Cavity
Left 0W3B
Right 0W39
Respiratory Tract 0W3Q
Retroperitoneum 0W3H
Shoulder Region
Left 0X33
Right 0X32
Control bleeding in — *continued*
Wrist Region
Left 0X3H
Right 0X3G
Control bleeding using Tourniquet, External *see* Compression, Anatomical Regions 2W1
Control, Epistaxis *see* Control bleeding in, Nasal Mucosa and Soft Tissue 093K
Conus arteriosus *use* Ventricle, Right
Conus medullaris *use* Lumbar Spinal Cord
Convalescent Plasma (Nonautologous) *see* New Technology, Anatomical Regions XW1
Conversion
Cardiac rhythm 5A2204Z
Gastrostomy to jejunostomy feeding device *see* Insertion of device in, Jejunum 0DHA
Cook Biodesign® Fistula Plug(s) *use* Nonautologous Tissue Substitute
Cook Biodesign® Hernia Graft(s) *use* Nonautologous Tissue Substitute
Cook Biodesign® Layered Graft(s) *use* Nonautologous Tissue Substitute
Cook Zenapro™ Layered Graft(s) *use* Nonautologous Tissue Substitute
Cook Zenith AAA Endovascular Graft *use* Intraluminal Device
Cook Zenith® Fenestrated AAA Endovascular Graft
use Intraluminal Device, Branched or Fenestrated, One or Two Arteries in 04V
use Intraluminal Device, Branched or Fenestrated, Three or More Arteries in 04V
Coracoacromial ligament
use Shoulder Bursa and Ligament, Left
use Shoulder Bursa and Ligament, Right
Coracobrachialis muscle
use Upper Arm Muscle, Left
use Upper Arm Muscle, Right
Coracoclavicular ligament
use Shoulder Bursa and Ligament, Left
use Shoulder Bursa and Ligament, Right
Coracohumeral ligament
use Shoulder Bursa and Ligament, Left
use Shoulder Bursa and Ligament, Right
Coracoid process
use Scapula, Left
use Scapula, Right
Cordotomy *see* Division, Central Nervous System and Cranial Nerves 008
Core needle biopsy *see* Excision with qualifier Diagnostic
CoreValve transcatheter aortic valve *use* Zooplastic Tissue in Heart and Great Vessels
Cormet Hip Resurfacing System *use* Resurfacing Device in Lower Joints
Corniculate cartilage *use* Larynx
CoRoent® XL *use* Interbody Fusion Device in Lower Joints
Coronary arteriography
see Fluoroscopy, Heart B21
see Plain Radiography, Heart B20
Corox (OTW) Bipolar Lead
use Cardiac Lead, Defibrillator in 02H
use Cardiac Lead, Pacemaker in 02H
Corpus callosum *use* Brain
Corpus cavernosum *use* Penis
Corpus spongiosum *use* Penis
Corpus striatum *use* Basal Ganglia
Corrugator supercilii muscle *use* Facial Muscle
Cortical strip neurostimulator lead *use* Neurostimulator Lead in Central Nervous System and Cranial Nerves
Corvia IASD® *use* Synthetic Substitute
COSELA™ *use* Trilaciclib
Costatectomy
see Excision, Upper Bones 0PB
see Resection, Upper Bones 0PT
Costectomy
see Excision, Upper Bones 0PB
see Resection, Upper Bones 0PT
Costocervical trunk
use Subclavian Artery, Left
use Subclavian Artery, Right
Costochondrectomy
see Excision, Upper Bones 0PB
see Resection, Upper Bones 0PT
Costoclavicular ligament
use Shoulder Bursa and Ligament, Left
Costoclavicular ligament — *continued*
use Shoulder Bursa and Ligament, Right
Costosternoplasty
see Repair, Upper Bones 0PQ
see Replacement, Upper Bones 0PR
see Supplement, Upper Bones 0PU
Costotomy
see Division, Upper Bones 0P8
see Drainage, Upper Bones 0P9
Costotransverse joint *use* Thoracic Vertebral Joint
Costotransverse ligament *use* Rib(s) Bursa and Ligament
Costovertebral joint *use* Thoracic Vertebral Joint
Costoxiphoid ligament *use* Sternum Bursa and Ligament
Counseling
Family, for substance abuse, Other Family Counseling HZ63ZZZ
Group
12-Step HZ43ZZZ
Behavioral HZ41ZZZ
Cognitive HZ40ZZZ
Cognitive-Behavioral HZ42ZZZ
Confrontational HZ48ZZZ
Continuing Care HZ49ZZZ
Infectious Disease
Post-Test HZ4CZZZ
Pre-Test HZ4CZZZ
Interpersonal HZ44ZZZ
Motivational Enhancement HZ47ZZZ
Psychoeducation HZ46ZZZ
Spiritual HZ4BZZZ
Vocational HZ45ZZZ
Individual
12-Step HZ33ZZZ
Behavioral HZ31ZZZ
Cognitive HZ30ZZZ
Cognitive-Behavioral HZ32ZZZ
Confrontational HZ38ZZZ
Continuing Care HZ39ZZZ
Infectious Disease
Post-Test HZ3CZZZ
Pre-Test HZ3CZZZ
Interpersonal HZ34ZZZ
Motivational Enhancement HZ37ZZZ
Psychoeducation HZ36ZZZ
Spiritual HZ3BZZZ
Vocational HZ35ZZZ
Mental Health Services
Educational GZ60ZZZ
Other Counseling GZ63ZZZ
Vocational GZ61ZZZ
Countershock, cardiac 5A2204Z
COVID-19 Vaccine XW0
COVID-19 Vaccine Dose 1 XW0
COVID-19 Vaccine Dose 2 XW0
Cowper's (bulbourethral) gland *use* Urethra
CPAP (continuous positive airway pressure) *see* Assistance, Respiratory 5A09
Craniectomy
see Excision, Head and Facial Bones 0NB
see Resection, Head and Facial Bones 0NT
Cranioplasty
see Repair, Head and Facial Bones 0NQ
see Replacement, Head and Facial Bones 0NR
see Supplement, Head and Facial Bones 0NU
Craniotomy
see Division, Head and Facial Bones 0N8
see Drainage, Central Nervous System and Cranial Nerves 009
see Drainage, Head and Facial Bones 0N9
Creation
Perineum
Female 0W4N0
Male 0W4M0
Valve
Aortic 024F0
Mitral 024G0
Tricuspid 024J0
Cremaster muscle *use* Perineum Muscle
CRESEMBA® (isavuconazonium sulfate) *use* Other Anti-infective
Cribriform plate
use Ethmoid Bone, Left
use Ethmoid Bone, Right
Cricoid cartilage *use* Trachea
Cricoidectomy *see* Excision, Larynx 0CBS

Cricothyroid artery
use Thyroid Artery, Left
use Thyroid Artery, Right
Cricothyroid muscle
use Neck Muscle, Left
use Neck Muscle, Right
Crisis Intervention GZ2ZZZZ
CRRT (Continuous renal replacement therapy) 5A1D90Z
Crural fascia
use Subcutaneous Tissue and Fascia, Left Upper Leg
use Subcutaneous Tissue and Fascia, Right Upper Leg
Crushing, nerve
Cranial *see* Destruction, Central Nervous System and Cranial Nerves 005
Peripheral *see* Destruction, Peripheral Nervous System 015
Cryoablation *see* Destruction
Cryotherapy *see* Destruction
Cryptorchidectomy
see Excision, Male Reproductive System 0VB
see Resection, Male Reproductive System 0VT
Cryptorchiectomy
see Excision, Male Reproductive System 0VB
see Resection, Male Reproductive System 0VT
Cryptotomy
see Division, Gastrointestinal System 0D8
see Drainage, Gastrointestinal System 0D9
CT scan *see* Computerized Tomography (CT Scan)
CT sialogram *see* Computerized Tomography (CT Scan), Ear, Nose, Mouth and Throat B92
Cubital lymph node
use Lymphatic, Left Upper Extremity
use Lymphatic, Right Upper Extremity
Cubital nerve *use* Ulnar Nerve
Cuboid bone
use Tarsal, Left
use Tarsal, Right
Cuboideonavicular joint
use Tarsal Joint, Left
use Tarsal Joint, Right
Culdocentesis *see* Drainage, Cul-de-sac 0U9F
Culdoplasty
see Repair, Cul-de-sac 0UQF
see Supplement, Cul-de-sac 0UUF
Culdoscopy 0UJH8ZZ
Culdotomy *see* Drainage, Cul-de-sac 0U9F
Culmen *use* Cerebellum
Cultured epidermal cell autograft *use* Autologous Tissue Substitute
Cuneiform cartilage *use* Larynx
Cuneonavicular joint
use Joint, Tarsal, Left
use Joint, Tarsal, Right
Cuneonavicular ligament
use Foot Bursa and Ligament, Left
use Foot Bursa and Ligament, Right
Curettage
see Excision
see Extraction
Cutaneous (transverse) cervical nerve *use* Cervical Plexus
CVP (central venous pressure) *see* Measurement, Venous 4A04
Cyclodiathermy *see* Destruction, Eye 085
Cyclophotocoagulation *see* Destruction, Eye 085
CYPHER® Stent *use* Intraluminal Device, Drug-eluting in Heart and Great Vessels
Cystectomy
see Excision, Bladder 0TBB
see Resection, Bladder 0TTB
Cystocele repair *see* Repair, Subcutaneous Tissue and Fascia, Pelvic Region 0JQC
Cystography
see Fluoroscopy, Urinary System BT1
see Plain Radiography, Urinary System BT0
Cystolithotomy *see* Extirpation, Bladder 0TCB
Cystopexy
see Repair, Bladder 0TQB
see Reposition, Bladder 0TSB
Cystoplasty
see Repair, Bladder 0TQB
see Replacement, Bladder 0TRB
see Supplement, Bladder 0TUB
Cystorrhaphy *see* Repair, Bladder 0TQB
Cystoscopy 0TJB8ZZ
Cystostomy *see* Bypass, Bladder 0T1B
Cystostomy Tube *use* Drainage Device
Cystotomy *see* Drainage, Bladder 0T9B
Cystourethrography
see Fluoroscopy, Urinary System BT1
see Plain Radiography, Urinary System BT0
Cystourethroplasty
see Repair, Urinary System 0TQ
see Replacement, Urinary System 0TR
see Supplement, Urinary System 0TU
Cytarabine and Daunorubicin Liposome Antineoplastic XW0

D

DBS lead *use* Neurostimulator Lead in Central Nervous System and Cranial Nerves
DeBakey Left Ventricular Assist Device *use* Implantable Heart Assist System in Heart and Great Vessels
Debridement
Excisional *see* Excision
Non-excisional *see* Extraction
Decompression, Circulatory 6A15
Decortication, lung
see Extirpation, Respiratory System 0BC
see Release, Respiratory System 0BN
Deep brain neurostimulator lead *use* Neurostimulator Lead in Central Nervous System and Cranial Nerves
Deep cervical fascia
use Subcutaneous Tissue and Fascia, Left Neck
use Subcutaneous Tissue and Fascia, Right Neck
Deep cervical vein
use Vertebral Vein, Left
use Vertebral Vein, Right
Deep circumflex iliac artery
use External Iliac Artery, Left
use External Iliac Artery, Right
Deep facial vein
use Face Vein, Left
use Face Vein, Right
Deep femoral artery
use Femoral Artery, Left
use Femoral Artery, Right
Deep femoral (profunda femoris) vein
use Femoral Vein, Left
use Femoral Vein, Right
Deep Inferior Epigastric Artery Perforator Flap
Replacement
Bilateral 0HRV077
Left 0HRU077
Right 0HRT077
Transfer
Left 0KXG
Right 0KXF
Deep palmar arch
use Hand Artery, Left
use Hand Artery, Right
Deep transverse perineal muscle *use* Perineum Muscle
Deferential artery
use Internal Iliac Artery, Left
use Internal Iliac Artery, Right
Defibrillator Generator
Abdomen 0JH8
Chest 0JH6
Defibrotide Sodium Anticoagulant XW0
Defibtech Automated Chest Compression (ACC) device 5A1221J
Defitelio *use* Defibrotide Sodium Anticoagulant
Delivery
Cesarean *see* Extraction, Products of Conception 10D0
Forceps *see* Extraction, Products of Conception 10D0
Manually assisted 10E0XZZ
Products of Conception 10E0XZZ
Vacuum assisted *see* Extraction, Products of Conception 10D0
Delta frame external fixator
use External Fixation Device, Hybrid in 0PH
use External Fixation Device, Hybrid in 0PS
use External Fixation Device, Hybrid in 0QH
Delta frame external fixator — *continued*
use External Fixation Device, Hybrid in 0QS
Delta III Reverse shoulder prosthesis *use* Synthetic Substitute, Reverse Ball and Socket in 0RR
Deltoid fascia
use Subcutaneous Tissue and Fascia, Left Upper Arm
use Subcutaneous Tissue and Fascia, Right Upper Arm
Deltoid ligament
use Ankle Bursa and Ligament, Left
use Ankle Bursa and Ligament, Right
Deltoid muscle
use Shoulder Muscle, Left
use Shoulder Muscle, Right
Deltopectoral (infraclavicular) lymph node
use Lymphatic, Left Upper Extremity
use Lymphatic, Right Upper Extremity
Denervation
Cranial nerve *see* Destruction, Central Nervous System and Cranial Nerves 005
Peripheral nerve *see* Destruction, Peripheral Nervous System 015
Dens *use* Cervical Vertebra
Densitometry
Plain Radiography
Femur
Left BQ04ZZ1
Right BQ03ZZ1
Hip
Left BQ01ZZ1
Right BQ00ZZ1
Spine
Cervical BR00ZZ1
Lumbar BR09ZZ1
Thoracic BR07ZZ1
Whole BR0GZZ1
Ultrasonography
Elbow
Left BP4HZZ1
Right BP4GZZ1
Hand
Left BP4PZZ1
Right BP4NZZ1
Shoulder
Left BP49ZZ1
Right BP48ZZ1
Wrist
Left BP4MZZ1
Right BP4LZZ1
Denticulate (dentate) ligament *use* Spinal Meninges
Depressor anguli oris muscle *use* Facial Muscle
Depressor labii inferioris muscle *use* Facial Muscle
Depressor septi nasi muscle *use* Facial Muscle
Depressor supercilii muscle *use* Facial Muscle
Dermabrasion *see* Extraction, Skin and Breast 0HD
Dermis *use* Skin
Descending genicular artery
use Femoral Artery, Left
use Femoral Artery, Right
Destruction
Acetabulum
Left 0Q55
Right 0Q54
Adenoids 0C5Q
Ampulla of Vater 0F5C
Anal Sphincter 0D5R
Anterior Chamber
Left 08533ZZ
Right 08523ZZ
Anus 0D5Q
Aorta
Abdominal
Thoracic
Ascending/Arch 025X
Descending 025W
Aortic Body 0G5D
Appendix 0D5J
Artery
Anterior Tibial
Left 045Q
Right 045P
Axillary
Left 0356
Right 0355
Brachial
Left 0358
Right 0357

Destruction — *continued*
- Artery — *continued*
  - Celiac Ø451
  - Colic
    - Left Ø457
    - Middle Ø458
    - Right Ø456
  - Common Carotid
    - Left Ø35J
    - Right Ø35H
  - Common Iliac
    - Left Ø45D
    - Right Ø45C
  - External Carotid
    - Left Ø35N
    - Right Ø35M
  - External Iliac
    - Left Ø45J
    - Right Ø45H
  - Face Ø35R
  - Femoral
    - Left Ø45L
    - Right Ø45K
  - Foot
    - Left Ø45W
    - Right Ø45V
  - Gastric Ø452
  - Hand
    - Left Ø35F
    - Right Ø35D
  - Hepatic Ø453
  - Inferior Mesenteric Ø45B
  - Innominate Ø352
  - Internal Carotid
    - Left Ø35L
    - Right Ø35K
  - Internal Iliac
    - Left Ø45F
    - Right Ø45E
  - Internal Mammary
    - Left Ø351
    - Right Ø35Ø
  - Intracranial Ø35G
  - Lower Ø45Y
  - Peroneal
    - Left Ø45U
    - Right Ø45T
  - Popliteal
    - Left Ø45N
    - Right Ø45M
  - Posterior Tibial
    - Left Ø45S
    - Right Ø45R
  - Pulmonary
    - Left Ø25R
    - Right Ø25Q
  - Pulmonary Trunk Ø25P
  - Radial
    - Left Ø35C
    - Right Ø35B
  - Renal
    - Left Ø45A
    - Right Ø459
  - Splenic Ø454
  - Subclavian
    - Left Ø354
    - Right Ø353
  - Superior Mesenteric Ø455
  - Temporal
    - Left Ø35T
    - Right Ø35S
  - Thyroid
    - Left Ø35V
    - Right Ø35U
  - Ulnar
    - Left Ø35A
    - Right Ø359
  - Upper Ø35Y
  - Vertebral
    - Left Ø35Q
    - Right Ø35P
- Atrium
  - Left Ø257
  - Right Ø256
- Auditory Ossicle
  - Left Ø95A
  - Right Ø959
- Basal Ganglia ØØ58
- Bladder ØT5B

Destruction — *continued*
- Bladder Neck ØT5C
- Bone
  - Ethmoid
    - Left ØN5G
    - Right ØN5F
  - Frontal ØN51
  - Hyoid ØN5X
  - Lacrimal
    - Left ØN5J
    - Right ØN5H
  - Nasal ØN5B
  - Occipital ØN57
  - Palatine
    - Left ØN5L
    - Right ØN5K
  - Parietal
    - Left ØN54
    - Right ØN53
  - Pelvic
    - Left ØQ53
    - Right ØQ52
  - Sphenoid ØN5C
  - Temporal
    - Left ØN56
    - Right ØN55
  - Zygomatic
    - Left ØN5N
    - Right ØN5M
- Brain ØØ5Ø
- Breast
  - Bilateral ØH5V
  - Left ØH5U
  - Right ØH5T
- Bronchus
  - Lingula ØB59
  - Lower Lobe
    - Left ØB5B
    - Right ØB56
  - Main
    - Left ØB57
    - Right ØB53
  - Middle Lobe, Right ØB55
  - Upper Lobe
    - Left ØB58
    - Right ØB54
- Buccal Mucosa ØC54
- Bursa and Ligament
  - Abdomen
    - Left ØM5J
    - Right ØM5H
  - Ankle
    - Left ØM5R
    - Right ØM5Q
  - Elbow
    - Left ØM54
    - Right ØM53
  - Foot
    - Left ØM5T
    - Right ØM5S
  - Hand
    - Left ØM58
    - Right ØM57
  - Head and Neck ØM5Ø
  - Hip
    - Left ØM5M
    - Right ØM5L
  - Knee
    - Left ØM5P
    - Right ØM5N
  - Lower Extremity
    - Left ØM5W
    - Right ØM5V
  - Perineum ØM5K
  - Rib(s) ØM5G
  - Shoulder
    - Left ØM52
    - Right ØM51
  - Spine
    - Lower ØM5D
    - Upper ØM5C
  - Sternum ØM5F
  - Upper Extremity
    - Left ØM5B
    - Right ØM59
  - Wrist
    - Left ØM56
    - Right ØM55
- Carina ØB52

Destruction — *continued*
- Carotid Bodies, Bilateral ØG58
- Carotid Body
  - Left ØG56
  - Right ØG57
- Carpal
  - Left ØP5N
  - Right ØP5M
- Cecum ØD5H
- Cerebellum ØØ5C
- Cerebral Hemisphere ØØ57
- Cerebral Meninges ØØ51
- Cerebral Ventricle ØØ56
- Cervix ØU5C
- Chordae Tendineae Ø259
- Choroid
  - Left Ø85B
  - Right Ø85A
- Cisterna Chyli Ø75L
- Clavicle
  - Left ØP5B
  - Right ØP59
- Clitoris ØU5J
- Coccygeal Glomus ØG5B
- Coccyx ØQ5S
- Colon
  - Ascending ØD5K
  - Descending ØD5M
  - Sigmoid ØD5N
  - Transverse ØD5L
- Conduction Mechanism Ø258
- Conjunctiva
  - Left Ø85TXZZ
  - Right Ø85SXZZ
- Cord
  - Bilateral ØV5H
  - Left ØV5G
  - Right ØV5F
- Cornea
  - Left Ø859XZZ
  - Right Ø858XZZ
- Cul-de-sac ØU5F
- Diaphragm ØB5T
- Disc
  - Cervical Vertebral ØR53
  - Cervicothoracic Vertebral ØR55
  - Lumbar Vertebral ØS52
  - Lumbosacral ØS54
  - Thoracic Vertebral ØR59
  - Thoracolumbar Vertebral ØR5B
- Duct
  - Common Bile ØF59
  - Cystic ØF58
  - Hepatic
    - Common ØF57
    - Left ØF56
    - Right ØF55
  - Lacrimal
    - Left Ø85Y
    - Right Ø85X
  - Pancreatic ØF5D
    - Accessory ØF5F
  - Parotid
    - Left ØC5C
    - Right ØC5B
- Duodenum ØD59
- Dura Mater ØØ52
- Ear
  - External
    - Left Ø951
    - Right Ø95Ø
  - External Auditory Canal
    - Left Ø954
    - Right Ø953
  - Inner
    - Left Ø95E
    - Right Ø95D
  - Middle
    - Left Ø956
    - Right Ø955
- Endometrium ØU5B
- Epididymis
  - Bilateral ØV5L
  - Left ØV5K
  - Right ØV5J
- Epiglottis ØC5R
- Esophagogastric Junction ØD54
- Esophagus ØD55
  - Lower ØD53

- **Destruction** — *continued*
  - Esophagus — *continued*
    - Middle ØD52
    - Upper ØD51
  - Eustachian Tube
    - Left Ø95G
    - Right Ø95F
  - Eye
    - Left Ø851XZZ
    - Right Ø85ØXZZ
  - Eyelid
    - Lower
      - Left Ø85R
      - Right Ø85Q
    - Upper
      - Left Ø85P
      - Right Ø85N
  - Fallopian Tube
    - Left ØU56
    - Right ØU55
  - Fallopian Tubes, Bilateral ØU57
  - Femoral Shaft
    - Left ØQ59
    - Right ØQ58
  - Femur
    - Lower
      - Left ØQ5C
      - Right ØQ5B
    - Upper
      - Left ØQ57
      - Right ØQ56
  - Fibula
    - Left ØQ5K
    - Right ØQ5J
  - Finger Nail ØH5QXZZ
  - Gallbladder ØF54
  - Gingiva
    - Lower ØC56
    - Upper ØC55
  - Gland
    - Adrenal
      - Bilateral ØG54
      - Left ØG52
      - Right ØG53
    - Lacrimal
      - Left Ø85W
      - Right Ø85V
    - Minor Salivary ØC5J
    - Parotid
      - Left ØC59
      - Right ØC58
    - Pituitary ØG5Ø
    - Sublingual
      - Left ØC5F
      - Right ØC5D
    - Submaxillary
      - Left ØC5H
      - Right ØC5G
    - Vestibular ØU5L
  - Glenoid Cavity
    - Left ØP58
    - Right ØP57
  - Glomus Jugulare ØG5C
  - Humeral Head
    - Left ØP5D
    - Right ØP5C
  - Humeral Shaft
    - Left ØP5G
    - Right ØP5F
  - Hymen ØU5K
  - Hypothalamus ØØ5A
  - Ileocecal Valve ØD5C
  - Ileum ØD5B
  - Intestine
    - Large ØD5E
      - Left ØD5G
      - Right ØD5F
    - Small ØD58
  - Iris
    - Left Ø85D3ZZ
    - Right Ø85C3ZZ
  - Jejunum ØD5A
  - Joint
    - Acromioclavicular
      - Left ØR5H
      - Right ØR5G
    - Ankle
      - Left ØS5G
      - Right ØS5F
- **Destruction** — *continued*
  - Joint — *continued*
    - Carpal
      - Left ØR5R
      - Right ØR5Q
    - Carpometacarpal
      - Left ØR5T
      - Right ØR5S
    - Cervical Vertebral ØR51
    - Cervicothoracic Vertebral ØR54
    - Coccygeal ØS56
    - Elbow
      - Left ØR5M
      - Right ØR5L
    - Finger Phalangeal
      - Left ØR5X
      - Right ØR5W
    - Hip
      - Left ØS5B
      - Right ØS59
    - Knee
      - Left ØS5D
      - Right ØS5C
    - Lumbar Vertebral ØS5Ø
    - Lumbosacral ØS53
    - Metacarpophalangeal
      - Left ØR5V
      - Right ØR5U
    - Metatarsal-Phalangeal
      - Left ØS5N
      - Right ØS5M
    - Occipital-cervical ØR5Ø
    - Sacrococcygeal ØS55
    - Sacroiliac
      - Left ØS58
      - Right ØS57
    - Shoulder
      - Left ØR5K
      - Right ØR5J
    - Sternoclavicular
      - Left ØR5F
      - Right ØR5E
    - Tarsal
      - Left ØS5J
      - Right ØS5H
    - Tarsometatarsal
      - Left ØS5L
      - Right ØS5K
    - Temporomandibular
      - Left ØR5D
      - Right ØR5C
    - Thoracic Vertebral ØR56
    - Thoracolumbar Vertebral ØR5A
    - Toe Phalangeal
      - Left ØS5Q
      - Right ØS5P
    - Wrist
      - Left ØR5P
      - Right ØR5N
  - Kidney
    - Left ØT51
    - Right ØT5Ø
  - Kidney Pelvis
    - Left ØT54
    - Right ØT53
  - Larynx ØC5S
  - Lens
    - Left Ø85K3ZZ
    - Right Ø85J3ZZ
  - Lip
    - Lower ØC51
    - Upper ØC5Ø
  - Liver ØF5Ø
    - Left Lobe ØF52
    - Right Lobe ØF51
  - Lung
    - Bilateral ØB5M
    - Left ØB5L
    - Lower Lobe
      - Left ØB5J
      - Right ØB5F
    - Middle Lobe, Right ØB5D
    - Right ØB5K
    - Upper Lobe
      - Left ØB5G
      - Right ØB5C
  - Lung Lingula ØB5H
  - Lymphatic
    - Aortic Ø75D
- **Destruction** — *continued*
  - Lymphatic — *continued*
    - Axillary
      - Left Ø756
      - Right Ø755
    - Head Ø75Ø
    - Inguinal
      - Left Ø75J
      - Right Ø75H
    - Internal Mammary
      - Left Ø759
      - Right Ø758
    - Lower Extremity
      - Left Ø75G
      - Right Ø75F
    - Mesenteric Ø75B
    - Neck
      - Left Ø752
      - Right Ø751
    - Pelvis Ø75C
    - Thoracic Duct Ø75K
    - Thorax Ø757
    - Upper Extremity
      - Left Ø754
      - Right Ø753
  - Mandible
    - Left ØN5V
    - Right ØN5T
  - Maxilla ØN5R
  - Medulla Oblongata ØØ5D
  - Mesentery ØD5V
  - Metacarpal
    - Left ØP5Q
    - Right ØP5P
  - Metatarsal
    - Left ØQ5P
    - Right ØQ5N
  - Muscle
    - Abdomen
      - Left ØK5L
      - Right ØK5K
    - Extraocular
      - Left Ø85M
      - Right Ø85L
    - Facial ØK51
    - Foot
      - Left ØK5W
      - Right ØK5V
    - Hand
      - Left ØK5D
      - Right ØK5C
    - Head ØK5Ø
    - Hip
      - Left ØK5P
      - Right ØK5N
    - Lower Arm and Wrist
      - Left ØK5B
      - Right ØK59
    - Lower Leg
      - Left ØK5T
      - Right ØK5S
    - Neck
      - Left ØK53
      - Right ØK52
    - Papillary Ø25D
    - Perineum ØK5M
    - Shoulder
      - Left ØK56
      - Right ØK55
    - Thorax
      - Left ØK5J
      - Right ØK5H
    - Tongue, Palate, Pharynx ØK54
    - Trunk
      - Left ØK5G
      - Right ØK5F
    - Upper Arm
      - Left ØK58
      - Right ØK57
    - Upper Leg
      - Left ØK5R
      - Right ØK5Q
  - Nasal Mucosa and Soft Tissue Ø95K
  - Nasopharynx Ø95N
  - Nerve
    - Abdominal Sympathetic Ø15M
    - Abducens ØØ5L
    - Accessory ØØ5R
    - Acoustic ØØ5N

Destruction — *continued*
- Nerve — *continued*
  - Brachial Plexus Ø153
  - Cervical Ø151
  - Cervical Plexus Ø15Ø
  - Facial ØØ5M
  - Femoral Ø15D
  - Glossopharyngeal ØØ5P
  - Head and Neck Sympathetic Ø15K
  - Hypoglossal ØØ5S
  - Lumbar Ø15B
  - Lumbar Plexus Ø159
  - Lumbar Sympathetic Ø15N
  - Lumbosacral Plexus Ø15A
  - Median Ø155
  - Oculomotor ØØ5H
  - Olfactory ØØ5F
  - Optic ØØ5G
  - Peroneal Ø15H
  - Phrenic Ø152
  - Pudendal Ø15C
  - Radial Ø156
  - Sacral Ø15R
  - Sacral Plexus Ø15Q
  - Sacral Sympathetic Ø15P
  - Sciatic Ø15F
  - Thoracic Ø158
  - Thoracic Sympathetic Ø15L
  - Tibial Ø15G
  - Trigeminal ØØ5K
  - Trochlear ØØ5J
  - Ulnar Ø154
  - Vagus ØØ5Q
- Nipple
  - Left ØH5X
  - Right ØH5W
- Omentum ØD5U
- Orbit
  - Left ØN5Q
  - Right ØN5P
- Ovary
  - Bilateral ØU52
  - Left ØU51
  - Right ØU5Ø
- Palate
  - Hard ØC52
  - Soft ØC53
- Pancreas ØF5G
- Para-aortic Body ØG59
- Paraganglion Extremity ØG5F
- Parathyroid Gland ØG5R
  - Inferior
    - Left ØG5P
    - Right ØG5N
  - Multiple ØG5Q
  - Superior
    - Left ØG5M
    - Right ØG5L
- Patella
  - Left ØQ5F
  - Right ØQ5D
- Penis ØV5S
- Pericardium Ø25N
- Peritoneum ØD5W
- Phalanx
  - Finger
    - Left ØP5V
    - Right ØP5T
  - Thumb
    - Left ØP5S
    - Right ØP5R
  - Toe
    - Left ØQ5R
    - Right ØQ5Q
- Pharynx ØC5M
- Pineal Body ØG51
- Pleura
  - Left ØB5P
  - Right ØB5N
- Pons ØØ5B
- Prepuce ØV5T
- Prostate ØV5Ø
  - Robotic Waterjet Ablation XV5Ø8A4
- Radius
  - Left ØP5J
  - Right ØP5H
- Rectum ØD5P
- Retina
  - Left Ø85F3ZZ
  - Right Ø85E3ZZ
- Retinal Vessel
  - Left Ø85H3ZZ
  - Right Ø85G3ZZ
- Ribs
  - 1 to 2 ØP51
  - 3 or More ØP52
- Sacrum ØQ51
- Scapula
  - Left ØP56
  - Right ØP55
- Sclera
  - Left Ø857XZZ
  - Right Ø856XZZ
- Scrotum ØV55
- Septum
  - Atrial Ø255
  - Nasal Ø95M
  - Ventricular Ø25M
- Sinus
  - Accessory Ø95P
  - Ethmoid
    - Left Ø95V
    - Right Ø95U
  - Frontal
    - Left Ø95T
    - Right Ø95S
  - Mastoid
    - Left Ø95C
    - Right Ø95B
  - Maxillary
    - Left Ø95R
    - Right Ø95Q
  - Sphenoid
    - Left Ø95X
    - Right Ø95W
- Skin
  - Abdomen ØH57XZ
  - Back ØH56XZ
  - Buttock ØH58XZ
  - Chest ØH55XZ
  - Ear
    - Left ØH53XZ
    - Right ØH52XZ
  - Face ØH51XZ
  - Foot
    - Left ØH5NXZ
    - Right ØH5MXZ
  - Hand
    - Left ØH5GXZ
    - Right ØH5FXZ
  - Inguinal ØH5AXZ
  - Lower Arm
    - Left ØH5EXZ
    - Right ØH5DXZ
  - Lower Leg
    - Left ØH5LXZ
    - Right ØH5KXZ
  - Neck ØH54XZ
  - Perineum ØH59XZ
  - Scalp ØH5ØXZ
  - Upper Arm
    - Left ØH5CXZ
    - Right ØH5BXZ
  - Upper Leg
    - Left ØH5JXZ
    - Right ØH5HXZ
- Skull ØN5Ø
- Spinal Cord
  - Cervical ØØ5W
  - Lumbar ØØ5Y
  - Thoracic ØØ5X
- Spinal Meninges ØØ5T
- Spleen Ø75P
- Sternum ØP5Ø
- Stomach ØD56
  - Pylorus ØD57
- Subcutaneous Tissue and Fascia
  - Abdomen ØJ58
  - Back ØJ57
  - Buttock ØJ59
  - Chest ØJ56
  - Face ØJ51
  - Foot
    - Left ØJ5R
    - Right ØJ5Q
  - Hand
    - Left ØJ5K
    - Right ØJ5J
  - Lower Arm
    - Left ØJ5H
    - Right ØJ5G
  - Lower Leg
    - Left ØJ5P
    - Right ØJ5N
  - Neck
    - Left ØJ55
    - Right ØJ54
  - Pelvic Region ØJ5C
  - Perineum ØJ5B
  - Scalp ØJ5Ø
  - Upper Arm
    - Left ØJ5F
    - Right ØJ5D
  - Upper Leg
    - Left ØJ5M
    - Right ØJ5L
- Tarsal
  - Left ØQ5M
  - Right ØQ5L
- Tendon
  - Abdomen
    - Left ØL5G
    - Right ØL5F
  - Ankle
    - Left ØL5T
    - Right ØL5S
  - Foot
    - Left ØL5W
    - Right ØL5V
  - Hand
    - Left ØL58
    - Right ØL57
  - Head and Neck ØL5Ø
  - Hip
    - Left ØL5K
    - Right ØL5J
  - Knee
    - Left ØL5R
    - Right ØL5Q
  - Lower Arm and Wrist
    - Left ØL56
    - Right ØL55
  - Lower Leg
    - Left ØL5P
    - Right ØL5N
  - Perineum ØL5H
  - Shoulder
    - Left ØL52
    - Right ØL51
  - Thorax
    - Left ØL5D
    - Right ØL5C
  - Trunk
    - Left ØL5B
    - Right ØL59
  - Upper Arm
    - Left ØL54
    - Right ØL53
  - Upper Leg
    - Left ØL5M
    - Right ØL5L
- Testis
  - Bilateral ØV5C
  - Left ØV5B
  - Right ØV59
- Thalamus ØØ59
- Thymus Ø75M
- Thyroid Gland ØG5K
  - Left Lobe ØG5G
  - Right Lobe ØG5H
- Tibia
  - Left ØQ5H
  - Right ØQ5G
- Toe Nail ØH5RXZZ
- Tongue ØC57
- Tonsils ØC5P
- Tooth
  - Lower ØC5X
  - Upper ØC5W
- Trachea ØB51
- Tunica Vaginalis
  - Left ØV57

- **Destruction** — *continued*
  - Tunica Vaginalis — *continued*
    - Right ØV56
  - Turbinate, Nasal Ø95L
  - Tympanic Membrane
    - Left Ø958
    - Right Ø957
  - Ulna
    - Left ØP5L
    - Right ØP5K
  - Ureter
    - Left ØT57
    - Right ØT56
  - Urethra ØT5D
  - Uterine Supporting Structure ØU54
  - Uterus ØU59
  - Uvula ØC5N
  - Vagina ØU5G
  - Valve
    - Aortic Ø25F
    - Mitral Ø25G
    - Pulmonary Ø25H
    - Tricuspid Ø25J
  - Vas Deferens
    - Bilateral ØV5Q
    - Left ØV5P
    - Right ØV5N
  - Vein
    - Axillary
      - Left Ø558
      - Right Ø557
    - Azygos Ø55Ø
    - Basilic
      - Left Ø55C
      - Right Ø55B
    - Brachial
      - Left Ø55A
      - Right Ø559
    - Cephalic
      - Left Ø55F
      - Right Ø55D
    - Colic Ø657
    - Common Iliac
      - Left Ø65D
      - Right Ø65C
    - Coronary Ø254
    - Esophageal Ø653
    - External Iliac
      - Left Ø65G
      - Right Ø65F
    - External Jugular
      - Left Ø55Q
      - Right Ø55P
    - Face
      - Left Ø55V
      - Right Ø55T
    - Femoral
      - Left Ø65N
      - Right Ø65M
    - Foot
      - Left Ø65V
      - Right Ø65T
    - Gastric Ø652
    - Hand
      - Left Ø55H
      - Right Ø55G
    - Hemiazygos Ø551
    - Hepatic Ø654
    - Hypogastric
      - Left Ø65J
      - Right Ø65H
    - Inferior Mesenteric Ø656
    - Innominate
      - Left Ø554
      - Right Ø553
    - Internal Jugular
      - Left Ø55N
      - Right Ø55M
    - Intracranial Ø55L
    - Lower Ø65Y
    - Portal Ø658
    - Pulmonary
      - Left Ø25T
      - Right Ø25S
    - Renal
      - Left Ø65B
      - Right Ø659
    - Saphenous
      - Left Ø65Q

- **Destruction** — *continued*
  - Vein — *continued*
    - Saphenous — *continued*
      - Right Ø65P
    - Splenic Ø651
    - Subclavian
      - Left Ø556
      - Right Ø555
    - Superior Mesenteric Ø655
    - Upper Ø55Y
    - Vertebral
      - Left Ø55S
      - Right Ø55R
  - Vena Cava
    - Inferior Ø65Ø
    - Superior Ø25V
  - Ventricle
    - Left Ø25L
    - Right Ø25K
  - Vertebra
    - Cervical ØP53
    - Lumbar ØQ5Ø
    - Thoracic ØP54
  - Vesicle
    - Bilateral ØV53
    - Left ØV52
    - Right ØV51
  - Vitreous
    - Left Ø8553ZZ
    - Right Ø8543ZZ
  - Vocal Cord
    - Left ØC5V
    - Right ØC5T
  - Vulva ØU5M
- **Detachment**
  - Arm
    - Lower
      - Left ØX6FØZ
      - Right ØX6DØZ
    - Upper
      - Left ØX69ØZ
      - Right ØX68ØZ
  - Elbow Region
    - Left ØX6CØZZ
    - Right ØX6BØZZ
  - Femoral Region
    - Left ØY68ØZZ
    - Right ØY67ØZZ
  - Finger
    - Index
      - Left ØX6PØZ
      - Right ØX6NØZ
    - Little
      - Left ØX6WØZ
      - Right ØX6VØZ
    - Middle
      - Left ØX6RØZ
      - Right ØX6QØZ
    - Ring
      - Left ØX6TØZ
      - Right ØX6SØZ
  - Foot
    - Left ØY6NØZ
    - Right ØY6MØZ
  - Forequarter
    - Left ØX61ØZZ
    - Right ØX6ØØZZ
  - Hand
    - Left ØX6KØZ
    - Right ØX6JØZ
  - Hindquarter
    - Bilateral ØY64ØZZ
    - Left ØY63ØZZ
    - Right ØY62ØZZ
  - Knee Region
    - Left ØY6GØZZ
    - Right ØY6FØZZ
  - Leg
    - Lower
      - Left ØY6JØZ
      - Right ØY6HØZ
    - Upper
      - Left ØY6DØZ
      - Right ØY6CØZ
  - Shoulder Region
    - Left ØX63ØZZ
    - Right ØX62ØZZ
  - Thumb
    - Left ØX6MØZ

- **Detachment** — *continued*
  - Thumb — *continued*
    - Right ØX6LØZ
  - Toe
    - 1st
      - Left ØY6QØZ
      - Right ØY6PØZ
    - 2nd
      - Left ØY6SØZ
      - Right ØY6RØZ
    - 3rd
      - Left ØY6UØZ
      - Right ØY6TØZ
    - 4th
      - Left ØY6WØZ
      - Right ØY6VØZ
    - 5th
      - Left ØY6YØZ
      - Right ØY6XØZ
- **Determination, Mental status** GZ14ZZZ
- **Detorsion**
  - *see* Release
  - *see* Reposition
- **Detoxification Services, for substance abuse** HZ2ZZZZ
- **Device Fitting** FØDZ
- **Diagnostic Audiology** *see* Audiology, Diagnostic
- **Diagnostic imaging** *see* Imaging, Diagnostic
- **Diagnostic radiology** *see* Imaging, Diagnostic
- **Dialysis**
  - Hemodialysis *see* Performance, Urinary 5A1D
  - Peritoneal 3E1M39Z
- **Diaphragma sellae** *use* Dura Mater
- **Diaphragmatic pacemaker generator** *use* Stimulator Generator in Subcutaneous Tissue and Fascia
- **Diaphragmatic Pacemaker Lead**
  - Insertion of device in, Diaphragm ØBHT
  - Removal of device from, Diaphragm ØBPT
  - Revision of device in, Diaphragm ØBWT
- **Digital radiography, plain** *see* Plain Radiography
- **Dilation**
  - Ampulla of Vater ØF7C
  - Anus ØD7Q
  - Aorta
    - Abdominal
    - Thoracic
      - Ascending/Arch Ø27X
      - Descending Ø27W
  - Artery
    - Anterior Tibial
      - Left Ø47Q
        - Sustained Release Drug-eluting Intraluminal Device X27Q385
          - Four or More X27Q3C5
          - Three X27Q3B5
          - Two X27Q395
      - Right Ø47P
        - Sustained Release Drug-eluting Intraluminal Device X27P385
          - Four or More X27P3C5
          - Three X27P3B5
          - Two X27P395
    - Axillary
      - Left Ø376
      - Right Ø375
    - Brachial
      - Left Ø378
      - Right Ø377
    - Celiac Ø471
    - Colic
      - Left Ø477
      - Middle Ø478
      - Right Ø476
    - Common Carotid
      - Left Ø37J
      - Right Ø37H
    - Common Iliac
      - Left Ø47D
      - Right Ø47C
    - Coronary
      - Four or More Arteries Ø273
      - One Artery Ø27Ø
      - Three Arteries Ø272
      - Two Arteries Ø271
    - External Carotid
      - Left Ø37N

Dilation — *continued*
Artery — *continued*
External Carotid — *continued*
Right Ø37M
External Iliac
Left Ø47J
Right Ø47H
Face Ø37R
Femoral
Left Ø47L
Sustained Release Drug-eluting Intraluminal Device X27J385
Four or More X27J3C5
Three X27J3B5
Two X27J395
Right Ø47K
Sustained Release Drug-eluting Intraluminal Device X27H385
Four or More X27H3C5
Three X27H3B5
Two X27H395
Foot
Left Ø47W
Right Ø47V
Gastric Ø472
Hand
Left Ø37F
Right Ø37D
Hepatic Ø473
Inferior Mesenteric Ø47B
Innominate Ø372
Internal Carotid
Left Ø37L
Right Ø37K
Internal Iliac
Left Ø47F
Right Ø47E
Internal Mammary
Left Ø371
Right Ø37Ø
Intracranial Ø37G
Lower Ø47Y
Peroneal
Left Ø47U
Sustained Release Drug-eluting Intraluminal Device X27U385
Four or More X27U3C5
Three X27U3B5
Two X27U395
Right Ø47T
Sustained Release Drug-eluting Intraluminal Device X27T385
Four or More X27T3C5
Three X27T3B5
Two X27T395
Popliteal
Left Ø47N
Left Distal
Sustained Release Drug-eluting Intraluminal Device X27N385
Four or More X27N3C5
Three X27N3B5
Two X27N395
Left Proximal
Sustained Release Drug-eluting Intraluminal Device X27L385
Four or More X27L3C5
Three X27L3B5
Two X27L395
Right Ø47M
Right Distal
Sustained Release Drug-eluting Intraluminal Device X27M385
Four or More X27M3C5
Three X27M3B5
Two X27M395
Right Proximal
Sustained Release Drug-eluting Intraluminal Device X27K385
Four or More X27K3C5
Three X27K3B5

Dilation — *continued*
Artery — *continued*
Popliteal — *continued*
Right Proximal — *continued*
Sustained Release Drug-eluting Intraluminal Device — *continued*
Two X27K395
Posterior Tibial
Left Ø47S
Sustained Release Drug-eluting Intraluminal Device X27S385
Four or More X27S3C5
Three X27S3B5
Two X27S395
Right Ø47R
Sustained Release Drug-eluting Intraluminal Device X27R385
Four or More X27R3C5
Three X27R3B5
Two X27R395
Pulmonary
Left Ø27R
Right Ø27Q
Pulmonary Trunk Ø27P
Radial
Left Ø37C
Right Ø37B
Renal
Left Ø47A
Right Ø479
Splenic Ø474
Subclavian
Left Ø374
Right Ø373
Superior Mesenteric Ø475
Temporal
Left Ø37T
Right Ø37S
Thyroid
Left Ø37V
Right Ø37U
Ulnar
Left Ø37A
Right Ø379
Upper Ø37Y
Vertebral
Left Ø37Q
Right Ø37P
Bladder ØT7B
Bladder Neck ØT7C
Bronchus
Lingula ØB79
Lower Lobe
Left ØB7B
Right ØB76
Main
Left ØB77
Right ØB73
Middle Lobe, Right ØB75
Upper Lobe
Left ØB78
Right ØB74
Carina ØB72
Cecum ØD7H
Cerebral Ventricle ØØ76
Cervix ØU7C
Colon
Ascending ØD7K
Descending ØD7M
Sigmoid ØD7N
Transverse ØD7L
Duct
Common Bile ØF79
Cystic ØF78
Hepatic
Common ØF77
Left ØF76
Right ØF75
Lacrimal
Left Ø87Y
Right Ø87X
Pancreatic ØF7D
Accessory ØF7F
Parotid
Left ØC7C
Right ØC7B

Dilation — *continued*
Duodenum ØD79
Esophagogastric Junction ØD74
Esophagus ØD75
Lower ØD73
Middle ØD72
Upper ØD71
Eustachian Tube
Left Ø97G
Right Ø97F
Fallopian Tube
Left ØU76
Right ØU75
Fallopian Tubes, Bilateral ØU77
Hymen ØU7K
Ileocecal Valve ØD7C
Ileum ØD7B
Intestine
Large ØD7E
Left ØD7G
Right ØD7F
Small ØD78
Jejunum ØD7A
Kidney Pelvis
Left ØT74
Right ØT73
Larynx ØC7S
Pharynx ØC7M
Rectum ØD7P
Stomach ØD76
Pylorus ØD77
Trachea ØB71
Ureter
Left ØT77
Right ØT76
Ureters, Bilateral ØT78
Urethra ØT7D
Uterus ØU79
Vagina ØU7G
Valve
Aortic Ø27F
Mitral Ø27G
Pulmonary Ø27H
Tricuspid Ø27J
Vas Deferens
Bilateral ØV7Q
Left ØV7P
Right ØV7N
Vein
Axillary
Left Ø578
Right Ø577
Azygos Ø57Ø
Basilic
Left Ø57C
Right Ø57B
Brachial
Left Ø57A
Right Ø579
Cephalic
Left Ø57F
Right Ø57D
Colic Ø677
Common Iliac
Left Ø67D
Right Ø67C
Esophageal Ø673
External Iliac
Left Ø67G
Right Ø67F
External Jugular
Left Ø57Q
Right Ø57P
Face
Left Ø57V
Right Ø57T
Femoral
Left Ø67N
Right Ø67M
Foot
Left Ø67V
Right Ø67T
Gastric Ø672
Hand
Left Ø57H
Right Ø57G
Hemiazygos Ø571
Hepatic Ø674

Dilation — *continued*
Vein — *continued*
Hypogastric
Left Ø67J
Right Ø67H
Inferior Mesenteric Ø676
Innominate
Left Ø574
Right Ø573
Internal Jugular
Left Ø57N
Right Ø57M
Intracranial Ø57L
Lower Ø67Y
Portal Ø678
Pulmonary
Left Ø27T
Right Ø27S
Renal
Left Ø67B
Right Ø679
Saphenous
Left Ø67Q
Right Ø67P
Splenic Ø671
Subclavian
Left Ø576
Right Ø575
Superior Mesenteric Ø675
Upper Ø57Y
Vertebral
Left Ø57S
Right Ø57R
Vena Cava
Inferior Ø670
Superior Ø27V
Ventricle
Left Ø27L
Right Ø27K
Direct Lateral Interbody Fusion (DLIF) device *use* Interbody Fusion Device in Lower Joints
Disarticulation *see* Detachment
Discectomy, diskectomy
see Excision, Lower Joints ØSB
see Excision, Upper Joints ØRB
see Resection, Lower Joints ØST
see Resection, Upper Joints ØRT
Discography
see Fluoroscopy, Axial Skeleton, Except Skull and Facial Bones BR1
see Plain Radiography, Axial Skeleton, Except Skull and Facial Bones BRØ
Dismembered pyeloplasty *see* Repair, Kidney Pelvis
Distal humerus
use Humeral Shaft, Left
use Humeral Shaft, Right
Distal humerus, involving joint
use Elbow Joint, Left
use Elbow Joint, Right
Distal radioulnar joint
use Wrist Joint, Left
use Wrist Joint, Right
Diversion *see* Bypass
Diverticulectomy *see* Excision, Gastrointestinal System ØDB
Division
Acetabulum
Left ØQ85
Right ØQ84
Anal Sphincter ØD8R
Basal Ganglia ØØ88
Bladder Neck ØT8C
Bone
Ethmoid
Left ØN8G
Right ØN8F
Frontal ØN81
Hyoid ØN8X
Lacrimal
Left ØN8J
Right ØN8H
Nasal ØN8B
Occipital ØN87
Palatine
Left ØN8L
Right ØN8K
Parietal
Left ØN84

Division — *continued*
Bone — *continued*
Parietal — *continued*
Right ØN83
Pelvic
Left ØQ83
Right ØQ82
Sphenoid ØN8C
Temporal
Left ØN86
Right ØN85
Zygomatic
Left ØN8N
Right ØN8M
Brain ØØ8Ø
Bursa and Ligament
Abdomen
Left ØM8J
Right ØM8H
Ankle
Left ØM8R
Right ØM8Q
Elbow
Left ØM84
Right ØM83
Foot
Left ØM8T
Right ØM8S
Hand
Left ØM88
Right ØM87
Head and Neck ØM8Ø
Hip
Left ØM8M
Right ØM8L
Knee
Left ØM8P
Right ØM8N
Lower Extremity
Left ØM8W
Right ØM8V
Perineum ØM8K
Rib(s) ØM8G
Shoulder
Left ØM82
Right ØM81
Spine
Lower ØM8D
Upper ØM8C
Sternum ØM8F
Upper Extremity
Left ØM8B
Right ØM89
Wrist
Left ØM86
Right ØM85
Carpal
Left ØP8N
Right ØP8M
Cerebral Hemisphere ØØ87
Chordae Tendineae Ø289
Clavicle
Left ØP8B
Right ØP89
Coccyx ØQ8S
Conduction Mechanism Ø288
Esophagogastric Junction ØD84
Femoral Shaft
Left ØQ89
Right ØQ88
Femur
Lower
Left ØQ8C
Right ØQ8B
Upper
Left ØQ87
Right ØQ86
Fibula
Left ØQ8K
Right ØQ8J
Gland, Pituitary ØG8Ø
Glenoid Cavity
Left ØP88
Right ØP87
Humeral Head
Left ØP8D
Right ØP8C
Humeral Shaft
Left ØP8G

Division — *continued*
Humeral Shaft — *continued*
Right ØP8F
Hymen ØU8K
Kidneys, Bilateral ØT82
Liver ØF8Ø
Left Lobe ØF82
Right Lobe ØF81
Mandible
Left ØN8V
Right ØN8T
Maxilla ØN8R
Metacarpal
Left ØP8Q
Right ØP8P
Metatarsal
Left ØQ8P
Right ØQ8N
Muscle
Abdomen
Left ØK8L
Right ØK8K
Facial ØK81
Foot
Left ØK8W
Right ØK8V
Hand
Left ØK8D
Right ØK8C
Head ØK8Ø
Hip
Left ØK8P
Right ØK8N
Lower Arm and Wrist
Left ØK8B
Right ØK89
Lower Leg
Left ØK8T
Right ØK8S
Neck
Left ØK83
Right ØK82
Papillary Ø28D
Perineum ØK8M
Shoulder
Left ØK86
Right ØK85
Thorax
Left ØK8J
Right ØK8H
Tongue, Palate, Pharynx ØK84
Trunk
Left ØK8G
Right ØK8F
Upper Arm
Left ØK88
Right ØK87
Upper Leg
Left ØK8R
Right ØK8Q
Nerve
Abdominal Sympathetic Ø18M
Abducens ØØ8L
Accessory ØØ8R
Acoustic ØØ8N
Brachial Plexus Ø183
Cervical Ø181
Cervical Plexus Ø18Ø
Facial ØØ8M
Femoral Ø18D
Glossopharyngeal ØØ8P
Head and Neck Sympathetic Ø18K
Hypoglossal ØØ8S
Lumbar Ø18B
Lumbar Plexus Ø189
Lumbar Sympathetic Ø18N
Lumbosacral Plexus Ø18A
Median Ø185
Oculomotor ØØ8H
Olfactory ØØ8F
Optic ØØ8G
Peroneal Ø18H
Phrenic Ø182
Pudendal Ø18C
Radial Ø186
Sacral Ø18R
Sacral Plexus Ø18Q
Sacral Sympathetic Ø18P
Sciatic Ø18F

Division — *continued*
Nerve — *continued*
Thoracic Ø188
Thoracic Sympathetic Ø18L
Tibial Ø18G
Trigeminal ØØ8K
Trochlear ØØ8J
Ulnar Ø184
Vagus ØØ8Q
Orbit
Left ØN8Q
Right ØN8P
Ovary
Bilateral ØU82
Left ØU81
Right ØU8Ø
Pancreas ØF8G
Patella
Left ØQ8F
Right ØQ8D
Perineum, Female ØW8NXZZ
Phalanx
Finger
Left ØP8V
Right ØP8T
Thumb
Left ØP8S
Right ØP8R
Toe
Left ØQ8R
Right ØQ8Q
Radius
Left ØP8J
Right ØP8H
Ribs
1 to 2 ØP81
3 or More ØP82
Sacrum ØQ81
Scapula
Left ØP86
Right ØP85
Skin
Abdomen ØH87XZZ
Back ØH86XZZ
Buttock ØH88XZZ
Chest ØH85XZZ
Ear
Left ØH83XZZ
Right ØH82XZZ
Face ØH81XZZ
Foot
Left ØH8NXZZ
Right ØH8MXZZ
Hand
Left ØH8GXZZ
Right ØH8FXZZ
Inguinal ØH8AXZZ
Lower Arm
Left ØH8EXZZ
Right ØH8DXZZ
Lower Leg
Left ØH8LXZZ
Right ØH8KXZZ
Neck ØH84XZZ
Perineum ØH89XZZ
Scalp ØH8ØXZZ
Upper Arm
Left ØH8CXZZ
Right ØH8BXZZ
Upper Leg
Left ØH8JXZZ
Right ØH8HXZZ
Skull ØN8Ø
Spinal Cord
Cervical ØØ8W
Lumbar ØØ8Y
Thoracic ØØ8X
Sternum ØP8Ø
Stomach, Pylorus ØD87
Subcutaneous Tissue and Fascia
Abdomen ØJ88
Back ØJ87
Buttock ØJ89
Chest ØJ86
Face ØJ81
Foot
Left ØJ8R
Right ØJ8Q

Division — *continued*
Subcutaneous Tissue and Fascia — *continued*
Hand
Left ØJ8K
Right ØJ8J
Head and Neck ØJ8S
Lower Arm
Left ØJ8H
Right ØJ8G
Lower Extremity ØJ8W
Lower Leg
Left ØJ8P
Right ØJ8N
Neck
Left ØJ85
Right ØJ84
Pelvic Region ØJ8C
Perineum ØJ8B
Scalp ØJ8Ø
Trunk ØJ8T
Upper Arm
Left ØJ8F
Right ØJ8D
Upper Extremity ØJ8V
Upper Leg
Left ØJ8M
Right ØJ8L
Tarsal
Left ØQ8M
Right ØQ8L
Tendon
Abdomen
Left ØL8G
Right ØL8F
Ankle
Left ØL8T
Right ØL8S
Foot
Left ØL8W
Right ØL8V
Hand
Left ØL88
Right ØL87
Head and Neck ØL8Ø
Hip
Left ØL8K
Right ØL8J
Knee
Left ØL8R
Right ØL8Q
Lower Arm and Wrist
Left ØL86
Right ØL85
Lower Leg
Left ØL8P
Right ØL8N
Perineum ØL8H
Shoulder
Left ØL82
Right ØL81
Thorax
Left ØL8D
Right ØL8C
Trunk
Left ØL8B
Right ØL89
Upper Arm
Left ØL84
Right ØL83
Upper Leg
Left ØL8M
Right ØL8L
Thyroid Gland Isthmus ØG8J
Tibia
Left ØQ8H
Right ØQ8G
Turbinate, Nasal Ø98L
Ulna
Left ØP8L
Right ØP8K
Uterine Supporting Structure ØU84
Vertebra
Cervical ØP83
Lumbar ØQ8Ø
Thoracic ØP84
Doppler study *see* Ultrasonography
Dorsal digital nerve *use* Radial Nerve
Dorsal metacarpal vein
use Hand Vein, Left

Dorsal metacarpal vein — *continued*
use Hand Vein, Right
Dorsal metatarsal artery
use Foot Artery, Left
use Foot Artery, Right
Dorsal metatarsal vein
use Foot Vein, Left
use Foot Vein, Right
Dorsal root ganglion
use Cervical Spinal Cord
use Lumbar Spinal Cord
use Spinal Cord
use Thoracic Spinal Cord
Dorsal scapular artery
use Subclavian Artery, Left
use Subclavian Artery, Right
Dorsal scapular nerve *use* Brachial Plexus
Dorsal venous arch
use Foot Vein, Left
use Foot Vein, Right
Dorsalis pedis artery
use Anterior Tibial Artery, Left
use Anterior Tibial Artery, Right
DownStream® System 5AØ512C, 5AØ522C
Drainage
Abdominal Wall ØW9F
Acetabulum
Left ØQ95
Right ØQ94
Adenoids ØC9Q
Ampulla of Vater ØF9C
Anal Sphincter ØD9R
Ankle Region
Left ØY9L
Right ØY9K
Anterior Chamber
Left Ø893
Right Ø892
Anus ØD9Q
Aorta, Abdominal Ø49Ø
Aortic Body ØG9D
Appendix ØD9J
Arm
Lower
Left ØX9F
Right ØX9D
Upper
Left ØX99
Right ØX98
Artery
Anterior Tibial
Left Ø49Q
Right Ø49P
Axillary
Left Ø396
Right Ø395
Brachial
Left Ø398
Right Ø397
Celiac Ø491
Colic
Left Ø497
Middle Ø498
Right Ø496
Common Carotid
Left Ø39J
Right Ø39H
Common Iliac
Left Ø49D
Right Ø49C
External Carotid
Left Ø39N
Right Ø39M
External Iliac
Left Ø49J
Right Ø49H
Face Ø39R
Femoral
Left Ø49L
Right Ø49K
Foot
Left Ø49W
Right Ø49V
Gastric Ø492
Hand
Left Ø39F
Right Ø39D
Hepatic Ø493

Drainage — *continued*
- Artery — *continued*
  - Inferior Mesenteric Ø49B
  - Innominate Ø392
  - Internal Carotid
    - Left Ø39L
    - Right Ø39K
  - Internal Iliac
    - Left Ø49F
    - Right Ø49E
  - Internal Mammary
    - Left Ø391
    - Right Ø39Ø
  - Intracranial Ø39G
  - Lower Ø49Y
  - Peroneal
    - Left Ø49U
    - Right Ø49T
  - Popliteal
    - Left Ø49N
    - Right Ø49M
  - Posterior Tibial
    - Left Ø49S
    - Right Ø49R
  - Radial
    - Left Ø39C
    - Right Ø39B
  - Renal
    - Left Ø49A
    - Right Ø499
  - Splenic Ø494
  - Subclavian
    - Left Ø394
    - Right Ø393
  - Superior Mesenteric Ø495
  - Temporal
    - Left Ø39T
    - Right Ø39S
  - Thyroid
    - Left Ø39V
    - Right Ø39U
  - Ulnar
    - Left Ø39A
    - Right Ø399
  - Upper Ø39Y
  - Vertebral
    - Left Ø39Q
    - Right Ø39P
- Auditory Ossicle
  - Left Ø99A
  - Right Ø999
- Axilla
  - Left ØX95
  - Right ØX94
- Back
  - Lower ØW9L
  - Upper ØW9K
- Basal Ganglia ØØ98
- Bladder ØT9B
- Bladder Neck ØT9C
- Bone
  - Ethmoid
    - Left ØN9G
    - Right ØN9F
  - Frontal ØN91
  - Hyoid ØN9X
  - Lacrimal
    - Left ØN9J
    - Right ØN9H
  - Nasal ØN9B
  - Occipital ØN97
  - Palatine
    - Left ØN9L
    - Right ØN9K
  - Parietal
    - Left ØN94
    - Right ØN93
  - Pelvic
    - Left ØQ93
    - Right ØQ92
  - Sphenoid ØN9C
  - Temporal
    - Left ØN96
    - Right ØN95
  - Zygomatic
    - Left ØN9N
    - Right ØN9M
- Bone Marrow Ø79T
- Brain ØØ9Ø

Drainage — *continued*
- Breast
  - Bilateral ØH9V
  - Left ØH9U
  - Right ØH9T
- Bronchus
  - Lingula ØB99
  - Lower Lobe
    - Left ØB9B
    - Right ØB96
  - Main
    - Left ØB97
    - Right ØB93
  - Middle Lobe, Right ØB95
  - Upper Lobe
    - Left ØB98
    - Right ØB94
- Buccal Mucosa ØC94
- Bursa and Ligament
  - Abdomen
    - Left ØM9J
    - Right ØM9H
  - Ankle
    - Left ØM9R
    - Right ØM9Q
  - Elbow
    - Left ØM94
    - Right ØM93
  - Foot
    - Left ØM9T
    - Right ØM9S
  - Hand
    - Left ØM98
    - Right ØM97
  - Head and Neck ØM9Ø
  - Hip
    - Left ØM9M
    - Right ØM9L
  - Knee
    - Left ØM9P
    - Right ØM9N
  - Lower Extremity
    - Left ØM9W
    - Right ØM9V
  - Perineum ØM9K
  - Rib(s) ØM9G
  - Shoulder
    - Left ØM92
    - Right ØM91
  - Spine
    - Lower ØM9D
    - Upper ØM9C
  - Sternum ØM9F
  - Upper Extremity
    - Left ØM9B
    - Right ØM99
  - Wrist
    - Left ØM96
    - Right ØM95
- Buttock
  - Left ØY91
  - Right ØY9Ø
- Carina ØB92
- Carotid Bodies, Bilateral ØG98
- Carotid Body
  - Left ØG96
  - Right ØG97
- Carpal
  - Left ØP9N
  - Right ØP9M
- Cavity, Cranial ØW91
- Cecum ØD9H
- Cerebellum ØØ9C
- Cerebral Hemisphere ØØ97
- Cerebral Meninges ØØ91
- Cerebral Ventricle ØØ96
- Cervix ØU9C
- Chest Wall ØW98
- Choroid
  - Left Ø89B
  - Right Ø89A
- Cisterna Chyli Ø79L
- Clavicle
  - Left ØP9B
  - Right ØP99
- Clitoris ØU9J
- Coccygeal Glomus ØG9B
- Coccyx ØQ9S

Drainage — *continued*
- Colon
  - Ascending ØD9K
  - Descending ØD9M
  - Sigmoid ØD9N
  - Transverse ØD9L
- Conjunctiva
  - Left Ø89T
  - Right Ø89S
- Cord
  - Bilateral ØV9H
  - Left ØV9G
  - Right ØV9F
- Cornea
  - Left Ø899
  - Right Ø898
- Cul-de-sac ØU9F
- Diaphragm ØB9T
- Disc
  - Cervical Vertebral ØR93
  - Cervicothoracic Vertebral ØR95
  - Lumbar Vertebral ØS92
  - Lumbosacral ØS94
  - Thoracic Vertebral ØR99
  - Thoracolumbar Vertebral ØR9B
- Duct
  - Common Bile ØF99
  - Cystic ØF98
  - Hepatic
    - Common ØF97
    - Left ØF96
    - Right ØF95
  - Lacrimal
    - Left Ø89Y
    - Right Ø89X
  - Pancreatic ØF9D
    - Accessory ØF9F
  - Parotid
    - Left ØC9C
    - Right ØC9B
- Duodenum ØD99
- Dura Mater ØØ92
- Ear
  - External
    - Left Ø991
    - Right Ø99Ø
  - External Auditory Canal
    - Left Ø994
    - Right Ø993
  - Inner
    - Left Ø99E
    - Right Ø99D
  - Middle
    - Left Ø996
    - Right Ø995
- Elbow Region
  - Left ØX9C
  - Right ØX9B
- Epididymis
  - Bilateral ØV9L
  - Left ØV9K
  - Right ØV9J
- Epidural Space, Intracranial ØØ93
- Epiglottis ØC9R
- Esophagogastric Junction ØD94
- Esophagus ØD95
  - Lower ØD93
  - Middle ØD92
  - Upper ØD91
- Eustachian Tube
  - Left Ø99G
  - Right Ø99F
- Extremity
  - Lower
    - Left ØY9B
    - Right ØY99
  - Upper
    - Left ØX97
    - Right ØX96
- Eye
  - Left Ø891
  - Right Ø89Ø
- Eyelid
  - Lower
    - Left Ø89R
    - Right Ø89Q
  - Upper
    - Left Ø89P
    - Right Ø89N

Drainage — *continued*
Face ØW92
Fallopian Tube
Left ØU96
Right ØU95
Fallopian Tubes, Bilateral ØU97
Femoral Region
Left ØY98
Right ØY97
Femoral Shaft
Left ØQ99
Right ØQ98
Femur
Lower
Left ØQ9C
Right ØQ9B
Upper
Left ØQ97
Right ØQ96
Fibula
Left ØQ9K
Right ØQ9J
Finger Nail ØH9Q
Foot
Left ØY9N
Right ØY9M
Gallbladder ØF94
Gingiva
Lower ØC96
Upper ØC95
Gland
Adrenal
Bilateral ØG94
Left ØG92
Right ØG93
Lacrimal
Left Ø89W
Right Ø89V
Minor Salivary ØC9J
Parotid
Left ØC99
Right ØC98
Pituitary ØG9Ø
Sublingual
Left ØC9F
Right ØC9D
Submaxillary
Left ØC9H
Right ØC9G
Vestibular ØU9L
Glenoid Cavity
Left ØP98
Right ØP97
Glomus Jugulare ØG9C
Hand
Left ØX9K
Right ØX9J
Head ØW9Ø
Humeral Head
Left ØP9D
Right ØP9C
Humeral Shaft
Left ØP9G
Right ØP9F
Hymen ØU9K
Hypothalamus ØØ9A
Ileocecal Valve ØD9C
Ileum ØD9B
Inguinal Region
Left ØY96
Right ØY95
Intestine
Large ØD9E
Left ØD9G
Right ØD9F
Small ØD98
Iris
Left Ø89D
Right Ø89C
Jaw
Lower ØW95
Upper ØW94
Jejunum ØD9A
Joint
Acromioclavicular
Left ØR9H
Right ØR9G
Ankle
Left ØS9G

Drainage — *continued*
Joint — *continued*
Ankle — *continued*
Right ØS9F
Carpal
Left ØR9R
Right ØR9Q
Carpometacarpal
Left ØR9T
Right ØR9S
Cervical Vertebral ØR91
Cervicothoracic Vertebral ØR94
Coccygeal ØS96
Elbow
Left ØR9M
Right ØR9L
Finger Phalangeal
Left ØR9X
Right ØR9W
Hip
Left ØS9B
Right ØS99
Knee
Left ØS9D
Right ØS9C
Lumbar Vertebral ØS9Ø
Lumbosacral ØS93
Metacarpophalangeal
Left ØR9V
Right ØR9U
Metatarsal-Phalangeal
Left ØS9N
Right ØS9M
Occipital-cervical ØR9Ø
Sacrococcygeal ØS95
Sacroiliac
Left ØS98
Right ØS97
Shoulder
Left ØR9K
Right ØR9J
Sternoclavicular
Left ØR9F
Right ØR9E
Tarsal
Left ØS9J
Right ØS9H
Tarsometatarsal
Left ØS9L
Right ØS9K
Temporomandibular
Left ØR9D
Right ØR9C
Thoracic Vertebral ØR96
Thoracolumbar Vertebral ØR9A
Toe Phalangeal
Left ØS9Q
Right ØS9P
Wrist
Left ØR9P
Right ØR9N
Kidney
Left ØT91
Right ØT9Ø
Kidney Pelvis
Left ØT94
Right ØT93
Knee Region
Left ØY9G
Right ØY9F
Larynx ØC9S
Leg
Lower
Left ØY9J
Right ØY9H
Upper
Left ØY9D
Right ØY9C
Lens
Left Ø89K
Right Ø89J
Lip
Lower ØC91
Upper ØC9Ø
Liver ØF9Ø
Left Lobe ØF92
Right Lobe ØF91
Lung
Bilateral ØB9M

Drainage — *continued*
Lung — *continued*
Left ØB9L
Lower Lobe
Left ØB9J
Right ØB9F
Middle Lobe, Right ØB9D
Right ØB9K
Upper Lobe
Left ØB9G
Right ØB9C
Lung Lingula ØB9H
Lymphatic
Aortic Ø79D
Axillary
Left Ø796
Right Ø795
Head Ø79Ø
Inguinal
Left Ø79J
Right Ø79H
Internal Mammary
Left Ø799
Right Ø798
Lower Extremity
Left Ø79G
Right Ø79F
Mesenteric Ø79B
Neck
Left Ø792
Right Ø791
Pelvis Ø79C
Thoracic Duct Ø79K
Thorax Ø797
Upper Extremity
Left Ø794
Right Ø793
Mandible
Left ØN9V
Right ØN9T
Maxilla ØN9R
Mediastinum ØW9C
Medulla Oblongata ØØ9D
Mesentery ØD9V
Metacarpal
Left ØP9Q
Right ØP9P
Metatarsal
Left ØQ9P
Right ØQ9N
Muscle
Abdomen
Left ØK9L
Right ØK9K
Extraocular
Left Ø89M
Right Ø89L
Facial ØK91
Foot
Left ØK9W
Right ØK9V
Hand
Left ØK9D
Right ØK9C
Head ØK9Ø
Hip
Left ØK9P
Right ØK9N
Lower Arm and Wrist
Left ØK9B
Right ØK99
Lower Leg
Left ØK9T
Right ØK9S
Neck
Left ØK93
Right ØK92
Perineum ØK9M
Shoulder
Left ØK96
Right ØK95
Thorax
Left ØK9J
Right ØK9H
Tongue, Palate, Pharynx ØK94
Trunk
Left ØK9G
Right ØK9F

Drainage — *continued*
Muscle — *continued*
Upper Arm
Left ØK98
Right ØK97
Upper Leg
Left ØK9R
Right ØK9Q
Nasal Mucosa and Soft Tissue Ø99K
Nasopharynx Ø99N
Neck ØW96
Nerve
Abdominal Sympathetic Ø19M
Abducens ØØ9L
Accessory ØØ9R
Acoustic ØØ9N
Brachial Plexus Ø193
Cervical Ø191
Cervical Plexus Ø19Ø
Facial ØØ9M
Femoral Ø19D
Glossopharyngeal ØØ9P
Head and Neck Sympathetic Ø19K
Hypoglossal ØØ9S
Lumbar Ø19B
Lumbar Plexus Ø199
Lumbar Sympathetic Ø19N
Lumbosacral Plexus Ø19A
Median Ø195
Oculomotor ØØ9H
Olfactory ØØ9F
Optic ØØ9G
Peroneal Ø19H
Phrenic Ø192
Pudendal Ø19C
Radial Ø196
Sacral Ø19R
Sacral Plexus Ø19Q
Sacral Sympathetic Ø19P
Sciatic Ø19F
Thoracic Ø198
Thoracic Sympathetic Ø19L
Tibial Ø19G
Trigeminal ØØ9K
Trochlear ØØ9J
Ulnar Ø194
Vagus ØØ9Q
Nipple
Left ØH9X
Right ØH9W
Omentum ØD9U
Oral Cavity and Throat ØW93
Orbit
Left ØN9Q
Right ØN9P
Ovary
Bilateral ØU92
Left ØU91
Right ØU9Ø
Palate
Hard ØC92
Soft ØC93
Pancreas ØF9G
Para-aortic Body ØG99
Paraganglion Extremity ØG9F
Parathyroid Gland ØG9R
Inferior
Left ØG9P
Right ØG9N
Multiple ØG9Q
Superior
Left ØG9M
Right ØG9L
Patella
Left ØQ9F
Right ØQ9D
Pelvic Cavity ØW9J
Penis ØV9S
Pericardial Cavity ØW9D
Perineum
Female ØW9N
Male ØW9M
Peritoneal Cavity ØW9G
Peritoneum ØD9W
Phalanx
Finger
Left ØP9V
Right ØP9T

Drainage — *continued*
Phalanx — *continued*
Thumb
Left ØP9S
Right ØP9R
Toe
Left ØQ9R
Right ØQ9Q
Pharynx ØC9M
Pineal Body ØG91
Pleura
Left ØB9P
Right ØB9N
Pleural Cavity
Left ØW9B
Right ØW99
Pons ØØ9B
Prepuce ØV9T
Products of Conception
Amniotic Fluid
Diagnostic 1Ø9Ø
Therapeutic 1Ø9Ø
Fetal Blood 1Ø9Ø
Fetal Cerebrospinal Fluid 1Ø9Ø
Fetal Fluid, Other 1Ø9Ø
Fluid, Other 1Ø9Ø
Prostate ØV9Ø
Radius
Left ØP9J
Right ØP9H
Rectum ØD9P
Retina
Left Ø89F
Right Ø89E
Retinal Vessel
Left Ø89H
Right Ø89G
Retroperitoneum ØW9H
Ribs
1 to 2 ØP91
3 or More ØP92
Sacrum ØQ91
Scapula
Left ØP96
Right ØP95
Sclera
Left Ø897
Right Ø896
Scrotum ØV95
Septum, Nasal Ø99M
Shoulder Region
Left ØX93
Right ØX92
Sinus
Accessory Ø99P
Ethmoid
Left Ø99V
Right Ø99U
Frontal
Left Ø99T
Right Ø99S
Mastoid
Left Ø99C
Right Ø99B
Maxillary
Left Ø99R
Right Ø99Q
Sphenoid
Left Ø99X
Right Ø99W
Skin
Abdomen ØH97
Back ØH96
Buttock ØH98
Chest ØH95
Ear
Left ØH93
Right ØH92
Face ØH91
Foot
Left ØH9N
Right ØH9M
Hand
Left ØH9G
Right ØH9F
Inguinal ØH9A
Lower Arm
Left ØH9E
Right ØH9D

Drainage — *continued*
Skin — *continued*
Lower Leg
Left ØH9L
Right ØH9K
Neck ØH94
Perineum ØH99
Scalp ØH9Ø
Upper Arm
Left ØH9C
Right ØH9B
Upper Leg
Left ØH9J
Right ØH9H
Skull ØN9Ø
Spinal Canal ØØ9U
Spinal Cord
Cervical ØØ9W
Lumbar ØØ9Y
Thoracic ØØ9X
Spinal Meninges ØØ9T
Spleen Ø79P
Sternum ØP9Ø
Stomach ØD96
Pylorus ØD97
Subarachnoid Space, Intracranial ØØ95
Subcutaneous Tissue and Fascia
Abdomen ØJ98
Back ØJ97
Buttock ØJ99
Chest ØJ96
Face ØJ91
Foot
Left ØJ9R
Right ØJ9Q
Hand
Left ØJ9K
Right ØJ9J
Lower Arm
Left ØJ9H
Right ØJ9G
Lower Leg
Left ØJ9P
Right ØJ9N
Neck
Left ØJ95
Right ØJ94
Pelvic Region ØJ9C
Perineum ØJ9B
Scalp ØJ9Ø
Upper Arm
Left ØJ9F
Right ØJ9D
Upper Leg
Left ØJ9M
Right ØJ9L
Subdural Space, Intracranial ØØ94
Tarsal
Left ØQ9M
Right ØQ9L
Tendon
Abdomen
Left ØL9G
Right ØL9F
Ankle
Left ØL9T
Right ØL9S
Foot
Left ØL9W
Right ØL9V
Hand
Left ØL98
Right ØL97
Head and Neck ØL9Ø
Hip
Left ØL9K
Right ØL9J
Knee
Left ØL9R
Right ØL9Q
Lower Arm and Wrist
Left ØL96
Right ØL95
Lower Leg
Left ØL9P
Right ØL9N
Perineum ØL9H
Shoulder
Left ØL92

- **Drainage** — *continued*
  - Tendon — *continued*
    - Shoulder — *continued*
      - Right ØL91
    - Thorax
      - Left ØL9D
      - Right ØL9C
    - Trunk
      - Left ØL9B
      - Right ØL99
    - Upper Arm
      - Left ØL94
      - Right ØL93
    - Upper Leg
      - Left ØL9M
      - Right ØL9L
  - Testis
    - Bilateral ØV9C
    - Left ØV9B
    - Right ØV99
  - Thalamus ØØ99
  - Thymus Ø79M
  - Thyroid Gland ØG9K
    - Left Lobe ØG9G
    - Right Lobe ØG9H
  - Tibia
    - Left ØQ9H
    - Right ØQ9G
  - Toe Nail ØH9R
  - Tongue ØC97
  - Tonsils ØC9P
  - Tooth
    - Lower ØC9X
    - Upper ØC9W
  - Trachea ØB91
  - Tunica Vaginalis
    - Left ØV97
    - Right ØV96
  - Turbinate, Nasal Ø99L
  - Tympanic Membrane
    - Left Ø998
    - Right Ø997
  - Ulna
    - Left ØP9L
    - Right ØP9K
  - Ureter
    - Left ØT97
    - Right ØT96
  - Ureters, Bilateral ØT98
  - Urethra ØT9D
  - Uterine Supporting Structure ØU94
  - Uterus ØU99
  - Uvula ØC9N
  - Vagina ØU9G
  - Vas Deferens
    - Bilateral ØV9Q
    - Left ØV9P
    - Right ØV9N
  - Vein
    - Axillary
      - Left Ø598
      - Right Ø597
    - Azygos Ø59Ø
    - Basilic
      - Left Ø59C
      - Right Ø59B
    - Brachial
      - Left Ø59A
      - Right Ø599
    - Cephalic
      - Left Ø59F
      - Right Ø59D
    - Colic Ø697
    - Common Iliac
      - Left Ø69D
      - Right Ø69C
    - Esophageal Ø693
    - External Iliac
      - Left Ø69G
      - Right Ø69F
    - External Jugular
      - Left Ø59Q
      - Right Ø59P
    - Face
      - Left Ø59V
      - Right Ø59T
    - Femoral
      - Left Ø69N
      - Right Ø69M
- **Drainage** — *continued*
  - Vein — *continued*
    - Foot
      - Left Ø69V
      - Right Ø69T
    - Gastric Ø692
    - Hand
      - Left Ø59H
      - Right Ø59G
    - Hemiazygos Ø591
    - Hepatic Ø694
    - Hypogastric
      - Left Ø69J
      - Right Ø69H
    - Inferior Mesenteric Ø696
    - Innominate
      - Left Ø594
      - Right Ø593
    - Internal Jugular
      - Left Ø59N
      - Right Ø59M
    - Intracranial Ø59L
    - Lower Ø69Y
    - Portal Ø698
    - Renal
      - Left Ø69B
      - Right Ø699
    - Saphenous
      - Left Ø69Q
      - Right Ø69P
    - Splenic Ø691
    - Subclavian
      - Left Ø596
      - Right Ø595
    - Superior Mesenteric Ø695
    - Upper Ø59Y
    - Vertebral
      - Left Ø59S
      - Right Ø59R
  - Vena Cava, Inferior Ø69Ø
  - Vertebra
    - Cervical ØP93
    - Lumbar ØQ9Ø
    - Thoracic ØP94
  - Vesicle
    - Bilateral ØV93
    - Left ØV92
    - Right ØV91
  - Vitreous
    - Left Ø895
    - Right Ø894
  - Vocal Cord
    - Left ØC9V
    - Right ØC9T
  - Vulva ØU9M
  - Wrist Region
    - Left ØX9H
    - Right ØX9G
- **Dressing**
  - Abdominal Wall 2W23X4Z
  - Arm
    - Lower
      - Left 2W2DX4Z
      - Right 2W2CX4Z
    - Upper
      - Left 2W2BX4Z
      - Right 2W2AX4Z
  - Back 2W25X4Z
  - Chest Wall 2W24X4Z
  - Extremity
    - Lower
      - Left 2W2MX4Z
      - Right 2W2LX4Z
    - Upper
      - Left 2W29X4Z
      - Right 2W28X4Z
  - Face 2W21X4Z
  - Finger
    - Left 2W2KX4Z
    - Right 2W2JX4Z
  - Foot
    - Left 2W2TX4Z
    - Right 2W2SX4Z
  - Hand
    - Left 2W2FX4Z
    - Right 2W2EX4Z
  - Head 2W2ØX4Z
  - Inguinal Region
    - Left 2W27X4Z
- **Dressing** — *continued*
  - Inguinal Region — *continued*
    - Right 2W26X4Z
  - Leg
    - Lower
      - Left 2W2RX4Z
      - Right 2W2QX4Z
    - Upper
      - Left 2W2PX4Z
      - Right 2W2NX4Z
  - Neck 2W22X4Z
  - Thumb
    - Left 2W2HX4Z
    - Right 2W2GX4Z
  - Toe
    - Left 2W2VX4Z
    - Right 2W2UX4Z
- **Driver stent (RX) (OTW)** *use* Intraluminal Device
- **Drotrecogin alfa, infusion** *see* Introduction of Recombinant Human-activated Protein C
- **Duct of Santorini** *use* Pancreatic Duct, Accessory
- **Duct of Wirsung** *use* Pancreatic Duct
- **Ductogram, mammary** *see* Plain Radiography, Skin, Subcutaneous Tissue and Breast BHØ
- **Ductography, mammary** *see* Plain Radiography, Skin, Subcutaneous Tissue and Breast BHØ
- **Ductus deferens**
  - *use* Vas Deferens
  - *use* Vas Deferens, Bilateral
  - *use* Vas Deferens, Left
  - *use* Vas Deferens, Right
- **Duodenal ampulla** *use* Ampulla of Vater
- **Duodenectomy**
  - *see* Excision, Duodenum ØDB9
  - *see* Resection, Duodenum ØDT9
- **Duodenocholedochotomy** *see* Drainage, Gallbladder ØF94
- **Duodenocystostomy**
  - *see* Bypass, Gallbladder ØF14
  - *see* Drainage, Gallbladder ØF94
- **Duodenoenterostomy**
  - *see* Bypass, Gastrointestinal System ØD1
  - *see* Drainage, Gastrointestinal System ØD9
- **Duodenojejunal flexure** *use* Jejunum
- **Duodenolysis** *see* Release, Duodenum ØDN9
- **Duodenorrhaphy** *see* Repair, Duodenum ØDQ9
- **Duodenoscopy, single-use (aScope™ Duodeno) (EXALT™ Model D)** *see* New Technology, Hepatobiliary System and Pancreas XFJ
- **Duodenostomy**
  - *see* Bypass, Duodenum ØD19
  - *see* Drainage, Duodenum ØD99
- **Duodenotomy** *see* Drainage, Duodenum ØD99
- **Dura mater, intracranial** *use* Dura Mater
- **Dura mater, spinal** *use* Spinal Meninges
- **DuraGraft® Endothelial Damage Inhibitor** *use* Endothelial Damage Inhibitor
- **DuraHeart Left Ventricular Assist System** *use* Implantable Heart Assist System in Heart and Great Vessels
- **Dural venous sinus** *use* Intracranial Vein
- **Durata® Defibrillation Lead** *use* Cardiac Lead, Defibrillator in Ø2H
- **Durvalumab Antineoplastic** XWØ
- **DynaNail Mini®**
  - *use* Internal Fixation Device, Sustained Compression in ØRG
  - *use* Internal Fixation Device, Sustained Compression in ØSG
- **DynaNail®**
  - *use* Internal Fixation Device, Sustained Compression in ØRG
  - *use* Internal Fixation Device, Sustained Compression in ØSG
- **Dynesys® Dynamic Stabilization System**
  - *use* Spinal Stabilization Device, Pedicle-Based in ØRH
  - *use* Spinal Stabilization Device, Pedicle-Based in ØSH

E

- **Earlobe**
  - *use* Ear, External, Bilateral
  - *use* Ear, External, Left
  - *use* Ear, External, Right

ECCO2R (Extracorporeal Carbon Dioxide Removal) 5A0920Z
Echocardiogram *see* Ultrasonography, Heart B24
Echography *see* Ultrasonography
EchoTip® Insight™ Portosystemic Pressure Gradient Measurement System 4A044B2
ECMO *see* Performance, Circulatory 5A15
ECMO, intraoperative *see* Performance, Circulatory 5A15A
Eculizumab XW0
EDWARDS INTUITY Elite valve system *use* Zooplastic Tissue, Rapid Deployment Technique in New Technology
EEG (electroencephalogram) *see* Measurement, Central Nervous 4A00
EGD (esophagogastroduodenoscopy) 0DJ08ZZ
Eighth cranial nerve *use* Acoustic Nerve
Ejaculatory duct
use Vas Deferens
use Vas Deferens, Bilateral
use Vas Deferens, Left
use Vas Deferens, Right
EKG (electrocardiogram) *see* Measurement, Cardiac 4A02
EKOS™ EkoSonic® Endovascular System *see* Fragmentation, Artery
Eladocagene exuparvovec XW0Q316
Electrical bone growth stimulator (EBGS)
use Bone Growth Stimulator in Head and Facial Bones
use Bone Growth Stimulator in Lower Bones
use Bone Growth Stimulator in Upper Bones
Electrical muscle stimulation (EMS) lead *use* Stimulator Lead in Muscles
Electrocautery
Destruction *see* Destruction
Repair *see* Repair
Electroconvulsive Therapy
Bilateral-Multiple Seizure GZB3ZZZ
Bilateral-Single Seizure GZB2ZZZ
Electroconvulsive Therapy, Other GZB4ZZZ
Unilateral-Multiple Seizure GZB1ZZZ
Unilateral-Single Seizure GZB0ZZZ
Electroencephalogram (EEG) *see* Measurement, Central Nervous 4A00
Electromagnetic Therapy
Central Nervous 6A22
Urinary 6A21
Electronic muscle stimulator lead *use* Stimulator Lead in Muscles
Electrophysiologic stimulation (EPS) *see* Measurement, Cardiac 4A02
Electroshock therapy *see* Electroconvulsive Therapy
Elevation, bone fragments, skull *see* Reposition, Head and Facial Bones 0NS
Eleventh cranial nerve *use* Accessory Nerve
Ellipsys® vascular access system *see* New Technology, Cardiovascular System X2K
E-Luminexx™ (Biliary) (Vascular) Stent *use* Intraluminal Device
Eluvia™ Drug-Eluting Vascular Stent System
use Intraluminal Device, Sustained Release Drug-eluting in New Technology
use Intraluminal Device, Sustained Release Drug-eluting, Two in New Technology
use Intraluminal Device, Sustained Release Drug-eluting, Three in New Technology
use Intraluminal Device, Sustained Release Drug-eluting, Four or More in New Technology
ELZONRIS™ *use* Tagraxofusp-erzs Antineoplastic
Embolectomy *see* Extirpation
Embolization
see Occlusion
see Restriction
Embolization coil(s) *use* Intraluminal Device
EMG (electromyogram) *see* Measurement, Musculoskeletal 4A0F
Encephalon *use* Brain
Endarterectomy
see Extirpation, Lower Arteries 04C
see Extirpation, Upper Arteries 03C
Endeavor® (III) (IV) (Sprint) Zotarolimus-eluting Coronary Stent System *use* Intraluminal Device, Drug-eluting in Heart and Great Vessels
EndoAVF procedure, using magnetic-guided radiofrequency *see* Bypass, Upper Arteries 031
EndoAVF procedure, using thermal resistance energy *see* New Technology, Cardiovascular System X2K
Endologix AFX® Endovascular AAA System *use* Intraluminal Device
EndoSure® sensor *use* Monitoring Device, Pressure Sensor in 02H
ENDOTAK RELIANCE® (G) Defibrillation Lead *use* Cardiac Lead, Defibrillator in 02H
Endothelial damage inhibitor, applied to vein graft XY0VX83
Endotracheal tube (cuffed) (double-lumen) *use* Intraluminal Device, Endotracheal Airway in Respiratory System
Endovascular fistula creation, using magnetic-guided radiofrequency *see* Bypass, Upper Arteries 031
Endovascular fistula creation, using thermal resistance energy *see* New Technology, Cardiovascular System X2K
Endurant® Endovascular Stent Graft *use* Intraluminal Device
Endurant® II AAA Stent Graft System *use* Intraluminal Device
Engineered Chimeric Antigen Receptor T-cell Immunotherapy
Allogeneic XW0
Autologous XW0
Enlargement
see Dilation
see Repair
EnRhythm *use* Pacemaker, Dual Chamber in 0JH
ENROUTE® Transcarotid Neuroprotection System *see* New Technology, Cardiovascular System X2A
ENSPRYNG™ *use* Satralizumab-mwge
Enterorrhaphy *see* Repair, Gastrointestinal System 0DQ
Enterra gastric neurostimulator *use* Stimulator Generator, Multiple Array in 0JH
Enucleation
Eyeball *see* Resection, Eye 08T
Eyeball with prosthetic implant *see* Replacement, Eye 08R
Ependyma *use* Cerebral Ventricle
Epicel® cultured epidermal autograft *use* Autologous Tissue Substitute
Epic™ Stented Tissue Valve (aortic) *use* Zooplastic Tissue in Heart and Great Vessels
Epidermis *use* Skin
Epididymectomy
see Excision, Male Reproductive System 0VB
see Resection, Male Reproductive System 0VT
Epididymoplasty
see Repair, Male Reproductive System 0VQ
see Supplement, Male Reproductive System 0VU
Epididymorrhaphy *see* Repair, Male Reproductive System 0VQ
Epididymotomy *see* Drainage, Male Reproductive System 0V9
Epidural space, spinal *use* Spinal Canal
Epiphysiodesis
see Insertion of device in, Lower Bones 0QH
see Insertion of device in, Upper Bones 0PH
see Repair, Lower Bones 0QQ
see Repair, Upper Bones 0PQ
Epiploic foramen *use* Peritoneum
Epiretinal Visual Prosthesis
Left 08H105Z
Right 08H005Z
Episiorrhaphy *see* Repair, Perineum, Female 0WQN
Episiotomy *see* Division, Perineum, Female 0W8N
Epithalamus *use* Thalamus
Epitrochlear lymph node
use Lymphatic, Left Upper Extremity
use Lymphatic, Right Upper Extremity
EPS (electrophysiologic stimulation) *see* Measurement, Cardiac 4A02
Eptifibatide, infusion *see* Introduction of Platelet Inhibitor
ERCP (endoscopic retrograde cholangiopancreatography) *see* Fluoroscopy, Hepatobiliary System and Pancreas BF1
Erdafitinib Antineoplastic XW0DXL5
Erector spinae muscle
use Trunk Muscle, Left
use Trunk Muscle, Right
ERLEADA™ *use* Apalutamide Antineoplastic
Esketamine Hydrochloride XW097M5
Esophageal artery *use* Upper Artery
Esophageal obturator airway (EOA) *use* Intraluminal Device, Airway in Gastrointestinal System
Esophageal plexus *use* Thoracic Sympathetic Nerve
Esophagectomy
see Excision, Gastrointestinal System 0DB
see Resection, Gastrointestinal System 0DT
Esophagocoloplasty
see Repair, Gastrointestinal System 0DQ
see Supplement, Gastrointestinal System 0DU
Esophagoenterostomy
see Bypass, Gastrointestinal System 0D1
see Drainage, Gastrointestinal System 0D9
Esophagoesophagostomy
see Bypass, Gastrointestinal System 0D1
see Drainage, Gastrointestinal System 0D9
Esophagogastrectomy
see Excision, Gastrointestinal System 0DB
see Resection, Gastrointestinal System 0DT
Esophagogastroduodenoscopy (EGD) 0DJ08ZZ
Esophagogastroplasty
see Repair, Gastrointestinal System 0DQ
see Supplement, Gastrointestinal System 0DU
Esophagogastroscopy 0DJ68ZZ
Esophagogastrostomy
see Bypass, Gastrointestinal System 0D1
see Drainage, Gastrointestinal System 0D9
Esophagojejunoplasty *see* Supplement, Gastrointestinal System 0DU
Esophagojejunostomy
see Bypass, Gastrointestinal System 0D1
see Drainage, Gastrointestinal System 0D9
Esophagomyotomy *see* Division, Esophagogastric Junction 0D84
Esophagoplasty
see Repair, Gastrointestinal System 0DQ
see Replacement, Esophagus 0DR5
see Supplement, Gastrointestinal System 0DU
Esophagoplication *see* Restriction, Gastrointestinal System 0DV
Esophagorrhaphy *see* Repair, Gastrointestinal System 0DQ
Esophagoscopy 0DJ08ZZ
Esophagotomy *see* Drainage, Gastrointestinal System 0D9
Esteem® implantable hearing system *use* Hearing Device in Ear, Nose, Sinus
ESWL (extracorporeal shock wave lithotripsy) *see* Fragmentation
Etesevimab Monoclonal Antibody XW0
Ethmoidal air cell
use Ethmoid Sinus, Left
use Ethmoid Sinus, Right
Ethmoidectomy
see Excision, Ear, Nose, Sinus 09B
see Excision, Head and Facial Bones 0NB
see Resection, Ear, Nose, Sinus 09T
see Resection, Head and Facial Bones 0NT
Ethmoidotomy *see* Drainage, Ear, Nose, Sinus 099
Evacuation
Hematoma *see* Extirpation
Other Fluid *see* Drainage
Evera (XT) (S) (DR/VR) *use* Defibrillator Generator in 0JH
Everolimus-eluting coronary stent *use* Intraluminal Device, Drug-eluting in Heart and Great Vessels
Evisceration
Eyeball *see* Resection, Eye 08T
Eyeball with prosthetic implant *see* Replacement, Eye 08R
EXALT™ Model D Single-Use Duodenoscope *see* New Technology, Hepatobiliary System and Pancreas XFJ
Examination *see* Inspection
Exchange *see* Change device in
Excision
Abdominal Wall 0WBF
Acetabulum
Left 0QB5
Right 0QB4
Adenoids 0CBQ
Ampulla of Vater 0FBC
Anal Sphincter 0DBR
Ankle Region
Left 0YBL
Right 0YBK

Excision — *continued*
Anus ØDBQ
Aorta
Abdominal
Thoracic
Ascending/Arch Ø2BX
Descending Ø2BW
Aortic Body ØGBD
Appendix ØDBJ
Arm
Lower
Left ØXBF
Right ØXBD
Upper
Left ØXB9
Right ØXB8
Artery
Anterior Tibial
Left Ø4BQ
Right Ø4BP
Axillary
Left Ø3B6
Right Ø3B5
Brachial
Left Ø3B8
Right Ø3B7
Celiac Ø4B1
Colic
Left Ø4B7
Middle Ø4B8
Right Ø4B6
Common Carotid
Left Ø3BJ
Right Ø3BH
Common Iliac
Left Ø4BD
Right Ø4BC
External Carotid
Left Ø3BN
Right Ø3BM
External Iliac
Left Ø4BJ
Right Ø4BH
Face Ø3BR
Femoral
Left Ø4BL
Right Ø4BK
Foot
Left Ø4BW
Right Ø4BV
Gastric Ø4B2
Hand
Left Ø3BF
Right Ø3BD
Hepatic Ø4B3
Inferior Mesenteric Ø4BB
Innominate Ø3B2
Internal Carotid
Left Ø3BL
Right Ø3BK
Internal Iliac
Left Ø4BF
Right Ø4BE
Internal Mammary
Left Ø3B1
Right Ø3BØ
Intracranial Ø3BG
Lower Ø4BY
Peroneal
Left Ø4BU
Right Ø4BT
Popliteal
Left Ø4BN
Right Ø4BM
Posterior Tibial
Left Ø4BS
Right Ø4BR
Pulmonary
Left Ø2BR
Right Ø2BQ
Pulmonary Trunk Ø2BP
Radial
Left Ø3BC
Right Ø3BB
Renal
Left Ø4BA
Right Ø4B9
Splenic Ø4B4

Excision — *continued*
Artery — *continued*
Subclavian
Left Ø3B4
Right Ø3B3
Superior Mesenteric Ø4B5
Temporal
Left Ø3BT
Right Ø3BS
Thyroid
Left Ø3BV
Right Ø3BU
Ulnar
Left Ø3BA
Right Ø3B9
Upper Ø3BY
Vertebral
Left Ø3BQ
Right Ø3BP
Atrium
Left Ø2B7
Right Ø2B6
Auditory Ossicle
Left Ø9BA
Right Ø9B9
Axilla
Left ØXB5
Right ØXB4
Back
Lower ØWBL
Upper ØWBK
Basal Ganglia ØØB8
Bladder ØTBB
Bladder Neck ØTBC
Bone
Ethmoid
Left ØNBG
Right ØNBF
Frontal ØNB1
Hyoid ØNBX
Lacrimal
Left ØNBJ
Right ØNBH
Nasal ØNBB
Occipital ØNB7
Palatine
Left ØNBL
Right ØNBK
Parietal
Left ØNB4
Right ØNB3
Pelvic
Left ØQB3
Right ØQB2
Sphenoid ØNBC
Temporal
Left ØNB6
Right ØNB5
Zygomatic
Left ØNBN
Right ØNBM
Brain ØØBØ
Breast
Bilateral ØHBV
Left ØHBU
Right ØHBT
Supernumerary ØHBY
Bronchus
Lingula ØBB9
Lower Lobe
Left ØBBB
Right ØBB6
Main
Left ØBB7
Right ØBB3
Middle Lobe, Right ØBB5
Upper Lobe
Left ØBB8
Right ØBB4
Buccal Mucosa ØCB4
Bursa and Ligament
Abdomen
Left ØMBJ
Right ØMBH
Ankle
Left ØMBR
Right ØMBQ
Elbow
Left ØMB4

Excision — *continued*
Bursa and Ligament — *continued*
Elbow — *continued*
Right ØMB3
Foot
Left ØMBT
Right ØMBS
Hand
Left ØMB8
Right ØMB7
Head and Neck ØMBØ
Hip
Left ØMBM
Right ØMBL
Knee
Left ØMBP
Right ØMBN
Lower Extremity
Left ØMBW
Right ØMBV
Perineum ØMBK
Rib(s) ØMBG
Shoulder
Left ØMB2
Right ØMB1
Spine
Lower ØMBD
Upper ØMBC
Sternum ØMBF
Upper Extremity
Left ØMBB
Right ØMB9
Wrist
Left ØMB6
Right ØMB5
Buttock
Left ØYB1
Right ØYBØ
Carina ØBB2
Carotid Bodies, Bilateral ØGB8
Carotid Body
Left ØGB6
Right ØGB7
Carpal
Left ØPBN
Right ØPBM
Cecum ØDBH
Cerebellum ØØBC
Cerebral Hemisphere ØØB7
Cerebral Meninges ØØB1
Cerebral Ventricle ØØB6
Cervix ØUBC
Chest Wall ØWB8
Chordae Tendineae Ø2B9
Choroid
Left Ø8BB
Right Ø8BA
Cisterna Chyli Ø7BL
Clavicle
Left ØPBB
Right ØPB9
Clitoris ØUBJ
Coccygeal Glomus ØGBB
Coccyx ØQBS
Colon
Ascending ØDBK
Descending ØDBM
Sigmoid ØDBN
Transverse ØDBL
Conduction Mechanism Ø2B8
Conjunctiva
Left Ø8BTXZ
Right Ø8BSXZ
Cord
Bilateral ØVBH
Left ØVBG
Right ØVBF
Cornea
Left Ø8B9XZ
Right Ø8B8XZ
Cul-de-sac ØUBF
Diaphragm ØBBT
Disc
Cervical Vertebral ØRB3
Cervicothoracic Vertebral ØRB5
Lumbar Vertebral ØSB2
Lumbosacral ØSB4
Thoracic Vertebral ØRB9
Thoracolumbar Vertebral ØRBB

Excision — *continued*
- Duct
  - Common Bile ØFB9
  - Cystic ØFB8
  - Hepatic
    - Common ØFB7
    - Left ØFB6
    - Right ØFB5
  - Lacrimal
    - Left Ø8BY
    - Right Ø8BX
  - Pancreatic ØFBD
    - Accessory ØFBF
  - Parotid
    - Left ØCBC
    - Right ØCBB
- Duodenum ØDB9
- Dura Mater ØØB2
- Ear
  - External
    - Left Ø9B1
    - Right Ø9BØ
  - External Auditory Canal
    - Left Ø9B4
    - Right Ø9B3
  - Inner
    - Left Ø9BE
    - Right Ø9BD
  - Middle
    - Left Ø9B6
    - Right Ø9B5
- Elbow Region
  - Left ØXBC
  - Right ØXBB
- Epididymis
  - Bilateral ØVBL
  - Left ØVBK
  - Right ØVBJ
- Epiglottis ØCBR
- Esophagogastric Junction ØDB4
- Esophagus ØDB5
  - Lower ØDB3
  - Middle ØDB2
  - Upper ØDB1
- Eustachian Tube
  - Left Ø9BG
  - Right Ø9BF
- Extremity
  - Lower
    - Left ØYBB
    - Right ØYB9
  - Upper
    - Left ØXB7
    - Right ØXB6
- Eye
  - Left Ø8B1
  - Right Ø8BØ
- Eyelid
  - Lower
    - Left Ø8BR
    - Right Ø8BQ
  - Upper
    - Left Ø8BP
    - Right Ø8BN
- Face ØWB2
- Fallopian Tube
  - Left ØUB6
  - Right ØUB5
- Fallopian Tubes, Bilateral ØUB7
- Femoral Region
  - Left ØYB8
  - Right ØYB7
- Femoral Shaft
  - Left ØQB9
  - Right ØQB8
- Femur
  - Lower
    - Left ØQBC
    - Right ØQBB
  - Upper
    - Left ØQB7
    - Right ØQB6
- Fibula
  - Left ØQBK
  - Right ØQBJ
- Finger Nail ØHBQXZ
- Floor of mouth *see* Excision, Oral Cavity and Throat ØWB3

Excision — *continued*
- Foot
  - Left ØYBN
  - Right ØYBM
- Gallbladder ØFB4
- Gingiva
  - Lower ØCB6
  - Upper ØCB5
- Gland
  - Adrenal
    - Bilateral ØGB4
    - Left ØGB2
    - Right ØGB3
  - Lacrimal
    - Left Ø8BW
    - Right Ø8BV
  - Minor Salivary ØCBJ
  - Parotid
    - Left ØCB9
    - Right ØCB8
  - Pituitary ØGBØ
  - Sublingual
    - Left ØCBF
    - Right ØCBD
  - Submaxillary
    - Left ØCBH
    - Right ØCBG
  - Vestibular ØUBL
- Glenoid Cavity
  - Left ØPB8
  - Right ØPB7
- Glomus Jugulare ØGBC
- Hand
  - Left ØXBK
  - Right ØXBJ
- Head ØWBØ
- Humeral Head
  - Left ØPBD
  - Right ØPBC
- Humeral Shaft
  - Left ØPBG
  - Right ØPBF
- Hymen ØUBK
- Hypothalamus ØØBA
- Ileocecal Valve ØDBC
- Ileum ØDBB
- Inguinal Region
  - Left ØYB6
  - Right ØYB5
- Intestine
  - Large ØDBE
    - Left ØDBG
    - Right ØDBF
  - Small ØDB8
- Iris
  - Left Ø8BD3Z
  - Right Ø8BC3Z
- Jaw
  - Lower ØWB5
  - Upper ØWB4
- Jejunum ØDBA
- Joint
  - Acromioclavicular
    - Left ØRBH
    - Right ØRBG
  - Ankle
    - Left ØSBG
    - Right ØSBF
  - Carpal
    - Left ØRBR
    - Right ØRBQ
  - Carpometacarpal
    - Left ØRBT
    - Right ØRBS
  - Cervical Vertebral ØRB1
  - Cervicothoracic Vertebral ØRB4
  - Coccygeal ØSB6
  - Elbow
    - Left ØRBM
    - Right ØRBL
  - Finger Phalangeal
    - Left ØRBX
    - Right ØRBW
  - Hip
    - Left ØSBB
    - Right ØSB9
  - Knee
    - Left ØSBD
    - Right ØSBC

Excision — *continued*
- Joint — *continued*
  - Lumbar Vertebral ØSBØ
  - Lumbosacral ØSB3
  - Metacarpophalangeal
    - Left ØRBV
    - Right ØRBU
  - Metatarsal-Phalangeal
    - Left ØSBN
    - Right ØSBM
  - Occipital-cervical ØRBØ
  - Sacrococcygeal ØSB5
  - Sacroiliac
    - Left ØSB8
    - Right ØSB7
  - Shoulder
    - Left ØRBK
    - Right ØRBJ
  - Sternoclavicular
    - Left ØRBF
    - Right ØRBE
  - Tarsal
    - Left ØSBJ
    - Right ØSBH
  - Tarsometatarsal
    - Left ØSBL
    - Right ØSBK
  - Temporomandibular
    - Left ØRBD
    - Right ØRBC
  - Thoracic Vertebral ØRB6
  - Thoracolumbar Vertebral ØRBA
  - Toe Phalangeal
    - Left ØSBQ
    - Right ØSBP
  - Wrist
    - Left ØRBP
    - Right ØRBN
- Kidney
  - Left ØTB1
  - Right ØTBØ
- Kidney Pelvis
  - Left ØTB4
  - Right ØTB3
- Knee Region
  - Left ØYBG
  - Right ØYBF
- Larynx ØCBS
- Leg
  - Lower
    - Left ØYBJ
    - Right ØYBH
  - Upper
    - Left ØYBD
    - Right ØYBC
- Lens
  - Left Ø8BK3Z
  - Right Ø8BJ3Z
- Lip
  - Lower ØCB1
  - Upper ØCBØ
- Liver ØFBØ
  - Left Lobe ØFB2
  - Right Lobe ØFB1
- Lung
  - Bilateral ØBBM
  - Left ØBBL
  - Lower Lobe
    - Left ØBBJ
    - Right ØBBF
  - Middle Lobe, Right ØBBD
  - Right ØBBK
  - Upper Lobe
    - Left ØBBG
    - Right ØBBC
- Lung Lingula ØBBH
- Lymphatic
  - Aortic Ø7BD
  - Axillary
    - Left Ø7B6
    - Right Ø7B5
  - Head Ø7BØ
  - Inguinal
    - Left Ø7BJ
    - Right Ø7BH
  - Internal Mammary
    - Left Ø7B9
    - Right Ø7B8

Excision — *continued*
Lymphatic — *continued*
Lower Extremity
Left Ø7BG
Right Ø7BF
Mesenteric Ø7BB
Neck
Left Ø7B2
Right Ø7B1
Pelvis Ø7BC
Thoracic Duct Ø7BK
Thorax Ø7B7
Upper Extremity
Left Ø7B4
Right Ø7B3
Mandible
Left ØNBV
Right ØNBT
Maxilla ØNBR
Mediastinum ØWBC
Medulla Oblongata ØØBD
Mesentery ØDBV
Metacarpal
Left ØPBQ
Right ØPBP
Metatarsal
Left ØQBP
Right ØQBN
Muscle
Abdomen
Left ØKBL
Right ØKBK
Extraocular
Left Ø8BM
Right Ø8BL
Facial ØKB1
Foot
Left ØKBW
Right ØKBV
Hand
Left ØKBD
Right ØKBC
Head ØKBØ
Hip
Left ØKBP
Right ØKBN
Lower Arm and Wrist
Left ØKBB
Right ØKB9
Lower Leg
Left ØKBT
Right ØKBS
Neck
Left ØKB3
Right ØKB2
Papillary Ø2BD
Perineum ØKBM
Shoulder
Left ØKB6
Right ØKB5
Thorax
Left ØKBJ
Right ØKBH
Tongue, Palate, Pharynx ØKB4
Trunk
Left ØKBG
Right ØKBF
Upper Arm
Left ØKB8
Right ØKB7
Upper Leg
Left ØKBR
Right ØKBQ
Nasal Mucosa and Soft Tissue Ø9BK
Nasopharynx Ø9BN
Neck ØWB6
Nerve
Abdominal Sympathetic Ø1BM
Abducens ØØBL
Accessory ØØBR
Acoustic ØØBN
Brachial Plexus Ø1B3
Cervical Ø1B1
Cervical Plexus Ø1BØ
Facial ØØBM
Femoral Ø1BD
Glossopharyngeal ØØBP
Head and Neck Sympathetic Ø1BK
Hypoglossal ØØBS

Excision — *continued*
Nerve — *continued*
Lumbar Ø1BB
Lumbar Plexus Ø1B9
Lumbar Sympathetic Ø1BN
Lumbosacral Plexus Ø1BA
Median Ø1B5
Oculomotor ØØBH
Olfactory ØØBF
Optic ØØBG
Peroneal Ø1BH
Phrenic Ø1B2
Pudendal Ø1BC
Radial Ø1B6
Sacral Ø1BR
Sacral Plexus Ø1BQ
Sacral Sympathetic Ø1BP
Sciatic Ø1BF
Thoracic Ø1B8
Thoracic Sympathetic Ø1BL
Tibial Ø1BG
Trigeminal ØØBK
Trochlear ØØBJ
Ulnar Ø1B4
Vagus ØØBQ
Nipple
Left ØHBX
Right ØHBW
Omentum ØDBU
Oral Cavity and Throat ØWB3
Orbit
Left ØNBQ
Right ØNBP
Ovary
Bilateral ØUB2
Left ØUB1
Right ØUBØ
Palate
Hard ØCB2
Soft ØCB3
Pancreas ØFBG
Para-aortic Body ØGB9
Paraganglion Extremity ØGBF
Parathyroid Gland ØGBR
Inferior
Left ØGBP
Right ØGBN
Multiple ØGBQ
Superior
Left ØGBM
Right ØGBL
Patella
Left ØQBF
Right ØQBD
Penis ØVBS
Pericardium Ø2BN
Perineum
Female ØWBN
Male ØWBM
Peritoneum ØDBW
Phalanx
Finger
Left ØPBV
Right ØPBT
Thumb
Left ØPBS
Right ØPBR
Toe
Left ØQBR
Right ØQBQ
Pharynx ØCBM
Pineal Body ØGB1
Pleura
Left ØBBP
Right ØBBN
Pons ØØBB
Prepuce ØVBT
Prostate ØVBØ
Radius
Left ØPBJ
Right ØPBH
Rectum ØDBP
Retina
Left Ø8BF3Z
Right Ø8BE3Z
Retroperitoneum ØWBH
Ribs
1 to 2 ØPB1
3 or More ØPB2

Excision — *continued*
Sacrum ØQB1
Scapula
Left ØPB6
Right ØPB5
Sclera
Left Ø8B7XZ
Right Ø8B6XZ
Scrotum ØVB5
Septum
Atrial Ø2B5
Nasal Ø9BM
Ventricular Ø2BM
Shoulder Region
Left ØXB3
Right ØXB2
Sinus
Accessory Ø9BP
Ethmoid
Left Ø9BV
Right Ø9BU
Frontal
Left Ø9BT
Right Ø9BS
Mastoid
Left Ø9BC
Right Ø9BB
Maxillary
Left Ø9BR
Right Ø9BQ
Sphenoid
Left Ø9BX
Right Ø9BW
Skin
Abdomen ØHB7XZ
Back ØHB6XZ
Buttock ØHB8XZ
Chest ØHB5XZ
Ear
Left ØHB3XZ
Right ØHB2XZ
Face ØHB1XZ
Foot
Left ØHBNXZ
Right ØHBMXZ
Hand
Left ØHBGXZ
Right ØHBFXZ
Inguinal ØHBAXZ
Lower Arm
Left ØHBEXZ
Right ØHBDXZ
Lower Leg
Left ØHBLXZ
Right ØHBKXZ
Neck ØHB4XZ
Perineum ØHB9XZ
Scalp ØHBØXZ
Upper Arm
Left ØHBCXZ
Right ØHBBXZ
Upper Leg
Left ØHBJXZ
Right ØHBHXZ
Skull ØNBØ
Spinal Cord
Cervical ØØBW
Lumbar ØØBY
Thoracic ØØBX
Spinal Meninges ØØBT
Spleen Ø7BP
Sternum ØPBØ
Stomach ØDB6
Pylorus ØDB7
Subcutaneous Tissue and Fascia
Abdomen ØJB8
Back ØJB7
Buttock ØJB9
Chest ØJB6
Face ØJB1
Foot
Left ØJBR
Right ØJBQ
Hand
Left ØJBK
Right ØJBJ
Lower Arm
Left ØJBH
Right ØJBG

Subterms under main terms may continue to next column or page

Excision — *continued*
Subcutaneous Tissue and Fascia — *continued*
Lower Leg
Left ØJBP
Right ØJBN
Neck
Left ØJB5
Right ØJB4
Pelvic Region ØJBC
Perineum ØJBB
Scalp ØJBØ
Upper Arm
Left ØJBF
Right ØJBD
Upper Leg
Left ØJBM
Right ØJBL
Tarsal
Left ØQBM
Right ØQBL
Tendon
Abdomen
Left ØLBG
Right ØLBF
Ankle
Left ØLBT
Right ØLBS
Foot
Left ØLBW
Right ØLBV
Hand
Left ØLB8
Right ØLB7
Head and Neck ØLBØ
Hip
Left ØLBK
Right ØLBJ
Knee
Left ØLBR
Right ØLBQ
Lower Arm and Wrist
Left ØLB6
Right ØLB5
Lower Leg
Left ØLBP
Right ØLBN
Perineum ØLBH
Shoulder
Left ØLB2
Right ØLB1
Thorax
Left ØLBD
Right ØLBC
Trunk
Left ØLBB
Right ØLB9
Upper Arm
Left ØLB4
Right ØLB3
Upper Leg
Left ØLBM
Right ØLBL
Testis
Bilateral ØVBC
Left ØVBB
Right ØVB9
Thalamus ØØB9
Thymus Ø7BM
Thyroid Gland
Left Lobe ØGBG
Right Lobe ØGBH
Thyroid Gland Isthmus ØGBJ
Tibia
Left ØQBH
Right ØQBG
Toe Nail ØHBRXZ
Tongue ØCB7
Tonsils ØCBP
Tooth
Lower ØCBX
Upper ØCBW
Trachea ØBB1
Tunica Vaginalis
Left ØVB7
Right ØVB6
Turbinate, Nasal Ø9BL
Tympanic Membrane
Left Ø9B8
Right Ø9B7

Excision — *continued*
Ulna
Left ØPBL
Right ØPBK
Ureter
Left ØTB7
Right ØTB6
Urethra ØTBD
Uterine Supporting Structure ØUB4
Uterus ØUB9
Uvula ØCBN
Vagina ØUBG
Valve
Aortic Ø2BF
Mitral Ø2BG
Pulmonary Ø2BH
Tricuspid Ø2BJ
Vas Deferens
Bilateral ØVBQ
Left ØVBP
Right ØVBN
Vein
Axillary
Left Ø5B8
Right Ø5B7
Azygos Ø5BØ
Basilic
Left Ø5BC
Right Ø5BB
Brachial
Left Ø5BA
Right Ø5B9
Cephalic
Left Ø5BF
Right Ø5BD
Colic Ø6B7
Common Iliac
Left Ø6BD
Right Ø6BC
Coronary Ø2B4
Esophageal Ø6B3
External Iliac
Left Ø6BG
Right Ø6BF
External Jugular
Left Ø5BQ
Right Ø5BP
Face
Left Ø5BV
Right Ø5BT
Femoral
Left Ø6BN
Right Ø6BM
Foot
Left Ø6BV
Right Ø6BT
Gastric Ø6B2
Hand
Left Ø5BH
Right Ø5BG
Hemiazygos Ø5B1
Hepatic Ø6B4
Hypogastric
Left Ø6BJ
Right Ø6BH
Inferior Mesenteric Ø6B6
Innominate
Left Ø5B4
Right Ø5B3
Internal Jugular
Left Ø5BN
Right Ø5BM
Intracranial Ø5BL
Lower Ø6BY
Portal Ø6B8
Pulmonary
Left Ø2BT
Right Ø2BS
Renal
Left Ø6BB
Right Ø6B9
Saphenous
Left Ø6BQ
Right Ø6BP
Splenic Ø6B1
Subclavian
Left Ø5B6
Right Ø5B5
Superior Mesenteric Ø6B5

Excision — *continued*
Vein — *continued*
Upper Ø5BY
Vertebral
Left Ø5BS
Right Ø5BR
Vena Cava
Inferior Ø6BØ
Superior Ø2BV
Ventricle
Left Ø2BL
Right Ø2BK
Vertebra
Cervical ØPB3
Lumbar ØQBØ
Thoracic ØPB4
Vesicle
Bilateral ØVB3
Left ØVB2
Right ØVB1
Vitreous
Left Ø8B53Z
Right Ø8B43Z
Vocal Cord
Left ØCBV
Right ØCBT
Vulva ØUBM
Wrist Region
Left ØXBH
Right ØXBG
EXCLUDER® AAA Endoprosthesis
use Intraluminal Device
use Intraluminal Device, Branched or Fenestrated, One or Two Arteries in Ø4V
use Intraluminal Device, Branched or Fenestrated, Three or More Arteries in Ø4V
EXCLUDER® IBE Endoprosthesis *use* Intraluminal Device, Branched or Fenestrated, One or Two Arteries in Ø4V
Exclusion, Left atrial appendage (LAA) *see* Occlusion, Atrium, Left Ø2L7
Exercise, rehabilitation *see* Motor Treatment, Rehabilitation FØ7
Exploration *see* Inspection
Express® Biliary SD Monorail® Premounted Stent System *use* Intraluminal Device
Express® (LD) Premounted Stent System *use* Intraluminal Device
Express® SD Renal Monorail® Premounted Stent System *use* Intraluminal Device
Ex-PRESS™ mini glaucoma shunt *use* Synthetic Substitute
Extensor carpi radialis muscle
use Lower Arm and Wrist Muscle, Left
use Lower Arm and Wrist Muscle, Right
Extensor carpi ulnaris muscle
use Lower Arm and Wrist Muscle, Left
use Lower Arm and Wrist Muscle, Right
Extensor digitorum brevis muscle
use Foot Muscle, Left
use Foot Muscle, Right
Extensor digitorum longus muscle
use Lower Leg Muscle, Left
use Lower Leg Muscle, Right
Extensor hallucis brevis muscle
use Foot Muscle, Left
use Foot Muscle, Right
Extensor hallucis longus muscle
use Lower Leg Muscle, Left
use Lower Leg Muscle, Right
External anal sphincter *use* Anal Sphincter
External auditory meatus
use External Auditory Canal, Left
use External Auditory Canal, Right
External fixator
use External Fixation Device in Head and Facial Bones
use External Fixation Device in Lower Bones
use External Fixation Device in Lower Joints
use External Fixation Device in Upper Bones
use External Fixation Device in Upper Joints
External maxillary artery *use* Face Artery
External naris *use* Nasal Mucosa and Soft Tissue
External oblique aponeurosis *use* Subcutaneous Tissue and Fascia, Trunk
External oblique muscle
use Abdomen Muscle, Left

Subterms under main terms may continue to next column or page

External oblique muscle — *continued*
use Abdomen Muscle, Right
External popliteal nerve *use* Peroneal Nerve
External pudendal artery
use Femoral Artery, Left
use Femoral Artery, Right
External pudendal vein
use Saphenous Vein, Left
use Saphenous Vein, Right
External urethral sphincter *use* Urethra
Extirpation
Acetabulum
Left ØQC5
Right ØQC4
Adenoids ØCCQ
Ampulla of Vater ØFCC
Anal Sphincter ØDCR
Anterior Chamber
Left Ø8C3
Right Ø8C2
Anus ØDCQ
Aorta
Abdominal Ø4CØ
Thoracic
Ascending/Arch Ø2CX
Descending Ø2CW
Aortic Body ØGCD
Appendix ØDCJ
Artery
Anterior Tibial
Left Ø4CQ
Right Ø4CP
Axillary
Left Ø3C6
Right Ø3C5
Brachial
Left Ø3C8
Right Ø3C7
Celiac Ø4C1
Colic
Left Ø4C7
Middle Ø4C8
Right Ø4C6
Common Carotid
Left Ø3CJ
Right Ø3CH
Common Iliac
Left Ø4CD
Right Ø4CC
Coronary
Four or More Arteries Ø2C3
One Artery Ø2CØ
Three Arteries Ø2C2
Two Arteries Ø2C1
External Carotid
Left Ø3CN
Right Ø3CM
External Iliac
Left Ø4CJ
Right Ø4CH
Face Ø3CR
Femoral
Left Ø4CL
Right Ø4CK
Foot
Left Ø4CW
Right Ø4CV
Gastric Ø4C2
Hand
Left Ø3CF
Right Ø3CD
Hepatic Ø4C3
Inferior Mesenteric Ø4CB
Innominate Ø3C2
Internal Carotid
Left Ø3CL
Right Ø3CK
Internal Iliac
Left Ø4CF
Right Ø4CE
Internal Mammary
Left Ø3C1
Right Ø3CØ
Intracranial Ø3CG
Lower Ø4CY
Peroneal
Left Ø4CU
Right Ø4CT

Extirpation — *continued*
Artery — *continued*
Popliteal
Left Ø4CN
Right Ø4CM
Posterior Tibial
Left Ø4CS
Right Ø4CR
Pulmonary
Left Ø2CR
Right Ø2CQ
Pulmonary Trunk Ø2CP
Radial
Left Ø3CC
Right Ø3CB
Renal
Left Ø4CA
Right Ø4C9
Splenic Ø4C4
Subclavian
Left Ø3C4
Right Ø3C3
Superior Mesenteric Ø4C5
Temporal
Left Ø3CT
Right Ø3CS
Thyroid
Left Ø3CV
Right Ø3CU
Ulnar
Left Ø3CA
Right Ø3C9
Upper Ø3CY
Vertebral
Left Ø3CQ
Right Ø3CP
Atrium
Left Ø2C7
Right Ø2C6
Auditory Ossicle
Left Ø9CA
Right Ø9C9
Basal Ganglia ØØC8
Bladder ØTCB
Bladder Neck ØTCC
Bone
Ethmoid
Left ØNCG
Right ØNCF
Frontal ØNC1
Hyoid ØNCX
Lacrimal
Left ØNCJ
Right ØNCH
Nasal ØNCB
Occipital ØNC7
Palatine
Left ØNCL
Right ØNCK
Parietal
Left ØNC4
Right ØNC3
Pelvic
Left ØQC3
Right ØQC2
Sphenoid ØNCC
Temporal
Left ØNC6
Right ØNC5
Zygomatic
Left ØNCN
Right ØNCM
Brain ØØCØ
Breast
Bilateral ØHCV
Left ØHCU
Right ØHCT
Bronchus
Lingula ØBC9
Lower Lobe
Left ØBCB
Right ØBC6
Main
Left ØBC7
Right ØBC3
Middle Lobe, Right ØBC5
Upper Lobe
Left ØBC8
Right ØBC4

Extirpation — *continued*
Buccal Mucosa ØCC4
Bursa and Ligament
Abdomen
Left ØMCJ
Right ØMCH
Ankle
Left ØMCR
Right ØMCQ
Elbow
Left ØMC4
Right ØMC3
Foot
Left ØMCT
Right ØMCS
Hand
Left ØMC8
Right ØMC7
Head and Neck ØMCØ
Hip
Left ØMCM
Right ØMCL
Knee
Left ØMCP
Right ØMCN
Lower Extremity
Left ØMCW
Right ØMCV
Perineum ØMCK
Rib(s) ØMCG
Shoulder
Left ØMC2
Right ØMC1
Spine
Lower ØMCD
Upper ØMCC
Sternum ØMCF
Upper Extremity
Left ØMCB
Right ØMC9
Wrist
Left ØMC6
Right ØMC5
Carina ØBC2
Carotid Bodies, Bilateral ØGC8
Carotid Body
Left ØGC6
Right ØGC7
Carpal
Left ØPCN
Right ØPCM
Cavity, Cranial ØWC1
Cecum ØDCH
Cerebellum ØØCC
Cerebral Hemisphere ØØC7
Cerebral Meninges ØØC1
Cerebral Ventricle ØØC6
Cervix ØUCC
Chordae Tendineae Ø2C9
Choroid
Left Ø8CB
Right Ø8CA
Cisterna Chyli Ø7CL
Clavicle
Left ØPCB
Right ØPC9
Clitoris ØUCJ
Coccygeal Glomus ØGCB
Coccyx ØQCS
Colon
Ascending ØDCK
Descending ØDCM
Sigmoid ØDCN
Transverse ØDCL
Computer-aided Mechanical Aspiration X2C
Conduction Mechanism Ø2C8
Conjunctiva
Left Ø8CTXZZ
Right Ø8CSXZZ
Cord
Bilateral ØVCH
Left ØVCG
Right ØVCF
Cornea
Left Ø8C9XZZ
Right Ø8C8XZZ
Cul-de-sac ØUCF
Diaphragm ØBCT

Extirpation — *continued*
Disc
Cervical Vertebral ØRC3
Cervicothoracic Vertebral ØRC5
Lumbar Vertebral ØSC2
Lumbosacral ØSC4
Thoracic Vertebral ØRC9
Thoracolumbar Vertebral ØRCB
Duct
Common Bile ØFC9
Cystic ØFC8
Hepatic
Common ØFC7
Left ØFC6
Right ØFC5
Lacrimal
Left Ø8CY
Right Ø8CX
Pancreatic ØFCD
Accessory ØFCF
Parotid
Left ØCCC
Right ØCCB
Duodenum ØDC9
Dura Mater ØØC2
Ear
External
Left Ø9C1
Right Ø9CØ
External Auditory Canal
Left Ø9C4
Right Ø9C3
Inner
Left Ø9CE
Right Ø9CD
Middle
Left Ø9C6
Right Ø9C5
Endometrium ØUCB
Epididymis
Bilateral ØVCL
Left ØVCK
Right ØVCJ
Epidural Space, Intracranial ØØC3
Epiglottis ØCCR
Esophagogastric Junction ØDC4
Esophagus ØDC5
Lower ØDC3
Middle ØDC2
Upper ØDC1
Eustachian Tube
Left Ø9CG
Right Ø9CF
Eye
Left Ø8C1XZZ
Right Ø8CØXZZ
Eyelid
Lower
Left Ø8CR
Right Ø8CQ
Upper
Left Ø8CP
Right Ø8CN
Fallopian Tube
Left ØUC6
Right ØUC5
Fallopian Tubes, Bilateral ØUC7
Femoral Shaft
Left ØQC9
Right ØQC8
Femur
Lower
Left ØQCC
Right ØQCB
Upper
Left ØQC7
Right ØQC6
Fibula
Left ØQCK
Right ØQCJ
Finger Nail ØHCQXZZ
Gallbladder ØFC4
Gastrointestinal Tract ØWCP
Genitourinary Tract ØWCR
Gingiva
Lower ØCC6
Upper ØCC5

Extirpation — *continued*
Gland
Adrenal
Bilateral ØGC4
Left ØGC2
Right ØGC3
Lacrimal
Left Ø8CW
Right Ø8CV
Minor Salivary ØCCJ
Parotid
Left ØCC9
Right ØCC8
Pituitary ØGCØ
Sublingual
Left ØCCF
Right ØCCD
Submaxillary
Left ØCCH
Right ØCCG
Vestibular ØUCL
Glenoid Cavity
Left ØPC8
Right ØPC7
Glomus Jugulare ØGCC
Humeral Head
Left ØPCD
Right ØPCC
Humeral Shaft
Left ØPCG
Right ØPCF
Hymen ØUCK
Hypothalamus ØØCA
Ileocecal Valve ØDCC
Ileum ØDCB
Intestine
Large ØDCE
Left ØDCG
Right ØDCF
Small ØDC8
Iris
Left Ø8CD
Right Ø8CC
Jaw
Lower ØWC5
Upper ØWC4
Jejunum ØDCA
Joint
Acromioclavicular
Left ØRCH
Right ØRCG
Ankle
Left ØSCG
Right ØSCF
Carpal
Left ØRCR
Right ØRCQ
Carpometacarpal
Left ØRCT
Right ØRCS
Cervical Vertebral ØRC1
Cervicothoracic Vertebral ØRC4
Coccygeal ØSC6
Elbow
Left ØRCM
Right ØRCL
Finger Phalangeal
Left ØRCX
Right ØRCW
Hip
Left ØSCB
Right ØSC9
Knee
Left ØSCD
Right ØSCC
Lumbar Vertebral ØSCØ
Lumbosacral ØSC3
Metacarpophalangeal
Left ØRCV
Right ØRCU
Metatarsal-Phalangeal
Left ØSCN
Right ØSCM
Occipital-cervical ØRCØ
Sacrococcygeal ØSC5
Sacroiliac
Left ØSC8
Right ØSC7

Extirpation — *continued*
Joint — *continued*
Shoulder
Left ØRCK
Right ØRCJ
Sternoclavicular
Left ØRCF
Right ØRCE
Tarsal
Left ØSCJ
Right ØSCH
Tarsometatarsal
Left ØSCL
Right ØSCK
Temporomandibular
Left ØRCD
Right ØRCC
Thoracic Vertebral ØRC6
Thoracolumbar Vertebral ØRCA
Toe Phalangeal
Left ØSCQ
Right ØSCP
Wrist
Left ØRCP
Right ØRCN
Kidney
Left ØTC1
Right ØTCØ
Kidney Pelvis
Left ØTC4
Right ØTC3
Larynx ØCCS
Lens
Left Ø8CK
Right Ø8CJ
Lip
Lower ØCC1
Upper ØCCØ
Liver ØFCØ
Left Lobe ØFC2
Right Lobe ØFC1
Lung
Bilateral ØBCM
Left ØBCL
Lower Lobe
Left ØBCJ
Right ØBCF
Middle Lobe, Right ØBCD
Right ØBCK
Upper Lobe
Left ØBCG
Right ØBCC
Lung Lingula ØBCH
Lymphatic
Aortic Ø7CD
Axillary
Left Ø7C6
Right Ø7C5
Head Ø7CØ
Inguinal
Left Ø7CJ
Right Ø7CH
Internal Mammary
Left Ø7C9
Right Ø7C8
Lower Extremity
Left Ø7CG
Right Ø7CF
Mesenteric Ø7CB
Neck
Left Ø7C2
Right Ø7C1
Pelvis Ø7CC
Thoracic Duct Ø7CK
Thorax Ø7C7
Upper Extremity
Left Ø7C4
Right Ø7C3
Mandible
Left ØNCV
Right ØNCT
Maxilla ØNCR
Mediastinum ØWCC
Medulla Oblongata ØØCD
Mesentery ØDCV
Metacarpal
Left ØPCQ
Right ØPCP

Extirpation — *continued*
Metatarsal
Left ØQCP
Right ØQCN
Muscle
Abdomen
Left ØKCL
Right ØKCK
Extraocular
Left Ø8CM
Right Ø8CL
Facial ØKC1
Foot
Left ØKCW
Right ØKCV
Hand
Left ØKCD
Right ØKCC
Head ØKCØ
Hip
Left ØKCP
Right ØKCN
Lower Arm and Wrist
Left ØKCB
Right ØKC9
Lower Leg
Left ØKCT
Right ØKCS
Neck
Left ØKC3
Right ØKC2
Papillary Ø2CD
Perineum ØKCM
Shoulder
Left ØKC6
Right ØKC5
Thorax
Left ØKCJ
Right ØKCH
Tongue, Palate, Pharynx ØKC4
Trunk
Left ØKCG
Right ØKCF
Upper Arm
Left ØKC8
Right ØKC7
Upper Leg
Left ØKCR
Right ØKCQ
Nasal Mucosa and Soft Tissue Ø9CK
Nasopharynx Ø9CN
Nerve
Abdominal Sympathetic Ø1CM
Abducens ØØCL
Accessory ØØCR
Acoustic ØØCN
Brachial Plexus Ø1C3
Cervical Ø1C1
Cervical Plexus Ø1CØ
Facial ØØCM
Femoral Ø1CD
Glossopharyngeal ØØCP
Head and Neck Sympathetic Ø1CK
Hypoglossal ØØCS
Lumbar Ø1CB
Lumbar Plexus Ø1C9
Lumbar Sympathetic Ø1CN
Lumbosacral Plexus Ø1CA
Median Ø1C5
Oculomotor ØØCH
Olfactory ØØCF
Optic ØØCG
Peroneal Ø1CH
Phrenic Ø1C2
Pudendal Ø1CC
Radial Ø1C6
Sacral Ø1CR
Sacral Plexus Ø1CQ
Sacral Sympathetic Ø1CP
Sciatic Ø1CF
Thoracic Ø1C8
Thoracic Sympathetic Ø1CL
Tibial Ø1CG
Trigeminal ØØCK
Trochlear ØØCJ
Ulnar Ø1C4
Vagus ØØCQ
Nipple
Left ØHCX

Extirpation — *continued*
Nipple — *continued*
Right ØHCW
Omentum ØDCU
Oral Cavity and Throat ØWC3
Orbit
Left ØNCQ
Right ØNCP
Orbital Atherectomy *see* Extirpation, Heart and Great Vessels Ø2C
Ovary
Bilateral ØUC2
Left ØUC1
Right ØUCØ
Palate
Hard ØCC2
Soft ØCC3
Pancreas ØFCG
Para-aortic Body ØGC9
Paraganglion Extremity ØGCF
Parathyroid Gland ØGCR
Inferior
Left ØGCP
Right ØGCN
Multiple ØGCQ
Superior
Left ØGCM
Right ØGCL
Patella
Left ØQCF
Right ØQCD
Pelvic Cavity ØWCJ
Penis ØVCS
Pericardial Cavity ØWCD
Pericardium Ø2CN
Peritoneal Cavity ØWCG
Peritoneum ØDCW
Phalanx
Finger
Left ØPCV
Right ØPCT
Thumb
Left ØPCS
Right ØPCR
Toe
Left ØQCR
Right ØQCQ
Pharynx ØCCM
Pineal Body ØGC1
Pleura
Left ØBCP
Right ØBCN
Pleural Cavity
Left ØWCB
Right ØWC9
Pons ØØCB
Prepuce ØVCT
Prostate ØVCØ
Radius
Left ØPCJ
Right ØPCH
Rectum ØDCP
Respiratory Tract ØWCQ
Retina
Left Ø8CF
Right Ø8CE
Retinal Vessel
Left Ø8CH
Right Ø8CG
Retroperitoneum ØWCH
Ribs
1 to 2 ØPC1
3 or More ØPC2
Sacrum ØQC1
Scapula
Left ØPC6
Right ØPC5
Sclera
Left Ø8C7XZZ
Right Ø8C6XZZ
Scrotum ØVC5
Septum
Atrial Ø2C5
Nasal Ø9CM
Ventricular Ø2CM
Sinus
Accessory Ø9CP
Ethmoid
Left Ø9CV

Extirpation — *continued*
Sinus — *continued*
Ethmoid — *continued*
Right Ø9CU
Frontal
Left Ø9CT
Right Ø9CS
Mastoid
Left Ø9CC
Right Ø9CB
Maxillary
Left Ø9CR
Right Ø9CQ
Sphenoid
Left Ø9CX
Right Ø9CW
Skin
Abdomen ØHC7XZZ
Back ØHC6XZZ
Buttock ØHC8XZZ
Chest ØHC5XZZ
Ear
Left ØHC3XZZ
Right ØHC2XZZ
Face ØHC1XZZ
Foot
Left ØHCNXZZ
Right ØHCMXZZ
Hand
Left ØHCGXZZ
Right ØHCFXZZ
Inguinal ØHCAXZZ
Lower Arm
Left ØHCEXZZ
Right ØHCDXZZ
Lower Leg
Left ØHCLXZZ
Right ØHCKXZZ
Neck ØHC4XZZ
Perineum ØHC9XZZ
Scalp ØHCØXZZ
Upper Arm
Left ØHCCXZZ
Right ØHCBXZZ
Upper Leg
Left ØHCJXZZ
Right ØHCHXZZ
Spinal Canal ØØCU
Spinal Cord
Cervical ØØCW
Lumbar ØØCY
Thoracic ØØCX
Spinal Meninges ØØCT
Spleen Ø7CP
Sternum ØPCØ
Stomach ØDC6
Pylorus ØDC7
Subarachnoid Space, Intracranial ØØC5
Subcutaneous Tissue and Fascia
Abdomen ØJC8
Back ØJC7
Buttock ØJC9
Chest ØJC6
Face ØJC1
Foot
Left ØJCR
Right ØJCQ
Hand
Left ØJCK
Right ØJCJ
Lower Arm
Left ØJCH
Right ØJCG
Lower Leg
Left ØJCP
Right ØJCN
Neck
Left ØJC5
Right ØJC4
Pelvic Region ØJCC
Perineum ØJCB
Scalp ØJCØ
Upper Arm
Left ØJCF
Right ØJCD
Upper Leg
Left ØJCM
Right ØJCL
Subdural Space, Intracranial ØØC4

Index
Extirpation — Extirpation

Extirpation — *continued*
- Tarsal
  - Left ØQCM
  - Right ØQCL
- Tendon
  - Abdomen
    - Left ØLCG
    - Right ØLCF
  - Ankle
    - Left ØLCT
    - Right ØLCS
  - Foot
    - Left ØLCW
    - Right ØLCV
  - Hand
    - Left ØLC8
    - Right ØLC7
  - Head and Neck ØLCØ
  - Hip
    - Left ØLCK
    - Right ØLCJ
  - Knee
    - Left ØLCR
    - Right ØLCQ
  - Lower Arm and Wrist
    - Left ØLC6
    - Right ØLC5
  - Lower Leg
    - Left ØLCP
    - Right ØLCN
  - Perineum ØLCH
  - Shoulder
    - Left ØLC2
    - Right ØLC1
  - Thorax
    - Left ØLCD
    - Right ØLCC
  - Trunk
    - Left ØLCB
    - Right ØLC9
  - Upper Arm
    - Left ØLC4
    - Right ØLC3
  - Upper Leg
    - Left ØLCM
    - Right ØLCL
- Testis
  - Bilateral ØVCC
  - Left ØVCB
  - Right ØVC9
- Thalamus ØØC9
- Thymus Ø7CM
- Thyroid Gland ØGCK
  - Left Lobe ØGCG
  - Right Lobe ØGCH
- Tibia
  - Left ØQCH
  - Right ØQCG
- Toe Nail ØHCRXZZ
- Tongue ØCC7
- Tonsils ØCCP
- Tooth
  - Lower ØCCX
  - Upper ØCCW
- Trachea ØBC1
- Tunica Vaginalis
  - Left ØVC7
  - Right ØVC6
- Turbinate, Nasal Ø9CL
- Tympanic Membrane
  - Left Ø9C8
  - Right Ø9C7
- Ulna
  - Left ØPCL
  - Right ØPCK
- Ureter
  - Left ØTC7
  - Right ØTC6
- Urethra ØTCD
- Uterine Supporting Structure ØUC4
- Uterus ØUC9
- Uvula ØCCN
- Vagina ØUCG
- Valve
  - Aortic Ø2CF
  - Mitral Ø2CG
  - Pulmonary Ø2CH
  - Tricuspid Ø2CJ

Extirpation — *continued*
- Vas Deferens
  - Bilateral ØVCQ
  - Left ØVCP
  - Right ØVCN
- Vein
  - Axillary
    - Left Ø5C8
    - Right Ø5C7
  - Azygos Ø5CØ
  - Basilic
    - Left Ø5CC
    - Right Ø5CB
  - Brachial
    - Left Ø5CA
    - Right Ø5C9
  - Cephalic
    - Left Ø5CF
    - Right Ø5CD
  - Colic Ø6C7
  - Common Iliac
    - Left Ø6CD
    - Right Ø6CC
  - Coronary Ø2C4
  - Esophageal Ø6C3
  - External Iliac
    - Left Ø6CG
    - Right Ø6CF
  - External Jugular
    - Left Ø5CQ
    - Right Ø5CP
  - Face
    - Left Ø5CV
    - Right Ø5CT
  - Femoral
    - Left Ø6CN
    - Right Ø6CM
  - Foot
    - Left Ø6CV
    - Right Ø6CT
  - Gastric Ø6C2
  - Hand
    - Left Ø5CH
    - Right Ø5CG
  - Hemiazygos Ø5C1
  - Hepatic Ø6C4
  - Hypogastric
    - Left Ø6CJ
    - Right Ø6CH
  - Inferior Mesenteric Ø6C6
  - Innominate
    - Left Ø5C4
    - Right Ø5C3
  - Internal Jugular
    - Left Ø5CN
    - Right Ø5CM
  - Intracranial Ø5CL
  - Lower Ø6CY
  - Portal Ø6C8
  - Pulmonary
    - Left Ø2CT
    - Right Ø2CS
  - Renal
    - Left Ø6CB
    - Right Ø6C9
  - Saphenous
    - Left Ø6CQ
    - Right Ø6CP
  - Splenic Ø6C1
  - Subclavian
    - Left Ø5C6
    - Right Ø5C5
  - Superior Mesenteric Ø6C5
  - Upper Ø5CY
  - Vertebral
    - Left Ø5CS
    - Right Ø5CR
- Vena Cava
  - Inferior Ø6CØ
  - Superior Ø2CV
- Ventricle
  - Left Ø2CL
  - Right Ø2CK
- Vertebra
  - Cervical ØPC3
  - Lumbar ØQCØ
  - Thoracic ØPC4
- Vesicle
  - Bilateral ØVC3

Extirpation — *continued*
- Vesicle — *continued*
  - Left ØVC2
  - Right ØVC1
- Vitreous
  - Left Ø8C5
  - Right Ø8C4
- Vocal Cord
  - Left ØCCV
  - Right ØCCT
- Vulva ØUCM

Extracorporeal Carbon Dioxide Removal (ECCO2R) 5AØ92ØZ

Extracorporeal shock wave lithotripsy *see* Fragmentation

Extracranial-intracranial bypass (EC-IC) *see* Bypass, Upper Arteries Ø31

Extraction
- Acetabulum
  - Left ØQD5ØZZ
  - Right ØQD4ØZZ
- Ampulla of Vater ØFDC
- Anus ØDDQ
- Appendix ØDDJ
- Auditory Ossicle
  - Left Ø9DAØZZ
  - Right Ø9D9ØZZ
- Bone
  - Ethmoid
    - Left ØNDGØZZ
    - Right ØNDFØZZ
  - Frontal ØND1ØZZ
  - Hyoid ØNDXØZZ
  - Lacrimal
    - Left ØNDJØZZ
    - Right ØNDHØZZ
  - Nasal ØNDBØZZ
  - Occipital ØND7ØZZ
  - Palatine
    - Left ØNDLØZZ
    - Right ØNDKØZZ
  - Parietal
    - Left ØND4ØZZ
    - Right ØND3ØZZ
  - Pelvic
    - Left ØQD3ØZZ
    - Right ØQD2ØZZ
  - Sphenoid ØNDCØZZ
  - Temporal
    - Left ØND6ØZZ
    - Right ØND5ØZZ
  - Zygomatic
    - Left ØNDNØZZ
    - Right ØNDMØZZ
- Bone Marrow Ø7DT
  - Iliac Ø7DR
  - Sternum Ø7DQ
  - Vertebral Ø7DS
- Brain ØØDØ
- Breast
  - Bilateral ØHDVØZZ
  - Left ØHDUØZZ
  - Right ØHDTØZZ
  - Supernumerary ØHDYØZZ
- Bronchus
  - Lingula ØBD9
  - Lower Lobe
    - Left ØBDB
    - Right ØBD6
  - Main
    - Left ØBD7
    - Right ØBD3
  - Middle Lobe, Right ØBD5
  - Upper Lobe
    - Left ØBD8
    - Right ØBD4
- Bursa and Ligament
  - Abdomen
    - Left ØMDJ
    - Right ØMDH
  - Ankle
    - Left ØMDR
    - Right ØMDQ
  - Elbow
    - Left ØMD4
    - Right ØMD3
  - Foot
    - Left ØMDT
    - Right ØMDS

Extraction — *continued*
- Bursa and Ligament — *continued*
  - Hand
    - Left ØMD8
    - Right ØMD7
  - Head and Neck ØMDØ
  - Hip
    - Left ØMDM
    - Right ØMDL
  - Knee
    - Left ØMDP
    - Right ØMDN
  - Lower Extremity
    - Left ØMDW
    - Right ØMDV
  - Perineum ØMDK
  - Rib(s) ØMDG
  - Shoulder
    - Left ØMD2
    - Right ØMD1
  - Spine
    - Lower ØMDD
    - Upper ØMDC
  - Sternum ØMDF
  - Upper Extremity
    - Left ØMDB
    - Right ØMD9
  - Wrist
    - Left ØMD6
    - Right ØMD5
- Carina ØBD2
- Carpal
  - Left ØPDNØZZ
  - Right ØPDMØZZ
- Cecum ØDDH
- Cerebral Hemisphere ØØD7
- Cerebral Meninges ØØD1
- Cisterna Chyli Ø7DL
- Clavicle
  - Left ØPDBØZZ
  - Right ØPD9ØZZ
- Coccyx ØQDSØZZ
- Colon
  - Ascending ØDDK
  - Descending ØDDM
  - Sigmoid ØDDN
  - Transverse ØDDL
- Cornea
  - Left Ø8D9XZ
  - Right Ø8D8XZ
- Duct
  - Common Bile ØFD9
  - Cystic ØFD8
  - Hepatic
    - Common ØFD7
    - Left ØFD6
    - Right ØFD5
  - Pancreatic ØFDD
    - Accessory ØFDF
- Duodenum ØDD9
- Dura Mater ØØD2
- Endometrium ØUDB
- Esophagogastric Junction ØDD4
- Esophagus ØDD5
  - Lower ØDD3
  - Middle ØDD2
  - Upper ØDD1
- Femoral Shaft
  - Left ØQD9ØZZ
  - Right ØQD8ØZZ
- Femur
  - Lower
    - Left ØQDCØZZ
    - Right ØQDBØZZ
  - Upper
    - Left ØQD7ØZZ
    - Right ØQD6ØZZ
- Fibula
  - Left ØQDKØZZ
  - Right ØQDJØZZ
- Finger Nail ØHDQXZZ
- Gallbladder ØFD4
- Glenoid Cavity
  - Left ØPD8ØZZ
  - Right ØPD7ØZZ
- Hair ØHDSXZZ
- Humeral Head
  - Left ØPDDØZZ
  - Right ØPDCØZZ

Extraction — *continued*
- Humeral Shaft
  - Left ØPDGØZZ
  - Right ØPDFØZZ
- Ileocecal Valve ØDDC
- Ileum ØDDB
- Intestine
  - Large ØDDE
    - Left ØDDG
    - Right ØDDF
  - Small ØDD8
- Jejunum ØDDA
- Kidney
  - Left ØTD1
  - Right ØTDØ
- Lens
  - Left Ø8DK3ZZ
  - Right Ø8DJ3ZZ
- Liver ØFDØ
  - Left Lobe ØFD2
  - Right Lobe ØFD1
- Lung
  - Bilateral ØBDM
  - Left ØBDL
  - Lower Lobe
    - Left ØBDJ
    - Right ØBDF
  - Middle Lobe, Right ØBDD
  - Right ØBDK
  - Upper Lobe
    - Left ØBDG
    - Right ØBDC
- Lung Lingula ØBDH
- Lymphatic
  - Aortic Ø7DD
  - Axillary
    - Left Ø7D6
    - Right Ø7D5
  - Head Ø7DØ
  - Inguinal
    - Left Ø7DJ
    - Right Ø7DH
  - Internal Mammary
    - Left Ø7D9
    - Right Ø7D8
  - Lower Extremity
    - Left Ø7DG
    - Right Ø7DF
  - Mesenteric Ø7DB
  - Neck
    - Left Ø7D2
    - Right Ø7D1
  - Pelvis Ø7DC
  - Thoracic Duct Ø7DK
  - Thorax Ø7D7
  - Upper Extremity
    - Left Ø7D4
    - Right Ø7D3
- Mandible
  - Left ØNDVØZZ
  - Right ØNDTØZZ
- Maxilla ØNDRØZZ
- Metacarpal
  - Left ØPDQØZZ
  - Right ØPDPØZZ
- Metatarsal
  - Left ØQDPØZZ
  - Right ØQDNØZZ
- Muscle
  - Abdomen
    - Left ØKDLØZZ
    - Right ØKDKØZZ
  - Facial ØKD1ØZZ
  - Foot
    - Left ØKDWØZZ
    - Right ØKDVØZZ
  - Hand
    - Left ØKDDØZZ
    - Right ØKDCØZZ
  - Head ØKDØØZZ
  - Hip
    - Left ØKDPØZZ
    - Right ØKDNØZZ
  - Lower Arm and Wrist
    - Left ØKDBØZZ
    - Right ØKD9ØZZ
  - Lower Leg
    - Left ØKDTØZZ
    - Right ØKDSØZZ

Extraction — *continued*
- Muscle — *continued*
  - Neck
    - Left ØKD3ØZZ
    - Right ØKD2ØZZ
  - Perineum ØKDMØZZ
  - Shoulder
    - Left ØKD6ØZZ
    - Right ØKD5ØZZ
  - Thorax
    - Left ØKDJØZZ
    - Right ØKDHØZZ
  - Tongue, Palate, Pharynx ØKD4ØZZ
  - Trunk
    - Left ØKDGØZZ
    - Right ØKDFØZZ
  - Upper Arm
    - Left ØKD8ØZZ
    - Right ØKD7ØZZ
  - Upper Leg
    - Left ØKDRØZZ
    - Right ØKDQØZZ
- Nerve
  - Abdominal Sympathetic Ø1DM
  - Abducens ØØDL
  - Accessory ØØDR
  - Acoustic ØØDN
  - Brachial Plexus Ø1D3
  - Cervical Ø1D1
  - Cervical Plexus Ø1DØ
  - Facial ØØDM
  - Femoral Ø1DD
  - Glossopharyngeal ØØDP
  - Head and Neck Sympathetic Ø1DK
  - Hypoglossal ØØDS
  - Lumbar Ø1DB
  - Lumbar Plexus Ø1D9
  - Lumbar Sympathetic Ø1DN
  - Lumbosacral Plexus Ø1DA
  - Median Ø1D5
  - Oculomotor ØØDH
  - Olfactory ØØDF
  - Optic ØØDG
  - Peroneal Ø1DH
  - Phrenic Ø1D2
  - Pudendal Ø1DC
  - Radial Ø1D6
  - Sacral Ø1DR
  - Sacral Plexus Ø1DQ
  - Sacral Sympathetic Ø1DP
  - Sciatic Ø1DF
  - Thoracic Ø1D8
  - Thoracic Sympathetic Ø1DL
  - Tibial Ø1DG
  - Trigeminal ØØDK
  - Trochlear ØØDJ
  - Ulnar Ø1D4
  - Vagus ØØDQ
- Orbit
  - Left ØNDQØZZ
  - Right ØNDPØZZ
- Ova ØUDN
- Pancreas ØFDG
- Patella
  - Left ØQDFØZZ
  - Right ØQDDØZZ
- Phalanx
  - Finger
    - Left ØPDVØZZ
    - Right ØPDTØZZ
  - Thumb
    - Left ØPDSØZZ
    - Right ØPDRØZZ
  - Toe
    - Left ØQDRØZZ
    - Right ØQDQØZZ
- Pleura
  - Left ØBDP
  - Right ØBDN
- Products of Conception
  - Ectopic 1ØD2
  - Extraperitoneal 1ØDØØZ2
  - High 1ØDØØZØ
  - High Forceps 1ØDØ7Z5
  - Internal Version 1ØDØ7Z7
  - Low 1ØDØØZ1
  - Low Forceps 1ØDØ7Z3
  - Mid Forceps 1ØDØ7Z4
  - Other 1ØDØ7Z8

Extraction — *continued*
- Products of Conception — *continued*
  - Retained 1ØD1
  - Vacuum 1ØDØ7Z6
- Radius
  - Left ØPDJØZZ
  - Right ØPDHØZZ
- Rectum ØDDP
- Ribs
  - 1 to 2 ØPD1ØZZ
  - 3 or More ØPD2ØZZ
- Sacrum ØQD1ØZZ
- Scapula
  - Left ØPD6ØZZ
  - Right ØPD5ØZZ
- Septum, Nasal Ø9DM
- Sinus
  - Accessory Ø9DP
  - Ethmoid
    - Left Ø9DV
    - Right Ø9DU
  - Frontal
    - Left Ø9DT
    - Right Ø9DS
  - Mastoid
    - Left Ø9DC
    - Right Ø9DB
  - Maxillary
    - Left Ø9DR
    - Right Ø9DQ
  - Sphenoid
    - Left Ø9DX
    - Right Ø9DW
- Skin
  - Abdomen ØHD7XZZ
  - Back ØHD6XZZ
  - Buttock ØHD8XZZ
  - Chest ØHD5XZZ
  - Ear
    - Left ØHD3XZZ
    - Right ØHD2XZZ
  - Face ØHD1XZZ
  - Foot
    - Left ØHDNXZZ
    - Right ØHDMXZZ
  - Hand
    - Left ØHDGXZZ
    - Right ØHDFXZZ
  - Inguinal ØHDAXZZ
  - Lower Arm
    - Left ØHDEXZZ
    - Right ØHDDXZZ
  - Lower Leg
    - Left ØHDLXZZ
    - Right ØHDKXZZ
  - Neck ØHD4XZZ
  - Perineum ØHD9XZZ
  - Scalp ØHDØXZZ
  - Upper Arm
    - Left ØHDCXZZ
    - Right ØHDBXZZ
  - Upper Leg
    - Left ØHDJXZZ
    - Right ØHDHXZZ
- Skull ØNDØØZZ
- Spinal Meninges ØØDT
- Spleen Ø7DP
- Sternum ØPDØØZZ
- Stomach ØDD6
  - Pylorus ØDD7
- Subcutaneous Tissue and Fascia
  - Abdomen ØJD8
  - Back ØJD7
  - Buttock ØJD9
  - Chest ØJD6
  - Face ØJD1
  - Foot
    - Left ØJDR
    - Right ØJDQ
  - Hand
    - Left ØJDK
    - Right ØJDJ
  - Lower Arm
    - Left ØJDH
    - Right ØJDG
  - Lower Leg
    - Left ØJDP
    - Right ØJDN

Extraction — *continued*
- Subcutaneous Tissue and Fascia — *continued*
  - Neck
    - Left ØJD5
    - Right ØJD4
  - Pelvic Region ØJDC
  - Perineum ØJDB
  - Scalp ØJDØ
  - Upper Arm
    - Left ØJDF
    - Right ØJDD
  - Upper Leg
    - Left ØJDM
    - Right ØJDL
- Tarsal
  - Left ØQDMØZZ
  - Right ØQDLØZZ
- Tendon
  - Abdomen
    - Left ØLDGØZZ
    - Right ØLDFØZZ
  - Ankle
    - Left ØLDTØZZ
    - Right ØLDSØZZ
  - Foot
    - Left ØLDWØZZ
    - Right ØLDVØZZ
  - Hand
    - Left ØLD8ØZZ
    - Right ØLD7ØZZ
  - Head and Neck ØLDØØZZ
  - Hip
    - Left ØLDKØZZ
    - Right ØLDJØZZ
  - Knee
    - Left ØLDRØZZ
    - Right ØLDQØZZ
  - Lower Arm and Wrist
    - Left ØLD6ØZZ
    - Right ØLD5ØZZ
  - Lower Leg
    - Left ØLDPØZZ
    - Right ØLDNØZZ
  - Perineum ØLDHØZZ
  - Shoulder
    - Left ØLD2ØZZ
    - Right ØLD1ØZZ
  - Thorax
    - Left ØLDDØZZ
    - Right ØLDCØZZ
  - Trunk
    - Left ØLDBØZZ
    - Right ØLD9ØZZ
  - Upper Arm
    - Left ØLD4ØZZ
    - Right ØLD3ØZZ
  - Upper Leg
    - Left ØLDMØZZ
    - Right ØDLLØZZ
- Thymus Ø7DM
- Tibia
  - Left ØQDHØZZ
  - Right ØQDGØZZ
- Toe Nail ØHDRXZZ
- Tooth
  - Lower ØCDXXZ
  - Upper ØCDWXZ
- Trachea ØBD1
- Turbinate, Nasal Ø9DL
- Tympanic Membrane
  - Left Ø9D8
  - Right Ø9D7
- Ulna
  - Left ØPDLØZZ
  - Right ØPDKØZZ
- Vein
  - Basilic
    - Left Ø5DC
    - Right Ø5DB
  - Brachial
    - Left Ø5DA
    - Right Ø5D9
  - Cephalic
    - Left Ø5DF
    - Right Ø5DD
  - Femoral
    - Left Ø6DN
    - Right Ø6DM

Extraction — *continued*
- Vein — *continued*
  - Foot
    - Left Ø6DV
    - Right Ø6DT
  - Hand
    - Left Ø5DH
    - Right Ø5DG
  - Lower Ø6DY
  - Saphenous
    - Left Ø6DQ
    - Right Ø6DP
  - Upper Ø5DY
- Vertebra
  - Cervical ØPD3ØZZ
  - Lumbar ØQDØØZZ
  - Thoracic ØPD4ØZZ
- Vocal Cord
  - Left ØCDV
  - Right ØCDT

Extradural space, intracranial *use* Epidural Space, Intracranial

Extradural space, spinal *use* Spinal Canal

EXtreme Lateral Interbody Fusion (XLIF) device *use* Interbody Fusion Device in Lower Joints

F

Face lift *see* Alteration, Face ØWØ2

Facet replacement spinal stabilization device
- *use* Spinal Stabilization Device, Facet Replacement in ØRH
- *use* Spinal Stabilization Device, Facet Replacement in ØSH

Facial artery *use* Face Artery

Factor Xa Inhibitor Reversal Agent, Andexanet Alfa *use* Coagulation Factor Xa, Inactivated

False vocal cord *use* Larynx

Falx cerebri *use* Dura Mater

Fascia lata
- *use* Subcutaneous Tissue and Fascia, Left Upper Leg
- *use* Subcutaneous Tissue and Fascia, Right Upper Leg

Fasciaplasty, fascioplasty
- *see* Repair, Subcutaneous Tissue and Fascia ØJQ
- *see* Replacement, Subcutaneous Tissue and Fascia ØJR

Fasciectomy *see* Excision, Subcutaneous Tissue and Fascia ØJB

Fasciorrhaphy *see* Repair, Subcutaneous Tissue and Fascia ØJQ

Fasciotomy
- *see* Division, Subcutaneous Tissue and Fascia ØJ8
- *see* Drainage, Subcutaneous Tissue and Fascia ØJ9
- *see* Release

Feeding Device
- Change device in
  - Lower ØD2DXUZ
  - Upper ØD2ØXUZ
- Insertion of device in
  - Duodenum ØDH9
  - Esophagus ØDH5
  - Ileum ØDHB
  - Intestine, Small ØDH8
  - Jejunum ØDHA
  - Stomach ØDH6
- Removal of device from
  - Esophagus ØDP5
  - Intestinal Tract
    - Lower ØDPD
    - Upper ØDPØ
  - Stomach ØDP6
- Revision of device in
  - Intestinal Tract
    - Lower ØDWD
    - Upper ØDWØ
  - Stomach ØDW6

Femoral head
- *use* Upper Femur, Left
- *use* Upper Femur, Right

Femoral lymph node
- *use* Lymphatic, Left Lower Extremity
- *use* Lymphatic, Right Lower Extremity

Femoropatellar joint
- *use* Knee Joint, Left
- *use* Knee Joint, Left, Tibial Surface

Femoropatellar joint — *continued*
use Knee Joint, Right
use Knee Joint, Right, Femoral Surface
Femorotibial joint
use Knee Joint, Left
use Knee Joint, Left, Tibial Surface
use Knee Joint, Right
use Knee Joint, Right, Tibial Surface
FETROJA® *use* Cefiderocol Anti-infective
FGS (fluorescence-guided surgery) *see* Fluorescence Guided Procedure
Fibular artery
use Peroneal Artery, Left
use Peroneal Artery, Right
Fibular sesamoid
use Metatarsal, Left
use Metatarsal, Right
Fibularis brevis muscle
use Lower Leg Muscle, Left
use Lower Leg Muscle, Right
Fibularis longus muscle
use Lower Leg Muscle, Left
use Lower Leg Muscle, Right
Fifth cranial nerve *use* Trigeminal Nerve
Filum terminale *use* Spinal Meninges
Fimbriectomy
see Excision, Female Reproductive System ØUB
see Resection, Female Reproductive System ØUT
Fine needle aspiration
Fluid or gas *see* Drainage
Tissue biopsy
see Excision
see Extraction
First cranial nerve *use* Olfactory Nerve
First intercostal nerve *use* Brachial Plexus
Fistulization
see Bypass
see Drainage
see Repair
Fitting
Arch bars, for fracture reduction *see* Reposition, Mouth and Throat ØCS
Arch bars, for immobilization *see* Immobilization, Face 2W31
Artificial limb *see* Device Fitting, Rehabilitation FØD
Hearing aid *see* Device Fitting, Rehabilitation FØD
Ocular prosthesis FØDZ8UZ
Prosthesis, limb *see* Device Fitting, Rehabilitation FØD
Prosthesis, ocular FØDZ8UZ
Fixation, bone
External, with fracture reduction *see* Reposition
External, without fracture reduction *see* Insertion
Internal, with fracture reduction *see* Reposition
Internal, without fracture reduction *see* Insertion
FLAIR® Endovascular Stent Graft *use* Intraluminal Device
Flexible Composite Mesh *use* Synthetic Substitute
Flexor carpi radialis muscle
use Lower Arm and Wrist Muscle, Left
use Lower Arm and Wrist Muscle, Right
Flexor carpi ulnaris muscle
use Lower Arm and Wrist Muscle, Left
use Lower Arm and Wrist Muscle, Right
Flexor digitorum brevis muscle
use Foot Muscle, Left
use Foot Muscle, Right
Flexor digitorum longus muscle
use Lower Leg Muscle, Left
use Lower Leg Muscle, Right
Flexor hallucis brevis muscle
use Foot Muscle, Left
use Foot Muscle, Right
Flexor hallucis longus muscle
use Lower Leg Muscle, Left
use Lower Leg Muscle, Right
Flexor pollicis longus muscle
use Lower Arm and Wrist Muscle, Left
use Lower Arm and Wrist Muscle, Right
Flow Diverter embolization device *use* Intraluminal Device, Flow Diverter in Ø3V
FlowSense Noninvasive Thermal Sensor *see* Measurement, Central Nervous Cerebrospinal Fluid Shunt

Fluorescence Guided Procedure
Extremity
Lower 8EØY
Upper 8EØX
Head and Neck Region 8EØ9
Aminolevulinic Acid 8EØ9ØEM
No Qualifier 8EØ9ØEZ
Trunk Region 8EØW
Fluorescent Pyrazine, Kidney XT25XE5
Fluoroscopy
Abdomen and Pelvis BW11
Airway, Upper BB1DZZZ
Ankle
Left BQ1H
Right BQ1G
Aorta
Abdominal B41Ø
Laser, Intraoperative B41Ø
Thoracic B31Ø
Laser, Intraoperative B31Ø
Thoraco-Abdominal B31P
Laser, Intraoperative B31P
Aorta and Bilateral Lower Extremity Arteries B41D
Laser, Intraoperative B41D
Arm
Left BP1FZZZ
Right BP1EZZZ
Artery
Brachiocephalic-Subclavian
Laser, Intraoperative B311
Right B311
Bronchial B31L
Laser, Intraoperative B31L
Bypass Graft, Other B21F
Cervico-Cerebral Arch B31Q
Laser, Intraoperative B31Q
Common Carotid
Bilateral B315
Laser, Intraoperative B315
Left B314
Laser, Intraoperative B314
Right B313
Laser, Intraoperative B313
Coronary
Bypass Graft
Multiple B213
Laser, Intraoperative B213
Single B212
Laser, Intraoperative B212
Multiple B211
Laser, Intraoperative B211
Single B21Ø
Laser, Intraoperative B21Ø
External Carotid
Bilateral B31C
Laser, Intraoperative B31C
Left B31B
Laser, Intraoperative B31B
Right B319
Laser, Intraoperative B319
Hepatic B412
Laser, Intraoperative B412
Inferior Mesenteric B415
Laser, Intraoperative B415
Intercostal B31L
Laser, Intraoperative B31L
Internal Carotid
Bilateral B318
Laser, Intraoperative B318
Left B317
Laser, Intraoperative B317
Right B316
Laser, Intraoperative B316
Internal Mammary Bypass Graft
Left B218
Right B217
Intra-Abdominal
Laser, Intraoperative B41B
Other B41B
Intracranial B31R
Laser, Intraoperative B31R
Lower
Laser, Intraoperative B41J
Other B41J
Lower Extremity
Bilateral and Aorta B41D
Laser, Intraoperative B41D
Left B41G
Laser, Intraoperative B41G

Fluoroscopy — *continued*
Artery — *continued*
Lower Extremity — *continued*
Right B41F
Laser, Intraoperative B41F
Lumbar B419
Laser, Intraoperative B419
Pelvic B41C
Laser, Intraoperative B41C
Pulmonary
Left B31T
Laser, Intraoperative B31T
Right B31S
Laser, Intraoperative B31S
Pulmonary Trunk B31U
Laser, Intraoperative B31U
Renal
Bilateral B418
Laser, Intraoperative B418
Left B417
Laser, Intraoperative B417
Right B416
Laser, Intraoperative B416
Spinal B31M
Laser, Intraoperative B31M
Splenic B413
Laser, Intraoperative B413
Subclavian
Laser, Intraoperative B312
Left B312
Superior Mesenteric B414
Laser, Intraoperative B414
Upper
Laser, Intraoperative B31N
Other B31N
Upper Extremity
Bilateral B31K
Laser, Intraoperative B31K
Left B31J
Laser, Intraoperative B31J
Right B31H
Laser, Intraoperative B31H
Vertebral
Bilateral B31G
Laser, Intraoperative B31G
Left B31F
Laser, Intraoperative B31F
Right B31D
Laser, Intraoperative B31D
Bile Duct BF1Ø
Pancreatic Duct and Gallbladder BF14
Bile Duct and Gallbladder BF13
Biliary Duct BF11
Bladder BT1Ø
Kidney and Ureter BT14
Left BT1F
Right BT1D
Bladder and Urethra BT1B
Bowel, Small BD1
Calcaneus
Left BQ1KZZZ
Right BQ1JZZZ
Clavicle
Left BP15ZZZ
Right BP14ZZZ
Coccyx BR1F
Colon BD14
Corpora Cavernosa BV1Ø
Dialysis Fistula B51W
Dialysis Shunt B51W
Diaphragm BB16ZZZ
Disc
Cervical BR11
Lumbar BR13
Thoracic BR12
Duodenum BD19
Elbow
Left BP1H
Right BP1G
Epiglottis B91G
Esophagus BD11
Extremity
Lower BW1C
Upper BW1J
Facet Joint
Cervical BR14
Lumbar BR16
Thoracic BR15

Fluoroscopy — *continued*
Fallopian Tube
Bilateral BU12
Left BU11
Right BU1Ø
Fallopian Tube and Uterus BU18
Femur
Left BQ14ZZZ
Right BQ13ZZZ
Finger
Left BP1SZZZ
Right BP1RZZZ
Foot
Left BQ1MZZZ
Right BQ1LZZZ
Forearm
Left BP1KZZZ
Right BP1JZZZ
Gallbladder BF12
Bile Duct and Pancreatic Duct BF14
Gallbladder and Bile Duct BF13
Gastrointestinal, Upper BD1
Hand
Left BP1PZZZ
Right BP1NZZZ
Head and Neck BW19
Heart
Left B215
Right B214
Right and Left B216
Hip
Left BQ11
Right BQ1Ø
Humerus
Left BP1BZZZ
Right BP1AZZZ
Ileal Diversion Loop BT1C
Ileal Loop, Ureters and Kidney BT1G
Intracranial Sinus B512
Joint
Acromioclavicular, Bilateral BP13ZZZ
Finger
Left BP1D
Right BP1C
Foot
Left BQ1Y
Right BQ1X
Hand
Left BP1D
Right BP1C
Lumbosacral BR1B
Sacroiliac BR1D
Sternoclavicular
Bilateral BP12ZZZ
Left BP11ZZZ
Right BP1ØZZZ
Temporomandibular
Bilateral BN19
Left BN18
Right BN17
Thoracolumbar BR18
Toe
Left BQ1Y
Right BQ1X
Kidney
Bilateral BT13
Ileal Loop and Ureter BT1G
Left BT12
Right BT11
Ureter and Bladder BT14
Left BT1F
Right BT1D
Knee
Left BQ18
Right BQ17
Larynx B91J
Leg
Left BQ1FZZZ
Right BQ1DZZZ
Liver BF15
Lung
Bilateral BB14ZZZ
Left BB13ZZZ
Right BB12ZZZ
Mediastinum BB1CZZZ
Mouth BD1B
Neck and Head BW19
Oropharynx BD1B
Pancreatic Duct BF1

Fluoroscopy — *continued*
Pancreatic Duct — *continued*
Gallbladder and Bile Buct BF14
Patella
Left BQ1WZZZ
Right BQ1VZZZ
Pelvis BR1C
Pelvis and Abdomen BW11
Pharynix B91G
Ribs
Left BP1YZZZ
Right BP1XZZZ
Sacrum BR1F
Scapula
Left BP17ZZZ
Right BP16ZZZ
Shoulder
Left BP19
Right BP18
Sinus, Intracranial B512
Spinal Cord BØ1B
Spine
Cervical BR1Ø
Lumbar BR19
Thoracic BR17
Whole BR1G
Sternum BR1H
Stomach BD12
Toe
Left BQ1QZZZ
Right BQ1PZZZ
Tracheobronchial Tree
Bilateral BB19YZZ
Left BB18YZZ
Right BB17YZZ
Ureter
Ileal Loop and Kidney BT1G
Kidney and Bladder BT14
Left BT1F
Right BT1D
Left BT17
Right BT16
Urethra BT15
Urethra and Bladder BT1B
Uterus BU16
Uterus and Fallopian Tube BU18
Vagina BU19
Vasa Vasorum BV18
Vein
Cerebellar B511
Cerebral B511
Epidural B51Ø
Jugular
Bilateral B515
Left B514
Right B513
Lower Extremity
Bilateral B51D
Left B51C
Right B51B
Other B51V
Pelvic (Iliac)
Left B51G
Right B51F
Pelvic (Iliac) Bilateral B51H
Portal B51T
Pulmonary
Bilateral B51S
Left B51R
Right B51Q
Renal
Bilateral B51L
Left B51K
Right B51J
Spanchnic B51T
Subclavian
Left B517
Right B516
Upper Extremity
Bilateral B51P
Left B51N
Right B51M
Vena Cava
Inferior B519
Superior B518
Wrist
Left BP1M
Right BP1L

Fluoroscopy, laser intraoperative
see Fluoroscopy, Heart B21
see Fluoroscopy, Lower Arteries B41
see Fluoroscopy, Upper Arteries B31
Flushing *see* Irrigation
Foley catheter *use* Drainage Device
Fontan completion procedure Stage II *see* Bypass, Vena Cava, Inferior Ø61Ø
Foramen magnum *use* Occipital Bone
Foramen of Monro (intraventricular) *use* Cerebral Ventricle
Foreskin *use* Prepuce
Formula™ Balloon-Expandable Renal Stent System *use* Intraluminal Device
Fosfomycin Anti-infective XWØ
Fosfomycin injection *use* Fosfomycin Anti-infective
Fossa of Rosenmuller *use* Nasopharynx
Fourth cranial nerve *use* Trochlear Nerve
Fourth ventricle *use* Cerebral Ventricle
Fovea
use Retina, Left
use Retina, Right
Fragmentation
Ampulla of Vater ØFFC
Anus ØDFQ
Appendix ØDFJ
Artery
Anterior Tibial
Left Ø4FQ3Z
Right Ø4FP3Z
Axillary
Left Ø3F63Z
Right Ø3F53Z
Brachial
Left Ø3F83Z
Right Ø3F73Z
Common Iliac
Left Ø4FD3Z
Right Ø4FC3Z
Coronary
Four or More Arteries Ø2F33ZZ
One Artery Ø2FØ3ZZ
Three Arteries Ø2F23ZZ
Two Arteries Ø2F13ZZ
External Iliac
Left Ø4FJ3Z
Right Ø4FH3Z
Femoral
Left Ø4FL3Z
Right Ø4FK3Z
Innominate Ø3F23Z
Internal Iliac
Left Ø4FF3Z
Right Ø4FE3Z
Intracranial Ø3FG3Z
Lower Ø4FY3Z
Peroneal
Left Ø4FU3Z
Right Ø4FT3Z
Popliteal
Left Ø4FN3Z
Right Ø4FM3Z
Posterior Tibial
Left Ø4FS3Z
Right Ø4FR3Z
Pulmonary
Left Ø2FR3Z
Right Ø2FQ3Z
Pulmonary Trunk Ø2FP3Z
Radial
Left Ø3FC3Z
Right Ø3FB3Z
Subclavian
Left Ø3F43Z
Right Ø3F33Z
Ulnar
Left Ø3FA3Z
Right Ø3F93Z
Upper Ø3FY3Z
Bladder ØTFB
Bladder Neck ØTFC
Bronchus
Lingula ØBF9
Lower Lobe
Left ØBFB
Right ØBF6
Main
Left ØBF7

Fragmentation — *continued*
Bronchus — *continued*
Main — *continued*
Right ØBF3
Middle Lobe, Right ØBF5
Upper Lobe
Left ØBF8
Right ØBF4
Carina ØBF2
Cavity, Cranial ØWF1
Cecum ØDFH
Cerebral Ventricle ØØF6
Colon
Ascending ØDFK
Descending ØDFM
Sigmoid ØDFN
Transverse ØDFL
Duct
Common Bile ØFF9
Cystic ØFF8
Hepatic
Common ØFF7
Left ØFF6
Right ØFF5
Pancreatic ØFFD
Accessory ØFFF
Parotid
Left ØCFC
Right ØCFB
Duodenum ØDF9
Epidural Space, Intracranial ØØF3
Esophagus ØDF5
Fallopian Tube
Left ØUF6
Right ØUF5
Fallopian Tubes, Bilateral ØUF7
Gallbladder ØFF4
Gastrointestinal Tract ØWFP
Genitourinary Tract ØWFR
Ileum ØDFB
Intestine
Large ØDFE
Left ØDFG
Right ØDFF
Small ØDF8
Jejunum ØDFA
Kidney Pelvis
Left ØTF4
Right ØTF3
Mediastinum ØWFC
Oral Cavity and Throat ØWF3
Pelvic Cavity ØWFJ
Pericardial Cavity ØWFD
Pericardium Ø2FN
Peritoneal Cavity ØWFG
Pleural Cavity
Left ØWFB
Right ØWF9
Rectum ØDFP
Respiratory Tract ØWFQ
Spinal Canal ØØFU
Stomach ØDF6
Subarachnoid Space, Intracranial ØØF5
Subdural Space, Intracranial ØØF4
Trachea ØBF1
Ureter
Left ØTF7
Right ØTF6
Urethra ØTFD
Uterus ØUF9
Vein
Axillary
Left Ø5F83Z
Right Ø5F73Z
Basilic
Left Ø5FC3Z
Right Ø5FB3Z
Brachial
Left Ø5FA3Z
Right Ø5F93Z
Cephalic
Left Ø5FF3Z
Right Ø5FD3Z
Common Iliac
Left Ø6FD3Z
Right Ø6FC3Z
External Iliac
Left Ø6FG3Z
Right Ø6FF3Z

Fragmentation — *continued*
Vein — *continued*
Femoral
Left Ø6FN3Z
Right Ø6FM3Z
Hypogastric
Left Ø6FJ3Z
Right Ø6FH3Z
Innominate
Left Ø5F43Z
Right Ø5F33Z
Lower Ø6FY3Z
Pulmonary
Left Ø2FT3Z
Right Ø2FS3Z
Saphenous
Left Ø6FQ3Z
Right Ø6FP3Z
Subclavian
Left Ø5F63Z
Right Ø5F53Z
Upper Ø5FY3Z
Vitreous
Left Ø8F5
Right Ø8F4
Fragmentation, Ultrasonic *see* Fragmentation, Artery
Freestyle (Stentless) Aortic Root Bioprosthesis *use* Zooplastic Tissue in Heart and Great Vessels
Frenectomy
see Excision, Mouth and Throat ØCB
see Resection, Mouth and Throat ØCT
Frenoplasty, frenuloplasty
see Repair, Mouth and Throat ØCQ
see Replacement, Mouth and Throat ØCR
see Supplement, Mouth and Throat ØCU
Frenotomy
see Drainage, Mouth and Throat ØC9
see Release, Mouth and Throat ØCN
Frenulotomy
see Drainage, Mouth and Throat ØC9
see Release, Mouth and Throat ØCN
Frenulum labii inferioris *use* Lower Lip
Frenulum labii superioris *use* Upper Lip
Frenulum linguae *use* Tongue
Frenulumectomy
see Excision, Mouth and Throat ØCB
see Resection, Mouth and Throat ØCT
Frontal lobe *use* Cerebral Hemisphere
Frontal vein
use Face Vein, Left
use Face Vein, Right
Frozen elephant trunk (FET) technique, aortic arch replacement
see New Technology, Cardiovascular System X2R
see Replacement, Heart and Great Vessels Ø2R
Frozen elephant trunk (FET) technique, thoracic aorta restriction
see New Technology, Cardiovascular System X2V
see Restriction, Heart and Great Vessels Ø2V
FUJIFILM EP-7ØØØX System for Oxygen Saturation Endoscopic Imaging (OXEI) *see* New Technology, Gastrointestinal System XD2
Fulguration *see* Destruction
Fundoplication, gastroesophageal *see* Restriction, Esophagogastric Junction ØDV4
Fundus uteri *use* Uterus
Fusion
Acromioclavicular
Left ØRGH
Right ØRGG
Ankle
Left ØSGG
Right ØSGF
Carpal
Left ØRGR
Right ØRGQ
Carpometacarpal
Left ØRGT
Right ØRGS
Cervical Vertebral ØRG1
2 or more ØRG2
Interbody Fusion Device
Nanotextured Surface XRG2Ø92
Radiolucent Porous XRG2ØF3
Interbody Fusion Device
Nanotextured Surface XRG1Ø92
Radiolucent Porous XRG1ØF3

Fusion — *continued*
Cervicothoracic Vertebral ØRG4
Interbody Fusion Device
Nanotextured Surface XRG4Ø92
Radiolucent Porous XRG4ØF3
Coccygeal ØSG6
Elbow
Left ØRGM
Right ØRGL
Finger Phalangeal
Left ØRGX
Right ØRGW
Hip
Left ØSGB
Right ØSG9
Knee
Left ØSGD
Right ØSGC
Lumbar Vertebral ØSGØ
2 or more ØSG1
Interbody Fusion Device
Customizable XRGC
Nanotextured Surface XRGCØ92
Radiolucent Porous XRGCØF3
Interbody Fusion Device
Customizable XRGB
Nanotextured Surface XRGBØ92
Radiolucent Porous XRGBØF3
Lumbosacral ØSG3
Interbody Fusion Device
Customizable XRGD
Nanotextured Surface XRGDØ92
Radiolucent Porous XRGDØF3
Metacarpophalangeal
Left ØRGV
Right ØRGU
Metatarsal-Phalangeal
Left ØSGN
Right ØSGM
Occipital-cervical ØRGØ
Interbody Fusion Device
Nanotextured Surface XRGØØ92
Radiolucent Porous XRGØØF3
Sacrococcygeal ØSG5
Sacroiliac
Left ØSG8
Right ØSG7
Shoulder
Left ØRGK
Right ØRGJ
Sternoclavicular
Left ØRGF
Right ØRGE
Tarsal
Left ØSGJ
Right ØSGH
Tarsometatarsal
Left ØSGL
Right ØSGK
Temporomandibular
Left ØRGD
Right ØRGC
Thoracic Vertebral ØRG6
2 to 7 ØRG7
Interbody Fusion Device
Nanotextured Surface XRG7Ø92
Radiolucent Porous XRG7ØF3
8 or more ØRG8
Interbody Fusion Device
Nanotextured Surface XRG8Ø92
Radiolucent Porous XRG8ØF3
Interbody Fusion Device
Nanotextured Surface XRG6Ø92
Radiolucent Porous XRG6ØF3
Thoracolumbar Vertebral ØRGA
Interbody Fusion Device
Customizable XRGA
Nanotextured Surface XRGAØ92
Radiolucent Porous XRGAØF3
Toe Phalangeal
Left ØSGQ
Right ØSGP
Wrist
Left ØRGP
Right ØRGN
Fusion screw (compression) (lag) (locking)
use Internal Fixation Device in Lower Joints
use Internal Fixation Device in Upper Joints

G

Gait training *see* Motor Treatment, Rehabilitation FØ7
Galea aponeurotica *use* Subcutaneous Tissue and Fascia, Scalp
Gammaglobulin *use* Globulin
GammaTile™ *use* Radioactive Element, Cesium-131 Collagen Implant in ØØH
GAMUNEX-C, for COVID-19 treatment *use* High-Dose Intravenous Immune Globulin
Ganglion impar (ganglion of Walther) *use* Sacral Sympathetic Nerve
Ganglionectomy
Destruction of lesion *see* Destruction
Excision of lesion *see* Excision
Gasserian ganglion *use* Trigeminal Nerve
Gastrectomy
Partial *see* Excision, Stomach ØDB6
Total *see* Resection, Stomach ØDT6
Vertical (sleeve) *see* Excision, Stomach ØDB6
Gastric electrical stimulation (GES) lead *use* Stimulator Lead in Gastrointestinal System
Gastric lymph node *use* Lymphatic, Aortic
Gastric pacemaker lead *use* Stimulator Lead in Gastrointestinal System
Gastric plexus *use* Abdominal Sympathetic Nerve
Gastrocnemius muscle
use Lower Leg Muscle, Left
use Lower Leg Muscle, Right
Gastrocolic ligament *use* Omentum
Gastrocolic omentum *use* Omentum
Gastrocolostomy
see Bypass, Gastrointestinal System ØD1
see Drainage, Gastrointestinal System ØD9
Gastroduodenal artery *use* Hepatic Artery
Gastroduodenectomy
see Excision, Gastrointestinal System ØDB
see Resection, Gastrointestinal System ØDT
Gastroduodenoscopy ØDJØ8ZZ
Gastroenteroplasty
see Repair, Gastrointestinal System ØDQ
see Supplement, Gastrointestinal System ØDU
Gastroenterostomy
see Bypass, Gastrointestinal System ØD1
see Drainage, Gastrointestinal System ØD9
Gastroesophageal (GE) junction *use* Esophagogastric Junction
Gastrogastrostomy
see Bypass, Stomach ØD16
see Drainage, Stomach ØD96
Gastrohepatic omentum *use* Omentum
Gastrojejunostomy
see Bypass, Stomach ØD16
see Drainage, Stomach ØD96
Gastrolysis *see* Release, Stomach ØDN6
Gastropexy
see Repair, Stomach ØDQ6
see Reposition, Stomach ØDS6
Gastrophrenic ligament *use* Omentum
Gastroplasty
see Repair, Stomach ØDQ6
see Supplement, Stomach ØDU6
Gastroplication *see* Restriction, Stomach ØDV6
Gastropylorectomy *see* Excision, Gastrointestinal System ØDB
Gastrorrhaphy *see* Repair, Stomach ØDQ6
Gastroscopy ØDJ68ZZ
Gastrosplenic ligament *use* Omentum
Gastrostomy
see Bypass, Stomach ØD16
see Drainage, Stomach ØD96
Gastrotomy *see* Drainage, Stomach ØD96
Gemellus muscle
use Hip Muscle, Left
use Hip Muscle, Right
Geniculate ganglion *use* Facial Nerve
Geniculate nucleus *use* Thalamus
Genioglossus muscle *use* Tongue, Palate, Pharynx Muscle
Genioplasty *see* Alteration, Jaw, Lower ØWØ5
Genitofemoral nerve *use* Lumbar Plexus
GIAPREZA™ *use* Synthetic Human Angiotensin II
Gilteritinib Antineoplastic XWØDXV5
Gingivectomy *see* Excision, Mouth and Throat ØCB
Gingivoplasty
see Repair, Mouth and Throat ØCQ
see Replacement, Mouth and Throat ØCR
see Supplement, Mouth and Throat ØCU
Glans penis *use* Prepuce
Glenohumeral joint
use Shoulder Joint, Left
use Shoulder Joint, Right
Glenohumeral ligament
use Shoulder Bursa and Ligament, Left
use Shoulder Bursa and Ligament, Right
Glenoid fossa (of scapula)
use Glenoid Cavity, Left
use Glenoid Cavity, Right
Glenoid ligament (labrum)
use Shoulder Joint, Left
use Shoulder Joint, Right
Globus pallidus *use* Basal Ganglia
Glomectomy
see Excision, Endocrine System ØGB
see Resection, Endocrine System ØGT
Glossectomy
see Excision, Tongue ØCB7
see Resection, Tongue ØCT7
Glossoepiglottic fold *use* Epiglottis
Glossopexy
see Repair, Tongue ØCQ7
see Reposition, Tongue ØCS7
Glossoplasty
see Repair, Tongue ØCQ7
see Replacement, Tongue ØCR7
see Supplement, Tongue ØCU7
Glossorrhaphy *see* Repair, Tongue ØCQ7
Glossotomy *see* Drainage, Tongue ØC97
Glottis *use* Larynx
Gluteal Artery Perforator Flap
Replacement
Bilateral ØHRVØ79
Left ØHRUØ79
Right ØHRTØ79
Transfer
Left ØKXG
Right ØKXF
Gluteal lymph node *use* Lymphatic, Pelvis
Gluteal vein
use Hypogastric Vein, Left
use Hypogastric Vein, Right
Gluteus maximus muscle
use Hip Muscle, Left
use Hip Muscle, Right
Gluteus medius muscle
use Hip Muscle, Left
use Hip Muscle, Right
Gluteus minimus muscle
use Hip Muscle, Left
use Hip Muscle, Right
GORE EXCLUDER® AAA Endoprosthesis
use Intraluminal Device
use Intraluminal Device, Branched or Fenestrated, One or Two Arteries in Ø4V
use Intraluminal Device, Branched or Fenestrated, Three or More Arteries in Ø4V
GORE EXCLUDER® IBE Endoprosthesis *use* Intraluminal Device, Branched or Fenestrated, One or Two Arteries in Ø4V
GORE TAG® Thoracic Endoprosthesis *use* Intraluminal Device
GORE® DUALMESH® *use* Synthetic Substitute
Gracilis muscle
use Upper Leg Muscle, Left
use Upper Leg Muscle, Right
Graft
see Replacement
see Supplement
Great auricular nerve *use* Cervical Plexus
Great cerebral vein *use* Intracranial Vein
Great(er) saphenous vein
use Saphenous Vein, Left
use Saphenous Vein, Right
Greater alar cartilage *use* Nasal Mucosa and Soft Tissue
Greater occipital nerve *use* Cervical Nerve
Greater Omentum *use* Omentum
Greater splanchnic nerve *use* Thoracic Sympathetic Nerve
Greater superficial petrosal nerve *use* Facial Nerve
Greater trochanter
use Upper Femur, Left
use Upper Femur, Right
Greater tuberosity
use Humeral Head, Left
use Humeral Head, Right
Greater vestibular (Bartholin's) gland *use* Vestibular Gland
Greater wing *use* Sphenoid Bone
GS-5734 *use* Remdesivir Anti-infective
Guedel airway *use* Intraluminal Device, Airway in Mouth and Throat
Guidance, catheter placement
EKG *see* Measurement, Physiological Systems 4AØ
Fluoroscopy *see* Fluoroscopy, Veins B51
Ultrasound *see* Ultrasonography, Veins B54

H

Hallux
use 1st Toe, Left
use 1st Toe, Right
Hamate bone
use Carpal, Left
use Carpal, Right
Hancock Bioprosthesis (aortic) (mitral) valve *use* Zooplastic Tissue in Heart and Great Vessels
Hancock Bioprosthetic Valved Conduit *use* Zooplastic Tissue in Heart and Great Vessels
Harmony™ transcatheter pulmonary valve (TPV) placement Ø2RH38M
Harvesting, Stem Cells *see* Pheresis, Circulatory 6A55
hdIVIG (high-dose intravenous immunoglobulin), for COVID-19 treatment *use* High-Dose Intravenous Immune Globulin
Head of fibula
use Fibula, Left
use Fibula, Right
Hearing Aid Assessment F14Z
Hearing Assessment F13Z
Hearing Device
Bone Conduction
Left Ø9HE
Right Ø9HD
Insertion of device in
Left ØNH6
Right ØNH5
Multiple Channel Cochlear Prosthesis
Left Ø9HE
Right Ø9HD
Removal of device from, Skull ØNPØ
Revision of device in, Skull ØNWØ
Single Channel Cochlear Prosthesis
Left Ø9HE
Right Ø9HD
Hearing Treatment FØ9Z
Heart Assist System
Implantable
Insertion of device in, Heart Ø2HA
Removal of device from, Heart Ø2PA
Revision of device in, Heart Ø2WA
Short-term External
Insertion of device in, Heart Ø2HA
Removal of device from, Heart Ø2PA
Revision of device in, Heart Ø2WA
HeartMate 3™ LVAS *use* Implantable Heart Assist System in Heart and Great Vessels
HeartMate II® Left Ventricular Assist Device (LVAD) *use* Implantable Heart Assist System in Heart and Great Vessels
HeartMate XVE® Left Ventricular Assist Device (LVAD) *use* Implantable Heart Assist System in Heart and Great Vessels
HeartMate® implantable heart assist system *see* Insertion of device in, Heart Ø2HA
Helix
use Ear, External, Bilateral
use Ear, External, Left
use Ear, External, Right
Hematopoietic cell transplant (HCT) *see* Transfusion, Circulatory 3Ø2
Hemicolectomy *see* Resection, Gastrointestinal System ØDT
Hemicystectomy *see* Excision, Urinary System ØTB
Hemigastrectomy *see* Excision, Gastrointestinal System ØDB

Hemiglossectomy *see* Excision, Mouth and Throat ØCB
Hemilaminectomy
see Excision, Lower Bones ØQB
see Excision, Upper Bones ØPB
Hemilaminotomy
see Drainage, Lower Bones ØQ9
see Drainage, Upper Bones ØP9
see Excision, Lower Bones ØQB
see Excision, Upper Bones ØPB
see Release, Central Nervous System and Cranial Nerves ØØN
see Release, Lower Bones ØQN
see Release, Peripheral Nervous System Ø1N
see Release, Upper Bones ØPN
Hemilaryngectomy *see* Excision, Larynx ØCBS
Hemimandibulectomy *see* Excision, Head and Facial Bones ØNB
Hemimaxillectomy *see* Excision, Head and Facial Bones ØNB
Hemipylorectomy *see* Excision, Gastrointestinal System ØDB
Hemispherectomy
see Excision, Central Nervous System and Cranial Nerves ØØB
see Resection, Central Nervous System and Cranial Nerves ØØT
Hemithyroidectomy
see Excision, Endocrine System ØGB
see Resection, Endocrine System ØGT
Hemodialysis *see* Performance, Urinary 5A1D
Hemolung® Respiratory Assist System (RAS) 5AØ92ØZ
Hemospray® Endoscopic Hemostat *use* Mineral-based Topical Hemostatic Agent
Hepatectomy
see Excision, Hepatobiliary System and Pancreas ØFB
see Resection, Hepatobiliary System and Pancreas ØFT
Hepatic artery proper *use* Hepatic Artery
Hepatic flexure *use* Transverse Colon
Hepatic lymph node *use* Lymphatic, Aortic
Hepatic plexus *use* Abdominal Sympathetic Nerve
Hepatic portal vein *use* Portal Vein
Hepaticoduodenostomy
see Bypass, Hepatobiliary System and Pancreas ØF1
see Drainage, Hepatobiliary System and Pancreas ØF9
Hepaticotomy *see* Drainage, Hepatobiliary System and Pancreas ØF9
Hepatocholedochostomy *see* Drainage, Duct, Common Bile ØF99
Hepatogastric ligament *use* Omentum
Hepatopancreatic ampulla *use* Ampulla of Vater
Hepatopexy
see Repair, Hepatobiliary System and Pancreas ØFQ
see Reposition, Hepatobiliary System and Pancreas ØFS
Hepatorrhaphy *see* Repair, Hepatobiliary System and Pancreas ØFQ
Hepatotomy *see* Drainage, Hepatobiliary System and Pancreas ØF9
Herculink (RX) Elite Renal Stent System *use* Intraluminal Device
Herniorrhaphy
see Repair, Anatomical Regions, General ØWQ
see Repair, Anatomical Regions, Lower Extremities ØYQ
With synthetic substitute
see Supplement, Anatomical Regions, General ØWU
see Supplement, Anatomical Regions, Lower Extremities ØYU
HIG (hyperimmune globulin), for COVID-19 treatment *use* Hyperimmune Globulin
High-Dose Intravenous Immune Globulin, for COVID-19 treatment XW1
High-dose intravenous immunoglobulin (hdIVIG), for COVID-19 treatment *use* High-Dose Intravenous Immune Globulin
Hip (joint) liner *use* Liner in Lower Joints
HIPEC (hyperthermic intraperitoneal chemotherapy) 3EØM3ØY
hIVIG (hyperimmune intravenous immunoglobulin), for COVID-19 treatment *use* Hyperimmune Globulin
Holter Monitoring 4A12X45
Holter valve ventricular shunt *use* Synthetic Substitute
Human angiotensin II, synthetic *use* Synthetic Human Angiotensin II
Humeroradial joint
use Elbow Joint, Left
use Elbow Joint, Right
Humeroulnar joint
use Elbow Joint, Left
use Elbow Joint, Right
Humerus, distal
use Humeral Shaft, Left
use Humeral Shaft, Right
Hydrocelectomy *see* Excision, Male Reproductive System ØVB
Hydrotherapy
Assisted exercise in pool *see* Motor Treatment, Rehabilitation FØ7
Whirlpool *see* Activities of Daily Living Treatment, Rehabilitation FØ8
Hymenectomy
see Excision, Hymen ØUBK
see Resection, Hymen ØUTK
Hymenoplasty
see Repair, Hymen ØUQK
see Supplement, Hymen ØUUK
Hymenorrhaphy *see* Repair, Hymen ØUQK
Hymenotomy
see Division, Hymen ØU8K
see Drainage, Hymen ØU9K
Hyoglossus muscle *use* Tongue, Palate, Pharynx Muscle
Hyoid artery
use Thyroid Artery, Left
use Thyroid Artery, Right
Hyperalimentation *see* Introduction of substance in or on
Hyperbaric oxygenation
Decompression sickness treatment *see* Decompression, Circulatory 6A15
Wound treatment *see* Assistance, Circulatory 5AØ5
Hyperimmune globulin *use* Globulin
Hyperimmune Globulin, for COVID-19 treatment XW1
Hyperimmune intravenous immunoglobulin (hIVIG), for COVID-19 treatment *use* Hyperimmune Globulin
Hyperthermia
Radiation Therapy
Abdomen DWY38ZZ
Adrenal Gland DGY28ZZ
Bile Ducts DFY28ZZ
Bladder DTY28ZZ
Bone Marrow D7YØ8ZZ
Bone, Other DPYC8ZZ
Brain DØYØ8ZZ
Brain Stem DØY18ZZ
Breast
Left DMYØ8ZZ
Right DMY18ZZ
Bronchus DBY18ZZ
Cervix DUY18ZZ
Chest DWY28ZZ
Chest Wall DBY78ZZ
Colon DDY58ZZ
Diaphragm DBY88ZZ
Duodenum DDY28ZZ
Ear D9YØ8ZZ
Esophagus DDYØ8ZZ
Eye D8YØ8ZZ
Femur DPY98ZZ
Fibula DPYB8ZZ
Gallbladder DFY18ZZ
Gland
Adrenal DGY28ZZ
Parathyroid DGY48ZZ
Pituitary DGYØ8ZZ
Thyroid DGY58ZZ
Glands, Salivary D9Y68ZZ
Head and Neck DWY18ZZ
Hemibody DWY48ZZ
Humerus DPY68ZZ
Hypopharynx D9Y38ZZ
Ileum DDY48ZZ
Jejunum DDY38ZZ
Kidney DTYØ8ZZ
Larynx D9YB8ZZ
Hyperthermia — *continued*
Radiation Therapy — *continued*
Liver DFYØ8ZZ
Lung DBY28ZZ
Lymphatics
Abdomen D7Y68ZZ
Axillary D7Y48ZZ
Inguinal D7Y88ZZ
Neck D7Y38ZZ
Pelvis D7Y78ZZ
Thorax D7Y58ZZ
Mandible DPY38ZZ
Maxilla DPY28ZZ
Mediastinum DBY68ZZ
Mouth D9Y48ZZ
Nasopharynx D9YD8ZZ
Neck and Head DWY18ZZ
Nerve, Peripheral DØY78ZZ
Nose D9Y18ZZ
Oropharynx D9YF8ZZ
Ovary DUYØ8ZZ
Palate
Hard D9Y88ZZ
Soft D9Y98ZZ
Pancreas DFY38ZZ
Parathyroid Gland DGY48ZZ
Pelvic Bones DPY88ZZ
Pelvic Region DWY68ZZ
Pineal Body DGY18ZZ
Pituitary Gland DGYØ8ZZ
Pleura DBY58ZZ
Prostate DVYØ8ZZ
Radius DPY78ZZ
Rectum DDY78ZZ
Rib DPY58ZZ
Sinuses D9Y78ZZ
Skin
Abdomen DHY88ZZ
Arm DHY48ZZ
Back DHY78ZZ
Buttock DHY98ZZ
Chest DHY68ZZ
Face DHY28ZZ
Leg DHYB8ZZ
Neck DHY38ZZ
Skull DPYØ8ZZ
Spinal Cord DØY68ZZ
Spleen D7Y28ZZ
Sternum DPY48ZZ
Stomach DDY18ZZ
Testis DVY18ZZ
Thymus D7Y18ZZ
Thyroid Gland DGY58ZZ
Tibia DPYB8ZZ
Tongue D9Y58ZZ
Trachea DBYØ8ZZ
Ulna DPY78ZZ
Ureter DTY18ZZ
Urethra DTY38ZZ
Uterus DUY28ZZ
Whole Body DWY58ZZ
Whole Body 6A3Z
Hyperthermic Intraperitoneal Chemotherapy (HIPEC) 3EØM3ØY
Hypnosis GZFZZZZ
Hypogastric artery
use Internal Iliac Artery, Left
use Internal Iliac Artery, Right
Hypopharynx *use* Pharynx
Hypophysectomy
see Excision, Gland, Pituitary ØGBØ
see Resection, Gland, Pituitary ØGTØ
Hypophysis *use* Pituitary Gland
Hypothalamotomy *see* Destruction, Thalamus ØØ59
Hypothenar muscle
use Hand Muscle, Left
use Hand Muscle, Right
Hypothermia, Whole Body 6A4Z
Hysterectomy
Supracervical *see* Resection, Uterus ØUT9
Total *see* Resection, Uterus ØUT9
Hysterolysis *see* Release, Uterus ØUN9
Hysteropexy
see Repair, Uterus ØUQ9
see Reposition, Uterus ØUS9
Hysteroplasty *see* Repair, Uterus ØUQ9
Hysterorrhaphy *see* Repair, Uterus ØUQ9
Hysteroscopy ØUJD8ZZ

Hysterotomy *see* Drainage, Uterus ØU9
Hysterotrachelectomy
see Resection, Cervix ØUTC
see Resection, Uterus ØUT9
Hysterotracheloplasty *see* Repair, Uterus ØUQ9
Hysterotrachelorrhaphy *see* Repair, Uterus ØUQ9

I

IABP (Intra-aortic balloon pump) *see* Assistance, Cardiac 5AØ2
IAEMT (Intraoperative anesthetic effect monitoring and titration) *see* Monitoring, Central Nervous 4A1Ø
IASD® (InterAtrial Shunt Device), Corvia *use* Synthetic Substitute
Idarucizumab, Pradaxa® (dabigatran) reversal agent *use* Other Therapeutic Substance
Idecabtagene Vicleucel *use* Idecabtagene Vicleucel Immunotherapy
Idecabtagene Vicleucel Immunotherapy XWØ
Ide-cel *use* Idecabtagene Vicleucel Immunotherapy
IGIV-C, for COVID-19 treatment *use* Hyperimmune Globulin
IHD (Intermittent hemodialysis) 5A1D7ØZ
Ileal artery *use* Superior Mesenteric Artery
Ileectomy
see Excision, Ileum ØDBB
see Resection, Ileum ØDTB
Ileocolic artery *use* Superior Mesenteric Artery
Ileocolic vein *use* Colic Vein
Ileopexy
see Repair, Ileum ØDQB
see Reposition, Ileum ØDSB
Ileorrhaphy *see* Repair, Ileum ØDQB
Ileoscopy ØDJD8ZZ
Ileostomy
see Bypass, Ileum ØD1B
see Drainage, Ileum ØD9B
Ileotomy *see* Drainage, Ileum ØD9B
Ileoureterostomy *see* Bypass, Urinary System ØT1
Iliac crest
use Pelvic Bone, Left
use Pelvic Bone, Right
Iliac fascia
use Subcutaneous Tissue and Fascia, Left Upper Leg
use Subcutaneous Tissue and Fascia, Right Upper Leg
Iliac lymph node *use* Lymphatic, Pelvis
Iliacus muscle
use Hip Muscle, Left
use Hip Muscle, Right
Iliofemoral ligament
use Hip Bursa and Ligament, Left
use Hip Bursa and Ligament, Right
Iliohypogastric nerve *use* Lumbar Plexus
Ilioinguinal nerve *use* Lumbar Plexus
Iliolumbar artery
use Internal Iliac Artery, Left
use Internal Iliac Artery, Right
Iliolumbar ligament *use* Lower Spine Bursa and Ligament
Iliotibial tract (band)
use Subcutaneous Tissue and Fascia, Left Upper Leg
use Subcutaneous Tissue and Fascia, Right Upper Leg
Ilium
use Pelvic Bone, Left
use Pelvic Bone, Right
Ilizarov external fixator
use External Fixation Device, Ring in ØPH
use External Fixation Device, Ring in ØPS
use External Fixation Device, Ring in ØQH
use External Fixation Device, Ring in ØQS
Ilizarov-Vecklich device
use External Fixation Device, Limb Lengthening in ØPH
use External Fixation Device, Limb Lengthening in ØQH
Imaging, diagnostic
see Computerized Tomography (CT Scan)
see Fluoroscopy
see Magnetic Resonance Imaging (MRI)
see Plain Radiography
Imaging, diagnostic — *continued*
see Ultrasonography
Imdevimab (REGN1Ø987) and Casirivimab (REGN1Ø933) *use* REGN-COV2 Monoclonal Antibody
IMFINZI® *use* Durvalumab Antineoplastic
Imipenem-cilastatin-relebactam Anti-infective XWØ
IMI/REL *use* Imipenem-cilastatin-relebactam Anti-infective
Immobilization
Abdominal Wall 2W33X
Arm
Lower
Left 2W3DX
Right 2W3CX
Upper
Left 2W3BX
Right 2W3AX
Back 2W35X
Chest Wall 2W34X
Extremity
Lower
Left 2W3MX
Right 2W3LX
Upper
Left 2W39X
Right 2W38X
Face 2W31X
Finger
Left 2W3KX
Right 2W3JX
Foot
Left 2W3TX
Right 2W3SX
Hand
Left 2W3FX
Right 2W3EX
Head 2W3ØX
Inguinal Region
Left 2W37X
Right 2W36X
Leg
Lower
Left 2W3RX
Right 2W3QX
Upper
Left 2W3PX
Right 2W3NX
Neck 2W32X
Thumb
Left 2W3HX
Right 2W3GX
Toe
Left 2W3VX
Right 2W3UX
Immunization *see* Introduction of Serum, Toxoid, and Vaccine
Immunoglobulin *use* Globulin
Immunotherapy *see* Introduction of Immunotherapeutic Substance
Immunotherapy, antineoplastic
Interferon *see* Introduction of Low-dose Interleukin-2
Interleukin-2, high-dose *see* Introduction of High-dose Interleukin-2
Interleukin-2, low-dose *see* Introduction of Low-dose Interleukin-2
Monoclonal antibody *see* Introduction of Monoclonal Antibody
Proleukin, high-dose *see* Introduction of High-dose Interleukin-2
Proleukin, low-dose *see* Introduction of Low-dose Interleukin-2
Impella® heart pump *use* Short-term External Heart Assist System in Heart and Great Vessels
Impeller Pump
Continuous, Output 5AØ221D
Intermittent, Output 5AØ211D
Implantable cardioverter-defibrillator (ICD) *use* Defibrillator Generator in ØJH
Implantable drug infusion pump (anti-spasmodic) (chemotherapy) (pain) *use* Infusion Device, Pump in Subcutaneous Tissue and Fascia
Implantable glucose monitoring device *use* Monitoring Device
Implantable hemodynamic monitor (IHM) *use* Monitoring Device, Hemodynamic in ØJH
Implantable hemodynamic monitoring system (IHMS) *use* Monitoring Device, Hemodynamic in ØJH
Implantable Miniature Telescope™ (IMT) *use* Synthetic Substitute, Intraocular Telescope in Ø8R
Implantation
see Insertion
see Replacement
Implanted (venous)(access) port *use* Vascular Access Device, Totally Implantable in Subcutaneous Tissue and Fascia
IMV (intermittent mandatory ventilation) *see* Assistance, Respiratory 5AØ9
In Vitro Fertilization 8EØZXY1
Incision, abscess *see* Drainage
Incudectomy
see Excision, Ear, Nose, Sinus Ø9B
see Resection, Ear, Nose, Sinus Ø9T
Incudopexy
see Repair, Ear, Nose, Sinus Ø9Q
see Reposition, Ear, Nose, Sinus Ø9S
Incus
use Auditory Ossicle, Left
use Auditory Ossicle, Right
Induction of labor
Artificial rupture of membranes *see* Drainage, Pregnancy 1Ø9
Oxytocin *see* Introduction of Hormone
InDura, intrathecal catheter (1P) (spinal) *use* Infusion Device
Inferior cardiac nerve *use* Thoracic Sympathetic Nerve
Inferior cerebellar vein *use* Intracranial Vein
Inferior cerebral vein *use* Intracranial Vein
Inferior epigastric artery
use External Iliac Artery, Left
use External Iliac Artery, Right
Inferior epigastric lymph node *use* Lymphatic, Pelvis
Inferior genicular artery
use Popliteal Artery, Left
use Popliteal Artery, Right
Inferior gluteal artery
use Internal Iliac Artery, Left
use Internal Iliac Artery, Right
Inferior gluteal nerve *use* Sacral Plexus
Inferior hypogastric plexus *use* Abdominal Sympathetic Nerve
Inferior labial artery *use* Face Artery
Inferior longitudinal muscle *use* Tongue, Palate, Pharynx Muscle
Inferior mesenteric ganglion *use* Abdominal Sympathetic Nerve
Inferior mesenteric lymph node *use* Lymphatic, Mesenteric
Inferior mesenteric plexus *use* Abdominal Sympathetic Nerve
Inferior oblique muscle
use Extraocular Muscle, Left
use Extraocular Muscle, Right
Inferior pancreaticoduodenal artery *use* Superior Mesenteric Artery
Inferior phrenic artery *use* Abdominal Aorta
Inferior rectus muscle
use Extraocular Muscle, Left
use Extraocular Muscle, Right
Inferior suprarenal artery
use Renal Artery, Left
use Renal Artery, Right
Inferior tarsal plate
use Lower Eyelid, Left
use Lower Eyelid, Right
Inferior thyroid vein
use Innominate Vein, Left
use Innominate Vein, Right
Inferior tibiofibular joint
use Ankle Joint, Left
use Ankle Joint, Right
Inferior turbinate *use* Nasal Turbinate
Inferior ulnar collateral artery
use Brachial Artery, Left
use Brachial Artery, Right
Inferior vesical artery
use Internal Iliac Artery, Left
use Internal Iliac Artery, Right
Infraauricular lymph node *use* Lymphatic, Head
Infraclavicular (deltopectoral) lymph node
use Lymphatic, Left Upper Extremity

Subterms under main terms may continue to next column or page

Infraclavicular (deltopectoral) lymph node — *continued*
use Lymphatic, Right Upper Extremity
Infrahyoid muscle
use Neck Muscle, Left
use Neck Muscle, Right
Infraparotid lymph node *use* Lymphatic, Head
Infraspinatus fascia
use Subcutaneous Tissue and Fascia, Left Upper Arm
use Subcutaneous Tissue and Fascia, Right Upper Arm
Infraspinatus muscle
use Shoulder Muscle, Left
use Shoulder Muscle, Right
Infundibulopelvic ligament *use* Uterine Supporting Structure
Infusion *see* Introduction of substance in or on
Infusion Device, Pump
Insertion of device in
Abdomen ØJH8
Back ØJH7
Chest ØJH6
Lower Arm
Left ØJHH
Right ØJHG
Lower Leg
Left ØJHP
Right ØJHN
Trunk ØJHT
Upper Arm
Left ØJHF
Right ØJHD
Upper Leg
Left ØJHM
Right ØJHL
Removal of device from
Lower Extremity ØJPW
Trunk ØJPT
Upper Extremity ØJPV
Revision of device in
Lower Extremity ØJWW
Trunk ØJWT
Upper Extremity ØJWV
Infusion, glucarpidase
Central Vein 3EØ43GQ
Peripheral Vein 3EØ33GQ
Inguinal canal
use Inguinal Region, Bilateral
use Inguinal Region, Left
use Inguinal Region, Right
Inguinal triangle
use Inguinal Region, Bilateral
use Inguinal Region, Left
use Inguinal Region, Right
Injection *see* Introduction of substance in or on
Injection, Concentrated Bone Marrow Aspirate (CBMA), intramuscular XKØ23Ø3
Injection reservoir, port *use* Vascular Access Device, Totally Implantable in Subcutaneous Tissue and Fascia
Injection reservoir, pump *use* Infusion Device, Pump in Subcutaneous Tissue and Fascia
Insemination, artificial 3EØP7LZ
Insertion
Antimicrobial envelope *see* Introduction of Anti-infective
Aqueous drainage shunt
see Bypass, Eye Ø81
see Drainage, Eye Ø89
Products of Conception 1ØHØ
Spinal Stabilization Device
see Insertion of device in, Lower Joints ØSH
see Insertion of device in, Upper Joints ØRH
Insertion of device in
Abdominal Wall ØWHF
Acetabulum
Left ØQH5
Right ØQH4
Anal Sphincter ØDHR
Ankle Region
Left ØYHL
Right ØYHK
Anus ØDHQ
Aorta
Abdominal Ø4HØ
Thoracic
Ascending/Arch Ø2HX

Insertion of device in — *continued*
Aorta — *continued*
Thoracic — *continued*
Descending Ø2HW
Arm
Lower
Left ØXHF
Right ØXHD
Upper
Left ØXH9
Right ØXH8
Artery
Anterior Tibial
Left Ø4HQ
Right Ø4HP
Axillary
Left Ø3H6
Right Ø3H5
Brachial
Left Ø3H8
Right Ø3H7
Celiac Ø4H1
Colic
Left Ø4H7
Middle Ø4H8
Right Ø4H6
Common Carotid
Left Ø3HJ
Right Ø3HH
Common Iliac
Left Ø4HD
Right Ø4HC
Coronary
Four or More Arteries Ø2H3
One Artery Ø2HØ
Three Arteries Ø2H2
Two Arteries Ø2H1
External Carotid
Left Ø3HN
Right Ø3HM
External Iliac
Left Ø4HJ
Right Ø4HH
Face Ø3HR
Femoral
Left Ø4HL
Right Ø4HK
Foot
Left Ø4HW
Right Ø4HV
Gastric Ø4H2
Hand
Left Ø3HF
Right Ø3HD
Hepatic Ø4H3
Inferior Mesenteric Ø4HB
Innominate Ø3H2
Internal Carotid
Left Ø3HL
Right Ø3HK
Internal Iliac
Left Ø4HF
Right Ø4HE
Internal Mammary
Left Ø3H1
Right Ø3HØ
Intracranial Ø3HG
Lower Ø4HY
Peroneal
Left Ø4HU
Right Ø4HT
Popliteal
Left Ø4HN
Right Ø4HM
Posterior Tibial
Left Ø4HS
Right Ø4HR
Pulmonary
Left Ø2HR
Right Ø2HQ
Pulmonary Trunk Ø2HP
Radial
Left Ø3HC
Right Ø3HB
Renal
Left Ø4HA
Right Ø4H9
Splenic Ø4H4

Insertion of device in — *continued*
Artery — *continued*
Subclavian
Left Ø3H4
Right Ø3H3
Superior Mesenteric Ø4H5
Temporal
Left Ø3HT
Right Ø3HS
Thyroid
Left Ø3HV
Right Ø3HU
Ulnar
Left Ø3HA
Right Ø3H9
Upper Ø3HY
Vertebral
Left Ø3HQ
Right Ø3HP
Atrium
Left Ø2H7
Right Ø2H6
Axilla
Left ØXH5
Right ØXH4
Back
Lower ØWHL
Upper ØWHK
Bladder ØTHB
Bladder Neck ØTHC
Bone
Ethmoid
Left ØNHG
Right ØNHF
Facial ØNHW
Frontal ØNH1
Hyoid ØNHX
Lacrimal
Left ØNHJ
Right ØNHH
Lower ØQHY
Nasal ØNHB
Occipital ØNH7
Palatine
Left ØNHL
Right ØNHK
Parietal
Left ØNH4
Right ØNH3
Pelvic
Left ØQH3
Right ØQH2
Sphenoid ØNHC
Temporal
Left ØNH6
Right ØNH5
Upper ØPHY
Zygomatic
Left ØNHN
Right ØNHM
Bone Marrow Ø7HT
Brain ØØHØ
Breast
Bilateral ØHHV
Left ØHHU
Right ØHHT
Bronchus
Lingula ØBH9
Lower Lobe
Left ØBHB
Right ØBH6
Main
Left ØBH7
Right ØBH3
Middle Lobe, Right ØBH5
Upper Lobe
Left ØBH8
Right ØBH4
Bursa and Ligament
Lower ØMHY
Upper ØMHX
Buttock
Left ØYH1
Right ØYHØ
Carpal
Left ØPHN
Right ØPHM
Cavity, Cranial ØWH1
Cerebral Ventricle ØØH6

Insertion of device in — *continued*
Cervix ØUHC
Chest Wall ØWH8
Cisterna Chyli Ø7HL
Clavicle
Left ØPHB
Right ØPH9
Coccyx ØQHS
Cul-de-sac ØUHF
Diaphragm ØBHT
Disc
Cervical Vertebral ØRH3
Cervicothoracic Vertebral ØRH5
Lumbar Vertebral ØSH2
Lumbosacral ØSH4
Thoracic Vertebral ØRH9
Thoracolumbar Vertebral ØRHB
Duct
Hepatobiliary ØFHB
Pancreatic ØFHD
Duodenum ØDH9
Ear
Inner
Left Ø9HE
Right Ø9HD
Left Ø9HJ
Right Ø9HH
Elbow Region
Left ØXHC
Right ØXHB
Epididymis and Spermatic Cord ØVHM
Esophagus ØDH5
Extremity
Lower
Left ØYHB
Right ØYH9
Upper
Left ØXH7
Right ØXH6
Eye
Left Ø8H1
Right Ø8HØ
Face ØWH2
Fallopian Tube ØUH8
Femoral Region
Left ØYH8
Right ØYH7
Femoral Shaft
Left ØQH9
Right ØQH8
Femur
Lower
Left ØQHC
Right ØQHB
Upper
Left ØQH7
Right ØQH6
Fibula
Left ØQHK
Right ØQHJ
Foot
Left ØYHN
Right ØYHM
Gallbladder ØFH4
Gastrointestinal Tract ØWHP
Genitourinary Tract ØWHR
Gland
Endocrine ØGHS
Salivary ØCHA
Glenoid Cavity
Left ØPH8
Right ØPH7
Hand
Left ØXHK
Right ØXHJ
Head ØWHØ
Heart Ø2HA
Humeral Head
Left ØPHD
Right ØPHC
Humeral Shaft
Left ØPHG
Right ØPHF
Ileum ØDHB
Inguinal Region
Left ØYH6
Right ØYH5
Intestinal Tract
Lower ØDHD

Insertion of device in — *continued*
Intestinal Tract — *continued*
Upper ØDHØ
Intestine
Large ØDHE
Small ØDH8
Jaw
Lower ØWH5
Upper ØWH4
Jejunum ØDHA
Joint
Acromioclavicular
Left ØRHH
Right ØRHG
Ankle
Left ØSHG
Right ØSHF
Carpal
Left ØRHR
Right ØRHQ
Carpometacarpal
Left ØRHT
Right ØRHS
Cervical Vertebral ØRH1
Cervicothoracic Vertebral ØRH4
Coccygeal ØSH6
Elbow
Left ØRHM
Right ØRHL
Finger Phalangeal
Left ØRHX
Right ØRHW
Hip
Left ØSHB
Right ØSH9
Knee
Left ØSHD
Right ØSHC
Lumbar Vertebral ØSHØ
Lumbosacral ØSH3
Metacarpophalangeal
Left ØRHV
Right ØRHU
Metatarsal-Phalangeal
Left ØSHN
Right ØSHM
Occipital-cervical ØRHØ
Sacrococcygeal ØSH5
Sacroiliac
Left ØSH8
Right ØSH7
Shoulder
Left ØRHK
Right ØRHJ
Sternoclavicular
Left ØRHF
Right ØRHE
Tarsal
Left ØSHJ
Right ØSHH
Tarsometatarsal
Left ØSHL
Right ØSHK
Temporomandibular
Left ØRHD
Right ØRHC
Thoracic Vertebral ØRH6
Thoracolumbar Vertebral ØRHA
Toe Phalangeal
Left ØSHQ
Right ØSHP
Wrist
Left ØRHP
Right ØRHN
Kidney ØTH5
Knee Region
Left ØYHG
Right ØYHF
Larynx ØCHS
Leg
Lower
Left ØYHJ
Right ØYHH
Upper
Left ØYHD
Right ØYHC
Liver ØFHØ
Left Lobe ØFH2
Right Lobe ØFH1

Insertion of device in — *continued*
Lung
Left ØBHL
Right ØBHK
Lymphatic Ø7HN
Thoracic Duct Ø7HK
Mandible
Left ØNHV
Right ØNHT
Maxilla ØNHR
Mediastinum ØWHC
Metacarpal
Left ØPHQ
Right ØPHP
Metatarsal
Left ØQHP
Right ØQHN
Mouth and Throat ØCHY
Muscle
Lower ØKHY
Upper ØKHX
Nasal Mucosa and Soft Tissue Ø9HK
Nasopharynx Ø9HN
Neck ØWH6
Nerve
Cranial ØØHE
Peripheral Ø1HY
Nipple
Left ØHHX
Right ØHHW
Oral Cavity and Throat ØWH3
Orbit
Left ØNHQ
Right ØNHP
Ovary ØUH3
Pancreas ØFHG
Patella
Left ØQHF
Right ØQHD
Pelvic Cavity ØWHJ
Penis ØVHS
Pericardial Cavity ØWHD
Pericardium Ø2HN
Perineum
Female ØWHN
Male ØWHM
Peritoneal Cavity ØWHG
Phalanx
Finger
Left ØPHV
Right ØPHT
Thumb
Left ØPHS
Right ØPHR
Toe
Left ØQHR
Right ØQHQ
Pleura ØBHQ
Pleural Cavity
Left ØWHB
Right ØWH9
Prostate ØVHØ
Prostate and Seminal Vesicles ØVH4
Radius
Left ØPHJ
Right ØPHH
Rectum ØDHP
Respiratory Tract ØWHQ
Retroperitoneum ØWHH
Ribs
1 to 2 ØPH1
3 or More ØPH2
Sacrum ØQH1
Scapula
Left ØPH6
Right ØPH5
Scrotum and Tunica Vaginalis ØVH8
Shoulder Region
Left ØXH3
Right ØXH2
Sinus Ø9HY
Skin ØHHPXYZ
Skull ØNHØ
Spinal Canal ØØHU
Spinal Cord ØØHV
Spleen Ø7HP
Sternum ØPHØ
Stomach ØDH6

Insertion of device in — *continued*
Subcutaneous Tissue and Fascia
Abdomen ØJH8
Back ØJH7
Buttock ØJH9
Chest ØJH6
Face ØJH1
Foot
Left ØJHR
Right ØJHQ
Hand
Left ØJHK
Right ØJHJ
Head and Neck ØJHS
Lower Arm
Left ØJHH
Right ØJHG
Lower Extremity ØJHW
Lower Leg
Left ØJHP
Right ØJHN
Neck
Left ØJH5
Right ØJH4
Pelvic Region ØJHC
Perineum ØJHB
Scalp ØJHØ
Trunk ØJHT
Upper Arm
Left ØJHF
Right ØJHD
Upper Extremity ØJHV
Upper Leg
Left ØJHM
Right ØJHL
Tarsal
Left ØQHM
Right ØQHL
Tendon
Lower ØLHY
Upper ØLHX
Testis ØVHD
Thymus Ø7HM
Tibia
Left ØQHH
Right ØQHG
Tongue ØCH7
Trachea ØBH1
Tracheobronchial Tree ØBHØ
Ulna
Left ØPHL
Right ØPHK
Ureter ØTH9
Urethra ØTHD
Uterus ØUH9
Uterus and Cervix ØUHD
Vagina ØUHG
Vagina and Cul-de-sac ØUHH
Vas Deferens ØVHR
Vein
Axillary
Left Ø5H8
Right Ø5H7
Azygos Ø5HØ
Basilic
Left Ø5HC
Right Ø5HB
Brachial
Left Ø5HA
Right Ø5H9
Cephalic
Left Ø5HF
Right Ø5HD
Colic Ø6H7
Common Iliac
Left Ø6HD
Right Ø6HC
Coronary Ø2H4
Esophageal Ø6H3
External Iliac
Left Ø6HG
Right Ø6HF
External Jugular
Left Ø5HQ
Right Ø5HP
Face
Left Ø5HV
Right Ø5HT

Insertion of device in — *continued*
Vein — *continued*
Femoral
Left Ø6HN
Right Ø6HM
Foot
Left Ø6HV
Right Ø6HT
Gastric Ø6H2
Hand
Left Ø5HH
Right Ø5HG
Hemiazygos Ø5H1
Hepatic Ø6H4
Hypogastric
Left Ø6HJ
Right Ø6HH
Inferior Mesenteric Ø6H6
Innominate
Left Ø5H4
Right Ø5H3
Internal Jugular
Left Ø5HN
Right Ø5HM
Intracranial Ø5HL
Lower Ø6HY
Portal Ø6H8
Pulmonary
Left Ø2HT
Right Ø2HS
Renal
Left Ø6HB
Right Ø6H9
Saphenous
Left Ø6HQ
Right Ø6HP
Splenic Ø6H1
Subclavian
Left Ø5H6
Right Ø5H5
Superior Mesenteric Ø6H5
Upper Ø5HY
Vertebral
Left Ø5HS
Right Ø5HR
Vena Cava
Inferior Ø6HØ
Superior Ø2HV
Ventricle
Left Ø2HL
Right Ø2HK
Vertebra
Cervical ØPH3
Lumbar ØQHØ
Thoracic ØPH4
Wrist Region
Left ØXHH
Right ØXHG
Inspection
Abdominal Wall ØWJF
Ankle Region
Left ØYJL
Right ØYJK
Arm
Lower
Left ØXJF
Right ØXJD
Upper
Left ØXJ9
Right ØXJ8
Artery
Lower Ø4JY
Upper Ø3JY
Axilla
Left ØXJ5
Right ØXJ4
Back
Lower ØWJL
Upper ØWJK
Bladder ØTJB
Bone
Facial ØNJW
Lower ØQJY
Nasal ØNJB
Upper ØPJY
Bone Marrow Ø7JT
Brain ØØJØ
Breast
Left ØHJU

Inspection — *continued*
Breast — *continued*
Right ØHJT
Bursa and Ligament
Lower ØMJY
Upper ØMJX
Buttock
Left ØYJ1
Right ØYJØ
Cavity, Cranial ØWJ1
Chest Wall ØWJ8
Cisterna Chyli Ø7JL
Diaphragm ØBJT
Disc
Cervical Vertebral ØRJ3
Cervicothoracic Vertebral ØRJ5
Lumbar Vertebral ØSJ2
Lumbosacral ØSJ4
Thoracic Vertebral ØRJ9
Thoracolumbar Vertebral ØRJB
Duct
Hepatobiliary ØFJB
Pancreatic ØFJD
Ear
Inner
Left Ø9JE
Right Ø9JD
Left Ø9JJ
Right Ø9JH
Elbow Region
Left ØXJC
Right ØXJB
Epididymis and Spermatic Cord ØVJM
Extremity
Lower
Left ØYJB
Right ØYJ9
Upper
Left ØXJ7
Right ØXJ6
Eye
Left Ø8J1XZZ
Right Ø8JØXZZ
Face ØWJ2
Fallopian Tube ØUJ8
Femoral Region
Bilateral ØYJE
Left ØYJ8
Right ØYJ7
Finger Nail ØHJQXZZ
Foot
Left ØYJN
Right ØYJM
Gallbladder ØFJ4
Gastrointestinal Tract ØWJP
Genitourinary Tract ØWJR
Gland
Adrenal ØGJ5
Endocrine ØGJS
Pituitary ØGJØ
Salivary ØCJA
Great Vessel Ø2JY
Hand
Left ØXJK
Right ØXJJ
Head ØWJØ
Heart Ø2JA
Inguinal Region
Bilateral ØYJA
Left ØYJ6
Right ØYJ5
Intestinal Tract
Lower ØDJD
Upper ØDJØ
Jaw
Lower ØWJ5
Upper ØWJ4
Joint
Acromioclavicular
Left ØRJH
Right ØRJG
Ankle
Left ØSJG
Right ØSJF
Carpal
Left ØRJR
Right ØRJQ
Carpometacarpal
Left ØRJT

Inspection — *continued*
Joint — *continued*
Carpometacarpal — *continued*
Right ØRJS
Cervical Vertebral ØRJ1
Cervicothoracic Vertebral ØRJ4
Coccygeal ØSJ6
Elbow
Left ØRJM
Right ØRJL
Finger Phalangeal
Left ØRJX
Right ØRJW
Hip
Left ØSJB
Right ØSJ9
Knee
Left ØSJD
Right ØSJC
Lumbar Vertebral ØSJØ
Lumbosacral ØSJ3
Metacarpophalangeal
Left ØRJV
Right ØRJU
Metatarsal-Phalangeal
Left ØSJN
Right ØSJM
Occipital-cervical ØRJØ
Sacrococcygeal ØSJ5
Sacroiliac
Left ØSJ8
Right ØSJ7
Shoulder
Left ØRJK
Right ØRJJ
Sternoclavicular
Left ØRJF
Right ØRJE
Tarsal
Left ØSJJ
Right ØSJH
Tarsometatarsal
Left ØSJL
Right ØSJK
Temporomandibular
Left ØRJD
Right ØRJC
Thoracic Vertebral ØRJ6
Thoracolumbar Vertebral ØRJA
Toe Phalangeal
Left ØSJQ
Right ØSJP
Wrist
Left ØRJP
Right ØRJN
Kidney ØTJ5
Knee Region
Left ØYJG
Right ØYJF
Larynx ØCJS
Leg
Lower
Left ØYJJ
Right ØYJH
Upper
Left ØYJD
Right ØYJC
Lens
Left Ø8JKXZZ
Right Ø8JJXZZ
Liver ØFJØ
Lung
Left ØBJL
Right ØBJK
Lymphatic Ø7JN
Thoracic Duct Ø7JK
Mediastinum ØWJC
Mesentery ØDJV
Mouth and Throat ØCJY
Muscle
Extraocular
Left Ø8JM
Right Ø8JL
Lower ØKJY
Upper ØKJX
Nasal Mucosa and Soft Tissue Ø9JK
Neck ØWJ6
Nerve
Cranial ØØJE

Inspection — *continued*
Nerve — *continued*
Peripheral Ø1JY
Omentum ØDJU
Oral Cavity and Throat ØWJ3
Ovary ØUJ3
Pancreas ØFJG
Parathyroid Gland ØGJR
Pelvic Cavity ØWJJ
Penis ØVJS
Pericardial Cavity ØWJD
Perineum
Female ØWJN
Male ØWJM
Peritoneal Cavity ØWJG
Peritoneum ØDJW
Pineal Body ØGJ1
Pleura ØBJQ
Pleural Cavity
Left ØWJB
Right ØWJ9
Products of Conception 1ØJØ
Ectopic 1ØJ2
Retained 1ØJ1
Prostate and Seminal Vesicles ØVJ4
Respiratory Tract ØWJQ
Retroperitoneum ØWJH
Scrotum and Tunica Vaginalis ØVJ8
Shoulder Region
Left ØXJ3
Right ØXJ2
Sinus Ø9JY
Skin ØHJPXZZ
Skull ØNJØ
Spinal Canal ØØJU
Spinal Cord ØØJV
Spleen Ø7JP
Stomach ØDJ6
Subcutaneous Tissue and Fascia
Head and Neck ØJJS
Lower Extremity ØJJW
Trunk ØJJT
Upper Extremity ØJJV
Tendon
Lower ØLJY
Upper ØLJX
Testis ØVJD
Thymus Ø7JM
Thyroid Gland ØGJK
Toe Nail ØHJRXZZ
Trachea ØBJ1
Tracheobronchial Tree ØBJØ
Tympanic Membrane
Left Ø9J8
Right Ø9J7
Ureter ØTJ9
Urethra ØTJD
Uterus and Cervix ØUJD
Vagina and Cul-de-sac ØUJH
Vas Deferens ØVJR
Vein
Lower Ø6JY
Upper Ø5JY
Vulva ØUJM
Wrist Region
Left ØXJH
Right ØXJG
Instillation *see* Introduction of substance in or on
Insufflation *see* Introduction of substance in or on
Interatrial septum *use* Atrial Septum
InterAtrial Shunt Device IASD®, Corvia *use* Synthetic Substitute
Interbody fusion (spine) cage
use Interbody Fusion Device in Lower Joints
use Interbody Fusion Device in Upper Joints
Interbody Fusion Device
Customizable
Lumbar Vertebral XRGB
2 or more XRGC
Lumbosacral XRGD
Thoracolumbar Vertebral XRGA
Nanotextured Surface
Cervical Vertebral XRG1Ø92
2 or more XRG2Ø92
Cervicothoracic Vertebral XRG4Ø92
Lumbar Vertebral XRGBØ92
2 or more XRGCØ92
Lumbosacral XRGDØ92

Interbody Fusion Device — *continued*
Nanotextured Surface — *continued*
Occipital-cervical XRGØØ92
Thoracic Vertebral XRG6Ø92
2 to 7 XRG7Ø92
8 or more XRG8Ø92
Thoracolumbar Vertebral XRGAØ92
Radiolucent Porous
Cervical Vertebral XRG1ØF3
2 or more XRG2ØF3
Cervicothoracic Vertebral XRG4ØF3
Lumbar Vertebral XRGBØF3
2 or more XRGCØF3
Lumbosacral XRGDØF3
Occipital-cervical XRGØØF3
Thoracic Vertebral XRG6ØF3
2 to 7 XRG7ØF3
8 or more XRG8ØF3
Thoracolumbar Vertebral XRGAØF3
Intercarpal joint
use Carpal Joint, Left
use Carpal Joint, Right
Intercarpal ligament
use Hand Bursa and Ligament, Left
use Hand Bursa and Ligament, Right
INTERCEPT Blood System for Plasma Pathogen Reduced Cryoprecipitated Fibrinogen Complex *use* Pathogen Reduced Cryoprecipitated Fibrinogen Complex
INTERCEPT Fibrinogen Complex *use* Pathogen Reduced Cryoprecipitated Fibrinogen Complex
Interclavicular ligament
use Shoulder Bursa and Ligament, Left
use Shoulder Bursa and Ligament, Right
Intercostal lymph node *use* Lymphatic, Thorax
Intercostal muscle
use Thorax Muscle, Left
use Thorax Muscle, Right
Intercostal nerve *use* Thoracic Nerve
Intercostobrachial nerve *use* Thoracic Nerve
Intercuneiform joint
use Tarsal Joint, Left
use Tarsal Joint, Right
Intercuneiform ligament
use Foot Bursa and Ligament, Left
use Foot Bursa and Ligament, Right
Intermediate bronchus *use* Main Bronchus, Right
Intermediate cuneiform bone
use Tarsal, Left
use Tarsal, Right
Intermittent hemodialysis (IHD) 5A1D70Z
Intermittent mandatory ventilation *see* Assistance, Respiratory 5AØ9
Intermittent Negative Airway Pressure
24-96 Consecutive Hours, Ventilation 5AØ945B
Greater than 96 Consecutive Hours, Ventilation 5AØ955B
Less than 24 Consecutive Hours, Ventilation 5AØ935B
Intermittent Positive Airway Pressure
24-96 Consecutive Hours, Ventilation 5AØ9458
Greater than 96 Consecutive Hours, Ventilation 5AØ9558
Less than 24 Consecutive Hours, Ventilation 5AØ9358
Intermittent positive pressure breathing *see* Assistance, Respiratory 5AØ9
Internal anal sphincter *use* Anal Sphincter
Internal carotid artery, intracranial portion *use* Intracranial Artery
Internal carotid plexus *use* Head and Neck Sympathetic Nerve
Internal (basal) cerebral vein *use* Intracranial Vein
Internal iliac vein
use Hypogastric Vein, Left
use Hypogastric Vein, Right
Internal maxillary artery
use External Carotid Artery, Left
use External Carotid Artery, Right
Internal naris *use* Nasal Mucosa and Soft Tissue
Internal oblique muscle
use Abdomen Muscle, Left
use Abdomen Muscle, Right
Internal pudendal artery
use Internal Iliac Artery, Left
use Internal Iliac Artery, Right

Internal pudendal vein
use Hypogastric Vein, Left
use Hypogastric Vein, Right
Internal thoracic artery
use Internal Mammary Artery, Left
use Internal Mammary Artery, Right
use Subclavian Artery, Left
use Subclavian Artery, Right
Internal urethral sphincter *use* Urethra
Interphalangeal (IP) joint
use Finger Phalangeal Joint, Left
use Finger Phalangeal Joint, Right
use Toe Phalangeal Joint, Left
use Toe Phalangeal Joint, Right
Interphalangeal ligament
use Foot Bursa and Ligament, Left
use Foot Bursa and Ligament, Right
use Hand Bursa and Ligament, Left
use Hand Bursa and Ligament, Right
Interrogation, cardiac rhythm related device
Interrogation only *see* Measurement, Cardiac 4B02
With cardiac function testing *see* Measurement, Cardiac 4A02
Interruption *see* Occlusion
Interspinalis muscle
use Trunk Muscle, Left
use Trunk Muscle, Right
Interspinous ligament, cervical *use* Head and Neck Bursa and Ligament
Interspinous ligament, lumbar *use* Lower Spine Bursa and Ligament
Interspinous ligament, thoracic *use* Upper Spine Bursa and Ligament
Interspinous process spinal stabilization device
use Spinal Stabilization Device, Interspinous Process in 0RH
use Spinal Stabilization Device, Interspinous Process in 0SH
InterStim® Therapy lead *use* Neurostimulator Lead in Peripheral Nervous System
InterStim™ II Therapy neurostimulator *use* Stimulator Generator, Single Array in 0JH
InterStim™ Micro Therapy neurostimulator *use* Stimulator Generator, Single Array Rechargeable in 0JH
Intertransversarius muscle
use Trunk Muscle, Left
use Trunk Muscle, Right
Intertransverse ligament, cervical *use* Head and Neck Bursa and Ligament
Intertransverse ligament, lumbar *use* Lower Spine Bursa and Ligament
Intertransverse ligament, thoracic *use* Upper Spine Bursa and Ligament
Interventricular foramen (Monro) *use* Cerebral Ventricle
Interventricular septum *use* Ventricular Septum
Intestinal lymphatic trunk *use* Cisterna Chyli
Intracranial Arterial Flow, Whole Blood mRNA XXE5XT7
Intraluminal Device
Airway
Esophagus 0DH5
Mouth and Throat 0CHY
Nasopharynx 09HN
Bioactive
Occlusion
Common Carotid
Left 03LJ
Right 03LH
External Carotid
Left 03LN
Right 03LM
Internal Carotid
Left 03LL
Right 03LK
Intracranial 03LG
Vertebral
Left 03LQ
Right 03LP
Restriction
Common Carotid
Left 03VJ
Right 03VH
External Carotid
Left 03VN
Right 03VM
Intraluminal Device — *continued*
Bioactive — *continued*
Restriction — *continued*
Internal Carotid
Left 03VL
Right 03VK
Intracranial 03VG
Vertebral
Left 03VQ
Right 03VP
Endobronchial Valve
Lingula 0BH9
Lower Lobe
Left 0BHB
Right 0BH6
Main
Left 0BH7
Right 0BH3
Middle Lobe, Right 0BH5
Upper Lobe
Left 0BH8
Right 0BH4
Endotracheal Airway
Change device in, Trachea 0B21XEZ
Insertion of device in, Trachea 0BH1
Pessary
Change device in, Vagina and Cul-de-sac 0U2HXGZ
Insertion of device in
Cul-de-sac 0UHF
Vagina 0UHG
Intramedullary (IM) rod (nail)
use Internal Fixation Device, Intramedullary in Lower Bones
use Internal Fixation Device, Intramedullary in Upper Bones
Intramedullary skeletal kinetic distractor (ISKD)
use Internal Fixation Device, Intramedullary in Lower Bones
use Internal Fixation Device, Intramedullary in Upper Bones
Intraocular Telescope
Left 08RK30Z
Right 08RJ30Z
Intraoperative Radiation Therapy (IORT)
Anus DDY8CZZ
Bile Ducts DFY2CZZ
Bladder DTY2CZZ
Brain D0Y0CZZ
Brain Stem D0Y1CZZ
Cervix DUY1CZZ
Colon DDY5CZZ
Duodenum DDY2CZZ
Gallbladder DFY1CZZ
Ileum DDY4CZZ
Jejunum DDY3CZZ
Kidney DTY0CZZ
Larynx D9YBCZZ
Liver DFY0CZZ
Mouth D9Y4CZZ
Nasopharynx D9YDCZZ
Nerve, Peripheral D0Y7CZZ
Ovary DUY0CZZ
Pancreas DFY3CZZ
Pharynx D9YCCZZ
Prostate DVY0CZZ
Rectum DDY7CZZ
Spinal Cord D0Y6CZZ
Stomach DDY1CZZ
Ureter DTY1CZZ
Urethra DTY3CZZ
Uterus DUY2CZZ
Intra.OX 8E02XDZ
Intrauterine Device (IUD) *use* Contraceptive Device in Female Reproductive System
Intravascular fluorescence angiography (IFA) *see* Monitoring, Physiological Systems 4A1
Intravascular Lithotripsy (IVL) *see* Fragmentation
Intravascular ultrasound assisted thrombolysis *see* Fragmentation, Artery
Introduction of substance in or on
Artery
Central 3E06
Analgesics 3E06
Anesthetic, Intracirculatory 3E06
Antiarrhythmic 3E06
Anti-infective 3E06
Anti-inflammatory 3E06
Introduction of substance in or on — *continued*
Artery — *continued*
Central — *continued*
Antineoplastic 3E06
Destructive Agent 3E06
Diagnostic Substance, Other 3E06
Electrolytic Substance 3E06
Hormone 3E06
Hypnotics 3E06
Immunotherapeutic 3E06
Nutritional Substance 3E06
Platelet Inhibitor 3E06
Radioactive Substance 3E06
Sedatives 3E06
Serum 3E06
Thrombolytic 3E06
Toxoid 3E06
Vaccine 3E06
Vasopressor 3E06
Water Balance Substance 3E06
Coronary 3E07
Diagnostic Substance, Other 3E07
Platelet Inhibitor 3E07
Thrombolytic 3E07
Peripheral 3E05
Analgesics 3E05
Anesthetic, Intracirculatory 3E05
Antiarrhythmic 3E05
Anti-infective 3E05
Anti-inflammatory 3E05
Antineoplastic 3E05
Destructive Agent 3E05
Diagnostic Substance, Other 3E05
Electrolytic Substance 3E05
Hormone 3E05
Hypnotics 3E05
Immunotherapeutic 3E05
Nutritional Substance 3E05
Platelet Inhibitor 3E05
Radioactive Substance 3E05
Sedatives 3E05
Serum 3E05
Thrombolytic 3E05
Toxoid 3E05
Vaccine 3E05
Vasopressor 3E05
Water Balance Substance 3E05
Biliary Tract 3E0J
Analgesics 3E0J
Anesthetic Agent 3E0J
Anti-infective 3E0J
Anti-inflammatory 3E0J
Antineoplastic 3E0J
Destructive Agent 3E0J
Diagnostic Substance, Other 3E0J
Electrolytic Substance 3E0J
Gas 3E0J
Hypnotics 3E0J
Islet Cells, Pancreatic 3E0J
Nutritional Substance 3E0J
Radioactive Substance 3E0J
Sedatives 3E0J
Water Balance Substance 3E0J
Bone 3E0V
Analgesics 3E0V3NZ
Anesthetic Agent 3E0V3BZ
Anti-infective 3E0V32
Anti-inflammatory 3E0V33Z
Antineoplastic 3E0V30
Destructive Agent 3E0V3TZ
Diagnostic Substance, Other 3E0V3KZ
Electrolytic Substance 3E0V37Z
Hypnotics 3E0V3NZ
Nutritional Substance 3E0V36Z
Radioactive Substance 3E0V3HZ
Sedatives 3E0V3NZ
Water Balance Substance 3E0V37Z
Bone Marrow 3E0A3GC
Antineoplastic 3E0A30
Brain 3E0Q
Analgesics 3E0Q
Anesthetic Agent 3E0Q
Anti-infective 3E0Q
Anti-inflammatory 3E0Q
Antineoplastic 3E0Q
Destructive Agent 3E0Q
Diagnostic Substance, Other 3E0Q
Electrolytic Substance 3E0Q
Gas 3E0Q

Introduction of substance in or on — *continued*
Brain — *continued*
Hypnotics 3E0Q
Nutritional Substance 3E0Q
Radioactive Substance 3E0Q
Sedatives 3E0Q
Stem Cells
Embryonic 3E0Q
Somatic 3E0Q
Water Balance Substance 3E0Q
Cranial Cavity 3E0Q
Analgesics 3E0Q
Anesthetic Agent 3E0Q
Anti-infective 3E0Q
Anti-inflammatory 3E0Q
Antineoplastic 3E0Q
Destructive Agent 3E0Q
Diagnostic Substance, Other 3E0Q
Electrolytic Substance 3E0Q
Gas 3E0Q
Hypnotics 3E0Q
Nutritional Substance 3E0Q
Radioactive Substance 3E0Q
Sedatives 3E0Q
Stem Cells
Embryonic 3E0Q
Somatic 3E0Q
Water Balance Substance 3E0Q
Ear 3E0B
Analgesics 3E0B
Anesthetic Agent 3E0B
Anti-infective 3E0B
Anti-inflammatory 3E0B
Antineoplastic 3E0B
Destructive Agent 3E0B
Diagnostic Substance, Other 3E0B
Hypnotics 3E0B
Radioactive Substance 3E0B
Sedatives 3E0B
Epidural Space 3E0S3GC
Analgesics 3E0S3NZ
Anesthetic Agent 3E0S3BZ
Anti-infective 3E0S32
Anti-inflammatory 3E0S33Z
Antineoplastic 3E0S30
Destructive Agent 3E0S3TZ
Diagnostic Substance, Other 3E0S3KZ
Electrolytic Substance 3E0S37Z
Gas 3E0S
Hypnotics 3E0S3NZ
Nutritional Substance 3E0S36Z
Radioactive Substance 3E0S3HZ
Sedatives 3E0S3NZ
Water Balance Substance 3E0S37Z
Eye 3E0C
Analgesics 3E0C
Anesthetic Agent 3E0C
Anti-infective 3E0C
Anti-inflammatory 3E0C
Antineoplastic 3E0C
Destructive Agent 3E0C
Diagnostic Substance, Other 3E0C
Gas 3E0C
Hypnotics 3E0C
Pigment 3E0C
Radioactive Substance 3E0C
Sedatives 3E0C
Gastrointestinal Tract
Lower 3E0H
Analgesics 3E0H
Anesthetic Agent 3E0H
Anti-infective 3E0H
Anti-inflammatory 3E0H
Antineoplastic 3E0H
Destructive Agent 3E0H
Diagnostic Substance, Other 3E0H
Electrolytic Substance 3E0H
Gas 3E0H
Hypnotics 3E0H
Nutritional Substance 3E0H
Radioactive Substance 3E0H
Sedatives 3E0H
Water Balance Substance 3E0H
Upper 3E0G
Analgesics 3E0G
Anesthetic Agent 3E0G
Anti-infective 3E0G
Anti-inflammatory 3E0G
Antineoplastic 3E0G

Introduction of substance in or on — *continued*
Gastrointestinal Tract — *continued*
Upper — *continued*
Destructive Agent 3E0G
Diagnostic Substance, Other 3E0G
Electrolytic Substance 3E0G
Gas 3E0G
Hypnotics 3E0G
Nutritional Substance 3E0G
Radioactive Substance 3E0G
Sedatives 3E0G
Water Balance Substance 3E0G
Genitourinary Tract 3E0K
Analgesics 3E0K
Anesthetic Agent 3E0K
Anti-infective 3E0K
Anti-inflammatory 3E0K
Antineoplastic 3E0K
Destructive Agent 3E0K
Diagnostic Substance, Other 3E0K
Electrolytic Substance 3E0K
Gas 3E0K
Hypnotics 3E0K
Nutritional Substance 3E0K
Radioactive Substance 3E0K
Sedatives 3E0K
Water Balance Substance 3E0K
Heart 3E08
Diagnostic Substance, Other 3E08
Platelet Inhibitor 3E08
Thrombolytic 3E08
Joint 3E0U
Analgesics 3E0U3NZ
Anesthetic Agent 3E0U3BZ
Anti-infective 3E0U
Anti-inflammatory 3E0U33Z
Antineoplastic 3E0U30
Destructive Agent 3E0U3TZ
Diagnostic Substance, Other 3E0U3KZ
Electrolytic Substance 3E0U37Z
Gas 3E0U3SF
Hypnotics 3E0U3NZ
Nutritional Substance 3E0U36Z
Radioactive Substance 3E0U3HZ
Sedatives 3E0U3NZ
Water Balance Substance 3E0U37Z
Lymphatic 3E0W3GC
Analgesics 3E0W3NZ
Anesthetic Agent 3E0W3BZ
Anti-infective 3E0W32
Anti-inflammatory 3E0W33Z
Antineoplastic 3E0W30
Destructive Agent 3E0W3TZ
Diagnostic Substance, Other 3E0W3KZ
Electrolytic Substance 3E0W37Z
Hypnotics 3E0W3NZ
Nutritional Substance 3E0W36Z
Radioactive Substance 3E0W3HZ
Sedatives 3E0W3NZ
Water Balance Substance 3E0W37Z
Mouth 3E0D
Analgesics 3E0D
Anesthetic Agent 3E0D
Antiarrhythmic 3E0D
Anti-infective 3E0D
Anti-inflammatory 3E0D
Antineoplastic 3E0D
Destructive Agent 3E0D
Diagnostic Substance, Other 3E0D
Electrolytic Substance 3E0D
Hypnotics 3E0D
Nutritional Substance 3E0D
Radioactive Substance 3E0D
Sedatives 3E0D
Serum 3E0D
Toxoid 3E0D
Vaccine 3E0D
Water Balance Substance 3E0D
Mucous Membrane 3E00XGC
Analgesics 3E00XNZ
Anesthetic Agent 3E00XBZ
Anti-infective 3E00X2
Anti-inflammatory 3E00X3Z
Antineoplastic 3E00X0
Destructive Agent 3E00XTZ
Diagnostic Substance, Other 3E00XKZ
Hypnotics 3E00XNZ
Pigment 3E00XMZ
Sedatives 3E00XNZ

Introduction of substance in or on — *continued*
Mucous Membrane — *continued*
Serum 3E00X4Z
Toxoid 3E00X4Z
Vaccine 3E00X4Z
Muscle 3E023GC
Analgesics 3E023NZ
Anesthetic Agent 3E023BZ
Anti-infective 3E0232
Anti-inflammatory 3E0233Z
Antineoplastic 3E0230
Destructive Agent 3E023TZ
Diagnostic Substance, Other 3E023KZ
Electrolytic Substance 3E0237Z
Hypnotics 3E023NZ
Nutritional Substance 3E0236Z
Radioactive Substance 3E023HZ
Sedatives 3E023NZ
Serum 3E0234Z
Toxoid 3E0234Z
Vaccine 3E0234Z
Water Balance Substance 3E0237Z
Nerve
Cranial 3E0X3GC
Anesthetic Agent 3E0X3BZ
Anti-inflammatory 3E0X33Z
Destructive Agent 3E0X3TZ
Peripheral 3E0T3GC
Anesthetic Agent 3E0T3BZ
Anti-inflammatory 3E0T33Z
Destructive Agent 3E0T3TZ
Plexus 3E0T3GC
Anesthetic Agent 3E0T3BZ
Anti-inflammatory 3E0T33Z
Destructive Agent 3E0T3TZ
Nose 3E09
Analgesics 3E09
Anesthetic Agent 3E09
Anti-infective 3E09
Anti-inflammatory 3E09
Antineoplastic 3E09
Destructive Agent 3E09
Diagnostic Substance, Other 3E09
Hypnotics 3E09
Radioactive Substance 3E09
Sedatives 3E09
Serum 3E09
Toxoid 3E09
Vaccine 3E09
Pancreatic Tract 3E0J
Analgesics 3E0J
Anesthetic Agent 3E0J
Anti-infective 3E0J
Anti-inflammatory 3E0J
Antineoplastic 3E0J
Destructive Agent 3E0J
Diagnostic Substance, Other 3E0J
Electrolytic Substance 3E0J
Gas 3E0J
Hypnotics 3E0J
Islet Cells, Pancreatic 3E0J
Nutritional Substance 3E0J
Radioactive Substance 3E0J
Sedatives 3E0J
Water Balance Substance 3E0J
Pericardial Cavity 3E0Y
Analgesics 3E0Y3NZ
Anesthetic Agent 3E0Y3BZ
Anti-infective 3E0Y32
Anti-inflammatory 3E0Y33Z
Antineoplastic 3E0Y
Destructive Agent 3E0Y3TZ
Diagnostic Substance, Other 3E0Y3KZ
Electrolytic Substance 3E0Y37Z
Gas 3E0Y
Hypnotics 3E0Y3NZ
Nutritional Substance 3E0Y36Z
Radioactive Substance 3E0Y3HZ
Sedatives 3E0Y3NZ
Water Balance Substance 3E0Y37Z
Peritoneal Cavity 3E0M
Adhesion Barrier 3E0M
Analgesics 3E0M3NZ
Anesthetic Agent 3E0M3BZ
Anti-infective 3E0M32
Anti-inflammatory 3E0M33Z
Antineoplastic 3E0M
Destructive Agent 3E0M3TZ
Diagnostic Substance, Other 3E0M3KZ

- **Introduction of substance in or on** — *continued*
  - Peritoneal Cavity — *continued*
    - Electrolytic Substance 3EØM37Z
    - Gas 3EØM
    - Hypnotics 3EØM3NZ
    - Nutritional Substance 3EØM36Z
    - Radioactive Substance 3EØM3HZ
    - Sedatives 3EØM3NZ
    - Water Balance Substance 3EØM37Z
  - Pharynx 3EØD
    - Analgesics 3EØD
    - Anesthetic Agent 3EØD
    - Antiarrhythmic 3EØD
    - Anti-infective 3EØD
    - Anti-inflammatory 3EØD
    - Antineoplastic 3EØD
    - Destructive Agent 3EØD
    - Diagnostic Substance, Other 3EØD
    - Electrolytic Substance 3EØD
    - Hypnotics 3EØD
    - Nutritional Substance 3EØD
    - Radioactive Substance 3EØD
    - Sedatives 3EØD
    - Serum 3EØD
    - Toxoid 3EØD
    - Vaccine 3EØD
    - Water Balance Substance 3EØD
  - Pleural Cavity 3EØL
    - Adhesion Barrier 3EØL
    - Analgesics 3EØL3NZ
    - Anesthetic Agent 3EØL3BZ
    - Anti-infective 3EØL32
    - Anti-inflammatory 3EØL33Z
    - Antineoplastic 3EØL
    - Destructive Agent 3EØL3TZ
    - Diagnostic Substance, Other 3EØL3KZ
    - Electrolytic Substance 3EØL37Z
    - Gas 3EØL
    - Hypnotics 3EØL3NZ
    - Nutritional Substance 3EØL36Z
    - Radioactive Substance 3EØL3HZ
    - Sedatives 3EØL3NZ
    - Water Balance Substance 3EØL37Z
  - Products of Conception 3EØE
    - Analgesics 3EØE
    - Anesthetic Agent 3EØE
    - Anti-infective 3EØE
    - Anti-inflammatory 3EØE
    - Antineoplastic 3EØE
    - Destructive Agent 3EØE
    - Diagnostic Substance, Other 3EØE
    - Electrolytic Substance 3EØE
    - Gas 3EØE
    - Hypnotics 3EØE
    - Nutritional Substance 3EØE
    - Radioactive Substance 3EØE
    - Sedatives 3EØE
    - Water Balance Substance 3EØE
  - Reproductive
    - Female 3EØP
      - Adhesion Barrier 3EØP
      - Analgesics 3EØP
      - Anesthetic Agent 3EØP
      - Anti-infective 3EØP
      - Anti-inflammatory 3EØP
      - Antineoplastic 3EØP
      - Destructive Agent 3EØP
      - Diagnostic Substance, Other 3EØP
      - Electrolytic Substance 3EØP
      - Gas 3EØP
      - Hormone 3EØP
      - Hypnotics 3EØP
      - Nutritional Substance 3EØP
      - Ovum, Fertilized 3EØP
      - Radioactive Substance 3EØP
      - Sedatives 3EØP
      - Sperm 3EØP
      - Water Balance Substance 3EØP
    - Male 3EØN
      - Analgesics 3EØN
      - Anesthetic Agent 3EØN
      - Anti-infective 3EØN
      - Anti-inflammatory 3EØN
      - Antineoplastic 3EØN
      - Destructive Agent 3EØN
      - Diagnostic Substance, Other 3EØN
      - Electrolytic Substance 3EØN
      - Gas 3EØN
      - Hypnotics 3EØN

- **Introduction of substance in or on** — *continued*
  - Reproductive — *continued*
    - Male — *continued*
      - Nutritional Substance 3EØN
      - Radioactive Substance 3EØN
      - Sedatives 3EØN
      - Water Balance Substance 3EØN
  - Respiratory Tract 3EØF
    - Analgesics 3EØF
    - Anesthetic Agent 3EØF
    - Anti-infective 3EØF
    - Anti-inflammatory 3EØF
    - Antineoplastic 3EØF
    - Destructive Agent 3EØF
    - Diagnostic Substance, Other 3EØF
    - Electrolytic Substance 3EØF
    - Gas 3EØF
    - Hypnotics 3EØF
    - Nutritional Substance 3EØF
    - Radioactive Substance 3EØF
    - Sedatives 3EØF
    - Water Balance Substance 3EØF
  - Skin 3EØØXGC
    - Analgesics 3EØØXNZ
    - Anesthetic Agent 3EØØXBZ
    - Anti-infective 3EØØX2
    - Anti-inflammatory 3EØØX3Z
    - Antineoplastic 3EØØXØ
    - Destructive Agent 3EØØXTZ
    - Diagnostic Substance, Other 3EØØXKZ
    - Hypnotics 3EØØXNZ
    - Pigment 3EØØXMZ
    - Sedatives 3EØØXNZ
    - Serum 3EØØX4Z
    - Toxoid 3EØØX4Z
    - Vaccine 3EØØX4Z
  - Spinal Canal 3EØR3GC
    - Analgesics 3EØR3NZ
    - Anesthetic Agent 3EØR3BZ
    - Anti-infective 3EØR32
    - Anti-inflammatory 3EØR33Z
    - Antineoplastic 3EØR3Ø
    - Destructive Agent 3EØR3TZ
    - Diagnostic Substance, Other 3EØR3KZ
    - Electrolytic Substance 3EØR37Z
    - Gas 3EØR
    - Hypnotics 3EØR3NZ
    - Nutritional Substance 3EØR36Z
    - Radioactive Substance 3EØR3HZ
    - Sedatives 3EØR3NZ
    - Stem Cells
      - Embryonic 3EØR
      - Somatic 3EØR
    - Water Balance Substance 3EØR37Z
  - Subcutaneous Tissue 3EØ13GC
    - Analgesics 3EØ13NZ
    - Anesthetic Agent 3EØ13BZ
    - Anti-infective 3EØ1
    - Anti-inflammatory 3EØ133Z
    - Antineoplastic 3EØ13Ø
    - Destructive Agent 3EØ13TZ
    - Diagnostic Substance, Other 3EØ13KZ
    - Electrolytic Substance 3EØ137Z
    - Hormone 3EØ13V
    - Hypnotics 3EØ13NZ
    - Nutritional Substance 3EØ136Z
    - Radioactive Substance 3EØ13HZ
    - Sedatives 3EØ13NZ
    - Serum 3EØ134Z
    - Toxoid 3EØ134Z
    - Vaccine 3EØ134Z
    - Water Balance Substance 3EØ137Z
  - Vein
    - Central 3EØ4
      - Analgesics 3EØ4
      - Anesthetic, Intracirculatory 3EØ4
      - Antiarrhythmic 3EØ4
      - Anti-infective 3EØ4
      - Anti-inflammatory 3EØ4
      - Antineoplastic 3EØ4
      - Destructive Agent 3EØ4
      - Diagnostic Substance, Other 3EØ4
      - Electrolytic Substance 3EØ4
      - Hormone 3EØ4
      - Hypnotics 3EØ4
      - Immunotherapeutic 3EØ4
      - Nutritional Substance 3EØ4
      - Platelet Inhibitor 3EØ4
      - Radioactive Substance 3EØ4

- **Introduction of substance in or on** — *continued*
  - Vein — *continued*
    - Central — *continued*
      - Sedatives 3EØ4
      - Serum 3EØ4
      - Thrombolytic 3EØ4
      - Toxoid 3EØ4
      - Vaccine 3EØ4
      - Vasopressor 3EØ4
      - Water Balance Substance 3EØ4
    - Peripheral 3EØ3
      - Analgesics 3EØ3
      - Anesthetic, Intracirculatory 3EØ3
      - Antiarrhythmic 3EØ3
      - Anti-infective 3EØ3
      - Anti-inflammatory 3EØ3
      - Antineoplastic 3EØ3
      - Destructive Agent 3EØ3
      - Diagnostic Substance, Other 3EØ3
      - Electrolytic Substance 3EØ3
      - Hormone 3EØ3
      - Hypnotics 3EØ3
      - Immunotherapeutic 3EØ3
      - Islet Cells, Pancreatic 3EØ3
      - Nutritional Substance 3EØ3
      - Platelet Inhibitor 3EØ3
      - Radioactive Substance 3EØ3
      - Sedatives 3EØ3
      - Serum 3EØ3
      - Thrombolytic 3EØ3
      - Toxoid 3EØ3
      - Vaccine 3EØ3
      - Vasopressor 3EØ3
      - Water Balance Substance 3EØ3
- **Intubation**
  - Airway
    - *see* Insertion of device in, Esophagus ØDH5
    - *see* Insertion of device in, Mouth and Throat ØCHY
    - *see* Insertion of device in, Trachea ØBH1
  - Drainage device *see* Drainage
  - Feeding Device *see* Insertion of device in, Gastrointestinal System ØDH
- **INTUITY Elite valve system, EDWARDS** *use* Zooplastic Tissue, Rapid Deployment Technique in New Technology
- **Iobenguane I-131 Antineoplastic** XWØ
- **Iobenguane I-131, High Specific Activity (HSA)** *use* Iobenguane I-131 Antineoplastic
- **IPPB (intermittent positive pressure breathing)** *see* Assistance, Respiratory 5AØ9
- **IRE (Irreversible Electroporation)** *see* Destruction, Hepatobiliary System and Pancreas ØF5
- **Iridectomy**
  - *see* Excision, Eye Ø8B
  - *see* Resection, Eye Ø8T
- **Iridoplasty**
  - *see* Repair, Eye Ø8Q
  - *see* Replacement, Eye Ø8R
  - *see* Supplement, Eye Ø8U
- **Iridotomy** *see* Drainage, Eye Ø89
- **Irreversible Electroporation (IRE)** *see* Destruction, Hepatobiliary System and Pancreas ØF5
- **Irrigation**
  - Biliary Tract, Irrigating Substance 3E1J
  - Brain, Irrigating Substance 3E1Q38Z
  - Cranial Cavity, Irrigating Substance 3E1Q38Z
  - Ear, Irrigating Substance 3E1B
  - Epidural Space, Irrigating Substance 3E1S38Z
  - Eye, Irrigating Substance 3E1C
  - Gastrointestinal Tract
    - Lower, Irrigating Substance 3E1H
    - Upper, Irrigating Substance 3E1G
  - Genitourinary Tract, Irrigating Substance 3E1K
  - Irrigating Substance 3C1ZX8Z
  - Joint, Irrigating Substance 3E1U
  - Mucous Membrane, Irrigating Substance 3E1Ø
  - Nose, Irrigating Substance 3E19
  - Pancreatic Tract, Irrigating Substance 3E1J
  - Pericardial Cavity, Irrigating Substance 3E1Y38Z
  - Peritoneal Cavity
    - Dialysate 3E1M39Z
    - Irrigating Substance 3E1M
  - Pleural Cavity, Irrigating Substance 3E1L38Z
  - Reproductive
    - Female, Irrigating Substance 3E1P
    - Male, Irrigating Substance 3E1N
  - Respiratory Tract, Irrigating Substance 3E1F

Irrigation — *continued*
Skin, Irrigating Substance 3E1Ø
Spinal Canal, Irrigating Substance 3E1R38Z
Isavuconazole (isavuconazonium sulfate) *use* Other Anti-infective
Ischiatic nerve *use* Sciatic Nerve
Ischiocavernosus muscle *use* Perineum Muscle
Ischiofemoral ligament
use Hip Bursa and Ligament, Left
use Hip Bursa and Ligament, Right
Ischium
use Pelvic Bone, Left
use Pelvic Bone, Right
ISC-REST kit
ISCDx XXE5XT7
QIAGEN Access Anti-SARS-CoV-2 Total Test XXE5XV7
QIAstat-Dx Respiratory SARS-CoV-2 Panel XXE97U7
Isolation 8EØZXY6
Isotope Administration, Other Radiation, Whole Body DWY5G
Itrel (3) (4) neurostimulator *use* Stimulator Generator, Single Array in ØJH

J

Jakafi® *use* Ruxolitinib
Jejunal artery *use* Superior Mesenteric Artery
Jejunectomy
see Excision, Jejunum ØDBA
see Resection, Jejunum ØDTA
Jejunocolostomy
see Bypass, Gastrointestinal System ØD1
see Drainage, Gastrointestinal System ØD9
Jejunopexy
see Repair, Jejunum ØDQA
see Reposition, Jejunum ØDSA
Jejunostomy
see Bypass, Jejunum ØD1A
see Drainage, Jejunum ØD9A
Jejunotomy *see* Drainage, Jejunum ØD9A
Joint fixation plate
use Internal Fixation Device in Lower Joints
use Internal Fixation Device in Upper Joints
Joint liner (insert) *use* Liner in Lower Joints
Joint spacer (antibiotic)
use Spacer in Lower Joints
use Spacer in Upper Joints
Jugular body *use* Glomus Jugulare
Jugular lymph node
use Lymphatic, Left Neck
use Lymphatic, Right Neck

K

Kappa *use* Pacemaker, Dual Chamber in ØJH
Kcentra *use* 4-Factor Prothrombin Complex Concentrate
Keratectomy, kerectomy
see Excision, Eye Ø8B
see Resection, Eye Ø8T
Keratocentesis *see* Drainage, Eye Ø89
Keratoplasty
see Repair, Eye Ø8Q
see Replacement, Eye Ø8R
see Supplement, Eye Ø8U
Keratotomy
see Drainage, Eye Ø89
see Repair, Eye Ø8Q
KEVZARA® *use* Sarilumab
Keystone Heart TriGuard 3™ CEPD (cerebral embolic protection device) X2A6325
Kirschner wire (K-wire)
use Internal Fixation Device in Head and Facial Bones
use Internal Fixation Device in Lower Bones
use Internal Fixation Device in Lower Joints
use Internal Fixation Device in Upper Bones
use Internal Fixation Device in Upper Joints
Knee (implant) insert *use* Liner in Lower Joints
KUB x-ray *see* Plain Radiography, Kidney, Ureter and Bladder BTØ4
Kuntscher nail
use Internal Fixation Device, Intramedullary in Lower Bones
Kuntscher nail — *continued*
use Internal Fixation Device, Intramedullary in Upper Bones
KYMRIAH® *use* Tisagenlecleucel Immunotherapy

L

Labia majora *use* Vulva
Labia minora *use* Vulva
Labial gland
use Lower Lip
use Upper Lip
Labiectomy
see Excision, Female Reproductive System ØUB
see Resection, Female Reproductive System ØUT
Lacrimal canaliculus
use Lacrimal Duct, Left
use Lacrimal Duct, Right
Lacrimal punctum
use Lacrimal Duct, Left
use Lacrimal Duct, Right
Lacrimal sac
use Lacrimal Duct, Left
use Lacrimal Duct, Right
LAGB (laparoscopic adjustable gastric banding)
Initial procedure ØDV64CZ
Surgical correction *see* Revision of device in, Stomach ØDW6
Laminectomy
see Excision, Lower Bones ØQB
see Excision, Upper Bones ØPB
see Release, Central Nervous System and Cranial Nerves ØØN
see Release, Peripheral Nervous System Ø1N
Laminotomy
see Drainage, Lower Bones ØQ9
see Drainage, Upper Bones ØP9
see Excision, Lower Bones ØQB
see Excision, Upper Bones ØPB
see Release, Central Nervous System and Cranial Nerves ØØN
see Release, Lower Bones ØQN
see Release, Peripheral Nervous System Ø1N
see Release, Upper Bones ØPN
Laparoscopic-assisted transanal pull-through
see Excision, Gastrointestinal System ØDB
see Resection, Gastrointestinal System ØDT
Laparoscopy *see* Inspection
Laparotomy
Drainage *see* Drainage, Peritoneal Cavity ØW9G
Exploratory *see* Inspection, Peritoneal Cavity ØWJG
LAP-BAND® adjustable gastric banding system *use* Extraluminal Device
Laryngectomy
see Excision, Larynx ØCBS
see Resection, Larynx ØCTS
Laryngocentesis *see* Drainage, Larynx ØC9S
Laryngogram *see* Fluoroscopy, Larynx B91J
Laryngopexy *see* Repair, Larynx ØCQS
Laryngopharynx *use* Pharynx
Laryngoplasty
see Repair, Larynx ØCQS
see Replacement, Larynx ØCRS
see Supplement, Larynx ØCUS
Laryngorrhaphy *see* Repair, Larynx ØCQS
Laryngoscopy ØCJS8ZZ
Laryngotomy *see* Drainage, Larynx ØC9S
Laser Interstitial Thermal Therapy
Adrenal Gland DGY2KZZ
Anus DDY8KZZ
Bile Ducts DFY2KZZ
Brain DØYØKZZ
Brain Stem DØY1KZZ
Breast
Left DMYØKZZ
Right DMY1KZZ
Bronchus DBY1KZZ
Chest Wall DBY7KZZ
Colon DDY5KZZ
Diaphragm DBY8KZZ
Duodenum DDY2KZZ
Esophagus DDYØKZZ
Gallbladder DFY1KZZ
Gland
Adrenal DGY2KZZ
Parathyroid DGY4KZZ
Laser Interstitial Thermal Therapy — *continued*
Gland — *continued*
Pituitary DGYØKZZ
Thyroid DGY5KZZ
Ileum DDY4KZZ
Jejunum DDY3KZZ
Liver DFYØKZZ
Lung DBY2KZZ
Mediastinum DBY6KZZ
Nerve, Peripheral DØY7KZZ
Pancreas DFY3KZZ
Parathyroid Gland DGY4KZZ
Pineal Body DGY1KZZ
Pituitary Gland DGYØKZZ
Pleura DBY5KZZ
Prostate DVYØKZZ
Rectum DDY7KZZ
Spinal Cord DØY6KZZ
Stomach DDY1KZZ
Thyroid Gland DGY5KZZ
Trachea DBYØKZZ
Lateral canthus
use Upper Eyelid, Left
use Upper Eyelid, Right
Lateral collateral ligament (LCL)
use Knee Bursa and Ligament, Left
use Knee Bursa and Ligament, Right
Lateral condyle of femur
use Lower Femur, Left
use Lower Femur, Right
Lateral condyle of tibia
use Tibia, Left
use Tibia, Right
Lateral cuneiform bone
use Tarsal, Left
use Tarsal, Right
Lateral epicondyle of femur
use Lower Femur, Left
use Lower Femur, Right
Lateral epicondyle of humerus
use Humeral Shaft, Left
use Humeral Shaft, Right
Lateral femoral cutaneous nerve *use* Lumbar Plexus
Lateral (brachial) lymph node
use Lymphatic, Left Axillary
use Lymphatic, Right Axillary
Lateral malleolus
use Fibula, Left
use Fibula, Right
Lateral meniscus
use Knee Joint, Left
use Knee Joint, Right
Lateral nasal cartilage *use* Nasal Mucosa and Soft Tissue
Lateral plantar artery
use Foot Artery, Left
use Foot Artery, Right
Lateral plantar nerve *use* Tibial Nerve
Lateral rectus muscle
use Extraocular Muscle, Left
use Extraocular Muscle, Right
Lateral sacral artery
use Internal Iliac Artery, Left
use Internal Iliac Artery, Right
Lateral sacral vein
use Hypogastric Vein, Left
use Hypogastric Vein, Right
Lateral sural cutaneous nerve *use* Peroneal Nerve
Lateral tarsal artery
use Foot Artery, Left
use Foot Artery, Right
Lateral temporomandibular ligament *use* Head and Neck Bursa and Ligament
Lateral thoracic artery
use Axillary Artery, Left
use Axillary Artery, Right
Latissimus dorsi muscle
use Trunk Muscle, Left
use Trunk Muscle, Right
Latissimus Dorsi Myocutaneous Flap
Replacement
Bilateral ØHRVØ75
Left ØHRUØ75
Right ØHRTØ75
Transfer
Left ØKXG
Right ØKXF

Subterms under main terms may continue to next column or page

Lavage
see Irrigation
Bronchial alveolar, diagnostic *see* Drainage, Respiratory System ØB9
Least splanchnic nerve *use* Thoracic Sympathetic Nerve
Lefamulin Anti-infective XWØ
Left ascending lumbar vein *use* Hemiazygos Vein
Left atrioventricular valve *use* Mitral Valve
Left auricular appendix *use* Atrium, Left
Left colic vein *use* Colic Vein
Left coronary sulcus *use* Heart, Left
Left gastric artery *use* Gastric Artery
Left gastroepiploic artery *use* Splenic Artery
Left gastroepiploic vein *use* Splenic Vein
Left inferior phrenic vein *use* Renal Vein, Left
Left inferior pulmonary vein *use* Pulmonary Vein, Left
Left jugular trunk *use* Thoracic Duct
Left lateral ventricle *use* Cerebral Ventricle
Left ovarian vein *use* Renal Vein, Left
Left second lumbar vein *use* Renal Vein, Left
Left subclavian trunk *use* Thoracic Duct
Left subcostal vein *use* Hemiazygos Vein
Left superior pulmonary vein *use* Pulmonary Vein, Left
Left suprarenal vein *use* Renal Vein, Left
Left testicular vein *use* Renal Vein, Left
Lengthening
Bone, with device *see* Insertion of Limb Lengthening Device
Muscle, by incision *see* Division, Muscles ØK8
Tendon, by incision *see* Division, Tendons ØL8
Leptomeninges, intracranial *use* Cerebral Meninges
Leptomeninges, spinal *use* Spinal Meninges
Leronlimab Monoclonal Antibody XWØ13K6
Lesser alar cartilage *use* Nasal Mucosa and Soft Tissue
Lesser occipital nerve *use* Cervical Plexus
Lesser Omentum *use* Omentum
Lesser saphenous vein
use Saphenous Vein, Left
use Saphenous Vein, Right
Lesser splanchnic nerve *use* Thoracic Sympathetic Nerve
Lesser trochanter
use Upper Femur, Left
use Upper Femur, Right
Lesser tuberosity
use Humeral Head, Left
use Humeral Head, Right
Lesser wing *use* Sphenoid Bone
Leukopheresis, therapeutic *see* Pheresis, Circulatory 6A55
Levator anguli oris muscle *use* Facial Muscle
Levator ani muscle *use* Perineum Muscle
Levator labii superioris alaeque nasi muscle *use* Facial Muscle
Levator labii superioris muscle *use* Facial Muscle
Levator palpebrae superioris muscle
use Upper Eyelid, Left
use Upper Eyelid, Right
Levator scapulae muscle
use Neck Muscle, Left
use Neck Muscle, Right
Levator veli palatini muscle *use* Tongue, Palate, Pharynx Muscle
Levatores costarum muscle
use Thorax Muscle, Left
use Thorax Muscle, Right
Lifeline ARM Automated Chest Compression (ACC) device 5A1221J
LifeStent® (Flexstar) (XL) Vascular Stent System
use Intraluminal Device
Lifileucel *use* Lifileucel Immunotherapy
Lifileucel Immunotherapy XWØ
Ligament of head of fibula
use Knee Bursa and Ligament, Left
use Knee Bursa and Ligament, Right
Ligament of the lateral malleolus
use Ankle Bursa and Ligament, Left
use Ankle Bursa and Ligament, Right
Ligamentum flavum, cervical *use* Head and Neck Bursa and Ligament
Ligamentum flavum, lumbar *use* Lower Spine Bursa and Ligament
Ligamentum flavum, thoracic *use* Upper Spine Bursa and Ligament
Ligation *see* Occlusion
Ligation, hemorrhoid *see* Occlusion, Lower Veins, Hemorrhoidal Plexus
Light Therapy GZJZZZZ
Liner
Removal of device from
Hip
Left ØSPBØ9Z
Right ØSP9Ø9Z
Knee
Left ØSPDØ9Z
Right ØSPCØ9Z
Revision of device in
Hip
Left ØSWBØ9Z
Right ØSW9Ø9Z
Knee
Left ØSWDØ9Z
Right ØSWCØ9Z
Supplement
Hip
Left ØSUBØ9Z
Acetabular Surface ØSUEØ9Z
Femoral Surface ØSUSØ9Z
Right ØSU9Ø9Z
Acetabular Surface ØSUAØ9Z
Femoral Surface ØSURØ9Z
Knee
Left ØSUDØ9
Femoral Surface ØSUUØ9Z
Tibial Surface ØSUWØ9Z
Right ØSUCØ9
Femoral Surface ØSUTØ9Z
Tibial Surface ØSUVØ9Z
Lingual artery
use External Carotid Artery, Left
use External Carotid Artery, Right
Lingual tonsil *use* Pharynx
Lingulectomy, lung
see Excision, Lung Lingula ØBBH
see Resection, Lung Lingula ØBTH
Lisocabtagene Maraleucel *use* Lisocabtagene Maraleucel Immunotherapy
Lisocabtagene Maraleucel Immunotherapy XWØ
Lithoplasty *see* Fragmentation
Lithotripsy
see Fragmentation
With removal of fragments *see* Extirpation
LITT (laser interstitial thermal therapy) *see* Laser Interstitial Thermal Therapy
LIVIAN™ CRT-D *use* Cardiac Resynchronization Defibrillator Pulse Generator in ØJH
Lobectomy
see Excision, Central Nervous System and Cranial Nerves ØØB
see Excision, Endocrine System ØGB
see Excision, Hepatobiliary System and Pancreas ØFB
see Excision, Respiratory System ØBB
see Resection, Endocrine System ØGT
see Resection, Hepatobiliary System and Pancreas ØFT
see Resection, Respiratory System ØBT
Lobotomy *see* Division, Brain ØØ8Ø
Localization
see Imaging
see Map
Locus ceruleus *use* Pons
Long thoracic nerve *use* Brachial Plexus
Loop ileostomy *see* Bypass, Ileum ØD1B
Loop recorder, implantable *use* Monitoring Device
Lower GI series *see* Fluoroscopy, Colon BD14
Lower Respiratory Fluid Nucleic Acid-base Microbial Detection XXEBXQ6
LTX Regional Anticoagulant *use* Nafamostat Anticoagulant
LUCAS® Chest Compression System 5A1221J
Lumbar artery *use* Abdominal Aorta
Lumbar facet joint *use* Lumbar Vertebral Joint
Lumbar ganglion *use* Lumbar Sympathetic Nerve
Lumbar lymph node *use* Lymphatic, Aortic
Lumbar lymphatic trunk *use* Cisterna Chyli
Lumbar splanchnic nerve *use* Lumbar Sympathetic Nerve
Lumbosacral facet joint *use* Lumbosacral Joint
Lumbosacral trunk *use* Lumbar Nerve
Lumpectomy *see* Excision
Lunate bone
use Carpal, Left
use Carpal, Right
Lunotriquetral ligament
use Hand Bursa and Ligament, Left
use Hand Bursa and Ligament, Right
Lurbinectedin XWØ
Lymphadenectomy
see Excision, Lymphatic and Hemic Systems Ø7B
see Resection, Lymphatic and Hemic Systems Ø7T
Lymphadenotomy *see* Drainage, Lymphatic and Hemic Systems Ø79
Lymphangiectomy
see Excision, Lymphatic and Hemic Systems Ø7B
see Resection, Lymphatic and Hemic Systems Ø7T
Lymphangiogram *see* Plain Radiography, Lymphatic System B7Ø
Lymphangioplasty
see Repair, Lymphatic and Hemic Systems Ø7Q
see Supplement, Lymphatic and Hemic Systems Ø7U
Lymphangiorrhaphy *see* Repair, Lymphatic and Hemic Systems Ø7Q
Lymphangiotomy *see* Drainage, Lymphatic and Hemic Systems Ø79
Lysis *see* Release

M

Macula XXE5XR7
use Retina, Left
use Retina, Right
MAGEC® Spinal Bracing and Distraction System
use Magnetically Controlled Growth Rod(s) in New Technology
Magnet extraction, ocular foreign body *see* Extirpation, Eye Ø8C
Magnetic Resonance Imaging (MRI)
Abdomen BW3Ø
Ankle
Left BQ3H
Right BQ3G
Aorta
Abdominal B43Ø
Thoracic B33Ø
Arm
Left BP3F
Right BP3E
Artery
Celiac B431
Cervico-Cerebral Arch B33Q
Common Carotid, Bilateral B335
Coronary
Bypass Graft, Multiple B233
Multiple B231
Internal Carotid, Bilateral B338
Intracranial B33R
Lower Extremity
Bilateral B43H
Left B43G
Right B43F
Pelvic B43C
Renal, Bilateral B438
Spinal B33M
Superior Mesenteric B434
Upper Extremity
Bilateral B33K
Left B33J
Right B33H
Vertebral, Bilateral B33G
Bladder BT3Ø
Brachial Plexus BW3P
Brain BØ3Ø
Breast
Bilateral BH32
Left BH31
Right BH3Ø
Calcaneus
Left BQ3K
Right BQ3J
Chest BW33Y
Coccyx BR3F
Connective Tissue
Lower Extremity BL31
Upper Extremity BL3Ø

Magnetic Resonance Imaging (MRI) — *continued*
Corpora Cavernosa BV3Ø
Disc
Cervical BR31
Lumbar BR33
Thoracic BR32
Ear B93Ø
Elbow
Left BP3H
Right BP3G
Eye
Bilateral B837
Left B836
Right B835
Femur
Left BQ34
Right BQ33
Fetal Abdomen BY33
Fetal Extremity BY35
Fetal Head BY3Ø
Fetal Heart BY31
Fetal Spine BY34
Fetal Thorax BY32
Fetus, Whole BY36
Foot
Left BQ3M
Right BQ3L
Forearm
Left BP3K
Right BP3J
Gland
Adrenal, Bilateral BG32
Parathyroid BG33
Parotid, Bilateral B936
Salivary, Bilateral B93D
Submandibular, Bilateral B939
Thyroid BG34
Head BW38
Heart, Right and Left B236
Hip
Left BQ31
Right BQ3Ø
Intracranial Sinus B532
Joint
Finger
Left BP3D
Right BP3C
Hand
Left BP3D
Right BP3C
Temporomandibular, Bilateral BN39
Kidney
Bilateral BT33
Left BT32
Right BT31
Transplant BT39
Knee
Left BQ38
Right BQ37
Larynx B93J
Leg
Left BQ3F
Right BQ3D
Liver BF35
Liver and Spleen BF36
Lung Apices BB3G
Nasopharynx B93F
Neck BW3F
Nerve
Acoustic BØ3C
Brachial Plexus BW3P
Oropharynx B93F
Ovary
Bilateral BU35
Left BU34
Right BU33
Ovary and Uterus BU3C
Pancreas BF37
Patella
Left BQ3W
Right BQ3V
Pelvic Region BW3G
Pelvis BR3C
Pituitary Gland BØ39
Plexus, Brachial BW3P
Prostate BV33
Retroperitoneum BW3H
Sacrum BR3F
Scrotum BV34

Magnetic Resonance Imaging (MRI) — *continued*
Sella Turcica BØ39
Shoulder
Left BP39
Right BP38
Sinus
Intracranial B532
Paranasal B932
Spinal Cord BØ3B
Spine
Cervical BR3Ø
Lumbar BR39
Thoracic BR37
Spleen and Liver BF36
Subcutaneous Tissue
Abdomen BH3H
Extremity
Lower BH3J
Upper BH3F
Head BH3D
Neck BH3D
Pelvis BH3H
Thorax BH3G
Tendon
Lower Extremity BL33
Upper Extremity BL32
Testicle
Bilateral BV37
Left BV36
Right BV35
Toe
Left BQ3Q
Right BQ3P
Uterus BU36
Pregnant BU3B
Uterus and Ovary BU3C
Vagina BU39
Vein
Cerebellar B531
Cerebral B531
Jugular, Bilateral B535
Lower Extremity
Bilateral B53D
Left B53C
Right B53B
Other B53V
Pelvic (Iliac) Bilateral B53H
Portal B53T
Pulmonary, Bilateral B53S
Renal, Bilateral B53L
Spanchnic B53T
Upper Extremity
Bilateral B53P
Left B53N
Right B53M
Vena Cava
Inferior B539
Superior B538
Wrist
Left BP3M
Right BP3L
Magnetically Controlled Growth Rod(s)
Cervical XNS3
Lumbar XNSØ
Thoracic XNS4
Magnetic-guided radiofrequency endovascular fistula
Radial Artery, Left Ø31C3ZF
Radial Artery, Right Ø31B3ZF
Ulnar Artery, Left Ø31A3ZF
Ulnar Artery, Right Ø3193ZF
Malleotomy *see* Drainage, Ear, Nose, Sinus Ø99
Malleus
use Auditory Ossicle, Left
use Auditory Ossicle, Right
Mammaplasty, mammoplasty
see Alteration, Skin and Breast ØHØ
see Repair, Skin and Breast ØHQ
see Replacement, Skin and Breast ØHR
see Supplement, Skin and Breast ØHU
Mammary duct
use Breast, Bilateral
use Breast, Left
use Breast, Right
Mammary gland
use Breast, Bilateral
use Breast, Left
use Breast, Right

Mammectomy
see Excision, Skin and Breast ØHB
see Resection, Skin and Breast ØHT
Mammillary body *use* Hypothalamus
Mammography *see* Plain Radiography, Skin, Subcutaneous Tissue and Breast BHØ
Mammotomy *see* Drainage, Skin and Breast ØH9
Mandibular nerve *use* Trigeminal Nerve
Mandibular notch
use Mandible, Left
use Mandible, Right
Mandibulectomy
see Excision, Head and Facial Bones ØNB
see Resection, Head and Facial Bones ØNT
Manipulation
Adhesions *see* Release
Chiropractic *see* Chiropractic Manipulation
Manual removal, retained placenta *see* Extraction, Products of Conception, Retained 1ØD1
Manubrium *use* Sternum
Map
Basal Ganglia ØØK8
Brain ØØKØ
Cerebellum ØØKC
Cerebral Hemisphere ØØK7
Conduction Mechanism Ø2K8
Hypothalamus ØØKA
Medulla Oblongata ØØKD
Pons ØØKB
Thalamus ØØK9
Mapping
Doppler ultrasound *see* Ultrasonography
Electrocardiogram only *see* Measurement, Cardiac 4AØ2
Mark IV Breathing Pacemaker System *use* Stimulator Generator in Subcutaneous Tissue and Fascia
Marsupialization
see Drainage
see Excision
Massage, cardiac
External 5A12Ø12
Open Ø2QAØZZ
Masseter muscle *use* Head Muscle
Masseteric fascia *use* Subcutaneous Tissue and Fascia, Face
Mastectomy
see Excision, Skin and Breast ØHB
see Resection, Skin and Breast ØHT
Mastoid air cells
use Mastoid Sinus, Left
use Mastoid Sinus, Right
Mastoid (postauricular) lymph node
use Lymphatic, Left Neck
use Lymphatic, Right Neck
Mastoid process
use Temporal Bone, Left
use Temporal Bone, Right
Mastoidectomy
see Excision, Ear, Nose, Sinus Ø9B
see Resection, Ear, Nose, Sinus Ø9T
Mastoidotomy *see* Drainage, Ear, Nose, Sinus Ø99
Mastopexy
see Repair, Skin and Breast ØHQ
see Reposition, Skin and Breast ØHS
Mastorrhaphy *see* Repair, Skin and Breast ØHQ
Mastotomy *see* Drainage, Skin and Breast ØH9
Maxillary artery
use External Carotid Artery, Left
use External Carotid Artery, Right
Maxillary nerve *use* Trigeminal Nerve
Maximo II DR (VR) *use* Defibrillator Generator in ØJH
Maximo II DR CRT-D *use* Cardiac Resynchronization Defibrillator Pulse Generator in ØJH
Measurement
Arterial
Flow
Coronary 4AØ3
Intracranial 4AØ3X5D
Peripheral 4AØ3
Pulmonary 4AØ3
Pressure
Coronary 4AØ3
Peripheral 4AØ3
Pulmonary 4AØ3
Thoracic, Other 4AØ3
Pulse
Coronary 4AØ3

Subterms under main terms may continue to next column or page

Measurement — *continued*
- Arterial — *continued*
  - Pulse — *continued*
    - Peripheral 4AØ3
    - Pulmonary 4AØ3
  - Saturation, Peripheral 4AØ3
  - Sound, Peripheral 4AØ3
- Biliary
  - Flow 4AØC
  - Pressure 4AØC
- Cardiac
  - Action Currents 4AØ2
  - Defibrillator 4BØ2XTZ
  - Electrical Activity 4AØ2
    - Guidance 4AØ2X4A
    - No Qualifier 4AØ2X4Z
  - Output 4AØ2
  - Pacemaker 4BØ2XSZ
  - Rate 4AØ2
  - Rhythm 4AØ2
  - Sampling and Pressure
    - Bilateral 4AØ2
    - Left Heart 4AØ2
    - Right Heart 4AØ2
  - Sound 4AØ2
  - Total Activity, Stress 4AØ2XM4
- Central Nervous
  - Cerebrospinal Fluid Shunt, Wireless Sensor 4BØØXWØ
  - Conductivity 4AØØ
  - Electrical Activity 4AØØ
  - Pressure 4AØØØBZ
    - Intracranial 4AØØ
  - Saturation, Intracranial 4AØØ
  - Stimulator 4BØØXVZ
  - Temperature, Intracranial 4AØØ
- Circulatory, Volume 4AØ5XLZ
- Gastrointestinal
  - Motility 4AØB
  - Pressure 4AØB
  - Secretion 4AØB
- Lower Respiratory Fluid Nucleic Acid-base Microbial Detection XXEBXQ6
- Lymphatic
  - Flow 4AØ6
  - Pressure 4AØ6
- Metabolism 4AØZ
- Musculoskeletal
  - Contractility 4AØF
  - Pressure 4AØF3BE
  - Stimulator 4BØFXVZ
- Olfactory, Acuity 4AØ8XØZ
- Peripheral Nervous
  - Conductivity
    - Motor 4AØ1
    - Sensory 4AØ1
  - Electrical Activity 4AØ1
  - Stimulator 4BØ1XVZ
- Positive Blood Culture Fluorescence Hybridization for Organism Identification, Concentration and Susceptibility XXE5XN6
- Products of Conception
  - Cardiac
    - Electrical Activity 4AØH
    - Rate 4AØH
    - Rhythm 4AØH
    - Sound 4AØH
  - Nervous
    - Conductivity 4AØJ
    - Electrical Activity 4AØJ
    - Pressure 4AØJ
- Respiratory
  - Capacity 4AØ9
  - Flow 4AØ9
  - Pacemaker 4BØ9XSZ
  - Rate 4AØ9
  - Resistance 4AØ9
  - Total Activity 4AØ9
  - Volume 4AØ9
- Sleep 4AØZXQZ
- Temperature 4AØZ
- Urinary
  - Contractility 4AØD
  - Flow 4AØD
  - Pressure 4AØD
  - Resistance 4AØD
  - Volume 4AØD

Measurement — *continued*
- Venous
  - Flow
    - Central 4AØ4
    - Peripheral 4AØ4
    - Portal 4AØ4
    - Pulmonary 4AØ4
  - Pressure
    - Central 4AØ4
    - Peripheral 4AØ4
    - Portal 4AØ4
    - Pulmonary 4AØ4
  - Pulse
    - Central 4AØ4
    - Peripheral 4AØ4
    - Portal 4AØ4
    - Pulmonary 4AØ4
  - Saturation, Peripheral 4AØ4
- Visual
  - Acuity 4AØ7XØZ
  - Mobility 4AØ7X7Z
  - Pressure 4AØ7XBZ
- Whole Blood Nucleic Acid-base Microbial Detection XXE5XM5

Meatoplasty, urethra *see* Repair, Urethra ØTQD

Meatotomy *see* Drainage, Urinary System ØT9

Mechanical chest compression (mCPR) 5A1221J

Mechanical Initial Specimen Diversion Technique Using Active Negative Pressure (blood collection) XXE5XR7

Mechanical ventilation *see* Performance, Respiratory 5A19

Medial canthus
- *use* Lower Eyelid, Left
- *use* Lower Eyelid, Right

Medial collateral ligament (MCL)
- *use* Knee Bursa and Ligament, Left
- *use* Knee Bursa and Ligament, Right

Medial condyle of femur
- *use* Lower Femur, Left
- *use* Lower Femur, Right

Medial condyle of tibia
- *use* Tibia, Left
- *use* Tibia, Right

Medial cuneiform bone
- *use* Tarsal, Left
- *use* Tarsal, Right

Medial epicondyle of femur
- *use* Lower Femur, Left
- *use* Lower Femur, Right

Medial epicondyle of humerus
- *use* Humeral Shaft, Left
- *use* Humeral Shaft, Right

Medial malleolus
- *use* Tibia, Left
- *use* Tibia, Right

Medial meniscus
- *use* Knee Joint, Left
- *use* Knee Joint, Right

Medial plantar artery
- *use* Foot Artery, Left
- *use* Foot Artery, Right

Medial plantar nerve *use* Tibial Nerve

Medial popliteal nerve *use* Tibial Nerve

Medial rectus muscle
- *use* Extraocular Muscle, Left
- *use* Extraocular Muscle, Right

Medial sural cutaneous nerve *use* Tibial Nerve

Median antebrachial vein
- *use* Basilic Vein, Left
- *use* Basilic Vein, Right

Median cubital vein
- *use* Basilic Vein, Left
- *use* Basilic Vein, Right

Median sacral artery *use* Abdominal Aorta

Mediastinal cavity *use* Mediastinum

Mediastinal lymph node *use* Lymphatic, Thorax

Mediastinal space *use* Mediastinum

Mediastinoscopy ØWJC4ZZ

Medication Management GZ3ZZZZ
- for substance abuse
  - Antabuse HZ83ZZZ
  - Bupropion HZ87ZZZ
  - Clonidine HZ86ZZZ
  - Levo-alpha-acetyl-methadol (LAAM) HZ82ZZZ
  - Methadone Maintenance HZ81ZZZ

Medication Management — *continued*
- for substance abuse — *continued*
  - Naloxone HZ85ZZZ
  - Naltrexone HZ84ZZZ
  - Nicotine Replacement HZ8ØZZZ
  - Other Replacement Medication HZ89ZZZ
  - Psychiatric Medication HZ88ZZZ

Meditation 8EØZXY5

Medtronic Endurant® II AAA stent graft system *use* Intraluminal Device

Meissner's (submucous) plexus *use* Abdominal Sympathetic Nerve

Melody® transcatheter pulmonary valve *use* Zooplastic Tissue in Heart and Great Vessels

Membranous urethra *use* Urethra

Meningeorrhaphy
- *see* Repair, Cerebral Meninges ØØQ1
- *see* Repair, Spinal Meninges ØØQT

Meniscectomy, knee
- *see* Excision, Joint, Knee, Left ØSBD
- *see* Excision, Joint, Knee, Right ØSBC

Mental foramen
- *use* Mandible, Left
- *use* Mandible, Right

Mentalis muscle *use* Facial Muscle

Mentoplasty *see* Alteration, Jaw, Lower ØWØ5

Meropenem-vaborbactam Anti-infective XWØ

Mesenterectomy *see* Excision, Mesentery ØDBV

Mesenteriorrhaphy, mesenterorrhaphy *see* Repair, Mesentery ØDQV

Mesenteriplication *see* Repair, Mesentery ØDQV

Mesoappendix *use* Mesentery

Mesocolon *use* Mesentery

Metacarpal ligament
- *use* Hand Bursa and Ligament, Left
- *use* Hand Bursa and Ligament, Right

Metacarpophalangeal ligament
- *use* Hand Bursa and Ligament, Left
- *use* Hand Bursa and Ligament, Right

Metal on metal bearing surface *use* Synthetic Substitute, Metal in ØSR

Metatarsal ligament
- *use* Foot Bursa and Ligament, Left
- *use* Foot Bursa and Ligament, Right

Metatarsectomy
- *see* Excision, Lower Bones ØQB
- *see* Resection, Lower Bones ØQT

Metatarsophalangeal (MTP) joint
- *use* Metatarsal-Phalangeal Joint, Left
- *use* Metatarsal-Phalangeal Joint, Right

Metatarsophalangeal ligament
- *use* Foot Bursa and Ligament, Left
- *use* Foot Bursa and Ligament, Right

Metathalamus *use* Thalamus

Micro-Driver stent (RX) (OTW) *use* Intraluminal Device

MicroMed HeartAssist *use* Implantable Heart Assist System in Heart and Great Vessels

Micrus CERECYTE Microcoil *use* Intraluminal Device, Bioactive in Upper Arteries

Midcarpal joint
- *use* Carpal Joint, Left
- *use* Carpal Joint, Right

Middle cardiac nerve *use* Thoracic Sympathetic Nerve

Middle cerebral artery *use* Intracranial Artery

Middle cerebral vein *use* Intracranial Vein

Middle colic vein *use* Colic Vein

Middle genicular artery
- *use* Popliteal Artery, Left
- *use* Popliteal Artery, Right

Middle hemorrhoidal vein
- *use* Hypogastric Vein, Left
- *use* Hypogastric Vein, Right

Middle rectal artery
- *use* Internal Iliac Artery, Left
- *use* Internal Iliac Artery, Right

Middle suprarenal artery *use* Abdominal Aorta

Middle temporal artery
- *use* Temporal Artery, Left
- *use* Temporal Artery, Right

Middle turbinate *use* Nasal Turbinate

Mineral-based Topical Hemostatic Agent XWØ

MIRODERM™ Biologic Wound Matrix *use* Skin Substitute, Porcine Liver Derived in New Technology

MitraClip valve repair system *use* Synthetic Substitute

Mitral annulus *use* Mitral Valve

Mitroflow® Aortic Pericardial Heart Valve *use* Zooplastic Tissue in Heart and Great Vessels
Mobilization, adhesions *see* Release
Molar gland *use* Buccal Mucosa
MolecuLight i:X® wound imaging *see* Other Imaging, Anatomical Regions BW5
Monitoring
Arterial
Flow
Coronary 4A13
Peripheral 4A13
Pulmonary 4A13
Pressure
Coronary 4A13
Peripheral 4A13
Pulmonary 4A13
Pulse
Coronary 4A13
Peripheral 4A13
Pulmonary 4A13
Saturation, Peripheral 4A13
Sound, Peripheral 4A13
Cardiac
Electrical Activity 4A12
Ambulatory 4A12X45
No Qualifier 4A12X4Z
Output 4A12
Rate 4A12
Rhythm 4A12
Sound 4A12
Total Activity, Stress 4A12XM4
Vascular Perfusion, Indocyanine Green Dye 4A12XSH
Central Nervous
Conductivity 4A1Ø
Electrical Activity
Intraoperative 4A1Ø
No Qualifier 4A1Ø
Pressure 4A1ØØBZ
Intracranial 4A1Ø
Saturation, Intracranial 4A1Ø
Temperature, Intracranial 4A1Ø
Gastrointestinal
Motility 4A1B
Pressure 4A1B
Secretion 4A1B
Vascular Perfusion, Indocyanine Green Dye 4A1BXSH
Kidney, Fluorescent Pyrazine XT25XE5
Lymphatic
Flow
Indocyanine Green Dye 4A16
No Qualifier 4A16
Pressure 4A16
Oxygen Saturation Endoscopic Imaging (OXEI) XD2
Peripheral Nervous
Conductivity
Motor 4A11
Sensory 4A11
Electrical Activity
Intraoperative 4A11
No Qualifier 4A11
Products of Conception
Cardiac
Electrical Activity 4A1H
Rate 4A1H
Rhythm 4A1H
Sound 4A1H
Nervous
Conductivity 4A1J
Electrical Activity 4A1J
Pressure 4A1J
Respiratory
Capacity 4A19
Flow 4A19
Rate 4A19
Resistance 4A19
Volume 4A19
Skin and Breast, Vascular Perfusion, Indocyanine Green Dye 4A1GXSH
Sleep 4A1ZXQZ
Temperature 4A1Z
Urinary
Contractility 4A1D
Flow 4A1D
Pressure 4A1D
Resistance 4A1D
Volume 4A1D
Monitoring — *continued*
Venous
Flow
Central 4A14
Peripheral 4A14
Portal 4A14
Pulmonary 4A14
Pressure
Central 4A14
Peripheral 4A14
Portal 4A14
Pulmonary 4A14
Pulse
Central 4A14
Peripheral 4A14
Portal 4A14
Pulmonary 4A14
Saturation
Central 4A14
Portal 4A14
Pulmonary 4A14
Monitoring Device, Hemodynamic
Abdomen ØJH8
Chest ØJH6
Mosaic Bioprosthesis (aortic) (mitral) valve *use* Zooplastic Tissue in Heart and Great Vessels
Motor Function Assessment FØ1
Motor Treatment FØ7
MR Angiography
see Magnetic Resonance Imaging (MRI), Heart B23
see Magnetic Resonance Imaging (MRI), Lower Arteries B43
see Magnetic Resonance Imaging (MRI), Upper Arteries B33
MULTI-LINK (VISION) (MINI-VISION) (ULTRA) Coronary Stent System *use* Intraluminal Device
Multiple sleep latency test 4AØZXQZ
Musculocutaneous nerve *use* Brachial Plexus
Musculopexy
see Repair, Muscles ØKQ
see Reposition, Muscles ØKS
Musculophrenic artery
use Internal Mammary Artery, Left
use Internal Mammary Artery, Right
Musculoplasty
see Repair, Muscles ØKQ
see Supplement, Muscles ØKU
Musculorrhaphy *see* Repair, Muscles ØKQ
Musculospiral nerve *use* Radial Nerve
Myectomy
see Excision, Muscles ØKB
see Resection, Muscles ØKT
Myelencephalon *use* Medulla Oblongata
Myelogram
CT *see* Computerized Tomography (CT Scan), Central Nervous System BØ2
MRI *see* Magnetic Resonance Imaging (MRI), Central Nervous System BØ3
Myenteric (Auerbach's) plexus *use* Abdominal Sympathetic Nerve
Myocardial Bridge Release *see* Release, Artery, Coronary
Myomectomy *see* Excision, Female Reproductive System ØUB
Myometrium *use* Uterus
Myopexy
see Repair, Muscles ØKQ
see Reposition, Muscles ØKS
Myoplasty
see Repair, Muscles ØKQ
see Supplement, Muscles ØKU
Myorrhaphy *see* Repair, Muscles ØKQ
Myoscopy *see* Inspection, Muscles ØKJ
Myotomy
see Division, Muscles ØK8
see Drainage, Muscles ØK9
Myringectomy
see Excision, Ear, Nose, Sinus Ø9B
see Resection, Ear, Nose, Sinus Ø9T
Myringoplasty
see Repair, Ear, Nose, Sinus Ø9Q
see Replacement, Ear, Nose, Sinus Ø9R
see Supplement, Ear, Nose, Sinus Ø9U
Myringostomy *see* Drainage, Ear, Nose, Sinus Ø99
Myringotomy *see* Drainage, Ear, Nose, Sinus Ø99

N

NA-1 (Nerinitide) *use* Nerinitide
Nafamostat Anticoagulant XYØYX37
Nail bed
use Finger Nail
use Toe Nail
Nail plate
use Finger Nail
use Toe Nail
nanoLOCK™ interbody fusion device *use* Interbody Fusion Device, Nanotextured Surface in New Technology
Narcosynthesis GZGZZZZ
Narsoplimab Monoclonal Antibody XWØ
Nasal cavity *use* Nasal Mucosa and Soft Tissue
Nasal concha *use* Nasal Turbinate
Nasalis muscle *use* Facial Muscle
Nasolacrimal duct
use Lacrimal Duct, Left
use Lacrimal Duct, Right
Nasopharyngeal airway (NPA) *use* Intraluminal Device, Airway in Ear, Nose, Sinus
Navicular bone
use Tarsal, Left
use Tarsal, Right
Near Infrared Spectroscopy, Circulatory System 8EØ2
Neck of femur
use Upper Femur, Left
use Upper Femur, Right
Neck of humerus (anatomical) (surgical)
use Humeral Head, Left
use Humeral Head, Right
Neovasc Reducer™ *use* Reduction Device in New Technology
Nephrectomy
see Excision, Urinary System ØTB
see Resection, Urinary System ØTT
Nephrolithotomy *see* Extirpation, Urinary System ØTC
Nephrolysis *see* Release, Urinary System ØTN
Nephropexy
see Repair, Urinary System ØTQ
see Reposition, Urinary System ØTS
Nephroplasty
see Repair, Urinary System ØTQ
see Supplement, Urinary System ØTU
Nephropyeloureterostomy
see Bypass, Urinary System ØT1
see Drainage, Urinary System ØT9
Nephrorrhaphy *see* Repair, Urinary System ØTQ
Nephroscopy, transurethral ØTJ58ZZ
Nephrostomy
see Bypass, Urinary System ØT1
see Drainage, Urinary System ØT9
Nephrotomography
see Fluoroscopy, Urinary System BT1
see Plain Radiography, Urinary System BTØ
Nephrotomy
see Division, Urinary System ØT8
see Drainage, Urinary System ØT9
Nerinitide XWØ
Nerve conduction study
see Measurement, Central Nervous 4AØØ
see Measurement, Peripheral Nervous 4AØ1
Nerve Function Assessment FØ1
Nerve to the stapedius *use* Facial Nerve
Nesiritide *use* Human B-Type Natriuretic Peptide
Neurectomy
see Excision, Central Nervous System and Cranial Nerves ØØB
see Excision, Peripheral Nervous System Ø1B
Neurexeresis
see Extraction, Central Nervous System and Cranial Nerves ØØD
see Extraction, Peripheral Nervous System Ø1D
Neurohypophysis *use* Pituitary Gland
Neurolysis
see Release, Central Nervous System and Cranial Nerves ØØN
see Release, Peripheral Nervous System Ø1N
Neuromuscular electrical stimulation (NEMS) lead *use* Stimulator Lead in Muscles
Neurophysiologic monitoring *see* Monitoring, Central Nervous 4A1Ø

Neuroplasty
- *see* Repair, Central Nervous System and Cranial Nerves ØØQ
- *see* Repair, Peripheral Nervous System Ø1Q
- *see* Supplement, Central Nervous System and Cranial Nerves ØØU
- *see* Supplement, Peripheral Nervous System Ø1U

Neurorrhaphy
- *see* Repair, Central Nervous System and Cranial Nerves ØØQ
- *see* Repair, Peripheral Nervous System Ø1Q

Neurostimulator Generator
- Insertion of device in, Skull ØNHØØNZ
- Removal of device from, Skull ØNPØØNZ
- Revision of device in, Skull ØNWØØNZ

Neurostimulator generator, multiple channel *use* Stimulator Generator, Multiple Array in ØJH

Neurostimulator generator, multiple channel rechargeable *use* Stimulator Generator, Multiple Array Rechargeable in ØJH

Neurostimulator generator, single channel *use* Stimulator Generator, Single Array in ØJH

Neurostimulator generator, single channel rechargeable *use* Stimulator Generator, Single Array Rechargeable in ØJH

Neurostimulator Lead
- Insertion of device in
  - Brain ØØHØ
  - Cerebral Ventricle ØØH6
  - Nerve
    - Cranial ØØHE
    - Peripheral Ø1HY
  - Spinal Canal ØØHU
  - Spinal Cord ØØHV
  - Vein
    - Azygos Ø5HØ
    - Innominate
      - Left Ø5H4
      - Right Ø5H3
- Removal of device from
  - Brain ØØPØ
  - Cerebral Ventricle ØØP6
  - Nerve
    - Cranial ØØPE
    - Peripheral Ø1PY
  - Spinal Canal ØØPU
  - Spinal Cord ØØPV
  - Vein
    - Azygos Ø5PØ
    - Innominate
      - Left Ø5P4
      - Right Ø5P3
- Revision of device in
  - Brain ØØWØ
  - Cerebral Ventricle ØØW6
  - Nerve
    - Cranial ØØWE
    - Peripheral Ø1WY
  - Spinal Canal ØØWU
  - Spinal Cord ØØWV
  - Vein
    - Azygos Ø5WØ
    - Innominate
      - Left Ø5W4
      - Right Ø5W3

Neurostimulator Lead in Oropharynx XWHD7Q7

Neurotomy
- *see* Division, Central Nervous System and Cranial Nerves ØØ8
- *see* Division, Peripheral Nervous System Ø18

Neurotripsy
- *see* Destruction, Central Nervous System and Cranial Nerves ØØ5
- *see* Destruction, Peripheral Nervous System Ø15

Neutralization plate
- *use* Internal Fixation Device in Head and Facial Bones
- *use* Internal Fixation Device in Lower Bones
- *use* Internal Fixation Device in Upper Bones

New Technology
- Amivantamab Monoclonal Antibody XWØ
- Antibiotic-eluting Bone Void Filler XWØVØP7
- Aorta
  - Thoracic Arch using Branched Synthetic Substitute with Intraluminal Device X2RXØN7

New Technology — *continued*
- Aorta — *continued*
  - Thoracic Descending using Branched Synthetic Substitute with Intraluminal Device X2VWØN7
- Apalutamide Antineoplastic XWØDXJ5
- Atezolizumab Antineoplastic XWØ
- Axicabtagene Ciloleucel Immunotherapy XWØ
- Bamlanivimab Monoclonal Antibody XWØ
- Baricitinib XWØ
- Bezlotoxumab Monoclonal Antibody XWØ
- Bioengineered Allogeneic Construct, Skin XHRPXF7
- Brexanolone XWØ
- Brexucabtagene Autoleucel Immunotherapy XWØ
- Bromelain-enriched Proteolytic Enzyme XWØ
- Caplacizumab XWØ
- CD24Fc Immunomodulator XWØ
- Cefiderocol Anti-infective XWØ
- Ceftolozane/Tazobactam Anti-infective XWØ
- Cerebral Embolic Filtration
  - Dual Filter X2A5312
  - Extracorporeal Flow Reversal Circuit X2A
  - Single Deflection Filter X2A6325
- Ciltacabtagene Autoleucel XWØ
- Coagulation Factor Xa, Inactivated XWØ
- Computer-aided Assessment, Intracranial Vascular Activity XXEØXØ7
- Computer-aided Guidance, Transthoracic Echocardiography X2JAX47
- Computer-aided Mechanical Aspiration X2C
- Computer-aided Triage and Notification, Pulmonary Artery Flow XXE3X27
- Concentrated Bone Marrow Aspirate XKØ23Ø3
- Coronary Sinus, Reduction Device X2V73Q7
- COVID-19 Vaccine XWØ
- COVID-19 Vaccine Dose 1 XWØ
- COVID-19 Vaccine Dose 2 XWØ
- Cytarabine and Daunorubicin Liposome Antineoplastic XWØ
- Defibrotide Sodium Anticoagulant XWØ
- Destruction, Prostate, Robotic Waterjet Ablation XV5Ø8A4
- Dilation
  - Anterior Tibial
    - Left
      - Sustained Release Drug-eluting Intraluminal Device X27Q385
      - Four or More X27Q3C5
      - Three X27Q3B5
      - Two X27Q395
    - Right
      - Sustained Release Drug-eluting Intraluminal Device X27P385
      - Four or More X27P3C5
      - Three X27P3B5
      - Two X27P395
  - Femoral
    - Left
      - Sustained Release Drug-eluting Intraluminal Device X27J385
      - Four or More X27J3C5
      - Three X27J3B5
      - Two X27J395
    - Right
      - Sustained Release Drug-eluting Intraluminal Device X27H385
      - Four or More X27H3C5
      - Three X27H3B5
      - Two X27H395
  - Peroneal
    - Left
      - Sustained Release Drug-eluting Intraluminal Device X27U385
      - Four or More X27U3C5
      - Three X27U3B5
      - Two X27U395
    - Right
      - Sustained Release Drug-eluting Intraluminal Device X27T385
      - Four or More X27T3C5
      - Three X27T3B5
      - Two X27T395

New Technology — *continued*
- Dilation — *continued*
  - Popliteal
    - Left Distal
      - Sustained Release Drug-eluting Intraluminal Device X27N385
      - Four or More X27N3C5
      - Three X27N3B5
      - Two X27N395
    - Left Proximal
      - Sustained Release Drug-eluting Intraluminal Device X27L385
      - Four or More X27L3C5
      - Three X27L3B5
      - Two X27L395
    - Right Distal
      - Sustained Release Drug-eluting Intraluminal Device X27M385
      - Four or More X27M3C5
      - Three X27M3B5
      - Two X27M395
    - Right Proximal
      - Sustained Release Drug-eluting Intraluminal Device X27K385
      - Four or More X27K3C5
      - Three X27K3B5
      - Two X27K395
  - Posterior Tibial
    - Left
      - Sustained Release Drug-eluting Intraluminal Device X27S385
      - Four or More X27S3C5
      - Three X27S3B5
      - Two X27S395
    - Right
      - Sustained Release Drug-eluting Intraluminal Device X27R385
      - Four or More X27R3C5
      - Three X27R3B5
      - Two X27R395
- Durvalumab Antineoplastic XWØ
- Eculizumab XWØ
- Eladocagene exuparvovec XWØQ316
- Endothelial Damage Inhibitor XYØVX83
- Engineered Chimeric Antigen Receptor T-cell Immunotherapy
  - Allogeneic XWØ
  - Autologous XWØ
- Erdafitinib Antineoplastic XWØDXL5
- Esketamine Hydrochloride XWØ97M5
- Etesevimab Monoclonal Antibody XWØ
- Fosfomycin Anti-infective XWØ
- Fusion
  - Cervical Vertebral
    - 2 or more
      - Nanotextured Surface XRG2Ø92
      - Radiolucent Porous XRG2ØF3
    - Interbody Fusion Device
      - Nanotextured Surface XRG1Ø92
      - Radiolucent Porous XRG1ØF3
  - Cervicothoracic Vertebral
    - Nanotextured Surface XRG4Ø92
    - Radiolucent Porous XRG4ØF3
  - Lumbar Vertebral
    - 2 or more
      - Customizable XRGC
      - Nanotextured Surface XRGCØ92
      - Radiolucent Porous XRGCØF3
    - Interbody Fusion Device
      - Customizable XRGB
      - Nanotextured Surface XRGBØ92
      - Radiolucent Porous XRGBØF3
  - Lumbosacral
    - Customizable XRGD
    - Nanotextured Surface XRGDØ92
    - Radiolucent Porous XRGDØF3
  - Occipital-cervical
    - Nanotextured Surface XRGØØ92
    - Radiolucent Porous XRGØØF3
  - Thoracic Vertebral
    - 2 to 7
      - Nanotextured Surface XRG7Ø92
      - Radiolucent Porous XRG7ØF3

New Technology — *continued*
Fusion — *continued*
Thoracic Vertebral — *continued*
8 or more
Nanotextured Surface XRG8Ø92
Radiolucent Porous XRG8ØF3
Interbody Fusion Device
Nanotextured Surface XRG6Ø92
Radiolucent Porous XRG6ØF3
Thoracolumbar Vertebral
Customizable XRGA
Nanotextured Surface XRGAØ92
Radiolucent Porous XRGAØF3
Gilteritinib Antineoplastic XWØDXV5
High-Dose Intravenous Immune Globulin, for COVID-19 treatment XW1
Hyperimmune Globulin, for COVID-19 treatment XW1
Idecabtagene Vicleucel Immunotherapy XWØ
Imipenem-cilastatin-relebactam Anti-infective XWØ
Intracranial Arterial Flow, Whole Blood mRNA XXE5XT7
Iobenguane I-131 Antineoplastic XWØ
Kidney, Fluorescent Pyrazine XT25XE5
Lefamulin Anti-infective XWØ
Leronlimab Monoclonal Antibody XWØ13K6
Lifileucel Immunotherapy XWØ
Lisocabtagene Maraleucel Immunotherapy XWØ
Lower Respiratory Fluid Nucleic Acid-base Microbial Detection XXEBXQ6
Lurbinectedin XWØ
Mechanical Initial Specimen Diversion Technique Using Active Negative Pressure (blood collection) XXE5XR7
Meropenem-vaborbactam Anti-infective XWØ
Mineral-based Topical Hemostatic Agent XWØ
Nafamostat Anticoagulant XYØYX37
Narsoplimab Monoclonal Antibody XWØ
Nerinitide XWØ
Neurostimulator Lead in Oropharynx XWHD7Q7
Omadacycline Anti-infective XWØ
Other New Technology Monoclonal Antibody XWØ
Other New Technology Therapeutic Substance XWØ
Oxygen Saturation Endoscopic Imaging (OXEI) XD2
Plasma, Convalescent (Nonautologous) XW1
Plazomicin Anti-infective XWØ
Positive Blood Culture Fluorescence Hybridization for Organism Identification, Concentration and Susceptibility XXE5XN6
Radial artery arteriovenous fistula, using Thermal Resistance Energy X2K
REGN-COV2 Monoclonal Antibody XWØ
Remdesivir Anti-infective XWØ
Replacement
Skin Substitute, Porcine Liver Derived XHRPXL2
Zooplastic Tissue, Rapid Deployment Technique X2RF
Reposition
Cervical, Magnetically Controlled Growth Rod(s) XNS3
Lumbar
Magnetically Controlled Growth Rod(s) XNSØ
Posterior (Dynamic) Distraction Device XNSØ
Thoracic
Magnetically Controlled Growth Rod(s) XNS4
Posterior (Dynamic) Distraction Device XNS4
Ruxolitinib XWØDXT5
Sarilumab XWØ
SARS-CoV-2 Antibody Detection, Serum/Plasma Nanoparticle Fluorescence XXE5XV7
SARS-CoV-2 Polymerase Chain Reaction, Nasopharyngeal Fluid XXE97U7
Satralizumab-mwge XWØ1397
Single-use Duodenoscope XFJ
Single-use Oversleeve with Intraoperative Colonic Irrigation XDPH8K7
Supplement
Lumbar, Mechanically Expandable (Paired) Synthetic Substitute XNUØ356
Thoracic, Mechanically Expandable (Paired) Synthetic Substitute XNU4356
Synthetic Human Angiotensin II XWØ

New Technology — *continued*
Tagraxofusp-erzs Antineoplastic XWØ
Terlipressin XWØ
Tisagenlecleucel Immunotherapy XWØ
Tocilizumab XWØ
Trilaciclib XWØ
Uridine Triacetate XWØDX82
Venetoclax Antineoplastic XWØDXR5
Whole Blood Nucleic Acid-base Microbial Detection XXE5XM5
NexoBrid™ *use* Bromelain-enriched Proteolytic Enzyme
Ninth cranial nerve *use* Glossopharyngeal Nerve
NIRS (Near Infrared Spectroscopy) *see* Physiological Systems and Anatomical Regions 8EØ
Nitinol framed polymer mesh *use* Synthetic Substitute
Niyad™ *use* Nafamostat Anticoagulant
Nonimaging Nuclear Medicine Assay
Bladder, Kidneys and Ureters CT63
Blood C763
Kidneys, Ureters and Bladder CT63
Lymphatics and Hematologic System C76YYZZ
Ureters, Kidneys and Bladder CT63
Urinary System CT6YYZZ
Nonimaging Nuclear Medicine Probe
Abdomen CW5Ø
Abdomen and Chest CW54
Abdomen and Pelvis CW51
Brain CØ5Ø
Central Nervous System CØ5YYZZ
Chest CW53
Chest and Abdomen CW54
Chest and Neck CW56
Extremity
Lower CP5PZZZ
Upper CP5NZZZ
Head and Neck CW5B
Heart C25YYZZ
Right and Left C256
Lymphatics
Head C75J
Head and Neck C755
Lower Extremity C75P
Neck C75K
Pelvic C75D
Trunk C75M
Upper Chest C75L
Upper Extremity C75N
Lymphatics and Hematologic System C75YYZZ
Musculoskeletal System, Other CP5YYZZ
Neck and Chest CW56
Neck and Head CW5B
Pelvic Region CW5J
Pelvis and Abdomen CW51
Spine CP55ZZZ
Nonimaging Nuclear Medicine Uptake
Endocrine System CG4YYZZ
Gland, Thyroid CG42
Non-tunneled central venous catheter *use* Infusion Device
Nostril *use* Nasal Mucosa and Soft Tissue
Novacor Left Ventricular Assist Device *use* Implantable Heart Assist System in Heart and Great Vessels
Novation® Ceramic AHS® (Articulation Hip System) *use* Synthetic Substitute, Ceramic in ØSR
Nuclear medicine
see Nonimaging Nuclear Medicine Assay
see Nonimaging Nuclear Medicine Probe
see Nonimaging Nuclear Medicine Uptake
see Planar Nuclear Medicine Imaging
see Positron Emission Tomographic (PET) Imaging
see Systemic Nuclear Medicine Therapy
see Tomographic (Tomo) Nuclear Medicine Imaging
Nuclear scintigraphy *see* Nuclear Medicine
Nutrition, concentrated substances
Enteral infusion 3EØG36Z
Parenteral (peripheral) infusion *see* Introduction of Nutritional Substance
NUZYRA™ *use* Omadacycline Anti-infective

O

Obliteration *see* Destruction
Obturator artery
use Internal Iliac Artery, Left

Obturator artery — *continued*
use Internal Iliac Artery, Right
Obturator lymph node *use* Lymphatic, Pelvis
Obturator muscle
use Hip Muscle, Left
use Hip Muscle, Right
Obturator nerve *use* Lumbar Plexus
Obturator vein
use Hypogastric Vein, Left
use Hypogastric Vein, Right
Obtuse margin *use* Heart, Left
Occipital artery
use External Carotid Artery, Left
use External Carotid Artery, Right
Occipital lobe *use* Cerebral Hemisphere
Occipital lymph node
use Lymphatic, Left Neck
use Lymphatic, Right Neck
Occipitofrontalis muscle *use* Facial Muscle
Occlusion
Ampulla of Vater ØFLC
Anus ØDLQ
Aorta
Abdominal Ø4LØ
Thoracic, Descending Ø2LW3DJ
Artery
Anterior Tibial
Left Ø4LQ
Right Ø4LP
Axillary
Left Ø3L6
Right Ø3L5
Brachial
Left Ø3L8
Right Ø3L7
Celiac Ø4L1
Colic
Left Ø4L7
Middle Ø4L8
Right Ø4L6
Common Carotid
Left Ø3LJ
Right Ø3LH
Common Iliac
Left Ø4LD
Right Ø4LC
External Carotid
Left Ø3LN
Right Ø3LM
External Iliac
Left Ø4LJ
Right Ø4LH
Face Ø3LR
Femoral
Left Ø4LL
Right Ø4LK
Foot
Left Ø4LW
Right Ø4LV
Gastric Ø4L2
Hand
Left Ø3LF
Right Ø3LD
Hepatic Ø4L3
Inferior Mesenteric Ø4LB
Innominate Ø3L2
Internal Carotid
Left Ø3LL
Right Ø3LK
Internal Iliac
Left Ø4LF
Right Ø4LE
Internal Mammary
Left Ø3L1
Right Ø3LØ
Intracranial Ø3LG
Lower Ø4LY
Peroneal
Left Ø4LU
Right Ø4LT
Popliteal
Left Ø4LN
Right Ø4LM
Posterior Tibial
Left Ø4LS
Right Ø4LR
Pulmonary
Left Ø2LR

Subterms under main terms may continue to next column or page

Occlusion — *continued*
Artery — *continued*
Pulmonary — *continued*
Right Ø2LQ
Pulmonary Trunk Ø2LP
Radial
Left Ø3LC
Right Ø3LB
Renal
Left Ø4LA
Right Ø4L9
Splenic Ø4L4
Subclavian
Left Ø3L4
Right Ø3L3
Superior Mesenteric Ø4L5
Temporal
Left Ø3LT
Right Ø3LS
Thyroid
Left Ø3LV
Right Ø3LU
Ulnar
Left Ø3LA
Right Ø3L9
Upper Ø3LY
Vertebral
Left Ø3LQ
Right Ø3LP
Atrium, Left Ø2L7
Bladder ØTLB
Bladder Neck ØTLC
Bronchus
Lingula ØBL9
Lower Lobe
Left ØBLB
Right ØBL6
Main
Left ØBL7
Right ØBL3
Middle Lobe, Right ØBL5
Upper Lobe
Left ØBL8
Right ØBL4
Carina ØBL2
Cecum ØDLH
Cisterna Chyli Ø7LL
Colon
Ascending ØDLK
Descending ØDLM
Sigmoid ØDLN
Transverse ØDLL
Cord
Bilateral ØVLH
Left ØVLG
Right ØVLF
Cul-de-sac ØULF
Duct
Common Bile ØFL9
Cystic ØFL8
Hepatic
Common ØFL7
Left ØFL6
Right ØFL5
Lacrimal
Left Ø8LY
Right Ø8LX
Pancreatic ØFLD
Accessory ØFLF
Parotid
Left ØCLC
Right ØCLB
Duodenum ØDL9
Esophagogastric Junction ØDL4
Esophagus ØDL5
Lower ØDL3
Middle ØDL2
Upper ØDL1
Fallopian Tube
Left ØUL6
Right ØUL5
Fallopian Tubes, Bilateral ØUL7
Ileocecal Valve ØDLC
Ileum ØDLB
Intestine
Large ØDLE
Left ØDLG
Right ØDLF
Small ØDL8

Occlusion — *continued*
Jejunum ØDLA
Kidney Pelvis
Left ØTL4
Right ØTL3
Left atrial appendage (LAA) *see* Occlusion, Atrium, Left Ø2L7
Lymphatic
Aortic Ø7LD
Axillary
Left Ø7L6
Right Ø7L5
Head Ø7LØ
Inguinal
Left Ø7LJ
Right Ø7LH
Internal Mammary
Left Ø7L9
Right Ø7L8
Lower Extremity
Left Ø7LG
Right Ø7LF
Mesenteric Ø7LB
Neck
Left Ø7L2
Right Ø7L1
Pelvis Ø7LC
Thoracic Duct Ø7LK
Thorax Ø7L7
Upper Extremity
Left Ø7L4
Right Ø7L3
Rectum ØDLP
Stomach ØDL6
Pylorus ØDL7
Trachea ØBL1
Ureter
Left ØTL7
Right ØTL6
Urethra ØTLD
Vagina ØULG
Valve, Pulmonary Ø2LH
Vas Deferens
Bilateral ØVLQ
Left ØVLP
Right ØVLN
Vein
Axillary
Left Ø5L8
Right Ø5L7
Azygos Ø5LØ
Basilic
Left Ø5LC
Right Ø5LB
Brachial
Left Ø5LA
Right Ø5L9
Cephalic
Left Ø5LF
Right Ø5LD
Colic Ø6L7
Common Iliac
Left Ø6LD
Right Ø6LC
Esophageal Ø6L3
External Iliac
Left Ø6LG
Right Ø6LF
External Jugular
Left Ø5LQ
Right Ø5LP
Face
Left Ø5LV
Right Ø5LT
Femoral
Left Ø6LN
Right Ø6LM
Foot
Left Ø6LV
Right Ø6LT
Gastric Ø6L2
Hand
Left Ø5LH
Right Ø5LG
Hemiazygos Ø5L1
Hepatic Ø6L4
Hypogastric
Left Ø6LJ
Right Ø6LH

Occlusion — *continued*
Vein — *continued*
Inferior Mesenteric Ø6L6
Innominate
Left Ø5L4
Right Ø5L3
Internal Jugular
Left Ø5LN
Right Ø5LM
Intracranial Ø5LL
Lower Ø6LY
Portal Ø6L8
Pulmonary
Left Ø2LT
Right Ø2LS
Renal
Left Ø6LB
Right Ø6L9
Saphenous
Left Ø6LQ
Right Ø6LP
Splenic Ø6L1
Subclavian
Left Ø5L6
Right Ø5L5
Superior Mesenteric Ø6L5
Upper Ø5LY
Vertebral
Left Ø5LS
Right Ø5LR
Vena Cava
Inferior Ø6LØ
Superior Ø2LV
Occlusion, REBOA (resuscitative endovascular balloon occlusion of the aorta)
Ø2LW3DJ
Ø4LØ3DJ
Occupational therapy *see* Activities of Daily Living Treatment, Rehabilitation FØ8
Octagam 10%, for COVID-19 treatment *use* High-Dose Intravenous Immune Globulin
Odentectomy
see Excision, Mouth and Throat ØCB
see Resection, Mouth and Throat ØCT
Odontoid process *use* Cervical Vertebra
Olecranon bursa
use Elbow Bursa and Ligament, Left
use Elbow Bursa and Ligament, Right
Olecranon process
use Ulna, Left
use Ulna, Right
Olfactory bulb *use* Olfactory Nerve
Olumiant® *use* Baricitinib
Omadacycline Anti-infective XWØ
Omentectomy, omentumectomy
see Excision, Gastrointestinal System ØDB
see Resection, Gastrointestinal System ØDT
Omentofixation *see* Repair, Gastrointestinal System ØDQ
Omentoplasty
see Repair, Gastrointestinal System ØDQ
see Replacement, Gastrointestinal System ØDR
see Supplement, Gastrointestinal System ØDU
Omentorrhaphy *see* Repair, Gastrointestinal System ØDQ
Omentotomy *see* Drainage, Gastrointestinal System ØD9
Omnilink Elite Vascular Balloon Expandable Stent System *use* Intraluminal Device
Onychectomy
see Excision, Skin and Breast ØHB
see Resection, Skin and Breast ØHT
Onychoplasty
see Repair, Skin and Breast ØHQ
see Replacement, Skin and Breast ØHR
Onychotomy *see* Drainage, Skin and Breast ØH9
Oophorectomy
see Excision, Female Reproductive System ØUB
see Resection, Female Reproductive System ØUT
Oophoropexy
see Repair, Female Reproductive System ØUQ
see Reposition, Female Reproductive System ØUS
Oophoroplasty
see Repair, Female Reproductive System ØUQ
see Supplement, Female Reproductive System ØUU
Oophororrhaphy *see* Repair, Female Reproductive System ØUQ

Oophorostomy *see* Drainage, Female Reproductive System ØU9
Oophorotomy
see Division, Female Reproductive System ØU8
see Drainage, Female Reproductive System ØU9
Oophorrhaphy *see* Repair, Female Reproductive System ØUQ
Open Pivot Aortic Valve Graft (AVG) *use* Synthetic Substitute
Open Pivot (mechanical) Valve *use* Synthetic Substitute
Ophthalmic artery *use* Intracranial Artery
Ophthalmic nerve *use* Trigeminal Nerve
Ophthalmic vein *use* Intracranial Vein
Opponensplasty
Tendon replacement *see* Replacement, Tendons ØLR
Tendon transfer *see* Transfer, Tendons ØLX
Optic chiasma *use* Optic Nerve
Optic disc
use Retina, Left
use Retina, Right
Optic foramen *use* Sphenoid Bone
Optical coherence tomography, intravascular *see* Computerized Tomography (CT Scan)
Optimizer™ III implantable pulse generator *use* Contractility Modulation Device in ØJH
Orbicularis oculi muscle
use Upper Eyelid, Left
use Upper Eyelid, Right
Orbicularis oris muscle *use* Facial Muscle
Orbital Atherectomy *see* Extirpation, Heart and Great Vessels Ø2C
Orbital fascia *use* Subcutaneous Tissue and Fascia, Face
Orbital portion of ethmoid bone
use Orbit, Left
use Orbit, Right
Orbital portion of frontal bone
use Orbit, Left
use Orbit, Right
Orbital portion of lacrimal bone
use Orbit, Left
use Orbit, Right
Orbital portion of maxilla
use Orbit, Left
use Orbit, Right
Orbital portion of palatine bone
use Orbit, Left
use Orbit, Right
Orbital portion of sphenoid bone
use Orbit, Left
use Orbit, Right
Orbital portion of zygomatic bone
use Orbit, Left
use Orbit, Right
Orchectomy, orchidectomy, orchiectomy
see Excision, Male Reproductive System ØVB
see Resection, Male Reproductive System ØVT
Orchidoplasty, orchioplasty
see Repair, Male Reproductive System ØVQ
see Replacement, Male Reproductive System ØVR
see Supplement, Male Reproductive System ØVU
Orchidorrhaphy, orchiorrhaphy *see* Repair, Male Reproductive System ØVQ
Orchidotomy, orchiotomy, orchotomy *see* Drainage, Male Reproductive System ØV9
Orchiopexy
see Repair, Male Reproductive System ØVQ
see Reposition, Male Reproductive System ØVS
Oropharyngeal airway (OPA) *use* Intraluminal Device, Airway in Mouth and Throat
Oropharynx *use* Pharynx
Ossiculectomy
see Excision, Ear, Nose, Sinus Ø9B
see Resection, Ear, Nose, Sinus Ø9T
Ossiculotomy *see* Drainage, Ear, Nose, Sinus Ø99
Ostectomy
see Excision, Head and Facial Bones ØNB
see Excision, Lower Bones ØQB
see Excision, Upper Bones ØPB
see Resection, Head and Facial Bones ØNT
see Resection, Lower Bones ØQT
see Resection, Upper Bones ØPT
Osteoclasis
see Division, Head and Facial Bones ØN8
Osteoclasis — *continued*
see Division, Lower Bones ØQ8
see Division, Upper Bones ØP8
Osteolysis
see Release, Head and Facial Bones ØNN
see Release, Lower Bones ØQN
see Release, Upper Bones ØPN
Osteopathic Treatment
Abdomen 7WØ9X
Cervical 7WØ1X
Extremity
Lower 7WØ6X
Upper 7WØ7X
Head 7WØØX
Lumbar 7WØ3X
Pelvis 7WØ5X
Rib Cage 7WØ8X
Sacrum 7WØ4X
Thoracic 7WØ2X
Osteopexy
see Repair, Head and Facial Bones ØNQ
see Repair, Lower Bones ØQQ
see Repair, Upper Bones ØPQ
see Reposition, Head and Facial Bones ØNS
see Reposition, Lower Bones ØQS
see Reposition, Upper Bones ØPS
Osteoplasty
see Repair, Head and Facial Bones ØNQ
see Repair, Lower Bones ØQQ
see Repair, Upper Bones ØPQ
see Replacement, Head and Facial Bones ØNR
see Replacement, Lower Bones ØQR
see Replacement, Upper Bones ØPR
see Supplement, Head and Facial Bones ØNU
see Supplement, Lower Bones ØQU
see Supplement, Upper Bones ØPU
Osteorrhaphy
see Repair, Head and Facial Bones ØNQ
see Repair, Lower Bones ØQQ
see Repair, Upper Bones ØPQ
Osteotomy, ostotomy
see Division, Head and Facial Bones ØN8
see Division, Lower Bones ØQ8
see Division, Upper Bones ØP8
see Drainage, Head and Facial Bones ØN9
see Drainage, Lower Bones ØQ9
see Drainage, Upper Bones ØP9
Other Imaging
Bile Duct and Gallbladder, Indocyanine Green Dye, Intraoperative BF532ØØ
Bile Duct, Indocyanine Green Dye, Intraoperative BF5Ø2ØØ
Extremity
Lower BW5CZ1Z
Upper BW5JZ1Z
Gallbladder and Bile Duct, Indocyanine Green Dye, Intraoperative BF532ØØ
Gallbladder, Indocyanine Green Dye, Intraoperative BF522ØØ
Head and Neck BW59Z1Z
Hepatobiliary System, All, Indocyanine Green Dye, Intraoperative BF5C2ØØ
Liver and Spleen, Indocyanine Green Dye, Intraoperative BF562ØØ
Liver, Indocyanine Green Dye, Intraoperative BF552ØØ
Neck and Head BW59Z1Z
Pancreas, Indocyanine Green Dye, Intraoperative BF572ØØ
Spleen and Liver, Indocyanine Green Dye, Intraoperative BF562ØØ
Trunk BW52Z1Z
Other New Technology Monoclonal Antibody XWØ
Other New Technology Therapeutic Substance XWØ
Otic ganglion *use* Head and Neck Sympathetic Nerve
OTL-1Ø1 *use* Hematopoietic Stem/Progenitor Cells, Genetically Modified
OTL-1Ø3 *use* Hematopoietic Stem/Progenitor Cells, Genetically Modified
OTL-2ØØ *use* Hematopoietic Stem/Progenitor Cells, Genetically Modified
Otoplasty
see Repair, Ear, Nose, Sinus Ø9Q
see Replacement, Ear, Nose, Sinus Ø9R
see Supplement, Ear, Nose, Sinus Ø9U
Otoscopy *see* Inspection, Ear, Nose, Sinus Ø9J
Oval window
use Middle Ear, Left
use Middle Ear, Right
Ovarian artery *use* Abdominal Aorta
Ovarian ligament *use* Uterine Supporting Structure
Ovariectomy
see Excision, Female Reproductive System ØUB
see Resection, Female Reproductive System ØUT
Ovariocentesis *see* Drainage, Female Reproductive System ØU9
Ovariopexy
see Repair, Female Reproductive System ØUQ
see Reposition, Female Reproductive System ØUS
Ovariotomy
see Division, Female Reproductive System ØU8
see Drainage, Female Reproductive System ØU9
Ovatio™ CRT-D *use* Cardiac Resynchronization Defibrillator Pulse Generator in ØJH
Oversewing
Gastrointestinal ulcer *see* Repair, Gastrointestinal System ØDQ
Pleural bleb *see* Repair, Respiratory System ØBQ
Oviduct
use Fallopian Tube, Left
use Fallopian Tube, Right
Oximetry, Fetal pulse 1ØHØ73Z
OXINIUM *use* Synthetic Substitute, Oxidized Zirconium on Polyethylene in ØSR
Oxygen Saturation Endoscopic Imaging (OXEI) XD2
Oxygenation
Extracorporeal membrane (ECMO) *see* Performance, Circulatory 5A15
Hyperbaric *see* Assistance, Circulatory 5AØ5
Supersaturated *see* Assistance, Circulatory 5AØ5

P

Pacemaker
Dual Chamber
Abdomen ØJH8
Chest ØJH6
Intracardiac
Insertion of device in
Atrium
Left Ø2H7
Right Ø2H6
Vein, Coronary Ø2H4
Ventricle
Left Ø2HL
Right Ø2HK
Removal of device from, Heart Ø2PA
Revision of device in, Heart Ø2WA
Single Chamber
Abdomen ØJH8
Chest ØJH6
Single Chamber Rate Responsive
Abdomen ØJH8
Chest ØJH6
Packing
Abdominal Wall 2W43X5Z
Anorectal 2Y43X5Z
Arm
Lower
Left 2W4DX5Z
Right 2W4CX5Z
Upper
Left 2W4BX5Z
Right 2W4AX5Z
Back 2W45X5Z
Chest Wall 2W44X5Z
Ear 2Y42X5Z
Extremity
Lower
Left 2W4MX5Z
Right 2W4LX5Z
Upper
Left 2W49X5Z
Right 2W48X5Z
Face 2W41X5Z
Finger
Left 2W4KX5Z
Right 2W4JX5Z
Foot
Left 2W4TX5Z
Right 2W4SX5Z
Genital Tract, Female 2Y44X5Z

Packing — *continued*
Hand
Left 2W4FX5Z
Right 2W4EX5Z
Head 2W40X5Z
Inguinal Region
Left 2W47X5Z
Right 2W46X5Z
Leg
Lower
Left 2W4RX5Z
Right 2W4QX5Z
Upper
Left 2W4PX5Z
Right 2W4NX5Z
Mouth and Pharynx 2Y40X5Z
Nasal 2Y41X5Z
Neck 2W42X5Z
Thumb
Left 2W4HX5Z
Right 2W4GX5Z
Toe
Left 2W4VX5Z
Right 2W4UX5Z
Urethra 2Y45X5Z
Paclitaxel-eluting coronary stent *use* Intraluminal Device, Drug-eluting in Heart and Great Vessels
Paclitaxel-eluting peripheral stent
use Intraluminal Device, Drug-eluting in Lower Arteries
use Intraluminal Device, Drug-eluting in Upper Arteries
Palatine gland *use* Buccal Mucosa
Palatine tonsil *use* Tonsils
Palatine uvula *use* Uvula
Palatoglossal muscle *use* Tongue, Palate, Pharynx Muscle
Palatopharyngeal muscle *use* Tongue, Palate, Pharynx Muscle
Palatoplasty
see Repair, Mouth and Throat 0CQ
see Replacement, Mouth and Throat 0CR
see Supplement, Mouth and Throat 0CU
Palatorrhaphy *see* Repair, Mouth and Throat 0CQ
Palmar cutaneous nerve
use Median Nerve
use Radial Nerve
Palmar (volar) digital vein
use Hand Vein, Left
use Hand Vein, Right
Palmar fascia (aponeurosis)
use Subcutaneous Tissue and Fascia, Left Hand
use Subcutaneous Tissue and Fascia, Right Hand
Palmar interosseous muscle
use Hand Muscle, Left
use Hand Muscle, Right
Palmar (volar) metacarpal vein
use Hand Vein, Left
use Hand Vein, Right
Palmar ulnocarpal ligament
use Wrist Bursa and Ligament, Left
use Wrist Bursa and Ligament, Right
Palmaris longus muscle
use Lower Arm and Wrist Muscle, Left
use Lower Arm and Wrist Muscle, Right
Pancreatectomy
see Excision, Pancreas 0FBG
see Resection, Pancreas 0FTG
Pancreatic artery *use* Splenic Artery
Pancreatic plexus *use* Abdominal Sympathetic Nerve
Pancreatic vein *use* Splenic Vein
Pancreaticoduodenostomy *see* Bypass, Hepatobiliary System and Pancreas 0F1
Pancreaticosplenic lymph node *use* Lymphatic, Aortic
Pancreatogram, endoscopic retrograde *see* Fluoroscopy, Pancreatic Duct BF18
Pancreatolithotomy *see* Extirpation, Pancreas 0FCG
Pancreatotomy
see Division, Pancreas 0F8G
see Drainage, Pancreas 0F9G
Panniculectomy
see Excision, Skin, Abdomen 0HB7
see Excision, Subcutaneous Tissue and Fascia, Abdomen 0JB8
Paraaortic lymph node *use* Lymphatic, Aortic
Paracentesis
Eye *see* Drainage, Eye 089
Peritoneal Cavity *see* Drainage, Peritoneal Cavity 0W9G
Tympanum *see* Drainage, Ear, Nose, Sinus 099
Parapharyngeal space *use* Neck
Pararectal lymph node *use* Lymphatic, Mesenteric
Parasternal lymph node *use* Lymphatic, Thorax
Parathyroidectomy
see Excision, Endocrine System 0GB
see Resection, Endocrine System 0GT
Paratracheal lymph node *use* Lymphatic, Thorax
Paraurethral (Skene's) gland *use* Vestibular Gland
Parenteral nutrition, total *see* Introduction of Nutritional Substance
Parietal lobe *use* Cerebral Hemisphere
Parotid lymph node *use* Lymphatic, Head
Parotid plexus *use* Facial Nerve
Parotidectomy
see Excision, Mouth and Throat 0CB
see Resection, Mouth and Throat 0CT
Pars flaccida
use Tympanic Membrane, Left
use Tympanic Membrane, Right
Partial joint replacement
Hip *see* Replacement, Lower Joints 0SR
Knee *see* Replacement, Lower Joints 0SR
Shoulder *see* Replacement, Upper Joints 0RR
Partially absorbable mesh *use* Synthetic Substitute
Patch, blood, spinal 3E0R3GC
Patellapexy
see Repair, Lower Bones 0QQ
see Reposition, Lower Bones 0QS
Patellaplasty
see Repair, Lower Bones 0QQ
see Replacement, Lower Bones 0QR
see Supplement, Lower Bones 0QU
Patellar ligament
use Knee Bursa and Ligament, Left
use Knee Bursa and Ligament, Right
Patellar tendon
use Knee Tendon, Left
use Knee Tendon, Right
Patellectomy
see Excision, Lower Bones 0QB
see Resection, Lower Bones 0QT
Patellofemoral joint
use Knee Joint, Left
use Knee Joint, Left, Femoral Surface
use Knee Joint, Right
use Knee Joint, Right, Femoral Surface
pAVF (percutaneous arteriovenous fistula), using magnetic-guided radiofrequency *see* Bypass, Upper Arteries 031
pAVF (percutaneous arteriovenous fistula), using thermal resistance energy *see* New Technology, Cardiovascular System X2K
Pectineus muscle
use Upper Leg Muscle, Left
use Upper Leg Muscle, Right
Pectoral fascia *use* Subcutaneous Tissue and Fascia, Chest
Pectoral (anterior) lymph node
use Lymphatic Left, Axillary
use Lymphatic Right, Axillary
Pectoralis major muscle
use Thorax Muscle, Left
use Thorax Muscle, Right
Pectoralis minor muscle
use Thorax Muscle, Left
use Thorax Muscle, Right
Pedicle-based dynamic stabilization device
use Spinal Stabilization Device, Pedicle-Based in 0SH
use Spinal Stabilization Device, Pedicle-Based in 0RH
PEEP (positive end expiratory pressure) *see* Assistance, Respiratory 5A09
PEG (percutaneous endoscopic gastrostomy) 0DH63UZ
PEJ (percutaneous endoscopic jejunostomy) 0DHA3UZ
Pelvic splanchnic nerve
use Abdominal Sympathetic Nerve
use Sacral Sympathetic Nerve
Penectomy
see Excision, Male Reproductive System 0VB
see Resection, Male Reproductive System 0VT
Penile urethra *use* Urethra
Penumbra Indigo® Aspiration System *see* New Technology, Cardiovascular System X2C
PERCEPT™ PC neurostimulator *use* Stimulator Generator, Multiple Array in 0JH
Perceval sutureless valve *use* Zooplastic Tissue, Rapid Deployment Technique in New Technology
Percutaneous endoscopic gastrojejunostomy (PEG/J) tube *use* Feeding Device in Gastrointestinal System
Percutaneous endoscopic gastrostomy (PEG) tube *use* Feeding Device in Gastrointestinal System
Percutaneous nephrostomy catheter *use* Drainage Device
Percutaneous transluminal coronary angioplasty (PTCA) *see* Dilation, Heart and Great Vessels 027
Performance
Biliary
Multiple, Filtration 5A1C60Z
Single, Filtration 5A1C00Z
Cardiac
Continuous
Output 5A1221Z
Pacing 5A1223Z
Intermittent, Pacing 5A1213Z
Single, Output, Manual 5A12012
Circulatory
Continuous
Central Membrane 5A1522F
Peripheral Veno-arterial Membrane 5A1522G
Peripheral Veno-venous Membrane 5A1522H
Intraoperative
Central Membrane 5A15A2F
Peripheral Veno-arterial Membrane 5A15A2G
Peripheral Veno-venous Membrane 5A15A2H
Respiratory
24-96 Consecutive Hours, Ventilation 5A1945Z
Greater than 96 Consecutive Hours, Ventilation 5A1955Z
Less than 24 Consecutive Hours, Ventilation 5A1935Z
Single, Ventilation, Nonmechanical 5A19054
Urinary
Continuous, Greater than 18 hours per day, Filtration 5A1D90Z
Intermittent, Less than 6 Hours Per Day, Filtration 5A1D70Z
Prolonged Intermittent, 6-18 hours per day, Filtration 5A1D80Z
Perfusion *see* Introduction of substance in or on
Perfusion, donor organ
Heart 6AB50BZ
Kidney(s) 6ABT0BZ
Liver 6ABF0BZ
Lung(s) 6ABB0BZ
Pericardiectomy
see Excision, Pericardium 02BN
see Resection, Pericardium 02TN
Pericardiocentesis *see* Drainage, Pericardial Cavity 0W9D
Pericardiolysis *see* Release, Pericardium 02NN
Pericardiophrenic artery
use Internal Mammary Artery, Left
use Internal Mammary Artery, Right
Pericardioplasty
see Repair, Pericardium 02QN
see Replacement, Pericardium 02RN
see Supplement, Pericardium 02UN
Pericardiorrhaphy *see* Repair, Pericardium 02QN
Pericardiostomy *see* Drainage, Pericardial Cavity 0W9D
Pericardiotomy *see* Drainage, Pericardial Cavity 0W9D
Perimetrium *use* Uterus
Peripheral Intravascular Lithotripsy (Peripheral IVL) *see* Fragmentation
Peripheral parenteral nutrition *see* Introduction of Nutritional Substance
Peripherally inserted central catheter (PICC) *use* Infusion Device
Peritoneal dialysis 3E1M39Z

Subterms under main terms may continue to next column or page

Peritoneocentesis
- *see* Drainage, Peritoneal Cavity ØW9G
- *see* Drainage, Peritoneum ØD9W

Peritoneoplasty
- *see* Repair, Peritoneum ØDQW
- *see* Replacement, Peritoneum ØDRW
- *see* Supplement, Peritoneum ØDUW

Peritoneoscopy ØDJW4ZZ

Peritoneotomy *see* Drainage, Peritoneum ØD9W

Peritoneumectomy *see* Excision, Peritoneum ØDBW

Peroneus brevis muscle
- *use* Lower Leg Muscle, Left
- *use* Lower Leg Muscle, Right

Peroneus longus muscle
- *use* Lower Leg Muscle, Left
- *use* Lower Leg Muscle, Right

Pessary ring *use* Intraluminal Device, Pessary in Female Reproductive System

PET scan *see* Positron Emission Tomographic (PET) Imaging

Petrous part of temoporal bone
- *use* Temporal Bone, Left
- *use* Temporal Bone, Right

Phacoemulsification, lens
- With IOL implant *see* Replacement, Eye Ø8R
- Without IOL implant *see* Extraction, Eye Ø8D

Phagenyx® System XWHD7Q7

Phalangectomy
- *see* Excision, Lower Bones ØQB
- *see* Excision, Upper Bones ØPB
- *see* Resection, Lower Bones ØQT
- *see* Resection, Upper Bones ØPT

Phallectomy
- *see* Excision, Penis ØVBS
- *see* Resection, Penis ØVTS

Phalloplasty
- *see* Repair, Penis ØVQS
- *see* Supplement, Penis ØVUS

Phallotomy *see* Drainage, Penis ØV9S

Pharmacotherapy, for substance abuse
- Antabuse HZ93ZZZ
- Bupropion HZ97ZZZ
- Clonidine HZ96ZZZ
- Levo-alpha-acetyl-methadol (LAAM) HZ92ZZZ
- Methadone Maintenance HZ91ZZZ
- Naloxone HZ95ZZZ
- Naltrexone HZ94ZZZ
- Nicotine Replacement HZ9ØZZZ
- Psychiatric Medication HZ98ZZZ
- Replacement Medication, Other HZ99ZZZ

Pharyngeal constrictor muscle *use* Tongue, Palate, Pharynx Muscle

Pharyngeal plexus *use* Vagus Nerve

Pharyngeal recess *use* Nasopharynx

Pharyngeal tonsil *use* Adenoids

Pharyngogram *see* Fluoroscopy, Pharynix B91G

Pharyngoplasty
- *see* Repair, Mouth and Throat ØCQ
- *see* Replacement, Mouth and Throat ØCR
- *see* Supplement, Mouth and Throat ØCU

Pharyngorrhaphy *see* Repair, Mouth and Throat ØCQ

Pharyngotomy *see* Drainage, Mouth and Throat ØC9

Pharyngotympanic tube
- *use* Eustachian Tube, Left
- *use* Eustachian Tube, Right

Pheresis
- Erythrocytes 6A55
- Leukocytes 6A55
- Plasma 6A55
- Platelets 6A55
- Stem Cells
  - Cord Blood 6A55
  - Hematopoietic 6A55

Phlebectomy
- *see* Excision, Lower Veins Ø6B
- *see* Excision, Upper Veins Ø5B
- *see* Extraction, Lower Veins Ø6D
- *see* Extraction, Upper Veins Ø5D

Phlebography
- *see* Plain Radiography, Veins B5Ø
- Impedance 4AØ4X51

Phleborrhaphy
- *see* Repair, Lower Veins Ø6Q
- *see* Repair, Upper Veins Ø5Q

Phlebotomy
- *see* Drainage, Lower Veins Ø69
- *see* Drainage, Upper Veins Ø59

Photocoagulation
- For Destruction *see* Destruction
- For Repair *see* Repair

Photopheresis, therapeutic *see* Phototherapy, Circulatory 6A65

Phototherapy
- Circulatory 6A65
- Skin 6A6Ø
- Ultraviolet light *see* Ultraviolet Light Therapy, Physiological Systems 6A8

Phrenectomy, phrenoneurectomy *see* Excision, Nerve, Phrenic Ø1B2

Phrenemphraxis *see* Destruction, Nerve, Phrenic Ø152

Phrenic nerve stimulator generator *use* Stimulator Generator in Subcutaneous Tissue and Fascia

Phrenic nerve stimulator lead *use* Diaphragmatic Pacemaker Lead in Respiratory System

Phreniclasis *see* Destruction, Nerve, Phrenic Ø152

Phrenicoexeresis *see* Extraction, Nerve, Phrenic Ø1D2

Phrenicotomy *see* Division, Nerve, Phrenic Ø182

Phrenicotripsy *see* Destruction, Nerve, Phrenic Ø152

Phrenoplasty
- *see* Repair, Respiratory System ØBQ
- *see* Supplement, Respiratory System ØBU

Phrenotomy *see* Drainage, Respiratory System ØB9

Physiatry *see* Motor Treatment, Rehabilitation FØ7

Physical medicine *see* Motor Treatment, Rehabilitation FØ7

Physical therapy *see* Motor Treatment, Rehabilitation FØ7

PHYSIOMESH™ Flexible Composite Mesh *use* Synthetic Substitute

Pia mater, intracranial *use* Cerebral Meninges

Pia mater, spinal *use* Spinal Meninges

Pinealectomy
- *see* Excision, Pineal Body ØGB1
- *see* Resection, Pineal Body ØGT1

Pinealoscopy ØGJ14ZZ

Pinealotomy *see* Drainage, Pineal Body ØG91

Pinna
- *use* External Ear, Bilateral
- *use* External Ear, Left
- *use* External Ear, Right

Pipeline™ (Flex) embolization device *use* Intraluminal Device, Flow Diverter in Ø3V

Piriform recess (sinus) *use* Pharynx

Piriformis muscle
- *use* Hip Muscle, Left
- *use* Hip Muscle, Right

PIRRT (Prolonged intermittent renal replacement therapy) 5A1D8ØZ

Pisiform bone
- *use* Carpal, Left
- *use* Carpal, Right

Pisohamate ligament
- *use* Hand Bursa and Ligament, Left
- *use* Hand Bursa and Ligament, Right

Pisometacarpal ligament
- *use* Hand Bursa and Ligament, Left
- *use* Hand Bursa and Ligament, Right

Pituitectomy
- *see* Excision, Gland, Pituitary ØGBØ
- *see* Resection, Gland, Pituitary ØGTØ

Plain film radiology *see* Plain Radiography

Plain Radiography
- Abdomen BWØØZZZ
- Abdomen and Pelvis BWØ1ZZZ
- Abdominal Lymphatic
  - Bilateral B7Ø1
  - Unilateral B7ØØ
- Airway, Upper BBØDZZZ
- Ankle
  - Left BQØH
  - Right BQØG
- Aorta
  - Abdominal B4ØØ
  - Thoracic B3ØØ
  - Thoraco-Abdominal B3ØP
- Aorta and Bilateral Lower Extremity Arteries B4ØD
- Arch
  - Bilateral BNØDZZZ
  - Left BNØCZZZ
  - Right BNØBZZZ
- Arm
  - Left BPØFZZZ
  - Right BPØEZZZ

Plain Radiography — *continued*
- Artery
  - Brachiocephalic-Subclavian, Right B3Ø1
  - Bronchial B3ØL
  - Bypass Graft, Other B2ØF
  - Cervico-Cerebral Arch B3ØQ
  - Common Carotid
    - Bilateral B3Ø5
    - Left B3Ø4
    - Right B3Ø3
  - Coronary
    - Bypass Graft
      - Multiple B2Ø3
      - Single B2Ø2
    - Multiple B2Ø1
    - Single B2ØØ
  - External Carotid
    - Bilateral B3ØC
    - Left B3ØB
    - Right B3Ø9
  - Hepatic B4Ø2
  - Inferior Mesenteric B4Ø5
  - Intercostal B3ØL
  - Internal Carotid
    - Bilateral B3Ø8
    - Left B3Ø7
    - Right B3Ø6
  - Internal Mammary Bypass Graft
    - Left B2Ø8
    - Right B2Ø7
  - Intra-Abdominal, Other B4ØB
  - Intracranial B3ØR
  - Lower Extremity
    - Bilateral and Aorta B4ØD
    - Left B4ØG
    - Right B4ØF
  - Lower, Other B4ØJ
  - Lumbar B4Ø9
  - Pelvic B4ØC
  - Pulmonary
    - Left B3ØT
    - Right B3ØS
  - Renal
    - Bilateral B4Ø8
    - Left B4Ø7
    - Right B4Ø6
    - Transplant B4ØM
  - Spinal B3ØM
  - Splenic B4Ø3
  - Subclavian, Left B3Ø2
  - Superior Mesenteric B4Ø4
  - Upper Extremity
    - Bilateral B3ØK
    - Left B3ØJ
    - Right B3ØH
  - Upper, Other B3ØN
  - Vertebral
    - Bilateral B3ØG
    - Left B3ØF
    - Right B3ØD
- Bile Duct BFØØ
- Bile Duct and Gallbladder BFØ3
- Bladder BTØØ
  - Kidney and Ureter BTØ4
- Bladder and Urethra BTØB
- Bone
  - Facial BNØ5ZZZ
  - Nasal BNØ4ZZZ
- Bones, Long, All BWØBZZZ
- Breast
  - Bilateral BHØ2ZZZ
  - Left BHØ1ZZZ
  - Right BHØØZZZ
- Calcaneus
  - Left BQØKZZZ
  - Right BQØJZZZ
- Chest BWØ3ZZZ
- Clavicle
  - Left BPØ5ZZZ
  - Right BPØ4ZZZ
- Coccyx BRØFZZZ
- Corpora Cavernosa BVØØ
- Dialysis Fistula B5ØW
- Dialysis Shunt B5ØW
- Disc
  - Cervical BRØ1
  - Lumbar BRØ3
  - Thoracic BRØ2

Plain Radiography — *continued*
Duct
Lacrimal
Bilateral B802
Left B801
Right B800
Mammary
Multiple
Left BH06
Right BH05
Single
Left BH04
Right BH03
Elbow
Left BP0H
Right BP0G
Epididymis
Left BV02
Right BV01
Extremity
Lower BW0CZZZ
Upper BW0JZZZ
Eye
Bilateral B807ZZZ
Left B806ZZZ
Right B805ZZZ
Facet Joint
Cervical BR04
Lumbar BR06
Thoracic BR05
Fallopian Tube
Bilateral BU02
Left BU01
Right BU00
Fallopian Tube and Uterus BU08
Femur
Left, Densitometry BQ04ZZ1
Right, Densitometry BQ03ZZ1
Finger
Left BP0SZZZ
Right BP0RZZZ
Foot
Left BQ0MZZZ
Right BQ0LZZZ
Forearm
Left BP0KZZZ
Right BP0JZZZ
Gallbladder and Bile Duct BF03
Gland
Parotid
Bilateral B906
Left B905
Right B904
Salivary
Bilateral B90D
Left B90C
Right B90B
Submandibular
Bilateral B909
Left B908
Right B907
Hand
Left BP0PZZZ
Right BP0NZZZ
Heart
Left B205
Right B204
Right and Left B206
Hepatobiliary System, All BF0C
Hip
Left BQ01
Densitometry BQ01ZZ1
Right BQ00
Densitometry BQ00ZZ1
Humerus
Left BP0BZZZ
Right BP0AZZZ
Ileal Diversion Loop BT0C
Intracranial Sinus B502
Joint
Acromioclavicular, Bilateral BP03ZZZ
Finger
Left BP0D
Right BP0C
Foot
Left BQ0Y
Right BQ0X
Hand
Left BP0D

Plain Radiography — *continued*
Joint — *continued*
Hand — *continued*
Right BP0C
Lumbosacral BR0BZZZ
Sacroiliac BR0D
Sternoclavicular
Bilateral BP02ZZZ
Left BP01ZZZ
Right BP00ZZZ
Temporomandibular
Bilateral BN09
Left BN08
Right BN07
Thoracolumbar BR08ZZZ
Toe
Left BQ0Y
Right BQ0X
Kidney
Bilateral BT03
Left BT02
Right BT01
Ureter and Bladder BT04
Knee
Left BQ08
Right BQ07
Leg
Left BQ0FZZZ
Right BQ0DZZZ
Lymphatic
Head B704
Lower Extremity
Bilateral B70B
Left B709
Right B708
Neck B704
Pelvic B70C
Upper Extremity
Bilateral B707
Left B706
Right B705
Mandible BN06ZZZ
Mastoid B90HZZZ
Nasopharynx B90FZZZ
Optic Foramina
Left B804ZZZ
Right B803ZZZ
Orbit
Bilateral BN03ZZZ
Left BN02ZZZ
Right BN01ZZZ
Oropharynx B90FZZZ
Patella
Left BQ0WZZZ
Right BQ0VZZZ
Pelvis BR0CZZZ
Pelvis and Abdomen BW01ZZZ
Prostate BV03
Retroperitoneal Lymphatic
Bilateral B701
Unilateral B700
Ribs
Left BP0YZZZ
Right BP0XZZZ
Sacrum BR0FZZZ
Scapula
Left BP07ZZZ
Right BP06ZZZ
Shoulder
Left BP09
Right BP08
Sinus
Intracranial B502
Paranasal B902ZZZ
Skull BN00ZZZ
Spinal Cord B00B
Spine
Cervical, Densitometry BR00ZZ1
Lumbar, Densitometry BR09ZZ1
Thoracic, Densitometry BR07ZZ1
Whole, Densitometry BR0GZZ1
Sternum BR0HZZZ
Teeth
All BN0JZZZ
Multiple BN0HZZZ
Testicle
Left BV06
Right BV05

Plain Radiography — *continued*
Toe
Left BQ0QZZZ
Right BQ0PZZZ
Tooth, Single BN0GZZZ
Tracheobronchial Tree
Bilateral BB09YZZ
Left BB08YZZ
Right BB07YZZ
Ureter
Bilateral BT08
Kidney and Bladder BT04
Left BT07
Right BT06
Urethra BT05
Urethra and Bladder BT0B
Uterus BU06
Uterus and Fallopian Tube BU08
Vagina BU09
Vasa Vasorum BV08
Vein
Cerebellar B501
Cerebral B501
Epidural B500
Jugular
Bilateral B505
Left B504
Right B503
Lower Extremity
Bilateral B50D
Left B50C
Right B50B
Other B50V
Pelvic (Iliac)
Left B50G
Right B50F
Pelvic (Iliac) Bilateral B50H
Portal B50T
Pulmonary
Bilateral B50S
Left B50R
Right B50Q
Renal
Bilateral B50L
Left B50K
Right B50J
Spanchnic B50T
Subclavian
Left B507
Right B506
Upper Extremity
Bilateral B50P
Left B50N
Right B50M
Vena Cava
Inferior B509
Superior B508
Whole Body BW0KZZZ
Infant BW0MZZZ
Whole Skeleton BW0LZZZ
Wrist
Left BP0M
Right BP0L
Planar Nuclear Medicine Imaging
Abdomen CW10
Abdomen and Chest CW14
Abdomen and Pelvis CW11
Anatomical Region, Other CW1ZZZZ
Anatomical Regions, Multiple CW1YYZZ
Bladder and Ureters CT1H
Bladder, Kidneys and Ureters CT13
Blood C713
Bone Marrow C710
Brain C010
Breast CH1YYZZ
Bilateral CH12
Left CH11
Right CH10
Bronchi and Lungs CB12
Central Nervous System C01YYZZ
Cerebrospinal Fluid C015
Chest CW13
Chest and Abdomen CW14
Chest and Neck CW16
Digestive System CD1YYZZ
Ducts, Lacrimal, Bilateral C819
Ear, Nose, Mouth and Throat C91YYZZ
Endocrine System CG1YYZZ

Planar Nuclear Medicine Imaging — *continued*
- Extremity
  - Lower CW1D
    - Bilateral CP1F
    - Left CP1D
    - Right CP1C
  - Upper CW1M
    - Bilateral CP1B
    - Left CP19
    - Right CP18
- Eye C81YYZZ
- Gallbladder CF14
- Gastrointestinal Tract CD17
  - Upper CD15
- Gland
  - Adrenal, Bilateral CG14
  - Parathyroid CG11
  - Thyroid CG12
- Glands, Salivary, Bilateral C91B
- Head and Neck CW1B
- Heart C21YYZZ
  - Right and Left C216
- Hepatobiliary System, All CF1C
- Hepatobiliary System and Pancreas CF1YYZZ
- Kidneys, Ureters and Bladder CT13
- Liver CF15
- Liver and Spleen CF16
- Lungs and Bronchi CB12
- Lymphatics
  - Head C71J
  - Head and Neck C715
  - Lower Extremity C71P
  - Neck C71K
  - Pelvic C71D
  - Trunk C71M
  - Upper Chest C71L
  - Upper Extremity C71N
- Lymphatics and Hematologic System C71YYZZ
- Musculoskeletal System
  - All CP1Z
  - Other CP1YYZZ
- Myocardium C21G
- Neck and Chest CW16
- Neck and Head CW1B
- Pancreas and Hepatobiliary System CF1YYZZ
- Pelvic Region CW1J
- Pelvis CP16
- Pelvis and Abdomen CW11
- Pelvis and Spine CP17
- Reproductive System, Male CV1YYZZ
- Respiratory System CB1YYZZ
- Skin CH1YYZZ
- Skull CP11
- Spine CP15
- Spine and Pelvis CP17
- Spleen C712
- Spleen and Liver CF16
- Subcutaneous Tissue CH1YYZZ
- Testicles, Bilateral CV19
- Thorax CP14
- Ureters and Bladder CT1H
- Ureters, Kidneys and Bladder CT13
- Urinary System CT1YYZZ
- Veins C51YYZZ
  - Central C51R
  - Lower Extremity
    - Bilateral C51D
    - Left C51C
    - Right C51B
  - Upper Extremity
    - Bilateral C51Q
    - Left C51P
    - Right C51N
- Whole Body CW1N

Plantar digital vein
- *use* Foot Vein, Left
- *use* Foot Vein, Right

Plantar fascia (aponeurosis)
- *use* Subcutaneous Tissue and Fascia, Left Foot
- *use* Subcutaneous Tissue and Fascia, Right Foot

Plantar metatarsal vein
- *use* Foot Vein, Left
- *use* Foot Vein, Right

Plantar venous arch
- *use* Foot Vein, Left
- *use* Foot Vein, Right

Plaque Radiation
- Abdomen DWY3FZZ

Plaque Radiation — *continued*
- Adrenal Gland DGY2FZZ
- Anus DDY8FZZ
- Bile Ducts DFY2FZZ
- Bladder DTY2FZZ
- Bone Marrow D7YØFZZ
- Bone, Other DPYCFZZ
- Brain DØYØFZZ
- Brain Stem DØY1FZZ
- Breast
  - Left DMYØFZZ
  - Right DMY1FZZ
- Bronchus DBY1FZZ
- Cervix DUY1FZZ
- Chest DWY2FZZ
- Chest Wall DBY7FZZ
- Colon DDY5FZZ
- Diaphragm DBY8FZZ
- Duodenum DDY2FZZ
- Ear D9YØFZZ
- Esophagus DDYØFZZ
- Eye D8YØFZZ
- Femur DPY9FZZ
- Fibula DPYBFZZ
- Gallbladder DFY1FZZ
- Gland
  - Adrenal DGY2FZZ
  - Parathyroid DGY4FZZ
  - Pituitary DGYØFZZ
  - Thyroid DGY5FZZ
- Glands, Salivary D9Y6FZZ
- Head and Neck DWY1FZZ
- Hemibody DWY4FZZ
- Humerus DPY6FZZ
- Ileum DDY4FZZ
- Jejunum DDY3FZZ
- Kidney DTYØFZZ
- Larynx D9YBFZZ
- Liver DFYØFZZ
- Lung DBY2FZZ
- Lymphatics
  - Abdomen D7Y6FZZ
  - Axillary D7Y4FZZ
  - Inguinal D7Y8FZZ
  - Neck D7Y3FZZ
  - Pelvis D7Y7FZZ
  - Thorax D7Y5FZZ
- Mandible DPY3FZZ
- Maxilla DPY2FZZ
- Mediastinum DBY6FZZ
- Mouth D9Y4FZZ
- Nasopharynx D9YDFZZ
- Neck and Head DWY1FZZ
- Nerve, Peripheral DØY7FZZ
- Nose D9Y1FZZ
- Ovary DUYØFZZ
- Palate
  - Hard D9Y8FZZ
  - Soft D9Y9FZZ
- Pancreas DFY3FZZ
- Parathyroid Gland DGY4FZZ
- Pelvic Bones DPY8FZZ
- Pelvic Region DWY6FZZ
- Pharynx D9YCFZZ
- Pineal Body DGY1FZZ
- Pituitary Gland DGYØFZZ
- Pleura DBY5FZZ
- Prostate DVYØFZZ
- Radius DPY7FZZ
- Rectum DDY7FZZ
- Rib DPY5FZZ
- Sinuses D9Y7FZZ
- Skin
  - Abdomen DHY8FZZ
  - Arm DHY4FZZ
  - Back DHY7FZZ
  - Buttock DHY9FZZ
  - Chest DHY6FZZ
  - Face DHY2FZZ
  - Foot DHYCFZZ
  - Hand DHY5FZZ
  - Leg DHYBFZZ
  - Neck DHY3FZZ
- Skull DPYØFZZ
- Spinal Cord DØY6FZZ
- Spleen D7Y2FZZ
- Sternum DPY4FZZ
- Stomach DDY1FZZ
- Testis DVY1FZZ

Plaque Radiation — *continued*
- Thymus D7Y1FZZ
- Thyroid Gland DGY5FZZ
- Tibia DPYBFZZ
- Tongue D9Y5FZZ
- Trachea DBYØFZZ
- Ulna DPY7FZZ
- Ureter DTY1FZZ
- Urethra DTY3FZZ
- Uterus DUY2FZZ
- Whole Body DWY5FZZ

Plasma, Convalescent (Nonautologous) XW1

Plasmapheresis, therapeutic *see* Pheresis, Physiological Systems 6A5

Plateletpheresis, therapeutic *see* Pheresis, Physiological Systems 6A5

Platysma muscle
- *use* Neck Muscle, Left
- *use* Neck Muscle, Right

Plazomicin Anti-infective XWØ

Pleurectomy
- *see* Excision, Respiratory System ØBB
- *see* Resection, Respiratory System ØBT

Pleurocentesis *see* Drainage, Anatomical Regions, General ØW9

Pleurodesis, pleurosclerosis
- Chemical injection *see* Introduction of Substance in or on, Pleural Cavity 3EØL
- Surgical *see* Destruction, Respiratory System ØB5

Pleurolysis *see* Release, Respiratory System ØBN

Pleuroscopy ØBJQ4ZZ

Pleurotomy *see* Drainage, Respiratory System ØB9

Plica semilunaris
- *use* Conjunctiva, Left
- *use* Conjunctiva, Right

Plication *see* Restriction

Pneumectomy
- *see* Excision, Respiratory System ØBB
- *see* Resection, Respiratory System ØBT

Pneumocentesis *see* Drainage, Respiratory System ØB9

Pneumogastric nerve *use* Vagus Nerve

Pneumolysis *see* Release, Respiratory System ØBN

Pneumonectomy *see* Resection, Respiratory System ØBT

Pneumonolysis *see* Release, Respiratory System ØBN

Pneumonopexy
- *see* Repair, Respiratory System ØBQ
- *see* Reposition, Respiratory System ØBS

Pneumonorrhaphy *see* Repair, Respiratory System ØBQ

Pneumonotomy *see* Drainage, Respiratory System ØB9

Pneumotaxic center *use* Pons

Pneumotomy *see* Drainage, Respiratory System ØB9

Pollicization *see* Transfer, Anatomical Regions, Upper Extremities ØXX

Polyclonal hyperimmune globulin *use* Globulin

Polyethylene socket *use* Synthetic Substitute, Polyethylene in ØSR

Polymethylmethacrylate (PMMA) *use* Synthetic Substitute

Polypectomy, gastrointestinal *see* Excision, Gastrointestinal System ØDB

Polypropylene mesh *use* Synthetic Substitute

Polysomnogram 4A1ZXQZ

Pontine tegmentum *use* Pons

Popliteal ligament
- *use* Knee Bursa and Ligament, Left
- *use* Knee Bursa and Ligament, Right

Popliteal lymph node
- *use* Lymphatic, Left Lower Extremity
- *use* Lymphatic, Right Lower Extremity

Popliteal vein
- *use* Femoral Vein, Left
- *use* Femoral Vein, Right

Popliteus muscle
- *use* Lower Leg Muscle, Left
- *use* Lower Leg Muscle, Right

Porcine (bioprosthetic) valve *use* Zooplastic Tissue in Heart and Great Vessels

Positive Blood Culture Fluorescence Hybridization for Organism Identification, Concentration and Susceptibility XXE5XN6

Positive end expiratory pressure *see* Performance, Respiratory 5A19

Positron Emission Tomographic (PET) Imaging
- Brain CØ3Ø

Positron Emission Tomographic (PET) Imaging — *continued*
Bronchi and Lungs CB32
Central Nervous System CØ3YYZZ
Heart C23YYZZ
Lungs and Bronchi CB32
Myocardium C23G
Respiratory System CB3YYZZ
Whole Body CW3NYZZ
Positron emission tomography *see* Positron Emission Tomographic (PET) Imaging
Postauricular (mastoid) lymph node
use Lymphatic, Left Neck
use Lymphatic, Right Neck
Postcava *use* Inferior Vena Cava
Posterior auricular artery
use External Carotid Artery, Left
use External Carotid Artery, Right
Posterior auricular nerve *use* Facial Nerve
Posterior auricular vein
use External Jugular Vein, Left
use External Jugular Vein, Right
Posterior cerebral artery *use* Intracranial Artery
Posterior chamber
use Eye, Left
use Eye, Right
Posterior circumflex humeral artery
use Axillary Artery, Left
use Axillary Artery, Right
Posterior communicating artery *use* Intracranial Artery
Posterior cruciate ligament (PCL)
use Knee Bursa and Ligament, Left
use Knee Bursa and Ligament, Right
Posterior (Dynamic) Distraction Device
Lumbar XNSØ
Thoracic XNS4
Posterior facial (retromandibular) vein
use Face Vein, Left
use Face Vein, Right
Posterior femoral cutaneous nerve *use* Sacral Plexus
Posterior inferior cerebellar artery (PICA) *use* Intracranial Artery
Posterior interosseous nerve *use* Radial Nerve
Posterior labial nerve *use* Pudendal Nerve
Posterior (subscapular) lymph node
use Lymphatic, Left Axillary
use Lymphatic, Right Axillary
Posterior scrotal nerve *use* Pudendal Nerve
Posterior spinal artery
use Vertebral Artery, Left
use Vertebral Artery, Right
Posterior tibial recurrent artery
use Anterior Tibial Artery, Left
use Anterior Tibial Artery, Right
Posterior ulnar recurrent artery
use Ulnar Artery, Left
use Ulnar Artery, Right
Posterior vagal trunk *use* Vagus Nerve
PPN (peripheral parenteral nutrition) *see* Introduction of Nutritional Substance
Praxbind® (idarucizumab), Pradaxa® (dabigatran) reversal agent *use* Other Therapeutic Substance
Preauricular lymph node *use* Lymphatic, Head
Precava *use* Superior Vena Cava
PRECICE intramedullary limb lengthening system
use Internal Fixation Device, Intramedullary Limb Lengthening in ØPH
use Internal Fixation Device, Intramedullary Limb Lengthening in ØQH
Prepatellar bursa
use Knee Bursa and Ligament, Left
use Knee Bursa and Ligament, Right
Preputiotomy *see* Drainage, Male Reproductive System ØV9
Pressure support ventilation *see* Performance, Respiratory 5A19
PRESTIGE® Cervical Disc *use* Synthetic Substitute
Pretracheal fascia
use Subcutaneous Tissue and Fascia, Left Neck
use Subcutaneous Tissue and Fascia, Right Neck
Prevertebral fascia
use Subcutaneous Tissue and Fascia, Left Neck
use Subcutaneous Tissue and Fascia, Right Neck
PrimeAdvanced neurostimulator (SureScan) (MRI Safe) *use* Stimulator Generator, Multiple Array in ØJH
Princeps pollicis artery
use Hand Artery, Left
use Hand Artery, Right
Probing, duct
Diagnostic *see* Inspection
Dilation *see* Dilation
PROCEED™ Ventral Patch *use* Synthetic Substitute
Procerus muscle *use* Facial Muscle
Proctectomy
see Excision, Rectum ØDBP
see Resection, Rectum ØDTP
Proctoclysis *see* Introduction of substance in or on, Gastrointestinal Tract, Lower 3EØH
Proctocolectomy
see Excision, Gastrointestinal System ØDB
see Resection, Gastrointestinal System ØDT
Proctocolpoplasty
see Repair, Gastrointestinal System ØDQ
see Supplement, Gastrointestinal System ØDU
Proctoperineoplasty
see Repair, Gastrointestinal System ØDQ
see Supplement, Gastrointestinal System ØDU
Proctoperineorrhaphy *see* Repair, Gastrointestinal System ØDQ
Proctopexy
see Repair, Rectum ØDQP
see Reposition, Rectum ØDSP
Proctoplasty
see Repair, Rectum ØDQP
see Supplement, Rectum ØDUP
Proctorrhaphy *see* Repair, Rectum ØDQP
Proctoscopy ØDJD8ZZ
Proctosigmoidectomy
see Excision, Gastrointestinal System ØDB
see Resection, Gastrointestinal System ØDT
Proctosigmoidoscopy ØDJD8ZZ
Proctostomy *see* Drainage, Rectum ØD9P
Proctotomy *see* Drainage, Rectum ØD9P
Prodisc-C *use* Synthetic Substitute
Prodisc-L *use* Synthetic Substitute
Production, atrial septal defect *see* Excision, Septum, Atrial Ø2B5
Profunda brachii
use Brachial Artery, Left
use Brachial Artery, Right
Profunda femoris (deep femoral) vein
use Femoral Vein, Left
use Femoral Vein, Right
PROLENE Polypropylene Hernia System (PHS) *use* Synthetic Substitute
Prolonged intermittent renal replacement therapy (PIRRT) 5A1D80Z
Pronator quadratus muscle
use Lower Arm and Wrist Muscle, Left
use Lower Arm and Wrist Muscle, Right
Pronator teres muscle
use Lower Arm and Wrist Muscle, Left
use Lower Arm and Wrist Muscle, Right
Prostatectomy
see Excision, Prostate ØVBØ
see Resection, Prostate ØVTØ
Prostatic urethra *use* Urethra
Prostatomy, prostatotomy *see* Drainage, Prostate ØV9Ø
Protecta XT CRT-D *use* Cardiac Resynchronization Defibrillator Pulse Generator in ØJH
Protecta XT DR (XT VR) *use* Defibrillator Generator in ØJH
Protege® RX Carotid Stent System *use* Intraluminal Device
Proximal radioulnar joint
use Elbow Joint, Left
use Elbow Joint, Right
Psoas muscle
use Hip Muscle, Left
use Hip Muscle, Right
PSV (pressure support ventilation) *see* Performance, Respiratory 5A19
Psychoanalysis GZ54ZZZ
Psychological Tests
Cognitive Status GZ14ZZZ
Developmental GZ1ØZZZ
Intellectual and Psychoeducational GZ12ZZZ
Neurobehavioral Status GZ14ZZZ
Neuropsychological GZ13ZZZ
Personality and Behavioral GZ11ZZZ
Psychotherapy
Family, Mental Health Services GZ72ZZZ
Group GZHZZZZ
Mental Health Services GZHZZZZ
Individual
see Psychotherapy, Individual, Mental Health Services
for substance abuse
12-Step HZ53ZZZ
Behavioral HZ51ZZZ
Cognitive HZ5ØZZZ
Cognitive-Behavioral HZ52ZZZ
Confrontational HZ58ZZZ
Interactive HZ55ZZZ
Interpersonal HZ54ZZZ
Motivational Enhancement HZ57ZZZ
Psychoanalysis HZ5BZZZ
Psychodynamic HZ5CZZZ
Psychoeducation HZ56ZZZ
Psychophysiological HZ5DZZZ
Supportive HZ59ZZZ
Mental Health Services
Behavioral GZ51ZZZ
Cognitive GZ52ZZZ
Cognitive-Behavioral GZ58ZZZ
Interactive GZ5ØZZZ
Interpersonal GZ53ZZZ
Psychoanalysis GZ54ZZZ
Psychodynamic GZ55ZZZ
Psychophysiological GZ59ZZZ
Supportive GZ56ZZZ
PTCA (percutaneous transluminal coronary angioplasty) *see* Dilation, Heart and Great Vessels Ø27
Pterygoid muscle *use* Head Muscle
Pterygoid process *use* Sphenoid Bone
Pterygopalatine (sphenopalatine) ganglion *use* Head and Neck Sympathetic Nerve
Pubis
use Pelvic Bone, Left
use Pelvic Bone, Right
Pubofemoral ligament
use Hip Bursa and Ligament, Left
use Hip Bursa and Ligament, Right
Pudendal nerve *use* Sacral Plexus
Pull-through, laparoscopic-assisted transanal
see Excision, Gastrointestinal System ØDB
see Resection, Gastrointestinal System ØDT
Pull-through, rectal *see* Resection, Rectum ØDTP
Pulmoaortic canal *use* Pulmonary Artery, Left
Pulmonary annulus *use* Pulmonary Valve
Pulmonary artery wedge monitoring *see* Monitoring, Arterial 4A13
Pulmonary plexus
use Thoracic Sympathetic Nerve
use Vagus Nerve
Pulmonic valve *use* Pulmonary Valve
Pulpectomy *see* Excision, Mouth and Throat ØCB
Pulverization *see* Fragmentation
Pulvinar *use* Thalamus
Pump reservoir *use* Infusion Device, Pump in Subcutaneous Tissue and Fascia
Punch biopsy *see* Excision with qualifier Diagnostic
Puncture *see* Drainage
Puncture, lumbar *see* Drainage, Spinal Canal ØØ9U
Pure-Vu® System XDPH8K7
Pyelography
see Fluoroscopy, Urinary System BT1
see Plain Radiography, Urinary System BTØ
Pyeloileostomy, urinary diversion *see* Bypass, Urinary System ØT1
Pyeloplasty
see Repair, Urinary System ØTQ
see Replacement, Urinary System ØTR
see Supplement, Urinary System ØTU
Pyeloplasty, dismembered *see* Repair, Kidney Pelvis
Pyelorrhaphy *see* Repair, Urinary System ØTQ
Pyeloscopy ØTJ58ZZ
Pyelostomy
see Bypass, Urinary System ØT1
see Drainage, Urinary System ØT9
Pyelotomy *see* Drainage, Urinary System ØT9
Pylorectomy
see Excision, Stomach, Pylorus ØDB7
see Resection, Stomach, Pylorus ØDT7
Pyloric antrum *use* Stomach, Pylorus
Pyloric canal *use* Stomach, Pylorus
Pyloric sphincter *use* Stomach, Pylorus

Pylorodiosis *see* Dilation, Stomach, Pylorus ØD77
Pylorogastrectomy
see Excision, Gastrointestinal System ØDB
see Resection, Gastrointestinal System ØDT
Pyloroplasty
see Repair, Stomach, Pylorus ØDQ7
see Supplement, Stomach, Pylorus ØDU7
Pyloroscopy ØDJ68ZZ
Pylorotomy *see* Drainage, Stomach, Pylorus ØD97
Pyramidalis muscle
use Abdomen Muscle, Left
use Abdomen Muscle, Right

Q

Quadrangular cartilage *use* Nasal Septum
Quadrant resection of breast *see* Excision, Skin and Breast ØHB
Quadrate lobe *use* Liver
Quadratus femoris muscle
use Hip Muscle, Left
use Hip Muscle, Right
Quadratus lumborum muscle
use Trunk Muscle, Left
use Trunk Muscle, Right
Quadratus plantae muscle
use Foot Muscle, Left
use Foot Muscle, Right
Quadriceps (femoris)
use Upper Leg Muscle, Left
use Upper Leg Muscle, Right
Quarantine 8EØZXY6

R

Radial artery arteriovenous fistula, using Thermal Resistance Energy X2K
Radial collateral carpal ligament
use Wrist Bursa and Ligament, Left
use Wrist Bursa and Ligament, Right
Radial collateral ligament
use Elbow Bursa and Ligament, Left
use Elbow Bursa and Ligament, Right
Radial notch
use Ulna, Left
use Ulna, Right
Radial recurrent artery
use Radial Artery, Left
use Radial Artery, Right
Radial vein
use Brachial Vein, Left
use Brachial Vein, Right
Radialis indicis
use Hand Artery, Left
use Hand Artery, Right
Radiation Therapy
see Beam Radiation
see Brachytherapy
see Other Radiation
see Stereotactic Radiosurgery
Radiation treatment *see* Radiation Therapy
Radiocarpal joint
use Wrist Joint, Left
use Wrist Joint, Right
Radiocarpal ligament
use Wrist Bursa and Ligament, Left
use Wrist Bursa and Ligament, Right
Radiography *see* Plain Radiography
Radiology, analog *see* Plain Radiography
Radiology, diagnostic *see* Imaging, Diagnostic
Radioulnar ligament
use Wrist Bursa and Ligament, Left
use Wrist Bursa and Ligament, Right
Range of motion testing *see* Motor Function Assessment, Rehabilitation FØ1
Rapid ASPECTS XXEØXØ7
REALIZE® Adjustable Gastric Band *use* Extraluminal Device
Reattachment
Abdominal Wall ØWMFØZZ
Ampulla of Vater ØFMC
Ankle Region
Left ØYMLØZZ
Right ØYMKØZZ

Reattachment — *continued*
Arm
Lower
Left ØXMFØZZ
Right ØXMDØZZ
Upper
Left ØXM9ØZZ
Right ØXM8ØZZ
Axilla
Left ØXM5ØZZ
Right ØXM4ØZZ
Back
Lower ØWMLØZZ
Upper ØWMKØZZ
Bladder ØTMB
Bladder Neck ØTMC
Breast
Bilateral ØHMVXZZ
Left ØHMUXZZ
Right ØHMTXZZ
Bronchus
Lingula ØBM9ØZZ
Lower Lobe
Left ØBMBØZZ
Right ØBM6ØZZ
Main
Left ØBM7ØZZ
Right ØBM3ØZZ
Middle Lobe, Right ØBM5ØZZ
Upper Lobe
Left ØBM8ØZZ
Right ØBM4ØZZ
Bursa and Ligament
Abdomen
Left ØMMJ
Right ØMMH
Ankle
Left ØMMR
Right ØMMQ
Elbow
Left ØMM4
Right ØMM3
Foot
Left ØMMT
Right ØMMS
Hand
Left ØMM8
Right ØMM7
Head and Neck ØMMØ
Hip
Left ØMMM
Right ØMML
Knee
Left ØMMP
Right ØMMN
Lower Extremity
Left ØMMW
Right ØMMV
Perineum ØMMK
Rib(s) ØMMG
Shoulder
Left ØMM2
Right ØMM1
Spine
Lower ØMMD
Upper ØMMC
Sternum ØMMF
Upper Extremity
Left ØMMB
Right ØMM9
Wrist
Left ØMM6
Right ØMM5
Buttock
Left ØYM1ØZZ
Right ØYMØØZZ
Carina ØBM2ØZZ
Cecum ØDMH
Cervix ØUMC
Chest Wall ØWM8ØZZ
Clitoris ØUMJXZZ
Colon
Ascending ØDMK
Descending ØDMM
Sigmoid ØDMN
Transverse ØDML
Cord
Bilateral ØVMH
Left ØVMG

Reattachment — *continued*
Cord — *continued*
Right ØVMF
Cul-de-sac ØUMF
Diaphragm ØBMTØZZ
Duct
Common Bile ØFM9
Cystic ØFM8
Hepatic
Common ØFM7
Left ØFM6
Right ØFM5
Pancreatic ØFMD
Accessory ØFMF
Duodenum ØDM9
Ear
Left Ø9M1XZZ
Right Ø9MØXZZ
Elbow Region
Left ØXMCØZZ
Right ØXMBØZZ
Esophagus ØDM5
Extremity
Lower
Left ØYMBØZZ
Right ØYM9ØZZ
Upper
Left ØXM7ØZZ
Right ØXM6ØZZ
Eyelid
Lower
Left Ø8MRXZZ
Right Ø8MQXZZ
Upper
Left Ø8MPXZZ
Right Ø8MNXZZ
Face ØWM2ØZZ
Fallopian Tube
Left ØUM6
Right ØUM5
Fallopian Tubes, Bilateral ØUM7
Femoral Region
Left ØYM8ØZZ
Right ØYM7ØZZ
Finger
Index
Left ØXMPØZZ
Right ØXMNØZZ
Little
Left ØXMWØZZ
Right ØXMVØZZ
Middle
Left ØXMRØZZ
Right ØXMQØZZ
Ring
Left ØXMTØZZ
Right ØXMSØZZ
Foot
Left ØYMNØZZ
Right ØYMMØZZ
Forequarter
Left ØXM1ØZZ
Right ØXMØØZZ
Gallbladder ØFM4
Gland
Left ØGM2
Right ØGM3
Hand
Left ØXMKØZZ
Right ØXMJØZZ
Hindquarter
Bilateral ØYM4ØZZ
Left ØYM3ØZZ
Right ØYM2ØZZ
Hymen ØUMK
Ileum ØDMB
Inguinal Region
Left ØYM6ØZZ
Right ØYM5ØZZ
Intestine
Large ØDME
Left ØDMG
Right ØDMF
Small ØDM8
Jaw
Lower ØWM5ØZZ
Upper ØWM4ØZZ
Jejunum ØDMA

Reattachment — *continued*
Kidney
Left ØTM1
Right ØTMØ
Kidney Pelvis
Left ØTM4
Right ØTM3
Kidneys, Bilateral ØTM2
Knee Region
Left ØYMGØZZ
Right ØYMFØZZ
Leg
Lower
Left ØYMJØZZ
Right ØYMHØZZ
Upper
Left ØYMDØZZ
Right ØYMCØZZ
Lip
Lower ØCM1ØZZ
Upper ØCMØØZZ
Liver ØFMØ
Left Lobe ØFM2
Right Lobe ØFM1
Lung
Left ØBMLØZZ
Lower Lobe
Left ØBMJØZZ
Right ØBMFØZZ
Middle Lobe, Right ØBMDØZZ
Right ØBMKØZZ
Upper Lobe
Left ØBMGØZZ
Right ØBMCØZZ
Lung Lingula ØBMHØZZ
Muscle
Abdomen
Left ØKML
Right ØKMK
Facial ØKM1
Foot
Left ØKMW
Right ØKMV
Hand
Left ØKMD
Right ØKMC
Head ØKMØ
Hip
Left ØKMP
Right ØKMN
Lower Arm and Wrist
Left ØKMB
Right ØKM9
Lower Leg
Left ØKMT
Right ØKMS
Neck
Left ØKM3
Right ØKM2
Perineum ØKMM
Shoulder
Left ØKM6
Right ØKM5
Thorax
Left ØKMJ
Right ØKMH
Tongue, Palate, Pharynx ØKM4
Trunk
Left ØKMG
Right ØKMF
Upper Arm
Left ØKM8
Right ØKM7
Upper Leg
Left ØKMR
Right ØKMQ
Nasal Mucosa and Soft Tissue Ø9MKXZZ
Neck ØWM6ØZZ
Nipple
Left ØHMXXZZ
Right ØHMWXZZ
Ovary
Bilateral ØUM2
Left ØUM1
Right ØUMØ
Palate, Soft ØCM3ØZZ
Pancreas ØFMG
Parathyroid Gland ØGMR

Reattachment — *continued*
Parathyroid Gland — *continued*
Inferior
Left ØGMP
Right ØGMN
Multiple ØGMQ
Superior
Left ØGMM
Right ØGML
Penis ØVMSXZZ
Perineum
Female ØWMNØZZ
Male ØWMMØZZ
Rectum ØDMP
Scrotum ØVM5XZZ
Shoulder Region
Left ØXM3ØZZ
Right ØXM2ØZZ
Skin
Abdomen ØHM7XZZ
Back ØHM6XZZ
Buttock ØHM8XZZ
Chest ØHM5XZZ
Ear
Left ØHM3XZZ
Right ØHM2XZZ
Face ØHM1XZZ
Foot
Left ØHMNXZZ
Right ØHMMXZZ
Hand
Left ØHMGXZZ
Right ØHMFXZZ
Inguinal ØHMAXZZ
Lower Arm
Left ØHMEXZZ
Right ØHMDXZZ
Lower Leg
Left ØHMLXZZ
Right ØHMKXZZ
Neck ØHM4XZZ
Perineum ØHM9XZZ
Scalp ØHMØXZZ
Upper Arm
Left ØHMCXZZ
Right ØHMBXZZ
Upper Leg
Left ØHMJXZZ
Right ØHMHXZZ
Stomach ØDM6
Tendon
Abdomen
Left ØLMG
Right ØLMF
Ankle
Left ØLMT
Right ØLMS
Foot
Left ØLMW
Right ØLMV
Hand
Left ØLM8
Right ØLM7
Head and Neck ØLMØ
Hip
Left ØLMK
Right ØLMJ
Knee
Left ØLMR
Right ØLMQ
Lower Arm and Wrist
Left ØLM6
Right ØLM5
Lower Leg
Left ØLMP
Right ØLMN
Perineum ØLMH
Shoulder
Left ØLM2
Right ØLM1
Thorax
Left ØLMD
Right ØLMC
Trunk
Left ØLMB
Right ØLM9
Upper Arm
Left ØLM4
Right ØLM3

Reattachment — *continued*
Tendon — *continued*
Upper Leg
Left ØLMM
Right ØLML
Testis
Bilateral ØVMC
Left ØVMB
Right ØVM9
Thumb
Left ØXMMØZZ
Right ØXMLØZZ
Thyroid Gland
Left Lobe ØGMG
Right Lobe ØGMH
Toe
1st
Left ØYMQØZZ
Right ØYMPØZZ
2nd
Left ØYMSØZZ
Right ØYMRØZZ
3rd
Left ØYMUØZZ
Right ØYMTØZZ
4th
Left ØYMWØZZ
Right ØYMVØZZ
5th
Left ØYMYØZZ
Right ØYMXØZZ
Tongue ØCM7ØZZ
Tooth
Lower ØCMX
Upper ØCMW
Trachea ØBM1ØZZ
Tunica Vaginalis
Left ØVM7
Right ØVM6
Ureter
Left ØTM7
Right ØTM6
Ureters, Bilateral ØTM8
Urethra ØTMD
Uterine Supporting Structure ØUM4
Uterus ØUM9
Uvula ØCMNØZZ
Vagina ØUMG
Vulva ØUMMXZZ
Wrist Region
Left ØXMHØZZ
Right ØXMGØZZ
REBOA (resuscitative endovascular balloon occlusion of the aorta)
Ø2LW3DJ
Ø4LØ3DJ
Rebound HRD® (Hernia Repair Device) *use* Synthetic Substitute
RECELL® cell suspension autograft *see* Replacement, Skin and Breast ØHR
Recession
see Repair
see Reposition
Reclosure, disrupted abdominal wall ØWQFXZZ
Reconstruction
see Repair
see Replacement
see Supplement
Rectectomy
see Excision, Rectum ØDBP
see Resection, Rectum ØDTP
Rectocele repair *see* Repair, Subcutaneous Tissue and Fascia, Pelvic Region ØJQC
Rectopexy
see Repair, Gastrointestinal System ØDQ
see Reposition, Gastrointestinal System ØDS
Rectoplasty
see Repair, Gastrointestinal System ØDQ
see Supplement, Gastrointestinal System ØDU
Rectorrhaphy *see* Repair, Gastrointestinal System ØDQ
Rectoscopy ØDJD8ZZ
Rectosigmoid junction *use* Sigmoid Colon
Rectosigmoidectomy
see Excision, Gastrointestinal System ØDB
see Resection, Gastrointestinal System ØDT
Rectostomy *see* Drainage, Rectum ØD9P
Rectotomy *see* Drainage, Rectum ØD9P

- **Rectus abdominis muscle**
  - *use* Abdomen Muscle, Left
  - *use* Abdomen Muscle, Right
- **Rectus femoris muscle**
  - *use* Upper Leg Muscle, Left
  - *use* Upper Leg Muscle, Right
- **Recurrent laryngeal nerve** *use* Vagus Nerve
- **Reducer™ System** *use* Reduction Device in New Technology
- **Reduction**
  - Dislocation *see* Reposition
  - Fracture *see* Reposition
  - Intussusception, intestinal *see* Reposition, Gastrointestinal System ØDS
  - Mammoplasty *see* Excision, Skin and Breast ØHB
  - Prolapse *see* Reposition
  - Torsion *see* Reposition
  - Volvulus, gastrointestinal *see* Reposition, Gastrointestinal System ØDS
- **Reduction Device, Coronary Sinus** X2V73Q7
- **Refusion** *see* Fusion
- **REGN-COV2 Monoclonal Antibody** XWØ
- **Rehabilitation**
  - *see* Activities of Daily Living Assessment, Rehabilitation FØ2
  - *see* Activities of Daily Living Treatment, Rehabilitation FØ8
  - *see* Caregiver Training, Rehabilitation FØF
  - *see* Cochlear Implant Treatment, Rehabilitation FØB
  - *see* Device Fitting, Rehabilitation FØD
  - *see* Hearing Treatment, Rehabilitation FØ9
  - *see* Motor Function Assessment, Rehabilitation FØ1
  - *see* Motor Treatment, Rehabilitation FØ7
  - *see* Speech Assessment, Rehabilitation FØØ
  - *see* Speech Treatment, Rehabilitation FØ6
  - *see* Vestibular Treatment, Rehabilitation FØC
- **Reimplantation**
  - *see* Reattachment
  - *see* Reposition
  - *see* Transfer
- **Reinforcement**
  - *see* Repair
  - *see* Supplement
- **Relaxation, scar tissue** *see* Release
- **Release**
  - Acetabulum
    - Left ØQN5
    - Right ØQN4
  - Adenoids ØCNQ
  - Ampulla of Vater ØFNC
  - Anal Sphincter ØDNR
  - Anterior Chamber
    - Left Ø8N33ZZ
    - Right Ø8N23ZZ
  - Anus ØDNQ
  - Aorta
    - Abdominal Ø4NØ
    - Thoracic
      - Ascending/Arch Ø2NX
      - Descending Ø2NW
  - Aortic Body ØGND
  - Appendix ØDNJ
  - Artery
    - Anterior Tibial
      - Left Ø4NQ
      - Right Ø4NP
    - Axillary
      - Left Ø3N6
      - Right Ø3N5
    - Brachial
      - Left Ø3N8
      - Right Ø3N7
    - Celiac Ø4N1
    - Colic
      - Left Ø4N7
      - Middle Ø4N8
      - Right Ø4N6
    - Common Carotid
      - Left Ø3NJ
      - Right Ø3NH
    - Common Iliac
      - Left Ø4ND
      - Right Ø4NC
    - Coronary
      - Four or More Arteries Ø2N3

- **Release** — *continued*
  - Artery — *continued*
    - Coronary — *continued*
      - One Artery Ø2NØ
      - Three Arteries Ø2N2
      - Two Arteries Ø2N1
    - External Carotid
      - Left Ø3NN
      - Right Ø3NM
    - External Iliac
      - Left Ø4NJ
      - Right Ø4NH
    - Face Ø3NR
    - Femoral
      - Left Ø4NL
      - Right Ø4NK
    - Foot
      - Left Ø4NW
      - Right Ø4NV
    - Gastric Ø4N2
    - Hand
      - Left Ø3NF
      - Right Ø3ND
    - Hepatic Ø4N3
    - Inferior Mesenteric Ø4NB
    - Innominate Ø3N2
    - Internal Carotid
      - Left Ø3NL
      - Right Ø3NK
    - Internal Iliac
      - Left Ø4NF
      - Right Ø4NE
    - Internal Mammary
      - Left Ø3N1
      - Right Ø3NØ
    - Intracranial Ø3NG
    - Lower Ø4NY
    - Peroneal
      - Left Ø4NU
      - Right Ø4NT
    - Popliteal
      - Left Ø4NN
      - Right Ø4NM
    - Posterior Tibial
      - Left Ø4NS
      - Right Ø4NR
    - Pulmonary
      - Left Ø2NR
      - Right Ø2NQ
    - Pulmonary Trunk Ø2NP
    - Radial
      - Left Ø3NC
      - Right Ø3NB
    - Renal
      - Left Ø4NA
      - Right Ø4N9
    - Splenic Ø4N4
    - Subclavian
      - Left Ø3N4
      - Right Ø3N3
    - Superior Mesenteric Ø4N5
    - Temporal
      - Left Ø3NT
      - Right Ø3NS
    - Thyroid
      - Left Ø3NV
      - Right Ø3NU
    - Ulnar
      - Left Ø3NA
      - Right Ø3N9
    - Upper Ø3NY
    - Vertebral
      - Left Ø3NQ
      - Right Ø3NP
  - Atrium
    - Left Ø2N7
    - Right Ø2N6
  - Auditory Ossicle
    - Left Ø9NA
    - Right Ø9N9
  - Basal Ganglia ØØN8
  - Bladder ØTNB
  - Bladder Neck ØTNC
  - Bone
    - Ethmoid
      - Left ØNNG
      - Right ØNNF
    - Frontal ØNN1
    - Hyoid ØNNX

- **Release** — *continued*
  - Bone — *continued*
    - Lacrimal
      - Left ØNNJ
      - Right ØNNH
    - Nasal ØNNB
    - Occipital ØNN7
    - Palatine
      - Left ØNNL
      - Right ØNNK
    - Parietal
      - Left ØNN4
      - Right ØNN3
    - Pelvic
      - Left ØQN3
      - Right ØQN2
    - Sphenoid ØNNC
    - Temporal
      - Left ØNN6
      - Right ØNN5
    - Zygomatic
      - Left ØNNN
      - Right ØNNM
  - Brain ØØNØ
  - Breast
    - Bilateral ØHNV
    - Left ØHNU
    - Right ØHNT
  - Bronchus
    - Lingula ØBN9
    - Lower Lobe
      - Left ØBNB
      - Right ØBN6
    - Main
      - Left ØBN7
      - Right ØBN3
    - Middle Lobe, Right ØBN5
    - Upper Lobe
      - Left ØBN8
      - Right ØBN4
  - Buccal Mucosa ØCN4
  - Bursa and Ligament
    - Abdomen
      - Left ØMNJ
      - Right ØMNH
    - Ankle
      - Left ØMNR
      - Right ØMNQ
    - Elbow
      - Left ØMN4
      - Right ØMN3
    - Foot
      - Left ØMNT
      - Right ØMNS
    - Hand
      - Left ØMN8
      - Right ØMN7
    - Head and Neck ØMNØ
    - Hip
      - Left ØMNM
      - Right ØMNL
    - Knee
      - Left ØMNP
      - Right ØMNN
    - Lower Extremity
      - Left ØMNW
      - Right ØMNV
    - Perineum ØMNK
    - Rib(s) ØMNG
    - Shoulder
      - Left ØMN2
      - Right ØMN1
    - Spine
      - Lower ØMND
      - Upper ØMNC
    - Sternum ØMNF
    - Upper Extremity
      - Left ØMNB
      - Right ØMN9
    - Wrist
      - Left ØMN6
      - Right ØMN5
  - Carina ØBN2
  - Carotid Bodies, Bilateral ØGN8
  - Carotid Body
    - Left ØGN6
    - Right ØGN7
  - Carpal
    - Left ØPNN

Release — *continued*
- Carpal — *continued*
  - Right ØPNM
- Cecum ØDNH
- Cerebellum ØØNC
- Cerebral Hemisphere ØØN7
- Cerebral Meninges ØØN1
- Cerebral Ventricle ØØN6
- Cervix ØUNC
- Chordae Tendineae Ø2N9
- Choroid
  - Left Ø8NB
  - Right Ø8NA
- Cisterna Chyli Ø7NL
- Clavicle
  - Left ØPNB
  - Right ØPN9
- Clitoris ØUNJ
- Coccygeal Glomus ØGNB
- Coccyx ØQNS
- Colon
  - Ascending ØDNK
  - Descending ØDNM
  - Sigmoid ØDNN
  - Transverse ØDNL
- Conduction Mechanism Ø2N8
- Conjunctiva
  - Left Ø8NTXZZ
  - Right Ø8NSXZZ
- Cord
  - Bilateral ØVNH
  - Left ØVNG
  - Right ØVNF
- Cornea
  - Left Ø8N9XZZ
  - Right Ø8N8XZZ
- Cul-de-sac ØUNF
- Diaphragm ØBNT
- Disc
  - Cervical Vertebral ØRN3
  - Cervicothoracic Vertebral ØRN5
  - Lumbar Vertebral ØSN2
  - Lumbosacral ØSN4
  - Thoracic Vertebral ØRN9
  - Thoracolumbar Vertebral ØRNB
- Duct
  - Common Bile ØFN9
  - Cystic ØFN8
  - Hepatic
    - Common ØFN7
    - Left ØFN6
    - Right ØFN5
  - Lacrimal
    - Left Ø8NY
    - Right Ø8NX
  - Pancreatic ØFND
    - Accessory ØFNF
  - Parotid
    - Left ØCNC
    - Right ØCNB
- Duodenum ØDN9
- Dura Mater ØØN2
- Ear
  - External
    - Left Ø9N1
    - Right Ø9NØ
  - External Auditory Canal
    - Left Ø9N4
    - Right Ø9N3
  - Inner
    - Left Ø9NE
    - Right Ø9ND
  - Middle
    - Left Ø9N6
    - Right Ø9N5
- Epididymis
  - Bilateral ØVNL
  - Left ØVNK
  - Right ØVNJ
- Epiglottis ØCNR
- Esophagogastric Junction ØDN4
- Esophagus ØDN5
  - Lower ØDN3
  - Middle ØDN2
  - Upper ØDN1
- Eustachian Tube
  - Left Ø9NG
  - Right Ø9NF

Release — *continued*
- Eye
  - Left Ø8N1XZZ
  - Right Ø8NØXZZ
- Eyelid
  - Lower
    - Left Ø8NR
    - Right Ø8NQ
  - Upper
    - Left Ø8NP
    - Right Ø8NN
- Fallopian Tube
  - Left ØUN6
  - Right ØUN5
- Fallopian Tubes, Bilateral ØUN7
- Femoral Shaft
  - Left ØQN9
  - Right ØQN8
- Femur
  - Lower
    - Left ØQNC
    - Right ØQNB
  - Upper
    - Left ØQN7
    - Right ØQN6
- Fibula
  - Left ØQNK
  - Right ØQNJ
- Finger Nail ØHNQXZZ
- Gallbladder ØFN4
- Gingiva
  - Lower ØCN6
  - Upper ØCN5
- Gland
  - Adrenal
    - Bilateral ØGN4
    - Left ØGN2
    - Right ØGN3
  - Lacrimal
    - Left Ø8NW
    - Right Ø8NV
  - Minor Salivary ØCNJ
  - Parotid
    - Left ØCN9
    - Right ØCN8
  - Pituitary ØGNØ
  - Sublingual
    - Left ØCNF
    - Right ØCND
  - Submaxillary
    - Left ØCNH
    - Right ØCNG
  - Vestibular ØUNL
- Glenoid Cavity
  - Left ØPN8
  - Right ØPN7
- Glomus Jugulare ØGNC
- Humeral Head
  - Left ØPND
  - Right ØPNC
- Humeral Shaft
  - Left ØPNG
  - Right ØPNF
- Hymen ØUNK
- Hypothalamus ØØNA
- Ileocecal Valve ØDNC
- Ileum ØDNB
- Intestine
  - Large ØDNE
    - Left ØDNG
    - Right ØDNF
  - Small ØDN8
- Iris
  - Left Ø8ND3ZZ
  - Right Ø8NC3ZZ
- Jejunum ØDNA
- Joint
  - Acromioclavicular
    - Left ØRNH
    - Right ØRNG
  - Ankle
    - Left ØSNG
    - Right ØSNF
  - Carpal
    - Left ØRNR
    - Right ØRNQ
  - Carpometacarpal
    - Left ØRNT
    - Right ØRNS

Release — *continued*
- Joint — *continued*
  - Cervical Vertebral ØRN1
  - Cervicothoracic Vertebral ØRN4
  - Coccygeal ØSN6
  - Elbow
    - Left ØRNM
    - Right ØRNL
  - Finger Phalangeal
    - Left ØRNX
    - Right ØRNW
  - Hip
    - Left ØSNB
    - Right ØSN9
  - Knee
    - Left ØSND
    - Right ØSNC
  - Lumbar Vertebral ØSNØ
  - Lumbosacral ØSN3
  - Metacarpophalangeal
    - Left ØRNV
    - Right ØRNU
  - Metatarsal-Phalangeal
    - Left ØSNN
    - Right ØSNM
  - Occipital-cervical ØRNØ
  - Sacrococcygeal ØSN5
  - Sacroiliac
    - Left ØSN8
    - Right ØSN7
  - Shoulder
    - Left ØRNK
    - Right ØRNJ
  - Sternoclavicular
    - Left ØRNF
    - Right ØRNE
  - Tarsal
    - Left ØSNJ
    - Right ØSNH
  - Tarsometatarsal
    - Left ØSNL
    - Right ØSNK
  - Temporomandibular
    - Left ØRND
    - Right ØRNC
  - Thoracic Vertebral ØRN6
  - Thoracolumbar Vertebral ØRNA
  - Toe Phalangeal
    - Left ØSNQ
    - Right ØSNP
  - Wrist
    - Left ØRNP
    - Right ØRNN
- Kidney
  - Left ØTN1
  - Right ØTNØ
- Kidney Pelvis
  - Left ØTN4
  - Right ØTN3
- Larynx ØCNS
- Lens
  - Left Ø8NK3ZZ
  - Right Ø8NJ3ZZ
- Lip
  - Lower ØCN1
  - Upper ØCNØ
- Liver ØFNØ
  - Left Lobe ØFN2
  - Right Lobe ØFN1
- Lung
  - Bilateral ØBNM
  - Left ØBNL
  - Lower Lobe
    - Left ØBNJ
    - Right ØBNF
  - Middle Lobe, Right ØBND
  - Right ØBNK
  - Upper Lobe
    - Left ØBNG
    - Right ØBNC
- Lung Lingula ØBNH
- Lymphatic
  - Aortic Ø7ND
  - Axillary
    - Left Ø7N6
    - Right Ø7N5
  - Head Ø7NØ
  - Inguinal
    - Left Ø7NJ

Release — *continued*
Lymphatic — *continued*
Inguinal — *continued*
Right Ø7NH
Internal Mammary
Left Ø7N9
Right Ø7N8
Lower Extremity
Left Ø7NG
Right Ø7NF
Mesenteric Ø7NB
Neck
Left Ø7N2
Right Ø7N1
Pelvis Ø7NC
Thoracic Duct Ø7NK
Thorax Ø7N7
Upper Extremity
Left Ø7N4
Right Ø7N3
Mandible
Left ØNNV
Right ØNNT
Maxilla ØNNR
Medulla Oblongata ØØND
Mesentery ØDNV
Metacarpal
Left ØPNQ
Right ØPNP
Metatarsal
Left ØQNP
Right ØQNN
Muscle
Abdomen
Left ØKNL
Right ØKNK
Extraocular
Left Ø8NM
Right Ø8NL
Facial ØKN1
Foot
Left ØKNW
Right ØKNV
Hand
Left ØKND
Right ØKNC
Head ØKNØ
Hip
Left ØKNP
Right ØKNN
Lower Arm and Wrist
Left ØKNB
Right ØKN9
Lower Leg
Left ØKNT
Right ØKNS
Neck
Left ØKN3
Right ØKN2
Papillary Ø2ND
Perineum ØKNM
Shoulder
Left ØKN6
Right ØKN5
Thorax
Left ØKNJ
Right ØKNH
Tongue, Palate, Pharynx ØKN4
Trunk
Left ØKNG
Right ØKNF
Upper Arm
Left ØKN8
Right ØKN7
Upper Leg
Left ØKNR
Right ØKNQ
Myocardial Bridge *see* Release, Artery, Coronary
Nasal Mucosa and Soft Tissue Ø9NK
Nasopharynx Ø9NN
Nerve
Abdominal Sympathetic Ø1NM
Abducens ØØNL
Accessory ØØNR
Acoustic ØØNN
Brachial Plexus Ø1N3
Cervical Ø1N1
Cervical Plexus Ø1NØ
Facial ØØNM

Release — *continued*
Nerve — *continued*
Femoral Ø1ND
Glossopharyngeal ØØNP
Head and Neck Sympathetic Ø1NK
Hypoglossal ØØNS
Lumbar Ø1NB
Lumbar Plexus Ø1N9
Lumbar Sympathetic Ø1NN
Lumbosacral Plexus Ø1NA
Median Ø1N5
Oculomotor ØØNH
Olfactory ØØNF
Optic ØØNG
Peroneal Ø1NH
Phrenic Ø1N2
Pudendal Ø1NC
Radial Ø1N6
Sacral Ø1NR
Sacral Plexus Ø1NQ
Sacral Sympathetic Ø1NP
Sciatic Ø1NF
Thoracic Ø1N8
Thoracic Sympathetic Ø1NL
Tibial Ø1NG
Trigeminal ØØNK
Trochlear ØØNJ
Ulnar Ø1N4
Vagus ØØNQ
Nipple
Left ØHNX
Right ØHNW
Omentum ØDNU
Orbit
Left ØNNQ
Right ØNNP
Ovary
Bilateral ØUN2
Left ØUN1
Right ØUNØ
Palate
Hard ØCN2
Soft ØCN3
Pancreas ØFNG
Para-aortic Body ØGN9
Paraganglion Extremity ØGNF
Parathyroid Gland ØGNR
Inferior
Left ØGNP
Right ØGNN
Multiple ØGNQ
Superior
Left ØGNM
Right ØGNL
Patella
Left ØQNF
Right ØQND
Penis ØVNS
Pericardium Ø2NN
Peritoneum ØDNW
Phalanx
Finger
Left ØPNV
Right ØPNT
Thumb
Left ØPNS
Right ØPNR
Toe
Left ØQNR
Right ØQNQ
Pharynx ØCNM
Pineal Body ØGN1
Pleura
Left ØBNP
Right ØBNN
Pons ØØNB
Prepuce ØVNT
Prostate ØVNØ
Radius
Left ØPNJ
Right ØPNH
Rectum ØDNP
Retina
Left Ø8NF3ZZ
Right Ø8NE3ZZ
Retinal Vessel
Left Ø8NH3ZZ
Right Ø8NG3ZZ

Release — *continued*
Ribs
1 to 2 ØPN1
3 or More ØPN2
Sacrum ØQN1
Scapula
Left ØPN6
Right ØPN5
Sclera
Left Ø8N7XZZ
Right Ø8N6XZZ
Scrotum ØVN5
Septum
Atrial Ø2N5
Nasal Ø9NM
Ventricular Ø2NM
Sinus
Accessory Ø9NP
Ethmoid
Left Ø9NV
Right Ø9NU
Frontal
Left Ø9NT
Right Ø9NS
Mastoid
Left Ø9NC
Right Ø9NB
Maxillary
Left Ø9NR
Right Ø9NQ
Sphenoid
Left Ø9NX
Right Ø9NW
Skin
Abdomen ØHN7XZZ
Back ØHN6XZZ
Buttock ØHN8XZZ
Chest ØHN5XZZ
Ear
Left ØHN3XZZ
Right ØHN2XZZ
Face ØHN1XZZ
Foot
Left ØHNNXZZ
Right ØHNMXZZ
Hand
Left ØHNGXZZ
Right ØHNFXZZ
Inguinal ØHNAXZZ
Lower Arm
Left ØHNEXZZ
Right ØHNDXZZ
Lower Leg
Left ØHNLXZZ
Right ØHNKXZZ
Neck ØHN4XZZ
Perineum ØHN9XZZ
Scalp ØHNØXZZ
Upper Arm
Left ØHNCXZZ
Right ØHNBXZZ
Upper Leg
Left ØHNJXZZ
Right ØHNHXZZ
Spinal Cord
Cervical ØØNW
Lumbar ØØNY
Thoracic ØØNX
Spinal Meninges ØØNT
Spleen Ø7NP
Sternum ØPNØ
Stomach ØDN6
Pylorus ØDN7
Subcutaneous Tissue and Fascia
Abdomen ØJN8
Back ØJN7
Buttock ØJN9
Chest ØJN6
Face ØJN1
Foot
Left ØJNR
Right ØJNQ
Hand
Left ØJNK
Right ØJNJ
Lower Arm
Left ØJNH
Right ØJNG

Subterms under main terms may continue to next column or page

Release — *continued*
- Subcutaneous Tissue and Fascia — *continued*
  - Lower Leg
    - Left ØJNP
    - Right ØJNN
  - Neck
    - Left ØJN5
    - Right ØJN4
  - Pelvic Region ØJNC
  - Perineum ØJNB
  - Scalp ØJNØ
  - Upper Arm
    - Left ØJNF
    - Right ØJND
  - Upper Leg
    - Left ØJNM
    - Right ØJNL
- Tarsal
  - Left ØQNM
  - Right ØQNL
- Tendon
  - Abdomen
    - Left ØLNG
    - Right ØLNF
  - Ankle
    - Left ØLNT
    - Right ØLNS
  - Foot
    - Left ØLNW
    - Right ØLNV
  - Hand
    - Left ØLN8
    - Right ØLN7
  - Head and Neck ØLNØ
  - Hip
    - Left ØLNK
    - Right ØLNJ
  - Knee
    - Left ØLNR
    - Right ØLNQ
  - Lower Arm and Wrist
    - Left ØLN6
    - Right ØLN5
  - Lower Leg
    - Left ØLNP
    - Right ØLNN
  - Perineum ØLNH
  - Shoulder
    - Left ØLN2
    - Right ØLN1
  - Thorax
    - Left ØLND
    - Right ØLNC
  - Trunk
    - Left ØLNB
    - Right ØLN9
  - Upper Arm
    - Left ØLN4
    - Right ØLN3
  - Upper Leg
    - Left ØLNM
    - Right ØLNL
- Testis
  - Bilateral ØVNC
  - Left ØVNB
  - Right ØVN9
- Thalamus ØØN9
- Thymus Ø7NM
- Thyroid Gland ØGNK
  - Left Lobe ØGNG
  - Right Lobe ØGNH
- Tibia
  - Left ØQNH
  - Right ØQNG
- Toe Nail ØHNRXZZ
- Tongue ØCN7
- Tonsils ØCNP
- Tooth
  - Lower ØCNX
  - Upper ØCNW
- Trachea ØBN1
- Tunica Vaginalis
  - Left ØVN7
  - Right ØVN6
- Turbinate, Nasal Ø9NL
- Tympanic Membrane
  - Left Ø9N8
  - Right Ø9N7

Release — *continued*
- Ulna
  - Left ØPNL
  - Right ØPNK
- Ureter
  - Left ØTN7
  - Right ØTN6
- Urethra ØTND
- Uterine Supporting Structure ØUN4
- Uterus ØUN9
- Uvula ØCNN
- Vagina ØUNG
- Valve
  - Aortic Ø2NF
  - Mitral Ø2NG
  - Pulmonary Ø2NH
  - Tricuspid Ø2NJ
- Vas Deferens
  - Bilateral ØVNQ
  - Left ØVNP
  - Right ØVNN
- Vein
  - Axillary
    - Left Ø5N8
    - Right Ø5N7
  - Azygos Ø5NØ
  - Basilic
    - Left Ø5NC
    - Right Ø5NB
  - Brachial
    - Left Ø5NA
    - Right Ø5N9
  - Cephalic
    - Left Ø5NF
    - Right Ø5ND
  - Colic Ø6N7
  - Common Iliac
    - Left Ø6ND
    - Right Ø6NC
  - Coronary Ø2N4
  - Esophageal Ø6N3
  - External Iliac
    - Left Ø6NG
    - Right Ø6NF
  - External Jugular
    - Left Ø5NQ
    - Right Ø5NP
  - Face
    - Left Ø5NV
    - Right Ø5NT
  - Femoral
    - Left Ø6NN
    - Right Ø6NM
  - Foot
    - Left Ø6NV
    - Right Ø6NT
  - Gastric Ø6N2
  - Hand
    - Left Ø5NH
    - Right Ø5NG
  - Hemiazygos Ø5N1
  - Hepatic Ø6N4
  - Hypogastric
    - Left Ø6NJ
    - Right Ø6NH
  - Inferior Mesenteric Ø6N6
  - Innominate
    - Left Ø5N4
    - Right Ø5N3
  - Internal Jugular
    - Left Ø5NN
    - Right Ø5NM
  - Intracranial Ø5NL
  - Lower Ø6NY
  - Portal Ø6N8
  - Pulmonary
    - Left Ø2NT
    - Right Ø2NS
  - Renal
    - Left Ø6NB
    - Right Ø6N9
  - Saphenous
    - Left Ø6NQ
    - Right Ø6NP
  - Splenic Ø6N1
  - Subclavian
    - Left Ø5N6
    - Right Ø5N5
  - Superior Mesenteric Ø6N5

Release — *continued*
- Vein — *continued*
  - Upper Ø5NY
  - Vertebral
    - Left Ø5NS
    - Right Ø5NR
- Vena Cava
  - Inferior Ø6NØ
  - Superior Ø2NV
- Ventricle
  - Left Ø2NL
  - Right Ø2NK
- Vertebra
  - Cervical ØPN3
  - Lumbar ØQNØ
  - Thoracic ØPN4
- Vesicle
  - Bilateral ØVN3
  - Left ØVN2
  - Right ØVN1
- Vitreous
  - Left Ø8N53ZZ
  - Right Ø8N43ZZ
- Vocal Cord
  - Left ØCNV
  - Right ØCNT
- Vulva ØUNM

Relocation *see* Reposition

Remdesivir Anti-infective XWØ

Removal
- Abdominal Wall 2W53X
- Anorectal 2Y53X5Z
- Arm
  - Lower
    - Left 2W5DX
    - Right 2W5CX
  - Upper
    - Left 2W5BX
    - Right 2W5AX
- Back 2W55X
- Chest Wall 2W54X
- Ear 2Y52X5Z
- Extremity
  - Lower
    - Left 2W5MX
    - Right 2W5LX
  - Upper
    - Left 2W59X
    - Right 2W58X
- Face 2W51X
- Finger
  - Left 2W5KX
  - Right 2W5JX
- Foot
  - Left 2W5TX
  - Right 2W5SX
- Genital Tract, Female 2Y54X5Z
- Hand
  - Left 2W5FX
  - Right 2W5EX
- Head 2W5ØX
- Inguinal Region
  - Left 2W57X
  - Right 2W56X
- Leg
  - Lower
    - Left 2W5RX
    - Right 2W5QX
  - Upper
    - Left 2W5PX
    - Right 2W5NX
- Mouth and Pharynx 2Y5ØX5Z
- Nasal 2Y51X5Z
- Neck 2W52X
- Thumb
  - Left 2W5HX
  - Right 2W5GX
- Toe
  - Left 2W5VX
  - Right 2W5UX
- Urethra 2Y55X5Z

Removal of device from
- Abdominal Wall ØWPF
- Acetabulum
  - Left ØQP5
  - Right ØQP4
- Anal Sphincter ØDPR
- Anus ØDPQ

Removal of device from — *continued*
Artery
Lower Ø4PY
Upper Ø3PY
Back
Lower ØWPL
Upper ØWPK
Bladder ØTPB
Bone
Facial ØNPW
Lower ØQPY
Nasal ØNPB
Pelvic
Left ØQP3
Right ØQP2
Upper ØPPY
Bone Marrow Ø7PT
Brain ØØPØ
Breast
Left ØHPU
Right ØHPT
Bursa and Ligament
Lower ØMPY
Upper ØMPX
Carpal
Left ØPPN
Right ØPPM
Cavity, Cranial ØWP1
Cerebral Ventricle ØØP6
Chest Wall ØWP8
Cisterna Chyli Ø7PL
Clavicle
Left ØPPB
Right ØPP9
Coccyx ØQPS
Diaphragm ØBPT
Disc
Cervical Vertebral ØRP3
Cervicothoracic Vertebral ØRP5
Lumbar Vertebral ØSP2
Lumbosacral ØSP4
Thoracic Vertebral ØRP9
Thoracolumbar Vertebral ØRPB
Duct
Hepatobiliary ØFPB
Pancreatic ØFPD
Ear
Inner
Left Ø9PJ
Right Ø9PD
Left Ø9PJ
Right Ø9PH
Epididymis and Spermatic Cord ØVPM
Esophagus ØDP5
Extremity
Lower
Left ØYPB
Right ØYP9
Upper
Left ØXP7
Right ØXP6
Eye
Left Ø8P1
Right Ø8PØ
Face ØWP2
Fallopian Tube ØUP8
Femoral Shaft
Left ØQP9
Right ØQP8
Femur
Lower
Left ØQPC
Right ØQPB
Upper
Left ØQP7
Right ØQP6
Fibula
Left ØQPK
Right ØQPJ
Finger Nail ØHPQX
Gallbladder ØFP4
Gastrointestinal Tract ØWPP
Genitourinary Tract ØWPR
Gland
Adrenal ØGP5
Endocrine ØGPS
Pituitary ØGPØ
Salivary ØCPA

Removal of device from — *continued*
Glenoid Cavity
Left ØPP8
Right ØPP7
Great Vessel Ø2PY
Hair ØHPSX
Head ØWPØ
Heart Ø2PA
Humeral Head
Left ØPPD
Right ØPPC
Humeral Shaft
Left ØPPG
Right ØPPF
Intestinal Tract
Lower ØDPD
Upper ØDPØ
Jaw
Lower ØWP5
Upper ØWP4
Joint
Acromioclavicular
Left ØRPH
Right ØRPG
Ankle
Left ØSPG
Right ØSPF
Carpal
Left ØRPR
Right ØRPQ
Carpometacarpal
Left ØRPT
Right ØRPS
Cervical Vertebral ØRP1
Cervicothoracic Vertebral ØRP4
Coccygeal ØSP6
Elbow
Left ØRPM
Right ØRPL
Finger Phalangeal
Left ØRPX
Right ØRPW
Hip
Left ØSPB
Acetabular Surface ØSPE
Femoral Surface ØSPS
Right ØSP9
Acetabular Surface ØSPA
Femoral Surface ØSPR
Knee
Left ØSPD
Femoral Surface ØSPU
Tibial Surface ØSPW
Right ØSPC
Femoral Surface ØSPT
Tibial Surface ØSPV
Lumbar Vertebral ØSPØ
Lumbosacral ØSP3
Metacarpophalangeal
Left ØRPV
Right ØRPU
Metatarsal-Phalangeal
Left ØSPN
Right ØSPM
Occipital-cervical ØRPØ
Sacrococcygeal ØSP5
Sacroiliac
Left ØSP8
Right ØSP7
Shoulder
Left ØRPK
Right ØRPJ
Sternoclavicular
Left ØRPF
Right ØRPE
Tarsal
Left ØSPJ
Right ØSPH
Tarsometatarsal
Left ØSPL
Right ØSPK
Temporomandibular
Left ØRPD
Right ØRPC
Thoracic Vertebral ØRP6
Thoracolumbar Vertebral ØRPA
Toe Phalangeal
Left ØSPQ
Right ØSPP

Removal of device from — *continued*
Joint — *continued*
Wrist
Left ØRPP
Right ØRPN
Kidney ØTP5
Larynx ØCPS
Lens
Left Ø8PK3
Right Ø8PJ3
Liver ØFPØ
Lung
Left ØBPL
Right ØBPK
Lymphatic Ø7PN
Thoracic Duct Ø7PK
Mediastinum ØWPC
Mesentery ØDPV
Metacarpal
Left ØPPQ
Right ØPPP
Metatarsal
Left ØQPP
Right ØQPN
Mouth and Throat ØCPY
Muscle
Extraocular
Left Ø8PM
Right Ø8PL
Lower ØKPY
Upper ØKPX
Nasal Mucosa and Soft Tissue Ø9PK
Neck ØWP6
Nerve
Cranial ØØPE
Peripheral Ø1PY
Omentum ØDPU
Ovary ØUP3
Pancreas ØFPG
Parathyroid Gland ØGPR
Patella
Left ØQPF
Right ØQPD
Pelvic Cavity ØWPJ
Penis ØVPS
Pericardial Cavity ØWPD
Perineum
Female ØWPN
Male ØWPM
Peritoneal Cavity ØWPG
Peritoneum ØDPW
Phalanx
Finger
Left ØPPV
Right ØPPT
Thumb
Left ØPPS
Right ØPPR
Toe
Left ØQPR
Right ØQPQ
Pineal Body ØGP1
Pleura ØBPQ
Pleural Cavity
Left ØWPB
Right ØWP9
Products of Conception 1ØPØ
Prostate and Seminal Vesicles ØVP4
Radius
Left ØPPJ
Right ØPPH
Rectum ØDPP
Respiratory Tract ØWPQ
Retroperitoneum ØWPH
Ribs
1 to 2 ØPP1
3 or More ØPP2
Sacrum ØQP1
Scapula
Left ØPP6
Right ØPP5
Scrotum and Tunica Vaginalis ØVP8
Sinus Ø9PY
Skin ØHPPX
Skull ØNPØ
Spinal Canal ØØPU
Spinal Cord ØØPV
Spleen Ø7PP
Sternum ØPPØ

Removal of device from — *continued*
- Stomach ØDP6
- Subcutaneous Tissue and Fascia
  - Head and Neck ØJPS
  - Lower Extremity ØJPW
  - Trunk ØJPT
  - Upper Extremity ØJPV
- Tarsal
  - Left ØQPM
  - Right ØQPL
- Tendon
  - Lower ØLPY
  - Upper ØLPX
- Testis ØVPD
- Thymus Ø7PM
- Thyroid Gland ØGPK
- Tibia
  - Left ØQPH
  - Right ØQPG
- Toe Nail ØHPRX
- Trachea ØBP1
- Tracheobronchial Tree ØBPØ
- Tympanic Membrane
  - Left Ø9P8
  - Right Ø9P7
- Ulna
  - Left ØPPL
  - Right ØPPK
- Ureter ØTP9
- Urethra ØTPD
- Uterus and Cervix ØUPD
- Vagina and Cul-de-sac ØUPH
- Vas Deferens ØVPR
- Vein
  - Azygos Ø5PØ
  - Innominate
    - Left Ø5P4
    - Right Ø5P3
  - Lower Ø6PY
  - Upper Ø5PY
- Vertebra
  - Cervical ØPP3
  - Lumbar ØQPØ
  - Thoracic ØPP4
- Vulva ØUPM

Renal calyx
- *use* Kidney
- *use* Kidney, Left
- *use* Kidney, Right
- *use* Kidneys, Bilateral

Renal capsule
- *use* Kidney
- *use* Kidney, Left
- *use* Kidney, Right
- *use* Kidneys, Bilateral

Renal cortex
- *use* Kidney
- *use* Kidney, Left
- *use* Kidney, Right
- *use* Kidneys, Bilateral

Renal dialysis *see* Performance, Urinary 5A1D

Renal nerve *use* Abdominal Sympathetic Nerve

Renal plexus *use* Abdominal Sympathetic Nerve

Renal segment
- *use* Kidney
- *use* Kidney, Left
- *use* Kidney, Right
- *use* Kidneys, Bilateral

Renal segmental artery
- *use* Renal Artery, Left
- *use* Renal Artery, Right

Reopening, operative site
- Control of bleeding *see* Control bleeding in
- Inspection only *see* Inspection

Repair
- Abdominal Wall ØWQF
- Acetabulum
  - Left ØQQ5
  - Right ØQQ4
- Adenoids ØCQQ
- Ampulla of Vater ØFQC
- Anal Sphincter ØDQR
- Ankle Region
  - Left ØYQL
  - Right ØYQK
- Anterior Chamber
  - Left Ø8Q33ZZ
  - Right Ø8Q23ZZ

Repair — *continued*
- Anus ØDQQ
- Aorta
  - Abdominal Ø4QØ
  - Thoracic
    - Ascending/Arch Ø2QX
    - Descending Ø2QW
- Aortic Body ØGQD
- Appendix ØDQJ
- Arm
  - Lower
    - Left ØXQF
    - Right ØXQD
  - Upper
    - Left ØXQ9
    - Right ØXQ8
- Artery
  - Anterior Tibial
    - Left Ø4QQ
    - Right Ø4QP
  - Axillary
    - Left Ø3Q6
    - Right Ø3Q5
  - Brachial
    - Left Ø3Q8
    - Right Ø3Q7
  - Celiac Ø4Q1
  - Colic
    - Left Ø4Q7
    - Middle Ø4Q8
    - Right Ø4Q6
  - Common Carotid
    - Left Ø3QJ
    - Right Ø3QH
  - Common Iliac
    - Left Ø4QD
    - Right Ø4QC
  - Coronary
    - Four or More Arteries Ø2Q3
    - One Artery Ø2QØ
    - Three Arteries Ø2Q2
    - Two Arteries Ø2Q1
  - External Carotid
    - Left Ø3QN
    - Right Ø3QM
  - External Iliac
    - Left Ø4QJ
    - Right Ø4QH
  - Face Ø3QR
  - Femoral
    - Left Ø4QL
    - Right Ø4QK
  - Foot
    - Left Ø4QW
    - Right Ø4QV
  - Gastric Ø4Q2
  - Hand
    - Left Ø3QF
    - Right Ø3QD
  - Hepatic Ø4Q3
  - Inferior Mesenteric Ø4QB
  - Innominate Ø3Q2
  - Internal Carotid
    - Left Ø3QL
    - Right Ø3QK
  - Internal Iliac
    - Left Ø4QF
    - Right Ø4QE
  - Internal Mammary
    - Left Ø3Q1
    - Right Ø3QØ
  - Intracranial Ø3QG
  - Lower Ø4QY
  - Peroneal
    - Left Ø4QU
    - Right Ø4QT
  - Popliteal
    - Left Ø4QN
    - Right Ø4QM
  - Posterior Tibial
    - Left Ø4QS
    - Right Ø4QR
  - Pulmonary
    - Left Ø2QR
    - Right Ø2QQ
  - Pulmonary Trunk Ø2QP
  - Radial
    - Left Ø3QC
    - Right Ø3QB

Repair — *continued*
- Artery — *continued*
  - Renal
    - Left Ø4QA
    - Right Ø4Q9
  - Splenic Ø4Q4
  - Subclavian
    - Left Ø3Q4
    - Right Ø3Q3
  - Superior Mesenteric Ø4Q5
  - Temporal
    - Left Ø3QT
    - Right Ø3QS
  - Thyroid
    - Left Ø3QV
    - Right Ø3QU
  - Ulnar
    - Left Ø3QA
    - Right Ø3Q9
  - Upper Ø3QY
  - Vertebral
    - Left Ø3QQ
    - Right Ø3QP
- Atrium
  - Left Ø2Q7
  - Right Ø2Q6
- Auditory Ossicle
  - Left Ø9QA
  - Right Ø9Q9
- Axilla
  - Left ØXQ5
  - Right ØXQ4
- Back
  - Lower ØWQL
  - Upper ØWQK
- Basal Ganglia ØØQ8
- Bladder ØTQB
- Bladder Neck ØTQC
- Bone
  - Ethmoid
    - Left ØNQG
    - Right ØNQF
  - Frontal ØNQ1
  - Hyoid ØNQX
  - Lacrimal
    - Left ØNQJ
    - Right ØNQH
  - Nasal ØNQB
  - Occipital ØNQ7
  - Palatine
    - Left ØNQL
    - Right ØNQK
  - Parietal
    - Left ØNQ4
    - Right ØNQ3
  - Pelvic
    - Left ØQQ3
    - Right ØQQ2
  - Sphenoid ØNQC
  - Temporal
    - Left ØNQ6
    - Right ØNQ5
  - Zygomatic
    - Left ØNQN
    - Right ØNQM
- Brain ØØQØ
- Breast
  - Bilateral ØHQV
  - Left ØHQU
  - Right ØHQT
  - Supernumerary ØHQY
- Bronchus
  - Lingula ØBQ9
  - Lower Lobe
    - Left ØBQB
    - Right ØBQ6
  - Main
    - Left ØBQ7
    - Right ØBQ3
  - Middle Lobe, Right ØBQ5
  - Upper Lobe
    - Left ØBQ8
    - Right ØBQ4
- Buccal Mucosa ØCQ4
- Bursa and Ligament
  - Abdomen
    - Left ØMQJ
    - Right ØMQH

- **Repair** — *continued*
  - Bursa and Ligament — *continued*
    - Ankle
      - Left ØMQR
      - Right ØMQQ
    - Elbow
      - Left ØMQ4
      - Right ØMQ3
    - Foot
      - Left ØMQT
      - Right ØMQS
    - Hand
      - Left ØMQ8
      - Right ØMQ7
    - Head and Neck ØMQØ
    - Hip
      - Left ØMQM
      - Right ØMQL
    - Knee
      - Left ØMQP
      - Right ØMQN
    - Lower Extremity
      - Left ØMQW
      - Right ØMQV
    - Perineum ØMQK
    - Rib(s) ØMQG
    - Shoulder
      - Left ØMQ2
      - Right ØMQ1
    - Spine
      - Lower ØMQD
      - Upper ØMQC
    - Sternum ØMQF
    - Upper Extremity
      - Left ØMQB
      - Right ØMQ9
    - Wrist
      - Left ØMQ6
      - Right ØMQ5
  - Buttock
    - Left ØYQ1
    - Right ØYQØ
  - Carina ØBQ2
  - Carotid Bodies, Bilateral ØGQ8
  - Carotid Body
    - Left ØGQ6
    - Right ØGQ7
  - Carpal
    - Left ØPQN
    - Right ØPQM
  - Cecum ØDQH
  - Cerebellum ØØQC
  - Cerebral Hemisphere ØØQ7
  - Cerebral Meninges ØØQ1
  - Cerebral Ventricle ØØQ6
  - Cervix ØUQC
  - Chest Wall ØWQ8
  - Chordae Tendineae Ø2Q9
  - Choroid
    - Left Ø8QB
    - Right Ø8QA
  - Cisterna Chyli Ø7QL
  - Clavicle
    - Left ØPQB
    - Right ØPQ9
  - Clitoris ØUQJ
  - Coccygeal Glomus ØGQB
  - Coccyx ØQQS
  - Colon
    - Ascending ØDQK
    - Descending ØDQM
    - Sigmoid ØDQN
    - Transverse ØDQL
  - Conduction Mechanism Ø2Q8
  - Conjunctiva
    - Left Ø8QTXZZ
    - Right Ø8QSXZZ
  - Cord
    - Bilateral ØVQH
    - Left ØVQG
    - Right ØVQF
  - Cornea
    - Left Ø8Q9XZZ
    - Right Ø8Q8XZZ
  - Cul-de-sac ØUQF
  - Diaphragm ØBQT
  - Disc
    - Cervical Vertebral ØRQ3
    - Cervicothoracic Vertebral ØRQ5
- **Repair** — *continued*
  - Disc — *continued*
    - Lumbar Vertebral ØSQ2
    - Lumbosacral ØSQ4
    - Thoracic Vertebral ØRQ9
    - Thoracolumbar Vertebral ØRQB
  - Duct
    - Common Bile ØFQ9
    - Cystic ØFQ8
    - Hepatic
      - Common ØFQ7
      - Left ØFQ6
      - Right ØFQ5
    - Lacrimal
      - Left Ø8QY
      - Right Ø8QX
    - Pancreatic ØFQD
      - Accessory ØFQF
    - Parotid
      - Left ØCQC
      - Right ØCQB
  - Duodenum ØDQ9
  - Dura Mater ØØQ2
  - Ear
    - External
      - Bilateral Ø9Q2
      - Left Ø9Q1
      - Right Ø9QØ
    - External Auditory Canal
      - Left Ø9Q4
      - Right Ø9Q3
    - Inner
      - Left Ø9QE
      - Right Ø9QD
    - Middle
      - Left Ø9Q6
      - Right Ø9Q5
  - Elbow Region
    - Left ØXQC
    - Right ØXQB
  - Epididymis
    - Bilateral ØVQL
    - Left ØVQK
    - Right ØVQJ
  - Epiglottis ØCQR
  - Esophagogastric Junction ØDQ4
  - Esophagus ØDQ5
    - Lower ØDQ3
    - Middle ØDQ2
    - Upper ØDQ1
  - Eustachian Tube
    - Left Ø9QG
    - Right Ø9QF
  - Extremity
    - Lower
      - Left ØYQB
      - Right ØYQ9
    - Upper
      - Left ØXQ7
      - Right ØXQ6
  - Eye
    - Left Ø8Q1XZZ
    - Right Ø8QØXZZ
  - Eyelid
    - Lower
      - Left Ø8QR
      - Right Ø8QQ
    - Upper
      - Left Ø8QP
      - Right Ø8QN
  - Face ØWQ2
  - Fallopian Tube
    - Left ØUQ6
    - Right ØUQ5
  - Fallopian Tubes, Bilateral ØUQ7
  - Femoral Region
    - Bilateral ØYQE
    - Left ØYQ8
    - Right ØYQ7
  - Femoral Shaft
    - Left ØQQ9
    - Right ØQQ8
  - Femur
    - Lower
      - Left ØQQC
      - Right ØQQB
    - Upper
      - Left ØQQ7
      - Right ØQQ6
- **Repair** — *continued*
  - Fibula
    - Left ØQQK
    - Right ØQQJ
  - Finger
    - Index
      - Left ØXQP
      - Right ØXQN
    - Little
      - Left ØXQW
      - Right ØXQV
    - Middle
      - Left ØXQR
      - Right ØXQQ
    - Ring
      - Left ØXQT
      - Right ØXQS
  - Finger Nail ØHQQXZZ
  - Floor of mouth *see* Repair, Oral Cavity and Throat ØWQ3
  - Foot
    - Left ØYQN
    - Right ØYQM
  - Gallbladder ØFQ4
  - Gingiva
    - Lower ØCQ6
    - Upper ØCQ5
  - Gland
    - Adrenal
      - Bilateral ØGQ4
      - Left ØGQ2
      - Right ØGQ3
    - Lacrimal
      - Left Ø8QW
      - Right Ø8QV
    - Minor Salivary ØCQJ
    - Parotid
      - Left ØCQ9
      - Right ØCQ8
    - Pituitary ØGQØ
    - Sublingual
      - Left ØCQF
      - Right ØCQD
    - Submaxillary
      - Left ØCQH
      - Right ØCQG
    - Vestibular ØUQL
  - Glenoid Cavity
    - Left ØPQ8
    - Right ØPQ7
  - Glomus Jugulare ØGQC
  - Hand
    - Left ØXQK
    - Right ØXQJ
  - Head ØWQØ
  - Heart Ø2QA
    - Left Ø2QC
    - Right Ø2QB
  - Humeral Head
    - Left ØPQD
    - Right ØPQC
  - Humeral Shaft
    - Left ØPQG
    - Right ØPQF
  - Hymen ØUQK
  - Hypothalamus ØØQA
  - Ileocecal Valve ØDQC
  - Ileum ØDQB
  - Inguinal Region
    - Bilateral ØYQA
    - Left ØYQ6
    - Right ØYQ5
  - Intestine
    - Large ØDQE
      - Left ØDQG
      - Right ØDQF
    - Small ØDQ8
  - Iris
    - Left Ø8QD3ZZ
    - Right Ø8QC3ZZ
  - Jaw
    - Lower ØWQ5
    - Upper ØWQ4
  - Jejunum ØDQA
  - Joint
    - Acromioclavicular
      - Left ØRQH
      - Right ØRQG

Repair — *continued*
Joint — *continued*
Ankle
Left ØSQG
Right ØSQF
Carpal
Left ØRQR
Right ØRQQ
Carpometacarpal
Left ØRQT
Right ØRQS
Cervical Vertebral ØRQ1
Cervicothoracic Vertebral ØRQ4
Coccygeal ØSQ6
Elbow
Left ØRQM
Right ØRQL
Finger Phalangeal
Left ØRQX
Right ØRQW
Hip
Left ØSQB
Right ØSQ9
Knee
Left ØSQD
Right ØSQC
Lumbar Vertebral ØSQØ
Lumbosacral ØSQ3
Metacarpophalangeal
Left ØRQV
Right ØRQU
Metatarsal-Phalangeal
Left ØSQN
Right ØSQM
Occipital-cervical ØRQØ
Sacrococcygeal ØSQ5
Sacroiliac
Left ØSQ8
Right ØSQ7
Shoulder
Left ØRQK
Right ØRQJ
Sternoclavicular
Left ØRQF
Right ØRQE
Tarsal
Left ØSQJ
Right ØSQH
Tarsometatarsal
Left ØSQL
Right ØSQK
Temporomandibular
Left ØRQD
Right ØRQC
Thoracic Vertebral ØRQ6
Thoracolumbar Vertebral ØRQA
Toe Phalangeal
Left ØSQQ
Right ØSQP
Wrist
Left ØRQP
Right ØRQN
Kidney
Left ØTQ1
Right ØTQØ
Kidney Pelvis
Left ØTQ4
Right ØTQ3
Knee Region
Left ØYQG
Right ØYQF
Larynx ØCQS
Leg
Lower
Left ØYQJ
Right ØYQH
Upper
Left ØYQD
Right ØYQC
Lens
Left Ø8QK3ZZ
Right Ø8QJ3ZZ
Lip
Lower ØCQ1
Upper ØCQØ
Liver ØFQØ
Left Lobe ØFQ2
Right Lobe ØFQ1

Repair — *continued*
Lung
Bilateral ØBQM
Left ØBQL
Lower Lobe
Left ØBQJ
Right ØBQF
Middle Lobe, Right ØBQD
Right ØBQK
Upper Lobe
Left ØBQG
Right ØBQC
Lung Lingula ØBQH
Lymphatic
Aortic Ø7QD
Axillary
Left Ø7Q6
Right Ø7Q5
Head Ø7QØ
Inguinal
Left Ø7QJ
Right Ø7QH
Internal Mammary
Left Ø7Q9
Right Ø7Q8
Lower Extremity
Left Ø7QG
Right Ø7QF
Mesenteric Ø7QB
Neck
Left Ø7Q2
Right Ø7Q1
Pelvis Ø7QC
Thoracic Duct Ø7QK
Thorax Ø7Q7
Upper Extremity
Left Ø7Q4
Right Ø7Q3
Mandible
Left ØNQV
Right ØNQT
Maxilla ØNQR
Mediastinum ØWQC
Medulla Oblongata ØØQD
Mesentery ØDQV
Metacarpal
Left ØPQQ
Right ØPQP
Metatarsal
Left ØQQP
Right ØQQN
Muscle
Abdomen
Left ØKQL
Right ØKQK
Extraocular
Left Ø8QM
Right Ø8QL
Facial ØKQ1
Foot
Left ØKQW
Right ØKQV
Hand
Left ØKQD
Right ØKQC
Head ØKQØ
Hip
Left ØKQP
Right ØKQN
Lower Arm and Wrist
Left ØKQB
Right ØKQ9
Lower Leg
Left ØKQT
Right ØKQS
Neck
Left ØKQ3
Right ØKQ2
Papillary Ø2QD
Perineum ØKQM
Shoulder
Left ØKQ6
Right ØKQ5
Thorax
Left ØKQJ
Right ØKQH
Tongue, Palate, Pharynx ØKQ4
Trunk
Left ØKQG

Repair — *continued*
Muscle — *continued*
Trunk — *continued*
Right ØKQF
Upper Arm
Left ØKQ8
Right ØKQ7
Upper Leg
Left ØKQR
Right ØKQQ
Nasal Mucosa and Soft Tissue Ø9QK
Nasopharynx Ø9QN
Neck ØWQ6
Nerve
Abdominal Sympathetic Ø1QM
Abducens ØØQL
Accessory ØØQR
Acoustic ØØQN
Brachial Plexus Ø1Q3
Cervical Ø1Q1
Cervical Plexus Ø1QØ
Facial ØØQM
Femoral Ø1QD
Glossopharyngeal ØØQP
Head and Neck Sympathetic Ø1QK
Hypoglossal ØØQS
Lumbar Ø1QB
Lumbar Plexus Ø1Q9
Lumbar Sympathetic Ø1QN
Lumbosacral Plexus Ø1QA
Median Ø1Q5
Oculomotor ØØQH
Olfactory ØØQF
Optic ØØQG
Peroneal Ø1QH
Phrenic Ø1Q2
Pudendal Ø1QC
Radial Ø1Q6
Sacral Ø1QR
Sacral Plexus Ø1QQ
Sacral Sympathetic Ø1QP
Sciatic Ø1QF
Thoracic Ø1Q8
Thoracic Sympathetic Ø1QL
Tibial Ø1QG
Trigeminal ØØQK
Trochlear ØØQJ
Ulnar Ø1Q4
Vagus ØØQQ
Nipple
Left ØHQX
Right ØHQW
Omentum ØDQU
Oral Cavity and Throat ØWQ3
Orbit
Left ØNQQ
Right ØNQP
Ovary
Bilateral ØUQ2
Left ØUQ1
Right ØUQØ
Palate
Hard ØCQ2
Soft ØCQ3
Pancreas ØFQG
Para-aortic Body ØGQ9
Paraganglion Extremity ØGQF
Parathyroid Gland ØGQR
Inferior
Left ØGQP
Right ØGQN
Multiple ØGQQ
Superior
Left ØGQM
Right ØGQL
Patella
Left ØQQF
Right ØQQD
Penis ØVQS
Pericardium Ø2QN
Perineum
Female ØWQN
Male ØWQM
Peritoneum ØDQW
Phalanx
Finger
Left ØPQV
Right ØPQT

Index

Repair — Repair

Repair — *continued*
Phalanx — *continued*
Thumb
Left ØPQS
Right ØPQR
Toe
Left ØQQR
Right ØQQQ
Pharynx ØCQM
Pineal Body ØGQ1
Pleura
Left ØBQP
Right ØBQN
Pons ØØQB
Prepuce ØVQT
Products of Conception 1ØQØ
Prostate ØVQØ
Radius
Left ØPQJ
Right ØPQH
Rectum ØDQP
Retina
Left Ø8QF3ZZ
Right Ø8QE3ZZ
Retinal Vessel
Left Ø8QH3ZZ
Right Ø8QG3ZZ
Ribs
1 to 2 ØPQ1
3 or More ØPQ2
Sacrum ØQQ1
Scapula
Left ØPQ6
Right ØPQ5
Sclera
Left Ø8Q7XZZ
Right Ø8Q6XZZ
Scrotum ØVQ5
Septum
Atrial Ø2Q5
Nasal Ø9QM
Ventricular Ø2QM
Shoulder Region
Left ØXQ3
Right ØXQ2
Sinus
Accessory Ø9QP
Ethmoid
Left Ø9QV
Right Ø9QU
Frontal
Left Ø9QT
Right Ø9QS
Mastoid
Left Ø9QC
Right Ø9QB
Maxillary
Left Ø9QR
Right Ø9QQ
Sphenoid
Left Ø9QX
Right Ø9QW
Skin
Abdomen ØHQ7XZZ
Back ØHQ6XZZ
Buttock ØHQ8XZZ
Chest ØHQ5XZZ
Ear
Left ØHQ3XZZ
Right ØHQ2XZZ
Face ØHQ1XZZ
Foot
Left ØHQNXZZ
Right ØHQMXZZ
Hand
Left ØHQGXZZ
Right ØHQFXZZ
Inguinal ØHQAXZZ
Lower Arm
Left ØHQEXZZ
Right ØHQDXZZ
Lower Leg
Left ØHQLXZZ
Right ØHQKXZZ
Neck ØHQ4XZZ
Perineum ØHQ9XZZ
Scalp ØHQØXZZ
Upper Arm
Left ØHQCXZZ

Repair — *continued*
Skin — *continued*
Upper Arm — *continued*
Right ØHQBXZZ
Upper Leg
Left ØHQJXZZ
Right ØHQHXZZ
Skull ØNQØ
Spinal Cord
Cervical ØØQW
Lumbar ØØQY
Thoracic ØØQX
Spinal Meninges ØØQT
Spleen Ø7QP
Sternum ØPQØ
Stomach ØDQ6
Pylorus ØDQ7
Subcutaneous Tissue and Fascia
Abdomen ØJQ8
Back ØJQ7
Buttock ØJQ9
Chest ØJQ6
Face ØJQ1
Foot
Left ØJQR
Right ØJQQ
Hand
Left ØJQK
Right ØJQJ
Lower Arm
Left ØJQH
Right ØJQG
Lower Leg
Left ØJQP
Right ØJQN
Neck
Left ØJQ5
Right ØJQ4
Pelvic Region ØJQC
Perineum ØJQB
Scalp ØJQØ
Upper Arm
Left ØJQF
Right ØJQD
Upper Leg
Left ØJQM
Right ØJQL
Tarsal
Left ØQQM
Right ØQQL
Tendon
Abdomen
Left ØLQG
Right ØLQF
Ankle
Left ØLQT
Right ØLQS
Foot
Left ØLQW
Right ØLQV
Hand
Left ØLQ8
Right ØLQ7
Head and Neck ØLQØ
Hip
Left ØLQK
Right ØLQJ
Knee
Left ØLQR
Right ØLQQ
Lower Arm and Wrist
Left ØLQ6
Right ØLQ5
Lower Leg
Left ØLQP
Right ØLQN
Perineum ØLQH
Shoulder
Left ØLQ2
Right ØLQ1
Thorax
Left ØLQD
Right ØLQC
Trunk
Left ØLQB
Right ØLQ9
Upper Arm
Left ØLQ4
Right ØLQ3

Repair — *continued*
Tendon — *continued*
Upper Leg
Left ØLQM
Right ØLQL
Testis
Bilateral ØVQC
Left ØVQB
Right ØVQ9
Thalamus ØØQ9
Thumb
Left ØXQM
Right ØXQL
Thymus Ø7QM
Thyroid Gland ØGQK
Left Lobe ØGQG
Right Lobe ØGQH
Thyroid Gland Isthmus ØGQJ
Tibia
Left ØQQH
Right ØQQG
Toe
1st
Left ØYQQ
Right ØYQP
2nd
Left ØYQS
Right ØYQR
3rd
Left ØYQU
Right ØYQT
4th
Left ØYQW
Right ØYQV
5th
Left ØYQY
Right ØYQX
Toe Nail ØHQRXZZ
Tongue ØCQ7
Tonsils ØCQP
Tooth
Lower ØCQX
Upper ØCQW
Trachea ØBQ1
Tunica Vaginalis
Left ØVQ7
Right ØVQ6
Turbinate, Nasal Ø9QL
Tympanic Membrane
Left Ø9Q8
Right Ø9Q7
Ulna
Left ØPQL
Right ØPQK
Ureter
Left ØTQ7
Right ØTQ6
Urethra ØTQD
Uterine Supporting Structure ØUQ4
Uterus ØUQ9
Uvula ØCQN
Vagina ØUQG
Valve
Aortic Ø2QF
Mitral Ø2QG
Pulmonary Ø2QH
Tricuspid Ø2QJ
Vas Deferens
Bilateral ØVQQ
Left ØVQP
Right ØVQN
Vein
Axillary
Left Ø5Q8
Right Ø5Q7
Azygos Ø5QØ
Basilic
Left Ø5QC
Right Ø5QB
Brachial
Left Ø5QA
Right Ø5Q9
Cephalic
Left Ø5QF
Right Ø5QD
Colic Ø6Q7
Common Iliac
Left Ø6QD
Right Ø6QC

Repair — *continued*
Vein — *continued*
Coronary Ø2Q4
Esophageal Ø6Q3
External Iliac
Left Ø6QG
Right Ø6QF
External Jugular
Left Ø5QQ
Right Ø5QP
Face
Left Ø5QV
Right Ø5QT
Femoral
Left Ø6QN
Right Ø6QM
Foot
Left Ø6QV
Right Ø6QT
Gastric Ø6Q2
Hand
Left Ø5QH
Right Ø5QG
Hemiazygos Ø5Q1
Hepatic Ø6Q4
Hypogastric
Left Ø6QJ
Right Ø6QH
Inferior Mesenteric Ø6Q6
Innominate
Left Ø5Q4
Right Ø5Q3
Internal Jugular
Left Ø5QN
Right Ø5QM
Intracranial Ø5QL
Lower Ø6QY
Portal Ø6Q8
Pulmonary
Left Ø2QT
Right Ø2QS
Renal
Left Ø6QB
Right Ø6Q9
Saphenous
Left Ø6QQ
Right Ø6QP
Splenic Ø6Q1
Subclavian
Left Ø5Q6
Right Ø5Q5
Superior Mesenteric Ø6Q5
Upper Ø5QY
Vertebral
Left Ø5QS
Right Ø5QR
Vena Cava
Inferior Ø6QØ
Superior Ø2QV
Ventricle
Left Ø2QL
Right Ø2QK
Vertebra
Cervical ØPQ3
Lumbar ØQQØ
Thoracic ØPQ4
Vesicle
Bilateral ØVQ3
Left ØVQ2
Right ØVQ1
Vitreous
Left Ø8Q53ZZ
Right Ø8Q43ZZ
Vocal Cord
Left ØCQV
Right ØCQT
Vulva ØUQM
Wrist Region
Left ØXQH
Right ØXQG
Repair, obstetric laceration, periurethral ØUQMXZZ
Replacement
Acetabulum
Left ØQR5
Right ØQR4
Ampulla of Vater ØFRC
Anal Sphincter ØDRR
Aorta
Abdominal Ø4RØ

Replacement — *continued*
Aorta — *continued*
Thoracic
Ascending/Arch Ø2RX
Descending Ø2RW
Artery
Anterior Tibial
Left Ø4RQ
Right Ø4RP
Axillary
Left Ø3R6
Right Ø3R5
Brachial
Left Ø3R8
Right Ø3R7
Celiac Ø4R1
Colic
Left Ø4R7
Middle Ø4R8
Right Ø4R6
Common Carotid
Left Ø3RJ
Right Ø3RH
Common Iliac
Left Ø4RD
Right Ø4RC
External Carotid
Left Ø3RN
Right Ø3RM
External Iliac
Left Ø4RJ
Right Ø4RH
Face Ø3RR
Femoral
Left Ø4RL
Right Ø4RK
Foot
Left Ø4RW
Right Ø4RV
Gastric Ø4R2
Hand
Left Ø3RF
Right Ø3RD
Hepatic Ø4R3
Inferior Mesenteric Ø4RB
Innominate Ø3R2
Internal Carotid
Left Ø3RL
Right Ø3RK
Internal Iliac
Left Ø4RF
Right Ø4RE
Internal Mammary
Left Ø3R1
Right Ø3RØ
Intracranial Ø3RG
Lower Ø4RY
Peroneal
Left Ø4RU
Right Ø4RT
Popliteal
Left Ø4RN
Right Ø4RM
Posterior Tibial
Left Ø4RS
Right Ø4RR
Pulmonary
Left Ø2RR
Right Ø2RQ
Pulmonary Trunk Ø2RP
Radial
Left Ø3RC
Right Ø3RB
Renal
Left Ø4RA
Right Ø4R9
Splenic Ø4R4
Subclavian
Left Ø3R4
Right Ø3R3
Superior Mesenteric Ø4R5
Temporal
Left Ø3RT
Right Ø3RS
Thyroid
Left Ø3RV
Right Ø3RU
Ulnar
Left Ø3RA

Replacement — *continued*
Artery — *continued*
Ulnar — *continued*
Right Ø3R9
Upper Ø3RY
Vertebral
Left Ø3RQ
Right Ø3RP
Atrium
Left Ø2R7
Right Ø2R6
Auditory Ossicle
Left Ø9RAØ
Right Ø9R9Ø
Bladder ØTRB
Bladder Neck ØTRC
Bone
Ethmoid
Left ØNRG
Right ØNRF
Frontal ØNR1
Hyoid ØNRX
Lacrimal
Left ØNRJ
Right ØNRH
Nasal ØNRB
Occipital ØNR7
Palatine
Left ØNRL
Right ØNRK
Parietal
Left ØNR4
Right ØNR3
Pelvic
Left ØQR3
Right ØQR2
Sphenoid ØNRC
Temporal
Left ØNR6
Right ØNR5
Zygomatic
Left ØNRN
Right ØNRM
Breast
Bilateral ØHRV
Left ØHRU
Right ØHRT
Bronchus
Lingula ØBR9
Lower Lobe
Left ØBRB
Right ØBR6
Main
Left ØBR7
Right ØBR3
Middle Lobe, Right ØBR5
Upper Lobe
Left ØBR8
Right ØBR4
Buccal Mucosa ØCR4
Bursa and Ligament
Abdomen
Left ØMRJ
Right ØMRH
Ankle
Left ØMRR
Right ØMRQ
Elbow
Left ØMR4
Right ØMR3
Foot
Left ØMRT
Right ØMRS
Hand
Left ØMR8
Right ØMR7
Head and Neck ØMRØ
Hip
Left ØMRM
Right ØMRL
Knee
Left ØMRP
Right ØMRN
Lower Extremity
Left ØMRW
Right ØMRV
Perineum ØMRK
Rib(s) ØMRG

Replacement — *continued*
Bursa and Ligament — *continued*
Shoulder
Left ØMR2
Right ØMR1
Spine
Lower ØMRD
Upper ØMRC
Sternum ØMRF
Upper Extremity
Left ØMRB
Right ØMR9
Wrist
Left ØMR6
Right ØMR5
Carina ØBR2
Carpal
Left ØPRN
Right ØPRM
Cerebral Meninges ØØR1
Cerebral Ventricle ØØR6
Chordae Tendineae Ø2R9
Choroid
Left Ø8RB
Right Ø8RA
Clavicle
Left ØPRB
Right ØPR9
Coccyx ØQRS
Conjunctiva
Left Ø8RTX
Right Ø8RSX
Cornea
Left Ø8R9
Right Ø8R8
Diaphragm ØBRT
Disc
Cervical Vertebral ØRR3Ø
Cervicothoracic Vertebral ØRR5Ø
Lumbar Vertebral ØSR2Ø
Lumbosacral ØSR4Ø
Thoracic Vertebral ØRR9Ø
Thoracolumbar Vertebral ØRRBØ
Duct
Common Bile ØFR9
Cystic ØFR8
Hepatic
Common ØFR7
Left ØFR6
Right ØFR5
Lacrimal
Left Ø8RY
Right Ø8RX
Pancreatic ØFRD
Accessory ØFRF
Parotid
Left ØCRC
Right ØCRB
Dura Mater ØØR2
Ear
External
Bilateral Ø9R2
Left Ø9R1
Right Ø9RØ
Inner
Left Ø9REØ
Right Ø9RDØ
Middle
Left Ø9R6Ø
Right Ø9R5Ø
Epiglottis ØCRR
Esophagus ØDR5
Eye
Left Ø8R1
Right Ø8RØ
Eyelid
Lower
Left Ø8RR
Right Ø8RQ
Upper
Left Ø8RP
Right Ø8RN
Femoral Shaft
Left ØQR9
Right ØQR8
Femur
Lower
Left ØQRC
Right ØQRB

Replacement — *continued*
Femur — *continued*
Upper
Left ØQR7
Right ØQR6
Fibula
Left ØQRK
Right ØQRJ
Finger Nail ØHRQX
Gingiva
Lower ØCR6
Upper ØCR5
Glenoid Cavity
Left ØPR8
Right ØPR7
Hair ØHRSX
Heart Ø2RAØ
Humeral Head
Left ØPRD
Right ØPRC
Humeral Shaft
Left ØPRG
Right ØPRF
Iris
Left Ø8RD3
Right Ø8RC3
Joint
Acromioclavicular
Left ØRRHØ
Right ØRRGØ
Ankle
Left ØSRG
Right ØSRF
Carpal
Left ØRRRØ
Right ØRRQØ
Carpometacarpal
Left ØRRTØ
Right ØRRSØ
Cervical Vertebral ØRR1Ø
Cervicothoracic Vertebral ØRR4Ø
Coccygeal ØSR6Ø
Elbow
Left ØRRMØ
Right ØRRLØ
Finger Phalangeal
Left ØRRXØ
Right ØRRWØ
Hip
Left ØSRB
Acetabular Surface ØSRE
Femoral Surface ØSRS
Right ØSR9
Acetabular Surface ØSRA
Femoral Surface ØSRR
Knee
Left ØSRD
Femoral Surface ØSRU
Tibial Surface ØSRW
Right ØSRC
Femoral Surface ØSRT
Tibial Surface ØSRV
Lumbar Vertebral ØSRØØ
Lumbosacral ØSR3Ø
Metacarpophalangeal
Left ØRRVØ
Right ØRRUØ
Metatarsal-Phalangeal
Left ØSRNØ
Right ØSRMØ
Occipital-cervical ØRRØØ
Sacrococcygeal ØSR5Ø
Sacroiliac
Left ØSR8Ø
Right ØSR7Ø
Shoulder
Left ØRRK
Right ØRRJ
Sternoclavicular
Left ØRRFØ
Right ØRREØ
Tarsal
Left ØSRJØ
Right ØSRHØ
Tarsometatarsal
Left ØSRLØ
Right ØSRKØ
Temporomandibular
Left ØRRDØ

Replacement — *continued*
Joint — *continued*
Temporomandibular — *continued*
Right ØRRCØ
Thoracic Vertebral ØRR6Ø
Thoracolumbar Vertebral ØRRAØ
Toe Phalangeal
Left ØSRQØ
Right ØSRPØ
Wrist
Left ØRRPØ
Right ØRRNØ
Kidney Pelvis
Left ØTR4
Right ØTR3
Larynx ØCRS
Lens
Left Ø8RK3ØZ
Right Ø8RJ3ØZ
Lip
Lower ØCR1
Upper ØCRØ
Mandible
Left ØNRV
Right ØNRT
Maxilla ØNRR
Mesentery ØDRV
Metacarpal
Left ØPRQ
Right ØPRP
Metatarsal
Left ØQRP
Right ØQRN
Muscle
Abdomen
Left ØKRL
Right ØKRK
Facial ØKR1
Foot
Left ØKRW
Right ØKRV
Hand
Left ØKRD
Right ØKRC
Head ØKRØ
Hip
Left ØKRP
Right ØKRN
Lower Arm and Wrist
Left ØKRB
Right ØKR9
Lower Leg
Left ØKRT
Right ØKRS
Neck
Left ØKR3
Right ØKR2
Papillary Ø2RD
Perineum ØKRM
Shoulder
Left ØKR6
Right ØKR5
Thorax
Left ØKRJ
Right ØKRH
Tongue, Palate, Pharynx ØKR4
Trunk
Left ØKRG
Right ØKRF
Upper Arm
Left ØKR8
Right ØKR7
Upper Leg
Left ØKRR
Right ØKRQ
Nasal Mucosa and Soft Tissue Ø9RK
Nasopharynx Ø9RN
Nerve
Abducens ØØRL
Accessory ØØRR
Acoustic ØØRN
Cervical Ø1R1
Facial ØØRM
Femoral Ø1RD
Glossopharyngeal ØØRP
Hypoglossal ØØRS
Lumbar Ø1RB
Median Ø1R5
Oculomotor ØØRH

Replacement — *continued*
Nerve — *continued*
Olfactory ØØRF
Optic ØØRG
Peroneal Ø1RH
Phrenic Ø1R2
Pudendal Ø1RC
Radial Ø1R6
Sacral Ø1RR
Sciatic Ø1RF
Thoracic Ø1R8
Tibial Ø1RG
Trigeminal ØØRK
Trochlear ØØRJ
Ulnar Ø1R4
Vagus ØØRQ
Nipple
Left ØHRX
Right ØHRW
Omentum ØDRU
Orbit
Left ØNRQ
Right ØNRP
Palate
Hard ØCR2
Soft ØCR3
Patella
Left ØQRF
Right ØQRD
Pericardium Ø2RN
Peritoneum ØDRW
Phalanx
Finger
Left ØPRV
Right ØPRT
Thumb
Left ØPRS
Right ØPRR
Toe
Left ØQRR
Right ØQRQ
Pharynx ØCRM
Radius
Left ØPRJ
Right ØPRH
Retinal Vessel
Left Ø8RH3
Right Ø8RG3
Ribs
1 to 2 ØPR1
3 or More ØPR2
Sacrum ØQR1
Scapula
Left ØPR6
Right ØPR5
Sclera
Left Ø8R7X
Right Ø8R6X
Septum
Atrial Ø2R5
Nasal Ø9RM
Ventricular Ø2RM
Skin
Abdomen ØHR7
Back ØHR6
Buttock ØHR8
Chest ØHR5
Ear
Left ØHR3
Right ØHR2
Face ØHR1
Foot
Left ØHRN
Right ØHRM
Hand
Left ØHRG
Right ØHRF
Inguinal ØHRA
Lower Arm
Left ØHRE
Right ØHRD
Lower Leg
Left ØHRL
Right ØHRK
Neck ØHR4
Perineum ØHR9
Scalp ØHRØ
Upper Arm
Left ØHRC

Replacement — *continued*
Skin — *continued*
Upper Arm — *continued*
Right ØHRB
Upper Leg
Left ØHRJ
Right ØHRH
Skin Substitute, Porcine Liver Derived XHRPXL2
Skull ØNRØ
Spinal Meninges ØØRT
Sternum ØPRØ
Subcutaneous Tissue and Fascia
Abdomen ØJR8
Back ØJR7
Buttock ØJR9
Chest ØJR6
Face ØJR1
Foot
Left ØJRR
Right ØJRQ
Hand
Left ØJRK
Right ØJRJ
Lower Arm
Left ØJRH
Right ØJRG
Lower Leg
Left ØJRP
Right ØJRN
Neck
Left ØJR5
Right ØJR4
Pelvic Region ØJRC
Perineum ØJRB
Scalp ØJRØ
Upper Arm
Left ØJRF
Right ØJRD
Upper Leg
Left ØJRM
Right ØJRL
Tarsal
Left ØQRM
Right ØQRL
Tendon
Abdomen
Left ØLRG
Right ØLRF
Ankle
Left ØLRT
Right ØLRS
Foot
Left ØLRW
Right ØLRV
Hand
Left ØLR8
Right ØLR7
Head and Neck ØLRØ
Hip
Left ØLRK
Right ØLRJ
Knee
Left ØLRR
Right ØLRQ
Lower Arm and Wrist
Left ØLR6
Right ØLR5
Lower Leg
Left ØLRP
Right ØLRN
Perineum ØLRH
Shoulder
Left ØLR2
Right ØLR1
Thorax
Left ØLRD
Right ØLRC
Trunk
Left ØLRB
Right ØLR9
Upper Arm
Left ØLR4
Right ØLR3
Upper Leg
Left ØLRM
Right ØLRL
Testis
Bilateral ØVRCØJZ
Left ØVRBØJZ

Replacement — *continued*
Testis — *continued*
Right ØVR9ØJZ
Thumb
Left ØXRM
Right ØXRL
Tibia
Left ØQRH
Right ØQRG
Toe Nail ØHRRX
Tongue ØCR7
Tooth
Lower ØCRX
Upper ØCRW
Trachea ØBR1
Turbinate, Nasal Ø9RL
Tympanic Membrane
Left Ø9R8
Right Ø9R7
Ulna
Left ØPRL
Right ØPRK
Ureter
Left ØTR7
Right ØTR6
Urethra ØTRD
Uvula ØCRN
Valve
Aortic Ø2RF
Mitral Ø2RG
Pulmonary Ø2RH
Tricuspid Ø2RJ
Vein
Axillary
Left Ø5R8
Right Ø5R7
Azygos Ø5RØ
Basilic
Left Ø5RC
Right Ø5RB
Brachial
Left Ø5RA
Right Ø5R9
Cephalic
Left Ø5RF
Right Ø5RD
Colic Ø6R7
Common Iliac
Left Ø6RD
Right Ø6RC
Esophageal Ø6R3
External Iliac
Left Ø6RG
Right Ø6RF
External Jugular
Left Ø5RQ
Right Ø5RP
Face
Left Ø5RV
Right Ø5RT
Femoral
Left Ø6RN
Right Ø6RM
Foot
Left Ø6RV
Right Ø6RT
Gastric Ø6R2
Hand
Left Ø5RH
Right Ø5RG
Hemiazygos Ø5R1
Hepatic Ø6R4
Hypogastric
Left Ø6RJ
Right Ø6RH
Inferior Mesenteric Ø6R6
Innominate
Left Ø5R4
Right Ø5R3
Internal Jugular
Left Ø5RN
Right Ø5RM
Intracranial Ø5RL
Lower Ø6RY
Portal Ø6R8
Pulmonary
Left Ø2RT
Right Ø2RS

Replacement — *continued*
Vein — *continued*
Renal
Left Ø6RB
Right Ø6R9
Saphenous
Left Ø6RQ
Right Ø6RP
Splenic Ø6R1
Subclavian
Left Ø5R6
Right Ø5R5
Superior Mesenteric Ø6R5
Upper Ø5RY
Vertebral
Left Ø5RS
Right Ø5RR
Vena Cava
Inferior Ø6RØ
Superior Ø2RV
Ventricle
Left Ø2RL
Right Ø2RK
Vertebra
Cervical ØPR3
Lumbar ØQRØ
Thoracic ØPR4
Vitreous
Left Ø8R53
Right Ø8R43
Vocal Cord
Left ØCRV
Right ØCRT
Zooplastic Tissue, Rapid Deployment Technique X2RF
Replacement, hip
Partial or total *see* Replacement, Lower Joints ØSR
Resurfacing only *see* Supplement, Lower Joints ØSU
Replantation *see* Reposition
Replantation, scalp *see* Reattachment, Skin, Scalp ØHMØ
Reposition
Acetabulum
Left ØQS5
Right ØQS4
Ampulla of Vater ØFSC
Anus ØDSQ
Aorta
Abdominal Ø4SØ
Thoracic
Ascending/Arch Ø2SXØZZ
Descending Ø2SWØZZ
Artery
Anterior Tibial
Left Ø4SQ
Right Ø4SP
Axillary
Left Ø3S6
Right Ø3S5
Brachial
Left Ø3S8
Right Ø3S7
Celiac Ø4S1
Colic
Left Ø4S7
Middle Ø4S8
Right Ø4S6
Common Carotid
Left Ø3SJ
Right Ø3SH
Common Iliac
Left Ø4SD
Right Ø4SC
Coronary
One Artery Ø2SØØZZ
Two Arteries Ø2S1ØZZ
External Carotid
Left Ø3SN
Right Ø3SM
External Iliac
Left Ø4SJ
Right Ø4SH
Face Ø3SR
Femoral
Left Ø4SL
Right Ø4SK
Foot
Left Ø4SW

Reposition — *continued*
Artery — *continued*
Foot — *continued*
Right Ø4SV
Gastric Ø4S2
Hand
Left Ø3SF
Right Ø3SD
Hepatic Ø4S3
Inferior Mesenteric Ø4SB
Innominate Ø3S2
Internal Carotid
Left Ø3SL
Right Ø3SK
Internal Iliac
Left Ø4SF
Right Ø4SE
Internal Mammary
Left Ø3S1
Right Ø3SØ
Intracranial Ø3SG
Lower Ø4SY
Peroneal
Left Ø4SU
Right Ø4ST
Popliteal
Left Ø4SN
Right Ø4SM
Posterior Tibial
Left Ø4SS
Right Ø4SR
Pulmonary
Left Ø2SRØZZ
Right Ø2SQØZZ
Pulmonary Trunk Ø2SPØZZ
Radial
Left Ø3SC
Right Ø3SB
Renal
Left Ø4SA
Right Ø4S9
Splenic Ø4S4
Subclavian
Left Ø3S4
Right Ø3S3
Superior Mesenteric Ø4S5
Temporal
Left Ø3ST
Right Ø3SS
Thyroid
Left Ø3SV
Right Ø3SU
Ulnar
Left Ø3SA
Right Ø3S9
Upper Ø3SY
Vertebral
Left Ø3SQ
Right Ø3SP
Auditory Ossicle
Left Ø9SA
Right Ø9S9
Bladder ØTSB
Bladder Neck ØTSC
Bone
Ethmoid
Left ØNSG
Right ØNSF
Frontal ØNS1
Hyoid ØNSX
Lacrimal
Left ØNSJ
Right ØNSH
Nasal ØNSB
Occipital ØNS7
Palatine
Left ØNSL
Right ØNSK
Parietal
Left ØNS4
Right ØNS3
Pelvic
Left ØQS3
Right ØQS2
Sphenoid ØNSC
Temporal
Left ØNS6
Right ØNS5

Reposition — *continued*
Bone — *continued*
Zygomatic
Left ØNSN
Right ØNSM
Breast
Bilateral ØHSVØZZ
Left ØHSUØZZ
Right ØHSTØZZ
Bronchus
Lingula ØBS9ØZZ
Lower Lobe
Left ØBSBØZZ
Right ØBS6ØZZ
Main
Left ØBS7ØZZ
Right ØBS3ØZZ
Middle Lobe, Right ØBS5ØZZ
Upper Lobe
Left ØBS8ØZZ
Right ØBS4ØZZ
Bursa and Ligament
Abdomen
Left ØMSJ
Right ØMSH
Ankle
Left ØMSR
Right ØMSQ
Elbow
Left ØMS4
Right ØMS3
Foot
Left ØMST
Right ØMSS
Hand
Left ØMS8
Right ØMS7
Head and Neck ØMSØ
Hip
Left ØMSM
Right ØMSL
Knee
Left ØMSP
Right ØMSN
Lower Extremity
Left ØMSW
Right ØMSV
Perineum ØMSK
Rib(s) ØMSG
Shoulder
Left ØMS2
Right ØMS1
Spine
Lower ØMSD
Upper ØMSC
Sternum ØMSF
Upper Extremity
Left ØMSB
Right ØMS9
Wrist
Left ØMS6
Right ØMS5
Carina ØBS2ØZZ
Carpal
Left ØPSN
Right ØPSM
Cecum ØDSH
Cervix ØUSC
Clavicle
Left ØPSB
Right ØPS9
Coccyx ØQSS
Colon
Ascending ØDSK
Descending ØDSM
Sigmoid ØDSN
Transverse ØDSL
Cord
Bilateral ØVSH
Left ØVSG
Right ØVSF
Cul-de-sac ØUSF
Diaphragm ØBSTØZZ
Duct
Common Bile ØFS9
Cystic ØFS8
Hepatic
Common ØFS7
Left ØFS6

Reposition — *continued*
Duct — *continued*
Hepatic — *continued*
Right ØFS5
Lacrimal
Left Ø8SY
Right Ø8SX
Pancreatic ØFSD
Accessory ØFSF
Parotid
Left ØCSC
Right ØCSB
Duodenum ØDS9
Ear
Bilateral Ø9S2
Left Ø9S1
Right Ø9SØ
Epiglottis ØCSR
Esophagus ØDS5
Eustachian Tube
Left Ø9SG
Right Ø9SF
Eyelid
Lower
Left Ø8SR
Right Ø8SQ
Upper
Left Ø8SP
Right Ø8SN
Fallopian Tube
Left ØUS6
Right ØUS5
Fallopian Tubes, Bilateral ØUS7
Femoral Shaft
Left ØQS9
Right ØQS8
Femur
Lower
Left ØQSC
Right ØQSB
Upper
Left ØQS7
Right ØQS6
Fibula
Left ØQSK
Right ØQSJ
Gallbladder ØFS4
Gland
Adrenal
Left ØGS2
Right ØGS3
Lacrimal
Left Ø8SW
Right Ø8SV
Glenoid Cavity
Left ØPS8
Right ØPS7
Hair ØHSSXZZ
Humeral Head
Left ØPSD
Right ØPSC
Humeral Shaft
Left ØPSG
Right ØPSF
Ileum ØDSB
Intestine
Large ØDSE
Small ØDS8
Iris
Left Ø8SD3ZZ
Right Ø8SC3ZZ
Jejunum ØDSA
Joint
Acromioclavicular
Left ØRSH
Right ØRSG
Ankle
Left ØSSG
Right ØSSF
Carpal
Left ØRSR
Right ØRSQ
Carpometacarpal
Left ØRST
Right ØRSS
Cervical Vertebral ØRS1
Cervicothoracic Vertebral ØRS4
Coccygeal ØSS6

Reposition — *continued*
Joint — *continued*
Elbow
Left ØRSM
Right ØRSL
Finger Phalangeal
Left ØRSX
Right ØRSW
Hip
Left ØSSB
Right ØSS9
Knee
Left ØSSD
Right ØSSC
Lumbar Vertebral ØSSØ
Lumbosacral ØSS3
Metacarpophalangeal
Left ØRSV
Right ØRSU
Metatarsal-Phalangeal
Left ØSSN
Right ØSSM
Occipital-cervical ØRSØ
Sacrococcygeal ØSS5
Sacroiliac
Left ØSS8
Right ØSS7
Shoulder
Left ØRSK
Right ØRSJ
Sternoclavicular
Left ØRSF
Right ØRSE
Tarsal
Left ØSSJ
Right ØSSH
Tarsometatarsal
Left ØSSL
Right ØSSK
Temporomandibular
Left ØRSD
Right ØRSC
Thoracic Vertebral ØRS6
Thoracolumbar Vertebral ØRSA
Toe Phalangeal
Left ØSSQ
Right ØSSP
Wrist
Left ØRSP
Right ØRSN
Kidney
Left ØTS1
Right ØTSØ
Kidney Pelvis
Left ØTS4
Right ØTS3
Kidneys, Bilateral ØTS2
Lens
Left Ø8SK3ZZ
Right Ø8SJ3ZZ
Lip
Lower ØCS1
Upper ØCSØ
Liver ØFSØ
Lung
Left ØBSLØZZ
Lower Lobe
Left ØBSJØZZ
Right ØBSFØZZ
Middle Lobe, Right ØBSDØZZ
Right ØBSKØZZ
Upper Lobe
Left ØBSGØZZ
Right ØBSCØZZ
Lung Lingula ØBSHØZZ
Mandible
Left ØNSV
Right ØNST
Maxilla ØNSR
Metacarpal
Left ØPSQ
Right ØPSP
Metatarsal
Left ØQSP
Right ØQSN
Muscle
Abdomen
Left ØKSL
Right ØKSK

Reposition — *continued*
Muscle — *continued*
Extraocular
Left Ø8SM
Right Ø8SL
Facial ØKS1
Foot
Left ØKSW
Right ØKSV
Hand
Left ØKSD
Right ØKSC
Head ØKSØ
Hip
Left ØKSP
Right ØKSN
Lower Arm and Wrist
Left ØKSB
Right ØKS9
Lower Leg
Left ØKST
Right ØKSS
Neck
Left ØKS3
Right ØKS2
Perineum ØKSM
Shoulder
Left ØKS6
Right ØKS5
Thorax
Left ØKSJ
Right ØKSH
Tongue, Palate, Pharynx ØKS4
Trunk
Left ØKSG
Right ØKSF
Upper Arm
Left ØKS8
Right ØKS7
Upper Leg
Left ØKSR
Right ØKSQ
Nasal Mucosa and Soft Tissue Ø9SK
Nerve
Abducens ØØSL
Accessory ØØSR
Acoustic ØØSN
Brachial Plexus Ø1S3
Cervical Ø1S1
Cervical Plexus Ø1SØ
Facial ØØSM
Femoral Ø1SD
Glossopharyngeal ØØSP
Hypoglossal ØØSS
Lumbar Ø1SB
Lumbar Plexus Ø1S9
Lumbosacral Plexus Ø1SA
Median Ø1S5
Oculomotor ØØSH
Olfactory ØØSF
Optic ØØSG
Peroneal Ø1SH
Phrenic Ø1S2
Pudendal Ø1SC
Radial Ø1S6
Sacral Ø1SR
Sacral Plexus Ø1SQ
Sciatic Ø1SF
Thoracic Ø1S8
Tibial Ø1SG
Trigeminal ØØSK
Trochlear ØØSJ
Ulnar Ø1S4
Vagus ØØSQ
Nipple
Left ØHSXXZZ
Right ØHSWXZZ
Orbit
Left ØNSQ
Right ØNSP
Ovary
Bilateral ØUS2
Left ØUS1
Right ØUSØ
Palate
Hard ØCS2
Soft ØCS3
Pancreas ØFSG
Parathyroid Gland ØGSR

Reposition — *continued*
Parathyroid Gland — *continued*
Inferior
Left ØGSP
Right ØGSN
Multiple ØGSQ
Superior
Left ØGSM
Right ØGSL
Patella
Left ØQSF
Right ØQSD
Phalanx
Finger
Left ØPSV
Right ØPST
Thumb
Left ØPSS
Right ØPSR
Toe
Left ØQSR
Right ØQSQ
Products of Conception 1ØSØ
Ectopic 1ØS2
Radius
Left ØPSJ
Right ØPSH
Rectum ØDSP
Retinal Vessel
Left Ø8SH3ZZ
Right Ø8SG3ZZ
Ribs
1 to 2 ØPS1
3 or More ØPS2
Sacrum ØQS1
Scapula
Left ØPS6
Right ØPS5
Septum, Nasal Ø9SM
Sesamoid Bone(s) 1st Toe
see Reposition, Metatarsal, Left ØQSP
see Reposition, Metatarsal, Right ØQSN
Skull ØNSØ
Spinal Cord
Cervical ØØSW
Lumbar ØØSY
Thoracic ØØSX
Spleen Ø7SPØZZ
Sternum ØPSØ
Stomach ØDS6
Tarsal
Left ØQSM
Right ØQSL
Tendon
Abdomen
Left ØLSG
Right ØLSF
Ankle
Left ØLST
Right ØLSS
Foot
Left ØLSW
Right ØLSV
Hand
Left ØLS8
Right ØLS7
Head and Neck ØLSØ
Hip
Left ØLSK
Right ØLSJ
Knee
Left ØLSR
Right ØLSQ
Lower Arm and Wrist
Left ØLS6
Right ØLS5
Lower Leg
Left ØLSP
Right ØLSN
Perineum ØLSH
Shoulder
Left ØLS2
Right ØLS1
Thorax
Left ØLSD
Right ØLSC
Trunk
Left ØLSB
Right ØLS9

Reposition — *continued*
Tendon — *continued*
Upper Arm
Left ØLS4
Right ØLS3
Upper Leg
Left ØLSM
Right ØLSL
Testis
Bilateral ØVSC
Left ØVSB
Right ØVS9
Thymus Ø7SMØZZ
Thyroid Gland
Left Lobe ØGSG
Right Lobe ØGSH
Tibia
Left ØQSH
Right ØQSG
Tongue ØCS7
Tooth
Lower ØCSX
Upper ØCSW
Trachea ØBS1ØZZ
Turbinate, Nasal Ø9SL
Tympanic Membrane
Left Ø9S8
Right Ø9S7
Ulna
Left ØPSL
Right ØPSK
Ureter
Left ØTS7
Right ØTS6
Ureters, Bilateral ØTS8
Urethra ØTSD
Uterine Supporting Structure ØUS4
Uterus ØUS9
Uvula ØCSN
Vagina ØUSG
Vein
Axillary
Left Ø5S8
Right Ø5S7
Azygos Ø5SØ
Basilic
Left Ø5SC
Right Ø5SB
Brachial
Left Ø5SA
Right Ø5S9
Cephalic
Left Ø5SF
Right Ø5SD
Colic Ø6S7
Common Iliac
Left Ø6SD
Right Ø6SC
Esophageal Ø6S3
External Iliac
Left Ø6SG
Right Ø6SF
External Jugular
Left Ø5SQ
Right Ø5SP
Face
Left Ø5SV
Right Ø5ST
Femoral
Left Ø6SN
Right Ø6SM
Foot
Left Ø6SV
Right Ø6ST
Gastric Ø6S2
Hand
Left Ø5SH
Right Ø5SG
Hemiazygos Ø5S1
Hepatic Ø6S4
Hypogastric
Left Ø6SJ
Right Ø6SH
Inferior Mesenteric Ø6S6
Innominate
Left Ø5S4
Right Ø5S3
Internal Jugular
Left Ø5SN

Reposition — *continued*
Vein — *continued*
Internal Jugular — *continued*
Right Ø5SM
Intracranial Ø5SL
Lower Ø6SY
Portal Ø6S8
Pulmonary
Left Ø2STØZZ
Right Ø2SSØZZ
Renal
Left Ø6SB
Right Ø6S9
Saphenous
Left Ø6SQ
Right Ø6SP
Splenic Ø6S1
Subclavian
Left Ø5S6
Right Ø5S5
Superior Mesenteric Ø6S5
Upper Ø5SY
Vertebral
Left Ø5SS
Right Ø5SR
Vena Cava
Inferior Ø6SØ
Superior Ø2SVØZZ
Vertebra
Cervical ØPS3
Magnetically Controlled Growth Rod(s) XNS3
Lumbar ØQSØ
Magnetically Controlled Growth Rod(s) XNSØ
Posterior (Dynamic) Distraction Device XNSØ
Thoracic ØPS4
Magnetically Controlled Growth Rod(s) XNS4
Posterior (Dynamic) Distraction Device XNS4
Vocal Cord
Left ØCSV
Right ØCST
Resection
Acetabulum
Left ØQT5ØZZ
Right ØQT4ØZZ
Adenoids ØCTQ
Ampulla of Vater ØFTC
Anal Sphincter ØDTR
Anus ØDTQ
Aortic Body ØGTD
Appendix ØDTJ
Auditory Ossicle
Left Ø9TA
Right Ø9T9
Bladder ØTTB
Bladder Neck ØTTC
Bone
Ethmoid
Left ØNTGØZZ
Right ØNTFØZZ
Frontal ØNT1ØZZ
Hyoid ØNTXØZZ
Lacrimal
Left ØNTJØZZ
Right ØNTHØZZ
Nasal ØNTBØZZ
Occipital ØNT7ØZZ
Palatine
Left ØNTLØZZ
Right ØNTKØZZ
Parietal
Left ØNT4ØZZ
Right ØNT3ØZZ
Pelvic
Left ØQT3ØZZ
Right ØQT2ØZZ
Sphenoid ØNTCØZZ
Temporal
Left ØNT6ØZZ
Right ØNT5ØZZ
Zygomatic
Left ØNTNØZZ
Right ØNTMØZZ
Breast
Bilateral ØHTVØZZ

Resection — *continued*
Breast — *continued*
Left ØHTUØZZ
Right ØHTTØZZ
Supernumerary ØHTYØZZ
Bronchus
Lingula ØBT9
Lower Lobe
Left ØBTB
Right ØBT6
Main
Left ØBT7
Right ØBT3
Middle Lobe, Right ØBT5
Upper Lobe
Left ØBT8
Right ØBT4
Bursa and Ligament
Abdomen
Left ØMTJ
Right ØMTH
Ankle
Left ØMTR
Right ØMTQ
Elbow
Left ØMT4
Right ØMT3
Foot
Left ØMTT
Right ØMTS
Hand
Left ØMT8
Right ØMT7
Head and Neck ØMTØ
Hip
Left ØMTM
Right ØMTL
Knee
Left ØMTP
Right ØMTN
Lower Extremity
Left ØMTW
Right ØMTV
Perineum ØMTK
Rib(s) ØMTG
Shoulder
Left ØMT2
Right ØMT1
Spine
Lower ØMTD
Upper ØMTC
Sternum ØMTF
Upper Extremity
Left ØMTB
Right ØMT9
Wrist
Left ØMT6
Right ØMT5
Carina ØBT2
Carotid Bodies, Bilateral ØGT8
Carotid Body
Left ØGT6
Right ØGT7
Carpal
Left ØPTNØZZ
Right ØPTMØZZ
Cecum ØDTH
Cerebral Hemisphere ØØT7
Cervix ØUTC
Chordae Tendineae Ø2T9
Cisterna Chyli Ø7TL
Clavicle
Left ØPTBØZZ
Right ØPT9ØZZ
Clitoris ØUTJ
Coccygeal Glomus ØGTB
Coccyx ØQTSØZZ
Colon
Ascending ØDTK
Descending ØDTM
Sigmoid ØDTN
Transverse ØDTL
Conduction Mechanism Ø2T8
Cord
Bilateral ØVTH
Left ØVTG
Right ØVTF
Cornea
Left Ø8T9XZZ

Resection — *continued*
Cornea — *continued*
Right Ø8T8XZZ
Cul-de-sac ØUTF
Diaphragm ØBTT
Disc
Cervical Vertebral ØRT3ØZZ
Cervicothoracic Vertebral ØRT5ØZZ
Lumbar Vertebral ØST2ØZZ
Lumbosacral ØST4ØZZ
Thoracic Vertebral ØRT9ØZZ
Thoracolumbar Vertebral ØRTBØZZ
Duct
Common Bile ØFT9
Cystic ØFT8
Hepatic
Common ØFT7
Left ØFT6
Right ØFT5
Lacrimal
Left Ø8TY
Right Ø8TX
Pancreatic ØFTD
Accessory ØFTF
Parotid
Left ØCTCØZZ
Right ØCTBØZZ
Duodenum ØDT9
Ear
External
Left Ø9T1
Right Ø9TØ
Inner
Left Ø9TE
Right Ø9TD
Middle
Left Ø9T6
Right Ø9T5
Epididymis
Bilateral ØVTL
Left ØVTK
Right ØVTJ
Epiglottis ØCTR
Esophagogastric Junction ØDT4
Esophagus ØDT5
Lower ØDT3
Middle ØDT2
Upper ØDT1
Eustachian Tube
Left Ø9TG
Right Ø9TF
Eye
Left Ø8T1XZZ
Right Ø8TØXZZ
Eyelid
Lower
Left Ø8TR
Right Ø8TQ
Upper
Left Ø8TP
Right Ø8TN
Fallopian Tube
Left ØUT6
Right ØUT5
Fallopian Tubes, Bilateral ØUT7
Femoral Shaft
Left ØQT9ØZZ
Right ØQT8ØZZ
Femur
Lower
Left ØQTCØZZ
Right ØQTBØZZ
Upper
Left ØQT7ØZZ
Right ØQT6ØZZ
Fibula
Left ØQTKØZZ
Right ØQTJØZZ
Finger Nail ØHTQXZZ
Gallbladder ØFT4
Gland
Adrenal
Bilateral ØGT4
Left ØGT2
Right ØGT3
Lacrimal
Left Ø8TW
Right Ø8TV
Minor Salivary ØCTJØZZ

Resection — *continued*
Gland — *continued*
Parotid
Left ØCT9ØZZ
Right ØCT8ØZZ
Pituitary ØGTØ
Sublingual
Left ØCTFØZZ
Right ØCTDØZZ
Submaxillary
Left ØCTHØZZ
Right ØCTGØZZ
Vestibular ØUTL
Glenoid Cavity
Left ØPT8ØZZ
Right ØPT7ØZZ
Glomus Jugulare ØGTC
Humeral Head
Left ØPTDØZZ
Right ØPTCØZZ
Humeral Shaft
Left ØPTGØZZ
Right ØPTFØZZ
Hymen ØUTK
Ileocecal Valve ØDTC
Ileum ØDTB
Intestine
Large ØDTE
Left ØDTG
Right ØDTF
Small ØDT8
Iris
Left Ø8TD3ZZ
Right Ø8TC3ZZ
Jejunum ØDTA
Joint
Acromioclavicular
Left ØRTHØZZ
Right ØRTGØZZ
Ankle
Left ØSTGØZZ
Right ØSTFØZZ
Carpal
Left ØRTRØZZ
Right ØRTQØZZ
Carpometacarpal
Left ØRTTØZZ
Right ØRTSØZZ
Cervicothoracic Vertebral ØRT4ØZZ
Coccygeal ØST6ØZZ
Elbow
Left ØRTMØZZ
Right ØRTLØZZ
Finger Phalangeal
Left ØRTXØZZ
Right ØRTWØZZ
Hip
Left ØSTBØZZ
Right ØST9ØZZ
Knee
Left ØSTDØZZ
Right ØSTCØZZ
Metacarpophalangeal
Left ØRTVØZZ
Right ØRTUØZZ
Metatarsal-Phalangeal
Left ØSTNØZZ
Right ØSTMØZZ
Sacrococcygeal ØST5ØZZ
Sacroiliac
Left ØST8ØZZ
Right ØST7ØZZ
Shoulder
Left ØRTKØZZ
Right ØRTJØZZ
Sternoclavicular
Left ØRTFØZZ
Right ØRTEØZZ
Tarsal
Left ØSTJØZZ
Right ØSTHØZZ
Tarsometatarsal
Left ØSTLØZZ
Right ØSTKØZZ
Temporomandibular
Left ØRTDØZZ
Right ØRTCØZZ
Toe Phalangeal
Left ØSTQØZZ

Resection — *continued*
Joint — *continued*
Toe Phalangeal — *continued*
Right ØSTPØZZ
Wrist
Left ØRTPØZZ
Right ØRTNØZZ
Kidney
Left ØTT1
Right ØTTØ
Kidney Pelvis
Left ØTT4
Right ØTT3
Kidneys, Bilateral ØTT2
Larynx ØCTS
Lens
Left Ø8TK3ZZ
Right Ø8TJ3ZZ
Lip
Lower ØCT1
Upper ØCTØ
Liver ØFTØ
Left Lobe ØFT2
Right Lobe ØFT1
Lung
Bilateral ØBTM
Left ØBTL
Lower Lobe
Left ØBTJ
Right ØBTF
Middle Lobe, Right ØBTD
Right ØBTK
Upper Lobe
Left ØBTG
Right ØBTC
Lung Lingula ØBTH
Lymphatic
Aortic Ø7TD
Axillary
Left Ø7T6
Right Ø7T5
Head Ø7TØ
Inguinal
Left Ø7TJ
Right Ø7TH
Internal Mammary
Left Ø7T9
Right Ø7T8
Lower Extremity
Left Ø7TG
Right Ø7TF
Mesenteric Ø7TB
Neck
Left Ø7T2
Right Ø7T1
Pelvis Ø7TC
Thoracic Duct Ø7TK
Thorax Ø7T7
Upper Extremity
Left Ø7T4
Right Ø7T3
Mandible
Left ØNTVØZZ
Right ØNTTØZZ
Maxilla ØNTRØZZ
Metacarpal
Left ØPTQØZZ
Right ØPTPØZZ
Metatarsal
Left ØQTPØZZ
Right ØQTNØZZ
Muscle
Abdomen
Left ØKTL
Right ØKTK
Extraocular
Left Ø8TM
Right Ø8TL
Facial ØKT1
Foot
Left ØKTW
Right ØKTV
Hand
Left ØKTD
Right ØKTC
Head ØKTØ
Hip
Left ØKTP
Right ØKTN

Resection — *continued*
Muscle — *continued*
Lower Arm and Wrist
Left ØKTB
Right ØKT9
Lower Leg
Left ØKTT
Right ØKTS
Neck
Left ØKT3
Right ØKT2
Papillary Ø2TD
Perineum ØKTM
Shoulder
Left ØKT6
Right ØKT5
Thorax
Left ØKTJ
Right ØKTH
Tongue, Palate, Pharynx ØKT4
Trunk
Left ØKTG
Right ØKTF
Upper Arm
Left ØKT8
Right ØKT7
Upper Leg
Left ØKTR
Right ØKTQ
Nasal Mucosa and Soft Tissue Ø9TK
Nasopharynx Ø9TN
Nipple
Left ØHTXXZZ
Right ØHTWXZZ
Omentum ØDTU
Orbit
Left ØNTQØZZ
Right ØNTPØZZ
Ovary
Bilateral ØUT2
Left ØUT1
Right ØUTØ
Palate
Hard ØCT2
Soft ØCT3
Pancreas ØFTG
Para-aortic Body ØGT9
Paraganglion Extremity ØGTF
Parathyroid Gland ØGTR
Inferior
Left ØGTP
Right ØGTN
Multiple ØGTQ
Superior
Left ØGTM
Right ØGTL
Patella
Left ØQTFØZZ
Right ØQTDØZZ
Penis ØVTS
Pericardium Ø2TN
Phalanx
Finger
Left ØPTVØZZ
Right ØPTTØZZ
Thumb
Left ØPTSØZZ
Right ØPTRØZZ
Toe
Left ØQTRØZZ
Right ØQTQØZZ
Pharynx ØCTM
Pineal Body ØGT1
Prepuce ØVTT
Products of Conception, Ectopic 1ØT2
Prostate ØVTØ
Radius
Left ØPTJØZZ
Right ØPTHØZZ
Rectum ØDTP
Ribs
1 to 2 ØPT1ØZZ
3 or More ØPT2ØZZ
Scapula
Left ØPT6ØZZ
Right ØPT5ØZZ
Scrotum ØVT5
Septum
Atrial Ø2T5

Resection — *continued*
Septum — *continued*
Nasal Ø9TM
Ventricular Ø2TM
Sinus
Accessory Ø9TP
Ethmoid
Left Ø9TV
Right Ø9TU
Frontal
Left Ø9TT
Right Ø9TS
Mastoid
Left Ø9TC
Right Ø9TB
Maxillary
Left Ø9TR
Right Ø9TQ
Sphenoid
Left Ø9TX
Right Ø9TW
Spleen Ø7TP
Sternum ØPTØØZZ
Stomach ØDT6
Pylorus ØDT7
Tarsal
Left ØQTMØZZ
Right ØQTLØZZ
Tendon
Abdomen
Left ØLTG
Right ØLTF
Ankle
Left ØLTT
Right ØLTS
Foot
Left ØLTW
Right ØLTV
Hand
Left ØLT8
Right ØLT7
Head and Neck ØLTØ
Hip
Left ØLTK
Right ØLTJ
Knee
Left ØLTR
Right ØLTQ
Lower Arm and Wrist
Left ØLT6
Right ØLT5
Lower Leg
Left ØLTP
Right ØLTN
Perineum ØLTH
Shoulder
Left ØLT2
Right ØLT1
Thorax
Left ØLTD
Right ØLTC
Trunk
Left ØLTB
Right ØLT9
Upper Arm
Left ØLT4
Right ØLT3
Upper Leg
Left ØLTM
Right ØLTL
Testis
Bilateral ØVTC
Left ØVTB
Right ØVT9
Thymus Ø7TM
Thyroid Gland ØGTK
Left Lobe ØGTG
Right Lobe ØGTH
Thyroid Gland Isthmus ØGTJ
Tibia
Left ØQTHØZZ
Right ØQTGØZZ
Toe Nail ØHTRXZZ
Tongue ØCT7
Tonsils ØCTP
Tooth
Lower ØCTXØZ
Upper ØCTWØZ
Trachea ØBT1

Resection — *continued*
Tunica Vaginalis
Left ØVT7
Right ØVT6
Turbinate, Nasal Ø9TL
Tympanic Membrane
Left Ø9T8
Right Ø9T7
Ulna
Left ØPTLØZZ
Right ØPTKØZZ
Ureter
Left ØTT7
Right ØTT6
Urethra ØTTD
Uterine Supporting Structure ØUT4
Uterus ØUT9
Uvula ØCTN
Vagina ØUTG
Valve, Pulmonary Ø2TH
Vas Deferens
Bilateral ØVTQ
Left ØVTP
Right ØVTN
Vesicle
Bilateral ØVT3
Left ØVT2
Right ØVT1
Vitreous
Left Ø8T53ZZ
Right Ø8T43ZZ
Vocal Cord
Left ØCTV
Right ØCTT
Vulva ØUTM
Resection, Left ventricular outflow tract obstruction (LVOT) *see* Dilation, Ventricle, Left Ø27L
Resection, Subaortic membrane (Left ventricular outflow tract obstruction) *see* Dilation, Ventricle, Left Ø27L
Restoration, Cardiac, Single, Rhythm 5A22Ø4Z
RestoreAdvanced neurostimulator (SureScan) (MRI Safe) *use* Stimulator Generator, Multiple Array Rechargeable in ØJH
RestoreSensor neurostimulator (SureScan) (MRI Safe) *use* Stimulator Generator, Multiple Array Rechargeable in ØJH
RestoreUltra neurostimulator (SureScan) (MRI Safe) *use* Stimulator Generator, Multiple Array Rechargeable in ØJH
Restriction
Ampulla of Vater ØFVC
Anus ØDVQ
Aorta
Abdominal Ø4VØ
Intraluminal Device, Branched or Fenestrated Ø4VØ
Thoracic
Ascending/Arch, Intraluminal Device, Branched or Fenestrated Ø2VX
Descending, Intraluminal Device, Branched or Fenestrated Ø2VW
Artery
Anterior Tibial
Left Ø4VQ
Right Ø4VP
Axillary
Left Ø3V6
Right Ø3V5
Brachial
Left Ø3V8
Right Ø3V7
Celiac Ø4V1
Colic
Left Ø4V7
Middle Ø4V8
Right Ø4V6
Common Carotid
Left Ø3VJ
Right Ø3VH
Common Iliac
Left Ø4VD
Right Ø4VC
External Carotid
Left Ø3VN
Right Ø3VM
External Iliac
Left Ø4VJ

Restriction — *continued*
Artery — *continued*
External Iliac — *continued*
Right Ø4VH
Face Ø3VR
Femoral
Left Ø4VL
Right Ø4VK
Foot
Left Ø4VW
Right Ø4VV
Gastric Ø4V2
Hand
Left Ø3VF
Right Ø3VD
Hepatic Ø4V3
Inferior Mesenteric Ø4VB
Innominate Ø3V2
Internal Carotid
Left Ø3VL
Right Ø3VK
Internal Iliac
Left Ø4VF
Right Ø4VE
Internal Mammary
Left Ø3V1
Right Ø3VØ
Intracranial Ø3VG
Lower Ø4VY
Peroneal
Left Ø4VU
Right Ø4VT
Popliteal
Left Ø4VN
Right Ø4VM
Posterior Tibial
Left Ø4VS
Right Ø4VR
Pulmonary
Left Ø2VR
Right Ø2VQ
Pulmonary Trunk Ø2VP
Radial
Left Ø3VC
Right Ø3VB
Renal
Left Ø4VA
Right Ø4V9
Splenic Ø4V4
Subclavian
Left Ø3V4
Right Ø3V3
Superior Mesenteric Ø4V5
Temporal
Left Ø3VT
Right Ø3VS
Thyroid
Left Ø3VV
Right Ø3VU
Ulnar
Left Ø3VA
Right Ø3V9
Upper Ø3VY
Vertebral
Left Ø3VQ
Right Ø3VP
Bladder ØTVB
Bladder Neck ØTVC
Bronchus
Lingula ØBV9
Lower Lobe
Left ØBVB
Right ØBV6
Main
Left ØBV7
Right ØBV3
Middle Lobe, Right ØBV5
Upper Lobe
Left ØBV8
Right ØBV4
Carina ØBV2
Cecum ØDVH
Cervix ØUVC
Cisterna Chyli Ø7VL
Colon
Ascending ØDVK
Descending ØDVM
Sigmoid ØDVN
Transverse ØDVL

Restriction — *continued*
Duct
Common Bile ØFV9
Cystic ØFV8
Hepatic
Common ØFV7
Left ØFV6
Right ØFV5
Lacrimal
Left Ø8VY
Right Ø8VX
Pancreatic ØFVD
Accessory ØFVF
Parotid
Left ØCVC
Right ØCVB
Duodenum ØDV9
Esophagogastric Junction ØDV4
Esophagus ØDV5
Lower ØDV3
Middle ØDV2
Upper ØDV1
Heart Ø2VA
Ileocecal Valve ØDVC
Ileum ØDVB
Intestine
Large ØDVE
Left ØDVG
Right ØDVF
Small ØDV8
Jejunum ØDVA
Kidney Pelvis
Left ØTV4
Right ØTV3
Lymphatic
Aortic Ø7VD
Axillary
Left Ø7V6
Right Ø7V5
Head Ø7VØ
Inguinal
Left Ø7VJ
Right Ø7VH
Internal Mammary
Left Ø7V9
Right Ø7V8
Lower Extremity
Left Ø7VG
Right Ø7VF
Mesenteric Ø7VB
Neck
Left Ø7V2
Right Ø7V1
Pelvis Ø7VC
Thoracic Duct Ø7VK
Thorax Ø7V7
Upper Extremity
Left Ø7V4
Right Ø7V3
Rectum ØDVP
Stomach ØDV6
Pylorus ØDV7
Trachea ØBV1
Ureter
Left ØTV7
Right ØTV6
Urethra ØTVD
Valve, Mitral Ø2VG
Vein
Axillary
Left Ø5V8
Right Ø5V7
Azygos Ø5VØ
Basilic
Left Ø5VC
Right Ø5VB
Brachial
Left Ø5VA
Right Ø5V9
Cephalic
Left Ø5VF
Right Ø5VD
Colic Ø6V7
Common Iliac
Left Ø6VD
Right Ø6VC
Esophageal Ø6V3
External Iliac
Left Ø6VG

Subterms under main terms may continue to next column or page

Restriction — *continued*
- Vein — *continued*
  - External Iliac — *continued*
    - Right Ø6VF
  - External Jugular
    - Left Ø5VQ
    - Right Ø5VP
  - Face
    - Left Ø5VV
    - Right Ø5VT
  - Femoral
    - Left Ø6VN
    - Right Ø6VM
  - Foot
    - Left Ø6VV
    - Right Ø6VT
  - Gastric Ø6V2
  - Hand
    - Left Ø5VH
    - Right Ø5VG
  - Hemiazygos Ø5V1
  - Hepatic Ø6V4
  - Hypogastric
    - Left Ø6VJ
    - Right Ø6VH
  - Inferior Mesenteric Ø6V6
  - Innominate
    - Left Ø5V4
    - Right Ø5V3
  - Internal Jugular
    - Left Ø5VN
    - Right Ø5VM
  - Intracranial Ø5VL
  - Lower Ø6VY
  - Portal Ø6V8
  - Pulmonary
    - Left Ø2VT
    - Right Ø2VS
  - Renal
    - Left Ø6VB
    - Right Ø6V9
  - Saphenous
    - Left Ø6VQ
    - Right Ø6VP
  - Splenic Ø6V1
  - Subclavian
    - Left Ø5V6
    - Right Ø5V5
  - Superior Mesenteric Ø6V5
  - Upper Ø5VY
  - Vertebral
    - Left Ø5VS
    - Right Ø5VR
- Vena Cava
  - Inferior Ø6VØ
  - Superior Ø2VV
- Ventricle, Left Ø2VL

Resurfacing Device
- Removal of device from
  - Left ØSPBØBZ
  - Right ØSP9ØBZ
- Revision of device in
  - Left ØSWBØBZ
  - Right ØSW9ØBZ
- Supplement
  - Left ØSUBØBZ
    - Acetabular Surface ØSUEØBZ
    - Femoral Surface ØSUSØBZ
  - Right ØSU9ØBZ
    - Acetabular Surface ØSUAØBZ
    - Femoral Surface ØSURØBZ

Resuscitation
- Cardiopulmonary *see* Assistance, Cardiac 5AØ2
- Cardioversion 5A22Ø4Z
- Defibrillation 5A22Ø4Z
- Endotracheal intubation *see* Insertion of device in, Trachea ØBH1
- External chest compression, manual 5A12Ø12
- External chest compression, mechanical 5A1221J
- Pulmonary 5A19Ø54

Resuscitative endovascular balloon occlusion of the aorta (REBOA)
- Ø2LW3DJ
- Ø4LØ3DJ

Resuture, Heart valve prosthesis *see* Revision of device in, Heart and Great Vessels Ø2W

Retained placenta, manual removal *see* Extraction, Products of Conception, Retained 1ØD1

Retraining
- Cardiac *see* Motor Treatment, Rehabilitation FØ7
- Vocational *see* Activities of Daily Living Treatment, Rehabilitation FØ8

Retrogasserian rhizotomy *see* Division, Nerve, Trigeminal ØØ8K

Retroperitoneal cavity *use* Retroperitoneum

Retroperitoneal lymph node *use* Lymphatic, Aortic

Retroperitoneal space *use* Retroperitoneum

Retropharyngeal lymph node
- *use* Lymphatic, Left Neck
- *use* Lymphatic, Right Neck

Retropharyngeal space *use* Neck

Retropubic space *use* Pelvic Cavity

Reveal (LINQ) (DX) (XT) *use* Monitoring Device

Reverse total shoulder replacement *see* Replacement, Upper Joints ØRR

Reverse® Shoulder Prosthesis *use* Synthetic Substitute, Reverse Ball and Socket in ØRR

Revision
- Correcting a portion of existing device *see* Revision of device in
- Removal of device without replacement *see* Removal of device from
- Replacement of existing device
  - *see* Removal of device from
  - *see* Root operation to place new device, e.g., Insertion, Replacement, Supplement

Revision of device in
- Abdominal Wall ØWWF
- Acetabulum
  - Left ØQW5
  - Right ØQW4
- Anal Sphincter ØDWR
- Anus ØDWQ
- Artery
  - Lower Ø4WY
  - Upper Ø3WY
- Auditory Ossicle
  - Left Ø9WA
  - Right Ø9W9
- Back
  - Lower ØWWL
  - Upper ØWWK
- Bladder ØTWB
- Bone
  - Facial ØNWW
  - Lower ØQWY
  - Nasal ØNWB
  - Pelvic
    - Left ØQW3
    - Right ØQW2
  - Upper ØPWY
- Bone Marrow Ø7WT
- Brain ØØWØ
- Breast
  - Left ØHWU
  - Right ØHWT
- Bursa and Ligament
  - Lower ØMWY
  - Upper ØMWX
- Carpal
  - Left ØPWN
  - Right ØPWM
- Cavity, Cranial ØWW1
- Cerebral Ventricle ØØW6
- Chest Wall ØWW8
- Cisterna Chyli Ø7WL
- Clavicle
  - Left ØPWB
  - Right ØPW9
- Coccyx ØQWS
- Diaphragm ØBWT
- Disc
  - Cervical Vertebral ØRW3
  - Cervicothoracic Vertebral ØRW5
  - Lumbar Vertebral ØSW2
  - Lumbosacral ØSW4
  - Thoracic Vertebral ØRW9
  - Thoracolumbar Vertebral ØRWB
- Duct
  - Hepatobiliary ØFWB
  - Pancreatic ØFWD
- Ear
  - Inner
    - Left Ø9WE
    - Right Ø9WD
  - Left Ø9WJ

Revision of device in — *continued*
- Ear — *continued*
  - Right Ø9WH
- Epididymis and Spermatic Cord ØVWM
- Esophagus ØDW5
- Extremity
  - Lower
    - Left ØYWB
    - Right ØYW9
  - Upper
    - Left ØXW7
    - Right ØXW6
- Eye
  - Left Ø8W1
  - Right Ø8WØ
- Face ØWW2
- Fallopian Tube ØUW8
- Femoral Shaft
  - Left ØQW9
  - Right ØQW8
- Femur
  - Lower
    - Left ØQWC
    - Right ØQWB
  - Upper
    - Left ØQW7
    - Right ØQW6
- Fibula
  - Left ØQWK
  - Right ØQWJ
- Finger Nail ØHWQX
- Gallbladder ØFW4
- Gastrointestinal Tract ØWWP
- Genitourinary Tract ØWWR
- Gland
  - Adrenal ØGW5
  - Endocrine ØGWS
  - Pituitary ØGWØ
  - Salivary ØCWA
- Glenoid Cavity
  - Left ØPW8
  - Right ØPW7
- Great Vessel Ø2WY
- Hair ØHWSX
- Head ØWWØ
- Heart Ø2WA
- Humeral Head
  - Left ØPWD
  - Right ØPWC
- Humeral Shaft
  - Left ØPWG
  - Right ØPWF
- Intestinal Tract
  - Lower ØDWD
  - Upper ØDWØ
- Intestine
  - Large ØDWE
  - Small ØDW8
- Jaw
  - Lower ØWW5
  - Upper ØWW4
- Joint
  - Acromioclavicular
    - Left ØRWH
    - Right ØRWG
  - Ankle
    - Left ØSWG
    - Right ØSWF
  - Carpal
    - Left ØRWR
    - Right ØRWQ
  - Carpometacarpal
    - Left ØRWT
    - Right ØRWS
  - Cervical Vertebral ØRW1
  - Cervicothoracic Vertebral ØRW4
  - Coccygeal ØSW6
  - Elbow
    - Left ØRWM
    - Right ØRWL
  - Finger Phalangeal
    - Left ØRWX
    - Right ØRWW
  - Hip
    - Left ØSWB
      - Acetabular Surface ØSWE
      - Femoral Surface ØSWS
    - Right ØSW9
      - Acetabular Surface ØSWA

Revision of device in — *continued*
Joint — *continued*
Hip — *continued*
Right — *continued*
Femoral Surface ØSWR
Knee
Left ØSWD
Femoral Surface ØSWU
Tibial Surface ØSWW
Right ØSWC
Femoral Surface ØSWT
Tibial Surface ØSWV
Lumbar Vertebral ØSWØ
Lumbosacral ØSW3
Metacarpophalangeal
Left ØRWV
Right ØRWU
Metatarsal-Phalangeal
Left ØSWN
Right ØSWM
Occipital-cervical ØRWØ
Sacrococcygeal ØSW5
Sacroiliac
Left ØSW8
Right ØSW7
Shoulder
Left ØRWK
Right ØRWJ
Sternoclavicular
Left ØRWF
Right ØRWE
Tarsal
Left ØSWJ
Right ØSWH
Tarsometatarsal
Left ØSWL
Right ØSWK
Temporomandibular
Left ØRWD
Right ØRWC
Thoracic Vertebral ØRW6
Thoracolumbar Vertebral ØRWA
Toe Phalangeal
Left ØSWQ
Right ØSWP
Wrist
Left ØRWP
Right ØRWN
Kidney ØTW5
Larynx ØCWS
Lens
Left Ø8WK
Right Ø8WJ
Liver ØFWØ
Lung
Left ØBWL
Right ØBWK
Lymphatic Ø7WN
Thoracic Duct Ø7WK
Mediastinum ØWWC
Mesentery ØDWV
Metacarpal
Left ØPWQ
Right ØPWP
Metatarsal
Left ØQWP
Right ØQWN
Mouth and Throat ØCWY
Muscle
Extraocular
Left Ø8WM
Right Ø8WL
Lower ØKWY
Upper ØKWX
Nasal Mucosa and Soft Tissue Ø9WK
Neck ØWW6
Nerve
Cranial ØØWE
Peripheral Ø1WY
Omentum ØDWU
Ovary ØUW3
Pancreas ØFWG
Parathyroid Gland ØGWR
Patella
Left ØQWF
Right ØQWD
Pelvic Cavity ØWWJ
Penis ØVWS
Pericardial Cavity ØWWD

Revision of device in — *continued*
Perineum
Female ØWWN
Male ØWWM
Peritoneal Cavity ØWWG
Peritoneum ØDWW
Phalanx
Finger
Left ØPWV
Right ØPWT
Thumb
Left ØPWS
Right ØPWR
Toe
Left ØQWR
Right ØQWQ
Pineal Body ØGW1
Pleura ØBWQ
Pleural Cavity
Left ØWWB
Right ØWW9
Prostate and Seminal Vesicles ØVW4
Radius
Left ØPWJ
Right ØPWH
Respiratory Tract ØWWQ
Retroperitoneum ØWWH
Ribs
1 to 2 ØPW1
3 or More ØPW2
Sacrum ØQW1
Scapula
Left ØPW6
Right ØPW5
Scrotum and Tunica Vaginalis ØVW8
Septum
Atrial Ø2W5
Ventricular Ø2WM
Sinus Ø9WY
Skin ØHWPX
Skull ØNWØ
Spinal Canal ØØWU
Spinal Cord ØØWV
Spleen Ø7WP
Sternum ØPWØ
Stomach ØDW6
Subcutaneous Tissue and Fascia
Head and Neck ØJWS
Lower Extremity ØJWW
Trunk ØJWT
Upper Extremity ØJWV
Tarsal
Left ØQWM
Right ØQWL
Tendon
Lower ØLWY
Upper ØLWX
Testis ØVWD
Thymus Ø7WM
Thyroid Gland ØGWK
Tibia
Left ØQWH
Right ØQWG
Toe Nail ØHWRX
Trachea ØBW1
Tracheobronchial Tree ØBWØ
Tympanic Membrane
Left Ø9W8
Right Ø9W7
Ulna
Left ØPWL
Right ØPWK
Ureter ØTW9
Urethra ØTWD
Uterus and Cervix ØUWD
Vagina and Cul-de-sac ØUWH
Valve
Aortic Ø2WF
Mitral Ø2WG
Pulmonary Ø2WH
Tricuspid Ø2WJ
Vas Deferens ØVWR
Vein
Azygos Ø5WØ
Innominate
Left Ø5W4
Right Ø5W3
Lower Ø6WY
Upper Ø5WY

Revision of device in — *continued*
Vertebra
Cervical ØPW3
Lumbar ØQWØ
Thoracic ØPW4
Vulva ØUWM
Revo MRI™ SureScan® pacemaker *use* Pacemaker, Dual Chamber in ØJH
rhBMP-2 *use* Recombinant Bone Morphogenetic Protein
Rheos® System device *use* Stimulator Generator in Subcutaneous Tissue and Fascia
Rheos® System lead *use* Stimulator Lead in Upper Arteries
Rhinopharynx *use* Nasopharynx
Rhinoplasty
see Alteration, Nasal Mucosa and Soft Tissue Ø9ØK
see Repair, Nasal Mucosa and Soft Tissue Ø9QK
see Replacement, Nasal Mucosa and Soft Tissue Ø9RK
see Supplement, Nasal Mucosa and Soft Tissue Ø9UK
Rhinorrhaphy *see* Repair, Nasal Mucosa and Soft Tissue Ø9QK
Rhinoscopy Ø9JKXZZ
Rhizotomy
see Division, Central Nervous System and Cranial Nerves ØØ8
see Division, Peripheral Nervous System Ø18
Rhomboid major muscle
use Trunk Muscle, Left
use Trunk Muscle, Right
Rhomboid minor muscle
use Trunk Muscle, Left
use Trunk Muscle, Right
Rhythm electrocardiogram *see* Measurement, Cardiac 4AØ2
Rhytidectomy *see* Alteration, Face ØWØ2
Right ascending lumbar vein *use* Azygos Vein
Right atrioventricular valve *use* Tricuspid Valve
Right auricular appendix *use* Atrium, Right
Right colic vein *use* Colic Vein
Right coronary sulcus *use* Heart, Right
Right gastric artery *use* Gastric Artery
Right gastroepiploic vein *use* Superior Mesenteric Vein
Right inferior phrenic vein *use* Inferior Vena Cava
Right inferior pulmonary vein *use* Pulmonary Vein, Right
Right jugular trunk *use* Lymphatic, Right Neck
Right lateral ventricle *use* Cerebral Ventricle
Right lymphatic duct *use* Lymphatic, Right Neck
Right ovarian vein *use* Inferior Vena Cava
Right second lumbar vein *use* Inferior Vena Cava
Right subclavian trunk *use* Lymphatic, Right Neck
Right subcostal vein *use* Azygos Vein
Right superior pulmonary vein *use* Pulmonary Vein, Right
Right suprarenal vein *use* Inferior Vena Cava
Right testicular vein *use* Inferior Vena Cava
Rima glottidis *use* Larynx
Risorius muscle *use* Facial Muscle
RNS System lead *use* Neurostimulator Lead in Central Nervous System and Cranial Nerves
RNS system neurostimulator generator *use* Neurostimulator Generator in Head and Facial Bones
Robotic Assisted Procedure
Extremity
Lower 8EØY
Upper 8EØX
Head and Neck Region 8EØ9
Trunk Region 8EØW
Robotic Waterjet Ablation, Destruction, Prostate XV5Ø8A4
Rotation of fetal head
Forceps 1ØSØ7ZZ
Manual 1ØSØXZZ
Round ligament of uterus *use* Uterine Supporting Structure
Round window
use Inner Ear, Left
use Inner Ear, Right
Roux-en-Y operation
see Bypass, Gastrointestinal System ØD1
see Bypass, Hepatobiliary System and Pancreas ØF1

Index

Revision of device in — Roux-en-Y operation

Rupture
Adhesions *see* Release
Fluid collection *see* Drainage
Ruxolitinib XWØDXT5

S

Sacral ganglion *use* Sacral Sympathetic Nerve
Sacral lymph node *use* Lymphatic, Pelvis
Sacral nerve modulation (SNM) lead *use* Stimulator Lead in Urinary System
Sacral neuromodulation lead *use* Stimulator Lead in Urinary System
Sacral splanchnic nerve *use* Sacral Sympathetic Nerve
Sacrectomy *see* Excision, Lower Bones ØQB
Sacrococcygeal ligament *use* Lower Spine Bursa and Ligament
Sacrococcygeal symphysis *use* Sacrococcygeal Joint
Sacroiliac ligament *use* Lower Spine Bursa and Ligament
Sacrospinous ligament *use* Lower Spine Bursa and Ligament
Sacrotuberous ligament *use* Lower Spine Bursa and Ligament
Salpingectomy
see Excision, Female Reproductive System ØUB
see Resection, Female Reproductive System ØUT
Salpingolysis *see* Release, Female Reproductive System ØUN
Salpingopexy
see Repair, Female Reproductive System ØUQ
see Reposition, Female Reproductive System ØUS
Salpingopharyngeus muscle *use* Tongue, Palate, Pharynx Muscle
Salpingoplasty
see Repair, Female Reproductive System ØUQ
see Supplement, Female Reproductive System ØUU
Salpingorrhaphy *see* Repair, Female Reproductive System ØUQ
Salpingoscopy ØUJ88ZZ
Salpingostomy *see* Drainage, Female Reproductive System ØU9
Salpingotomy *see* Drainage, Female Reproductive System ØU9
Salpinx
use Fallopian Tube, Left
use Fallopian Tube, Right
Saphenous nerve *use* Femoral Nerve
SAPIEN transcatheter aortic valve *use* Zooplastic Tissue in Heart and Great Vessels
Sarilumab XWØ
SARS-CoV-2 Antibody Detection, Serum/Plasma Nanoparticle Fluorescence XXE5XV7
SARS-CoV-2 Polymerase Chain Reaction, Nasopharyngeal Fluid XXE97U7
Sartorius muscle
use Upper Leg Muscle, Left
use Upper Leg Muscle, Right
Satralizumab-mwge XWØ1397
SAVAL below-the-knee (BTK) drug-eluting stent system
use Intraluminal Device, Sustained Release Drug-eluting in New Technology
use Intraluminal Device, Sustained Release Drug-eluting, Two in New Technology
use Intraluminal Device, Sustained Release Drug-eluting, Three in New Technology
use Intraluminal Device, Sustained Release Drug-eluting, Four or More in New Technology
Scalene muscle
use Neck Muscle, Left
use Neck Muscle, Right
Scan
Computerized Tomography (CT) *see* Computerized Tomography (CT Scan)
Radioisotope *see* Planar Nuclear Medicine Imaging
Scaphoid bone
use Carpal, Left
use Carpal, Right
Scapholunate ligament
use Wrist Bursa and Ligament, Left
use Wrist Bursa and Ligament, Right
Scaphotrapezium ligament
use Hand Bursa and Ligament, Left
use Hand Bursa and Ligament, Right
Scapulectomy
see Excision, Upper Bones ØPB
see Resection, Upper Bones ØPT
Scapulopexy
see Repair, Upper Bones ØPQ
see Reposition, Upper Bones ØPS
Scarpa's (vestibular) ganglion *use* Acoustic Nerve
Sclerectomy *see* Excision, Eye Ø8B
Sclerotherapy, mechanical *see* Destruction
Sclerotherapy, via injection of sclerosing agent *see* Introduction, Destructive Agent
Sclerotomy *see* Drainage, Eye Ø89
Scrotectomy
see Excision, Male Reproductive System ØVB
see Resection, Male Reproductive System ØVT
Scrotoplasty
see Repair, Male Reproductive System ØVQ
see Supplement, Male Reproductive System ØVU
Scrotorrhaphy *see* Repair, Male Reproductive System ØVQ
Scrototomy *see* Drainage, Male Reproductive System ØV9
Sebaceous gland *use* Skin
Second cranial nerve *use* Optic Nerve
Section, cesarean *see* Extraction, Pregnancy 1ØD
Secura (DR) (VR) *use* Defibrillator Generator in ØJH
Sella turcica *use* Sphenoid Bone
Semicircular canal
use Inner Ear, Left
use Inner Ear, Right
Semimembranosus muscle
use Upper Leg Muscle, Left
use Upper Leg Muscle, Right
Semitendinosus muscle
use Upper Leg Muscle, Left
use Upper Leg Muscle, Right
Sentinel™ Cerebral Protection System (CPS) X2A5312
Seprafilm *use* Adhesion Barrier
Septal cartilage *use* Nasal Septum
Septectomy
see Excision, Ear, Nose, Sinus Ø9B
see Excision, Heart and Great Vessels Ø2B
see Resection, Ear, Nose, Sinus Ø9T
see Resection, Heart and Great Vessels Ø2T
Septoplasty
see Repair, Ear, Nose, Sinus Ø9Q
see Repair, Heart and Great Vessels Ø2Q
see Replacement, Ear, Nose, Sinus Ø9R
see Replacement, Heart and Great Vessels Ø2R
see Reposition, Ear, Nose, Sinus Ø9S
see Supplement, Ear, Nose, Sinus Ø9U
see Supplement, Heart and Great Vessels Ø2U
Septostomy, balloon atrial Ø2163Z7
Septotomy *see* Drainage, Ear, Nose, Sinus Ø99
Sequestrectomy, bone *see* Extirpation
Serratus anterior muscle
use Thorax Muscle, Left
use Thorax Muscle, Right
Serratus posterior muscle
use Trunk Muscle, Left
use Trunk Muscle, Right
Seventh cranial nerve *use* Facial Nerve
Shapshot_NIR 8EØ2XDZ
Sheffield hybrid external fixator
use External Fixation Device, Hybrid in ØPH
use External Fixation Device, Hybrid in ØPS
use External Fixation Device, Hybrid in ØQH
use External Fixation Device, Hybrid in ØQS
Sheffield ring external fixator
use External Fixation Device, Ring in ØPH
use External Fixation Device, Ring in ØPS
use External Fixation Device, Ring in ØQH
use External Fixation Device, Ring in ØQS
Shirodkar cervical cerclage ØUVC7ZZ
Shock Wave Therapy, Musculoskeletal 6A93
Shockwave Intravascular Lithotripsy (Shockwave IVL) *see* Fragmentation
Short gastric artery *use* Splenic Artery
Shortening
see Excision
see Repair
see Reposition
Shunt creation *see* Bypass
Sialoadenectomy
Complete *see* Resection, Mouth and Throat ØCT
Sialoadenectomy — *continued*
Partial *see* Excision, Mouth and Throat ØCB
Sialodochoplasty
see Repair, Mouth and Throat ØCQ
see Replacement, Mouth and Throat ØCR
see Supplement, Mouth and Throat ØCU
Sialoectomy
see Excision, Mouth and Throat ØCB
see Resection, Mouth and Throat ØCT
Sialography *see* Plain Radiography, Ear, Nose, Mouth and Throat B9Ø
Sialolithotomy *see* Extirpation, Mouth and Throat ØCC
S-ICD™ lead *use* Subcutaneous Defibrillator Lead in Subcutaneous Tissue and Fascia
Sigmoid artery *use* Inferior Mesenteric Artery
Sigmoid flexure *use* Sigmoid Colon
Sigmoid vein *use* Inferior Mesenteric Vein
Sigmoidectomy
see Excision, Gastrointestinal System ØDB
see Resection, Gastrointestinal System ØDT
Sigmoidorrhaphy *see* Repair, Gastrointestinal System ØDQ
Sigmoidoscopy ØDJD8ZZ
Sigmoidotomy *see* Drainage, Gastrointestinal System ØD9
Single lead pacemaker (atrium) (ventricle) *use* Pacemaker, Single Chamber in ØJH
Single lead rate responsive pacemaker (atrium) (ventricle) *use* Pacemaker, Single Chamber Rate Responsive in ØJH
Single-use Duodenoscope XFJ
Single-use Oversleeve with Intraoperative Colonic Irrigation XDPH8K7
Sinoatrial node *use* Conduction Mechanism
Sinogram
Abdominal Wall *see* Fluoroscopy, Abdomen and Pelvis BW11
Chest Wall *see* Plain Radiography, Chest BWØ3
Retroperitoneum *see* Fluoroscopy, Abdomen and Pelvis BW11
Sinus venosus *use* Atrium, Right
Sinusectomy
see Excision, Ear, Nose, Sinus Ø9B
see Resection, Ear, Nose, Sinus Ø9T
Sinusoscopy Ø9JY4ZZ
Sinusotomy *see* Drainage, Ear, Nose, Sinus Ø99
Sirolimus-eluting coronary stent *use* Intraluminal Device, Drug-eluting in Heart and Great Vessels
Sixth cranial nerve *use* Abducens Nerve
Size reduction, breast *see* Excision, Skin and Breast ØHB
SJM Biocor® Stented Valve System *use* Zooplastic Tissue in Heart and Great Vessels
Skene's (paraurethral) gland *use* Vestibular Gland
Skin Substitute, Porcine Liver Derived, Replacement XHRPXL2
Sling
Fascial, orbicularis muscle (mouth) *see* Supplement, Muscle, Facial ØKU1
Levator muscle, for urethral suspension *see* Reposition, Bladder Neck ØTSC
Pubococcygeal, for urethral suspension *see* Reposition, Bladder Neck ØTSC
Rectum *see* Reposition, Rectum ØDSP
Small bowel series *see* Fluoroscopy, Bowel, Small BD13
Small saphenous vein
use Saphenous Vein, Left
use Saphenous Vein, Right
Snapshot_NIR 8EØ2XDZ
Snaring, polyp, colon *see* Excision, Gastrointestinal System ØDB
Solar (celiac) plexus *use* Abdominal Sympathetic Nerve
Soleus muscle
use Lower Leg Muscle, Left
use Lower Leg Muscle, Right
Soliris® *use* Eculizumab
Spacer
Insertion of device in
Disc
Lumbar Vertebral ØSH2
Lumbosacral ØSH4
Joint
Acromioclavicular
Left ØRHH
Right ØRHG

Spacer — *continued*
Insertion of device in — *continued*
Joint — *continued*
Ankle
Left ØSHG
Right ØSHF
Carpal
Left ØRHR
Right ØRHQ
Carpometacarpal
Left ØRHT
Right ØRHS
Cervical Vertebral ØRH1
Cervicothoracic Vertebral ØRH4
Coccygeal ØSH6
Elbow
Left ØRHM
Right ØRHL
Finger Phalangeal
Left ØRHX
Right ØRHW
Hip
Left ØSHB
Right ØSH9
Knee
Left ØSHD
Right ØSHC
Lumbar Vertebral ØSHØ
Lumbosacral ØSH3
Metacarpophalangeal
Left ØRHV
Right ØRHU
Metatarsal-Phalangeal
Left ØSHN
Right ØSHM
Occipital-cervical ØRHØ
Sacrococcygeal ØSH5
Sacroiliac
Left ØSH8
Right ØSH7
Shoulder
Left ØRHK
Right ØRHJ
Sternoclavicular
Left ØRHF
Right ØRHE
Tarsal
Left ØSHJ
Right ØSHH
Tarsometatarsal
Left ØSHL
Right ØSHK
Temporomandibular
Left ØRHD
Right ØRHC
Thoracic Vertebral ØRH6
Thoracolumbar Vertebral ØRHA
Toe Phalangeal
Left ØSHQ
Right ØSHP
Wrist
Left ØRHP
Right ØRHN
Removal of device from
Acromioclavicular
Left ØRPH
Right ØRPG
Ankle
Left ØSPG
Right ØSPF
Carpal
Left ØRPR
Right ØRPQ
Carpometacarpal
Left ØRPT
Right ØRPS
Cervical Vertebral ØRP1
Cervicothoracic Vertebral ØRP4
Coccygeal ØSP6
Elbow
Left ØRPM
Right ØRPL
Finger Phalangeal
Left ØRPX
Right ØRPW
Hip
Left ØSPB
Right ØSP9

Spacer — *continued*
Removal of device from — *continued*
Knee
Left ØSPD
Right ØSPC
Lumbar Vertebral ØSPØ
Lumbosacral ØSP3
Metacarpophalangeal
Left ØRPV
Right ØRPU
Metatarsal-Phalangeal
Left ØSPN
Right ØSPM
Occipital-cervical ØRPØ
Sacrococcygeal ØSP5
Sacroiliac
Left ØSP8
Right ØSP7
Shoulder
Left ØRPK
Right ØRPJ
Sternoclavicular
Left ØRPF
Right ØRPE
Tarsal
Left ØSPJ
Right ØSPH
Tarsometatarsal
Left ØSPL
Right ØSPK
Temporomandibular
Left ØRPD
Right ØRPC
Thoracic Vertebral ØRP6
Thoracolumbar Vertebral ØRPA
Toe Phalangeal
Left ØSPQ
Right ØSPP
Wrist
Left ØRPP
Right ØRPN
Revision of device in
Acromioclavicular
Left ØRWH
Right ØRWG
Ankle
Left ØSWG
Right ØSWF
Carpal
Left ØRWR
Right ØRWQ
Carpometacarpal
Left ØRWT
Right ØRWS
Cervical Vertebral ØRW1
Cervicothoracic Vertebral ØRW4
Coccygeal ØSW6
Elbow
Left ØRWM
Right ØRWL
Finger Phalangeal
Left ØRWX
Right ØRWW
Hip
Left ØSWB
Right ØSW9
Knee
Left ØSWD
Right ØSWC
Lumbar Vertebral ØSWØ
Lumbosacral ØSW3
Metacarpophalangeal
Left ØRWV
Right ØRWU
Metatarsal-Phalangeal
Left ØSWN
Right ØSWM
Occipital-cervical ØRWØ
Sacrococcygeal ØSW5
Sacroiliac
Left ØSW8
Right ØSW7
Shoulder
Left ØRWK
Right ØRWJ
Sternoclavicular
Left ØRWF
Right ØRWE

Spacer — *continued*
Revision of device in — *continued*
Tarsal
Left ØSWJ
Right ØSWH
Tarsometatarsal
Left ØSWL
Right ØSWK
Temporomandibular
Left ØRWD
Right ØRWC
Thoracic Vertebral ØRW6
Thoracolumbar Vertebral ØRWA
Toe Phalangeal
Left ØSWQ
Right ØSWP
Wrist
Left ØRWP
Right ØRWN
Spacer, Articulating (Antibiotic) *use* Articulating Spacer in Lower Joints
Spacer, Static (Antibiotic) *use* Spacer in Lower Joints
Spectroscopy
Intravascular Near Infrared 8EØ23DZ
Near Infrared *see* Physiological Systems and Anatomical Regions 8EØ
Speech Assessment FØØ
Speech therapy *see* Speech Treatment, Rehabilitation FØ6
Speech Treatment FØ6
Sphenoidectomy
see Excision, Ear, Nose, Sinus Ø9B
see Excision, Head and Facial Bones ØNB
see Resection, Ear, Nose, Sinus Ø9T
see Resection, Head and Facial Bones ØNT
Sphenoidotomy *see* Drainage, Ear, Nose, Sinus Ø99
Sphenomandibular ligament *use* Head and Neck Bursa and Ligament
Sphenopalatine (pterygopalatine) ganglion *use* Head and Neck Sympathetic Nerve
Sphincterorrhaphy, anal *see* Repair, Anal Sphincter ØDQR
Sphincterotomy, anal
see Division, Anal Sphincter ØD8R
see Drainage, Anal Sphincter ØD9R
Spinal cord neurostimulator lead *use* Neurostimulator Lead in Central Nervous System and Cranial Nerves
Spinal growth rods, magnetically controlled *use* Magnetically Controlled Growth Rod(s) in New Technology
Spinal nerve, cervical *use* Cervical Nerve
Spinal nerve, lumbar *use* Lumbar Nerve
Spinal nerve, sacral *use* Sacral Nerve
Spinal nerve, thoracic *use* Thoracic Nerve
Spinal Stabilization Device
Facet Replacement
Cervical Vertebral ØRH1
Cervicothoracic Vertebral ØRH4
Lumbar Vertebral ØSHØ
Lumbosacral ØSH3
Occipital-cervical ØRHØ
Thoracic Vertebral ØRH6
Thoracolumbar Vertebral ØRHA
Interspinous Process
Cervical Vertebral ØRH1
Cervicothoracic Vertebral ØRH4
Lumbar Vertebral ØSHØ
Lumbosacral ØSH3
Occipital-cervical ØRHØ
Thoracic Vertebral ØRH6
Thoracolumbar Vertebral ØRHA
Pedicle-Based
Cervical Vertebral ØRH1
Cervicothoracic Vertebral ØRH4
Lumbar Vertebral ØSHØ
Lumbosacral ØSH3
Occipital-cervical ØRHØ
Thoracic Vertebral ØRH6
Thoracolumbar Vertebral ØRHA
SpineJack® system *use* Synthetic Substitute, Mechanically Expandable (Paired) in New Technology
Spinous process
use Cervical Vertebra
use Lumbar Vertebra
use Thoracic Vertebra
Spiral ganglion *use* Acoustic Nerve

Spiration IBV™ Valve System *use* Intraluminal Device, Endobronchial Valve in Respiratory System
Splenectomy
see Excision, Lymphatic and Hemic Systems Ø7B
see Resection, Lymphatic and Hemic Systems Ø7T
Splenic flexure *use* Transverse Colon
Splenic plexus *use* Abdominal Sympathetic Nerve
Splenius capitis muscle *use* Head Muscle
Splenius cervicis muscle
use Neck Muscle, Left
use Neck Muscle, Right
Splenolysis *see* Release, Lymphatic and Hemic Systems Ø7N
Splenopexy
see Repair, Lymphatic and Hemic Systems Ø7Q
see Reposition, Lymphatic and Hemic Systems Ø7S
Splenoplasty *see* Repair, Lymphatic and Hemic Systems Ø7Q
Splenorrhaphy *see* Repair, Lymphatic and Hemic Systems Ø7Q
Splenotomy *see* Drainage, Lymphatic and Hemic Systems Ø79
Splinting, musculoskeletal *see* Immobilization, Anatomical Regions 2W3
SPRAVATO™ *use* Esketamine Hydrochloride
SPY PINPOINT fluorescence imaging system
see Monitoring, Physiological Systems 4A1
see Other Imaging, Hepatobiliary System and Pancreas BF5
SPY system intraoperative fluorescence cholangiography *see* Other Imaging, Hepatobiliary System and Pancreas BF5
SPY system intravascular fluorescence angiography *see* Monitoring, Physiological Systems 4A1
Staged hepatectomy
see Division, Hepatobiliary System and Pancreas ØF8
see Resection, Hepatobiliary System and Pancreas ØFT
Stapedectomy
see Excision, Ear, Nose, Sinus Ø9B
see Resection, Ear, Nose, Sinus Ø9T
Stapediolysis *see* Release, Ear, Nose, Sinus Ø9N
Stapedioplasty
see Repair, Ear, Nose, Sinus Ø9Q
see Replacement, Ear, Nose, Sinus Ø9R
see Supplement, Ear, Nose, Sinus Ø9U
Stapedotomy *see* Drainage, Ear, Nose, Sinus Ø99
Stapes
use Auditory Ossicle, Left
use Auditory Ossicle, Right
Static Spacer (Antibiotic) *use* Spacer in Lower Joints
STELARA® *use* Other New Technology Therapeutic Substance
Stellate ganglion *use* Head and Neck Sympathetic Nerve
Stem cell transplant *see* Transfusion, Circulatory 3Ø2
Stensen's duct
use Parotid Duct, Left
use Parotid Duct, Right
Stent, intraluminal (cardiovascular) (gastrointestinal) (hepatobiliary) (urinary) *use* Intraluminal Device
Stent retriever thrombectomy *see* Extirpation, Upper Arteries Ø3C
Stented tissue valve *use* Zooplastic Tissue in Heart and Great Vessels
Stereotactic Radiosurgery
Abdomen DW23
Adrenal Gland DG22
Bile Ducts DF22
Bladder DT22
Bone Marrow D72Ø
Brain DØ2Ø
Brain Stem DØ21
Breast
Left DM2Ø
Right DM21
Bronchus DB21
Cervix DU21
Chest DW22
Chest Wall DB27
Colon DD25
Diaphragm DB28
Duodenum DD22
Ear D92Ø
Esophagus DD2Ø

Stereotactic Radiosurgery — *continued*
Eye D82Ø
Gallbladder DF21
Gamma Beam
Abdomen DW23JZZ
Adrenal Gland DG22JZZ
Bile Ducts DF22JZZ
Bladder DT22JZZ
Bone Marrow D72ØJZZ
Brain DØ2ØJZZ
Brain Stem DØ21JZZ
Breast
Left DM2ØJZZ
Right DM21JZZ
Bronchus DB21JZZ
Cervix DU21JZZ
Chest DW22JZZ
Chest Wall DB27JZZ
Colon DD25JZZ
Diaphragm DB28JZZ
Duodenum DD22JZZ
Ear D92ØJZZ
Esophagus DD2ØJZZ
Eye D82ØJZZ
Gallbladder DF21JZZ
Gland
Adrenal DG22JZZ
Parathyroid DG24JZZ
Pituitary DG2ØJZZ
Thyroid DG25JZZ
Glands, Salivary D926JZZ
Head and Neck DW21JZZ
Ileum DD24JZZ
Jejunum DD23JZZ
Kidney DT2ØJZZ
Larynx D92BJZZ
Liver DF2ØJZZ
Lung DB22JZZ
Lymphatics
Abdomen D726JZZ
Axillary D724JZZ
Inguinal D728JZZ
Neck D723JZZ
Pelvis D727JZZ
Thorax D725JZZ
Mediastinum DB26JZZ
Mouth D924JZZ
Nasopharynx D92DJZZ
Neck and Head DW21JZZ
Nerve, Peripheral DØ27JZZ
Nose D921JZZ
Ovary DU2ØJZZ
Palate
Hard D928JZZ
Soft D929JZZ
Pancreas DF23JZZ
Parathyroid Gland DG24JZZ
Pelvic Region DW26JZZ
Pharynx D92CJZZ
Pineal Body DG21JZZ
Pituitary Gland DG2ØJZZ
Pleura DB25JZZ
Prostate DV2ØJZZ
Rectum DD27JZZ
Sinuses D927JZZ
Spinal Cord DØ26JZZ
Spleen D722JZZ
Stomach DD21JZZ
Testis DV21JZZ
Thymus D721JZZ
Thyroid Gland DG25JZZ
Tongue D925JZZ
Trachea DB2ØJZZ
Ureter DT21JZZ
Urethra DT23JZZ
Uterus DU22JZZ
Gland
Adrenal DG22
Parathyroid DG24
Pituitary DG2Ø
Thyroid DG25
Glands, Salivary D926
Head and Neck DW21
Ileum DD24
Jejunum DD23
Kidney DT2Ø
Larynx D92B
Liver DF2Ø
Lung DB22

Stereotactic Radiosurgery — *continued*
Lymphatics
Abdomen D726
Axillary D724
Inguinal D728
Neck D723
Pelvis D727
Thorax D725
Mediastinum DB26
Mouth D924
Nasopharynx D92D
Neck and Head DW21
Nerve, Peripheral DØ27
Nose D921
Other Photon
Abdomen DW23DZZ
Adrenal Gland DG22DZZ
Bile Ducts DF22DZZ
Bladder DT22DZZ
Bone Marrow D72ØDZZ
Brain DØ2ØDZZ
Brain Stem DØ21DZZ
Breast
Left DM2ØDZZ
Right DM21DZZ
Bronchus DB21DZZ
Cervix DU21DZZ
Chest DW22DZZ
Chest Wall DB27DZZ
Colon DD25DZZ
Diaphragm DB28DZZ
Duodenum DD22DZZ
Ear D92ØDZZ
Esophagus DD2ØDZZ
Eye D82ØDZZ
Gallbladder DF21DZZ
Gland
Adrenal DG22DZZ
Parathyroid DG24DZZ
Pituitary DG2ØDZZ
Thyroid DG25DZZ
Glands, Salivary D926DZZ
Head and Neck DW21DZZ
Ileum DD24DZZ
Jejunum DD23DZZ
Kidney DT2ØDZZ
Larynx D92BDZZ
Liver DF2ØDZZ
Lung DB22DZZ
Lymphatics
Abdomen D726DZZ
Axillary D724DZZ
Inguinal D728DZZ
Neck D723DZZ
Pelvis D727DZZ
Thorax D725DZZ
Mediastinum DB26DZZ
Mouth D924DZZ
Nasopharynx D92DDZZ
Neck and Head DW21DZZ
Nerve, Peripheral DØ27DZZ
Nose D921DZZ
Ovary DU2ØDZZ
Palate
Hard D928DZZ
Soft D929DZZ
Pancreas DF23DZZ
Parathyroid Gland DG24DZZ
Pelvic Region DW26DZZ
Pharynx D92CDZZ
Pineal Body DG21DZZ
Pituitary Gland DG2ØDZZ
Pleura DB25DZZ
Prostate DV2ØDZZ
Rectum DD27DZZ
Sinuses D927DZZ
Spinal Cord DØ26DZZ
Spleen D722DZZ
Stomach DD21DZZ
Testis DV21DZZ
Thymus D721DZZ
Thyroid Gland DG25DZZ
Tongue D925DZZ
Trachea DB2ØDZZ
Ureter DT21DZZ
Urethra DT23DZZ
Uterus DU22DZZ
Ovary DU2Ø

Stereotactic Radiosurgery — *continued*
- Palate
  - Hard D928
  - Soft D929
- Pancreas DF23
- Parathyroid Gland DG24
- Particulate
  - Abdomen DW23HZZ
  - Adrenal Gland DG22HZZ
  - Bile Ducts DF22HZZ
  - Bladder DT22HZZ
  - Bone Marrow D720HZZ
  - Brain DØ2ØHZZ
  - Brain Stem DØ21HZZ
  - Breast
    - Left DM2ØHZZ
    - Right DM21HZZ
  - Bronchus DB21HZZ
  - Cervix DU21HZZ
  - Chest DW22HZZ
  - Chest Wall DB27HZZ
  - Colon DD25HZZ
  - Diaphragm DB28HZZ
  - Duodenum DD22HZZ
  - Ear D92ØHZZ
  - Esophagus DD2ØHZZ
  - Eye D82ØHZZ
  - Gallbladder DF21HZZ
  - Gland
    - Adrenal DG22HZZ
    - Parathyroid DG24HZZ
    - Pituitary DG2ØHZZ
    - Thyroid DG25HZZ
  - Glands, Salivary D926HZZ
  - Head and Neck DW21HZZ
  - Ileum DD24HZZ
  - Jejunum DD23HZZ
  - Kidney DT2ØHZZ
  - Larynx D92BHZZ
  - Liver DF2ØHZZ
  - Lung DB22HZZ
  - Lymphatics
    - Abdomen D726HZZ
    - Axillary D724HZZ
    - Inguinal D728HZZ
    - Neck D723HZZ
    - Pelvis D727HZZ
    - Thorax D725HZZ
  - Mediastinum DB26HZZ
  - Mouth D924HZZ
  - Nasopharynx D92DHZZ
  - Neck and Head DW21HZZ
  - Nerve, Peripheral DØ27HZZ
  - Nose D921HZZ
  - Ovary DU2ØHZZ
  - Palate
    - Hard D928HZZ
    - Soft D929HZZ
  - Pancreas DF23HZZ
  - Parathyroid Gland DG24HZZ
  - Pelvic Region DW26HZZ
  - Pharynx D92CHZZ
  - Pineal Body DG21HZZ
  - Pituitary Gland DG2ØHZZ
  - Pleura DB25HZZ
  - Prostate DV2ØHZZ
  - Rectum DD27HZZ
  - Sinuses D927HZZ
  - Spinal Cord DØ26HZZ
  - Spleen D722HZZ
  - Stomach DD21HZZ
  - Testis DV21HZZ
  - Thymus D721HZZ
  - Thyroid Gland DG25HZZ
  - Tongue D925HZZ
  - Trachea DB2ØHZZ
  - Ureter DT21HZZ
  - Urethra DT23HZZ
  - Uterus DU22HZZ
- Pelvic Region DW26
- Pharynx D92C
- Pineal Body DG21
- Pituitary Gland DG2Ø
- Pleura DB25
- Prostate DV2Ø
- Rectum DD27
- Sinuses D927
- Spinal Cord DØ26
- Spleen D722

Stereotactic Radiosurgery — *continued*
- Stomach DD21
- Testis DV21
- Thymus D721
- Thyroid Gland DG25
- Tongue D925
- Trachea DB2Ø
- Ureter DT21
- Urethra DT23
- Uterus DU22

Steripath® Micro™ Blood Collection System XXE5XR7

Sternoclavicular ligament
- *use* Shoulder Bursa and Ligament, Left
- *use* Shoulder Bursa and Ligament, Right

Sternocleidomastoid artery
- *use* Thyroid Artery, Left
- *use* Thyroid Artery, Right

Sternocleidomastoid muscle
- *use* Neck Muscle, Left
- *use* Neck Muscle, Right

Sternocostal ligament *use* Sternum Bursa and Ligament

Sternotomy
- *see* Division, Sternum ØP8Ø
- *see* Drainage, Sternum ØP9Ø

Stimulation, cardiac
- Cardioversion 5A22Ø4Z
- Electrophysiologic testing *see* Measurement, Cardiac 4AØ2

Stimulator Generator
- Insertion of device in
  - Abdomen ØJH8
  - Back ØJH7
  - Chest ØJH6
- Multiple Array
  - Abdomen ØJH8
  - Back ØJH7
  - Chest ØJH6
- Multiple Array Rechargeable
  - Abdomen ØJH8
  - Back ØJH7
  - Chest ØJH6
- Removal of device from, Subcutaneous Tissue and Fascia, Trunk ØJPT
- Revision of device in, Subcutaneous Tissue and Fascia, Trunk ØJWT
- Single Array
  - Abdomen ØJH8
  - Back ØJH7
  - Chest ØJH6
- Single Array Rechargeable
  - Abdomen ØJH8
  - Back ØJH7
  - Chest ØJH6

Stimulator Lead
- Insertion of device in
  - Anal Sphincter ØDHR
  - Artery
    - Left Ø3HL
    - Right Ø3HK
  - Bladder ØTHB
  - Muscle
    - Lower ØKHY
    - Upper ØKHX
  - Stomach ØDH6
  - Ureter ØTH9
- Removal of device from
  - Anal Sphincter ØDPR
  - Artery, Upper Ø3PY
  - Bladder ØTPB
  - Muscle
    - Lower ØKPY
    - Upper ØKPX
  - Stomach ØDP6
  - Ureter ØTP9
- Revision of device in
  - Anal Sphincter ØDWR
  - Artery, Upper Ø3WY
  - Bladder ØTWB
  - Muscle
    - Lower ØKWY
    - Upper ØKWX
  - Stomach ØDW6
  - Ureter ØTW9

Stoma
- Excision
  - Abdominal Wall ØWBFXZ2

Stoma — *continued*
- Excision — *continued*
  - Neck ØWB6XZ2
- Repair
  - Abdominal Wall ØWQFXZ2
  - Neck ØWQ6XZ2

Stomatoplasty
- *see* Repair, Mouth and Throat ØCQ
- *see* Replacement, Mouth and Throat ØCR
- *see* Supplement, Mouth and Throat ØCU

Stomatorrhaphy *see* Repair, Mouth and Throat ØCQ

StrataGraft® *use* Bioengineered Allogeneic Construct

Stratos LV *use* Cardiac Resynchronization Pacemaker Pulse Generator in ØJH

Stress test 4AØ2XM4, 4A12XM4

Stripping *see* Extraction

Study
- Electrophysiologic stimulation, cardiac *see* Measurement, Cardiac 4AØ2
- Ocular motility 4AØ7X7Z
- Pulmonary airway flow measurement *see* Measurement, Respiratory 4AØ9
- Visual acuity 4AØ7XØZ

Styloglossus muscle *use* Tongue, Palate, Pharynx Muscle

Stylomandibular ligament *use* Head and Neck Bursa and Ligament

Stylopharyngeus muscle *use* Tongue, Palate, Pharynx Muscle

Subacromial bursa
- *use* Shoulder Bursa and Ligament, Left
- *use* Shoulder Bursa and Ligament, Right

Subaortic (common iliac) lymph node *use* Lymphatic, Pelvis

Subarachnoid space, spinal *use* Spinal Canal

Subclavicular (apical) lymph node
- *use* Lymphatic, Left Axillary
- *use* Lymphatic, Right Axillary

Subclavius muscle
- *use* Thorax Muscle, Left
- *use* Thorax Muscle, Right

Subclavius nerve *use* Brachial Plexus

Subcostal artery *use* Upper Artery

Subcostal muscle
- *use* Thorax Muscle, Left
- *use* Thorax Muscle, Right

Subcostal nerve *use* Thoracic Nerve

Subcutaneous Defibrillator Lead
- Insertion of device in, Subcutaneous Tissue and Fascia, Chest ØJH6
- Removal of device from, Subcutaneous Tissue and Fascia, Trunk ØJPT
- Revision of device in, Subcutaneous Tissue and Fascia, Trunk ØJWT

Subcutaneous injection reservoir, port *use* Vascular Access Device, Totally Implantable in Subcutaneous Tissue and Fascia

Subcutaneous injection reservoir, pump *use* Infusion Device, Pump in Subcutaneous Tissue and Fascia

Subdermal progesterone implant *use* Contraceptive Device in Subcutaneous Tissue and Fascia

Subdural space, spinal *use* Spinal Canal

Submandibular ganglion
- *use* Facial Nerve
- *use* Head and Neck Sympathetic Nerve

Submandibular gland
- *use* Submaxillary Gland, Left
- *use* Submaxillary Gland, Right

Submandibular lymph node *use* Lymphatic, Head

Submandibular space *use* Subcutaneous Tissue and Fascia, Face

Submaxillary ganglion *use* Head and Neck Sympathetic Nerve

Submaxillary lymph node *use* Lymphatic, Head

Submental artery *use* Face Artery

Submental lymph node *use* Lymphatic, Head

Submucous (Meissner's) plexus *use* Abdominal Sympathetic Nerve

Suboccipital nerve *use* Cervical Nerve

Suboccipital venous plexus
- *use* Vertebral Vein, Left
- *use* Vertebral Vein, Right

Subparotid lymph node *use* Lymphatic, Head

Subscapular aponeurosis
- *use* Subcutaneous Tissue and Fascia, Left Upper Arm

Subscapular aponeurosis — *continued*
- *use* Subcutaneous Tissue and Fascia, Right Upper Arm

Subscapular artery
- *use* Axillary Artery, Left
- *use* Axillary Artery, Right

Subscapular (posterior) lymph node
- *use* Lymphatic, Axillary, Left
- *use* Lymphatic, Axillary, Right

Subscapularis muscle
- *use* Shoulder Muscle, Left
- *use* Shoulder Muscle, Right

Substance Abuse Treatment
- Counseling
  - Family, for substance abuse, Other Family Counseling HZ63ZZZ
  - Group
    - 12-Step HZ43ZZZ
    - Behavioral HZ41ZZZ
    - Cognitive HZ40ZZZ
    - Cognitive-Behavioral HZ42ZZZ
    - Confrontational HZ48ZZZ
    - Continuing Care HZ49ZZZ
    - Infectious Disease
      - Post-Test HZ4CZZZ
      - Pre-Test HZ4CZZZ
    - Interpersonal HZ44ZZZ
    - Motivational Enhancement HZ47ZZZ
    - Psychoeducation HZ46ZZZ
    - Spiritual HZ4BZZZ
    - Vocational HZ45ZZZ
  - Individual
    - 12-Step HZ33ZZZ
    - Behavioral HZ31ZZZ
    - Cognitive HZ30ZZZ
    - Cognitive-Behavioral HZ32ZZZ
    - Confrontational HZ38ZZZ
    - Continuing Care HZ39ZZZ
    - Infectious Disease
      - Post-Test HZ3CZZZ
      - Pre-Test HZ3CZZZ
    - Interpersonal HZ34ZZZ
    - Motivational Enhancement HZ37ZZZ
    - Psychoeducation HZ36ZZZ
    - Spiritual HZ3BZZZ
    - Vocational HZ35ZZZ
- Detoxification Services, for substance abuse HZ2ZZZZ
- Medication Management
  - Antabuse HZ83ZZZ
  - Bupropion HZ87ZZZ
  - Clonidine HZ86ZZZ
  - Levo-alpha-acetyl-methadol (LAAM) HZ82ZZZ
  - Methadone Maintenance HZ81ZZZ
  - Naloxone HZ85ZZZ
  - Naltrexone HZ84ZZZ
  - Nicotine Replacement HZ80ZZZ
  - Other Replacement Medication HZ89ZZZ
  - Psychiatric Medication HZ88ZZZ
- Pharmacotherapy
  - Antabuse HZ93ZZZ
  - Bupropion HZ97ZZZ
  - Clonidine HZ96ZZZ
  - Levo-alpha-acetyl-methadol (LAAM) HZ92ZZZ
  - Methadone Maintenance HZ91ZZZ
  - Naloxone HZ95ZZZ
  - Naltrexone HZ94ZZZ
  - Nicotine Replacement HZ90ZZZ
  - Psychiatric Medication HZ98ZZZ
  - Replacement Medication, Other HZ99ZZZ
- Psychotherapy
  - 12-Step HZ53ZZZ
  - Behavioral HZ51ZZZ
  - Cognitive HZ50ZZZ
  - Cognitive-Behavioral HZ52ZZZ
  - Confrontational HZ58ZZZ
  - Interactive HZ55ZZZ
  - Interpersonal HZ54ZZZ
  - Motivational Enhancement HZ57ZZZ
  - Psychoanalysis HZ5BZZZ
  - Psychodynamic HZ5CZZZ
  - Psychoeducation HZ56ZZZ
  - Psychophysiological HZ5DZZZ
  - Supportive HZ59ZZZ

Substantia nigra *use* Basal Ganglia

Subtalar (talocalcaneal) joint
- *use* Tarsal Joint, Left
- *use* Tarsal Joint, Right

Subtalar ligament
- *use* Foot Bursa and Ligament, Left
- *use* Foot Bursa and Ligament, Right

Subthalamic nucleus *use* Basal Ganglia

Suction curettage (D&C), nonobstetric *see* Extraction, Endometrium ØUDB

Suction curettage, obstetric post-delivery *see* Extraction, Products of Conception, Retained 1ØD1

Superficial circumflex iliac vein
- *use* Saphenous Vein, Left
- *use* Saphenous Vein, Right

Superficial epigastric artery
- *use* Femoral Artery, Left
- *use* Femoral Artery, Right

Superficial epigastric vein
- *use* Saphenous Vein, Left
- *use* Saphenous Vein, Right

Superficial Inferior Epigastric Artery Flap
- Replacement
  - Bilateral ØHRVØ78
  - Left ØHRUØ78
  - Right ØHRTØ78
- Transfer
  - Left ØKXG
  - Right ØKXF

Superficial palmar arch
- *use* Hand Artery, Left
- *use* Hand Artery, Right

Superficial palmar venous arch
- *use* Hand Vein, Left
- *use* Hand Vein, Right

Superficial temporal artery
- *use* Temporal Artery, Left
- *use* Temporal Artery, Right

Superficial transverse perineal muscle *use* Perineum Muscle

Superior cardiac nerve *use* Thoracic Sympathetic Nerve

Superior cerebellar vein *use* Intracranial Vein

Superior cerebral vein *use* Intracranial Vein

Superior clunic (cluneal) nerve *use* Lumbar Nerve

Superior epigastric artery
- *use* Internal Mammary Artery, Left
- *use* Internal Mammary Artery, Right

Superior genicular artery
- *use* Popliteal Artery, Left
- *use* Popliteal Artery, Right

Superior gluteal artery
- *use* Internal Iliac Artery, Left
- *use* Internal Iliac Artery, Right

Superior gluteal nerve *use* Lumbar Plexus

Superior hypogastric plexus *use* Abdominal Sympathetic Nerve

Superior labial artery *use* Face Artery

Superior laryngeal artery
- *use* Thyroid Artery, Left
- *use* Thyroid Artery, Right

Superior laryngeal nerve *use* Vagus Nerve

Superior longitudinal muscle *use* Tongue, Palate, Pharynx Muscle

Superior mesenteric ganglion *use* Abdominal Sympathetic Nerve

Superior mesenteric lymph node *use* Lymphatic, Mesenteric

Superior mesenteric plexus *use* Abdominal Sympathetic Nerve

Superior oblique muscle
- *use* Extraocular Muscle, Left
- *use* Extraocular Muscle, Right

Superior olivary nucleus *use* Pons

Superior rectal artery *use* Inferior Mesenteric Artery

Superior rectal vein *use* Inferior Mesenteric Vein

Superior rectus muscle
- *use* Extraocular Muscle, Left
- *use* Extraocular Muscle, Right

Superior tarsal plate
- *use* Upper Eyelid, Left
- *use* Upper Eyelid, Right

Superior thoracic artery
- *use* Axillary Artery, Left
- *use* Axillary Artery, Right

Superior thyroid artery
- *use* External Carotid Artery, Left
- *use* External Carotid Artery, Right

Superior thyroid artery — *continued*
- *use* Thyroid Artery, Left
- *use* Thyroid Artery, Right

Superior turbinate *use* Nasal Turbinate

Superior ulnar collateral artery
- *use* Brachial Artery, Left
- *use* Brachial Artery, Right

Supersaturated Oxygen therapy 5AØ512C, 5AØ522C

Supplement
- Abdominal Wall ØWUF
- Acetabulum
  - Left ØQU5
  - Right ØQU4
- Ampulla of Vater ØFUC
- Anal Sphincter ØDUR
- Ankle Region
  - Left ØYUL
  - Right ØYUK
- Anus ØDUQ
- Aorta
  - Abdominal Ø4UØ
  - Thoracic
    - Ascending/Arch Ø2UX
    - Descending Ø2UW
- Arm
  - Lower
    - Left ØXUF
    - Right ØXUD
  - Upper
    - Left ØXU9
    - Right ØXU8
- Artery
  - Anterior Tibial
    - Left Ø4UQ
    - Right Ø4UP
  - Axillary
    - Left Ø3U6
    - Right Ø3U5
  - Brachial
    - Left Ø3U8
    - Right Ø3U7
  - Celiac Ø4U1
  - Colic
    - Left Ø4U7
    - Middle Ø4U8
    - Right Ø4U6
  - Common Carotid
    - Left Ø3UJ
    - Right Ø3UH
  - Common Iliac
    - Left Ø4UD
    - Right Ø4UC
  - Coronary
    - Four or More Arteries Ø2U3
    - One Artery Ø2UØ
    - Three Arteries Ø2U2
    - Two Arteries Ø2U1
  - External Carotid
    - Left Ø3UN
    - Right Ø3UM
  - External Iliac
    - Left Ø4UJ
    - Right Ø4UH
  - Face Ø3UR
  - Femoral
    - Left Ø4UL
    - Right Ø4UK
  - Foot
    - Left Ø4UW
    - Right Ø4UV
  - Gastric Ø4U2
  - Hand
    - Left Ø3UF
    - Right Ø3UD
  - Hepatic Ø4U3
  - Inferior Mesenteric Ø4UB
  - Innominate Ø3U2
  - Internal Carotid
    - Left Ø3UL
    - Right Ø3UK
  - Internal Iliac
    - Left Ø4UF
    - Right Ø4UE
  - Internal Mammary
    - Left Ø3U1
    - Right Ø3UØ
  - Intracranial Ø3UG
  - Lower Ø4UY

Supplement — *continued*
- Artery — *continued*
  - Peroneal
    - Left Ø4UU
    - Right Ø4UT
  - Popliteal
    - Left Ø4UN
    - Right Ø4UM
  - Posterior Tibial
    - Left Ø4US
    - Right Ø4UR
  - Pulmonary
    - Left Ø2UR
    - Right Ø2UQ
  - Pulmonary Trunk Ø2UP
  - Radial
    - Left Ø3UC
    - Right Ø3UB
  - Renal
    - Left Ø4UA
    - Right Ø4U9
  - Splenic Ø4U4
  - Subclavian
    - Left Ø3U4
    - Right Ø3U3
  - Superior Mesenteric Ø4U5
  - Temporal
    - Left Ø3UT
    - Right Ø3US
  - Thyroid
    - Left Ø3UV
    - Right Ø3UU
  - Ulnar
    - Left Ø3UA
    - Right Ø3U9
  - Upper Ø3UY
  - Vertebral
    - Left Ø3UQ
    - Right Ø3UP
- Atrium
  - Left Ø2U7
  - Right Ø2U6
- Auditory Ossicle
  - Left Ø9UA
  - Right Ø9U9
- Axilla
  - Left ØXU5
  - Right ØXU4
- Back
  - Lower ØWUL
  - Upper ØWUK
- Bladder ØTUB
- Bladder Neck ØTUC
- Bone
  - Ethmoid
    - Left ØNUG
    - Right ØNUF
  - Frontal ØNU1
  - Hyoid ØNUX
  - Lacrimal
    - Left ØNUJ
    - Right ØNUH
  - Nasal ØNUB
  - Occipital ØNU7
  - Palatine
    - Left ØNUL
    - Right ØNUK
  - Parietal
    - Left ØNU4
    - Right ØNU3
  - Pelvic
    - Left ØQU3
    - Right ØQU2
  - Sphenoid ØNUC
  - Temporal
    - Left ØNU6
    - Right ØNU5
  - Zygomatic
    - Left ØNUN
    - Right ØNUM
- Breast
  - Bilateral ØHUV
  - Left ØHUU
  - Right ØHUT
- Bronchus
  - Lingula ØBU9
  - Lower Lobe
    - Left ØBUB
    - Right ØBU6

Supplement — *continued*
- Bronchus — *continued*
  - Main
    - Left ØBU7
    - Right ØBU3
  - Middle Lobe, Right ØBU5
  - Upper Lobe
    - Left ØBU8
    - Right ØBU4
- Buccal Mucosa ØCU4
- Bursa and Ligament
  - Abdomen
    - Left ØMUJ
    - Right ØMUH
  - Ankle
    - Left ØMUR
    - Right ØMUQ
  - Elbow
    - Left ØMU4
    - Right ØMU3
  - Foot
    - Left ØMUT
    - Right ØMUS
  - Hand
    - Left ØMU8
    - Right ØMU7
  - Head and Neck ØMUØ
  - Hip
    - Left ØMUM
    - Right ØMUL
  - Knee
    - Left ØMUP
    - Right ØMUN
  - Lower Extremity
    - Left ØMUW
    - Right ØMUV
  - Perineum ØMUK
  - Rib(s) ØMUG
  - Shoulder
    - Left ØMU2
    - Right ØMU1
  - Spine
    - Lower ØMUD
    - Upper ØMUC
  - Sternum ØMUF
  - Upper Extremity
    - Left ØMUB
    - Right ØMU9
  - Wrist
    - Left ØMU6
    - Right ØMU5
- Buttock
  - Left ØYU1
  - Right ØYUØ
- Carina ØBU2
- Carpal
  - Left ØPUN
  - Right ØPUM
- Cecum ØDUH
- Cerebral Meninges ØØU1
- Cerebral Ventricle ØØU6
- Chest Wall ØWU8
- Chordae Tendineae Ø2U9
- Cisterna Chyli Ø7UL
- Clavicle
  - Left ØPUB
  - Right ØPU9
- Clitoris ØUUJ
- Coccyx ØQUS
- Colon
  - Ascending ØDUK
  - Descending ØDUM
  - Sigmoid ØDUN
  - Transverse ØDUL
- Cord
  - Bilateral ØVUH
  - Left ØVUG
  - Right ØVUF
- Cornea
  - Left Ø8U9
  - Right Ø8U8
- Cul-de-sac ØUUF
- Diaphragm ØBUT
- Disc
  - Cervical Vertebral ØRU3
  - Cervicothoracic Vertebral ØRU5
  - Lumbar Vertebral ØSU2
  - Lumbosacral ØSU4
  - Thoracic Vertebral ØRU9

Supplement — *continued*
- Disc — *continued*
  - Thoracolumbar Vertebral ØRUB
- Duct
  - Common Bile ØFU9
  - Cystic ØFU8
  - Hepatic
    - Common ØFU7
    - Left ØFU6
    - Right ØFU5
  - Lacrimal
    - Left Ø8UY
    - Right Ø8UX
  - Pancreatic ØFUD
    - Accessory ØFUF
- Duodenum ØDU9
- Dura Mater ØØU2
- Ear
  - External
    - Bilateral Ø9U2
    - Left Ø9U1
    - Right Ø9UØ
  - Inner
    - Left Ø9UE
    - Right Ø9UD
  - Middle
    - Left Ø9U6
    - Right Ø9U5
- Elbow Region
  - Left ØXUC
  - Right ØXUB
- Epididymis
  - Bilateral ØVUL
  - Left ØVUK
  - Right ØVUJ
- Epiglottis ØCUR
- Esophagogastric Junction ØDU4
- Esophagus ØDU5
  - Lower ØDU3
  - Middle ØDU2
  - Upper ØDU1
- Extremity
  - Lower
    - Left ØYUB
    - Right ØYU9
  - Upper
    - Left ØXU7
    - Right ØXU6
- Eye
  - Left Ø8U1
  - Right Ø8UØ
- Eyelid
  - Lower
    - Left Ø8UR
    - Right Ø8UQ
  - Upper
    - Left Ø8UP
    - Right Ø8UN
- Face ØWU2
- Fallopian Tube
  - Left ØUU6
  - Right ØUU5
- Fallopian Tubes, Bilateral ØUU7
- Femoral Region
  - Bilateral ØYUE
  - Left ØYU8
  - Right ØYU7
- Femoral Shaft
  - Left ØQU9
  - Right ØQU8
- Femur
  - Lower
    - Left ØQUC
    - Right ØQUB
  - Upper
    - Left ØQU7
    - Right ØQU6
- Fibula
  - Left ØQUK
  - Right ØQUJ
- Finger
  - Index
    - Left ØXUP
    - Right ØXUN
  - Little
    - Left ØXUW
    - Right ØXUV
  - Middle
    - Left ØXUR

Supplement — *continued*
Finger — *continued*
Middle — *continued*
Right ØXUQ
Ring
Left ØXUT
Right ØXUS
Foot
Left ØYUN
Right ØYUM
Gingiva
Lower ØCU6
Upper ØCU5
Glenoid Cavity
Left ØPU8
Right ØPU7
Hand
Left ØXUK
Right ØXUJ
Head ØWUØ
Heart Ø2UA
Humeral Head
Left ØPUD
Right ØPUC
Humeral Shaft
Left ØPUG
Right ØPUF
Hymen ØUUK
Ileocecal Valve ØDUC
Ileum ØDUB
Inguinal Region
Bilateral ØYUA
Left ØYU6
Right ØYU5
Intestine
Large ØDUE
Left ØDUG
Right ØDUF
Small ØDU8
Iris
Left Ø8UD
Right Ø8UC
Jaw
Lower ØWU5
Upper ØWU4
Jejunum ØDUA
Joint
Acromioclavicular
Left ØRUH
Right ØRUG
Ankle
Left ØSUG
Right ØSUF
Carpal
Left ØRUR
Right ØRUQ
Carpometacarpal
Left ØRUT
Right ØRUS
Cervical Vertebral ØRU1
Cervicothoracic Vertebral ØRU4
Coccygeal ØSU6
Elbow
Left ØRUM
Right ØRUL
Finger Phalangeal
Left ØRUX
Right ØRUW
Hip
Left ØSUB
Acetabular Surface ØSUE
Femoral Surface ØSUS
Right ØSU9
Acetabular Surface ØSUA
Femoral Surface ØSUR
Knee
Left ØSUD
Femoral Surface ØSUUØ9Z
Tibial Surface ØSUWØ9Z
Right ØSUC
Femoral Surface ØSUTØ9Z
Tibial Surface ØSUVØ9Z
Lumbar Vertebral ØSUØ
Lumbosacral ØSU3
Metacarpophalangeal
Left ØRUV
Right ØRUU
Metatarsal-Phalangeal
Left ØSUN

Supplement — *continued*
Joint — *continued*
Metatarsal-Phalangeal — *continued*
Right ØSUM
Occipital-cervical ØRUØ
Sacrococcygeal ØSU5
Sacroiliac
Left ØSU8
Right ØSU7
Shoulder
Left ØRUK
Right ØRUJ
Sternoclavicular
Left ØRUF
Right ØRUE
Tarsal
Left ØSUJ
Right ØSUH
Tarsometatarsal
Left ØSUL
Right ØSUK
Temporomandibular
Left ØRUD
Right ØRUC
Thoracic Vertebral ØRU6
Thoracolumbar Vertebral ØRUA
Toe Phalangeal
Left ØSUQ
Right ØSUP
Wrist
Left ØRUP
Right ØRUN
Kidney Pelvis
Left ØTU4
Right ØTU3
Knee Region
Left ØYUG
Right ØYUF
Larynx ØCUS
Leg
Lower
Left ØYUJ
Right ØYUH
Upper
Left ØYUD
Right ØYUC
Lip
Lower ØCU1
Upper ØCUØ
Lymphatic
Aortic Ø7UD
Axillary
Left Ø7U6
Right Ø7U5
Head Ø7UØ
Inguinal
Left Ø7UJ
Right Ø7UH
Internal Mammary
Left Ø7U9
Right Ø7U8
Lower Extremity
Left Ø7UG
Right Ø7UF
Mesenteric Ø7UB
Neck
Left Ø7U2
Right Ø7U1
Pelvis Ø7UC
Thoracic Duct Ø7UK
Thorax Ø7U7
Upper Extremity
Left Ø7U4
Right Ø7U3
Mandible
Left ØNUV
Right ØNUT
Maxilla ØNUR
Mediastinum ØWUC
Mesentery ØDUV
Metacarpal
Left ØPUQ
Right ØPUP
Metatarsal
Left ØQUP
Right ØQUN
Muscle
Abdomen
Left ØKUL

Supplement — *continued*
Muscle — *continued*
Abdomen — *continued*
Right ØKUK
Extraocular
Left Ø8UM
Right Ø8UL
Facial ØKU1
Foot
Left ØKUW
Right ØKUV
Hand
Left ØKUD
Right ØKUC
Head ØKUØ
Hip
Left ØKUP
Right ØKUN
Lower Arm and Wrist
Left ØKUB
Right ØKU9
Lower Leg
Left ØKUT
Right ØKUS
Neck
Left ØKU3
Right ØKU2
Papillary Ø2UD
Perineum ØKUM
Shoulder
Left ØKU6
Right ØKU5
Thorax
Left ØKUJ
Right ØKUH
Tongue, Palate, Pharynx ØKU4
Trunk
Left ØKUG
Right ØKUF
Upper Arm
Left ØKU8
Right ØKU7
Upper Leg
Left ØKUR
Right ØKUQ
Nasal Mucosa and Soft Tissue Ø9UK
Nasopharynx Ø9UN
Neck ØWU6
Nerve
Abducens ØØUL
Accessory ØØUR
Acoustic ØØUN
Cervical Ø1U1
Facial ØØUM
Femoral Ø1UD
Glossopharyngeal ØØUP
Hypoglossal ØØUS
Lumbar Ø1UB
Median Ø1U5
Oculomotor ØØUH
Olfactory ØØUF
Optic ØØUG
Peroneal Ø1UH
Phrenic Ø1U2
Pudendal Ø1UC
Radial Ø1U6
Sacral Ø1UR
Sciatic Ø1UF
Thoracic Ø1U8
Tibial Ø1UG
Trigeminal ØØUK
Trochlear ØØUJ
Ulnar Ø1U4
Vagus ØØUQ
Nipple
Left ØHUX
Right ØHUW
Omentum ØDUU
Orbit
Left ØNUQ
Right ØNUP
Palate
Hard ØCU2
Soft ØCU3
Patella
Left ØQUF
Right ØQUD
Penis ØVUS
Pericardium Ø2UN

Supplement — *continued*
Perineum
Female ØWUN
Male ØWUM
Peritoneum ØDUW
Phalanx
Finger
Left ØPUV
Right ØPUT
Thumb
Left ØPUS
Right ØPUR
Toe
Left ØQUR
Right ØQUQ
Pharynx ØCUM
Prepuce ØVUT
Radius
Left ØPUJ
Right ØPUH
Rectum ØDUP
Retina
Left Ø8UF
Right Ø8UE
Retinal Vessel
Left Ø8UH
Right Ø8UG
Ribs
1 to 2 ØPU1
3 or More ØPU2
Sacrum ØQU1
Scapula
Left ØPU6
Right ØPU5
Scrotum ØVU5
Septum
Atrial Ø2U5
Nasal Ø9UM
Ventricular Ø2UM
Shoulder Region
Left ØXU3
Right ØXU2
Sinus
Accessory Ø9UP
Ethmoid
Left Ø9UV
Right Ø9UU
Frontal
Left Ø9UT
Right Ø9US
Mastoid
Left Ø9UC
Right Ø9UB
Maxillary
Left Ø9UR
Right Ø9UQ
Sphenoid
Left Ø9UX
Right Ø9UW
Skull ØNUØ
Spinal Meninges ØØUT
Sternum ØPUØ
Stomach ØDU6
Pylorus ØDU7
Subcutaneous Tissue and Fascia
Abdomen ØJU8
Back ØJU7
Buttock ØJU9
Chest ØJU6
Face ØJU1
Foot
Left ØJUR
Right ØJUQ
Hand
Left ØJUK
Right ØJUJ
Lower Arm
Left ØJUH
Right ØJUG
Lower Leg
Left ØJUP
Right ØJUN
Neck
Left ØJU5
Right ØJU4
Pelvic Region ØJUC
Perineum ØJUB
Scalp ØJUØ

Supplement — *continued*
Subcutaneous Tissue and Fascia — *continued*
Upper Arm
Left ØJUF
Right ØJUD
Upper Leg
Left ØJUM
Right ØJUL
Tarsal
Left ØQUM
Right ØQUL
Tendon
Abdomen
Left ØLUG
Right ØLUF
Ankle
Left ØLUT
Right ØLUS
Foot
Left ØLUW
Right ØLUV
Hand
Left ØLU8
Right ØLU7
Head and Neck ØLUØ
Hip
Left ØLUK
Right ØLUJ
Knee
Left ØLUR
Right ØLUQ
Lower Arm and Wrist
Left ØLU6
Right ØLU5
Lower Leg
Left ØLUP
Right ØLUN
Perineum ØLUH
Shoulder
Left ØLU2
Right ØLU1
Thorax
Left ØLUD
Right ØLUC
Trunk
Left ØLUB
Right ØLU9
Upper Arm
Left ØLU4
Right ØLU3
Upper Leg
Left ØLUM
Right ØLUL
Testis
Bilateral ØVUCØ
Left ØVUBØ
Right ØVU9Ø
Thumb
Left ØXUM
Right ØXUL
Tibia
Left ØQUH
Right ØQUG
Toe
1st
Left ØYUQ
Right ØYUP
2nd
Left ØYUS
Right ØYUR
3rd
Left ØYUU
Right ØYUT
4th
Left ØYUW
Right ØYUV
5th
Left ØYUY
Right ØYUX
Tongue ØCU7
Trachea ØBU1
Tunica Vaginalis
Left ØVU7
Right ØVU6
Turbinate, Nasal Ø9UL
Tympanic Membrane
Left Ø9U8
Right Ø9U7

Supplement — *continued*
Ulna
Left ØPUL
Right ØPUK
Ureter
Left ØTU7
Right ØTU6
Urethra ØTUD
Uterine Supporting Structure ØUU4
Uvula ØCUN
Vagina ØUUG
Valve
Aortic Ø2UF
Mitral Ø2UG
Pulmonary Ø2UH
Tricuspid Ø2UJ
Vas Deferens
Bilateral ØVUQ
Left ØVUP
Right ØVUN
Vein
Axillary
Left Ø5U8
Right Ø5U7
Azygos Ø5UØ
Basilic
Left Ø5UC
Right Ø5UB
Brachial
Left Ø5UA
Right Ø5U9
Cephalic
Left Ø5UF
Right Ø5UD
Colic Ø6U7
Common Iliac
Left Ø6UD
Right Ø6UC
Esophageal Ø6U3
External Iliac
Left Ø6UG
Right Ø6UF
External Jugular
Left Ø5UQ
Right Ø5UP
Face
Left Ø5UV
Right Ø5UT
Femoral
Left Ø6UN
Right Ø6UM
Foot
Left Ø6UV
Right Ø6UT
Gastric Ø6U2
Hand
Left Ø5UH
Right Ø5UG
Hemiazygos Ø5U1
Hepatic Ø6U4
Hypogastric
Left Ø6UJ
Right Ø6UH
Inferior Mesenteric Ø6U6
Innominate
Left Ø5U4
Right Ø5U3
Internal Jugular
Left Ø5UN
Right Ø5UM
Intracranial Ø5UL
Lower Ø6UY
Portal Ø6U8
Pulmonary
Left Ø2UT
Right Ø2US
Renal
Left Ø6UB
Right Ø6U9
Saphenous
Left Ø6UQ
Right Ø6UP
Splenic Ø6U1
Subclavian
Left Ø5U6
Right Ø5U5
Superior Mesenteric Ø6U5
Upper Ø5UY

Supplement — *continued*
Vein — *continued*
Vertebral
Left Ø5US
Right Ø5UR
Vena Cava
Inferior Ø6UØ
Superior Ø2UV
Ventricle
Left Ø2UL
Right Ø2UK
Vertebra
Cervical ØPU3
Lumbar ØQUØ
Mechanically Expandable (Paired) Synthetic Substitute XNUØ356
Thoracic ØPU4
Mechanically Expandable (Paired) Synthetic Substitute XNU4356
Vesicle
Bilateral ØVU3
Left ØVU2
Right ØVU1
Vocal Cord
Left ØCUV
Right ØCUT
Vulva ØUUM
Wrist Region
Left ØXUH
Right ØXUG
Supraclavicular (Virchow's) lymph node
use Lymphatic, Left Neck
use Lymphatic, Right Neck
Supraclavicular nerve *use* Cervical Plexus
Suprahyoid lymph node *use* Lymphatic, Head
Suprahyoid muscle
use Neck Muscle, Left
use Neck Muscle, Right
Suprainguinal lymph node *use* Lymphatic, Pelvis
Supraorbital vein
use Face Vein, Left
use Face Vein, Right
Suprarenal gland
use Adrenal Gland
use Adrenal Gland, Bilateral
use Adrenal Gland, Left
use Adrenal Gland, Right
Suprarenal plexus *use* Abdominal Sympathetic Nerve
Suprascapular nerve *use* Brachial Plexus
Supraspinatus fascia
use Subcutaneous Tissue and Fascia, Left Upper Arm
use Subcutaneous Tissue and Fascia, Right Upper Arm
Supraspinatus muscle
use Shoulder Muscle, Left
use Shoulder Muscle, Right
Supraspinous ligament
use Lower Spine Bursa and Ligament
use Upper Spine Bursa and Ligament
Suprasternal notch *use* Sternum
Supratrochlear lymph node
use Lymphatic, Left Upper Extremity
use Lymphatic, Right Upper Extremity
Sural artery
use Popliteal Artery, Left
use Popliteal Artery, Right
Surpass Streamline™ Flow Diverter *use* Intraluminal Device, Flow Diverter in Ø3V
Suspension
Bladder Neck *see* Reposition, Bladder Neck ØTSC
Kidney *see* Reposition, Urinary System ØTS
Urethra *see* Reposition, Urinary System ØTS
Urethrovesical *see* Reposition, Bladder Neck ØTSC
Uterus *see* Reposition, Uterus ØUS9
Vagina *see* Reposition, Vagina ØUSG
Sustained Release Drug-eluting Intraluminal Device
Dilation
Anterior Tibial
Left X27Q385
Right X27P385
Femoral
Left X27J385
Right X27H385
Peroneal
Left X27U385
Sustained Release Drug-eluting Intraluminal Device — *continued*
Dilation — *continued*
Peroneal — *continued*
Right X27T385
Popliteal
Left Distal X27N385
Left Proximal X27L385
Right Distal X27M385
Right Proximal X27K385
Posterior Tibial
Left X27S385
Right X27R385
Four or More
Anterior Tibial
Left X27Q3C5
Right X27P3C5
Femoral
Left X27J3C5
Right X27H3C5
Peroneal
Left X27U3C5
Right X27T3C5
Popliteal
Left Distal X27N3C5
Left Proximal X27L3C5
Right Distal X27M3C5
Right Proximal X27K3C5
Posterior Tibial
Left X27S3C5
Right X27R3C5
Three
Anterior Tibial
Left X27Q3B5
Right X27P3B5
Femoral
Left X27J3B5
Right X27H3B5
Peroneal
Left X27U3B5
Right X27T3B5
Popliteal
Left Distal X27N3B5
Left Proximal X27L3B5
Right Distal X27M3B5
Right Proximal X27K3B5
Posterior Tibial
Left X27S3B5
Right X27R3B5
Two
Anterior Tibial
Left X27Q395
Right X27P395
Femoral
Left X27J395
Right X27H395
Peroneal
Left X27U395
Right X27T395
Popliteal
Left Distal X27N395
Left Proximal X27L395
Right Distal X27M395
Right Proximal X27K395
Posterior Tibial
Left X27S395
Right X27R395
Suture
Laceration repair *see* Repair
Ligation *see* Occlusion
Suture Removal
Extremity
Lower 8EØYXY8
Upper 8EØXXY8
Head and Neck Region 8EØ9XY8
Trunk Region 8EØWXY8
Sutureless valve, Perceval *use* Zooplastic Tissue, Rapid Deployment Technique in New Technology
Sweat gland *use* Skin
Sympathectomy *see* Excision, Peripheral Nervous System Ø1B
SynCardia (temporary) total artificial heart (TAH)
use Synthetic Substitute, Pneumatic in Ø2R
SynCardia Total Artificial Heart *use* Synthetic Substitute
Synchra CRT-P *use* Cardiac Resynchronization Pacemaker Pulse Generator in ØJH
SynchroMed pump *use* Infusion Device, Pump in Subcutaneous Tissue and Fascia
Synechiotomy, iris *see* Release, Eye Ø8N
Synovectomy
Lower joint *see* Excision, Lower Joints ØSB
Upper joint *see* Excision, Upper Joints ØRB
Synthetic Human Angiotensin II XWØ
Systemic Nuclear Medicine Therapy
Abdomen CW7Ø
Anatomical Regions, Multiple CW7YYZZ
Chest CW73
Thyroid CW7G
Whole Body CW7N

T

Tagraxofusp-erzs Antineoplastic XWØ
Takedown
Arteriovenous shunt *see* Removal of device from, Upper Arteries Ø3P
Arteriovenous shunt, with creation of new shunt *see* Bypass, Upper Arteries Ø31
Stoma
see Excision
see Reposition
Talent® Converter *use* Intraluminal Device
Talent® Occluder *use* Intraluminal Device
Talent® Stent Graft (abdominal) (thoracic) *use* Intraluminal Device
Talocalcaneal (subtalar) joint
use Tarsal Joint, Left
use Tarsal Joint, Right
Talocalcaneal ligament
use Foot Bursa and Ligament, Left
use Foot Bursa and Ligament, Right
Talocalcaneonavicular joint
use Tarsal Joint, Left
use Tarsal Joint, Right
Talocalcaneonavicular ligament
use Foot Bursa and Ligament, Left
use Foot Bursa and Ligament, Right
Talocrural joint
use Ankle Joint, Left
use Joint, Ankle, Right
Talofibular ligament
use Ankle Bursa and Ligament, Left
use Ankle Bursa and Ligament, Right
Talus bone
use Tarsal, Left
use Tarsal, Right
TandemHeart® System *use* Short-term External Heart Assist System in Heart and Great Vessels
Tarsectomy
see Excision, Lower Bones ØQB
see Resection, Lower Bones ØQT
Tarsometatarsal ligament
use Foot Bursa and Ligament, Left
use Foot Bursa and Ligament, Right
Tarsorrhaphy *see* Repair, Eye Ø8Q
Tattooing
Cornea 3EØCXMZ
Skin *see* Introduction of substance in or on, Skin 3EØØ
TAXUS® Liberte® Paclitaxel-eluting Coronary Stent System *use* Intraluminal Device, Drug-eluting in Heart and Great Vessels
TBNA (transbronchial needle aspiration)
Fluid or gas *see* Drainage, Respiratory System ØB9
Tissue biopsy *see* Extraction, Respiratory System ØBD
Tecartus™ *use* Brexucabtagene Autoleucel Immunotherapy
TECENTRIQ® *use* Atezolizumab Antineoplastic
Telemetry 4A12X4Z
Ambulatory 4A12X45
Temperature gradient study 4AØZXKZ
Temporal lobe *use* Cerebral Hemisphere
Temporalis muscle *use* Head Muscle
Temporoparietalis muscle *use* Head Muscle
Tendolysis *see* Release, Tendons ØLN
Tendonectomy
see Excision, Tendons ØLB
see Resection, Tendons ØLT
Tendonoplasty, tenoplasty
see Repair, Tendons ØLQ
see Replacement, Tendons ØLR

Tendonoplasty, tenoplasty — *continued*
see Supplement, Tendons ØLU
Tendorrhaphy *see* Repair, Tendons ØLQ
Tendototomy
see Division, Tendons ØL8
see Drainage, Tendons ØL9
Tenectomy, tenonectomy
see Excision, Tendons ØLB
see Resection, Tendons ØLT
Tenolysis *see* Release, Tendons ØLN
Tenontorrhaphy *see* Repair, Tendons ØLQ
Tenontotomy
see Division, Tendons ØL8
see Drainage, Tendons ØL9
Tenorrhaphy *see* Repair, Tendons ØLQ
Tenosynovectomy
see Excision, Tendons ØLB
see Resection, Tendons ØLT
Tenotomy
see Division, Tendons ØL8
see Drainage, Tendons ØL9
Tensor fasciae latae muscle
use Hip Muscle, Left
use Hip Muscle, Right
Tensor veli palatini muscle *use* Tongue, Palate, Pharynx Muscle
Tenth cranial nerve *use* Vagus Nerve
Tentorium cerebelli *use* Dura Mater
Teres major muscle
use Shoulder Muscle, Left
use Shoulder Muscle, Right
Teres minor muscle
use Shoulder Muscle, Left
use Shoulder Muscle, Right
Terlipressin XWØ
TERLIVAZ® *use* Terlipressin
Termination of pregnancy
Aspiration curettage 1ØAØ7ZZ
Dilation and curettage 1ØAØ7ZZ
Hysterotomy 1ØAØØZZ
Intra-amniotic injection 1ØAØ3ZZ
Laminaria 1ØAØ7ZW
Vacuum 1ØAØ7Z6
Testectomy
see Excision, Male Reproductive System ØVB
see Resection, Male Reproductive System ØVT
Testicular artery *use* Abdominal Aorta
Testing
Glaucoma 4AØ7XBZ
Hearing *see* Hearing Assessment, Diagnostic Audiology F13
Mental health *see* Psychological Tests
Muscle function, electromyography (EMG) *see* Measurement, Musculoskeletal 4AØF
Muscle function, manual *see* Motor Function Assessment, Rehabilitation FØ1
Neurophysiologic monitoring, intra-operative *see* Monitoring, Physiological Systems 4A1
Range of motion *see* Motor Function Assessment, Rehabilitation FØ1
Vestibular function *see* Vestibular Assessment, Diagnostic Audiology F15
Thalamectomy *see* Excision, Thalamus ØØB9
Thalamotomy *see* Drainage, Thalamus ØØ99
Thenar muscle
use Hand Muscle, Left
use Hand Muscle, Right
Therapeutic Massage
Musculoskeletal System 8EØKX1Z
Reproductive System
Prostate 8EØVX1C
Rectum 8EØVX1D
Therapeutic occlusion coil(s) *use* Intraluminal Device
Thermography 4AØZXKZ
Thermotherapy, prostate *see* Destruction, Prostate ØV5Ø
Third cranial nerve *use* Oculomotor Nerve
Third occipital nerve *use* Cervical Nerve
Third ventricle *use* Cerebral Ventricle
Thoracectomy *see* Excision, Anatomical Regions, General ØWB
Thoracentesis *see* Drainage, Anatomical Regions, General ØW9
Thoracic aortic plexus *use* Thoracic Sympathetic Nerve
Thoracic esophagus *use* Esophagus, Middle
Thoracic facet joint *use* Thoracic Vertebral Joint
Thoracic ganglion *use* Thoracic Sympathetic Nerve
Thoracoacromial artery
use Axillary Artery, Left
use Axillary Artery, Right
Thoracocentesis *see* Drainage, Anatomical Regions, General ØW9
Thoracolumbar facet joint *use* Thoracolumbar Vertebral Joint
Thoracoplasty
see Repair, Anatomical Regions, General ØWQ
see Supplement, Anatomical Regions, General ØWU
Thoracostomy, for lung collapse *see* Drainage, Respiratory System ØB9
Thoracostomy tube *use* Drainage Device
Thoracotomy *see* Drainage, Anatomical Regions, General ØW9
Thoraflex™ Hybrid device *use* Branched Synthetic Substitute with Intraluminal Device in New Technology
Thoratec IVAD (Implantable Ventricular Assist Device) *use* Implantable Heart Assist System in Heart and Great Vessels
Thoratec Paracorporeal Ventricular Assist Device *use* Short-term External Heart Assist System in Heart and Great Vessels
Thrombectomy *see* Extirpation
Thrombolysis, Ultrasound assisted *see* Fragmentation, Artery
Thymectomy
see Excision, Lymphatic and Hemic Systems Ø7B
see Resection, Lymphatic and Hemic Systems Ø7T
Thymopexy
see Repair, Lymphatic and Hemic Systems Ø7Q
see Reposition, Lymphatic and Hemic Systems Ø7S
Thymus gland *use* Thymus
Thyroarytenoid muscle
use Neck Muscle, Left
use Neck Muscle, Right
Thyrocervical trunk
use Thyroid Artery, Left
use Thyroid Artery, Right
Thyroid cartilage *use* Larynx
Thyroidectomy
see Excision, Endocrine System ØGB
see Resection, Endocrine System ØGT
Thyroidorrhaphy *see* Repair, Endocrine System ØGQ
Thyroidoscopy ØGJK4ZZ
Thyroidotomy *see* Drainage, Endocrine System ØG9
Tibial insert *use* Liner in Lower Joints
Tibial sesamoid
use Metatarsal, Left
use Metatarsal, Right
Tibialis anterior muscle
use Lower Leg Muscle, Left
use Lower Leg Muscle, Right
Tibialis posterior muscle
use Lower Leg Muscle, Left
use Lower Leg Muscle, Right
Tibiofemoral joint
use Knee Joint, Left
use Knee Joint, Right
use Knee Joint, Tibial Surface, Left
use Knee Joint, Tibial Surface, Right
Tibioperoneal trunk
use Popliteal Artery, Left
use Popliteal Artery, Right
Tisagenlecleucel *use* Tisagenlecleucel Immunotherapy
Tisagenlecleucel Immunotherapy XWØ
Tissue bank graft *use* Nonautologous Tissue Substitute
Tissue expander (inflatable) (injectable)
use Tissue Expander in Skin and Breast
use Tissue Expander in Subcutaneous Tissue and Fascia
Tissue Expander
Insertion of device in
Breast
Bilateral ØHHV
Left ØHHU
Right ØHHT
Nipple
Left ØHHX
Right ØHHW
Subcutaneous Tissue and Fascia
Abdomen ØJH8
Back ØJH7
Buttock ØJH9
Chest ØJH6
Face ØJH1
Tissue Expander — *continued*
Insertion of device in — *continued*
Subcutaneous Tissue and Fascia — *continued*
Foot
Left ØJHR
Right ØJHQ
Hand
Left ØJHK
Right ØJHJ
Lower Arm
Left ØJHH
Right ØJHG
Lower Leg
Left ØJHP
Right ØJHN
Neck
Left ØJH5
Right ØJH4
Pelvic Region ØJHC
Perineum ØJHB
Scalp ØJHØ
Upper Arm
Left ØJHF
Right ØJHD
Upper Leg
Left ØJHM
Right ØJHL
Removal of device from
Breast
Left ØHPU
Right ØHPT
Subcutaneous Tissue and Fascia
Head and Neck ØJPS
Lower Extremity ØJPW
Trunk ØJPT
Upper Extremity ØJPV
Revision of device in
Breast
Left ØHWU
Right ØHWT
Subcutaneous Tissue and Fascia
Head and Neck ØJWS
Lower Extremity ØJWW
Trunk ØJWT
Upper Extremity ØJWV
Tissue Plasminogen Activator (tPA) (r-tPA) *use* Other Thrombolytic
Titanium Sternal Fixation System (TSFS)
use Internal Fixation Device, Rigid Plate in ØPS
use Internal Fixation Device, Rigid Plate in ØPH
Tocilizumab XWØ
Tomographic (Tomo) Nuclear Medicine Imaging
Abdomen CW2Ø
Abdomen and Chest CW24
Abdomen and Pelvis CW21
Anatomical Regions, Multiple CW2YYZZ
Bladder, Kidneys and Ureters CT23
Brain CØ2Ø
Breast CH2YYZZ
Bilateral CH22
Left CH21
Right CH2Ø
Bronchi and Lungs CB22
Central Nervous System CØ2YYZZ
Cerebrospinal Fluid CØ25
Chest CW23
Chest and Abdomen CW24
Chest and Neck CW26
Digestive System CD2YYZZ
Endocrine System CG2YYZZ
Extremity
Lower CW2D
Bilateral CP2F
Left CP2D
Right CP2C
Upper CW2M
Bilateral CP2B
Left CP29
Right CP28
Gallbladder CF24
Gastrointestinal Tract CD27
Gland, Parathyroid CG21
Head and Neck CW2B
Heart C22YYZZ
Right and Left C226
Hepatobiliary System and Pancreas CF2YYZZ
Kidneys, Ureters and Bladder CT23
Liver CF25

Tomographic (Tomo) Nuclear Medicine Imaging — *continued*
  Liver and Spleen CF26
  Lungs and Bronchi CB22
  Lymphatics and Hematologic System C72YYZZ
  Musculoskeletal System, Other CP2YYZZ
  Myocardium C22G
  Neck and Chest CW26
  Neck and Head CW2B
  Pancreas and Hepatobiliary System CF2YYZZ
  Pelvic Region CW2J
  Pelvis CP26
  Pelvis and Abdomen CW21
  Pelvis and Spine CP27
  Respiratory System CB2YYZZ
  Skin CH2YYZZ
  Skull CP21
  Skull and Cervical Spine CP23
  Spine
    Cervical CP22
    Cervical and Skull CP23
    Lumbar CP2H
    Thoracic CP2G
    Thoracolumbar CP2J
  Spine and Pelvis CP27
  Spleen C722
  Spleen and Liver CF26
  Subcutaneous Tissue CH2YYZZ
  Thorax CP24
  Ureters, Kidneys and Bladder CT23
  Urinary System CT2YYZZ
Tomography, computerized *see* Computerized Tomography (CT Scan)
Tongue, base of *use* Pharynx
Tonometry 4AØ7XBZ
Tonsillectomy
  see Excision, Mouth and Throat ØCB
  see Resection, Mouth and Throat ØCT
Tonsillotomy *see* Drainage, Mouth and Throat ØC9
Total Anomalous Pulmonary Venous Return (TAPVR) repair
  see Bypass, Atrium, Left Ø217
  see Bypass, Vena Cava, Superior Ø21V
Total artificial (replacement) heart *use* Synthetic Substitute
Total parenteral nutrition (TPN) *see* Introduction of Nutritional Substance
Tourniquet, External *see* Compression, Anatomical Regions 2W1
Trachectomy
  see Excision, Trachea ØBB1
  see Resection, Trachea ØBT1
Trachelectomy
  see Excision, Cervix ØUBC
  see Resection, Cervix ØUTC
Trachelopexy
  see Repair, Cervix ØUQC
  see Reposition, Cervix ØUSC
Tracheloplasty *see* Repair, Cervix ØUQC
Trachelorrhaphy *see* Repair, Cervix ØUQC
Trachelotomy *see* Drainage, Cervix ØU9C
Tracheobronchial lymph node *use* Lymphatic, Thorax
Tracheoesophageal fistulization ØB11ØD6
Tracheolysis *see* Release, Respiratory System ØBN
Tracheoplasty
  see Repair, Respiratory System ØBQ
  see Supplement, Respiratory System ØBU
Tracheorrhaphy *see* Repair, Respiratory System ØBQ
Tracheoscopy ØBJ18ZZ
Tracheostomy *see* Bypass, Respiratory System ØB1
Tracheostomy Device
  Bypass, Trachea ØB11
  Change device in, Trachea ØB21XFZ
  Removal of device from, Trachea ØBP1
  Revision of device in, Trachea ØBW1
Tracheostomy tube *use* Tracheostomy Device in Respiratory System
Tracheotomy *see* Drainage, Respiratory System ØB9
Traction
  Abdominal Wall 2W63X
  Arm
    Lower
      Left 2W6DX
      Right 2W6CX
    Upper
      Left 2W6BX
      Right 2W6AX
Traction — *continued*
  Back 2W65X
  Chest Wall 2W64X
  Extremity
    Lower
      Left 2W6MX
      Right 2W6LX
    Upper
      Left 2W69X
      Right 2W68X
  Face 2W61X
  Finger
    Left 2W6KX
    Right 2W6JX
  Foot
    Left 2W6TX
    Right 2W6SX
  Hand
    Left 2W6FX
    Right 2W6EX
  Head 2W6ØX
  Inguinal Region
    Left 2W67X
    Right 2W66X
  Leg
    Lower
      Left 2W6RX
      Right 2W6QX
    Upper
      Left 2W6PX
      Right 2W6NX
  Neck 2W62X
  Thumb
    Left 2W6HX
    Right 2W6GX
  Toe
    Left 2W6VX
    Right 2W6UX
Tractotomy *see* Division, Central Nervous System and Cranial Nerves ØØ8
Tragus
  use External Ear, Bilateral
  use External Ear, Left
  use External Ear, Right
Training, caregiver *see* Caregiver Training
TRAM (transverse rectus abdominis myocutaneous) flap reconstruction
  Free *see* Replacement, Skin and Breast ØHR
  Pedicled *see* Transfer, Muscles ØKX
Transcatheter Pulmonary Valve (TPV) placement
  In conduit Ø2RH38L
  Native site Ø2RH38M
Transdermal Glomerular Filtration Rate (GFR) Measurement System XT25XE5
Transection *see* Division
Transfer
  Buccal Mucosa ØCX4
  Bursa and Ligament
    Abdomen
      Left ØMXJ
      Right ØMXH
    Ankle
      Left ØMXR
      Right ØMXQ
    Elbow
      Left ØMX4
      Right ØMX3
    Foot
      Left ØMXT
      Right ØMXS
    Hand
      Left ØMX8
      Right ØMX7
    Head and Neck ØMXØ
    Hip
      Left ØMXM
      Right ØMXL
    Knee
      Left ØMXP
      Right ØMXN
    Lower Extremity
      Left ØMXW
      Right ØMXV
    Perineum ØMXK
    Rib(s) ØMXG
    Shoulder
      Left ØMX2
      Right ØMX1
Transfer — *continued*
  Bursa and Ligament — *continued*
    Spine
      Lower ØMXD
      Upper ØMXC
    Sternum ØMXF
    Upper Extremity
      Left ØMXB
      Right ØMX9
    Wrist
      Left ØMX6
      Right ØMX5
  Finger
    Left ØXXPØZM
    Right ØXXNØZL
  Gingiva
    Lower ØCX6
    Upper ØCX5
  Intestine
    Large ØDXE
    Small ØDX8
  Lip
    Lower ØCX1
    Upper ØCXØ
  Muscle
    Abdomen
      Left ØKXL
      Right ØKXK
    Extraocular
      Left Ø8XM
      Right Ø8XL
    Facial ØKX1
    Foot
      Left ØKXW
      Right ØKXV
    Hand
      Left ØKXD
      Right ØKXC
    Head ØKXØ
    Hip
      Left ØKXP
      Right ØKXN
    Lower Arm and Wrist
      Left ØKXB
      Right ØKX9
    Lower Leg
      Left ØKXT
      Right ØKXS
    Neck
      Left ØKX3
      Right ØKX2
    Perineum ØKXM
    Shoulder
      Left ØKX6
      Right ØKX5
    Thorax
      Left ØKXJ
      Right ØKXH
    Tongue, Palate, Pharynx ØKX4
    Trunk
      Left ØKXG
      Right ØKXF
    Upper Arm
      Left ØKX8
      Right ØKX7
    Upper Leg
      Left ØKXR
      Right ØKXQ
  Nerve
    Abducens ØØXL
    Accessory ØØXR
    Acoustic ØØXN
    Cervical Ø1X1
    Facial ØØXM
    Femoral Ø1XD
    Glossopharyngeal ØØXP
    Hypoglossal ØØXS
    Lumbar Ø1XB
    Median Ø1X5
    Oculomotor ØØXH
    Olfactory ØØXF
    Optic ØØXG
    Peroneal Ø1XH
    Phrenic Ø1X2
    Pudendal Ø1XC
    Radial Ø1X6
    Sciatic Ø1XF
    Thoracic Ø1X8
    Tibial Ø1XG

- **Transfer** — *continued*
  - Nerve — *continued*
    - Trigeminal ØØXK
    - Trochlear ØØXJ
    - Ulnar Ø1X4
    - Vagus ØØXQ
  - Palate, Soft ØCX3
  - Prepuce ØVXT
  - Skin
    - Abdomen ØHX7XZZ
    - Back ØHX6XZZ
    - Buttock ØHX8XZZ
    - Chest ØHX5XZZ
    - Ear
      - Left ØHX3XZZ
      - Right ØHX2XZZ
    - Face ØHX1XZZ
    - Foot
      - Left ØHXNXZZ
      - Right ØHXMXZZ
    - Hand
      - Left ØHXGXZZ
      - Right ØHXFXZZ
    - Inguinal ØHXAXZZ
    - Lower Arm
      - Left ØHXEXZZ
      - Right ØHXDXZZ
    - Lower Leg
      - Left ØHXLXZZ
      - Right ØHXKXZZ
    - Neck ØHX4XZZ
    - Perineum ØHX9XZZ
    - Scalp ØHXØXZZ
    - Upper Arm
      - Left ØHXCXZZ
      - Right ØHXBXZZ
    - Upper Leg
      - Left ØHXJXZZ
      - Right ØHXHXZZ
  - Stomach ØDX6
  - Subcutaneous Tissue and Fascia
    - Abdomen ØJX8
    - Back ØJX7
    - Buttock ØJX9
    - Chest ØJX6
    - Face ØJX1
    - Foot
      - Left ØJXR
      - Right ØJXQ
    - Hand
      - Left ØJXK
      - Right ØJXJ
    - Lower Arm
      - Left ØJXH
      - Right ØJXG
    - Lower Leg
      - Left ØJXP
      - Right ØJXN
    - Neck
      - Left ØJX5
      - Right ØJX4
    - Pelvic Region ØJXC
    - Perineum ØJXB
    - Scalp ØJXØ
    - Upper Arm
      - Left ØJXF
      - Right ØJXD
    - Upper Leg
      - Left ØJXM
      - Right ØJXL
  - Tendon
    - Abdomen
      - Left ØLXG
      - Right ØLXF
    - Ankle
      - Left ØLXT
      - Right ØLXS
    - Foot
      - Left ØLXW
      - Right ØLXV
    - Hand
      - Left ØLX8
      - Right ØLX7
    - Head and Neck ØLXØ
    - Hip
      - Left ØLXK
      - Right ØLXJ
    - Knee
      - Left ØLXR

- **Transfer** — *continued*
  - Tendon — *continued*
    - Knee — *continued*
      - Right ØLXQ
    - Lower Arm and Wrist
      - Left ØLX6
      - Right ØLX5
    - Lower Leg
      - Left ØLXP
      - Right ØLXN
    - Perineum ØLXH
    - Shoulder
      - Left ØLX2
      - Right ØLX1
    - Thorax
      - Left ØLXD
      - Right ØLXC
    - Trunk
      - Left ØLXB
      - Right ØLX9
    - Upper Arm
      - Left ØLX4
      - Right ØLX3
    - Upper Leg
      - Left ØLXM
      - Right ØLXL
  - Tongue ØCX7
- **Transfusion**
  - Immunotherapy *see* New Technology, Anatomical Regions XW2
  - Products of Conception
    - Antihemophilic Factors 3Ø27
    - Blood
      - Platelets 3Ø27
      - Red Cells 3Ø27
        - Frozen 3Ø27
      - White Cells 3Ø27
      - Whole 3Ø27
    - Factor IX 3Ø27
    - Fibrinogen 3Ø27
    - Globulin 3Ø27
    - Plasma
      - Fresh 3Ø27
      - Frozen 3Ø27
    - Plasma Cryoprecipitate 3Ø27
    - Serum Albumin 3Ø27
  - Vein
    - 4-Factor Prothrombin Complex Concentrate 3Ø283B1
    - Central
      - Antihemophilic Factors 3Ø243V
      - Blood
        - Platelets 3Ø243R
        - Red Cells 3Ø243N
          - Frozen 3Ø243P
        - White Cells 3Ø243Q
        - Whole 3Ø243H
      - Bone Marrow 3Ø243G
      - Factor IX 3Ø243W
      - Fibrinogen 3Ø243T
      - Globulin 3Ø243S
      - Hematopoietic Stem/Progenitor Cells (HSPC), Genetically Modified 3Ø243CØ
      - Pathogen Reduced Cryoprecipitated Fibrinogen Complex 3Ø243D1
      - Plasma
        - Fresh 3Ø243L
        - Frozen 3Ø243K
      - Plasma Cryoprecipitate 3Ø243M
      - Serum Albumin 3Ø243J
      - Stem Cells
        - Cord Blood 3Ø243X
        - Embryonic 3Ø243AZ
        - Hematopoietic 3Ø243Y
        - T-cell Depleted Hematopoietic 3Ø243U
    - Peripheral
      - Antihemophilic Factors 3Ø233V
      - Blood
        - Platelets 3Ø233R
        - Red Cells 3Ø233N
          - Frozen 3Ø233P
        - White Cells 3Ø233Q
        - Whole 3Ø233H
      - Bone Marrow 3Ø233G
      - Factor IX 3Ø233W
      - Fibrinogen 3Ø233T
      - Globulin 3Ø233S

- **Transfusion** — *continued*
  - Vein — *continued*
    - Peripheral — *continued*
      - Hematopoietic Stem/Progenitor Cells (HSPC), Genetically Modified 3Ø233CØ
      - Pathogen Reduced Cryoprecipitated Fibrinogen Complex 3Ø233D1
      - Plasma
        - Fresh 3Ø233L
        - Frozen 3Ø233K
      - Plasma Cryoprecipitate 3Ø233M
      - Serum Albumin 3Ø233J
      - Stem Cells
        - Cord Blood 3Ø233X
        - Embryonic 3Ø233AZ
        - Hematopoietic 3Ø233Y
        - T-cell Depleted Hematopoietic 3Ø233U
- **Transplant** *see* Transplantation
- **Transplantation**
  - Bone marrow *see* Transfusion, Circulatory 3Ø2
  - Esophagus ØDY5ØZ
  - Face ØWY2ØZ
  - Hand
    - Left ØXYKØZ
    - Right ØXYJØZ
  - Heart Ø2YAØZ
  - Hematopoietic cell *see* Transfusion, Circulatory 3Ø2
  - Intestine
    - Large ØDYEØZ
    - Small ØDY8ØZ
  - Kidney
    - Left ØTY1ØZ
    - Right ØTYØØZ
  - Liver ØFYØØZ
  - Lung
    - Bilateral ØBYMØZ
    - Left ØBYLØZ
    - Lower Lobe
      - Left ØBYJØZ
      - Right ØBYFØZ
    - Middle Lobe, Right ØBYDØZ
    - Right ØBYKØZ
    - Upper Lobe
      - Left ØBYGØZ
      - Right ØBYCØZ
  - Lung Lingula ØBYHØZ
  - Ovary
    - Left ØUY1ØZ
    - Right ØUYØØZ
  - Pancreas ØFYGØZ
  - Penis ØVYSØZ
  - Products of Conception 1ØYØ
  - Scrotum ØVY5ØZ
  - Spleen Ø7YPØZ
  - Stem cell *see* Transfusion, Circulatory 3Ø2
  - Stomach ØDY6ØZ
  - Thymus Ø7YMØZ
  - Uterus ØUY9ØZ
- **Transposition**
  - *see* Bypass
  - *see* Reposition
  - *see* Transfer
- **Transversalis fascia** *use* Subcutaneous Tissue and Fascia, Trunk
- **Transverse acetabular ligament**
  - *use* Hip Bursa and Ligament, Left
  - *use* Hip Bursa and Ligament, Right
- **Transverse (cutaneous) cervical nerve** *use* Cervical Plexus
- **Transverse facial artery**
  - *use* Temporal Artery, Left
  - *use* Temporal Artery, Right
- **Transverse foramen** *use* Cervical Vertebra
- **Transverse humeral ligament**
  - *use* Shoulder Bursa and Ligament, Left
  - *use* Shoulder Bursa and Ligament, Right
- **Transverse ligament of atlas** *use* Head and Neck Bursa and Ligament
- **Transverse process**
  - *use* Cervical Vertebra
  - *use* Lumbar Vertebra
  - *use* Thoracic Vertebra
- **Transverse Rectus Abdominis Myocutaneous Flap**
  - Replacement
    - Bilateral ØHRVØ76

Transverse Rectus Abdominis Myocutaneous Flap — *continued*
Replacement — *continued*
Left ØHRUØ76
Right ØHRTØ76
Transfer
Left ØKXL
Right ØKXK
Transverse scapular ligament
use Shoulder Bursa and Ligament, Left
use Shoulder Bursa and Ligament, Right
Transverse thoracis muscle
use Thorax Muscle, Left
use Thorax Muscle, Right
Transversospinalis muscle
use Trunk Muscle, Left
use Trunk Muscle, Right
Transversus abdominis muscle
use Abdomen Muscle, Left
use Abdomen Muscle, Right
Trapezium bone
use Carpal, Left
use Carpal, Right
Trapezius muscle
use Trunk Muscle, Left
use Trunk Muscle, Right
Trapezoid bone
use Carpal, Left
use Carpal, Right
Triceps brachii muscle
use Upper Arm Muscle, Left
use Upper Arm Muscle, Right
Tricuspid annulus *use* Tricuspid Valve
Trifacial nerve *use* Trigeminal Nerve
Trifecta™ Valve (aortic) *use* Zooplastic Tissue in Heart and Great Vessels
Trigone of bladder *use* Bladder
TriGuard 3™ CEPD (cerebral embolic protection device) X2A6325
Trilaciclib XWØ
Trimming, excisional *see* Excision
Triquetral bone
use Carpal, Left
use Carpal, Right
Trochanteric bursa
use Hip Bursa and Ligament, Left
use Hip Bursa and Ligament, Right
TUMT (transurethral microwave thermotherapy of prostate) ØV5Ø7ZZ
TUNA (transurethral needle ablation of prostate) ØV5Ø7ZZ
Tunneled central venous catheter *use* Vascular Access Device, Tunneled in Subcutaneous Tissue and Fascia
Tunneled spinal (intrathecal) catheter *use* Infusion Device
Turbinectomy
see Excision, Ear, Nose, Sinus Ø9B
see Resection, Ear, Nose, Sinus Ø9T
Turbinoplasty
see Repair, Ear, Nose, Sinus Ø9Q
see Replacement, Ear, Nose, Sinus Ø9R
see Supplement, Ear, Nose, Sinus Ø9U
Turbinotomy
see Division, Ear, Nose, Sinus Ø98
see Drainage, Ear, Nose, Sinus Ø99
TURP (transurethral resection of prostate) ØVBØ7ZZ
see Excision, Prostate ØVBØ
see Resection, Prostate ØVTØ
Twelfth cranial nerve *use* Hypoglossal Nerve
Two lead pacemaker *use* Pacemaker, Dual Chamber in ØJH
Tympanic cavity
use Middle Ear, Left
use Middle Ear, Right
Tympanic nerve *use* Glossopharyngeal Nerve
Tympanic part of temoporal bone
use Temporal Bone, Left
use Temporal Bone, Right
Tympanogram *see* Hearing Assessment, Diagnostic Audiology F13
Tympanoplasty
see Repair, Ear, Nose, Sinus Ø9Q
see Replacement, Ear, Nose, Sinus Ø9R
see Supplement, Ear, Nose, Sinus Ø9U
Tympanosympathectomy *see* Excision, Nerve, Head and Neck Sympathetic Ø1BK
Tympanotomy *see* Drainage, Ear, Nose, Sinus Ø99
TYRX Antibacterial Envelope *use* Anti-Infective Envelope

U

Ulnar collateral carpal ligament
use Wrist Bursa and Ligament, Left
use Wrist Bursa and Ligament, Right
Ulnar collateral ligament
use Elbow Bursa and Ligament, Left
use Elbow Bursa and Ligament, Right
Ulnar notch
use Radius, Left
use Radius, Right
Ulnar vein
use Brachial Vein, Left
use Brachial Vein, Right
Ultrafiltration
Hemodialysis *see* Performance, Urinary 5A1D
Therapeutic plasmapheresis *see* Pheresis, Circulatory 6A55
Ultraflex™ Precision Colonic Stent System *use* Intraluminal Device
ULTRAPRO Hernia System (UHS) *use* Synthetic Substitute
ULTRAPRO Partially Absorbable Lightweight Mesh *use* Synthetic Substitute
ULTRAPRO Plug *use* Synthetic Substitute
Ultrasonic osteogenic stimulator
use Bone Growth Stimulator in Head and Facial Bones
use Bone Growth Stimulator in Lower Bones
use Bone Growth Stimulator in Upper Bones
Ultrasonography
Abdomen BW4ØZZZ
Abdomen and Pelvis BW41ZZZ
Abdominal Wall BH49ZZZ
Aorta
Abdominal, Intravascular B44ØZZ3
Thoracic, Intravascular B34ØZZ3
Appendix BD48ZZZ
Artery
Brachiocephalic-Subclavian, Right, Intravascular B341ZZ3
Celiac and Mesenteric, Intravascular B44KZZ3
Common Carotid
Bilateral, Intravascular B345ZZ3
Left, Intravascular B344ZZ3
Right, Intravascular B343ZZ3
Coronary
Multiple B241YZZ
Intravascular B241ZZ3
Transesophageal B241ZZ4
Single B24ØYZZ
Intravascular B24ØZZ3
Transesophageal B24ØZZ4
Femoral, Intravascular B44LZZ3
Inferior Mesenteric, Intravascular B445ZZ3
Internal Carotid
Bilateral, Intravascular B348ZZ3
Left, Intravascular B347ZZ3
Right, Intravascular B346ZZ3
Intra-Abdominal, Other, Intravascular B44BZZ3
Intracranial, Intravascular B34RZZ3
Lower Extremity
Bilateral, Intravascular B44HZZ3
Left, Intravascular B44GZZ3
Right, Intravascular B44FZZ3
Mesenteric and Celiac, Intravascular B44KZZ3
Ophthalmic, Intravascular B34VZZ3
Penile, Intravascular B44NZZ3
Pulmonary
Left, Intravascular B34TZZ3
Right, Intravascular B34SZZ3
Renal
Bilateral, Intravascular B448ZZ3
Left, Intravascular B447ZZ3
Right, Intravascular B446ZZ3
Subclavian, Left, Intravascular B342ZZ3
Superior Mesenteric, Intravascular B444ZZ3
Upper Extremity
Bilateral, Intravascular B34KZZ3
Left, Intravascular B34JZZ3
Ultrasonography — *continued*
Artery — *continued*
Upper Extremity — *continued*
Right, Intravascular B34HZZ3
Bile Duct BF4ØZZZ
Bile Duct and Gallbladder BF43ZZZ
Bladder BT4ØZZZ
and Kidney BT4JZZZ
Brain BØ4ØZZZ
Breast
Bilateral BH42ZZZ
Left BH41ZZZ
Right BH4ØZZZ
Chest Wall BH4BZZZ
Coccyx BR4FZZZ
Connective Tissue
Lower Extremity BL41ZZZ
Upper Extremity BL4ØZZZ
Duodenum BD49ZZZ
Elbow
Left, Densitometry BP4HZZ1
Right, Densitometry BP4GZZ1
Esophagus BD41ZZZ
Extremity
Lower BH48ZZZ
Upper BH47ZZZ
Eye
Bilateral B847ZZZ
Left B846ZZZ
Right B845ZZZ
Fallopian Tube
Bilateral BU42
Left BU41
Right BU4Ø
Fetal Umbilical Cord BY47ZZZ
Fetus
First Trimester, Multiple Gestation BY4BZZZ
Second Trimester, Multiple Gestation BY4DZZZ
Single
First Trimester BY49ZZZ
Second Trimester BY4CZZZ
Third Trimester BY4FZZZ
Third Trimester, Multiple Gestation BY4GZZZ
Gallbladder BF42ZZZ
Gallbladder and Bile Duct BF43ZZZ
Gastrointestinal Tract BD47ZZZ
Gland
Adrenal
Bilateral BG42ZZZ
Left BG41ZZZ
Right BG4ØZZZ
Parathyroid BG43ZZZ
Thyroid BG44ZZZ
Hand
Left, Densitometry BP4PZZ1
Right, Densitometry BP4NZZ1
Head and Neck BH4CZZZ
Heart
Left B245YZZ
Intravascular B245ZZ3
Transesophageal B245ZZ4
Pediatric B24DYZZ
Intravascular B24DZZ3
Transesophageal B24DZZ4
Right B244YZZ
Intravascular B244ZZ3
Transesophageal B244ZZ4
Right and Left B246YZZ
Intravascular B246ZZ3
Transesophageal B246ZZ4
Heart with Aorta B24BYZZ
Intravascular B24BZZ3
Transesophageal B24BZZ4
Hepatobiliary System, All BF4CZZZ
Hip
Bilateral BQ42ZZZ
Left BQ41ZZZ
Right BQ4ØZZZ
Kidney
and Bladder BT4JZZZ
Bilateral BT43ZZZ
Left BT42ZZZ
Right BT41ZZZ
Transplant BT49ZZZ
Knee
Bilateral BQ49ZZZ
Left BQ48ZZZ
Right BQ47ZZZ

Ultrasonography — *continued*
Liver BF45ZZZ
Liver and Spleen BF46ZZZ
Mediastinum BB4CZZZ
Neck BW4FZZZ
Ovary
Bilateral BU45
Left BU44
Right BU43
Ovary and Uterus BU4C
Pancreas BF47ZZZ
Pelvic Region BW4GZZZ
Pelvis and Abdomen BW41ZZZ
Penis BV4BZZZ
Pericardium B24CYZZ
Intravascular B24CZZ3
Transesophageal B24CZZ4
Placenta BY48ZZZ
Pleura BB4BZZZ
Prostate and Seminal Vesicle BV49ZZZ
Rectum BD4CZZZ
Sacrum BR4FZZZ
Scrotum BV44ZZZ
Seminal Vesicle and Prostate BV49ZZZ
Shoulder
Left, Densitometry BP49ZZ1
Right, Densitometry BP48ZZ1
Spinal Cord BØ4BZZZ
Spine
Cervical BR4ØZZZ
Lumbar BR49ZZZ
Thoracic BR47ZZZ
Spleen and Liver BF46ZZZ
Stomach BD42ZZZ
Tendon
Lower Extremity BL43ZZZ
Upper Extremity BL42ZZZ
Ureter
Bilateral BT48ZZZ
Left BT47ZZZ
Right BT46ZZZ
Urethra BT45ZZZ
Uterus BU46
Uterus and Ovary BU4C
Vein
Jugular
Left, Intravascular B544ZZ3
Right, Intravascular B543ZZ3
Lower Extremity
Bilateral, Intravascular B54DZZ3
Left, Intravascular B54CZZ3
Right, Intravascular B54BZZ3
Portal, Intravascular B54TZZ3
Renal
Bilateral, Intravascular B54LZZ3
Left, Intravascular B54KZZ3
Right, Intravascular B54JZZ3
Spanchnic, Intravascular B54TZZ3
Subclavian
Left, Intravascular B547ZZ3
Right, Intravascular B546ZZ3
Upper Extremity
Bilateral, Intravascular B54PZZ3
Left, Intravascular B54NZZ3
Right, Intravascular B54MZZ3
Vena Cava
Inferior, Intravascular B549ZZ3
Superior, Intravascular B548ZZ3
Wrist
Left, Densitometry BP4MZZ1
Right, Densitometry BP4LZZ1
Ultrasound bone healing system
use Bone Growth Stimulator in Head and Facial Bones
use Bone Growth Stimulator in Lower Bones
use Bone Growth Stimulator in Upper Bones
Ultrasound Therapy
Heart 6A75
No Qualifier 6A75
Vessels
Head and Neck 6A75
Other 6A75
Peripheral 6A75
Ultraviolet Light Therapy, Skin 6A8Ø
Umbilical artery
use Internal Iliac Artery, Left
use Internal Iliac Artery, Right
use Lower Artery
Uniplanar external fixator
use External Fixation Device, Monoplanar in ØPH
use External Fixation Device, Monoplanar in ØPS
use External Fixation Device, Monoplanar in ØQH
use External Fixation Device, Monoplanar in ØQS
Upper GI series *see* Fluoroscopy, Gastrointestinal, Upper BD15
Ureteral orifice
use Ureter
use Ureter, Left
use Ureter, Right
use Ureters, Bilateral
Ureterectomy
see Excision, Urinary System ØTB
see Resection, Urinary System ØTT
Ureterocolostomy *see* Bypass, Urinary System ØT1
Ureterocystostomy *see* Bypass, Urinary System ØT1
Ureteroenterostomy *see* Bypass, Urinary System ØT1
Ureteroileostomy *see* Bypass, Urinary System ØT1
Ureterolithotomy *see* Extirpation, Urinary System ØTC
Ureterolysis *see* Release, Urinary System ØTN
Ureteroneocystostomy
see Bypass, Urinary System ØT1
see Reposition, Urinary System ØTS
Ureteropelvic junction (UPJ)
use Kidney Pelvis, Left
use Kidney Pelvis, Right
Ureteropexy
see Repair, Urinary System ØTQ
see Reposition, Urinary System ØTS
Ureteroplasty
see Repair, Urinary System ØTQ
see Replacement, Urinary System ØTR
see Supplement, Urinary System ØTU
Ureteroplication *see* Restriction, Urinary System ØTV
Ureteropyelography *see* Fluoroscopy, Urinary System BT1
Ureterorrhaphy *see* Repair, Urinary System ØTQ
Ureteroscopy ØTJ98ZZ
Ureterostomy
see Bypass, Urinary System ØT1
see Drainage, Urinary System ØT9
Ureterotomy *see* Drainage, Urinary System ØT9
Ureteroureterostomy *see* Bypass, Urinary System ØT1
Ureterovesical orifice
use Ureter
use Ureter, Left
use Ureter, Right
use Ureters, Bilateral
Urethral catheterization, indwelling ØT9B7ØZ
Urethrectomy
see Excision, Urethra ØTBD
see Resection, Urethra ØTTD
Urethrolithotomy *see* Extirpation, Urethra ØTCD
Urethrolysis *see* Release, Urethra ØTND
Urethropexy
see Repair, Urethra ØTQD
see Reposition, Urethra ØTSD
Urethroplasty
see Repair, Urethra ØTQD
see Replacement, Urethra ØTRD
see Supplement, Urethra ØTUD
Urethrorrhaphy *see* Repair, Urethra ØTQD
Urethroscopy ØTJD8ZZ
Urethrotomy *see* Drainage, Urethra ØT9D
Uridine Triacetate XWØDX82
Urinary incontinence stimulator lead *use* Stimulator Lead in Urinary System
Urography *see* Fluoroscopy, Urinary System BT1
Ustekinumab *use* Other New Technology Therapeutic Substance
Uterine Artery
use Internal Iliac Artery, Left
use Internal Iliac Artery, Right
Uterine artery embolization (UAE) *see* Occlusion, Lower Arteries Ø4L
Uterine cornu *use* Uterus
Uterine tube
use Fallopian Tube, Left
use Fallopian Tube, Right
Uterine vein
use Hypogastric Vein, Left
use Hypogastric Vein, Right
Uvulectomy
see Excision, Uvula ØCBN
see Resection, Uvula ØCTN
Uvulorrhaphy *see* Repair, Uvula ØCQN
Uvulotomy *see* Drainage, Uvula ØC9N

V

Vabomere™ *use* Meropenem-vaborbactam Anti-infective
Vaccination *see* Introduction of Serum, Toxoid, and Vaccine
Vacuum extraction, obstetric 1ØDØ7Z6
Vaginal artery
use Internal Iliac Artery, Left
use Internal Iliac Artery, Right
Vaginal pessary *use* Intraluminal Device, Pessary in Female Reproductive System
Vaginal vein
use Hypogastric Vein, Left
use Hypogastric Vein, Right
Vaginectomy
see Excision, Vagina ØUBG
see Resection, Vagina ØUTG
Vaginofixation
see Repair, Vagina ØUQG
see Reposition, Vagina ØUSG
Vaginoplasty
see Repair, Vagina ØUQG
see Supplement, Vagina ØUUG
Vaginorrhaphy *see* Repair, Vagina ØUQG
Vaginoscopy ØUJH8ZZ
Vaginotomy *see* Drainage, Female Reproductive System ØU9
Vagotomy *see* Division, Nerve, Vagus ØØ8Q
Valiant Thoracic Stent Graft *use* Intraluminal Device
Valvotomy, valvulotomy
see Division, Heart and Great Vessels Ø28
see Release, Heart and Great Vessels Ø2N
Valvuloplasty
see Repair, Heart and Great Vessels Ø2Q
see Replacement, Heart and Great Vessels Ø2R
see Supplement, Heart and Great Vessels Ø2U
Valvuloplasty, Alfieri Stitch *see* Restriction, Valve, Mitral Ø2VG
Vascular Access Device
Totally Implantable
Insertion of device in
Abdomen ØJH8
Chest ØJH6
Lower Arm
Left ØJHH
Right ØJHG
Lower Leg
Left ØJHP
Right ØJHN
Upper Arm
Left ØJHF
Right ØJHD
Upper Leg
Left ØJHM
Right ØJHL
Removal of device from
Lower Extremity ØJPW
Trunk ØJPT
Upper Extremity ØJPV
Revision of device in
Lower Extremity ØJWW
Trunk ØJWT
Upper Extremity ØJWV
Tunneled
Insertion of device in
Abdomen ØJH8
Chest ØJH6
Lower Arm
Left ØJHH
Right ØJHG
Lower Leg
Left ØJHP
Right ØJHN
Upper Arm
Left ØJHF
Right ØJHD
Upper Leg
Left ØJHM
Right ØJHL
Removal of device from
Lower Extremity ØJPW
Trunk ØJPT
Upper Extremity ØJPV

Vascular Access Device — *continued*
Tunneled — *continued*
Revision of device in
Lower Extremity ØJWW
Trunk ØJWT
Upper Extremity ØJWV
Vasectomy *see* Excision, Male Reproductive System ØVB
Vasography
see Fluoroscopy, Male Reproductive System BV1
see Plain Radiography, Male Reproductive System BVØ
Vasoligation *see* Occlusion, Male Reproductive System ØVL
Vasorrhaphy *see* Repair, Male Reproductive System ØVQ
Vasostomy *see* Bypass, Male Reproductive System ØV1
Vasotomy
Drainage *see* Drainage, Male Reproductive System ØV9
With ligation *see* Occlusion, Male Reproductive System ØVL
Vasovasostomy *see* Repair, Male Reproductive System ØVQ
Vastus intermedius muscle
use Upper Leg Muscle, Left
use Upper Leg Muscle, Right
Vastus lateralis muscle
use Upper Leg Muscle, Left
use Upper Leg Muscle, Right
Vastus medialis muscle
use Upper Leg Muscle, Left
use Upper Leg Muscle, Right
VCG (vectorcardiogram) *see* Measurement, Cardiac 4AØ2
Vectra® Vascular Access Graft *use* Vascular Access Device, Tunneled in Subcutaneous Tissue and Fascia
Veklury *use* Remdesivir Anti-infective
Venclexta® *use* Venetoclax Antineoplastic
Venectomy
see Excision, Lower Veins Ø6B
see Excision, Upper Veins Ø5B
Venetoclax Antineoplastic XWØDXR5
Venography
see Fluoroscopy, Veins B51
see Plain Radiography, Veins B5Ø
Venorrhaphy
see Repair, Lower Veins Ø6Q
see Repair, Upper Veins Ø5Q
Venotripsy
see Occlusion, Lower Veins Ø6L
see Occlusion, Upper Veins Ø5L
Ventricular fold *use* Larynx
Ventriculoatriostomy *see* Bypass, Central Nervous System and Cranial Nerves ØØ1
Ventriculocisternostomy *see* Bypass, Central Nervous System and Cranial Nerves ØØ1
Ventriculogram, cardiac
Combined left and right heart *see* Fluoroscopy, Heart, Right and Left B216
Left ventricle *see* Fluoroscopy, Heart, Left B215
Right ventricle *see* Fluoroscopy, Heart, Right B214
Ventriculopuncture, through previously implanted catheter 8CØ1X6J
Ventriculoscopy ØØJØ4ZZ
Ventriculostomy
External drainage *see* Drainage, Cerebral Ventricle ØØ96
Internal shunt *see* Bypass, Cerebral Ventricle ØØ16
Ventriculovenostomy *see* Bypass, Cerebral Ventricle ØØ16
Ventrio™ Hernia Patch *use* Synthetic Substitute
VEP (visual evoked potential) 4AØ7XØZ
Vermiform appendix *use* Appendix
Vermilion border
use Lower Lip
use Upper Lip
Versa *use* Pacemaker, Dual Chamber in ØJH
Version, obstetric
External 1ØSØXZZ
Internal 1ØSØ7ZZ
Vertebral arch
use Cervical Vertebra
use Lumbar Vertebra
use Thoracic Vertebra
Vertebral body
use Cervical Vertebra
use Lumbar Vertebra
use Thoracic Vertebra
Vertebral canal *use* Spinal Canal
Vertebral foramen
use Cervical Vertebra
use Lumbar Vertebra
use Thoracic Vertebra
Vertebral lamina
use Cervical Vertebra
use Lumbar Vertebra
use Thoracic Vertebra
Vertebral pedicle
use Cervical Vertebra
use Lumbar Vertebra
use Thoracic Vertebra
Vesical vein
use Hypogastric Vein, Left
use Hypogastric Vein, Right
Vesicotomy *see* Drainage, Urinary System ØT9
Vesiculectomy
see Excision, Male Reproductive System ØVB
see Resection, Male Reproductive System ØVT
Vesiculogram, seminal *see* Plain Radiography, Male Reproductive System BVØ
Vesiculotomy *see* Drainage, Male Reproductive System ØV9
Vestibular Assessment F15Z
Vestibular (Scarpa's) ganglion *use* Acoustic Nerve
Vestibular nerve *use* Acoustic Nerve
Vestibular Treatment FØC
Vestibulocochlear nerve *use* Acoustic Nerve
VH-IVUS (virtual histology intravascular ultrasound) *see* Ultrasonography, Heart B24
Virchow's (supraclavicular) lymph node
use Lymphatic, Left Neck
use Lymphatic, Right Neck
Virtuoso (II) (DR) (VR) *use* Defibrillator Generator in ØJH
Vistogard(R) *use* Uridine Triacetate
Vitrectomy
see Excision, Eye Ø8B
see Resection, Eye Ø8T
Vitreous body
use Vitreous, Left
use Vitreous, Right
Viva (XT) (S) *use* Cardiac Resynchronization Defibrillator Pulse Generator in ØJH
Vocal fold
use Vocal Cord, Left
use Vocal Cord, Right
Vocational
Assessment *see* Activities of Daily Living Assessment, Rehabilitation FØ2
Retraining *see* Activities of Daily Living Treatment, Rehabilitation FØ8
Volar (palmar) digital vein
use Hand Vein, Left
use Hand Vein, Right
Volar (palmar) metacarpal vein
use Hand Vein, Left
use Hand Vein, Right
Vomer bone *use* Nasal Septum
Vomer of nasal septum *use* Nasal Bone
Voraxaze *use* Glucarpidase
Vulvectomy
see Excision, Female Reproductive System ØUB
see Resection, Female Reproductive System ØUT
V-Wave Interatrial Shunt System *use* Synthetic Substitute
VYXEOS™ *use* Cytarabine and Daunorubicin Liposome Antineoplastic

W

WALLSTENT® Endoprosthesis *use* Intraluminal Device
Washing *see* Irrigation
WavelinQ EndoAVF system
Radial Artery, Left Ø31C3ZF
Radial Artery, Right Ø31B3ZF
Ulnar Artery, Left Ø31A3ZF
Ulnar Artery, Right Ø3193ZF
Wedge resection, pulmonary *see* Excision, Respiratory System ØBB
Whole Blood Nucleic Acid-base Microbial Detection XXE5XM5
Window *see* Drainage
Wiring, dental 2W31X9Z

X

Xact Carotid Stent System *use* Intraluminal Device
XENLETA™ *use* Lefamulin Anti-infective
Xenograft *use* Zooplastic Tissue in Heart and Great Vessels
XIENCE Everolimus Eluting Coronary Stent System *use* Intraluminal Device, Drug-eluting in Heart and Great Vessels
Xiphoid process *use* Sternum
XLIF® System *use* Interbody Fusion Device in Lower Joints
XOSPATA® *use* Gilteritinib Antineoplastic
X-ray *see* Plain Radiography
X-STOP® Spacer
use Spinal Stabilization Device, Interspinous Process in ØRH
use Spinal Stabilization Device, Interspinous Process in ØSH

Y

Yescarta® *use* Axicabtagene Ciloleucel Immunotherapy
Yoga Therapy 8EØZXY4

Z

Zenith AAA Endovascular Graft *use* Intraluminal Device
Zenith Flex® AAA Endovascular Graft *use* Intraluminal Device
Zenith TX2® TAA Endovascular Graft *use* Intraluminal Device
Zenith® Fenestrated AAA Endovascular Graft
use Intraluminal Device, Branched or Fenestrated, One or Two Arteries in Ø4V
use Intraluminal Device, Branched or Fenestrated, Three or More Arteries in Ø4V
Zenith® Renu™ AAA Ancillary Graft *use* Intraluminal Device
ZEPZELCA™ *use* Lurbinectedin
ZERBAXA® *use* Ceftolozane/Tazobactam Anti-infective
Zilver® PTX® (paclitaxel) Drug-Eluting Peripheral Stent
use Intraluminal Device, Drug-eluting in Lower Arteries
use Intraluminal Device, Drug-eluting in Upper Arteries
Zimmer® NexGen® LPS Mobile Bearing Knee *use* Synthetic Substitute
Zimmer® NexGen® LPS-Flex Mobile Knee *use* Synthetic Substitute
ZINPLAVA™ use Bezlotoxumab Monoclonal Antibody
Zonule of Zinn
use Lens, Left
use Lens, Right
Zooplastic Tissue, Rapid Deployment Technique, Replacement X2RF
Zotarolimus-eluting Coronary Stent *use* Intraluminal Device, Drug-eluting in Heart and Great Vessels
Z-plasty, skin for scar contracture *see* Release, Skin and Breast ØHN
ZULRESSO™ use Brexanolone
Zygomatic process of frontal bone *use* Frontal Bone
Zygomatic process of temporal bone
use Temporal Bone, Left
use Temporal Bone, Right
Zygomaticus muscle *use* Facial Muscle
Zyvox *use* Oxazolidinones

ICD-10-PCS Tables

Central Nervous System and Cranial Nerves ØØ1–ØØX

Character Meanings

This Character Meaning table is provided as a guide to assist the user in the identification of character members that may be found in this section of code tables. It **SHOULD NOT** be used to build a PCS code.

Operation–Character 3	Body Part–Character 4	Approach–Character 5	Device–Character 6	Qualifier–Character 7
1 Bypass	Ø Brain	Ø Open	Ø Drainage Device	Ø Nasopharynx
2 Change	1 Cerebral Meninges	3 Percutaneous	1 Radioactive Element	1 Mastoid Sinus
5 Destruction	2 Dura Mater	4 Percutaneous Endoscopic	2 Monitoring Device	2 Atrium
7 Dilation	3 Epidural Space, Intracranial	X External	3 Infusion Device	3 Blood Vessel
8 Division	4 Subdural Space, Intracranial		4 Radioactive Element, Cesium-131 Collagen Implant	4 Pleural Cavity
9 Drainage	5 Subarachnoid Space, Intracranial		7 Autologous Tissue Substitute	5 Intestine
B Excision	6 Cerebral Ventricle		J Synthetic Substitute	6 Peritoneal Cavity
C Extirpation	7 Cerebral Hemisphere		K Nonautologous Tissue Substitute	7 Urinary Tract
D Extraction	8 Basal Ganglia		M Neurostimulator Lead	8 Bone Marrow
F Fragmentation	9 Thalamus		Y Other Device	9 Fallopian Tube
H Insertion	A Hypothalamus		Z No Device	A Subgaleal Space
J Inspection	B Pons			B Cerebral Cisterns
K Map	C Cerebellum			F Olfactory Nerve
N Release	D Medulla Oblongata			G Optic Nerve
P Removal	E Cranial Nerve			H Oculomotor Nerve
Q Repair	F Olfactory Nerve			J Trochlear Nerve
R Replacement	G Optic Nerve			K Trigeminal Nerve
S Reposition	H Oculomotor Nerve			L Abducens Nerve
T Resection	J Trochlear Nerve			M Facial Nerve
U Supplement	K Trigeminal Nerve			N Acoustic Nerve
W Revision	L Abducens Nerve			P Glossopharyngeal Nerve
X Transfer	M Facial Nerve			Q Vagus Nerve
	N Acoustic Nerve			R Accessory Nerve
	P Glossopharyngeal Nerve			S Hypoglossal Nerve
	Q Vagus Nerve			X Diagnostic
	R Accessory Nerve			Z No Qualifier
	S Hypoglossal Nerve			
	T Spinal Meninges			
	U Spinal Canal			
	V Spinal Cord			
	W Cervical Spinal Cord			
	X Thoracic Spinal Cord			
	Y Lumbar Spinal Cord			

AHA Coding Clinic for table ØØ1

2021, 2Q, 19	Electromagnetic stealth guided ventriculoperitoneal shunt insertion with endoscopy
2019, 4Q, 21-22	Cerebral ventricle bypass Qualifier
2018, 4Q, 86	Placement of lumboatrial shunt
2017, 4Q, 39-41	Dilation and bypass of cerebral ventricle
2015, 2Q, 9	Revision of ventriculoperitoneal (VP) shunt
2013, 2Q, 36	Insertion of ventriculoperitoneal shunt with laparoscopic assistance

AHA Coding Clinic for table ØØ5

2021, 2Q, 17	Dorsal root entry zone procedure

AHA Coding Clinic for table ØØ7

2017, 4Q, 39-41	Dilation and bypass of cerebral ventricle

AHA Coding Clinic for table ØØ9

2018, 4Q, 85	Externalization of lumboatrial shunt
2017, 1Q, 50	Failed lumbar puncture
2015, 3Q, 10	Open evacuation of subdural hematoma
2015, 3Q, 11	Percutaneous drainage of subdural hematoma
2015, 3Q, 12	Subdural evacuation portal system (SEPS) placement
2015, 3Q, 12	Placement of ventriculostomy catheter via burr hole
2015, 2Q, 30	Drainage of syrinx
2015, 1Q, 31	Intrathecal chemotherapy
2014, 1Q, 8	Diagnostic lumbar tap
2014, 1Q, 8	Lumbar drainage port aspiration

AHA Coding Clinic for table ØØB

2017, 3Q, 17	Resection of schwannoma and placement of DuraGen and Lorenz cranial plating system
2016, 2Q, 12	Resection of malignant neoplasm of infratemporal fossa
2016, 2Q, 18	Amygdalohippocampectomy
2014, 4Q, 34	Resection of brain malignancy with implantation of chemotherapeutic wafer
2014, 3Q, 24	Repair of lipomyelomeningocele and tethered cord

AHA Coding Clinic for table ØØC

2019, 3Q, 4	Evacuation of subdural hematoma and control of bleeding artery
2019, 2Q, 36	Evacuation of hematoma using NICO Brainpath® technology
2017, 4Q, 48	New and revised body part values - Extirpation spinal canal
2016, 2Q, 29	Decompressive craniectomy with cryopreservation and storage of bone flap
2015, 3Q, 10	Open evacuation of subdural hematoma
2015, 3Q, 11	Percutaneous drainage of subdural hematoma
2015, 3Q, 13	Evacuation of intracerebral hematoma

AHA Coding Clinic for table ØØD

2015, 3Q, 13	Nonexcisional debridement of cranial wound with removal and replacement of hardware

AHA Coding Clinic for table ØØH

2020, 4Q, 43-44	Insertion of radioactive element
2020, 2Q, 15	Ommaya Reservoir with Ventricular Catheter Placement
2020, 2Q, 16	Ommaya Reservoir Placement for Cerebrospinal Fluid Infusion Therapy
2017, 4Q, 30-31	Radiotherapeutic brain implant
2017, 3Q, 13	Implantation of bilateral neurostimulator electrodes
2014, 3Q, 19	End of life replacement of Baclofen pump

AHA Coding Clinic for table ØØJ

2021, 2Q, 19	Electromagnetic stealth guided ventriculoperitoneal shunt insertion with endoscopy
2019, 2Q, 36	Evacuation of hematoma using NICO Brainpath® technology
2017, 1Q, 50	Failed lumbar puncture

AHA Coding Clinic for table ØØN

2019, 2Q, 19	Cervical spinal fusion, decompression and placement of interfacet stabilization device
2019, 1Q, 28	Decompressive laminectomy of both spinal cord and nerve roots
2018, 3Q, 30	Decompressive laminectomy (release of spinal cord versus release of spinal meninges)
2017, 3Q, 10	Repair of Chiari malformation
2017, 2Q, 23	Decompression of spinal cord and placement of instrumentation
2016, 2Q, 29	Decompressive craniectomy with cryopreservation and storage of bone flap
2015, 2Q, 20	Cervical laminoplasty
2015, 2Q, 21	Multiple decompressive cervical laminectomies
2015, 2Q, 34	Decompressive laminectomy
2014, 3Q, 24	Repair of lipomyelomeningocele and tethered cord

AHA Coding Clinic for table ØØP

2014, 3Q, 19	End of life replacement of Baclofen pump

AHA Coding Clinic for table ØØQ

2014, 3Q, 7	Hemi-cranioplasty for repair of cranial defect
2013, 3Q, 25	Fracture of frontal bone with repair and coagulation for hemostasis

AHA Coding Clinic for table ØØS

2014, 4Q, 35	Reimplantation of buccal nerve

AHA Coding Clinic for table ØØU

2018, 1Q, 9	Craniectomy with DuraGaurd placement
2017, 4Q, 62	Added and revised device values - Nerve substitutes
2017, 3Q, 10	Repair of Chiari malformation
2017, 3Q, 17	Resection of schwannoma and placement of DuraGen and Lorenz cranial plating system
2015, 4Q, 39	Dural patch graft
2014, 3Q, 24	Repair of lipomyelomeningocele and tethered cord

AHA Coding Clinic for table ØØW

2018, 4Q, 86	Placement of lumboatrial shunt

Brain

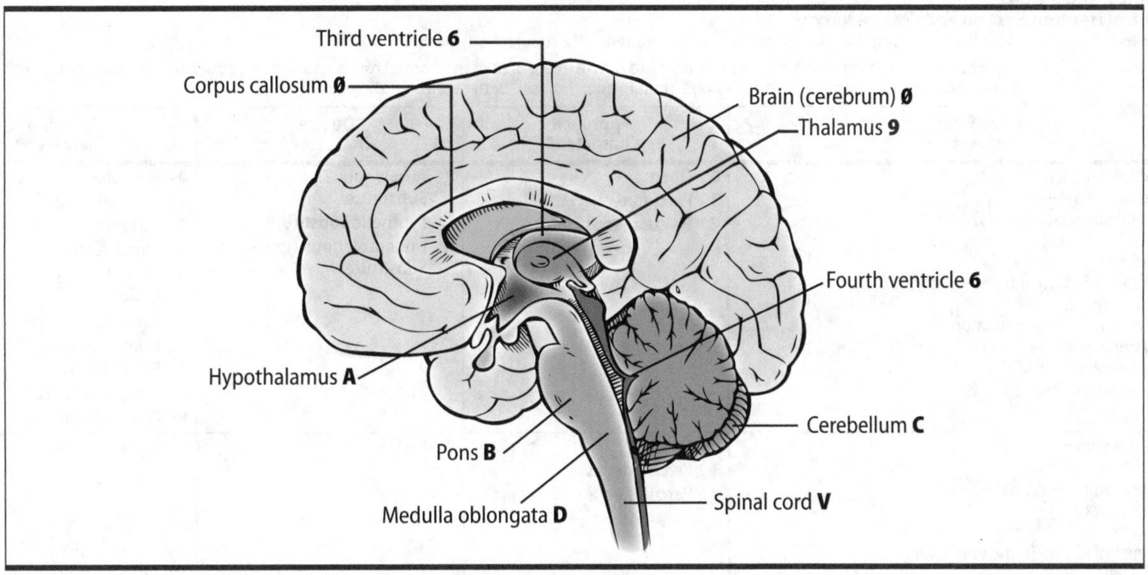

Cranial Nerves

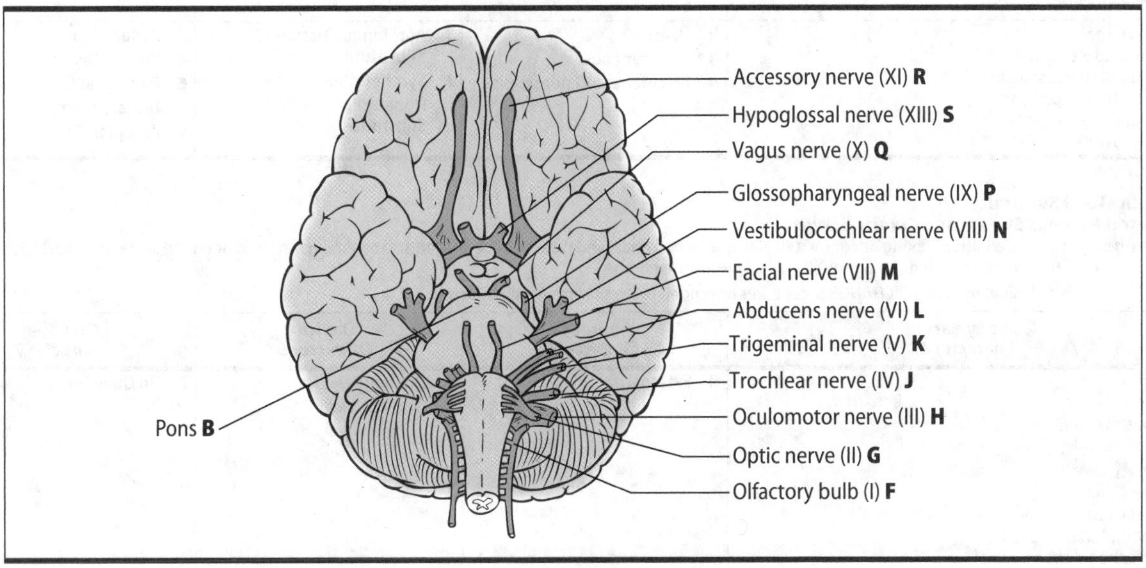

0 Medical and Surgical
0 Central Nervous System and Cranial Nerves
1 Bypass Definition: Altering the route of passage of the contents of a tubular body part

Explanation: Rerouting contents of a body part to a downstream area of the normal route, to a similar route and body part, or to an abnormal route and dissimilar body part. Includes one or more anastomoses, with or without the use of a device.

Body Part Character 4	Approach Character 5	Device Character 6	Qualifier Character 7
6 Cerebral Ventricle Aqueduct of Sylvius Cerebral aqueduct (Sylvius) Choroid plexus Ependyma Foramen of Monro (intraventricular) Fourth ventricle Interventricular foramen (Monro) Left lateral ventricle Right lateral ventricle Third ventricle	**0 Open** **3 Percutaneous** **4 Percutaneous Endoscopic**	**7 Autologous Tissue Substitute** **J Synthetic Substitute** **K Nonautologous Tissue Substitute**	**0 Nasopharynx** **1 Mastoid Sinus** **2 Atrium** **3 Blood Vessel** **4 Pleural Cavity** **5 Intestine** **6 Peritoneal Cavity** **7 Urinary Tract** **8 Bone Marrow** **A Subgaleal Space** **B Cerebral Cisterns**
6 Cerebral Ventricle Aqueduct of Sylvius Cerebral aqueduct (Sylvius) Choroid plexus Ependyma Foramen of Monro (intraventricular) Fourth ventricle Interventricular foramen (Monro) Left lateral ventricle Right lateral ventricle Third ventricle	**0 Open** **3 Percutaneous** **4 Percutaneous Endoscopic**	**Z No Device**	**B Cerebral Cisterns**
U Spinal Canal Epidural space, spinal Extradural space, spinal Subarachnoid space, spinal Subdural space, spinal Vertebral canal	**0 Open** **3 Percutaneous** **4 Percutaneous Endoscopic**	**7 Autologous Tissue Substitute** **J Synthetic Substitute** **K Nonautologous Tissue Substitute**	**2 Atrium** **4 Pleural Cavity** **6 Peritoneal Cavity** **7 Urinary Tract** **9 Fallopian Tube**

0 Medical and Surgical
0 Central Nervous System and Cranial Nerves
2 Change Definition: Taking out or off a device from a body part and putting back an identical or similar device in or on the same body part without cutting or puncturing the skin or a mucous membrane

Explanation: All CHANGE procedures are coded using the approach EXTERNAL

Body Part Character 4	Approach Character 5	Device Character 6	Qualifier Character 7
0 Brain Cerebrum Corpus callosum Encephalon **E Cranial Nerve** **U Spinal Canal** Epidural space, spinal Extradural space, spinal Subarachnoid space, spinal Subdural space, spinal Vertebral canal	**X External**	**0 Drainage Device** **Y Other Device**	**Z No Qualifier**

Non-OR All body part, approach, device, and qualifier values

0 Medical and Surgical
0 Central Nervous System and Cranial Nerves
5 Destruction Definition: Physical eradication of all or a portion of a body part by the direct use of energy, force, or a destructive agent
Explanation: None of the body part is physically taken out

Body Part Character 4	Approach Character 5	Device Character 6	Qualifier Character 7
0 Brain Cerebrum, Corpus callosum, Encephalon **1 Cerebral Meninges** Arachnoid mater, intracranial; Leptomeninges, intracranial; Pia mater, intracranial **2 Dura Mater** Diaphragma sellae; Dura mater, intracranial; Falx cerebri; Tentorium cerebelli **6 Cerebral Ventricle** Aqueduct of Sylvius; Cerebral aqueduct (Sylvius); Choroid plexus; Ependyma; Foramen of Monro (intraventricular); Fourth ventricle; Interventricular foramen (Monro); Left lateral ventricle; Right lateral ventricle; Third ventricle **7 Cerebral Hemisphere** Frontal lobe; Occipital lobe; Parietal lobe; Temporal lobe **8 Basal Ganglia** Basal nuclei; Claustrum; Corpus striatum; Globus pallidus; Substantia nigra; Subthalamic nucleus **9 Thalamus** Epithalamus; Geniculate nucleus; Metathalamus; Pulvinar **A Hypothalamus** Mammillary body **B Pons** Apneustic center; Basis pontis; Locus ceruleus; Pneumotaxic center; Pontine tegmentum; Superior olivary nucleus **C Cerebellum** Culmen **D Medulla Oblongata** Myelencephalon **F Olfactory Nerve** First cranial nerve; Olfactory bulb **G Optic Nerve** Optic chiasma; Second cranial nerve **H Oculomotor Nerve** Third cranial nerve **J Trochlear Nerve** Fourth cranial nerve **K Trigeminal Nerve** Fifth cranial nerve; Gasserian ganglion; Mandibular nerve; Maxillary nerve; Ophthalmic nerve; Trifacial nerve **L Abducens Nerve** Sixth cranial nerve **M Facial Nerve** Chorda tympani; Geniculate ganglion; Greater superficial petrosal nerve; Nerve to the stapedius; Parotid plexus; Posterior auricular nerve; Seventh cranial nerve; Submandibular ganglion **N Acoustic Nerve** Cochlear nerve; Eighth cranial nerve; Scarpa's (vestibular) ganglion; Spiral ganglion; Vestibular (Scarpa's) ganglion; Vestibular nerve; Vestibulocochlear nerve **P Glossopharyngeal Nerve** Carotid sinus nerve; Ninth cranial nerve; Tympanic nerve **Q Vagus Nerve** Anterior vagal trunk; Pharyngeal plexus; Pneumogastric nerve; Posterior vagal trunk; Pulmonary plexus; Recurrent laryngeal nerve; Superior laryngeal nerve; Tenth cranial nerve **R Accessory Nerve** Eleventh cranial nerve **S Hypoglossal Nerve** Twelfth cranial nerve **T Spinal Meninges** Arachnoid mater, spinal; Denticulate (dentate) ligament; Dura mater, spinal; Filum terminale; Leptomeninges, spinal; Pia mater, spinal **W Cervical Spinal Cord** Dorsal root ganglion **X Thoracic Spinal Cord** Dorsal root ganglion **Y Lumbar Spinal Cord** Cauda equina; Conus medullaris; Dorsal root ganglion	**0 Open** **3 Percutaneous** **4 Percutaneous Endoscopic**	**Z No Device**	**Z No Qualifier**

Non-OR 005[F,G,H,J,K,L,M,N,P,Q,R,S][0,3,4]ZZ

Ø Medical and Surgical
Ø Central Nervous System and Cranial Nerves
7 Dilation Definition: Expanding an orifice or the lumen of a tubular body part

Explanation: The orifice can be a natural orifice or an artificially created orifice. Accomplished by stretching a tubular body part using intraluminal pressure or by cutting part of the orifice or wall of the tubular body part.

Body Part Character 4	Approach Character 5	Device Character 6	Qualifier Character 7
6 Cerebral Ventricle Aqueduct of Sylvius Cerebral aqueduct (Sylvius) Choroid plexus Ependyma Foramen of Monro (intraventricular) Fourth ventricle Interventricular foramen (Monro) Left lateral ventricle Right lateral ventricle Third ventricle	**Ø Open** **3 Percutaneous** **4 Percutaneous Endoscopic**	**Z No Device**	**Z No Qualifier**

Ø Medical and Surgical
Ø Central Nervous System and Cranial Nerves
8 Division Definition: Cutting into a body part, without draining fluids and/or gases from the body part, in order to separate or transect a body part

Explanation: All or a portion of the body part is separated into two or more portions

Body Part Character 4		Approach Character 5	Device Character 6	Qualifier Character 7
Ø Brain Cerebrum Corpus callosum Encephalon **7 Cerebral Hemisphere** Frontal lobe Occipital lobe Parietal lobe Temporal lobe **8 Basal Ganglia** Basal nuclei Claustrum Corpus striatum Globus pallidus Substantia nigra Subthalamic nucleus **F Olfactory Nerve** First cranial nerve Olfactory bulb **G Optic Nerve** Optic chiasma Second cranial nerve **H Oculomotor Nerve** Third cranial nerve **J Trochlear Nerve** Fourth cranial nerve **K Trigeminal Nerve** Fifth cranial nerve Gasserian ganglion Mandibular nerve Maxillary nerve Ophthalmic nerve Trifacial nerve **L Abducens Nerve** Sixth cranial nerve **M Facial Nerve** Chorda tympani Geniculate ganglion Greater superficial petrosal nerve Nerve to the stapedius Parotid plexus Posterior auricular nerve Seventh cranial nerve Submandibular ganglion	**N Acoustic Nerve** Cochlear nerve Eighth cranial nerve Scarpa's (vestibular) ganglion Spiral ganglion Vestibular (Scarpa's) ganglion Vestibular nerve Vestibulocochlear nerve **P Glossopharyngeal Nerve** Carotid sinus nerve Ninth cranial nerve Tympanic nerve **Q Vagus Nerve** Anterior vagal trunk Pharyngeal plexus Pneumogastric nerve Posterior vagal trunk Pulmonary plexus Recurrent laryngeal nerve Superior laryngeal nerve Tenth cranial nerve **R Accessory Nerve** Eleventh cranial nerve **S Hypoglossal Nerve** Twelfth cranial nerve **W Cervical Spinal Cord** Dorsal root ganglion **X Thoracic Spinal Cord** Dorsal root ganglion **Y Lumbar Spinal Cord** Cauda equina Conus medullaris Dorsal root ganglion	**Ø Open** **3 Percutaneous** **4 Percutaneous Endoscopic**	**Z No Device**	**Z No Qualifier**

Ø Medical and Surgical
Ø Central Nervous System and Cranial Nerves
9 Drainage Definition: Taking or letting out fluids and/or gases from a body part

Explanation: The qualifier DIAGNOSTIC is used to identify drainage procedures that are biopsies

Body Part Character 4		Approach Character 5	Device Character 6	Qualifier Character 7
Ø Brain Cerebrum Corpus callosum Encephalon **1 Cerebral Meninges** Arachnoid mater, intracranial Leptomeninges, intracranial Pia mater, intracranial **2 Dura Mater** Diaphragma sellae Dura mater, intracranial Falx cerebri Tentorium cerebelli **3 Epidural Space, Intracranial** Extradural space, intracranial **4 Subdural Space, Intracranial** **5 Subarachnoid Space, Intracranial** **6 Cerebral Ventricle** Aqueduct of Sylvius Cerebral aqueduct (Sylvius) Choroid plexus Ependyma Foramen of Monro (intraventricular) Fourth ventricle Interventricular foramen (Monro) Left lateral ventricle Right lateral ventricle Third ventricle **7 Cerebral Hemisphere** Frontal lobe Occipital lobe Parietal lobe Temporal lobe **8 Basal Ganglia** Basal nuclei Claustrum Corpus striatum Globus pallidus Substantia nigra Subthalamic nucleus **9 Thalamus** Epithalamus Geniculate nucleus Metathalamus Pulvinar **A Hypothalamus** Mammillary body **B Pons** Apneustic center Basis pontis Locus ceruleus Pneumotaxic center Pontine tegmentum Superior olivary nucleus **C Cerebellum** Culmen **D Medulla Oblongata** Myelencephalon **F Olfactory Nerve** First cranial nerve Olfactory bulb	**G Optic Nerve** Optic chiasma Second cranial nerve **H Oculomotor Nerve** Third cranial nerve **J Trochlear Nerve** Fourth cranial nerve **K Trigeminal Nerve** Fifth cranial nerve Gasserian ganglion Mandibular nerve Maxillary nerve Ophthalmic nerve Trifacial nerve **L Abducens Nerve** Sixth cranial nerve **M Facial Nerve** Chorda tympani Geniculate ganglion Greater superficial petrosal nerve Nerve to the stapedius Parotid plexus Posterior auricular nerve Seventh cranial nerve Submandibular ganglion **N Acoustic Nerve** Cochlear nerve Eighth cranial nerve Scarpa's (vestibular) ganglion Spiral ganglion Vestibular (Scarpa's) ganglion Vestibular nerve Vestibulocochlear nerve **P Glossopharyngeal Nerve** Carotid sinus nerve Ninth cranial nerve Tympanic nerve **Q Vagus Nerve** Anterior vagal trunk Pharyngeal plexus Pneumogastric nerve Posterior vagal trunk Pulmonary plexus Recurrent laryngeal nerve Superior laryngeal nerve Tenth cranial nerve **R Accessory Nerve** Eleventh cranial nerve **S Hypoglossal Nerve** Twelfth cranial nerve **T Spinal Meninges** Arachnoid mater, spinal Denticulate (dentate) ligament Dura mater, spinal Filum terminale Leptomeninges, spinal Pia mater, spinal **U Spinal Canal** Epidural space, spinal Extradural space, spinal Subarachnoid space, spinal Subdural space, spinal Vertebral canal **W Cervical Spinal Cord** Dorsal root ganglion **X Thoracic Spinal Cord** Dorsal root ganglion **Y Lumbar Spinal Cord** Cauda equina Conus medullaris Dorsal root ganglion	**Ø Open** **3 Percutaneous** **4 Percutaneous Endoscopic**	**Ø Drainage Device**	**Z No Qualifier**

Non-OR ØØ9[T,W,X,Y]3ØZ
Non-OR ØØ9U[3,4]ØZ

ØØ9 Continued on next page

Ø Medical and Surgical
Ø Central Nervous System and Cranial Nerves
9 Drainage Definition: Taking or letting out fluids and/or gases from a body part
Explanation: The qualifier DIAGNOSTIC is used to identify drainage procedures that are biopsies

ØØ9 Continued

Body Part Character 4	Approach Character 5	Device Character 6	Qualifier Character 7
Ø **Brain** Cerebrum Corpus callosum Encephalon 1 **Cerebral Meninges** Arachnoid mater, intracranial Leptomeninges, intracranial Pia mater, intracranial 2 **Dura Mater** Diaphragma sellae Dura mater, intracranial Falx cerebri Tentorium cerebelli 3 **Epidural Space, Intracranial** Extradural space, intracranial 4 **Subdural Space, Intracranial** 5 **Subarachnoid Space, Intracranial** 6 **Cerebral Ventricle** Aqueduct of Sylvius Cerebral aqueduct (Sylvius) Choroid plexus Ependyma Foramen of Monro (intraventricular) Fourth ventricle Interventricular foramen (Monro) Left lateral ventricle Right lateral ventricle Third ventricle 7 **Cerebral Hemisphere** Frontal lobe Occipital lobe Parietal lobe Temporal lobe 8 **Basal Ganglia** Basal nuclei Claustrum Corpus striatum Globus pallidus Substantia nigra Subthalamic nucleus 9 **Thalamus** Epithalamus Geniculate nucleus Metathalamus Pulvinar A **Hypothalamus** Mammillary body B **Pons** Apneustic center Basis pontis Locus ceruleus Pneumotaxic center Pontine tegmentum Superior olivary nucleus C **Cerebellum** Culmen D **Medulla Oblongata** Myelencephalon F **Olfactory Nerve** First cranial nerve Olfactory bulb G **Optic Nerve** Optic chiasma Second cranial nerve H **Oculomotor Nerve** Third cranial nerve J **Trochlear Nerve** Fourth cranial nerve K **Trigeminal Nerve** Fifth cranial nerve Gasserian ganglion Mandibular nerve Maxillary nerve Ophthalmic nerve Trifacial nerve L **Abducens Nerve** Sixth cranial nerve M **Facial Nerve** Chorda tympani Geniculate ganglion Greater superficial petrosal nerve Nerve to the stapedius Parotid plexus Posterior auricular nerve Seventh cranial nerve Submandibular ganglion N **Acoustic Nerve** Cochlear nerve Eighth cranial nerve Scarpa's (vestibular) ganglion Spiral ganglion Vestibular (Scarpa's) ganglion Vestibular nerve Vestibulocochlear nerve P **Glossopharyngeal Nerve** Carotid sinus nerve Ninth cranial nerve Tympanic nerve Q **Vagus Nerve** Anterior vagal trunk Pharyngeal plexus Pneumogastric nerve Posterior vagal trunk Pulmonary plexus Recurrent laryngeal nerve Superior laryngeal nerve Tenth cranial nerve R **Accessory Nerve** Eleventh cranial nerve S **Hypoglossal Nerve** Twelfth cranial nerve T **Spinal Meninges** Arachnoid mater, spinal Denticulate (dentate) ligament Dura mater, spinal Filum terminale Leptomeninges, spinal Pia mater, spinal U **Spinal Canal** Epidural space, spinal Extradural space, spinal Subarachnoid space, spinal Subdural space, spinal Vertebral canal W **Cervical Spinal Cord** Dorsal root ganglion X **Thoracic Spinal Cord** Dorsal root ganglion Y **Lumbar Spinal Cord** Cauda equina Conus medullaris Dorsal root ganglion	Ø Open 3 Percutaneous 4 Percutaneous Endoscopic	Z No Device	X Diagnostic Z No Qualifier

Non-OR ØØ9[Ø,1,2,3,4,5,6,7,8,9,A,B,C,D,F,G,H,J,K,L,M,N,P,Q,R,S][3,4]ZX
Non-OR ØØ9[T,W,X,Y]3Z[X,Z]
Non-OR ØØ9U[3,4]Z[X,Z]

Non-OR Procedure DRG Non-OR Procedure Valid OR Procedure HAC Associated Procedure Combination Only New/Revised GREEN

Ø Medical and Surgical
Ø Central Nervous System and Cranial Nerves
B Excision Definition: Cutting out or off, without replacement, a portion of a body part
Explanation: The qualifier DIAGNOSTIC is used to identify excision procedures that are biopsies

Body Part Character 4	Approach Character 5	Device Character 6	Qualifier Character 7
Ø Brain Cerebrum Corpus callosum Encephalon **1 Cerebral Meninges** Arachnoid mater, intracranial Leptomeninges, intracranial Pia mater, intracranial **2 Dura Mater** Diaphragma sellae Dura mater, intracranial Falx cerebri Tentorium cerebelli **6 Cerebral Ventricle** Aqueduct of Sylvius Cerebral aqueduct (Sylvius) Choroid plexus Ependyma Foramen of Monro (intraventricular) Fourth ventricle Interventricular foramen (Monro) Left lateral ventricle Right lateral ventricle Third ventricle **7 Cerebral Hemisphere** Frontal lobe Occipital lobe Parietal lobe Temporal lobe **8 Basal Ganglia** Basal nuclei Claustrum Corpus striatum Globus pallidus Substantia nigra Subthalamic nucleus **9 Thalamus** Epithalamus Geniculate nucleus Metathalamus Pulvinar **A Hypothalamus** Mammillary body **B Pons** Apneustic center Basis pontis Locus ceruleus Pneumotaxic center Pontine tegmentum Superior olivary nucleus **C Cerebellum** Culmen **D Medulla Oblongata** Myelencephalon **F Olfactory Nerve** First cranial nerve Olfactory bulb **G Optic Nerve** Optic chiasma Second cranial nerve **H Oculomotor Nerve** Third cranial nerve **J Trochlear Nerve** Fourth cranial nerve **K Trigeminal Nerve** Fifth cranial nerve Gasserian ganglion Mandibular nerve Maxillary nerve Ophthalmic nerve Trifacial nerve **L Abducens Nerve** Sixth cranial nerve **M Facial Nerve** Chorda tympani Geniculate ganglion Greater superficial petrosal nerve Nerve to the stapedius Parotid plexus Posterior auricular nerve Seventh cranial nerve Submandibular ganglion **N Acoustic Nerve** Cochlear nerve Eighth cranial nerve Scarpa's (vestibular) ganglion Spiral ganglion Vestibular (Scarpa's) ganglion Vestibular nerve Vestibulocochlear nerve **P Glossopharyngeal Nerve** Carotid sinus nerve Ninth cranial nerve Tympanic nerve **Q Vagus Nerve** Anterior vagal trunk Pharyngeal plexus Pneumogastric nerve Posterior vagal trunk Pulmonary plexus Recurrent laryngeal nerve Superior laryngeal nerve Tenth cranial nerve **R Accessory Nerve** Eleventh cranial nerve **S Hypoglossal Nerve** Twelfth cranial nerve **T Spinal Meninges** Arachnoid mater, spinal Denticulate (dentate) ligament Dura mater, spinal Filum terminale Leptomeninges, spinal Pia mater, spinal **W Cervical Spinal Cord** Dorsal root ganglion **X Thoracic Spinal Cord** Dorsal root ganglion **Y Lumbar Spinal Cord** Cauda equina Conus medullaris Dorsal root ganglion	**Ø Open** **3 Percutaneous** **4 Percutaneous Endoscopic**	**Z No Device**	**X Diagnostic** **Z No Qualifier**

Non-OR ØØB[F,G,H,J,K,L,M,N,P,Q,R,S][3,4]ZX

Ø Medical and Surgical
Ø Central Nervous System and Cranial Nerves
C Extirpation Definition: Taking or cutting out solid matter from a body part

Explanation: The solid matter may be an abnormal byproduct of a biological function or a foreign body; it may be imbedded in a body part or in the lumen of a tubular body part. The solid matter may or may not have been previously broken into pieces.

Body Part Character 4	Approach Character 5	Device Character 6	Qualifier Character 7
Ø Brain Cerebrum Corpus callosum Encephalon **1 Cerebral Meninges** Arachnoid mater, intracranial Leptomeninges, intracranial Pia mater, intracranial **2 Dura Mater** Diaphragma sellae Dura mater, intracranial Falx cerebri Tentorium cerebelli **3 Epidural Space, Intracranial** Extradural space, intracranial **4 Subdural Space, Intracranial** **5 Subarachnoid Space, Intracranial** **6 Cerebral Ventricle** Aqueduct of Sylvius Cerebral aqueduct (Sylvius) Choroid plexus Ependyma Foramen of Monro (intraventricular) Fourth ventricle Interventricular foramen (Monro) Left lateral ventricle Right lateral ventricle Third ventricle **7 Cerebral Hemisphere** Frontal lobe Occipital lobe Parietal lobe Temporal lobe **8 Basal Ganglia** Basal nuclei Claustrum Corpus striatum Globus pallidus Substantia nigra Subthalamic nucleus **9 Thalamus** Epithalamus Geniculate nucleus Metathalamus Pulvinar **A Hypothalamus** Mammillary body **B Pons** Apneustic center Basis pontis Locus ceruleus Pneumotaxic center Pontine tegmentum Superior olivary nucleus **C Cerebellum** Culmen **D Medulla Oblongata** Myelencephalon **F Olfactory Nerve** First cranial nerve Olfactory bulb **G Optic Nerve** Optic chiasma Second cranial nerve **H Oculomotor Nerve** Third cranial nerve **J Trochlear Nerve** Fourth cranial nerve **K Trigeminal Nerve** Fifth cranial nerve Gasserian ganglion Mandibular nerve Maxillary nerve Ophthalmic nerve Trifacial nerve **L Abducens Nerve** Sixth cranial nerve **M Facial Nerve** Chorda tympani Geniculate ganglion Greater superficial petrosal nerve Nerve to the stapedius Parotid plexus Posterior auricular nerve Seventh cranial nerve Submandibular ganglion **N Acoustic Nerve** Cochlear nerve Eighth cranial nerve Scarpa's (vestibular) ganglion Spiral ganglion Vestibular (Scarpa's) ganglion Vestibular nerve Vestibulocochlear nerve **P Glossopharyngeal Nerve** Carotid sinus nerve Ninth cranial nerve Tympanic nerve **Q Vagus Nerve** Anterior vagal trunk Pharyngeal plexus Pneumogastric nerve Posterior vagal trunk Pulmonary plexus Recurrent laryngeal nerve Superior laryngeal nerve Tenth cranial nerve **R Accessory Nerve** Eleventh cranial nerve **S Hypoglossal Nerve** Twelfth cranial nerve **T Spinal Meninges** Arachnoid mater, spinal Denticulate (dentate) ligament Dura mater, spinal Filum terminale Leptomeninges, spinal Pia mater, spinal **U Spinal Canal** **W Cervical Spinal Cord** Dorsal root ganglion **X Thoracic Spinal Cord** Dorsal root ganglion **Y Lumbar Spinal Cord** Cauda equina Conus medullaris Dorsal root ganglion	**Ø Open** **3 Percutaneous** **4 Percutaneous Endoscopic**	**Z No Device**	**Z No Qualifier**

Ø Medical and Surgical
Ø Central Nervous System and Cranial Nerves
D Extraction Definition: Pulling or stripping out or off all or a portion of a body part by the use of force
Explanation: The qualifier DIAGNOSTIC is used to identify extraction procedures that are biopsies

Body Part Character 4		Approach Character 5	Device Character 6	Qualifier Character 7
Ø Brain Cerebrum Corpus callosum Encephalon **1 Cerebral Meninges** Arachnoid mater, intracranial Leptomeninges, intracranial Pia mater, intracranial **2 Dura Mater** Diaphragma sellae Dura mater, intracranial Falx cerebri Tentorium cerebelli 7 Cerebral Hemisphere Frontal lobe Occipital lobe Parietal lobe Temporal lobe **F Olfactory Nerve** First cranial nerve Olfactory bulb **G Optic Nerve** Optic chiasma Second cranial nerve **H Oculomotor Nerve** Third cranial nerve **J Trochlear Nerve** Fourth cranial nerve **K Trigeminal Nerve** Fifth cranial nerve Gasserian ganglion Mandibular nerve Maxillary nerve Ophthalmic nerve Trifacial nerve **L Abducens Nerve** Sixth cranial nerve	**M Facial Nerve** Chorda tympani Geniculate ganglion Greater superficial petrosal nerve Nerve to the stapedius Parotid plexus Posterior auricular nerve Seventh cranial nerve Submandibular ganglion **N Acoustic Nerve** Cochlear nerve Eighth cranial nerve Scarpa's (vestibular) ganglion Spiral ganglion Vestibular (Scarpa's) ganglion Vestibular nerve Vestibulocochlear nerve **P Glossopharyngeal Nerve** Carotid sinus nerve Ninth cranial nerve Tympanic nerve **Q Vagus Nerve** Anterior vagal trunk Pharyngeal plexus Pneumogastric nerve Posterior vagal trunk Pulmonary plexus Recurrent laryngeal nerve Superior laryngeal nerve Tenth cranial nerve **R Accessory Nerve** Eleventh cranial nerve **S Hypoglossal Nerve** Twelfth cranial nerve **T Spinal Meninges** Arachnoid mater, spinal Denticulate (dentate) ligament Dura mater, spinal Filum terminale Leptomeninges, spinal Pia mater, spinal	**Ø Open** **3 Percutaneous** **4 Percutaneous Endoscopic**	**Z No Device**	**Z No Qualifier**

Central Nervous System and Cranial Nerves

ØØD–ØØD

Ø Medical and Surgical
Ø Central Nervous System and Cranial Nerves
F Fragmentation Definition: Breaking solid matter in a body part into pieces

Explanation: Physical force (e.g., manual, ultrasonic) applied directly or indirectly is used to break the solid matter into pieces. The solid matter may be an abnormal byproduct of a biological function or a foreign body. The pieces of solid matter are not taken out.

Body Part Character 4	Approach Character 5	Device Character 6	Qualifier Character 7
3 Epidural Space, Intracranial NC Extradural space, intracranial **4 Subdural Space, Intracranial** NC **5 Subarachnoid Space, Intracranial** NC **6 Cerebral Ventricle** NC Aqueduct of Sylvius Cerebral aqueduct (Sylvius) Choroid plexus Ependyma Foramen of Monro (intraventricular) Fourth ventricle Interventricular foramen (Monro) Left lateral ventricle Right lateral ventricle Third ventricle **U Spinal Canal** Epidural space, spinal Extradural space, spinal Subarachnoid space, spinal Subdural space, spinal Vertebral canal	**Ø Open** **3 Percutaneous** **4 Percutaneous Endoscopic** **X External**	**Z No Device**	**Z No Qualifier**

Non-OR ØØF[3,4,5,6]XZZ
NC ØØF[3,4,5,6]XZZ

Ø Medical and Surgical
Ø Central Nervous System and Cranial Nerves
H Insertion Definition: Putting in a nonbiological appliance that monitors, assists, performs, or prevents a physiological function but does not physically take the place of a body part

Explanation: None

Body Part Character 4	Approach Character 5	Device Character 6	Qualifier Character 7
Ø Brain ⊞ Cerebrum Corpus callosum Encephalon	**Ø Open**	**1 Radioactive Element** **2 Monitoring Device** **3 Infusion Device** **4 Radioactive Element, Cesium-131 Collagen Implant** **M Neurostimulator Lead** **Y Other Device**	**Z No Qualifier**
Ø Brain ⊞ Cerebrum Corpus callosum Encephalon	**3 Percutaneous** **4 Percutaneous Endoscopic**	**1 Radioactive Element** **2 Monitoring Device** **3 Infusion Device** **M Neurostimulator Lead** **Y Other Device**	**Z No Qualifier**
6 Cerebral Ventricle ⊞ Aqueduct of Sylvius Cerebral aqueduct (Sylvius) Choroid plexus Ependyma Foramen of Monro (intraventricular) Fourth ventricle Interventricular foramen (Monro) Left lateral ventricle Right lateral ventricle Third ventricle **E Cranial Nerve** ⊞ **U Spinal Canal** ⊞ Epidural space, spinal Extradural space, spinal Subarachnoid space, spinal Subdural space, spinal Vertebral canal **V Spinal Cord** ⊞ Dorsal root ganglion	**Ø Open** **3 Percutaneous** **4 Percutaneous Endoscopic**	**1 Radioactive Element** **2 Monitoring Device** **3 Infusion Device** **M Neurostimulator Lead** **Y Other Device**	**Z No Qualifier**

DRG Non-OR ØØHØØ4Z
Non-OR ØØH[E,U,V]32Z
Non-OR ØØH[E,U][3,4]YZ
Non-OR ØØH[U,V][Ø,3,4]3Z

See Appendix L for Procedure Combinations
⊞ ØØHØØMZ
⊞ ØØHØ[3,4]MZ
⊞ ØØH[6,E,U,V][Ø,3,4]MZ

Ø Medical and Surgical
Ø Central Nervous System and Cranial Nerves
J Inspection Definition: Visually and/or manually exploring a body part

Explanation: Visual exploration may be performed with or without optical instrumentation. Manual exploration may be performed directly or through intervening body layers.

Body Part Character 4	Approach Character 5	Device Character 6	Qualifier Character 7
Ø Brain Cerebrum Corpus callosum Encephalon **E Cranial Nerve** **U Spinal Canal** Epidural space, spinal Extradural space, spinal Subarachnoid space, spinal Subdural space, spinal Vertebral canal **V Spinal Cord** Dorsal root ganglion	**Ø Open** **3 Percutaneous** **4 Percutaneous Endoscopic**	**Z** No Device	**Z** No Qualifier

Non-OR ØØJ[Ø,E,U,V]3ZZ

Ø Medical and Surgical
Ø Central Nervous System and Cranial Nerves
K Map Definition: Locating the route of passage of electrical impulses and/or locating functional areas in a body part

Explanation: Applicable only to the cardiac conduction mechanism and the central nervous system

Body Part Character 4	Approach Character 5	Device Character 6	Qualifier Character 7
Ø Brain Cerebrum Corpus callosum Encephalon **7 Cerebral Hemisphere** Frontal lobe Occipital lobe Parietal lobe Temporal lobe **8 Basal Ganglia** Basal nuclei Claustrum Corpus striatum Globus pallidus Substantia nigra Subthalamic nucleus **9 Thalamus** Epithalamus Geniculate nucleus Metathalamus Pulvinar **A Hypothalamus** Mammillary body **B Pons** Apneustic center Basis pontis Locus ceruleus Pneumotaxic center Pontine tegmentum Superior olivary nucleus **C Cerebellum** Culmen **D Medulla Oblongata** Myelencephalon	**Ø Open** **3 Percutaneous** **4 Percutaneous Endoscopic**	**Z** No Device	**Z** No Qualifier

Ø Medical and Surgical
Ø Central Nervous System and Cranial Nerves
N Release Definition: Freeing a body part from an abnormal physical constraint by cutting or by the use of force
Explanation: Some of the restraining tissue may be taken out but none of the body part is taken out

Body Part Character 4	Approach Character 5	Device Character 6	Qualifier Character 7
Ø Brain Cerebrum Corpus callosum Encephalon **1 Cerebral Meninges** Arachnoid mater, intracranial Leptomeninges, intracranial Pia mater, intracranial **2 Dura Mater** Diaphragma sellae Dura mater, intracranial Falx cerebri Tentorium cerebelli **6 Cerebral Ventricle** Aqueduct of Sylvius Cerebral aqueduct (Sylvius) Choroid plexus Ependyma Foramen of Monro (intraventricular) Fourth ventricle Interventricular foramen (Monro) Left lateral ventricle Right lateral ventricle Third ventricle **7 Cerebral Hemisphere** Frontal lobe Occipital lobe Parietal lobe Temporal lobe **8 Basal Ganglia** Basal nuclei Claustrum Corpus striatum Globus pallidus Substantia nigra Subthalamic nucleus **9 Thalamus** Epithalamus Geniculate nucleus Metathalamus Pulvinar **A Hypothalamus** Mammillary body **B Pons** Apneustic center Basis pontis Locus ceruleus Pneumotaxic center Pontine tegmentum Superior olivary nucleus **C Cerebellum** Culmen **D Medulla Oblongata** Myelencephalon **F Olfactory Nerve** First cranial nerve Olfactory bulb **G Optic Nerve** Optic chiasma Second cranial nerve **H Oculomotor Nerve** Third cranial nerve **J Trochlear Nerve** Fourth cranial nerve **K Trigeminal Nerve** Fifth cranial nerve Gasserian ganglion Mandibular nerve Maxillary nerve Ophthalmic nerve Trifacial nerve **L Abducens Nerve** Sixth cranial nerve **M Facial Nerve** Chorda tympani Geniculate ganglion Greater superficial petrosal nerve Nerve to the stapedius Parotid plexus Posterior auricular nerve Seventh cranial nerve Submandibular ganglion **N Acoustic Nerve** Cochlear nerve Eighth cranial nerve Scarpa's (vestibular) ganglion Spiral ganglion Vestibular (Scarpa's) ganglion Vestibular nerve Vestibulocochlear nerve **P Glossopharyngeal Nerve** Carotid sinus nerve Ninth cranial nerve Tympanic nerve **Q Vagus Nerve** Anterior vagal trunk Pharyngeal plexus Pneumogastric nerve Posterior vagal trunk Pulmonary plexus Recurrent laryngeal nerve Superior laryngeal nerve Tenth cranial nerve **R Accessory Nerve** Eleventh cranial nerve **S Hypoglossal Nerve** Twelfth cranial nerve **T Spinal Meninges** Arachnoid mater, spinal Denticulate (dentate) ligament Dura mater, spinal Filum terminale Leptomeninges, spinal Pia mater, spinal **W Cervical Spinal Cord** Dorsal root ganglion **X Thoracic Spinal Cord** Dorsal root ganglion **Y Lumbar Spinal Cord** Cauda equina Conus medullaris Dorsal root ganglion	**Ø Open** **3 Percutaneous** **4 Percutaneous Endoscopic**	**Z No Device**	**Z No Qualifier**

Ø Medical and Surgical
Ø Central Nervous System and Cranial Nerves
P Removal Definition: Taking out or off a device from a body part

Explanation: If a device is taken out and a similar device put in without cutting or puncturing the skin or mucous membrane, the procedure is coded to the root operation CHANGE. Otherwise, the procedure for taking out a device is coded to the root operation REMOVAL.

Body Part Character 4	Approach Character 5	Device Character 6	Qualifier Character 7
Ø Brain Cerebrum Corpus callosum Encephalon **V Spinal Cord** Dorsal root ganglion	**Ø Open** **3 Percutaneous** **4 Percutaneous Endoscopic**	**Ø Drainage Device** **2 Monitoring Device** **3 Infusion Device** **7 Autologous Tissue Substitute** **J Synthetic Substitute** **K Nonautologous Tissue Substitute** **M Neurostimulator Lead** **Y Other Device**	**Z No Qualifier**
Ø Brain Cerebrum Corpus callosum Encephalon **V Spinal Cord** Dorsal root ganglion	**X External**	**Ø Drainage Device** **2 Monitoring Device** **3 Infusion Device** **M Neurostimulator Lead**	**Z No Qualifier**
6 Cerebral Ventricle Aqueduct of Sylvius Cerebral aqueduct (Sylvius) Choroid plexus Ependyma Foramen of Monro (intraventricular) Fourth ventricle Interventricular foramen (Monro) Left lateral ventricle Right lateral ventricle Third ventricle **U Spinal Canal** Epidural space, spinal Extradural space, spinal Subarachnoid space, spinal Subdural space, spinal Vertebral canal	**Ø Open** **3 Percutaneous** **4 Percutaneous Endoscopic**	**Ø Drainage Device** **2 Monitoring Device** **3 Infusion Device** **J Synthetic Substitute** **M Neurostimulator Lead** **Y Other Device**	**Z No Qualifier**
6 Cerebral Ventricle Aqueduct of Sylvius Cerebral aqueduct (Sylvius) Choroid plexus Ependyma Foramen of Monro (intraventricular) Fourth ventricle Interventricular foramen (Monro) Left lateral ventricle Right lateral ventricle Third ventricle **U Spinal Canal** Epidural space, spinal Extradural space, spinal Subarachnoid space, spinal Subdural space, spinal Vertebral canal	**X External**	**Ø Drainage Device** **2 Monitoring Device** **3 Infusion Device** **M Neurostimulator Lead**	**Z No Qualifier**
E Cranial Nerve	**Ø Open** **3 Percutaneous** **4 Percutaneous Endoscopic**	**Ø Drainage Device** **2 Monitoring Device** **3 Infusion Device** **7 Autologous Tissue Substitute** **M Neurostimulator Lead** **Y Other Device**	**Z No Qualifier**
E Cranial Nerve	**X External**	**Ø Drainage Device** **2 Monitoring Device** **3 Infusion Device** **M Neurostimulator Lead**	**Z No Qualifier**

Non-OR ØØP[Ø,V]3[Ø,2,3]Z
Non-OR ØØP[Ø,V][3,4]YZ
Non-OR ØØP[Ø,V]X[Ø,2,3,M]Z
Non-OR ØØP[6,U]3[Ø,2,3]Z
Non-OR ØØP[6,U][3,4]YZ
Non-OR ØØP[6,U]X[Ø,2,3,M]Z
Non-OR ØØPE3[Ø,2,3]Z
Non-OR ØØPE[3,4]YZ
Non-OR ØØPEX[Ø,2,3,M]Z

Ø Medical and Surgical
Ø Central Nervous System and Cranial Nerves
Q Repair Definition: Restoring, to the extent possible, a body part to its normal anatomic structure and function

Explanation: Used only when the method to accomplish the repair is not one of the other root operations

Body Part Character 4		Approach Character 5	Device Character 6	Qualifier Character 7
Ø Brain Cerebrum Corpus callosum Encephalon **1 Cerebral Meninges** Arachnoid mater, intracranial Leptomeninges, intracranial Pia mater, intracranial **2 Dura Mater** Diaphragma sellae Dura mater, intracranial Falx cerebri Tentorium cerebelli **6 Cerebral Ventricle** Aqueduct of Sylvius Cerebral aqueduct (Sylvius) Choroid plexus Ependyma Foramen of Monro (intraventricular) Fourth ventricle Interventricular foramen (Monro) Left lateral ventricle Right lateral ventricle Third ventricle **7 Cerebral Hemisphere** Frontal lobe Occipital lobe Parietal lobe Temporal lobe **8 Basal Ganglia** Basal nuclei Claustrum Corpus striatum Globus pallidus Substantia nigra Subthalamic nucleus **9 Thalamus** Epithalamus Geniculate nucleus Metathalamus Pulvinar **A Hypothalamus** Mammillary body **B Pons** Apneustic center Basis pontis Locus ceruleus Pneumotaxic center Pontine tegmentum Superior olivary nucleus **C Cerebellum** Culmen **D Medulla Oblongata** Myelencephalon **F Olfactory Nerve** First cranial nerve Olfactory bulb **G Optic Nerve** Optic chiasma Second cranial nerve	**H Oculomotor Nerve** Third cranial nerve **J Trochlear Nerve** Fourth cranial nerve **K Trigeminal Nerve** Fifth cranial nerve Gasserian ganglion Mandibular nerve Maxillary nerve Ophthalmic nerve Trifacial nerve **L Abducens Nerve** Sixth cranial nerve **M Facial Nerve** Chorda tympani Geniculate ganglion Greater superficial petrosal nerve Nerve to the stapedius Parotid plexus Posterior auricular nerve Seventh cranial nerve Submandibular ganglion **N Acoustic Nerve** Cochlear nerve Eighth cranial nerve Scarpa's (vestibular) ganglion Spiral ganglion Vestibular (Scarpa's) ganglion Vestibular nerve Vestibulocochlear nerve **P Glossopharyngeal Nerve** Carotid sinus nerve Ninth cranial nerve Tympanic nerve **Q Vagus Nerve** Anterior vagal trunk Pharyngeal plexus Pneumogastric nerve Posterior vagal trunk Pulmonary plexus Recurrent laryngeal nerve Superior laryngeal nerve Tenth cranial nerve **R Accessory Nerve** Eleventh cranial nerve **S Hypoglossal Nerve** Twelfth cranial nerve **T Spinal Meninges** Arachnoid mater, spinal Denticulate (dentate) ligament Dura mater, spinal Filum terminale Leptomeninges, spinal Pia mater, spinal **W Cervical Spinal Cord** Dorsal root ganglion **X Thoracic Spinal Cord** Dorsal root ganglion **Y Lumbar Spinal Cord** Cauda equina Conus medullaris Dorsal root ganglion	**Ø Open** **3 Percutaneous** **4 Percutaneous Endoscopic**	**Z No Device**	**Z No Qualifier**

Ø Medical and Surgical
Ø Central Nervous System and Cranial Nerves
R Replacement Definition: Putting in or on biological or synthetic material that physically takes the place and/or function of all or a portion of a body part

Explanation: The body part may have been taken out or replaced, or may be taken out, physically eradicated, or rendered nonfunctional during the REPLACEMENT procedure. A REMOVAL procedure is coded for taking out the device used in a previous replacement procedure.

Body Part Character 4	Approach Character 5	Device Character 6	Qualifier Character 7
1 Cerebral Meninges Arachnoid mater, intracranial; Leptomeninges, intracranial; Pia mater, intracranial **2 Dura Mater** Diaphragma sellae; Dura mater, intracranial; Falx cerebri; Tentorium cerebelli **6 Cerebral Ventricle** Aqueduct of Sylvius; Cerebral aqueduct (Sylvius); Choroid plexus; Ependyma; Foramen of Monro (intraventricular); Fourth ventricle; Interventricular foramen (Monro); Left lateral ventricle; Right lateral ventricle; Third ventricle **F Olfactory Nerve** First cranial nerve; Olfactory bulb **G Optic Nerve** Optic chiasma; Second cranial nerve **H Oculomotor Nerve** Third cranial nerve **J Trochlear Nerve** Fourth cranial nerve **K Trigeminal Nerve** Fifth cranial nerve; Gasserian ganglion; Mandibular nerve; Maxillary nerve; Ophthalmic nerve; Trifacial nerve **L Abducens Nerve** Sixth cranial nerve **M Facial Nerve** Chorda tympani; Geniculate ganglion; Greater superficial petrosal nerve; Nerve to the stapedius; Parotid plexus; Posterior auricular nerve; Seventh cranial nerve; Submandibular ganglion **N Acoustic Nerve** Cochlear nerve; Eighth cranial nerve; Scarpa's (vestibular) ganglion; Spiral ganglion; Vestibular (Scarpa's) ganglion; Vestibular nerve; Vestibulocochlear nerve **P Glossopharyngeal Nerve** Carotid sinus nerve; Ninth cranial nerve; Tympanic nerve **Q Vagus Nerve** Anterior vagal trunk; Pharyngeal plexus; Pneumogastric nerve; Posterior vagal trunk; Pulmonary plexus; Recurrent laryngeal nerve; Superior laryngeal nerve; Tenth cranial nerve **R Accessory Nerve** Eleventh cranial nerve **S Hypoglossal Nerve** Twelfth cranial nerve **T Spinal Meninges** Arachnoid mater, spinal; Denticulate (dentate) ligament; Dura mater, spinal; Filum terminale; Leptomeninges, spinal; Pia mater, spinal	**Ø Open** **4 Percutaneous Endoscopic**	**7 Autologous Tissue Substitute** **J Synthetic Substitute** **K Nonautologous Tissue Substitute**	**Z No Qualifier**

Ø Medical and Surgical
Ø Central Nervous System and Cranial Nerves
S Reposition Definition: Moving to its normal location, or other suitable location, all or a portion of a body part

Explanation: The body part is moved to a new location from an abnormal location, or from a normal location where it is not functioning correctly. The body part may or may not be cut out or off to be moved to the new location.

Body Part Character 4	Approach Character 5	Device Character 6	Qualifier Character 7
F Olfactory Nerve First cranial nerve Olfactory bulb **G Optic Nerve** Optic chiasma Second cranial nerve **H Oculomotor Nerve** Third cranial nerve **J Trochlear Nerve** Fourth cranial nerve **K Trigeminal Nerve** Fifth cranial nerve Gasserian ganglion Mandibular nerve Maxillary nerve Ophthalmic nerve Trifacial nerve **L Abducens Nerve** Sixth cranial nerve **M Facial Nerve** Chorda tympani Geniculate ganglion Greater superficial petrosal nerve Nerve to the stapedius Parotid plexus Posterior auricular nerve Seventh cranial nerve Submandibular ganglion **N Acoustic Nerve** Cochlear nerve Eighth cranial nerve Scarpa's (vestibular) ganglion Spiral ganglion Vestibular (Scarpa's) ganglion Vestibular nerve Vestibulocochlear nerve **P Glossopharyngeal Nerve** Carotid sinus nerve Ninth cranial nerve Tympanic nerve **Q Vagus Nerve** Anterior vagal trunk Pharyngeal plexus Pneumogastric nerve Posterior vagal trunk Pulmonary plexus Recurrent laryngeal nerve Superior laryngeal nerve Tenth cranial nerve **R Accessory Nerve** Eleventh cranial nerve **S Hypoglossal Nerve** Twelfth cranial nerve **W Cervical Spinal Cord** Dorsal root ganglion **X Thoracic Spinal Cord** Dorsal root ganglion **Y Lumbar Spinal Cord** Cauda equina Conus medullaris Dorsal root ganglion	**Ø Open** **3 Percutaneous** **4 Percutaneous Endoscopic**	**Z No Device**	**Z No Qualifier**

Ø Medical and Surgical
Ø Central Nervous System and Cranial Nerves
T Resection Definition: Cutting out or off, without replacement, all of a body part

Explanation: None

Body Part Character 4	Approach Character 5	Device Character 6	Qualifier Character 7
7 Cerebral Hemisphere Frontal lobe Occipital lobe Parietal lobe Temporal lobe	**Ø Open** **3 Percutaneous** **4 Percutaneous Endoscopic**	**Z No Device**	**Z No Qualifier**

Ø Medical and Surgical
Ø Central Nervous System and Cranial Nerves
U Supplement Definition: Putting in or on biological or synthetic material that physically reinforces and/or augments the function of a portion of a body part

Explanation: The biological material is non-living, or is living and from the same individual. The body part may have been previously replaced, and the SUPPLEMENT procedure is performed to physically reinforce and/or augment the function of the replaced body part.

Body Part Character 4		Approach Character 5	Device Character 6	Qualifier Character 7
1 Cerebral Meninges Arachnoid mater, intracranial Leptomeninges, intracranial Pia mater, intracranial **2 Dura Mater** Diaphragma sellae Dura mater, intracranial Falx cerebri Tentorium cerebelli **6 Cerebral Ventricle** Aqueduct of Sylvius Cerebral aqueduct (Sylvius) Choroid plexus Ependyma Foramen of Monro (intraventricular) Fourth ventricle Interventricular foramen (Monro) Left lateral ventricle Right lateral ventricle Third ventricle **F Olfactory Nerve** First cranial nerve Olfactory bulb **G Optic Nerve** Optic chiasma Second cranial nerve **H Oculomotor Nerve** Third cranial nerve **J Trochlear Nerve** Fourth cranial nerve **K Trigeminal Nerve** Fifth cranial nerve Gasserian ganglion Mandibular nerve Maxillary nerve Ophthalmic nerve Trifacial nerve **L Abducens Nerve** Sixth cranial nerve	**M Facial Nerve** Chorda tympani Geniculate ganglion Greater superficial petrosal nerve Nerve to the stapedius Parotid plexus Posterior auricular nerve Seventh cranial nerve Submandibular ganglion **N Acoustic Nerve** Cochlear nerve Eighth cranial nerve Scarpa's (vestibular) ganglion Spiral ganglion Vestibular (Scarpa's) ganglion Vestibular nerve Vestibulocochlear nerve **P Glossopharyngeal Nerve** Carotid sinus nerve Ninth cranial nerve Tympanic nerve **Q Vagus Nerve** Anterior vagal trunk Pharyngeal plexus Pneumogastric nerve Posterior vagal trunk Pulmonary plexus Recurrent laryngeal nerve Superior laryngeal nerve Tenth cranial nerve **R Accessory Nerve** Eleventh cranial nerve **S Hypoglossal Nerve** Twelfth cranial nerve **T Spinal Meninges** Arachnoid mater, spinal Denticulate (dentate) ligament Dura mater, spinal Filum terminale Leptomeninges, spinal Pia mater, spinal	**Ø Open** **3 Percutaneous** **4 Percutaneous Endoscopic**	**7 Autologous Tissue Substitute** **J Synthetic Substitute** **K Nonautologous Tissue Substitute**	**Z No Qualifier**

Central Nervous System and Cranial Nerves

ØØU–ØØU

Ø Medical and Surgical
Ø Central Nervous System and Cranial Nerves
W Revision Definition: Correcting, to the extent possible, a portion of a malfunctioning device or the position of a displaced device

Explanation: Revision can include correcting a malfunctioning or displaced device by taking out or putting in components of the device such as a screw or pin

Body Part Character 4	Approach Character 5	Device Character 6	Qualifier Character 7
Ø Brain Cerebrum Corpus callosum Encephalon V Spinal Cord Dorsal root ganglion	Ø Open 3 Percutaneous 4 Percutaneous Endoscopic	Ø Drainage Device 2 Monitoring Device 3 Infusion Device 7 Autologous Tissue Substitute J Synthetic Substitute K Nonautologous Tissue Substitute M Neurostimulator Lead Y Other Device	Z No Qualifier
Ø Brain Cerebrum Corpus callosum Encephalon V Spinal Cord Dorsal root ganglion	X External	Ø Drainage Device 2 Monitoring Device 3 Infusion Device 7 Autologous Tissue Substitute J Synthetic Substitute K Nonautologous Tissue Substitute M Neurostimulator Lead	Z No Qualifier
6 Cerebral Ventricle Aqueduct of Sylvius Cerebral aqueduct (Sylvius) Choroid plexus Ependyma Foramen of Monro (intraventricular) Fourth ventricle Interventricular foramen (Monro) Left lateral ventricle Right lateral ventricle Third ventricle U Spinal Canal Epidural space, spinal Extradural space, spinal Subarachnoid space, spinal Subdural space, spinal Vertebral canal	Ø Open 3 Percutaneous 4 Percutaneous Endoscopic	Ø Drainage Device 2 Monitoring Device 3 Infusion Device J Synthetic Substitute M Neurostimulator Lead Y Other Device	Z No Qualifier
6 Cerebral Ventricle Aqueduct of Sylvius Cerebral aqueduct (Sylvius) Choroid plexus Ependyma Foramen of Monro (intraventricular) Fourth ventricle Interventricular foramen (Monro) Left lateral ventricle Right lateral ventricle Third ventricle U Spinal Canal Epidural space, spinal Extradural space, spinal Subarachnoid space, spinal Subdural space, spinal Vertebral canal	X External	Ø Drainage Device 2 Monitoring Device 3 Infusion Device J Synthetic Substitute M Neurostimulator Lead	Z No Qualifier
E Cranial Nerve	Ø Open 3 Percutaneous 4 Percutaneous Endoscopic	Ø Drainage Device 2 Monitoring Device 3 Infusion Device 7 Autologous Tissue Substitute M Neurostimulator Lead Y Other Device	Z No Qualifier
E Cranial Nerve	X External	Ø Drainage Device 2 Monitoring Device 3 Infusion Device 7 Autologous Tissue Substitute M Neurostimulator Lead	Z No Qualifier

Non-OR ØØW[Ø,V][3,4]YZ
Non-OR ØØW[Ø,V]X[Ø,2,3,7,J,K,M]Z
Non-OR ØØW[6,U][3,4]YZ
Non-OR ØØW[6,U]X[Ø,2,3,J,M]Z
Non-OR ØØWE[3,4]YZ
Non-OR ØØWEX[Ø,2,3,7,M]Z

Ø Medical and Surgical
Ø Central Nervous System and Cranial Nerves
X Transfer Definition: Moving, without taking out, all or a portion of a body part to another location to take over the function of all or a portion of a body part
Explanation: The body part transferred remains connected to its vascular and nervous supply

Body Part Character 4	Approach Character 5	Device Character 6	Qualifier Character 7
F Olfactory Nerve First cranial nerve Olfactory bulb **G Optic Nerve** Optic chiasma Second cranial nerve **H Oculomotor Nerve** Third cranial nerve **J Trochlear Nerve** Fourth cranial nerve **K Trigeminal Nerve** Fifth cranial nerve Gasserian ganglion Mandibular nerve Maxillary nerve Ophthalmic nerve Trifacial nerve **L Abducens Nerve** Sixth cranial nerve **M Facial Nerve** Chorda tympani Geniculate ganglion Greater superficial petrosal nerve Nerve to the stapedius Parotid plexus Posterior auricular nerve Seventh cranial nerve Submandibular ganglion **N Acoustic Nerve** Cochlear nerve Eighth cranial nerve Scarpa's (vestibular) ganglion Spiral ganglion Vestibular (Scarpa's) ganglion Vestibular nerve Vestibulocochlear nerve **P Glossopharyngeal Nerve** Carotid sinus nerve Ninth cranial nerve Tympanic nerve **Q Vagus Nerve** Anterior vagal trunk Pharyngeal plexus Pneumogastric nerve Posterior vagal trunk Pulmonary plexus Recurrent laryngeal nerve Superior laryngeal nerve Tenth cranial nerve **R Accessory Nerve** Eleventh cranial nerve **S Hypoglossal Nerve** Twelfth cranial nerve	**Ø Open** **4 Percutaneous Endoscopic**	**Z No Device**	**F Olfactory Nerve** **G Optic Nerve** **H Oculomotor Nerve** **J Trochlear Nerve** **K Trigeminal Nerve** **L Abducens Nerve** **M Facial Nerve** **N Acoustic Nerve** **P Glossopharyngeal Nerve** **Q Vagus Nerve** **R Accessory Nerve** **S Hypoglossal Nerve**

Peripheral Nervous System Ø12–Ø1X

Character Meanings

This Character Meaning table is provided as a guide to assist the user in the identification of character members that may be found in this section of code tables. It **SHOULD NOT** be used to build a PCS code.

Operation–Character 3	Body Part–Character 4	Approach–Character 5	Device–Character 6	Qualifier–Character 7
2 Change	Ø Cervical Plexus	Ø Open	Ø Drainage Device	1 Cervical Nerve
5 Destruction	1 Cervical Nerve	3 Percutaneous	1 Radioactive Element	2 Phrenic Nerve
8 Division	2 Phrenic Nerve	4 Percutaneous Endoscopic	2 Monitoring Device	4 Ulnar Nerve
9 Drainage	3 Brachial Plexus	X External	7 Autologous Tissue Substitute	5 Median Nerve
B Excision	4 Ulnar Nerve		J Synthetic Substitute	6 Radial Nerve
C Extirpation	5 Median Nerve		K Nonautologous Tissue Substitute	8 Thoracic Nerve
D Extraction	6 Radial Nerve		M Neurostimulator Lead	B Lumbar Nerve
H Insertion	8 Thoracic Nerve		Y Other Device	C Perineal Nerve
J Inspection	9 Lumbar Plexus		Z No Device	D Femoral Nerve
N Release	A Lumbosacral Plexus			F Sciatic Nerve
P Removal	B Lumbar Nerve			G Tibial Nerve
Q Repair	C Pudendal Nerve			H Peroneal Nerve
R Replacement	D Femoral Nerve			X Diagnostic
S Reposition	F Sciatic Nerve			Z No Qualifier
U Supplement	G Tibial Nerve			
W Revision	H Peroneal Nerve			
X Transfer	K Head and Neck Sympathetic Nerve			
	L Thoracic Sympathetic Nerve			
	M Abdominal Sympathetic Nerve			
	N Lumbar Sympathetic Nerve			
	P Sacral Sympathetic Nerve			
	Q Sacral Plexus			
	R Sacral Nerve			
	Y Peripheral Nerve			

AHA Coding Clinic for table Ø1B
2018, 2Q, 22 Excision of synovial cyst
2017, 2Q, 19 Thoracic outlet decompression with sympathectomy

AHA Coding Clinic for table Ø1H
2020, 4Q, 43-44 Insertion of radioactive element

AHA Coding Clinic for table Ø1N
2019, 1Q, 28 Decompressive laminectomy of both spinal cord and nerve roots
2018, 2Q, 22 Excision of synovial cyst
2017, 2Q, 19 Thoracic outlet decompression with sympathectomy
2016, 2Q, 16 Decompressive laminectomy/foraminotomy and lumbar discectomy
2016, 2Q, 17 Removal of longitudinal ligament to decompress cervical nerve root
2016, 2Q, 23 Thoracic outlet syndrome and release of brachial plexus
2015, 2Q, 34 Decompressive laminectomy
2014, 3Q, 33 Radial fracture treatment with open reduction internal fixation, and release of carpal ligament

AHA Coding Clinic for table Ø1Q
2019, 3Q, 32 Breast reconstruction with neurotization

AHA Coding Clinic for table Ø1U
2019, 3Q, 32 Breast reconstruction with neurotization
2017, 4Q, 62 Added and revised device values - Nerve substitutes

Median and Ulnar Nerves

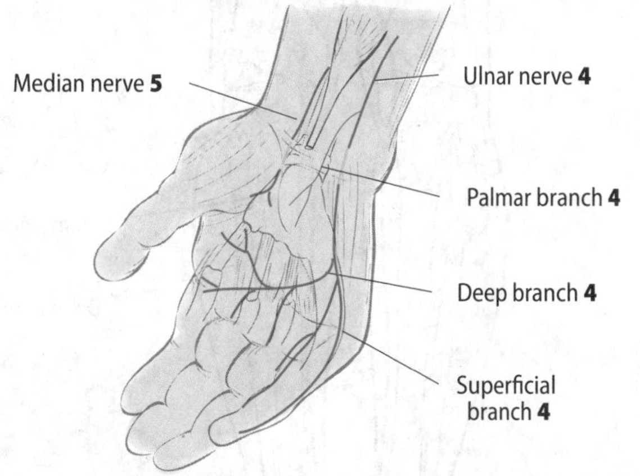

Peripheral Nervous System

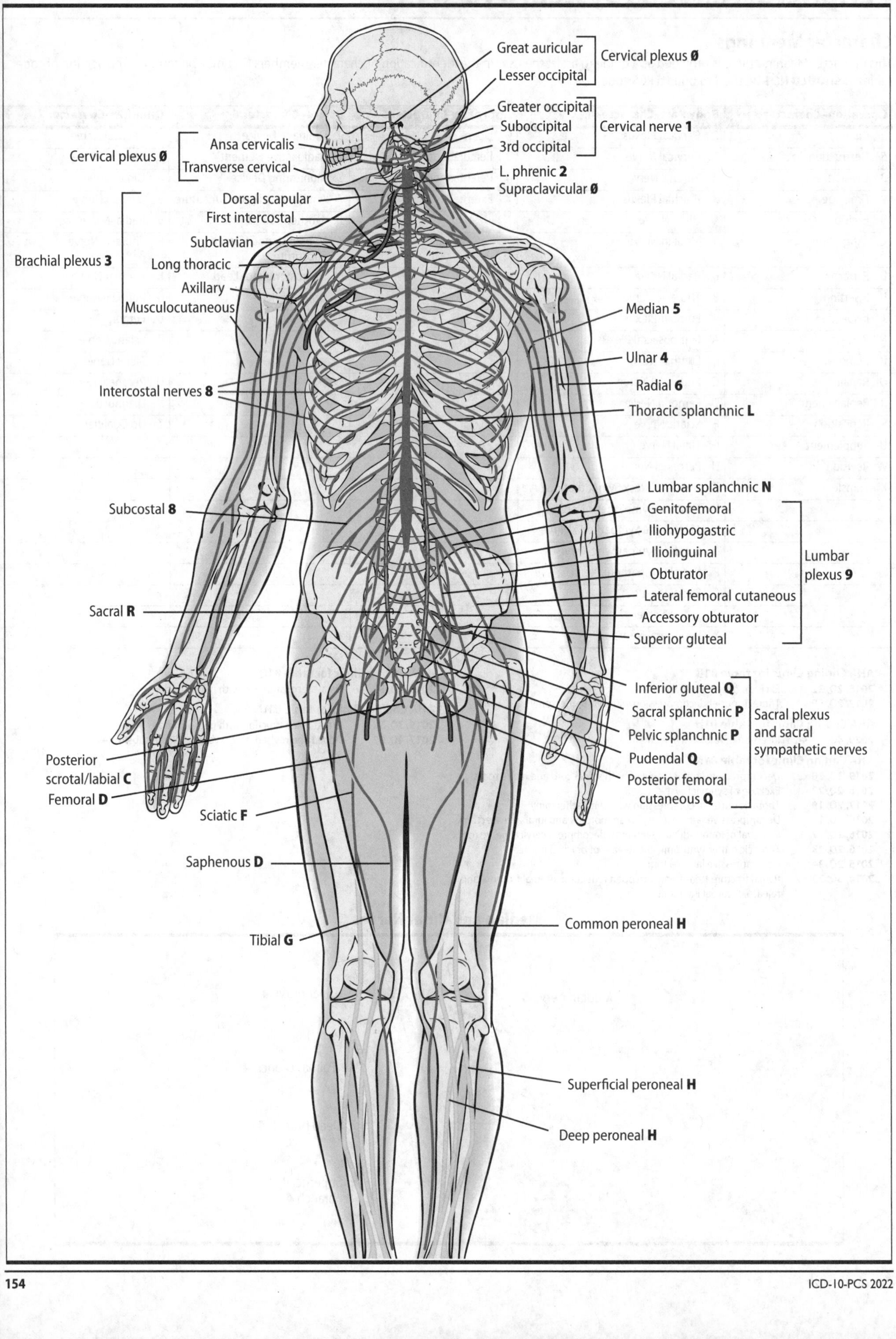

Ø Medical and Surgical
1 Peripheral Nervous System
2 Change Definition: Taking out or off a device from a body part and putting back an identical or similar device in or on the same body part without cutting or puncturing the skin or a mucous membrane

Explanation: All CHANGE procedures are coded using the approach EXTERNAL

Body Part Character 4	Approach Character 5	Device Character 6	Qualifier Character 7
Y Peripheral Nerve	X External	Ø Drainage Device Y Other Device	Z No Qualifier

Non-OR All body part, approach, device, and qualifier values

Ø Medical and Surgical
1 Peripheral Nervous System
5 Destruction

Definition: Physical eradication of all or a portion of a body part by the direct use of energy, force, or a destructive agent
Explanation: None of the body part is physically taken out

Body Part Character 4	Approach Character 5	Device Character 6	Qualifier Character 7
Ø Cervical Plexus Ansa cervicalis Cutaneous (transverse) cervical nerve Great auricular nerve Lesser occipital nerve Supraclavicular nerve Transverse (cutaneous) cervical nerve 1 Cervical Nerve Greater occipital nerve Spinal nerve, cervical Suboccipital nerve Third occipital nerve 2 Phrenic Nerve Accessory phrenic nerve 3 Brachial Plexus Axillary nerve Dorsal scapular nerve First intercostal nerve Long thoracic nerve Musculocutaneous nerve Subclavius nerve Suprascapular nerve 4 Ulnar Nerve Cubital nerve 5 Median Nerve Anterior interosseous nerve Palmar cutaneous nerve 6 Radial Nerve Dorsal digital nerve Musculospiral nerve Palmar cutaneous nerve Posterior interosseous nerve 8 Thoracic Nerve Intercostal nerve Intercostobrachial nerve Spinal nerve, thoracic Subcostal nerve 9 Lumbar Plexus Accessory obturator nerve Genitofemoral nerve Iliohypogastric nerve Ilioinguinal nerve Lateral femoral cutaneous nerve Obturator nerve Superior gluteal nerve A Lumbosacral Plexus B Lumbar Nerve Lumbosacral trunk Spinal nerve, lumbar Superior clunic (cluneal) nerve C Pudendal Nerve Posterior labial nerve Posterior scrotal nerve D Femoral Nerve Anterior crural nerve Saphenous nerve F Sciatic Nerve Ischiatic nerve G Tibial Nerve Lateral plantar nerve Medial plantar nerve Medial popliteal nerve Medial sural cutaneous nerve H Peroneal Nerve Common fibular nerve Common peroneal nerve External popliteal nerve Lateral sural cutaneous nerve K Head and Neck Sympathetic Nerve Cavernous plexus Cervical ganglion Ciliary ganglion Internal carotid plexus Otic ganglion Pterygopalatine (sphenopalatine) ganglion Sphenopalatine (pterygopalatine) ganglion Stellate ganglion Submandibular ganglion Submaxillary ganglion L Thoracic Sympathetic Nerve Cardiac plexus Esophageal plexus Greater splanchnic nerve Inferior cardiac nerve Least splanchnic nerve Lesser splanchnic nerve Middle cardiac nerve Pulmonary plexus Superior cardiac nerve Thoracic aortic plexus Thoracic ganglion M Abdominal Sympathetic Nerve Abdominal aortic plexus Auerbach's (myenteric) plexus Celiac (solar) plexus Celiac ganglion Gastric plexus Hepatic plexus Inferior hypogastric plexus Inferior mesenteric ganglion Inferior mesenteric plexus Meissner's (submucous) plexus Myenteric (Auerbach's) plexus Pancreatic plexus Pelvic splanchnic nerve Renal nerve Renal plexus Solar (celiac) plexus Splenic plexus Submucous (Meissner's) plexus Superior hypogastric plexus Superior mesenteric ganglion Superior mesenteric plexus Suprarenal plexus N Lumbar Sympathetic Nerve Lumbar ganglion Lumbar splanchnic nerve P Sacral Sympathetic Nerve Ganglion impar (ganglion of Walther) Pelvic splanchnic nerve Sacral ganglion Sacral splanchnic nerve Q Sacral Plexus Inferior gluteal nerve Posterior femoral cutaneous nerve Pudendal nerve R Sacral Nerve Spinal nerve, sacral	Ø Open 3 Percutaneous 4 Percutaneous Endoscopic	Z No Device	Z No Qualifier

Non-OR Ø15[Ø,2,3,4,5,6,9,A,C,D,F,G,H,Q][Ø,3,4]ZZ Non-OR Ø15[1,8,B,R]3ZZ

Ø Medical and Surgical
1 Peripheral Nervous System
8 Division Definition: Cutting into a body part, without draining fluids and/or gases from the body part, in order to separate or transect a body part

Explanation: All or a portion of the body part is separated into two or more portions

Body Part Character 4		Approach Character 5	Device Character 6	Qualifier Character 7
Ø Cervical Plexus Ansa cervicalis Cutaneous (transverse) cervical nerve Great auricular nerve Lesser occipital nerve Supraclavicular nerve Transverse (cutaneous) cervical nerve **1 Cervical Nerve** Greater occipital nerve Spinal nerve, cervical Suboccipital nerve Third occipital nerve **2 Phrenic Nerve** Accessory phrenic nerve **3 Brachial Plexus** Axillary nerve Dorsal scapular nerve First intercostal nerve Long thoracic nerve Musculocutaneous nerve Subclavius nerve Suprascapular nerve **4 Ulnar Nerve** Cubital nerve **5 Median Nerve** Anterior interosseous nerve Palmar cutaneous nerve **6 Radial Nerve** Dorsal digital nerve Musculospiral nerve Palmar cutaneous nerve Posterior interosseous nerve **8 Thoracic Nerve** Intercostal nerve Intercostobrachial nerve Spinal nerve, thoracic Subcostal nerve **9 Lumbar Plexus** Accessory obturator nerve Genitofemoral nerve Iliohypogastric nerve Ilioinguinal nerve Lateral femoral cutaneous nerve Obturator nerve Superior gluteal nerve **A Lumbosacral Plexus** **B Lumbar Nerve** Lumbosacral trunk Spinal nerve, lumbar Superior clunic (cluneal) nerve **C Pudendal Nerve** Posterior labial nerve Posterior scrotal nerve **D Femoral Nerve** Anterior crural nerve Saphenous nerve **F Sciatic Nerve** Ischiatic nerve **G Tibial Nerve** Lateral plantar nerve Medial plantar nerve Medial popliteal nerve Medial sural cutaneous nerve	**H Peroneal Nerve** Common fibular nerve Common peroneal nerve External popliteal nerve Lateral sural cutaneous nerve **K Head and Neck Sympathetic Nerve** Cavernous plexus Cervical ganglion Ciliary ganglion Internal carotid plexus Otic ganglion Pterygopalatine (sphenopalatine) ganglion Sphenopalatine (pterygopalatine) ganglion Stellate ganglion Submandibular ganglion Submaxillary ganglion **L Thoracic Sympathetic Nerve** Cardiac plexus Esophageal plexus Greater splanchnic nerve Inferior cardiac nerve Least splanchnic nerve Lesser splanchnic nerve Middle cardiac nerve Pulmonary plexus Superior cardiac nerve Thoracic aortic plexus Thoracic ganglion **M Abdominal Sympathetic Nerve** Abdominal aortic plexus Auerbach's (myenteric) plexus Celiac (solar) plexus Celiac ganglion Gastric plexus Hepatic plexus Inferior hypogastric plexus Inferior mesenteric ganglion Inferior mesenteric plexus Meissner's (submucous) plexus Myenteric (Auerbach's) plexus Pancreatic plexus Pelvic splanchnic nerve Renal nerve Renal plexus Solar (celiac) plexus Splenic plexus Submucous (Meissner's) plexus Superior hypogastric plexus Superior mesenteric ganglion Superior mesenteric plexus Suprarenal plexus **N Lumbar Sympathetic Nerve** Lumbar ganglion Lumbar splanchnic nerve **P Sacral Sympathetic Nerve** Ganglion impar (ganglion of Walther) Pelvic splanchnic nerve Sacral ganglion Sacral splanchnic nerve **Q Sacral Plexus** Inferior gluteal nerve Posterior femoral cutaneous nerve Pudendal nerve **R Sacral Nerve** Spinal nerve, sacral	**Ø Open** **3 Percutaneous** **4 Percutaneous Endoscopic**	**Z No Device**	**Z No Qualifier**

Ø Medical and Surgical
1 Peripheral Nervous System
9 Drainage Definition: Taking or letting out fluids and/or gases from a body part
Explanation: The qualifier DIAGNOSTIC is used to identify drainage procedures that are biopsies

Body Part Character 4		Approach Character 5	Device Character 6	Qualifier Character 7
Ø Cervical Plexus Ansa cervicalis Cutaneous (transverse) cervical nerve Great auricular nerve Lesser occipital nerve Supraclavicular nerve Transverse (cutaneous) cervical nerve **1 Cervical Nerve** Greater occipital nerve Spinal nerve, cervical Suboccipital nerve Third occipital nerve **2 Phrenic Nerve** Accessory phrenic nerve **3 Brachial Plexus** Axillary nerve Dorsal scapular nerve First intercostal nerve Long thoracic nerve Musculocutaneous nerve Subclavius nerve Suprascapular nerve **4 Ulnar Nerve** Cubital nerve **5 Median Nerve** Anterior interosseous nerve Palmar cutaneous nerve **6 Radial Nerve** Dorsal digital nerve Musculospiral nerve Palmar cutaneous nerve Posterior interosseous nerve **8 Thoracic Nerve** Intercostal nerve Intercostobrachial nerve Spinal nerve, thoracic Subcostal nerve **9 Lumbar Plexus** Accessory obturator nerve Genitofemoral nerve Iliohypogastric nerve Ilioinguinal nerve Lateral femoral cutaneous nerve Obturator nerve Superior gluteal nerve **A Lumbosacral Plexus** **B Lumbar Nerve** Lumbosacral trunk Spinal nerve, lumbar Superior clunic (cluneal) nerve **C Pudendal Nerve** Posterior labial nerve Posterior scrotal nerve **D Femoral Nerve** Anterior crural nerve Saphenous nerve **F Sciatic Nerve** Ischiatic nerve **G Tibial Nerve** Lateral plantar nerve Medial plantar nerve Medial popliteal nerve Medial sural cutaneous nerve	**H Peroneal Nerve** Common fibular nerve Common peroneal nerve External popliteal nerve Lateral sural cutaneous nerve **K Head and Neck Sympathetic Nerve** Cavernous plexus Cervical ganglion Ciliary ganglion Internal carotid plexus Otic ganglion Pterygopalatine (sphenopalatine) ganglion Sphenopalatine (pterygopalatine) ganglion Stellate ganglion Submandibular ganglion Submaxillary ganglion **L Thoracic Sympathetic Nerve** Cardiac plexus Esophageal plexus Greater splanchnic nerve Inferior cardiac nerve Least splanchnic nerve Lesser splanchnic nerve Middle cardiac nerve Pulmonary plexus Superior cardiac nerve Thoracic aortic plexus Thoracic ganglion **M Abdominal Sympathetic Nerve** Abdominal aortic plexus Auerbach's (myenteric) plexus Celiac (solar) plexus Celiac ganglion Gastric plexus Hepatic plexus Inferior hypogastric plexus Inferior mesenteric ganglion Inferior mesenteric plexus Meissner's (submucous) plexus Myenteric (Auerbach's) plexus Pancreatic plexus Pelvic splanchnic nerve Renal nerve Renal plexus Solar (celiac) plexus Splenic plexus Submucous (Meissner's) plexus Superior hypogastric plexus Superior mesenteric ganglion Superior mesenteric plexus Suprarenal plexus **N Lumbar Sympathetic Nerve** Lumbar ganglion Lumbar splanchnic nerve **P Sacral Sympathetic Nerve** Ganglion impar (ganglion of Walther) Pelvic splanchnic nerve Sacral ganglion Sacral splanchnic nerve **Q Sacral Plexus** Inferior gluteal nerve Posterior femoral cutaneous nerve Pudendal nerve **R Sacral Nerve** Spinal nerve, sacral	**Ø Open** **3 Percutaneous** **4 Percutaneous Endoscopic**	**Ø Drainage Device**	**Z No Qualifier**

Non-OR Ø19[Ø,1,2,3,4,5,6,8,9,A,B,C,D,F,G,H,K,L,M,N,P,Q,R]3ØZ

Ø19 Continued on next page

Ø19 Continued

Ø Medical and Surgical
1 Peripheral Nervous System
9 Drainage Definition: Taking or letting out fluids and/or gases from a body part
Explanation: The qualifier DIAGNOSTIC is used to identify drainage procedures that are biopsies

Body Part Character 4	Approach Character 5	Device Character 6	Qualifier Character 7
Ø Cervical Plexus Ansa cervicalis Cutaneous (transverse) cervical nerve Great auricular nerve Lesser occipital nerve Supraclavicular nerve Transverse (cutaneous) cervical nerve **1 Cervical Nerve** Greater occipital nerve Spinal nerve, cervical Suboccipital nerve Third occipital nerve **2 Phrenic Nerve** Accessory phrenic nerve **3 Brachial Plexus** Axillary nerve Dorsal scapular nerve First intercostal nerve Long thoracic nerve Musculocutaneous nerve Subclavius nerve Suprascapular nerve **4 Ulnar Nerve** Cubital nerve **5 Median Nerve** Anterior interosseous nerve Palmar cutaneous nerve **6 Radial Nerve** Dorsal digital nerve Musculospiral nerve Palmar cutaneous nerve Posterior interosseous nerve **8 Thoracic Nerve** Intercostal nerve Intercostobrachial nerve Spinal nerve, thoracic Subcostal nerve **9 Lumbar Plexus** Accessory obturator nerve Genitofemoral nerve Iliohypogastric nerve Ilioinguinal nerve Lateral femoral cutaneous nerve Obturator nerve Superior gluteal nerve **A Lumbosacral Plexus** **B Lumbar Nerve** Lumbosacral trunk Spinal nerve, lumbar Superior clunic (cluneal) nerve **C Pudendal Nerve** Posterior labial nerve Posterior scrotal nerve **D Femoral Nerve** Anterior crural nerve Saphenous nerve **F Sciatic Nerve** Ischiatic nerve **G Tibial Nerve** Lateral plantar nerve Medial plantar nerve Medial popliteal nerve Medial sural cutaneous nerve **H Peroneal Nerve** Common fibular nerve Common peroneal nerve External popliteal nerve Lateral sural cutaneous nerve **K Head and Neck Sympathetic Nerve** Cavernous plexus Cervical ganglion Ciliary ganglion Internal carotid plexus Otic ganglion Pterygopalatine (sphenopalatine) ganglion Sphenopalatine (pterygopalatine) ganglion Stellate ganglion Submandibular ganglion Submaxillary ganglion **L Thoracic Sympathetic Nerve** Cardiac plexus Esophageal plexus Greater splanchnic nerve Inferior cardiac nerve Least splanchnic nerve Lesser splanchnic nerve Middle cardiac nerve Pulmonary plexus Superior cardiac nerve Thoracic aortic plexus Thoracic ganglion **M Abdominal Sympathetic Nerve** Abdominal aortic plexus Auerbach's (myenteric) plexus Celiac (solar) plexus Celiac ganglion Gastric plexus Hepatic plexus Inferior hypogastric plexus Inferior mesenteric ganglion Inferior mesenteric plexus Meissner's (submucous) plexus Myenteric (Auerbach's) plexus Pancreatic plexus Pelvic splanchnic nerve Renal nerve Renal plexus Solar (celiac) plexus Splenic plexus Submucous (Meissner's) plexus Superior hypogastric plexus Superior mesenteric ganglion Superior mesenteric plexus Suprarenal plexus **N Lumbar Sympathetic Nerve** Lumbar ganglion Lumbar splanchnic nerve **P Sacral Sympathetic Nerve** Ganglion impar (ganglion of Walther) Pelvic splanchnic nerve Sacral ganglion Sacral splanchnic nerve **Q Sacral Plexus** Inferior gluteal nerve Posterior femoral cutaneous nerve Pudendal nerve **R Sacral Nerve** Spinal nerve, sacral	Ø Open 3 Percutaneous 4 Percutaneous Endoscopic	Z No Device	X Diagnostic Z No Qualifier

Non-OR Ø19[Ø,1,2,3,4,5,6,8,9,A,B,C,D,F,G,H,Q,R][3,4]ZX
Non-OR Ø19[Ø,1,2,3,4,5,6,8,9,A,B,C,D,F,G,H,K,L,M,N,P,Q,R]3ZZ

Ø Medical and Surgical
1 Peripheral Nervous System
B Excision Definition: Cutting out or off, without replacement, a portion of a body part
Explanation: The qualifier DIAGNOSTIC is used to identify excision procedures that are biopsies

Body Part Character 4		Approach Character 5	Device Character 6	Qualifier Character 7
Ø Cervical Plexus Ansa cervicalis Cutaneous (transverse) cervical nerve Great auricular nerve Lesser occipital nerve Supraclavicular nerve Transverse (cutaneous) cervical nerve **1 Cervical Nerve** Greater occipital nerve Spinal nerve, cervical Suboccipital nerve Third occipital nerve **2 Phrenic Nerve** Accessory phrenic nerve **3 Brachial Plexus** Axillary nerve Dorsal scapular nerve First intercostal nerve Long thoracic nerve Musculocutaneous nerve Subclavius nerve Suprascapular nerve **4 Ulnar Nerve** Cubital nerve **5 Median Nerve** Anterior interosseous nerve Palmar cutaneous nerve **6 Radial Nerve** Dorsal digital nerve Musculospiral nerve Palmar cutaneous nerve Posterior interosseous nerve **8 Thoracic Nerve** Intercostal nerve Intercostobrachial nerve Spinal nerve, thoracic Subcostal nerve **9 Lumbar Plexus** Accessory obturator nerve Genitofemoral nerve Iliohypogastric nerve Ilioinguinal nerve Lateral femoral cutaneous nerve Obturator nerve Superior gluteal nerve **A Lumbosacral Plexus** **B Lumbar Nerve** Lumbosacral trunk Spinal nerve, lumbar Superior clunic (cluneal) nerve **C Pudendal Nerve** Posterior labial nerve Posterior scrotal nerve **D Femoral Nerve** Anterior crural nerve Saphenous nerve **F Sciatic Nerve** Ischiatic nerve **G Tibial Nerve** Lateral plantar nerve Medial plantar nerve Medial popliteal nerve Medial sural cutaneous nerve	**H Peroneal Nerve** Common fibular nerve Common peroneal nerve External popliteal nerve Lateral sural cutaneous nerve **K Head and Neck Sympathetic Nerve** Cavernous plexus Cervical ganglion Ciliary ganglion Internal carotid plexus Otic ganglion Pterygopalatine (sphenopalatine) ganglion Sphenopalatine (pterygopalatine) ganglion Stellate ganglion Submandibular ganglion Submaxillary ganglion **L Thoracic Sympathetic Nerve** Cardiac plexus Esophageal plexus Greater splanchnic nerve Inferior cardiac nerve Least splanchnic nerve Lesser splanchnic nerve Middle cardiac nerve Pulmonary plexus Superior cardiac nerve Thoracic aortic plexus Thoracic ganglion **M Abdominal Sympathetic Nerve** Abdominal aortic plexus Auerbach's (myenteric) plexus Celiac (solar) plexus Celiac ganglion Gastric plexus Hepatic plexus Inferior hypogastric plexus Inferior mesenteric ganglion Inferior mesenteric plexus Meissner's (submucous) plexus Myenteric (Auerbach's) plexus Pancreatic plexus Pelvic splanchnic nerve Renal nerve Renal plexus Solar (celiac) plexus Splenic plexus Submucous (Meissner's) plexus Superior hypogastric plexus Superior mesenteric ganglion Superior mesenteric plexus Suprarenal plexus **N Lumbar Sympathetic Nerve** Lumbar ganglion Lumbar splanchnic nerve **P Sacral Sympathetic Nerve** Ganglion impar (ganglion of Walther) Pelvic splanchnic nerve Sacral ganglion Sacral splanchnic nerve **Q Sacral Plexus** Inferior gluteal nerve Posterior femoral cutaneous nerve Pudendal nerve **R Sacral Nerve** Spinal nerve, sacral	**Ø Open** **3 Percutaneous** **4 Percutaneous Endoscopic**	**Z No Device**	**X Diagnostic** **Z No Qualifier**

Non-OR Ø1B[Ø,1,2,3,4,5,6,8,9,A,B,C,D,F,G,H,Q,R][3,4]ZX

Ø Medical and Surgical
1 Peripheral Nervous System
C Extirpation Definition: Taking or cutting out solid matter from a body part

Explanation: The solid matter may be an abnormal byproduct of a biological function or a foreign body; it may be imbedded in a body part or in the lumen of a tubular body part. The solid matter may or may not have been previously broken into pieces.

Body Part Character 4	Approach Character 5	Device Character 6	Qualifier Character 7
Ø Cervical Plexus Ansa cervicalis Cutaneous (transverse) cervical nerve Great auricular nerve Lesser occipital nerve Supraclavicular nerve Transverse (cutaneous) cervical nerve **1 Cervical Nerve** Greater occipital nerve Spinal nerve, cervical Suboccipital nerve Third occipital nerve **2 Phrenic Nerve** Accessory phrenic nerve **3 Brachial Plexus** Axillary nerve Dorsal scapular nerve First intercostal nerve Long thoracic nerve Musculocutaneous nerve Subclavius nerve Suprascapular nerve **4 Ulnar Nerve** Cubital nerve **5 Median Nerve** Anterior interosseous nerve Palmar cutaneous nerve **6 Radial Nerve** Dorsal digital nerve Musculospiral nerve Palmar cutaneous nerve Posterior interosseous nerve **8 Thoracic Nerve** Intercostal nerve Intercostobrachial nerve Spinal nerve, thoracic Subcostal nerve **9 Lumbar Plexus** Accessory obturator nerve Genitofemoral nerve Iliohypogastric nerve Ilioinguinal nerve Lateral femoral cutaneous nerve Obturator nerve Superior gluteal nerve **A Lumbosacral Plexus** **B Lumbar Nerve** Lumbosacral trunk Spinal nerve, lumbar Superior clunic (cluneal) nerve **C Pudendal Nerve** Posterior labial nerve Posterior scrotal nerve **D Femoral Nerve** Anterior crural nerve Saphenous nerve **F Sciatic Nerve** Ischiatic nerve **G Tibial Nerve** Lateral plantar nerve Medial plantar nerve Medial popliteal nerve Medial sural cutaneous nerve **H Peroneal Nerve** Common fibular nerve Common peroneal nerve External popliteal nerve Lateral sural cutaneous nerve **K Head and Neck Sympathetic Nerve** Cavernous plexus Cervical ganglion Ciliary ganglion Internal carotid plexus Otic ganglion Pterygopalatine (sphenopalatine) ganglion Sphenopalatine (pterygopalatine) ganglion Stellate ganglion Submandibular ganglion Submaxillary ganglion **L Thoracic Sympathetic Nerve** Cardiac plexus Esophageal plexus Greater splanchnic nerve Inferior cardiac nerve Least splanchnic nerve Lesser splanchnic nerve Middle cardiac nerve Pulmonary plexus Superior cardiac nerve Thoracic aortic plexus Thoracic ganglion **M Abdominal Sympathetic Nerve** Abdominal aortic plexus Auerbach's (myenteric) plexus Celiac (solar) plexus Celiac ganglion Gastric plexus Hepatic plexus Inferior hypogastric plexus Inferior mesenteric ganglion Inferior mesenteric plexus Meissner's (submucous) plexus Myenteric (Auerbach's) plexus Pancreatic plexus Pelvic splanchnic nerve Renal nerve Renal plexus Solar (celiac) plexus Splenic plexus Submucous (Meissner's) plexus Superior hypogastric plexus Superior mesenteric ganglion Superior mesenteric plexus Suprarenal plexus **N Lumbar Sympathetic Nerve** Lumbar ganglion Lumbar splanchnic nerve **P Sacral Sympathetic Nerve** Ganglion impar (ganglion of Walther) Pelvic splanchnic nerve Sacral ganglion Sacral splanchnic nerve **Q Sacral Plexus** Inferior gluteal nerve Posterior femoral cutaneous nerve Pudendal nerve **R Sacral Nerve** Spinal nerve, sacral	**Ø Open** **3 Percutaneous** **4 Percutaneous Endoscopic**	**Z No Device**	**Z No Qualifier**

Ø Medical and Surgical
1 Peripheral Nervous System
D Extraction Definition: Pulling or stripping out or off all or a portion of a body part by the use of force
Explanation: The qualifier DIAGNOSTIC is used to identify extraction procedures that are biopsies

Body Part Character 4	Approach Character 5	Device Character 6	Qualifier Character 7
Ø Cervical Plexus Ansa cervicalis; Cutaneous (transverse) cervical nerve; Great auricular nerve; Lesser occipital nerve; Supraclavicular nerve; Transverse (cutaneous) cervical nerve **1 Cervical Nerve** Greater occipital nerve; Spinal nerve, cervical; Suboccipital nerve; Third occipital nerve **2 Phrenic Nerve** Accessory phrenic nerve **3 Brachial Plexus** Axillary nerve; Dorsal scapular nerve; First intercostal nerve; Long thoracic nerve; Musculocutaneous nerve; Subclavius nerve; Suprascapular nerve **4 Ulnar Nerve** Cubital nerve **5 Median Nerve** Anterior interosseous nerve; Palmar cutaneous nerve **6 Radial Nerve** Dorsal digital nerve; Musculospiral nerve; Palmar cutaneous nerve; Posterior interosseous nerve **8 Thoracic Nerve** Intercostal nerve; Intercostobrachial nerve; Spinal nerve, thoracic; Subcostal nerve **9 Lumbar Plexus** Accessory obturator nerve; Genitofemoral nerve; Iliohypogastric nerve; Ilioinguinal nerve; Lateral femoral cutaneous nerve; Obturator nerve; Superior gluteal nerve **A Lumbosacral Plexus** **B Lumbar Nerve** Lumbosacral trunk; Spinal nerve, lumbar; Superior clunic (cluneal) nerve **C Pudendal Nerve]** Posterior labial nerve; Posterior scrotal nerve **D Femoral Nerve** Anterior crural nerve; Saphenous nerve **F Sciatic Nerve** Ischiatic nerve **G Tibial Nerve** Lateral plantar nerve; Medial plantar nerve; Medial popliteal nerve; Medial sural cutaneous nerve **H Peroneal Nerve** Common fibular nerve; Common peroneal nerve; External popliteal nerve; Lateral sural cutaneous nerve **K Head and Neck Sympathetic Nerve** Cavernous plexus; Cervical ganglion; Ciliary ganglion; Internal carotid plexus; Otic ganglion; Pterygopalatine (sphenopalatine) ganglion; Sphenopalatine (pterygopalatine) ganglion; Stellate ganglion; Submandibular ganglion; Submaxillary ganglion **L Thoracic Sympathetic Nerve** Cardiac plexus; Esophageal plexus; Greater splanchnic nerve; Inferior cardiac nerve; Least splanchnic nerve; Lesser splanchnic nerve; Middle cardiac nerve; Pulmonary plexus; Superior cardiac nerve; Thoracic aortic plexus; Thoracic ganglion **M Abdominal Sympathetic Nerve** Abdominal aortic plexus; Auerbach's (myenteric) plexus; Celiac (solar) plexus; Celiac ganglion; Gastric plexus; Hepatic plexus; Inferior hypogastric plexus; Inferior mesenteric ganglion; Inferior mesenteric plexus; Meissner's (submucous) plexus; Myenteric (Auerbach's) plexus; Pancreatic plexus; Pelvic splanchnic nerve; Renal nerve; Renal plexus; Solar (celiac) plexus; Splenic plexus; Submucous (Meissner's) plexus; Superior hypogastric plexus; Superior mesenteric ganglion; Superior mesenteric plexus; Suprarenal plexus **N Lumbar Sympathetic Nerve** Lumbar ganglion; Lumbar splanchnic nerve **P Sacral Sympathetic Nerve** Ganglion impar (ganglion of Walther); Pelvic splanchnic nerve; Sacral ganglion; Sacral splanchnic nerve **Q Sacral Plexus** Inferior gluteal nerve; Posterior femoral cutaneous nerve; Pudendal nerve **R Sacral Nerve** Spinal nerve, sacral	**Ø Open** **3 Percutaneous** **4 Percutaneous Endoscopic**	**Z No Device**	**Z No Qualifier**

Ø1D–Ø1D

Ø Medical and Surgical
1 Peripheral Nervous System
H Insertion Definition: Putting in a nonbiological appliance that monitors, assists, performs, or prevents a physiological function but does not physically take the place of a body part

Explanation: None

Body Part Character 4	Approach Character 5	Device Character 6	Qualifier Character 7
Y Peripheral Nerve	Ø Open 3 Percutaneous 4 Percutaneous Endoscopic	1 Radioactive Element 2 Monitoring Device M Neurostimulator Lead Y Other Device	Z No Qualifier

Non-OR Ø1HY31Z
Non-OR Ø1HY[3,4]YZ

See Appendix L for Procedure Combinations
Ø1HY[Ø,3,4]MZ

Ø Medical and Surgical
1 Peripheral Nervous System
J Inspection Definition: Visually and/or manually exploring a body part

Explanation: Visual exploration may be performed with or without optical instrumentation. Manual exploration may be performed directly or through intervening body layers.

Body Part Character 4	Approach Character 5	Device Character 6	Qualifier Character 7
Y Peripheral Nerve	Ø Open 3 Percutaneous 4 Percutaneous Endoscopic	Z No Device	Z No Qualifier

Non-OR Ø1JY3ZZ

Ø Medical and Surgical
1 Peripheral Nervous System
N Release Definition: Freeing a body part from an abnormal physical constraint by cutting or by the use of force
Explanation: Some of the restraining tissue may be taken out but none of the body part is taken out

Body Part Character 4	Approach Character 5	Device Character 6	Qualifier Character 7
Ø Cervical Plexus Ansa cervicalis; Cutaneous (transverse) cervical nerve; Great auricular nerve; Lesser occipital nerve; Supraclavicular nerve; Transverse (cutaneous) cervical nerve **1 Cervical Nerve** Greater occipital nerve; Spinal nerve, cervical; Suboccipital nerve; Third occipital nerve **2 Phrenic Nerve** Accessory phrenic nerve **3 Brachial Plexus** Axillary nerve; Dorsal scapular nerve; First intercostal nerve; Long thoracic nerve; Musculocutaneous nerve; Subclavius nerve; Suprascapular nerve **4 Ulnar Nerve** Cubital nerve **5 Median Nerve** Anterior interosseous nerve; Palmar cutaneous nerve **6 Radial Nerve** Dorsal digital nerve; Musculospiral nerve; Palmar cutaneous nerve; Posterior interosseous nerve **8 Thoracic Nerve** Intercostal nerve; Intercostobrachial nerve; Spinal nerve, thoracic; Subcostal nerve **9 Lumbar Plexus** Accessory obturator nerve; Genitofemoral nerve; Iliohypogastric nerve; Ilioinguinal nerve; Lateral femoral cutaneous nerve; Obturator nerve; Superior gluteal nerve **A Lumbosacral Plexus** **B Lumbar Nerve** Lumbosacral trunk; Spinal nerve, lumbar; Superior clunic (cluneal) nerve **C Pudendal Nerve** Posterior labial nerve; Posterior scrotal nerve **D Femoral Nerve** Anterior crural nerve; Saphenous nerve **F Sciatic Nerve** Ischiatic nerve **G Tibial Nerve** Lateral plantar nerve; Medial plantar nerve; Medial popliteal nerve; Medial sural cutaneous nerve **H Peroneal Nerve** Common fibular nerve; Common peroneal nerve; External popliteal nerve; Lateral sural cutaneous nerve **K Head and Neck Sympathetic Nerve** Cavernous plexus; Cervical ganglion; Ciliary ganglion; Internal carotid plexus; Otic ganglion; Pterygopalatine (sphenopalatine) ganglion; Sphenopalatine (pterygopalatine) ganglion; Stellate ganglion; Submandibular ganglion; Submaxillary ganglion **L Thoracic Sympathetic Nerve** Cardiac plexus; Esophageal plexus; Greater splanchnic nerve; Inferior cardiac nerve; Least splanchnic nerve; Lesser splanchnic nerve; Middle cardiac nerve; Pulmonary plexus; Superior cardiac nerve; Thoracic aortic plexus; Thoracic ganglion **M Abdominal Sympathetic Nerve** Abdominal aortic plexus; Auerbach's (myenteric) plexus; Celiac (solar) plexus; Celiac ganglion; Gastric plexus; Hepatic plexus; Inferior hypogastric plexus; Inferior mesenteric ganglion; Inferior mesenteric plexus; Meissner's (submucous) plexus; Myenteric (Auerbach's) plexus; Pancreatic plexus; Pelvic splanchnic nerve; Renal nerve; Renal plexus; Solar (celiac) plexus; Splenic plexus; Submucous (Meissner's) plexus; Superior hypogastric plexus; Superior mesenteric ganglion; Superior mesenteric plexus; Suprarenal plexus **N Lumbar Sympathetic Nerve** Lumbar ganglion; Lumbar splanchnic nerve **P Sacral Sympathetic Nerve** Ganglion impar (ganglion of Walther); Pelvic splanchnic nerve; Sacral ganglion; Sacral splanchnic nerve **Q Sacral Plexus** Inferior gluteal nerve; Posterior femoral cutaneous nerve; Pudendal nerve **R Sacral Nerve** Spinal nerve, sacral	**Ø Open** **3 Percutaneous** **4 Percutaneous Endoscopic**	**Z No Device**	**Z No Qualifier**

Ø Medical and Surgical
1 Peripheral Nervous System
P Removal Definition: Taking out or off a device from a body part

Explanation: If a device is taken out and a similar device put in without cutting or puncturing the skin or mucous membrane, the procedure is coded to the root operation CHANGE. Otherwise, the procedure for taking out a device is coded to the root operation REMOVAL.

Body Part Character 4	Approach Character 5	Device Character 6	Qualifier Character 7
Y Peripheral Nerve	Ø Open 3 Percutaneous 4 Percutaneous Endoscopic	Ø Drainage Device 2 Monitoring Device 7 Autologous Tissue Substitute M Neurostimulator Lead Y Other Device	Z No Qualifier
Y Peripheral Nerve	X External	Ø Drainage Device 2 Monitoring Device M Neurostimulator Lead	Z No Qualifier

Non-OR Ø1PY3[Ø,2]Z
Non-OR Ø1PY[3,4]YZ
Non-OR Ø1PYX[Ø,2,M]Z

Ø Medical and Surgical
1 Peripheral Nervous System
Q Repair Definition: Restoring, to the extent possible, a body part to its normal anatomic structure and function
Explanation: Used only when the method to accomplish the repair is not one of the other root operations

Body Part Character 4	Approach Character 5	Device Character 6	Qualifier Character 7
Ø Cervical Plexus Ansa cervicalis; Cutaneous (transverse) cervical nerve; Great auricular nerve; Lesser occipital nerve; Supraclavicular nerve; Transverse (cutaneous) cervical nerve **1 Cervical Nerve** Greater occipital nerve; Spinal nerve, cervical; Suboccipital nerve; Third occipital nerve **2 Phrenic Nerve** Accessory phrenic nerve **3 Brachial Plexus** Axillary nerve; Dorsal scapular nerve; First intercostal nerve; Long thoracic nerve; Musculocutaneous nerve; Subclavius nerve; Suprascapular nerve **4 Ulnar Nerve** Cubital nerve **5 Median Nerve** Anterior interosseous nerve; Palmar cutaneous nerve **6 Radial Nerve** Dorsal digital nerve; Musculospiral nerve; Palmar cutaneous nerve; Posterior interosseous nerve **8 Thoracic Nerve** Intercostal nerve; Intercostobrachial nerve; Spinal nerve, thoracic; Subcostal nerve **9 Lumbar Plexus** Accessory obturator nerve; Genitofemoral nerve; Iliohypogastric nerve; Ilioinguinal nerve; Lateral femoral cutaneous nerve; Obturator nerve; Superior gluteal nerve **A Lumbosacral Plexus** **B Lumbar Nerve** Lumbosacral trunk; Spinal nerve, lumbar; Superior clunic (cluneal) nerve **C Pudendal Nerve** Posterior labial nerve; Posterior scrotal nerve **D Femoral Nerve** Anterior crural nerve; Saphenous nerve **F Sciatic Nerve** Ischiatic nerve **G Tibial Nerve** Lateral plantar nerve; Medial plantar nerve; Medial popliteal nerve; Medial sural cutaneous nerve **H Peroneal Nerve** Common fibular nerve; Common peroneal nerve; External popliteal nerve; Lateral sural cutaneous nerve **K Head and Neck Sympathetic Nerve** Cavernous plexus; Cervical ganglion; Ciliary ganglion; Internal carotid plexus; Otic ganglion; Pterygopalatine (sphenopalatine) ganglion; Sphenopalatine (pterygopalatine) ganglion; Stellate ganglion; Submandibular ganglion; Submaxillary ganglion **L Thoracic Sympathetic Nerve** Cardiac plexus; Esophageal plexus; Greater splanchnic nerve; Inferior cardiac nerve; Least splanchnic nerve; Lesser splanchnic nerve; Middle cardiac nerve; Pulmonary plexus; Superior cardiac nerve; Thoracic aortic plexus; Thoracic ganglion **M Abdominal Sympathetic Nerve** Abdominal aortic plexus; Auerbach's (myenteric) plexus; Celiac (solar) plexus; Celiac ganglion; Gastric plexus; Hepatic plexus; Inferior hypogastric plexus; Inferior mesenteric ganglion; Inferior mesenteric plexus; Meissner's (submucous) plexus; Myenteric (Auerbach's) plexus; Pancreatic plexus; Pelvic splanchnic nerve; Renal nerve; Renal plexus; Solar (celiac) plexus; Splenic plexus; Submucous (Meissner's) plexus; Superior hypogastric plexus; Superior mesenteric ganglion; Superior mesenteric plexus; Suprarenal plexus **N Lumbar Sympathetic Nerve** Lumbar ganglion; Lumbar splanchnic nerve **P Sacral Sympathetic Nerve** Ganglion impar (ganglion of Walther); Pelvic splanchnic nerve; Sacral ganglion; Sacral splanchnic nerve **Q Sacral Plexus** Inferior gluteal nerve; Posterior femoral cutaneous nerve; Pudendal nerve **R Sacral Nerve** Spinal nerve, sacral	**Ø Open** **3 Percutaneous** **4 Percutaneous Endoscopic**	**Z No Device**	**Z No Qualifier**

Ø Medical and Surgical
1 Peripheral Nervous System
R Replacement Definition: Putting in or on biological or synthetic material that physically takes the place and/or function of all or a portion of a body part

Explanation: The body part may have been taken out or replaced, or may be taken out, physically eradicated, or rendered nonfunctional during the REPLACEMENT procedure. A REMOVAL procedure is coded for taking out the device used in a previous replacement procedure.

Body Part Character 4	Approach Character 5	Device Character 6	Qualifier Character 7
1 Cervical Nerve Greater occipital nerve Spinal nerve, cervical Suboccipital nerve Third occipital nerve **2 Phrenic Nerve** Accessory phrenic nerve **4 Ulnar Nerve** Cubital nerve **5 Median Nerve** Anterior interosseous nerve Palmar cutaneous nerve **6 Radial Nerve** Dorsal digital nerve Musculospiral nerve Palmar cutaneous nerve Posterior interosseous nerve **8 Thoracic Nerve** Intercostal nerve Intercostobrachial nerve Spinal nerve, thoracic Subcostal nerve **B Lumbar Nerve** Lumbosacral trunk Spinal nerve, lumbar Superior clunic (cluneal) nerve **C Pudendal Nerve** Posterior labial nerve Posterior scrotal nerve **D Femoral Nerve** Anterior crural nerve Saphenous nerve **F Sciatic Nerve** Ischiatic nerve **G Tibial Nerve** Lateral plantar nerve Medial plantar nerve Medial popliteal nerve Medial sural cutaneous nerve **H Peroneal Nerve** Common fibular nerve Common peroneal nerve External popliteal nerve Lateral sural cutaneous nerve **R Sacral Nerve** Spinal nerve, sacral	**Ø Open** **4 Percutaneous Endoscopic**	**7 Autologous Tissue Substitute** **J Synthetic Substitute** **K Nonautologous Tissue Substitute**	**Z No Qualifier**

Ø Medical and Surgical
1 Peripheral Nervous System
S Reposition Definition: Moving to its normal location, or other suitable location, all or a portion of a body part

Explanation: The body part is moved to a new location from an abnormal location, or from a normal location where it is not functioning correctly. The body part may or may not be cut out or off to be moved to the new location.

Body Part Character 4	Approach Character 5	Device Character 6	Qualifier Character 7
Ø Cervical Plexus Ansa cervicalis Cutaneous (transverse) cervical nerve Great auricular nerve Lesser occipital nerve Supraclavicular nerve Transverse (cutaneous) cervical nerve **1 Cervical Nerve** Greater occipital nerve Spinal nerve, cervical Suboccipital nerve Third occipital nerve **2 Phrenic Nerve** Accessory phrenic nerve **3 Brachial Plexus** Axillary nerve Dorsal scapular nerve First intercostal nerve Long thoracic nerve Musculocutaneous nerve Subclavius nerve Suprascapular nerve **4 Ulnar Nerve** Cubital nerve **5 Median Nerve** Anterior interosseous nerve Palmar cutaneous nerve **6 Radial Nerve** Dorsal digital nerve Musculospiral nerve Palmar cutaneous nerve Posterior interosseous nerve **8 Thoracic Nerve** Intercostal nerve Intercostobrachial nerve Spinal nerve, thoracic Subcostal nerve **9 Lumbar Plexus** Accessory obturator nerve Genitofemoral nerve Iliohypogastric nerve Ilioinguinal nerve Lateral femoral cutaneous nerve Obturator nerve Superior gluteal nerve **A Lumbosacral Plexus** **B Lumbar Nerve** Lumbosacral trunk Spinal nerve, lumbar Superior clunic (cluneal) nerve **C Pudendal Nerve** Posterior labial nerve Posterior scrotal nerve **D Femoral Nerve** Anterior crural nerve Saphenous nerve **F Sciatic Nerve** Ischiatic nerve **G Tibial Nerve** Lateral plantar nerve Medial plantar nerve Medial popliteal nerve Medial sural cutaneous nerve **H Peroneal Nerve** Common fibular nerve Common peroneal nerve External popliteal nerve Lateral sural cutaneous nerve **Q Sacral Plexus** Inferior gluteal nerve Posterior femoral cutaneous nerve Pudendal nerve **R Sacral Nerve** Spinal nerve, sacral	**Ø Open** **3 Percutaneous** **4 Percutaneous Endoscopic**	**Z No Device**	**Z No Qualifier**

Ø Medical and Surgical
1 Peripheral Nervous System
U Supplement Definition: Putting in or on biological or synthetic material that physically reinforces and/or augments the function of a portion of a body part

Explanation: The biological material is non-living, or is living and from the same individual. The body part may have been previously replaced, and the SUPPLEMENT procedure is performed to physically reinforce and/or augment the function of the replaced body part.

Body Part Character 4	Approach Character 5	Device Character 6	Qualifier Character 7
1 Cervical Nerve Greater occipital nerve Spinal nerve, cervical Suboccipital nerve Third occipital nerve **2 Phrenic Nerve** Accessory phrenic nerve **4 Ulnar Nerve** Cubital nerve **5 Median Nerve** Anterior interosseous nerve Palmar cutaneous nerve **6 Radial Nerve** Dorsal digital nerve Musculospiral nerve Palmar cutaneous nerve Posterior interosseous nerve **8 Thoracic Nerve** Intercostal nerve Intercostobrachial nerve Spinal nerve, thoracic Subcostal nerve **B Lumbar Nerve** Lumbosacral trunk Spinal nerve, lumbar Superior clunic (cluneal) nerve **C Pudendal Nerve** Posterior labial nerve Posterior scrotal nerve **D Femoral Nerve** Anterior crural nerve Saphenous nerve **F Sciatic Nerve** Ischiatic nerve **G Tibial Nerve** Lateral plantar nerve Medial plantar nerve Medial popliteal nerve Medial sural cutaneous nerve **H Peroneal Nerve** Common fibular nerve Common peroneal nerve External popliteal nerve Lateral sural cutaneous nerve **R Sacral Nerve** Spinal nerve, sacral	**Ø Open** **3 Percutaneous** **4 Percutaneous Endoscopic**	**7 Autologous Tissue Substitute** **J Synthetic Substitute** **K Nonautologous Tissue Substitute**	**Z No Qualifier**

Ø Medical and Surgical
1 Peripheral Nervous System
W Revision Definition: Correcting, to the extent possible, a portion of a malfunctioning device or the position of a displaced device

Explanation: Revision can include correcting a malfunctioning or displaced device by taking out or putting in components of the device such as a screw or pin

Body Part Character 4	Approach Character 5	Device Character 6	Qualifier Character 7
Y Peripheral Nerve	**Ø Open** **3 Percutaneous** **4 Percutaneous Endoscopic**	**Ø Drainage Device** **2 Monitoring Device** **7 Autologous Tissue Substitute** **M Neurostimulator Lead** **Y Other Device**	**Z No Qualifier**
Y Peripheral Nerve	**X External**	**Ø Drainage Device** **2 Monitoring Device** **7 Autologous Tissue Substitute** **M Neurostimulator Lead**	**Z No Qualifier**

Non-OR Ø1WY[3,4]YZ
Non-OR Ø1WYX[Ø,2,7,M]Z

Ø Medical and Surgical
1 Peripheral Nervous System
X Transfer Definition: Moving, without taking out, all or a portion of a body part to another location to take over the function of all or a portion of a body part
Explanation: The body part transferred remains connected to its vascular and nervous supply

Body Part Character 4	Approach Character 5	Device Character 6	Qualifier Character 7
1 Cervical Nerve Greater occipital nerve Spinal nerve, cervical Suboccipital nerve Third occipital nerve **2 Phrenic Nerve** Accessory phrenic nerve	**Ø Open** **4 Percutaneous Endoscopic**	**Z No Device**	**1 Cervical Nerve** **2 Phrenic Nerve**
4 Ulnar Nerve Cubital nerve **5 Median Nerve** Anterior interosseous nerve Palmar cutaneous nerve **6 Radial Nerve** Dorsal digital nerve Musculospiral nerve Palmar cutaneous nerve Posterior interosseous nerve	**Ø Open** **4 Percutaneous Endoscopic**	**Z No Device**	**4 Ulnar Nerve** **5 Median Nerve** **6 Radial Nerve**
8 Thoracic Nerve Intercostal nerve Intercostobrachial nerve Spinal nerve, thoracic Subcostal nerve	**Ø Open** **4 Percutaneous Endoscopic**	**Z No Device**	**8 Thoracic Nerve**
B Lumbar Nerve Lumbosacral trunk Spinal nerve, lumbar Superior clunic (cluneal) nerve **C Pudendal Nerve** Posterior labial nerve Posterior scrotal nerve	**Ø Open** **4 Percutaneous Endoscopic**	**Z No Device**	**B Lumbar Nerve** **C Perineal Nerve**
D Femoral Nerve Anterior crural nerve Saphenous nerve **F Sciatic Nerve** Ischiatic nerve **G Tibial Nerve** Lateral plantar nerve Medial plantar nerve Medial popliteal nerve Medial sural cutaneous nerve **H Peroneal Nerve** Common fibular nerve Common peroneal nerve External popliteal nerve Lateral sural cutaneous nerve	**Ø Open** **4 Percutaneous Endoscopic**	**Z No Device**	**D Femoral Nerve** **F Sciatic Nerve** **G Tibial Nerve** **H Peroneal Nerve**

Heart and Great Vessels Ø21–Ø2Y

Character Meanings

This Character Meaning table is provided as a guide to assist the user in the identification of character members that may be found in this section of code tables. It **SHOULD NOT** be used to build a PCS code.

Operation–Character 3	Body Part–Character 4	Approach–Character 5	Device–Character 6	Qualifier–Character 7
1 Bypass	Ø Coronary Artery, One Artery	Ø Open	Ø Monitoring Device, Pressure Sensor	Ø Allogeneic OR Ultrasonic
4 Creation	1 Coronary Artery, Two Arteries	3 Percutaneous	2 Monitoring Device	1 Syngeneic
5 Destruction	2 Coronary Artery, Three Arteries	4 Percutaneous Endoscopic	3 Infusion Device	2 Zooplastic OR Common Atrioventricular Valve
7 Dilation	3 Coronary Artery, Four or More Arteries	X External	4 Intraluminal Device, Drug-eluting	3 Coronary Artery
8 Division	4 Coronary Vein		5 Intraluminal Device, Drug-eluting, Two	4 Coronary Vein
B Excision	5 Atrial Septum		6 Intraluminal Device, Drug-eluting, Three	5 Coronary Circulation
C Extirpation	6 Atrium, Right		7 Intraluminal Device, Drug-eluting, Four or More OR Autologous Tissue Substitute	6 Bifurcation OR Atrium, Right
F Fragmentation	7 Atrium, Left		8 Zooplastic Tissue	7 Atrium, Left OR Orbital Atherectomy Technique
H Insertion	8 Conduction Mechanism		9 Autologous Venous Tissue	8 Internal Mammary, Right
J Inspection	9 Chordae Tendineae		A Autologous Arterial Tissue	9 Internal Mammary, Left
K Map	A Heart		C Extraluminal Device	A Innominate Artery
L Occlusion	B Heart, Right		D Intraluminal Device	B Subclavian
N Release	C Heart, Left		E Intraluminal Device, Two OR Intraluminal Device, Branched or Fenestrated, One or Two Arteries	C Thoracic Artery
P Removal	D Papillary Muscle		F Intraluminal Device, Three OR Intraluminal Device, Branched or Fenestrated, Three or More Arteries	D Carotid
Q Repair	F Aortic Valve		G Intraluminal Device, Four or More	E Atrioventricular Valve, Left
R Replacement	G Mitral Valve		J Synthetic Substitute OR Cardiac Lead, Pacemaker	F Abdominal Artery
S Reposition	H Pulmonary Valve		K Nonautologous Tissue Substitute OR Cardiac Lead, Defibrillator	G Atrioventricular Valve, Right OR Axillary Artery
T Resection	J Tricuspid Valve		L Biologic with Synthetic Substitute, Autoregulated Electrohydraulic	H Transapical OR Brachial Artery
U Supplement	K Ventricle, Right		M Cardiac Lead OR Synthetic Substitute, Pneumatic	J Truncal Valve OR Temporary OR Intraoperative
V Restriction	L Ventricle, Left		N Intracardiac Pacemaker	K Left Atrial Appendage
			Q Implantable Heart Assist System	L In Existing Conduit
			R Short-term External Heart Assist System	M Native Site
W Revision	M Ventricular Septum		T Intraluminal Device, Radioactive	P Pulmonary Trunk
Y Transplantation	N Pericardium		Y Other Device	Q Pulmonary Artery, Right
	P Pulmonary Trunk		Z No Device	R Pulmonary Artery, Left
	Q Pulmonary Artery, Right			S Pulmonary Vein, Right OR Biventricular
	R Pulmonary Artery, Left			T Pulmonary Vein, Left OR Ductus Arteriosus
	S Pulmonary Vein, Right			U Pulmonary Vein, Confluence
	T Pulmonary Vein, Left			V Lower Extremity Artery
	V Superior Vena Cava			W Aorta
	W Thoracic Aorta, Descending			X Diagnostic
	X Thoracic Aorta, Ascending/Arch			Z No Qualifier
	Y Great Vessel			

AHA Coding Clinic for table Ø21

2020, 4Q, 44-45	Atrium bypass qualifier
2020, 1Q, 24	Pulmonary artery unifocalization
2020, 1Q, 37	Bypass of ascending aorta to brachiocephalic artery
2019, 4Q, 23	Bypass thoracic aorta to innominate artery
2019, 3Q, 30	Aortic aneurysm repair with debranching of common carotid and brachiocephalic arteries
2018, 4Q, 45-46	Descending thoracic aorta bypass
2018, 3Q, 8	Coronary artery bypass graft surgery (revision versus total redo)
2018, 3Q, 26	Coronary artery bypass graft surgery with endarterectomy
2017, 4Q, 56	Added approach values - Percutaneous heart valve procedures
2017, 1Q, 19	Norwood Sano procedure
2016, 4Q, 80-81	Thoracic aorta, ascending/arch and descending
2016, 4Q, 82-83	Coronary artery, number of arteries
2016, 4Q, 102-109	Correction of congenital heart defects
2016, 4Q, 144	Repair of atrial septal defect and anomalous pulmonary venous return
2016, 4Q, 145	Modified Warden procedure for repair of septal defect and right partial anomalous pulmonary venous return
2016, 1Q, 27	Aortocoronary bypass graft utilizing Y-graft
2015, 4Q, 22, 24	Congenital heart corrective procedures
2015, 3Q, 16	Revision of previous truncus arteriosus surgery with ventricle to pulmonary artery conduit
2014, 3Q, 3	Blalock-Taussig shunt procedure
2014, 3Q, 8	Coronary artery bypass graft utilizing internal mammary as pedicle graft
2014, 3Q, 20	MAZE procedure performed with coronary artery bypass graft
2014, 3Q, 29	Fontan completion procedure stage II
2014, 3Q, 30	Creation of conduit from right ventricle to pulmonary artery
2014, 1Q, 10	Repair of thoracic aortic aneurysm & coronary artery bypass graft
2013, 2Q, 37	Coronary artery release performed during coronary artery bypass graft

AHA Coding Clinic for table Ø24

2016, 4Q, 101	Root operation Creation
2016, 4Q, 102-109	Correction of congenital heart defects

AHA Coding Clinic for table Ø25

2020, 1Q, 32	Ablation convergent procedure (catheter-based and thoracoscopic ablations)
2018, 3Q, 27	Alcohol septal ablation
2016, 4Q, 80-81	Thoracic aorta, ascending/arch and descending
2016, 3Q, 43-44	Peri-pulmonary catheter ablation
2016, 3Q, 44-45	Maze procedure
2016, 2Q, 17	Photodynamic therapy for treatment of malignant mesothelioma
2014, 4Q, 47	Catheter ablation of peripulmonary veins
2014, 3Q, 19	Ablation of ventricular tachycardia with Impella® support
2014, 3Q, 20	MAZE procedure performed with coronary artery bypass graft
2013, 2Q, 38	Catheter ablation to treat atrial fibrillation

AHA Coding Clinic for table Ø27

2018, 3Q, 7	Coronary brachytherapy with angioplasty
2018, 3Q, 10	Disruption of perma-catheter fibrin sheath via angioplasty of superior vena cava
2018, 2Q, 24	Coronary artery bifurcation
2017, 4Q, 32-33	Corrective surgery of left ventricular outflow tract obstruction
2016, 4Q, 80-81	Thoracic aorta, ascending/arch and descending
2016, 4Q, 82-83	Coronary artery, number of arteries
2016, 4Q, 84-85	Coronary Artery, number of stents
2016, 4Q, 86-88	Coronary and peripheral artery bifurcation
2016, 1Q, 16	Pulmonary valvotomy and dilation of annulus
2015, 4Q, 13	New Section X codes—New Technology procedures
2015, 3Q, 9	Failed attempt to treat coronary artery occlusion
2015, 3Q, 10	Coronary angioplasty with unsuccessful stent insertion
2015, 3Q, 16	Revision of previous truncus arteriosus surgery with ventricle to pulmonary artery conduit
2015, 2Q, 3-5	Coronary artery intervention site
2014, 2Q, 4	Coronary angioplasty of bypassed vessel

AHA Coding Clinic for table Ø2B

2019, 3Q, 32	Endomyocardial biopsy and right heart catheterization
2019, 2Q, 20	Pericardiectomy for constrictive pericarditis
2017, 1Q, 38	Mitral valve repair and chordae tendineae transfer
2016, 4Q, 80-81	Thoracic aorta, ascending/arch and descending
2015, 2Q, 23	Annuloplasty ring

AHA Coding Clinic for table Ø2C

2019, 4Q, 25	Coronary artery to root operation Supplement
2018, 3Q, 26	Coronary artery bypass graft surgery with endarterectomy
2018, 2Q, 24	Coronary artery bifurcation
2017, 2Q, 23	Thrombectomy via Fogarty catheter
2016, 4Q, 80-81	Thoracic aorta, ascending/arch and descending
2016, 4Q, 82-83	Coronary artery, number of arteries
2016, 4Q, 86-87	Coronary and peripheral artery bifurcation
2016, 2Q, 24	Repair/decalcification of mitral valve
2016, 2Q, 25	Aortic valve surgery with excision of calcium deposits

AHA Coding Clinic for table Ø2F

2020, 4Q, 45-49	New fragmentation tables
2020, 4Q, 49-50	Intravascular ultrasound assisted thrombolysis
2020, 4Q, 50	Intravascular lithotripsy

AHA Coding Clinic for table Ø2H

2021, 2Q, 23	Clarification of lead placement in bundle of HIS
2019, 4Q, 23-24	Coronary artery Body Part to root operation Insertion
2019, 3Q, 19	Insertion of left ventricular catheter
2019, 3Q, 23	Placement of pacemaker lead in Bundle of HIS
2019, 1Q, 24	Replacement of left ventricular assist device with retention of outflow graft
2018, 4Q, 94	Insertion and removal of failed Watchman™ device
2018, 2Q, 3-5	Intra-aortic balloon pump
2018, 2Q, 19	Pacing lead attached to automatic implantable cardioverter defibrillator
2017, 4Q, 42-45	Insertion of external heart assist devices
2017, 4Q, 63-64	Added and revised device values - Vascular access reservoir
2017, 4Q, 104	Placement of Watchman™ left atrial appendage device
2017, 3Q, 11	Placement of peripherally inserted central catheter using 3CG ECG technology
2017, 2Q, 24	Tunneled catheter versus totally implantable catheter
2017, 2Q, 26	Exchange of tunneled catheter
2017, 1Q, 10-11	External heart assist device
2016, 4Q, 80-81	Thoracic aorta, ascending/arch and descending
2016, 4Q, 95	Intracardiac pacemaker
2016, 4Q, 137-138	Heart assist device systems
2016, 2Q, 15	Removal and replacement of tunneled internal jugular catheter
2015, 4Q, 14	New Section X codes—New Technology procedures
2015, 4Q, 26-31	Vascular access devices
2015, 3Q, 35	Swan Ganz catheterization
2015, 2Q, 31	Leadless pacemaker insertion
2015, 2Q, 33	Totally implantable central venous access device (Port-a-Cath)
2013, 3Q, 18	Placement of peripherally inserted central catheter (PICC)

AHA Coding Clinic for table Ø2J

2015, 3Q, 9	Failed attempt to treat coronary artery occlusion

AHA Coding Clinic for table Ø2K

2020, 1Q, 32	Ablation convergent procedure (catheter-based and thoracoscopic ablations)

AHA Coding Clinic for table Ø2L

2018, 4Q, 94	Insertion and removal of failed Watchman™ device
2017, 4Q, 31	Resuscitative endovascular balloon occlusion of the aorta
2017, 4Q, 33-34	Occlusion/ligation of pulmonary trunk & right pulmonary artery
2016, 4Q, 102-109	Correction of congenital heart defects
2016, 2Q, 26	Embolization of pulmonary arteriovenous fistula
2015, 4Q, 23	Congenital heart corrective procedures
2014, 3Q, 20	MAZE procedure performed with coronary artery bypass graft

AHA Coding Clinic for table Ø2N

2019, 2Q, 13	Unroofing of anomalous coronary artery
2019, 2Q, 20	Pericardiectomy for constrictive pericarditis
2017, 4Q, 35	Release of myocardial bridge
2016, 4Q, 80-81	Thoracic aorta, ascending/arch and descending
2014, 3Q, 16	Repair of Tetralogy of Fallot

AHA Coding Clinic for table Ø2P

2019, 1Q, 24	Replacement of left ventricular assist device with retention of outflow graft
2018, 4Q, 52-54	Percutaneous extracorporeal membrane oxygenation
2018, 4Q, 85	Externalization of lumboatrial shunt
2018, 4Q, 94	Insertion and removal of failed Watchman™ device
2018, 2Q, 3-5	Intra-aortic balloon pump
2017, 4Q, 42-45	Insertion of external heart assist devices
2017, 4Q, 104	Placement of Watchman™ left atrial appendage device
2017, 3Q, 18	Intra-aortic balloon pump removal
2017, 2Q, 24	Tunneled catheter versus totally implantable catheter
2017, 2Q, 26	Exchange of tunneled catheter
2017, 1Q, 11	External heart assist device
2017, 1Q, 13	SynCardia total artificial heart
2016, 4Q, 95-96	Intracardiac pacemaker
2016, 4Q, 137-139	Heart assist device systems
2016, 3Q, 19	Nonoperative removal of peripherally inserted central catheter
2016, 2Q, 15	Removal and replacement of tunneled internal jugular catheter
2015, 4Q, 31	Vascular access devices
2015, 3Q, 33	Approach values for repositioning and removal of cardiac lead

AHA Coding Clinic for table Ø2Q

2018, 1Q, 12	Percutaneous balloon valvuloplasty & cardiac catheterization with ventriculogram
2017, 1Q, 18	Sutureless repair of pulmonary vein stenosis
2016, 4Q, 80-81	Thoracic aorta, ascending/arch and descending
2016, 4Q, 82-83	Coronary artery, number of arteries
2016, 4Q, 101	Root operation Creation
2016, 4Q, 102-109	Correction of congenital heart defects
2015, 4Q, 23	Congenital heart corrective procedures
2015, 3Q, 16	Vascular ring surgery and double aortic arch
2015, 2Q, 23	Annuloplasty ring
2013, 3Q, 26	Transcatheter replacement of heart valve (TAVR) with measurements

AHA Coding Clinic for table Ø2R

2020, 1Q, 25	Elephant trunk repair of aortic dissection
2019, 4Q, 24	Coronary artery Body Part to root operation Insertion
2019, 4Q, 46	Cerebral embolic filtration
2019, 3Q, 23	Replacement of atrioventricular valve
2019, 3Q, 24	Valve sparing aortic root replacement with modified Gleason Vascutek® graft to ascending aorta
2019, 1Q, 31	Transcatheter aortic valve in valve replacement
2018, 3Q, 11	Transcatheter aortic valve replacement via transaortic approach
2018, 1Q, 12	Percutaneous balloon valvuloplasty & cardiac catheterization with ventriculogram
2017, 4Q, 55-56	Added approach values - Percutaneous heart valve procedures
2017, 1Q, 13	SynCardia total artificial heart
2016, 4Q, 80-81	Thoracic aorta, ascending/arch and descending
2016, 3Q, 32	Transcatheter tricuspid valve replacement
2014, 1Q, 10	Repair of thoracic aortic aneurysm & coronary artery bypass graft

AHA Coding Clinic for table Ø2S

2016, 4Q, 80-81	Thoracic aorta, ascending/arch and descending
2016, 4Q, 82-83	Coronary artery, number of arteries
2016, 4Q, 102-109	Correction of congenital heart defects
2015, 4Q, 23	Congenital heart corrective procedures

AHA Coding Clinic for table Ø2U

2020, 4Q, 52	Transapical mitral valve repair with device
2020, 1Q, 24	Pulmonary artery unifocalization
2019, 4Q, 25	Coronary artery to root operation Supplement
2018, 1Q, 12	Percutaneous balloon valvuloplasty & cardiac catheterization with ventriculogram
2017, 4Q, 36	Alfieri stitch procedure
2017, 3Q, 7	Senning procedure (arterial switch)
2017, 1Q, 19	Norwood Sano procedure
2016, 4Q, 80-81	Thoracic aorta, ascending/arch and descending
2016, 4Q, 101	Root operation Creation
2016, 4Q, 102-109	Correction of congenital heart defects
2016, 2Q, 23	Repair of tetralogy of Fallot with autologous pericardial patch graft
2016, 2Q, 26	Aortic valve replacement with aortic root enlargement
2015, 4Q, 22-24	Congenital heart corrective procedures
2015, 3Q, 16	Revision of previous truncus arteriosus surgery with ventricle to pulmonary artery conduit
2015, 2Q, 23	Annuloplasty ring
2014, 3Q, 16	Repair of Tetralogy of Fallot

AHA Coding Clinic for table Ø2V

2020, 1Q, 25	Elephant trunk repair of aortic dissection
2017, 4Q, 35-36	Alfieri stitch procedure
2016, 4Q, 80-81	Thoracic aorta, ascending/arch and descending
2016, 4Q, 89-92	Branched and fenestrated endograft repair of aneurysms

AHA Coding Clinic for table Ø2W

2019, 1Q, 24	Replacement of left ventricular assist device with retention of outflow graft
2018, 3Q, 8	Coronary artery bypass graft surgery (revision versus total redo)
2018, 3Q, 9	Fibrin sheath stripping of malfunctioning port-a-cath
2018, 1Q, 17	Repositioning of Impella short-term external heart assist device
2017, 4Q, 42-45	Insertion of external heart assist devices
2017, 4Q, 55-56	Added approach values - Percutaneous heart valve procedures
2016, 4Q, 85	Coronary Artery, number of stents
2016, 4Q, 95-96	Intracardiac pacemaker
2015, 3Q, 32	Approach values for repositioning and removal of cardiac lead
2014, 3Q, 31	Closure of paravalvular leak using Amplatzer® vascular plug

AHA Coding Clinic for table Ø2Y

2013, 3Q, 18	Heart transplant surgery

Coronary Arteries

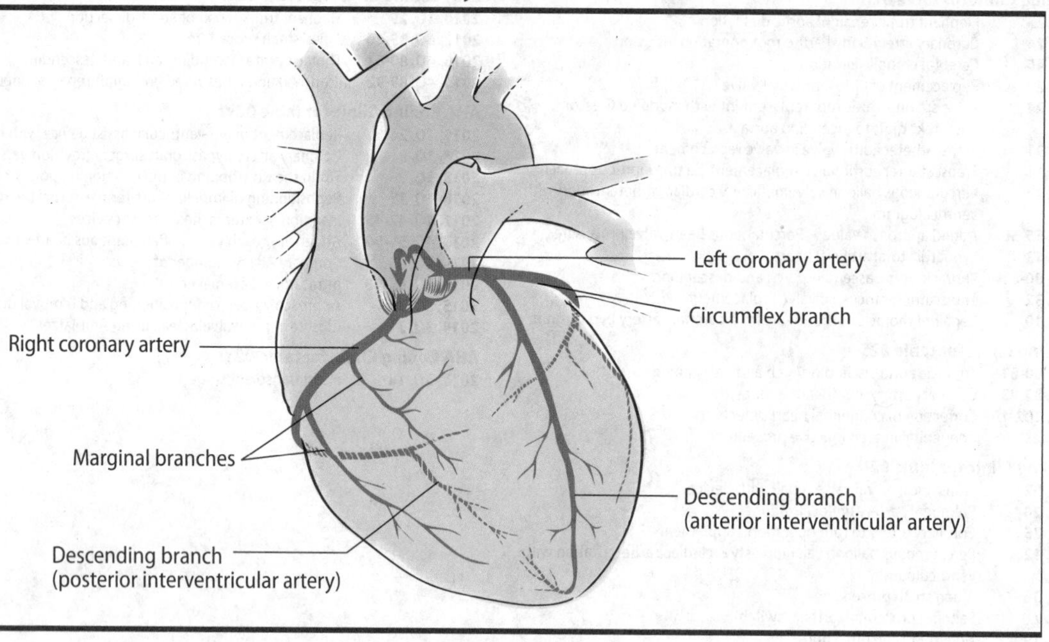

Heart Anatomy

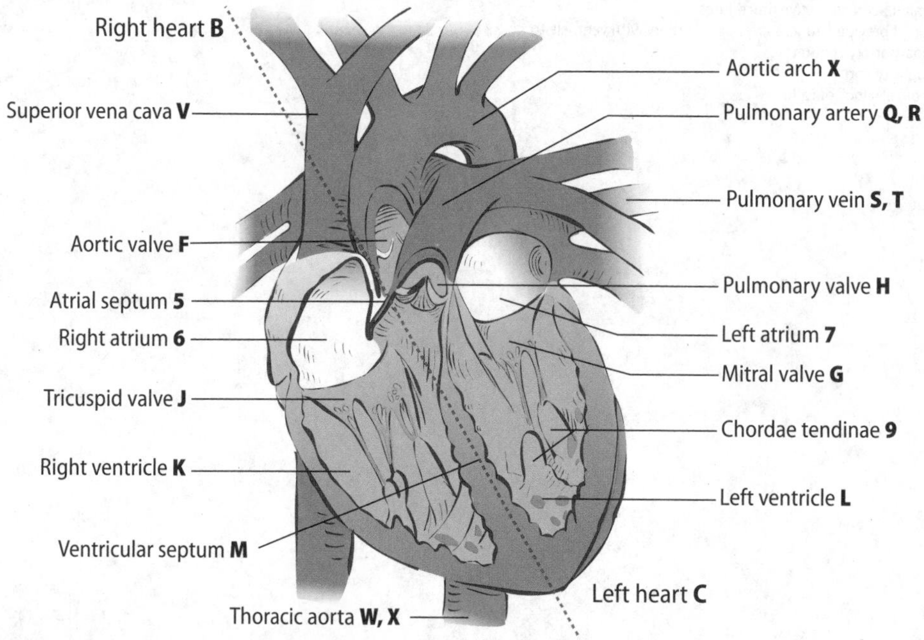

Ø Medical and Surgical
2 Heart and Great Vessels
1 Bypass Definition: Altering the route of passage of the contents of a tubular body part
Explanation: Rerouting contents of a body part to a downstream area of the normal route, to a similar route and body part, or to an abnormal route and dissimilar body part. Includes one or more anastomoses, with or without the use of a device.

Body Part Character 4	Approach Character 5	Device Character 6	Qualifier Character 7
Ø Coronary Artery, One Artery **1 Coronary Artery, Two Arteries** **2 Coronary Artery, Three Arteries** **3 Coronary Artery, Four or More Arteries**	**Ø Open**	**8 Zooplastic Tissue** **9 Autologous Venous Tissue** **A Autologous Arterial Tissue** **J Synthetic Substitute** **K Nonautologous Tissue Substitute**	**3 Coronary Artery** **8 Internal Mammary, Right** **9 Internal Mammary, Left** **C Thoracic Artery** **F Abdominal Artery** **W Aorta**
Ø Coronary Artery, One Artery **1 Coronary Artery, Two Arteries** **2 Coronary Artery, Three Arteries** **3 Coronary Artery, Four or More Arteries**	**Ø Open**	**Z No Device**	**3 Coronary Artery** **8 Internal Mammary, Right** **9 Internal Mammary, Left** **C Thoracic Artery** **F Abdominal Artery**
Ø Coronary Artery, One Artery **1 Coronary Artery, Two Arteries** **2 Coronary Artery, Three Arteries** **3 Coronary Artery, Four or More Arteries**	**3 Percutaneous**	**4 Intraluminal Device, Drug-eluting** **D Intraluminal Device**	**4 Coronary Vein**
Ø Coronary Artery, One Artery **1 Coronary Artery, Two Arteries** **2 Coronary Artery, Three Arteries** **3 Coronary Artery, Four or More Arteries**	**4 Percutaneous Endoscopic**	**4 Intraluminal Device, Drug-eluting** **D Intraluminal Device**	**4 Coronary Vein**
Ø Coronary Artery, One Artery **1 Coronary Artery, Two Arteries** **2 Coronary Artery, Three Arteries** **3 Coronary Artery, Four or More Arteries**	**4 Percutaneous Endoscopic**	**8 Zooplastic Tissue** **9 Autologous Venous Tissue** **A Autologous Arterial Tissue** **J Synthetic Substitute** **K Nonautologous Tissue Substitute**	**3 Coronary Artery** **8 Internal Mammary, Right** **9 Internal Mammary, Left** **C Thoracic Artery** **F Abdominal Artery** **W Aorta**
Ø Coronary Artery, One Artery **1 Coronary Artery, Two Arteries** **2 Coronary Artery, Three Arteries** **3 Coronary Artery, Four or More Arteries**	**4 Percutaneous Endoscopic**	**Z No Device**	**3 Coronary Artery** **8 Internal Mammary, Right** **9 Internal Mammary, Left** **C Thoracic Artery** **F Abdominal Artery**
6 Atrium, Right Atrium dextrum cordis Right auricular appendix Sinus venosus	**Ø Open** **4 Percutaneous Endoscopic**	**8 Zooplastic Tissue** **9 Autologous Venous Tissue** **A Autologous Arterial Tissue** **J Synthetic Substitute** **K Nonautologous Tissue Substitute**	**P Pulmonary Trunk** **Q Pulmonary Artery, Right** **R Pulmonary Artery, Left**
6 Atrium, Right Atrium dextrum cordis Right auricular appendix Sinus venosus	**Ø Open** **4 Percutaneous Endoscopic**	**Z No Device**	**7 Atrium, Left** **P Pulmonary Trunk** **Q Pulmonary Artery, Right** **R Pulmonary Artery, Left**
6 Atrium, Right Atrium dextrum cordis Right auricular appendix Sinus venosus	**3 Percutaneous**	**Z No Device**	**7 Atrium, Left**
7 Atrium, Left Atrium pulmonale Left auricular appendix	**Ø Open** **4 Percutaneous Endoscopic**	**8 Zooplastic Tissue** **9 Autologous Venous Tissue** **A Autologous Arterial Tissue** **J Synthetic Substitute** **K Nonautologous Tissue Substitute** **Z No Device**	**P Pulmonary Trunk** **Q Pulmonary Artery, Right** **R Pulmonary Artery, Left** **S Pulmonary Vein, Right** **T Pulmonary Vein, Left** **U Pulmonary Vein, Confluence**
7 Atrium, Left Atrium pulmonale Left auricular appendix	**3 Percutaneous**	**J Synthetic Substitute**	**6 Atrium, Right**
K Ventricle, Right Conus arteriosus **L Ventricle, Left**	**Ø Open** **4 Percutaneous Endoscopic**	**8 Zooplastic Tissue** **9 Autologous Venous Tissue** **A Autologous Arterial Tissue** **J Synthetic Substitute** **K Nonautologous Tissue Substitute**	**P Pulmonary Trunk** **Q Pulmonary Artery, Right** **R Pulmonary Artery, Left**

HAC Ø21[Ø,1,2,3]Ø[8,9,A,J,K][3,8,9,C,F,W] when reported with SDx J98.51 or J98.59
HAC Ø21[Ø,1,2,3]ØZ[3,8,9,C,F] when reported with SDx J98.51 or J98.59
HAC Ø21[Ø,1,2,3]4[8,9,A,J,K][3,8,9,C,F,W] when reported with SDx J98.51 or J98.59
HAC Ø21[Ø,1,2,3]4Z[3,8,9,C,F] when reported with SDx J98.51 or J98.59

Ø21 Continued on next page

Ø Medical and Surgical
2 Heart and Great Vessels
1 Bypass Definition: Altering the route of passage of the contents of a tubular body part

Ø21 Continued

Explanation: Rerouting contents of a body part to a downstream area of the normal route, to a similar route and body part, or to an abnormal route and dissimilar body part. Includes one or more anastomoses, with or without the use of a device.

Body Part Character 4	Approach Character 5	Device Character 6	Qualifier Character 7
K Ventricle, Right Conus arteriosus **L Ventricle, Left**	**Ø Open** **4 Percutaneous Endoscopic**	**Z No Device**	**5 Coronary Circulation** **8 Internal Mammary, Right** **9 Internal Mammary, Left** **C Thoracic Artery** **F Abdominal Artery** **P Pulmonary Trunk** **Q Pulmonary Artery, Right** **R Pulmonary Artery, Left** **W Aorta**
P Pulmonary Trunk **Q Pulmonary Artery, Right** **R Pulmonary Artery, Left** Arterial canal (duct) Botallo's duct Pulmoaortic canal	**Ø Open** **4 Percutaneous Endoscopic**	**8 Zooplastic Tissue** **9 Autologous Venous Tissue** **A Autologous Arterial Tissue** **J Synthetic Substitute** **K Nonautologous Tissue Substitute** **Z No Device**	**A Innominate Artery** **B Subclavian** **D Carotid**
V Superior Vena Cava Precava	**Ø Open** **4 Percutaneous Endoscopic**	**8 Zooplastic Tissue** **9 Autologous Venous Tissue** **A Autologous Arterial Tissue** **J Synthetic Substitute** **K Nonautologous Tissue Substitute** **Z No Device**	**P Pulmonary Trunk** **Q Pulmonary Artery, Right** **R Pulmonary Artery, Left** **S Pulmonary Vein, Right** **T Pulmonary Vein, Left** **U Pulmonary Vein, Confluence**
W Thoracic Aorta, Descending	**Ø Open**	**8 Zooplastic Tissue** **9 Autologous Venous Tissue** **A Autologous Arterial Tissue** **J Synthetic Substitute** **K Nonautologous Tissue Substitute**	**A Innominate Artery** **B Subclavian** **D Carotid** **F Abdominal Artery** **G Axillary Artery** **H Brachial Artery** **P Pulmonary Trunk** **Q Pulmonary Artery, Right** **R Pulmonary Artery, Left** **V Lower Extremity Artery**
W Thoracic Aorta, Descending	**Ø Open**	**Z No Device**	**A Innominate Artery** **B Subclavian** **D Carotid** **P Pulmonary Trunk** **Q Pulmonary Artery, Right** **R Pulmonary Artery, Left**
W Thoracic Aorta, Descending	**4 Percutaneous Endoscopic**	**8 Zooplastic Tissue** **9 Autologous Venous Tissue** **A Autologous Arterial Tissue** **J Synthetic Substitute** **K Nonautologous Tissue Substitute** **Z No Device**	**A Innominate Artery** **B Subclavian** **D Carotid** **P Pulmonary Trunk** **Q Pulmonary Artery, Right** **R Pulmonary Artery, Left**
X Thoracic Aorta, Ascending/Arch Aortic arch Ascending aorta	**Ø Open** **4 Percutaneous Endoscopic**	**8 Zooplastic Tissue** **9 Autologous Venous Tissue** **A Autologous Arterial Tissue** **J Synthetic Substitute** **K Nonautologous Tissue Substitute** **Z No Device**	**A Innominate Artery** **B Subclavian** **D Carotid** **P Pulmonary Trunk** **Q Pulmonary Artery, Right** **R Pulmonary Artery, Left**

Ø Medical and Surgical
2 Heart and Great Vessels
4 Creation Definition: Putting in or on biological or synthetic material to form a new body part that to the extent possible replicates the anatomic structure or function of an absent body part

Explanation: Used for gender reassignment surgery and corrective procedures in individuals with congenital anomalies

Body Part Character 4	Approach Character 5	Device Character 6	Qualifier Character 7
F Aortic Valve Aortic annulus	**Ø Open**	**7 Autologous Tissue** **8 Zooplastic Tissue** **J Synthetic Substitute** **K Nonautologous Tissue Substitute**	**J Truncal Valve**
G Mitral Valve Bicuspid valve Left atrioventricular valve Mitral annulus **J Tricuspid Valve** Right atrioventricular valve Tricuspid annulus	**Ø Open**	**7 Autologous Tissue** **8 Zooplastic Tissue** **J Synthetic Substitute** **K Nonautologous Tissue Substitute**	**2 Common Atrioventricular Valve**

Ø Medical and Surgical
2 Heart and Great Vessels
5 Destruction Definition: Physical eradication of all or a portion of a body part by the direct use of energy, force, or a destructive agent
Explanation: None of the body part is physically taken out

Body Part Character 4	Approach Character 5	Device Character 6	Qualifier Character 7
4 Coronary Vein **5 Atrial Septum** Interatrial septum **6 Atrium, Right** Atrium dextrum cordis Right auricular appendix Sinus venosus **8 Conduction Mechanism** Atrioventricular node Bundle of His Bundle of Kent Sinoatrial node **9 Chordae Tendineae** **D Papillary Muscle** **F Aortic Valve** Aortic annulus **G Mitral Valve** Bicuspid valve Left atrioventricular valve Mitral annulus **H Pulmonary Valve** Pulmonary annulus Pulmonic valve **J Tricuspid Valve** Right atrioventricular valve Tricuspid annulus **K Ventricle, Right** Conus arteriosus **L Ventricle, Left** **M Ventricular Septum** Interventricular septum **N Pericardium** **P Pulmonary Trunk** **Q Pulmonary Artery, Right** **R Pulmonary Artery, Left** Arterial canal (duct) Botallo's duct Pulmoaortic canal **S Pulmonary Vein, Right** Right inferior pulmonary vein Right superior pulmonary vein **T Pulmonary Vein, Left** Left inferior pulmonary vein Left superior pulmonary vein **V Superior Vena Cava** Precava **W Thoracic Aorta, Descending** **X Thoracic Aorta, Ascending/Arch** Aortic arch Ascending aorta	**Ø Open** **3 Percutaneous** **4 Percutaneous Endoscopic**	**Z No Device**	**Z No Qualifier**
7 Atrium, Left Atrium pulmonale Left auricular appendix	**Ø Open** **3 Percutaneous** **4 Percutaneous Endoscopic**	**Z No Device**	**K Left Atrial Appendage** **Z No Qualifier**

DRG Non-OR Ø257[Ø,3,4]ZK

Ø Medical and Surgical
2 Heart and Great Vessels
7 Dilation Definition: Expanding an orifice or the lumen of a tubular body part

Explanation: The orifice can be a natural orifice or an artificially created orifice. Accomplished by stretching a tubular body part using intraluminal pressure or by cutting part of the orifice or wall of the tubular body part.

Body Part Character 4	Approach Character 5	Device Character 6	Qualifier Character 7
Ø Coronary Artery, One Artery **1** Coronary Artery, Two Arteries **2** Coronary Artery, Three Arteries **3** Coronary Artery, Four or More Arteries	**Ø** Open **3** Percutaneous **4** Percutaneous Endoscopic	**4** Intraluminal Device, Drug-eluting **5** Intraluminal Device, Drug-eluting, Two **6** Intraluminal Device, Drug-eluting, Three **7** Intraluminal Device, Drug-eluting, Four or More **D** Intraluminal Device **E** Intraluminal Device, Two **F** Intraluminal Device, Three **G** Intraluminal Device, Four or More **T** Intraluminal Device, Radioactive **Z** No Device	**6** Bifurcation **Z** No Qualifier
F Aortic Valve Aortic annulus **G** Mitral Valve Bicuspid valve Left atrioventricular valve Mitral annulus **H** Pulmonary Valve Pulmonary annulus Pulmonic valve **J** Tricuspid Valve Right atrioventricular valve Tricuspid annulus **K** Ventricle, Right Conus arteriosus **L** Ventricle, Left **P** Pulmonary Trunk **Q** Pulmonary Artery, Right **S** Pulmonary Vein, Right Right inferior pulmonary vein Right superior pulmonary vein **T** Pulmonary Vein, Left Left inferior pulmonary vein Left superior pulmonary vein **V** Superior Vena Cava Precava **W** Thoracic Aorta, Descending **X** Thoracic Aorta, Ascending/Arch Aortic arch Ascending aorta	**Ø** Open **3** Percutaneous **4** Percutaneous Endoscopic	**4** Intraluminal Device, Drug-eluting **D** Intraluminal Device **Z** No Device	**Z** No Qualifier
R Pulmonary Artery, Left Arterial canal (duct) Botallo's duct Pulmoaortic canal	**Ø** Open **3** Percutaneous **4** Percutaneous Endoscopic	**4** Intraluminal Device, Drug-eluting **D** Intraluminal Device **Z** No Device	**T** Ductus Arteriosus **Z** No Qualifier

Ø Medical and Surgical
2 Heart and Great Vessels
8 Division Definition: Cutting into a body part, without draining fluids and/or gases from the body part, in order to separate or transect a body part

Explanation: All or a portion of the body part is separated into two or more portions

Body Part Character 4	Approach Character 5	Device Character 6	Qualifier Character 7
8 Conduction Mechanism Atrioventricular node Bundle of His Bundle of Kent Sinoatrial node **9** Chordae Tendineae **D** Papillary Muscle	**Ø** Open **3** Percutaneous **4** Percutaneous Endoscopic	**Z** No Device	**Z** No Qualifier

Ø Medical and Surgical
2 Heart and Great Vessels
B Excision Definition: Cutting out or off, without replacement, a portion of a body part
Explanation: The qualifier DIAGNOSTIC is used to identify excision procedures that are biopsies

Body Part Character 4	Approach Character 5	Device Character 6	Qualifier Character 7
4 Coronary Vein **5 Atrial Septum** Interatrial septum **6 Atrium, Right** Atrium dextrum cordis Right auricular appendix Sinus venosus **8 Conduction Mechanism** Atrioventricular node Bundle of His Bundle of Kent Sinoatrial node **9 Chordae Tendineae** **D Papillary Muscle** **F Aortic Valve** Aortic annulus **G Mitral Valve** Bicuspid valve Left atrioventricular valve Mitral annulus **H Pulmonary Valve** Pulmonary annulus Pulmonic valve **J Tricuspid Valve** Right atrioventricular valve Tricuspid annulus **K Ventricle, Right** NC Conus arteriosus **L Ventricle, Left** NC **M Ventricular Septum** Interventricular septum **N Pericardium** **P Pulmonary Trunk** **Q Pulmonary Artery, Right** **R Pulmonary Artery, Left** Arterial canal (duct) Botallo's duct Pulmoaortic canal **S Pulmonary Vein, Right** Right inferior pulmonary vein Right superior pulmonary vein **T Pulmonary Vein, Left** Left inferior pulmonary vein Left superior pulmonary vein **V Superior Vena Cava** Precava **W Thoracic Aorta, Descending** **X Thoracic Aorta, Ascending/Arch** Aortic arch Ascending aorta	**Ø Open** **3 Percutaneous** **4 Percutaneous Endoscopic**	**Z No Device**	**X Diagnostic** **Z No Qualifier**
7 Atrium, Left Atrium pulmonale Left auricular appendix	**Ø Open** **3 Percutaneous** **4 Percutaneous Endoscopic**	**Z No Device**	**K Left Atrial Appendage** **X Diagnostic** **Z No Qualifier**

DRG Non-OR Ø2B7[Ø,3,4]ZK
Non-OR Ø2B[4,5,6,8,9,D,F,G,H,J,K,L,M][Ø,3,4]ZX
NC Ø2B[K,L][Ø,3,4]ZZ

Ø Medical and Surgical
2 Heart and Great Vessels
C Extirpation Definition: Taking or cutting out solid matter from a body part

Explanation: The solid matter may be an abnormal byproduct of a biological function or a foreign body; it may be imbedded in a body part or in the lumen of a tubular body part. The solid matter may or may not have been previously broken into pieces.

Body Part Character 4	Approach Character 5	Device Character 6	Qualifier Character 7
Ø Coronary Artery, One Artery **1** Coronary Artery, Two Arteries **2** Coronary Artery, Three Arteries **3** Coronary Artery, Four or More Arteries	**Ø** Open **4** Percutaneous Endoscopic	**Z** No Device	**6** Bifurcation **Z** No Qualifier
Ø Coronary Artery, One Artery **1** Coronary Artery, Two Arteries **2** Coronary Artery, Three Arteries **3** Coronary Artery, Four or More Arteries	**3** Percutaneous	**Z** No Device	**6** Bifurcation **7** Orbital Atherectomy Technique **Z** No Qualifier
4 Coronary Vein **5** Atrial Septum Interatrial septum **6** Atrium, Right Atrium dextrum cordis Right auricular appendix Sinus venosus **7** Atrium, Left Atrium pulmonale Left auricular appendix **8** Conduction Mechanism Atrioventricular node Bundle of His Bundle of Kent Sinoatrial node **9** Chordae Tendineae **D** Papillary Muscle **F** Aortic Valve Aortic annulus **G** Mitral Valve Bicuspid valve Left atrioventricular valve Mitral annulus **H** Pulmonary Valve Pulmonary annulus Pulmonic valve **J** Tricuspid Valve Right atrioventricular valve Tricuspid annulus **K** Ventricle, Right Conus arteriosus **L** Ventricle, Left **M** Ventricular Septum Interventricular septum **N** Pericardium **P** Pulmonary Trunk **Q** Pulmonary Artery, Right **R** Pulmonary Artery, Left Arterial canal (duct) Botallo's duct Pulmoaortic canal **S** Pulmonary Vein, Right Right inferior pulmonary vein Right superior pulmonary vein **T** Pulmonary Vein, Left Left inferior pulmonary vein Left superior pulmonary vein **V** Superior Vena Cava Precava **W** Thoracic Aorta, Descending **X** Thoracic Aorta, Ascending/Arch Aortic arch Ascending aorta	**Ø** Open **3** Percutaneous **4** Percutaneous Endoscopic	**Z** No Device	**Z** No Qualifier

Ø Medical and Surgical
2 Heart and Great Vessels
F Fragmentation Definition: Breaking solid matter in a body part into pieces

Explanation: Physical force (e.g., manual, ultrasonic) applied directly or indirectly is used to break the solid matter into pieces. The solid matter may be an abnormal byproduct of a biological function or a foreign body. The pieces of solid matter are not taken out.

Body Part Character 4	Approach Character 5	Device Character 6	Qualifier Character 7
Ø Coronary Artery, One Artery 1 Coronary Artery, Two Arteries 2 Coronary Artery, Three Arteries 3 Coronary Artery, Four or More Arteries	3 Percutaneous	Z No Device	Z No Qualifier
N Pericardium NC	**Ø Open** **3 Percutaneous** **4 Percutaneous Endoscopic** **X External**	Z No Device	Z No Qualifier
P Pulmonary Trunk **Q Pulmonary Artery, Right** **R Pulmonary Artery, Left** Arterial canal (duct) Botallo's duct Pulmoaortic canal **S Pulmonary Vein, Right** Right inferior pulmonary vein Right superior pulmonary vein **T Pulmonary Vein, Left** Left inferior pulmonary vein Left superior pulmonary vein	3 Percutaneous	Z No Device	Ø Ultrasonic Z No Qualifier

Non-OR Ø2FNXZZ
NC Ø2FNXZZ

Heart and Great Vessels

Ø2F–Ø2F

Ø Medical and Surgical
2 Heart and Great Vessels
H Insertion Definition: Putting in a nonbiological appliance that monitors, assists, performs, or prevents a physiological function but does not physically take the place of a body part
Explanation: None

Body Part Character 4	Approach Character 5	Device Character 6	Qualifier Character 7
Ø Coronary Artery, One Artery **1** Coronary Artery, Two Arteries **2** Coronary Artery, Three Arteries **3** Coronary Artery, Four or More Arteries	**Ø** Open **3** Percutaneous **4** Percutaneous Endoscopic	**D** Intraluminal Device **Y** Other Device	**Z** No Qualifier
4 Coronary Vein ⊞ **6** Atrium, Right ⊞ Atrium dextrum cordis Right auricular appendix Sinus venosus **7** Atrium, Left ⊞ Atrium pulmonale Left auricular appendix **K** Ventricle, Right ⊞ Conus arteriosus **L** Ventricle, Left ⊞	**Ø** Open **3** Percutaneous **4** Percutaneous Endoscopic	**Ø** Monitoring Device, Pressure Sensor **2** Monitoring Device **3** Infusion Device **D** Intraluminal Device **J** Cardiac Lead, Pacemaker **K** Cardiac Lead, Defibrillator **M** Cardiac Lead **N** Intracardiac Pacemaker **Y** Other Device	**Z** No Qualifier
A Heart LC NC	**Ø** Open **3** Percutaneous **4** Percutaneous Endoscopic	**Q** Implantable Heart Assist System **Y** Other Device	**Z** No Qualifier
A Heart ⊞	**Ø** Open **3** Percutaneous **4** Percutaneous Endoscopic	**R** Short-term External Heart Assist System	**J** Intraoperative **S** Biventricular **Z** No Qualifier
N Pericardium ⊞	**Ø** Open **3** Percutaneous **4** Percutaneous Endoscopic	**Ø** Monitoring Device, Pressure Sensor **2** Monitoring Device **J** Cardiac Lead, Pacemaker **K** Cardiac Lead, Defibrillator **M** Cardiac Lead **Y** Other Device	**Z** No Qualifier
P Pulmonary Trunk **Q** Pulmonary Artery, Right **R** Pulmonary Artery, Left Arterial canal (duct) Botallo's duct Pulmoaortic canal **S** Pulmonary Vein, Right Right inferior pulmonary vein Right superior pulmonary vein **T** Pulmonary Vein, Left Left inferior pulmonary vein Left superior pulmonary vein **V** Superior Vena Cava Precava **W** Thoracic Aorta, Descending	**Ø** Open **3** Percutaneous **4** Percutaneous Endoscopic	**Ø** Monitoring Device, Pressure Sensor **2** Monitoring Device **3** Infusion Device **D** Intraluminal Device **Y** Other Device	**Z** No Qualifier
X Thoracic Aorta, Ascending/Arch Aortic arch Ascending aorta	**Ø** Open **3** Percutaneous **4** Percutaneous Endoscopic	**Ø** Monitoring Device, Pressure Sensor **2** Monitoring Device **3** Infusion Device **D** Intraluminal Device	**Z** No Qualifier

DRG Non-OR Ø2H[4,6,7,K,L][Ø,3,4][J,M]Z
DRG Non-OR Ø2HK32Z
DRG Non-OR Ø2HN[Ø,3,4][J,M]Z
Non-OR Ø2H[4,6,7,L]3[2,3]Z
Non-OR Ø2H[6,7]3MZ
Non-OR Ø2HK3[Ø,3]Z
Non-OR Ø2HN32Z
Non-OR Ø2HP[Ø,3,4][Ø,2,3]Z
Non-OR Ø2H[Q,R][Ø,3,4][2,3]Z
Non-OR Ø2H[S,T,V,W][Ø,3,4]3Z
Non-OR Ø2H[S,T,V,W]32Z
Non-OR Ø2HW[Ø,3]ØZ
Non-OR Ø2HX[Ø,3,4][Ø,3]Z

HAC Ø2H43[J,K,M]Z when reported with SDx K68.11 or T81.4Ø-T81.49, T82.6-T82.7 with 7th character A
HAC Ø2H[6,K]33Z when reported with SDx J95.811
HAC Ø2H[6,7]3[J,M]Z when reported with SDx K68.11 or T81.4Ø-T81.49, T82.6-T82.7 with 7th character A
HAC Ø2H[K,L]3JZ when reported with SDx K68.11 or T81.4Ø-T81.49, T82.6-T82.7 with 7th character A
HAC Ø2HN[Ø,3,4][J,M]Z when reported with SDx K68.11 or T81.4Ø-T81.49, T82.6-T82.7 with 7th character A
HAC Ø2H[S,T,V][3,4]3Z when reported with SDx J95.811
LC Ø2HAØQZ
NC Ø2HA[3,4]QZ

See Appendix L for Procedure Combinations
⊞ Ø2H[4,6,7,K,L][Ø,3,4][J,K,M]Z
⊞ Ø2HA[Ø,4]R[S,Z]
⊞ Ø2HA3RS
⊞ Ø2HN[Ø,3,4][J,K,M]Z

Ø Medical and Surgical
2 Heart and Great Vessels
J Inspection Definition: Visually and/or manually exploring a body part

Explanation: Visual exploration may be performed with or without optical instrumentation. Manual exploration may be performed directly or through intervening body layers.

Body Part Character 4	Approach Character 5	Device Character 6	Qualifier Character 7
A Heart Y Great Vessel	Ø Open 3 Percutaneous 4 Percutaneous Endoscopic	Z No Device	Z No Qualifier

Non-OR Ø2J[A,Y]3ZZ

Ø Medical and Surgical
2 Heart and Great Vessels
K Map Definition: Locating the route of passage of electrical impulses and/or locating functional areas in a body part

Explanation: Applicable only to the cardiac conduction mechanism and the central nervous system

Body Part Character 4	Approach Character 5	Device Character 6	Qualifier Character 7
8 Conduction Mechanism Atrioventricular node Bundle of His Bundle of Kent Sinoatrial node	Ø Open 3 Percutaneous 4 Percutaneous Endoscopic	Z No Device	Z No Qualifier

DRG Non-OR Ø2K8[Ø,3,4]ZZ

Ø Medical and Surgical
2 Heart and Great Vessels
L Occlusion Definition: Completely closing an orifice or the lumen of a tubular body part

Explanation: The orifice can be a natural orifice or an artificially created orifice

Body Part Character 4	Approach Character 5	Device Character 6	Qualifier Character 7
7 Atrium, Left Atrium pulmonale Left auricular appendix	Ø Open 3 Percutaneous 4 Percutaneous Endoscopic	C Extraluminal Device D Intraluminal Device Z No Device	K Left Atrial Appendage
H Pulmonary Valve Pulmonary annulus Pulmonic valve P Pulmonary Trunk Q Pulmonary Artery, Right S Pulmonary Vein, Right Right inferior pulmonary vein Right superior pulmonary vein T Pulmonary Vein, Left Left inferior pulmonary vein Left superior pulmonary vein V Superior Vena Cava Precava	Ø Open 3 Percutaneous 4 Percutaneous Endoscopic	C Extraluminal Device D Intraluminal Device Z No Device	Z No Qualifier
R Pulmonary Artery, Left Arterial canal (duct) Botallo's duct Pulmoaortic canal	Ø Open 3 Percutaneous 4 Percutaneous Endoscopic	C Extraluminal Device D Intraluminal Device Z No Device	T Ductus Arteriosus Z No Qualifier
W Thoracic Aorta, Descending	3 Percutaneous	D Intraluminal Device	J Temporary

DRG Non-OR Ø2L7[Ø,3,4][C,D,Z]K

Ø Medical and Surgical
2 Heart and Great Vessels
N Release Definition: Freeing a body part from an abnormal physical constraint by cutting or by the use of force
Explanation: Some of the restraining tissue may be taken out but none of the body part is taken out

Body Part Character 4	Approach Character 5	Device Character 6	Qualifier Character 7
Ø Coronary Artery, One Artery **1 Coronary Artery, Two Arteries** **2 Coronary Artery, Three Arteries** **3 Coronary Artery, Four or More Arteries** **4 Coronary Vein** **5 Atrial Septum** Interatrial septum **6 Atrium, Right** Atrium dextrum cordis Right auricular appendix Sinus venosus **7 Atrium, Left** Atrium pulmonale Left auricular appendix **8 Conduction Mechanism** Atrioventricular node Bundle of His Bundle of Kent Sinoatrial node **9 Chordae Tendineae** **D Papillary Muscle** **F Aortic Valve** Aortic annulus **G Mitral Valve** Bicuspid valve Left atrioventricular valve Mitral annulus **H Pulmonary Valve** Pulmonary annulus Pulmonic valve **J Tricuspid Valve** Right atrioventricular valve Tricuspid annulus **K Ventricle, Right** Conus arteriosus **L Ventricle, Left** **M Ventricular Septum** Interventricular septum **N Pericardium** **P Pulmonary Trunk** **Q Pulmonary Artery, Right** **R Pulmonary Artery, Left** Arterial canal (duct) Botallo's duct Pulmoaortic canal **S Pulmonary Vein, Right** Right inferior pulmonary vein Right superior pulmonary vein **T Pulmonary Vein, Left** Left inferior pulmonary vein Left superior pulmonary vein **V Superior Vena Cava** Precava **W Thoracic Aorta, Descending** **X Thoracic Aorta, Ascending/Arch** Aortic arch Ascending aorta	**Ø Open** **3 Percutaneous** **4 Percutaneous Endoscopic**	**Z No Device**	**Z No Qualifier**

Ø Medical and Surgical
2 Heart and Great Vessels
P Removal Definition: Taking out or off a device from a body part

Explanation: If a device is taken out and a similar device put in without cutting or puncturing the skin or mucous membrane, the procedure is coded to the root operation CHANGE. Otherwise, the procedure for taking out a device is coded to the root operation REMOVAL.

Body Part Character 4	Approach Character 5	Device Character 6	Qualifier Character 7
A Heart	Ø Open 3 Percutaneous 4 Percutaneous Endoscopic	2 Monitoring Device 3 Infusion Device 7 Autologous Tissue Substitute 8 Zooplastic Tissue C Extraluminal Device D Intraluminal Device J Synthetic Substitute K Nonautologous Tissue Substitute M Cardiac Lead N Intracardiac Pacemaker Q Implantable Heart Assist System Y Other Device	Z No Qualifier
A Heart ⊞	Ø Open 3 Percutaneous 4 Percutaneous Endoscopic	R Short-term External Heart Assist System	S Biventricular Z No Qualifier
A Heart	X External	2 Monitoring Device 3 Infusion Device D Intraluminal Device M Cardiac Lead	Z No Qualifier
Y Great Vessel	Ø Open 3 Percutaneous 4 Percutaneous Endoscopic	2 Monitoring Device 3 Infusion Device 7 Autologous Tissue Substitute 8 Zooplastic Tissue C Extraluminal Device D Intraluminal Device J Synthetic Substitute K Nonautologous Tissue Substitute Y Other Device	Z No Qualifier
Y Great Vessel	X External	2 Monitoring Device 3 Infusion Device D Intraluminal Device	Z No Qualifier

Non-OR Ø2PA3[2,3,D]Z
Non-OR Ø2PA[3,4]YZ
Non-OR Ø2PAX[2,3,D,M]Z
Non-OR Ø2PY3[2,3,D]Z
Non-OR Ø2PY[3,4]YZ
Non-OR Ø2PYX[2,3,D]Z
HAC Ø2PA[Ø,3,4]MZ when reported with SDx K68.11 or T81.4Ø-T81.49, T82.6-T82.7 with 7th character A
HAC Ø2PAXMZ when reported with SDx K68.11 or T81.4Ø-T81.49, T82.6-T82.7 with 7th character A

See Appendix L for Procedure Combinations
⊞ Ø2PA[Ø,3,4]RZ

0 Medical and Surgical
2 Heart and Great Vessels
Q Repair Definition: Restoring, to the extent possible, a body part to its normal anatomic structure and function
Explanation: Used only when the method to accomplish the repair is not one of the other root operations

Body Part Character 4	Approach Character 5	Device Character 6	Qualifier Character 7
0 Coronary Artery, One Artery **1 Coronary Artery, Two Arteries** **2 Coronary Artery, Three Arteries** **3 Coronary Artery, Four or More Arteries** **4 Coronary Vein** **5 Atrial Septum** Interatrial septum **6 Atrium, Right** Atrium dextrum cordis Right auricular appendix Sinus venosus **7 Atrium, Left** Atrium pulmonale Left auricular appendix **8 Conduction Mechanism** Atrioventricular node Bundle of His Bundle of Kent Sinoatrial node **9 Chordae Tendineae** **A Heart** **B Heart, Right** Right coronary sulcus **C Heart, Left** Left coronary sulcus Obtuse margin **D Papillary Muscle** **H Pulmonary Valve** Pulmonary annulus Pulmonic valve **K Ventricle, Right** Conus arteriosus **L Ventricle, Left** **M Ventricular Septum** Interventricular septum **N Pericardium** **P Pulmonary Trunk** **Q Pulmonary Artery, Right** **R Pulmonary Artery, Left** Arterial canal (duct) Botallo's duct Pulmoaortic canal **S Pulmonary Vein, Right** Right inferior pulmonary vein Right superior pulmonary vein **T Pulmonary Vein, Left** Left inferior pulmonary vein Left superior pulmonary vein **V Superior Vena Cava** Precava **W Thoracic Aorta, Descending** **X Thoracic Aorta, Ascending/Arch** Aortic arch Ascending aorta	**0 Open** **3 Percutaneous** **4 Percutaneous Endoscopic**	**Z No Device**	**Z No Qualifier**
F Aortic Valve Aortic annulus	**0 Open** **3 Percutaneous** **4 Percutaneous Endoscopic**	**Z No Device**	**J Truncal Valve** **Z No Qualifier**
G Mitral Valve Bicuspid valve Left atrioventricular valve Mitral annulus	**0 Open** **3 Percutaneous** **4 Percutaneous Endoscopic**	**Z No Device**	**E Atrioventricular Valve, Left** **Z No Qualifier**
J Tricuspid Valve Right atrioventricular valve Tricuspid annulus	**0 Open** **3 Percutaneous** **4 Percutaneous Endoscopic**	**Z No Device**	**G Atrioventricular Valve, Right** **Z No Qualifier**

Ø Medical and Surgical
2 Heart and Great Vessels
R Replacement Definition: Putting in or on biological or synthetic material that physically takes the place and/or function of all or a portion of a body part

Explanation: The body part may have been taken out or replaced, or may be taken out, physically eradicated, or rendered nonfunctional during the REPLACEMENT procedure. A REMOVAL procedure is coded for taking out the device used in a previous replacement procedure.

Body Part Character 4	Approach Character 5	Device Character 6	Qualifier Character 7
5 Atrial Septum Interatrial septum **6 Atrium, Right** Atrium dextrum cordis Right auricular appendix Sinus venosus **7 Atrium, Left** Atrium pulmonale Left auricular appendix **9 Chordae Tendineae** **D Papillary Muscle** **K Ventricle, Right** LC NC ⊞ Conus arteriosus **L Ventricle, Left** LC NC ⊞ **M Ventricular Septum** Interventricular septum **N Pericardium** **P Pulmonary Trunk** **Q Pulmonary Artery, Right** **R Pulmonary Artery, Left** Arterial canal (duct) Botallo's duct Pulmoaortic canal **S Pulmonary Vein, Right** Right inferior pulmonary vein Right superior pulmonary vein **T Pulmonary Vein, Left** Left inferior pulmonary vein Left superior pulmonary vein **V Superior Vena Cava** Precava **W Thoracic Aorta, Descending** **X Thoracic Aorta, Ascending/Arch** Aortic arch Ascending aorta	**Ø Open** **4 Percutaneous Endoscopic**	**7 Autologous Tissue Substitute** **8 Zooplastic Tissue** **J Synthetic Substitute** **K Nonautologous Tissue Substitute**	**Z No Qualifier**
A Heart	Ø Open	L Biologic with Synthetic Substitute, Autoregulated Electrohydraulic M Synthetic Substitute, Pneumatic	Z No Qualifier
F Aortic Valve Aortic annulus **G Mitral Valve** Bicuspid valve Left atrioventricular valve Mitral annulus **J Tricuspid Valve** Right atrioventricular valve Tricuspid annulus	**Ø Open** **4 Percutaneous Endoscopic**	**7 Autologous Tissue Substitute** **8 Zooplastic Tissue** **J Synthetic Substitute** **K Nonautologous Tissue Substitute**	**Z No Qualifier**
F Aortic Valve Aortic annulus **G Mitral Valve** Bicuspid valve Left atrioventricular valve Mitral annulus **J Tricuspid Valve** Right atrioventricular valve Tricuspid annulus	**3 Percutaneous**	**7 Autologous Tissue Substitute** **8 Zooplastic Tissue** **J Synthetic Substitute** **K Nonautologous Tissue Substitute**	**H Transapical** **Z No Qualifier**
H Pulmonary Valve Pulmonary annulus Pulmonic valve	**Ø Open** **4 Percutaneous Endoscopic**	**7 Autologous Tissue Substitute** **8 Zooplastic Tissue** **J Synthetic Substitute** **K Nonautologous Tissue Substitute**	**Z No Qualifier**
H Pulmonary Valve Pulmonary annulus Pulmonic valve	**3 Percutaneous**	**7 Autologous Tissue Substitute** **J Synthetic Substitute** **K Nonautologous Tissue Substitute**	**H Transapical** **Z No Qualifier**
H Pulmonary Valve Pulmonary annulus Pulmonic valve	**3 Percutaneous**	**8 Zooplastic Tissue**	**H Transapical** L In Existing Conduit M Native Site **Z No Qualifier**

LC Ø2RKØJZ with Ø2RLØJZ with diagnosis code ZØØ.6
NC Ø2RKØJZ with Ø2RLØJZ without diagnosis code ZØØ.6

See Appendix L for Procedure Combinations
⊞ Ø2R[K,L]ØJZ

Ø Medical and Surgical
2 Heart and Great Vessels
S Reposition Definition: Moving to its normal location, or other suitable location, all or a portion of a body part

Explanation: The body part is moved to a new location from an abnormal location, or from a normal location where it is not functioning correctly. The body part may or may not be cut out or off to be moved to the new location.

Body Part Character 4	Approach Character 5	Device Character 6	Qualifier Character 7
Ø Coronary Artery, One Artery **1 Coronary Artery, Two Arteries** **P Pulmonary Trunk** **Q Pulmonary Artery, Right** **R Pulmonary Artery, Left** Arterial canal (duct) Botallo's duct Pulmoaortic canal **S Pulmonary Vein, Right** Right inferior pulmonary vein Right superior pulmonary vein **T Pulmonary Vein, Left** Left inferior pulmonary vein Left superior pulmonary vein **V Superior Vena Cava** Precava **W Thoracic Aorta, Descending** **X Thoracic Aorta, Ascending/Arch** Aortic arch Ascending aorta	**Ø Open**	**Z No Device**	**Z No Qualifier**

Ø Medical and Surgical
2 Heart and Great Vessels
T Resection Definition: Cutting out or off, without replacement, all of a body part

Explanation: None

Body Part Character 4	Approach Character 5	Device Character 6	Qualifier Character 7
5 Atrial Septum Interatrial septum **8 Conduction Mechanism** Atrioventricular node Bundle of His Bundle of Kent Sinoatrial node **9 Chordae Tendineae** **D Papillary Muscle** **H Pulmonary Valve** Pulmonary annulus Pulmonic valve **M Ventricular Septum** Interventricular septum **N Pericardium**	**Ø Open** **3 Percutaneous** **4 Percutaneous Endoscopic**	**Z No Device**	**Z No Qualifier**

0 Medical and Surgical
2 Heart and Great Vessels
U Supplement Definition: Putting in or on biological or synthetic material that physically reinforces and/or augments the function of a portion of a body part

Explanation: The biological material is non-living, or is living and from the same individual. The body part may have been previously replaced, and the SUPPLEMENT procedure is performed to physically reinforce and/or augment the function of the replaced body part.

Body Part Character 4	Approach Character 5	Device Character 6	Qualifier Character 7
0 Coronary Artery, One Artery **1 Coronary Artery, Two Arteries** **2 Coronary Artery, Three Arteries** **3 Coronary Artery, Four or More Arteries** **5 Atrial Septum** Interatrial septum **6 Atrium, Right** Atrium dextrum cordis Right auricular appendix Sinus venosus **7 Atrium, Left** Atrium pulmonale Left auricular appendix **9 Chordae Tendineae** **A Heart** **D Papillary Muscle** **H Pulmonary Valve** Pulmonary annulus Pulmonic valve **K Ventricle, Right** Conus arteriosus **L Ventricle, Left** **M Ventricular Septum** Interventricular septum **N Pericardium** **P Pulmonary Trunk** **Q Pulmonary Artery, Right** **R Pulmonary Artery, Left** Arterial canal (duct) Botallo's duct Pulmoaortic canal **S Pulmonary Vein, Right** Right inferior pulmonary vein Right superior pulmonary vein **T Pulmonary Vein, Left** Left inferior pulmonary vein Left superior pulmonary vein **V Superior Vena Cava** Precava **W Thoracic Aorta, Descending** **X Thoracic Aorta, Ascending/Arch** Aortic arch Ascending aorta	**0 Open** **3 Percutaneous** **4 Percutaneous Endoscopic**	**7 Autologous Tissue Substitute** **8 Zooplastic Tissue** **J Synthetic Substitute** **K Nonautologous Tissue Substitute**	**Z No Qualifier**
F Aortic Valve Aortic annulus	**0 Open** **3 Percutaneous** **4 Percutaneous Endoscopic**	**7 Autologous Tissue Substitute** **8 Zooplastic Tissue** **J Synthetic Substitute** **K Nonautologous Tissue Substitute**	**J Truncal Valve** **Z No Qualifier**
G Mitral Valve Bicuspid valve Left atrioventricular valve Mitral annulus	**0 Open** **4 Percutaneous Endoscopic**	**7 Autologous Tissue Substitute** **8 Zooplastic Tissue** **J Synthetic Substitute** **K Nonautologous Tissue Substitute**	**E Atrioventricular Valve, Left** **Z No Qualifier**
G Mitral Valve Bicuspid valve Left atrioventricular valve Mitral annulus	**3 Percutaneous**	**7 Autologous Tissue Substitute** **8 Zooplastic Tissue** **K Nonautologous Tissue Substitute**	**E Atrioventricular Valve, Left** **Z No Qualifier**
G Mitral Valve Bicuspid valve Left atrioventricular valve Mitral annulus	**3 Percutaneous**	**J Synthetic Substitute**	**E Atrioventricular Valve, Left** **H Transapical** **Z No Qualifier**
J Tricuspid Valve Right atrioventricular valve Tricuspid annulus	**0 Open** **3 Percutaneous** **4 Percutaneous Endoscopic**	**7 Autologous Tissue Substitute** **8 Zooplastic Tissue** **J Synthetic Substitute** **K Nonautologous Tissue Substitute**	**G Atrioventricular Valve, Right** **Z No Qualifier**

DRG Non-OR 02U7[3,4]JZ

Ø Medical and Surgical
2 Heart and Great Vessels
V Restriction Definition: Partially closing an orifice or the lumen of a tubular body part
Explanation: The orifice can be a natural orifice or an artificially created orifice

Body Part Character 4	Approach Character 5	Device Character 6	Qualifier Character 7
A Heart	**Ø Open** **3 Percutaneous** **4 Percutaneous Endoscopic**	**C Extraluminal Device** **Z No Device**	**Z No Qualifier**
G Mitral Valve Bicuspid valve Left atrioventricular valve Mitral annulus	**Ø Open** **3 Percutaneous** **4 Percutaneous Endoscopic**	**Z No Device**	**Z No Qualifier**
L Ventricle, Left **P Pulmonary Trunk** **Q Pulmonary Artery, Right** **S Pulmonary Vein, Right** Right inferior pulmonary vein Right superior pulmonary vein **T Pulmonary Vein, Left** Left inferior pulmonary vein Left superior pulmonary vein **V Superior Vena Cava** Precava	**Ø Open** **3 Percutaneous** **4 Percutaneous Endoscopic**	**C Extraluminal Device** **D Intraluminal Device** **Z No Device**	**Z No Qualifier**
R Pulmonary Artery, Left Arterial canal (duct) Botallo's duct Pulmoaortic canal	**Ø Open** **3 Percutaneous** **4 Percutaneous Endoscopic**	**C Extraluminal Device** **D Intraluminal Device** **Z No Device**	**T Ductus Arteriosus** **Z No Qualifier**
W Thoracic Aorta, Descending **X Thoracic Aorta, Ascending/Arch** Aortic arch Ascending aorta	**Ø Open** **3 Percutaneous** **4 Percutaneous Endoscopic**	**C Extraluminal Device** **D Intraluminal Device** **E Intraluminal Device, Branched or Fenestrated, One or Two Arteries** **F Intraluminal Device, Branched or Fenestrated, Three or More Arteries** **Z No Device**	**Z No Qualifier**

Ø Medical and Surgical
2 Heart and Great Vessels
W Revision Definition: Correcting, to the extent possible, a portion of a malfunctioning device or the position of a displaced device

Explanation: Revision can include correcting a malfunctioning or displaced device by taking out or putting in components of the device such as a screw or pin

Body Part Character 4	Approach Character 5	Device Character 6	Qualifier Character 7
5 Atrial Septum Interatrial septum **M Ventricular Septum** Interventricular septum	**Ø Open** **4 Percutaneous Endoscopic**	**J Synthetic Substitute**	**Z No Qualifier**
A Heart LC NC ⊞	**Ø Open** **3 Percutaneous** **4 Percutaneous Endoscopic**	**2 Monitoring Device** **3 Infusion Device** **7 Autologous Tissue Substitute** **8 Zooplastic Tissue** **C Extraluminal Device** **D Intraluminal Device** **J Synthetic Substitute** **K Nonautologous Tissue Substitute** **M Cardiac Lead** **N Intracardiac Pacemaker** **Q Implantable Heart Assist System** **Y Other Device**	**Z No Qualifier**
A Heart ⊞	**Ø Open** **3 Percutaneous** **4 Percutaneous Endoscopic**	**R Short-term External Heart Assist System**	**S Biventricular** **Z No Qualifier**
A Heart	**X External**	**2 Monitoring Device** **3 Infusion Device** **7 Autologous Tissue Substitute** **8 Zooplastic Tissue** **C Extraluminal Device** **D Intraluminal Device** **J Synthetic Substitute** **K Nonautologous Tissue Substitute** **M Cardiac Lead** **N Intracardiac Pacemaker** **Q Implantable Heart Assist System**	**Z No Qualifier**
A Heart	**X External**	**R Short-term External Heart Assist System**	**S Biventricular** **Z No Qualifier**
F Aortic Valve Aortic annulus **G Mitral Valve** Bicuspid valve, Left atrioventricular valve, Mitral annulus **H Pulmonary Valve** Pulmonary annulus, Pulmonic valve **J Tricuspid Valve** Right atrioventricular valve, Tricuspid annulus	**Ø Open** **3 Percutaneous** **4 Percutaneous Endoscopic**	**7 Autologous Tissue Substitute** **8 Zooplastic Tissue** **J Synthetic Substitute** **K Nonautologous Tissue Substitute**	**Z No Qualifier**
Y Great Vessel	**Ø Open** **3 Percutaneous** **4 Percutaneous Endoscopic**	**2 Monitoring Device** **3 Infusion Device** **7 Autologous Tissue Substitute** **8 Zooplastic Tissue** **C Extraluminal Device** **D Intraluminal Device** **J Synthetic Substitute** **K Nonautologous Tissue Substitute** **Y Other Device**	**Z No Qualifier**
Y Great Vessel	**X External**	**2 Monitoring Device** **3 Infusion Device** **7 Autologous Tissue Substitute** **8 Zooplastic Tissue** **C Extraluminal Device** **D Intraluminal Device** **J Synthetic Substitute** **K Nonautologous Tissue Substitute**	**Z No Qualifier**

Non-OR Ø2WA3[2,3,D]Z
Non-OR Ø2WA[3,4]YZ
Non-OR Ø2WAX[2,3,7,8,C,D,J,K,M,N,Q]Z
Non-OR Ø2WAXRZ
Non-OR Ø2WY3[2,3,D]Z
Non-OR Ø2WY[3,4]YZ
Non-OR Ø2WYX[2,3,7,8,C,D,J,K]Z

HAC Ø2WA[Ø,3,4]MZ when reported with T81.4Ø–T81.49, T82.6–T82.7 with 7th character A
LC Ø2WAØ[J,Q]Z
NC Ø2WA[3,4]QZ

See Appendix L for Procedure Combinations
⊞ Ø2WA[Ø,3,4]QZ
⊞ Ø2WA[Ø,3,4]RZ

NC Noncovered Procedure LC Limited Coverage QA Questionable OB Admit NT New Tech Add-on ⊞ Combination Member ♂ Male ♀ Female

Ø Medical and Surgical
2 Heart and Great Vessels
Y Transplantation Definition: Putting in or on all or a portion of a living body part taken from another individual or animal to physically take the place and/or function of all or a portion of a similar body part

Explanation: The native body part may or may not be taken out, and the transplanted body part may take over all or a portion of its function

Body Part Character 4	Approach Character 5	Device Character 6	Qualifier Character 7
A Heart LC	Ø Open	Z No Device	Ø Allogeneic 1 Syngeneic 2 Zooplastic

LC Ø2YAØZ[Ø,1,2]

Upper Arteries Ø31–Ø3W

Character Meanings

This Character Meaning table is provided as a guide to assist the user in the identification of character members that may be found in this section of code tables. It **SHOULD NOT** be used to build a PCS code.

Operation–Character 3	Body Part–Character 4	Approach–Character 5	Device–Character 6	Qualifier–Character 7
1 Bypass	Ø Internal Mammary Artery, Right	Ø Open	Ø Drainage Device	Ø Upper Arm Artery, Right OR Ultrasonic
5 Destruction	1 Internal Mammary Artery, Left	3 Percutaneous	2 Monitoring Device	1 Upper Arm Artery, Left OR Drug-Coated Balloon
7 Dilation	2 Innominate Artery	4 Percutaneous Endoscopic	3 Infusion Device	2 Upper Arm Artery, Bilateral
9 Drainage	3 Subclavian Artery, Right	X External	4 Intraluminal Device, Drug-eluting	3 Lower Arm Artery, Right
B Excision	4 Subclavian Artery, Left		5 Intraluminal Device, Drug-eluting, Two	4 Lower Arm Artery, Left
C Extirpation	5 Axillary Artery, Right		6 Intraluminal Device, Drug-eluting, Three	5 Lower Arm Artery, Bilateral
F Fragmentation	6 Axillary Artery, Left		7 Intraluminal Device, Drug-eluting, Four or More OR Autologous Tissue Substitute	6 Upper Leg Artery, Right
H Insertion	7 Brachial Artery, Right		9 Autologous Venous Tissue	7 Upper Leg Artery, Left OR Stent Retriever
J Inspection	8 Brachial Artery, Left		A Autologous Arterial Tissue	8 Upper Leg Artery, Bilateral
L Occlusion	9 Ulnar Artery, Right		B Intraluminal Device, Bioactive	9 Lower Leg Artery, Right
N Release	A Ulnar Artery, Left		C Extraluminal Device	B Lower Leg Artery, Left
P Removal	B Radial Artery, Right		D Intraluminal Device	C Lower Leg Artery, Bilateral
Q Repair	C Radial Artery, Left		E Intraluminal Device, Two	D Upper Arm Vein
R Replacement	D Hand Artery, Right		F Intraluminal Device, Three	F Lower Arm Vein
S Reposition	F Hand Artery, Left		G Intraluminal Device, Four or More	G Intracranial Artery
U Supplement	G Intracranial Artery		H Intraluminal Device, Flow Diverter	J Extracranial Artery, Right
V Restriction	H Common Carotid Artery, Right		J Synthetic Substitute	K Extracranial Artery, Left
W Revision	J Common Carotid Artery, Left		K Nonautologous Tissue Substitute	M Pulmonary Artery, Right
	K Internal Carotid Artery, Right		M Stimulator Lead	N Pulmonary Artery, Left
	L Internal Carotid Artery, Left		Y Other Device	T Abdominal Artery
	M External Carotid Artery, Right		Z No Device	V Superior Vena Cava
	N External Carotid Artery, Left			W Lower Extremity Vein
	P Vertebral Artery, Right			X Diagnostic
	Q Vertebral Artery, Left			Y Upper Artery
	R Face Artery			Z No Qualifier
	S Temporal Artery, Right			
	T Temporal Artery, Left			
	U Thyroid Artery, Right			
	V Thyroid Artery, Left			
	Y Upper Artery			

AHA Coding Clinic for table Ø31

2019, 4Q, 26	Upper artery bypass Qualifier
2019, 4Q, 26	Percutaneous approach upper artery bypass
2017, 4Q, 64-65	New qualifier values - Left to right carotid bypass
2017, 2Q, 22	Carotid artery to subclavian artery transposition
2017, 1Q, 31	Left to right common carotid artery bypass
2016, 3Q, 37	Insertion of arteriovenous graft using HeRO device
2016, 3Q, 39	Revision of arteriovenous graft
2013, 4Q, 125	Stage II cephalic vein transposition (superficialization) of arteriovenous fistula
2013, 1Q, 27	Creation of radial artery fistula

AHA Coding Clinic for table Ø37

2020, 4Q, 70-71	Cerebral embolic filtration extracorporeal flow reversal circuit
2019, 4Q, 27	Bifurcation Qualifier
2019, 3Q, 29	Transcarotid arterial catheterization
2018, 2Q, 24	Coronary artery bifurcation
2016, 4Q, 86	Peripheral artery, number of stents
2016, 4Q, 86-87	Coronary and peripheral artery bifurcation
2015, 1Q, 32	Deployment of stent for herniated/migrated coil in basilar artery

AHA Coding Clinic for table Ø3B

2016, 2Q, 12	Resection of malignant neoplasm of infratemporal fossa

AHA Coding Clinic for table Ø3C

2021, 2Q, 13	Thromboendarterectomy with deconstruction of internal carotid artery
2020, 3Q, 38	Thrombectomy of arteriovenous fistula with angioplasty and stent placement
2019, 4Q, 27	Bifurcation Qualifier
2018, 4Q, 47-48	Endovascular thrombectomy with stent retriever
2018, 2Q, 24	Coronary artery bifurcation
2017, 4Q, 64-65	New qualifier values - Left to right carotid bypass
2017, 2Q, 23	Thrombectomy via Fogarty catheter
2016, 4Q, 86-87	Coronary and peripheral artery bifurcation
2016, 2Q, 11	Carotid endarterectomy with patch angioplasty
2015, 1Q, 29	Discontinued carotid endarterectomy

AHA Coding Clinic for table Ø3F

2020, 4Q, 45-49	New fragmentation tables
2020, 4Q, 49-50	Intravascular ultrasound assisted thrombolysis
2020, 4Q, 50	Intravascular lithotripsy

AHA Coding Clinic for table Ø3H

2020, 1Q, 25	Elephant trunk repair of aortic dissection
2016, 2Q, 32	Arterial catheter placement

AHA Coding Clinic for table Ø3J

2021, 1Q, 16	Placement of Sentinel™ embolic protection device with deployment of single filter
2015, 1Q, 29	Discontinued carotid endarterectomy

AHA Coding Clinic for table Ø3L

2021, 2Q, 13	Thromboendarterectomy with deconstruction of internal carotid artery
2016, 2Q, 30	Clipping (occlusion) of cerebral artery, decompressive craniectomy and storage of bone flap in abdominal wall
2014, 4Q, 20	Control of epistaxis
2014, 4Q, 37	Endovascular embolization of arteriovenous malformation using Onyx-18 liquid

AHA Coding Clinic for table Ø3Q

2017, 1Q, 31	Left to right common carotid artery bypass

AHA Coding Clinic for table Ø3S

2017, 2Q, 22	Carotid artery to subclavian artery transposition
2015, 3Q, 27	Moyamoya disease and hemispheric pial synagiosis with craniotomy

AHA Coding Clinic for table Ø3U

2019, 1Q, 22	Cerebral artery fusiform aneurysm repair via wrapping
2016, 2Q, 11	Carotid endarterectomy with patch angioplasty

AHA Coding Clinic for table Ø3V

2019, 4Q, 27-28	Aneurysm treatment using flow diverter stent
2019, 1Q, 22	Cerebral artery fusiform aneurysm repair via wrapping
2016, 1Q, 19	Embolization of superior hypophyseal aneurysm using stent-assisted coil

AHA Coding Clinic for table Ø3W

2016, 3Q, 39	Revision of arteriovenous graft
2015, 1Q, 32	Deployment of stent for herniated/migrated coil in basilar artery

Upper Arteries

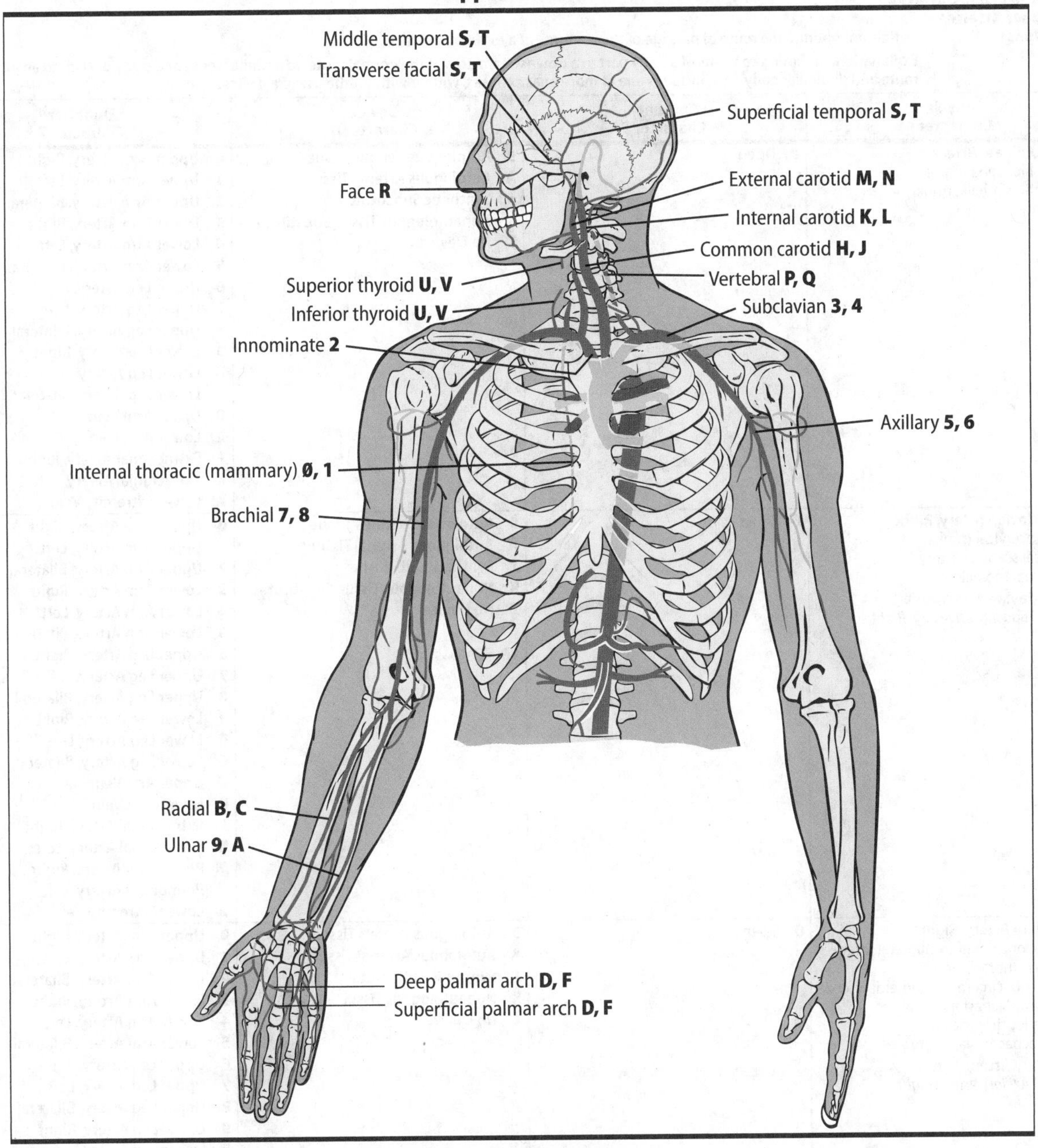

Head and Neck Arteries

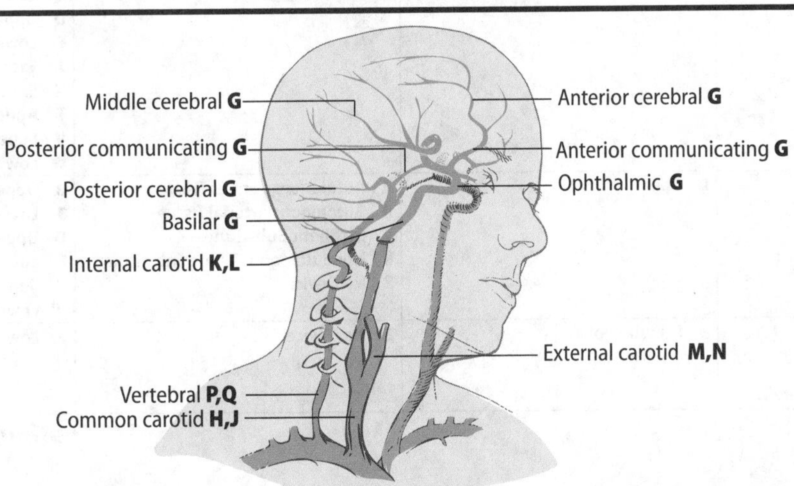

Ø Medical and Surgical
3 Upper Arteries
1 Bypass Definition: Altering the route of passage of the contents of a tubular body part

Explanation: Rerouting contents of a body part to a downstream area of the normal route, to a similar route and body part, or to an abnormal route and dissimilar body part. Includes one or more anastomoses, with or without the use of a device.

Body Part Character 4	Approach Character 5	Device Character 6	Qualifier Character 7
2 Innominate Artery Brachiocephalic artery Brachiocephalic trunk	**Ø Open**	**9 Autologous Venous Tissue** **A Autologous Arterial Tissue** **J Synthetic Substitute** **K Nonautologous Tissue Substitute** **Z No Device**	**Ø Upper Arm Artery, Right** **1 Upper Arm Artery, Left** **2 Upper Arm Artery, Bilateral** **3 Lower Arm Artery, Right** **4 Lower Arm Artery, Left** **5 Lower Arm Artery, Bilateral** **6 Upper Leg Artery, Right** **7 Upper Leg Artery, Left** **8 Upper Leg Artery, Bilateral** **9 Lower Leg Artery, Right** **B Lower Leg Artery, Left** **C Lower Leg Artery, Bilateral** **D Upper Arm Vein** **F Lower Arm Vein** **J Extracranial Artery, Right** **K Extracranial Artery, Left** **W Lower Extremity Vein**
3 Subclavian Artery, Right Costocervical trunk Dorsal scapular artery Internal thoracic artery **4 Subclavian Artery, Left** *See 3 Subclavian Artery, Right*	**Ø Open**	**9 Autologous Venous Tissue** **A Autologous Arterial Tissue** **J Synthetic Substitute** **K Nonautologous Tissue Substitute** **Z No Device**	**Ø Upper Arm Artery, Right** **1 Upper Arm Artery, Left** **2 Upper Arm Artery, Bilateral** **3 Lower Arm Artery, Right** **4 Lower Arm Artery, Left** **5 Lower Arm Artery, Bilateral** **6 Upper Leg Artery, Right** **7 Upper Leg Artery, Left** **8 Upper Leg Artery, Bilateral** **9 Lower Leg Artery, Right** **B Lower Leg Artery, Left** **C Lower Leg Artery, Bilateral** **D Upper Arm Vein** **F Lower Arm Vein** **J Extracranial Artery, Right** **K Extracranial Artery, Left** **M Pulmonary Artery, Right** **N Pulmonary Artery, Left** **W Lower Extremity Vein**
5 Axillary Artery, Right Anterior circumflex humeral artery Lateral thoracic artery Posterior circumflex humeral artery Subscapular artery Superior thoracic artery Thoracoacromial artery **6 Axillary Artery, Left** *See 5 Axillary Artery, Right*	**Ø Open**	**9 Autologous Venous Tissue** **A Autologous Arterial Tissue** **J Synthetic Substitute** **K Nonautologous Tissue Substitute** **Z No Device**	**Ø Upper Arm Artery, Right** **1 Upper Arm Artery, Left** **2 Upper Arm Artery, Bilateral** **3 Lower Arm Artery, Right** **4 Lower Arm Artery, Left** **5 Lower Arm Artery, Bilateral** **6 Upper Leg Artery, Right** **7 Upper Leg Artery, Left** **8 Upper Leg Artery, Bilateral** **9 Lower Leg Artery, Right** **B Lower Leg Artery, Left** **C Lower Leg Artery, Bilateral** **D Upper Arm Vein** **F Lower Arm Vein** **J Extracranial Artery, Right** **K Extracranial Artery, Left** **T Abdominal Artery** **V Superior Vena Cava** **W Lower Extremity Vein**
7 Brachial Artery, Right Inferior ulnar collateral artery Profunda brachii Superior ulnar collateral artery	**Ø Open**	**9 Autologous Venous Tissue** **A Autologous Arterial Tissue** **J Synthetic Substitute** **K Nonautologous Tissue Substitute** **Z No Device**	**Ø Upper Arm Artery, Right** **3 Lower Arm Artery, Right** **D Upper Arm Vein** **F Lower Arm Vein** **V Superior Vena Cava** **W Lower Extremity Vein**
7 Brachial Artery, Right Inferior ulnar collateral artery Profunda brachii Superior ulnar collateral artery	**3 Percutaneous**	**Z No Device**	**F Lower Arm Vein**

Ø31 Continued on next page

Ø31 Continued

Ø Medical and Surgical
3 Upper Arteries
1 Bypass Definition: Altering the route of passage of the contents of a tubular body part

Explanation: Rerouting contents of a body part to a downstream area of the normal route, to a similar route and body part, or to an abnormal route and dissimilar body part. Includes one or more anastomoses, with or without the use of a device.

Body Part Character 4	Approach Character 5	Device Character 6	Qualifier Character 7
8 Brachial Artery, Left Inferior ulnar collateral artery Profunda brachii Superior ulnar collateral artery	**Ø Open**	**9 Autologous Venous Tissue** **A Autologous Arterial Tissue** **J Synthetic Substitute** **K Nonautologous Tissue Substitute** **Z No Device**	**1 Upper Arm Artery, Left** **4 Lower Arm Artery, Left** **D Upper Arm Vein** **F Lower Arm Vein** **V Superior Vena Cava** **W Lower Extremity Vein**
8 Brachial Artery, Left Inferior ulnar collateral artery Profunda brachii Superior ulnar collateral artery	3 Percutaneous	Z No Device	F Lower Arm Vein
9 Ulnar Artery, Right Anterior ulnar recurrent artery Common interosseous artery Posterior ulnar recurrent artery **B Radial Artery, Right** Radial recurrent artery	**Ø Open**	**9 Autologous Venous Tissue** **A Autologous Arterial Tissue** **J Synthetic Substitute** **K Nonautologous Tissue Substitute** **Z No Device**	**3 Lower Arm Artery, Right** **F Lower Arm Vein**
9 Ulnar Artery, Right Anterior ulnar recurrent artery Common interosseous artery Posterior ulnar recurrent artery **B Radial Artery, Right** Radial recurrent artery	**3 Percutaneous**	**Z No Device**	**F Lower Arm Vein**
A Ulnar Artery, Left Anterior ulnar recurrent artery Common interosseous artery Posterior ulnar recurrent artery **C Radial Artery, Left** Radial recurrent artery	**Ø Open**	**9 Autologous Venous Tissue** **A Autologous Arterial Tissue** **J Synthetic Substitute** **K Nonautologous Tissue Substitute** **Z No Device**	**4 Lower Arm Artery, Left** **F Lower Arm Vein**
A Ulnar Artery, Left Anterior ulnar recurrent artery Common interosseous artery Posterior ulnar recurrent artery **C Radial Artery, Left** Radial recurrent artery	**3 Percutaneous**	**Z No Device**	**F Lower Arm Vein**
G Intracranial Artery Anterior cerebral artery Anterior choroidal artery Anterior communicating artery Basilar artery Circle of Willis Internal carotid artery, intracranial portion Middle cerebral artery Ophthalmic artery Posterior cerebral artery Posterior communicating artery Posterior inferior cerebellar artery (PICA) **S Temporal Artery, Right** Middle temporal artery Superficial temporal artery Transverse facial artery **T Temporal Artery, Left** ***See*** *S Temporal Artery, Right*	**Ø Open**	**9 Autologous Venous Tissue** **A Autologous Arterial Tissue** **J Synthetic Substitute** **K Nonautologous Tissue Substitute** **Z No Device**	**G Intracranial Artery**
H Common Carotid Artery, Right **J Common Carotid Artery, Left**	**Ø Open**	**9 Autologous Venous Tissue** **A Autologous Arterial Tissue** **J Synthetic Substitute** **K Nonautologous Tissue Substitute** **Z No Device**	**G Intracranial Artery** **J Extracranial Artery, Right** **K Extracranial Artery, Left** **Y Upper Artery**

Ø31 Continued on next page

Ø31 Continued

Ø Medical and Surgical
3 Upper Arteries
1 Bypass Definition: Altering the route of passage of the contents of a tubular body part

Explanation: Rerouting contents of a body part to a downstream area of the normal route, to a similar route and body part, or to an abnormal route and dissimilar body part. Includes one or more anastomoses, with or without the use of a device.

Body Part Character 4	Approach Character 5	Device Character 6	Qualifier Character 7
K Internal Carotid Artery, Right Caroticotympanic artery Carotid sinus **L Internal Carotid Artery, Left** Caroticotympanic artery Carotid sinus **M External Carotid Artery, Right** Ascending pharyngeal artery Internal maxillary artery Lingual artery Maxillary artery Occipital artery Posterior auricular artery Superior thyroid artery **N External Carotid Artery, Left** Ascending pharyngeal artery Internal maxillary artery Lingual artery Maxillary artery Occipital artery Posterior auricular artery Superior thyroid artery	**Ø Open**	**9 Autologous Venous Tissue** **A Autologous Arterial Tissue** **J Synthetic Substitute** **K Nonautologous Tissue Substitute** **Z No Device**	**J Extracranial Artery, Right** **K Extracranial Artery, Left**

Ø Medical and Surgical
3 Upper Arteries
5 Destruction Definition: Physical eradication of all or a portion of a body part by the direct use of energy, force, or a destructive agent

Explanation: None of the body part is physically taken out

Body Part Character 4	Approach Character 5	Device Character 6	Qualifier Character 7
Ø Internal Mammary Artery, Right Anterior intercostal artery Internal thoracic artery Musculophrenic artery Pericardiophrenic artery Superior epigastric artery	**Ø Open**	**Z No Device**	**Z No Qualifier**
1 Internal Mammary Artery, Left *See Ø Internal Mammary Artery, Right*	**3 Percutaneous**		
2 Innominate Artery Brachiocephalic artery Brachiocephalic trunk	**4 Percutaneous Endoscopic**		
3 Subclavian Artery, Right Costocervical trunk Dorsal scapular artery Internal thoracic artery			
4 Subclavian Artery, Left *See 3 Subclavian Artery, Right*			
5 Axillary Artery, Right Anterior circumflex humeral artery Lateral thoracic artery Posterior circumflex humeral artery Subscapular artery Superior thoracic artery Thoracoacromial artery			
6 Axillary Artery, Left *See 5 Axillary Artery, Right*			
7 Brachial Artery, Right Inferior ulnar collateral artery Profunda brachii Superior ulnar collateral artery			
8 Brachial Artery, Left *See 7 Brachial Artery, Right*			
9 Ulnar Artery, Right Anterior ulnar recurrent artery Common interosseous artery Posterior ulnar recurrent artery			
A Ulnar Artery, Left *See 9 Ulnar Artery, Right*			
B Radial Artery, Right Radial recurrent artery			
C Radial Artery, Left *See B Radial Artery, Right*			
D Hand Artery, Right Deep palmar arch Princeps pollicis artery Radialis indicis Superficial palmar arch			
F Hand Artery, Left *See D Hand Artery, Right*			
G Intracranial Artery Anterior cerebral artery Anterior choroidal artery Anterior communicating artery Basilar artery Circle of Willis Internal carotid artery, intracranial portion Middle cerebral artery Ophthalmic artery Posterior cerebral artery Posterior communicating artery Posterior inferior cerebellar artery (PICA)			
H Common Carotid Artery, Right			
J Common Carotid Artery, Left			
K Internal Carotid Artery, Right Caroticotympanic artery Carotid sinus			
L Internal Carotid Artery, Left *See K Internal Carotid Artery, Right*			
M External Carotid Artery, Right Ascending pharyngeal artery Internal maxillary artery Lingual artery Maxillary artery Occipital artery Posterior auricular artery Superior thyroid artery			
N External Carotid Artery, Left *See M External Carotid Artery, Right*			
P Vertebral Artery, Right Anterior spinal artery Posterior spinal artery			
Q Vertebral Artery, Left *See P Vertebral Artery, Right*			
R Face Artery Angular artery Ascending palatine artery External maxillary artery Facial artery Inferior labial artery Submental artery Superior labial artery			
S Temporal Artery, Right Middle temporal artery Superficial temporal artery Transverse facial artery			
T Temporal Artery, Left *See S Temporal Artery, Right*			
U Thyroid Artery, Right Cricothyroid artery Hyoid artery Sternocleidomastoid artery Superior laryngeal artery Superior thyroid artery Thyrocervical trunk			
V Thyroid Artery, Left *See U Thyroid Artery, Right*			
Y Upper Artery Aortic intercostal artery Bronchial artery Esophageal artery Subcostal artery			

Ø Medical and Surgical
3 Upper Arteries
7 Dilation Definition: Expanding an orifice or the lumen of a tubular body part

Explanation: The orifice can be a natural orifice or an artificially created orifice. Accomplished by stretching a tubular body part using intraluminal pressure or by cutting part of the orifice or wall of the tubular body part.

Body Part Character 4		Approach Character 5	Device Character 6	Qualifier Character 7
Ø Internal Mammary Artery, Right Anterior intercostal artery Internal thoracic artery Musculophrenic artery Pericardiophrenic artery Superior epigastric artery **1 Internal Mammary Artery, Left** *See Ø Internal Mammary Artery, Right* **2 Innominate Artery** Brachiocephalic artery Brachiocephalic trunk **3 Subclavian Artery, Right** Costocervical trunk Dorsal scapular artery Internal thoracic artery **4 Subclavian Artery, Left** *See 3 Subclavian Artery, Right* **5 Axillary Artery, Right** Anterior circumflex humeral artery Lateral thoracic artery Posterior circumflex humeral artery Subscapular artery Superior thoracic artery Thoracoacromial artery	**6 Axillary Artery, Left** *See 5 Axillary Artery, Right* **7 Brachial Artery, Right** Inferior ulnar collateral artery Profunda brachii Superior ulnar collateral artery **8 Brachial Artery, Left** *See 7 Brachial Artery, Right* **9 Ulnar Artery, Right** Anterior ulnar recurrent artery Common interosseous artery Posterior ulnar recurrent artery **A Ulnar Artery, Left** *See 9 Ulnar Artery, Right* **B Radial Artery, Right** Radial recurrent artery **C Radial Artery, Left** *See B Radial Artery, Right*	**Ø Open** **3 Percutaneous** **4 Percutaneous Endoscopic**	**4 Intraluminal Device, Drug-eluting** **5 Intraluminal Device, Drug-eluting, Two** **6 Intraluminal Device, Drug-eluting, Three** **7 Intraluminal Device, Drug-eluting, Four or More** **E Intraluminal Device, Two** **F Intraluminal Device, Three** **G Intraluminal Device, Four or More**	**Z No Qualifier**
Ø Internal Mammary Artery, Right Anterior intercostal artery Internal thoracic artery Musculophrenic artery Pericardiophrenic artery Superior epigastric artery **1 Internal Mammary Artery, Left** *See Ø Internal Mammary Artery, Right* **2 Innominate Artery** Brachiocephalic artery Brachiocephalic trunk **3 Subclavian Artery, Right** Costocervical trunk Dorsal scapular artery Internal thoracic artery **4 Subclavian Artery, Left** *See 3 Subclavian Artery, Right* **5 Axillary Artery, Right** Anterior circumflex humeral artery Lateral thoracic artery Posterior circumflex humeral artery Subscapular artery Superior thoracic artery Thoracoacromial artery	**6 Axillary Artery, Left** *See 5 Axillary Artery, Right* **7 Brachial Artery, Right** Inferior ulnar collateral artery Profunda brachii Superior ulnar collateral artery **8 Brachial Artery, Left** *See 7 Brachial Artery, Right* **9 Ulnar Artery, Right** Anterior ulnar recurrent artery Common interosseous artery Posterior ulnar recurrent artery **A Ulnar Artery, Left** *See 9 Ulnar Artery, Right* **B Radial Artery, Right** Radial recurrent artery **C Radial Artery, Left** *See B Radial Artery, Right*	**Ø Open** **3 Percutaneous** **4 Percutaneous Endoscopic**	**D Intraluminal Device** **Z No Device**	**1 Drug-Coated Balloon** **Z No Qualifier**

Ø37 Continued on next page

Ø37 Continued

Ø Medical and Surgical
3 Upper Arteries
7 Dilation Definition: Expanding an orifice or the lumen of a tubular body part

Explanation: The orifice can be a natural orifice or an artificially created orifice. Accomplished by stretching a tubular body part using intraluminal pressure or by cutting part of the orifice or wall of the tubular body part.

Body Part Character 4		Approach Character 5	Device Character 6	Qualifier Character 7
D Hand Artery, Right Deep palmar arch Princeps pollicis artery Radialis indicis Superficial palmar arch **F Hand Artery, Left** *See D Hand Artery, Right* **G Intracranial Artery** NC Anterior cerebral artery Anterior choroidal artery Anterior communicating artery Basilar artery Circle of Willis Internal carotid artery, intracranial portion Middle cerebral artery Ophthalmic artery Posterior cerebral artery Posterior communicating artery Posterior inferior cerebellar artery (PICA) **H Common Carotid Artery, Right** **J Common Carotid Artery, Left** **K Internal Carotid Artery, Right** Caroticotympanic artery Carotid sinus **L Internal Carotid Artery, Left** *See K Internal Carotid Artery, Right* **M External Carotid Artery, Right** Ascending pharyngeal artery Internal maxillary artery Lingual artery Maxillary artery Occipital artery Posterior auricular artery Superior thyroid artery	**N External Carotid Artery, Left** *See M External Carotid Artery, Right* **P Vertebral Artery, Right** Anterior spinal artery Posterior spinal artery **Q Vertebral Artery, Left** *See P Vertebral Artery, Right* **R Face Artery** Angular artery Ascending palatine artery External maxillary artery Facial artery Inferior labial artery Submental artery Superior labial artery **S Temporal Artery, Right** Middle temporal artery Superficial temporal artery Transverse facial artery **T Temporal Artery, Left** *See S Temporal Artery, Right* **U Thyroid Artery, Right** Cricothyroid artery Hyoid artery Sternocleidomastoid artery Superior laryngeal artery Superior thyroid artery Thyrocervical trunk **V Thyroid Artery, Left** *See U Thyroid Artery, Right* **Y Upper Artery** Aortic intercostal artery Bronchial artery Esophageal artery Subcostal artery	**Ø Open** **3 Percutaneous** **4 Percutaneous Endoscopic**	**4 Intraluminal Device, Drug-eluting** **5 Intraluminal Device, Drug-eluting, Two** **6 Intraluminal Device, Drug-eluting, Three** **7 Intraluminal Device, Drug-eluting, Four or More** **D Intraluminal Device** **E Intraluminal Device, Two** **F Intraluminal Device, Three** **G Intraluminal Device, Four or More** **Z No Device**	**Z No Qualifier**

NC Ø37G[3,4]ZZ

Ø Medical and Surgical
3 Upper Arteries
9 Drainage Definition: Taking or letting out fluids and/or gases from a body part

Explanation: The qualifier DIAGNOSTIC is used to identify drainage procedures that are biopsies

Body Part Character 4	Approach Character 5	Device Character 6	Qualifier Character 7
Ø **Internal Mammary Artery, Right** Anterior intercostal artery Internal thoracic artery Musculophrenic artery Pericardiophrenic artery Superior epigastric artery	Ø Open 3 Percutaneous 4 Percutaneous Endoscopic	Ø Drainage Device	Z No Qualifier
1 **Internal Mammary Artery, Left** *See Ø Internal Mammary Artery, Right above*			
2 **Innominate Artery** Brachiocephalic artery Brachiocephalic trunk			
3 **Subclavian Artery, Right** Costocervical trunk Dorsal scapular artery Internal thoracic artery			
4 **Subclavian Artery, Left** *See 3 Subclavian Artery, Right*			
5 **Axillary Artery, Right** Anterior circumflex humeral artery Lateral thoracic artery Posterior circumflex humeral artery Subscapular artery Superior thoracic artery Thoracoacromial artery			
6 **Axillary Artery, Left** *See 5 Axillary Artery, Right*			
7 **Brachial Artery, Right** Inferior ulnar collateral artery Profunda brachii Superior ulnar collateral artery			
8 **Brachial Artery, Left** *See 7 Brachial Artery, Right*			
9 **Ulnar Artery, Right** Anterior ulnar recurrent artery Common interosseous artery Posterior ulnar recurrent artery			
A **Ulnar Artery, Left** *See 9 Ulnar Artery, Right*			
B **Radial Artery, Right** Radial recurrent artery			
C **Radial Artery, Left** *See B Radial Artery, Right*			
D **Hand Artery, Right** Deep palmar arch Princeps pollicis artery Radialis indicis Superficial palmar arch			
F **Hand Artery, Left** *See D Hand Artery, Right*			
G **Intracranial Artery** Anterior cerebral artery Anterior choroidal artery Anterior communicating artery Basilar artery Circle of Willis Internal carotid artery, intracranial portion Middle cerebral artery Ophthalmic artery Posterior cerebral artery Posterior communicating artery Posterior inferior cerebellar artery (PICA)			
H **Common Carotid Artery, Right**			
J **Common Carotid Artery, Left**			
K **Internal Carotid Artery, Right** Caroticotympanic artery Carotid sinus			
L **Internal Carotid Artery, Left** *See K Internal Carotid Artery, Right*			
M **External Carotid Artery, Right** Ascending pharyngeal artery Internal maxillary artery Lingual artery Maxillary artery Occipital artery Posterior auricular artery Superior thyroid artery			
N **External Carotid Artery, Left** *See M External Carotid Artery, Right*			
P **Vertebral Artery, Right** Anterior spinal artery Posterior spinal artery			
Q **Vertebral Artery, Left** *See P Vertebral Artery, Right*			
R **Face Artery** Angular artery Ascending palatine artery External maxillary artery Facial artery Inferior labial artery Submental artery Superior labial artery			
S **Temporal Artery, Right** Middle temporal artery Superficial temporal artery Transverse facial artery			
T **Temporal Artery, Left** *See S Temporal Artery, Right*			
U **Thyroid Artery, Right** Cricothyroid artery Hyoid artery Sternocleidomastoid artery Superior laryngeal artery Superior thyroid artery Thyrocervical trunk			
V **Thyroid Artery, Left** *See U Thyroid Artery, Right*			
Y **Upper Artery** Aortic intercostal artery Bronchial artery Esophageal artery Subcostal artery			

Non-OR Ø39[Ø,1,2,3,4,5,6,7,8,9,A,B,C,D,F,G,H,J,K,L,M,N,P,Q,R,S,T,U,V,Y][Ø,3,4]ØZ

Ø39 Continued on next page

Ø Medical and Surgical
3 Upper Arteries
9 Drainage Definition: Taking or letting out fluids and/or gases from a body part
Explanation: The qualifier DIAGNOSTIC is used to identify drainage procedures that are biopsies

Ø39 Continued

Body Part Character 4	Approach Character 5	Device Character 6	Qualifier Character 7
Ø Internal Mammary Artery, Right Anterior intercostal artery Internal thoracic artery Musculophrenic artery Pericardiophrenic artery Superior epigastric artery **1 Internal Mammary Artery, Left** *See Ø Internal Mammary Artery, Right* **2 Innominate Artery** Brachiocephalic artery Brachiocephalic trunk **3 Subclavian Artery, Right** Costocervical trunk Dorsal scapular artery Internal thoracic artery **4 Subclavian Artery, Left** *See 3 Subclavian Artery, Right* **5 Axillary Artery, Right** Anterior circumflex humeral artery Lateral thoracic artery Posterior circumflex humeral artery Subscapular artery Superior thoracic artery Thoracoacromial artery **6 Axillary Artery, Left** *See 5 Axillary Artery, Right* **7 Brachial Artery, Right** Inferior ulnar collateral artery Profunda brachii Superior ulnar collateral artery **8 Brachial Artery, Left** *See 7 Brachial Artery, Right* **9 Ulnar Artery, Right** Anterior ulnar recurrent artery Common interosseous artery Posterior ulnar recurrent artery **A Ulnar Artery, Left** *See 9 Ulnar Artery, Right* **B Radial Artery, Right** Radial recurrent artery **C Radial Artery, Left** *See B Radial Artery, Right* **D Hand Artery, Right** Deep palmar arch Princeps pollicis artery Radialis indicis Superficial palmar arch **F Hand Artery, Left** *See D Hand Artery, Right* **G Intracranial Artery** Anterior cerebral artery Anterior choroidal artery Anterior communicating artery Basilar artery Circle of Willis Internal carotid artery, intracranial portion Middle cerebral artery Ophthalmic artery Posterior cerebral artery Posterior communicating artery Posterior inferior cerebellar artery (PICA) **H Common Carotid Artery, Right** **J Common Carotid Artery, Left** **K Internal Carotid Artery, Right** Caroticotympanic artery Carotid sinus **L Internal Carotid Artery, Left** *See K Internal Carotid Artery, Right* **M External Carotid Artery, Right** Ascending pharyngeal artery Internal maxillary artery Lingual artery Maxillary artery Occipital artery Posterior auricular artery Superior thyroid artery **N External Carotid Artery, Left** *See M External Carotid Artery, Right* **P Vertebral Artery, Right** Anterior spinal artery Posterior spinal artery **Q Vertebral Artery, Left** *See P Vertebral Artery, Right* **R Face Artery** Angular artery Ascending palatine artery External maxillary artery Facial artery Inferior labial artery Submental artery Superior labial artery **S Temporal Artery, Right** Middle temporal artery Superficial temporal artery Transverse facial artery **T Temporal Artery, Left** *See S Temporal Artery, Right* **U Thyroid Artery, Right** Cricothyroid artery Hyoid artery Sternocleidomastoid artery Superior laryngeal artery Superior thyroid artery Thyrocervical trunk **V Thyroid Artery, Left** *See U Thyroid Artery, Right* **Y Upper Artery** Aortic intercostal artery Bronchial artery Esophageal artery Subcostal artery	**Ø** Open **3** Percutaneous **4** Percutaneous Endoscopic	**Z** No Device	**X** Diagnostic **Z** No Qualifier

Non-OR Ø39[Ø,1,2,3,4,5,6,7,8,9,A,B,C,D,F,G,H,J,K,L,M,N,P,Q,R,S,T,U,V,Y]3ZX
Non-OR Ø39[Ø,1,2,3,4,5,6,7,8,9,A,B,C,D,F,G,H,J,K,L,M,N,P,Q,R,S,T,U,V,Y][Ø,3,4]ZZ

Ø Medical and Surgical
3 Upper Arteries
B Excision Definition: Cutting out or off, without replacement, a portion of a body part

Explanation: The qualifier DIAGNOSTIC is used to identify excision procedures that are biopsies

Body Part Character 4	Approach Character 5	Device Character 6	Qualifier Character 7
Ø Internal Mammary Artery, Right Anterior intercostal artery Internal thoracic artery Musculophrenic artery Pericardiophrenic artery Superior epigastric artery **1 Internal Mammary Artery, Left** ***See*** *Ø Internal Mammary Artery, Right* **2 Innominate Artery** Brachiocephalic artery Brachiocephalic trunk **3 Subclavian Artery, Right** Costocervical trunk Dorsal scapular artery Internal thoracic artery **4 Subclavian Artery, Left** ***See*** *3 Subclavian Artery, Right* **5 Axillary Artery, Right** Anterior circumflex humeral artery Lateral thoracic artery Posterior circumflex humeral artery Subscapular artery Superior thoracic artery Thoracoacromial artery **6 Axillary Artery, Left** ***See*** *5 Axillary Artery, Right* **7 Brachial Artery, Right** Inferior ulnar collateral artery Profunda brachii Superior ulnar collateral artery **8 Brachial Artery, Left** ***See*** *7 Brachial Artery, Right* **9 Ulnar Artery, Right** Anterior ulnar recurrent artery Common interosseous artery Posterior ulnar recurrent artery **A Ulnar Artery, Left** ***See*** *9 Ulnar Artery, Right* **B Radial Artery, Right** Radial recurrent artery **C Radial Artery, Left** ***See*** *B Radial Artery, Right* **D Hand Artery, Right** Deep palmar arch Princeps pollicis artery Radialis indicis Superficial palmar arch **F Hand Artery, Left** ***See*** *D Hand Artery, Right* **G Intracranial Artery** Anterior cerebral artery Anterior choroidal artery Anterior communicating artery Basilar artery Circle of Willis Internal carotid artery, intracranial portion Middle cerebral artery Ophthalmic artery Posterior cerebral artery Posterior communicating artery Posterior inferior cerebellar artery (PICA) **H Common Carotid Artery, Right** **J Common Carotid Artery, Left** **K Internal Carotid Artery, Right** Caroticotympanic artery Carotid sinus **L Internal Carotid Artery, Left** ***See*** *K Internal Carotid Artery, Right* **M External Carotid Artery, Right** Ascending pharyngeal artery Internal maxillary artery Lingual artery Maxillary artery Occipital artery Posterior auricular artery Superior thyroid artery **N External Carotid Artery, Left** ***See*** *M External Carotid Artery, Right* **P Vertebral Artery, Right** Anterior spinal artery Posterior spinal artery **Q Vertebral Artery, Left** ***See*** *P Vertebral Artery, Right* **R Face Artery** Angular artery Ascending palatine artery External maxillary artery Facial artery Inferior labial artery Submental artery Superior labial artery **S Temporal Artery, Right** Middle temporal artery Superficial temporal artery Transverse facial artery **T Temporal Artery, Left** ***See*** *S Temporal Artery, Right* **U Thyroid Artery, Right** Cricothyroid artery Hyoid artery Sternocleidomastoid artery Superior laryngeal artery Superior thyroid artery Thyrocervical trunk **V Thyroid Artery, Left** ***See*** *U Thyroid Artery, Right* **Y Upper Artery** Aortic intercostal artery Bronchial artery Esophageal artery Subcostal artery	**Ø** Open **3** Percutaneous **4** Percutaneous Endoscopic	**Z** No Device	**X** Diagnostic **Z** No Qualifier

Ø Medical and Surgical
3 Upper Arteries
C Extirpation Definition: Taking or cutting out solid matter from a body part

Explanation: The solid matter may be an abnormal byproduct of a biological function or a foreign body; it may be imbedded in a body part or in the lumen of a tubular body part. The solid matter may or may not have been previously broken into pieces.

Body Part Character 4		Approach Character 5	Device Character 6	Qualifier Character 7
Ø Internal Mammary Artery, Right Anterior intercostal artery Internal thoracic artery Musculophrenic artery Pericardiophrenic artery Superior epigastric artery **1 Internal Mammary Artery, Left** *See Ø Internal Mammary Artery, Right* **2 Innominate Artery** Brachiocephalic artery Brachiocephalic trunk **3 Subclavian Artery, Right** Costocervical trunk Dorsal scapular artery Internal thoracic artery **4 Subclavian Artery, Left** *See 3 Subclavian Artery, Right* **5 Axillary Artery, Right** Anterior circumflex humeral artery Lateral thoracic artery Posterior circumflex humeral artery Subscapular artery Superior thoracic artery Thoracoacromial artery **6 Axillary Artery, Left** *See 5 Axillary Artery, Right* **7 Brachial Artery, Right** Inferior ulnar collateral artery Profunda brachii Superior ulnar collateral artery **8 Brachial Artery, Left** *See 7 Brachial Artery, Right* **9 Ulnar Artery, Right** Anterior ulnar recurrent artery Common interosseous artery Posterior ulnar recurrent artery	**A Ulnar Artery, Left** *See 9 Ulnar Artery, Right* **B Radial Artery, Right** Radial recurrent artery **C Radial Artery, Left** *See B Radial Artery, Right* **D Hand Artery, Right** Deep palmar arch Princeps pollicis artery Radialis indicis Superficial palmar arch **F Hand Artery, Left** *See D Hand Artery, Right* **R Face Artery** Angular artery Ascending palatine artery External maxillary artery Facial artery Inferior labial artery Submental artery Superior labial artery **S Temporal Artery, Right** Middle temporal artery Superficial temporal artery Transverse facial artery **T Temporal Artery, Left** *See S Temporal Artery, Right* **U Thyroid Artery, Right** Cricothyroid artery Hyoid artery Sternocleidomastoid artery Superior laryngeal artery Superior thyroid artery Thyrocervical trunk **V Thyroid Artery, Left** *See U Thyroid Artery, Right* **Y Upper Artery** Aortic intercostal artery Bronchial artery Esophageal artery Subcostal artery	**Ø Open** **3 Percutaneous** **4 Percutaneous Endoscopic**	**Z No Device**	**Z No Qualifier**
G Intracranial Artery Anterior cerebral artery Anterior choroidal artery Anterior communicating artery Basilar artery Circle of Willis Internal carotid artery, intracranial portion Middle cerebral artery Ophthalmic artery Posterior cerebral artery Posterior communicating artery Posterior inferior cerebellar artery (PICA) **H Common Carotid Artery, Right** **J Common Carotid Artery, Left** **K Internal Carotid Artery, Right** Caroticotympanic artery Carotid sinus	**L Internal Carotid Artery, Left** *See K Internal Carotid Artery, Right* **M External Carotid Artery, Right** Ascending pharyngeal artery Internal maxillary artery Lingual artery Maxillary artery Occipital artery Posterior auricular artery Superior thyroid artery **N External Carotid Artery, Left** *See M External Carotid Artery, Right* **P Vertebral Artery, Right** Anterior spinal artery Posterior spinal artery **Q Vertebral Artery, Left** *See P Vertebral Artery, Right*	**Ø Open** **4 Percutaneous Endoscopic**	**Z No Device**	**Z No Qualifier**

Ø3C Continued on next page

Ø Medical and Surgical
3 Upper Arteries
C Extirpation Definition: Taking or cutting out solid matter from a body part

Ø3C Continued

Explanation: The solid matter may be an abnormal byproduct of a biological function or a foreign body; it may be imbedded in a body part or in the lumen of a tubular body part. The solid matter may or may not have been previously broken into pieces.

Body Part Character 4	Approach Character 5	Device Character 6	Qualifier Character 7
G Intracranial Artery Anterior cerebral artery Anterior choroidal artery Anterior communicating artery Basilar artery Circle of Willis Internal carotid artery, intracranial portion Middle cerebral artery Ophthalmic artery Posterior cerebral artery Posterior communicating artery Posterior inferior cerebellar artery (PICA) **H Common Carotid Artery, Right** **J Common Carotid Artery, Left** **K Internal Carotid Artery, Right** Caroticotympanic artery Carotid sinus **L Internal Carotid Artery, Left** *See K Internal Carotid Artery, Right* **M External Carotid Artery, Right** Ascending pharyngeal artery Internal maxillary artery Lingual artery Maxillary artery Occipital artery Posterior auricular artery Superior thyroid artery **N External Carotid Artery, Left** *See M External Carotid Artery, Right* **P Vertebral Artery, Right** Anterior spinal artery Posterior spinal artery **Q Vertebral Artery, Left** *See P Vertebral Artery, Right*	**3 Percutaneous**	**Z No Device**	**7 Stent Retriever** **Z No Qualifier**

Ø Medical and Surgical
3 Upper Arteries
F Fragmentation Definition: Breaking solid matter in a body part into pieces

Explanation: Physical force (e.g., manual, ultrasonic) applied directly or indirectly is used to break the solid matter into pieces. The solid matter may be an abnormal byproduct of a biological function or a foreign body. The pieces of solid matter are not taken out.

Body Part Character 4	Approach Character 5	Device Character 6	Qualifier Character 7
2 Innominate Artery Brachiocephalic artery Brachiocephalic trunk **3 Subclavian Artery, Right** Costocervical trunk Dorsal scapular artery Internal thoracic artery **4 Subclavian Artery, Left** *See 3 Subclavian Artery, Right* **5 Axillary Artery, Right** Anterior circumflex humeral artery Lateral thoracic artery Posterior circumflex humeral artery Subscapular artery Superior thoracic artery Thoracoacromial artery **6 Axillary Artery, Left** *See 5 Axillary Artery, Right* **7 Brachial Artery, Right** Inferior ulnar collateral artery Profunda brachii Superior ulnar collateral artery **8 Brachial Artery, Left** *See 7 Brachial Artery, Right* **9 Ulnar Artery, Right** Anterior ulnar recurrent artery Common interosseous artery Posterior ulnar recurrent artery **A Ulnar Artery, Left** *See 9 Ulnar Artery, Right* **B Radial Artery, Right** Radial recurrent artery **C Radial Artery, Left** *See B Radial Artery, Right* **G Intracranial Artery** Anterior cerebral artery Anterior choroidal artery Anterior communicating artery Basilar artery Circle of Willis Internal carotid artery, intracranial portion Middle cerebral artery Ophthalmic artery Posterior cerebral artery Posterior communicating artery Posterior inferior cerebellar artery (PICA) **Y Upper Artery** Aortic intercostal artery Bronchial artery Esophageal artery Subcostal artery	**3 Percutaneous**	**Z No Device**	**Ø Ultrasonic** **Z No Qualifier**

Ø Medical and Surgical
3 Upper Arteries
H Insertion Definition: Putting in a nonbiological appliance that monitors, assists, performs, or prevents a physiological function but does not physically take the place of a body part

Explanation: None

Body Part Character 4		Approach Character 5	Device Character 6	Qualifier Character 7
Ø Internal Mammary Artery, Right Anterior intercostal artery Internal thoracic artery Musculophrenic artery Pericardiophrenic artery Superior epigastric artery **1 Internal Mammary Artery, Left** *See Ø Internal Mammary Artery, Right* **2 Innominate Artery** Brachiocephalic artery Brachiocephalic trunk **3 Subclavian Artery, Right** Costocervical trunk Dorsal scapular artery Internal thoracic artery **4 Subclavian Artery, Left** *See 3 Subclavian Artery, Right* **5 Axillary Artery, Right** Anterior circumflex humeral artery Lateral thoracic artery Posterior circumflex humeral artery Subscapular artery Superior thoracic artery Thoracoacromial artery **6 Axillary Artery, Left** *See 5 Axillary Artery, Right* **7 Brachial Artery, Right** Inferior ulnar collateral artery Profunda brachii Superior ulnar collateral artery **8 Brachial Artery, Left** *See 7 Brachial Artery, Right* **9 Ulnar Artery, Right** Anterior ulnar recurrent artery Common interosseous artery Posterior ulnar recurrent artery **A Ulnar Artery, Left** *See 9 Ulnar Artery, Right* **B Radial Artery, Right** Radial recurrent artery **C Radial Artery, Left** *See B Radial Artery, Right* **D Hand Artery, Right** Deep palmar arch Princeps pollicis artery Radialis indicis Superficial palmar arch **F Hand Artery, Left** *See D Hand Artery, Right*	**G Intracranial Artery** Anterior cerebral artery Anterior choroidal artery Anterior communicating artery Basilar artery Circle of Willis Internal carotid artery, intracranial portion Middle cerebral artery Ophthalmic artery Posterior cerebral artery Posterior communicating artery Posterior inferior cerebellar artery (PICA) **H Common Carotid Artery, Right** **J Common Carotid Artery, Left** **M External Carotid Artery, Right** Ascending pharyngeal artery Internal maxillary artery Lingual artery Maxillary artery Occipital artery Posterior auricular artery Superior thyroid artery **N External Carotid Artery, Left** *See M External Carotid Artery, Right* **P Vertebral Artery, Right** Anterior spinal artery Posterior spinal artery **Q Vertebral Artery, Left** *See P Vertebral Artery, Right* **R Face Artery** Angular artery Ascending palatine artery External maxillary artery Facial artery Inferior labial artery Submental artery Superior labial artery **S Temporal Artery, Right** Middle temporal artery Superficial temporal artery Transverse facial artery **T Temporal Artery, Left** *See S Temporal Artery, Right* **U Thyroid Artery, Right** Cricothyroid artery Hyoid artery Sternocleidomastoid artery Superior laryngeal artery Superior thyroid artery Thyrocervical trunk **V Thyroid Artery, Left** *See U Thyroid Artery, Right*	**Ø Open** **3 Percutaneous** **4 Percutaneous Endoscopic**	**3 Infusion Device** **D Intraluminal Device**	**Z No Qualifier**
K Internal Carotid Artery, Right Caroticotympanic artery Carotid sinus **L Internal Carotid Artery, Left** *See K Internal Carotid Artery, Right*		**Ø Open** **3 Percutaneous** **4 Percutaneous Endoscope**	**3 Infusion Device** **D Intraluminal Device** **M Stimulator Lead** NT	**Z No Qualifier**
Y Upper Artery Aortic intercostal artery Bronchial artery Esophageal artery Subcostal artery		**Ø Open** **3 Percutaneous** **4 Percutaneous Endoscopic**	**2 Monitoring Device** **3 Infusion Device** **D Intraluminal Device** **Y Other Device**	**Z No Qualifier**

Non-OR Ø3H[Ø,1,2,3,4,5,6,7,8,9,A,B,C,D,F,G,H,J,M,N,P,Q,R,S,T,U,V][Ø,3,4]3Z
Non-OR Ø3H[K,L][Ø,3,4]3Z
Non-OR Ø3HY[Ø,3,4]3Z
Non-OR Ø3HY32Z
Non-OR Ø3HY[3,4]YZ
NT Ø3HK3MZ or Ø3HL3MZ in combination with ØJH6ØMZ *See* Appendix H for applicable device trade name

NC Noncovered Procedure LC Limited Coverage QA Questionable OB Admit NT New Tech Add-on ⊞ Combination Member ♂ Male ♀ Female

Ø Medical and Surgical
3 Upper Arteries
J Inspection Definition: Visually and/or manually exploring a body part

Explanation: Visual exploration may be performed with or without optical instrumentation. Manual exploration may be performed directly or through intervening body layers.

Body Part Character 4	Approach Character 5	Device Character 6	Qualifier Character 7
Y Upper Artery Aortic intercostal artery Bronchial artery Esophageal artery Subcostal artery	**Ø** Open **3** Percutaneous **4** Percutaneous Endoscopic **X** External	**Z** No Device	**Z** No Qualifier

Non-OR Ø3JY[3,4,X]ZZ

Ø Medical and Surgical
3 Upper Arteries
L Occlusion Definition: Completely closing an orifice or the lumen of a tubular body part
Explanation: The orifice can be a natural orifice or an artificially created orifice

Body Part Character 4		Approach Character 5	Device Character 6	Qualifier Character 7
Ø Internal Mammary Artery, Right Anterior intercostal artery Internal thoracic artery Musculophrenic artery Pericardiophrenic artery Superior epigastric artery **1 Internal Mammary Artery, Left** *See Ø Internal Mammary Artery, Left* **2 Innominate Artery** Brachiocephalic artery Brachiocephalic trunk **3 Subclavian Artery, Right** Costocervical trunk Dorsal scapular artery Internal thoracic artery **4 Subclavian Artery, Left** *See 3 Subclavian Artery, Right* **5 Axillary Artery, Right** Anterior circumflex humeral artery Lateral thoracic artery Posterior circumflex humeral artery Subscapular artery Superior thoracic artery Thoracoacromial artery **6 Axillary Artery, Left** *See 5 Axillary Artery, Right* **7 Brachial Artery, Right** Inferior ulnar collateral artery Profunda brachii Superior ulnar collateral artery **8 Brachial Artery, Left** *See 7 Brachial Artery, Right* **9 Ulnar Artery, Right** Anterior ulnar recurrent artery Common interosseous artery Posterior ulnar recurrent artery	**A Ulnar Artery, Left** *See 9 Ulnar Artery, Right* **B Radial Artery, Right** Radial recurrent artery **C Radial Artery, Left** *See B Radial Artery, Right* **D Hand Artery, Right** Deep palmar arch Princeps pollicis artery Radialis indicis Superficial palmar arch **F Hand Artery, Left** *See D Hand Artery, Right* **R Face Artery** Angular artery Ascending palatine artery External maxillary artery Facial artery Inferior labial artery Submental artery Superior labial artery **S Temporal Artery, Right** Middle temporal artery Superficial temporal artery Transverse facial artery **T Temporal Artery, Left** *See S Temporal Artery, Right* **U Thyroid Artery, Right** Cricothyroid artery Hyoid artery Sternocleidomastoid artery Superior laryngeal artery Superior thyroid artery Thyrocervical trunk **V Thyroid Artery, Left** *See U Thyroid Artery, Right* **Y Upper Artery** Aortic intercostal artery Bronchial artery Esophageal artery Subcostal artery	**Ø Open** **3 Percutaneous** **4 Percutaneous Endoscopic**	**C Extraluminal Device** **D Intraluminal Device** **Z No Device**	**Z No Qualifier**
G Intracranial Artery Anterior cerebral artery Anterior choroidal artery Anterior communicating artery Basilar artery Circle of Willis Internal carotid artery, intracranial portion Middle cerebral artery Ophthalmic artery Posterior cerebral artery Posterior communicating artery Posterior inferior cerebellar artery (PICA) **H Common Carotid Artery, Right** **J Common Carotid Artery, Left** **K Internal Carotid Artery, Right** Caroticotympanic artery Carotid sinus	**L Internal Carotid Artery, Left** *See K Internal Carotid Artery, Right* **M External Carotid Artery, Right** Ascending pharyngeal artery Internal maxillary artery Lingual artery Maxillary artery Occipital artery Posterior auricular artery Superior thyroid artery **N External Carotid Artery, Left** *See M External Carotid Artery, Right* **P Vertebral Artery, Right** Anterior spinal artery Posterior spinal artery **Q Vertebral Artery, Left** *See P Vertebral Artery, Right*	**Ø Open** **3 Percutaneous** **4 Percutaneous Endoscopic**	**B Intraluminal Device, Bioactive** **C Extraluminal Device** **D Intraluminal Device** **Z No Device**	**Z No Qualifier**

Ø Medical and Surgical
3 Upper Arteries
N Release Definition: Freeing a body part from an abnormal physical constraint by cutting or by the use of force
Explanation: Some of the restraining tissue may be taken out but none of the body part is taken out

Body Part Character 4	Approach Character 5	Device Character 6	Qualifier Character 7
Ø Internal Mammary Artery, Right Anterior intercostal artery Internal thoracic artery Musculophrenic artery Pericardiophrenic artery Superior epigastric artery **1 Internal Mammary Artery, Left** *See Ø Internal Mammary Artery, Right* **2 Innominate Artery** Brachiocephalic artery Brachiocephalic trunk **3 Subclavian Artery, Right** Costocervical trunk Dorsal scapular artery Internal thoracic artery **4 Subclavian Artery, Left** *See 3 Subclavian Artery, Right* **5 Axillary Artery, Right** Anterior circumflex humeral artery Lateral thoracic artery Posterior circumflex humeral artery Subscapular artery Superior thoracic artery Thoracoacromial artery **6 Axillary Artery, Left** *See 5 Axillary Artery, Right* **7 Brachial Artery, Right** Inferior ulnar collateral artery Profunda brachii Superior ulnar collateral artery **8 Brachial Artery, Left** *See 7 Brachial Artery, Right* **9 Ulnar Artery, Right** Anterior ulnar recurrent artery Common interosseous artery Posterior ulnar recurrent artery **A Ulnar Artery, Left** *See 9 Ulnar Artery, Right* **B Radial Artery, Right** Radial recurrent artery **C Radial Artery, Left** *See B Radial Artery, Right* **D Hand Artery, Right** Deep palmar arch Princeps pollicis artery Radialis indicis Superficial palmar arch **F Hand Artery, Left** *See D Hand Artery, Right* **G Intracranial Artery** Anterior cerebral artery Anterior choroidal artery Anterior communicating artery Basilar artery Circle of Willis Internal carotid artery, intracranial portion Middle cerebral artery Ophthalmic artery Posterior cerebral artery Posterior communicating artery Posterior inferior cerebellar artery (PICA) **H Common Carotid Artery, Right** **J Common Carotid Artery, Left** **K Internal Carotid Artery, Right** Caroticotympanic artery Carotid sinus **L Internal Carotid Artery, Left** *See K Internal Carotid Artery, Right* **M External Carotid Artery, Right** Ascending pharyngeal artery Internal maxillary artery Lingual artery Maxillary artery Occipital artery Posterior auricular artery Superior thyroid artery **N External Carotid Artery, Left** *See M External Carotid Artery, Right* **P Vertebral Artery, Right** Anterior spinal artery Posterior spinal artery **Q Vertebral Artery, Left** *See P Vertebral Artery, Right* **R Face Artery** Angular artery Ascending palatine artery External maxillary artery Facial artery Inferior labial artery Submental artery Superior labial artery **S Temporal Artery, Right** Middle temporal artery Superficial temporal artery Transverse facial artery **T Temporal Artery, Left** *See S Temporal Artery, Right* **U Thyroid Artery, Right** Cricothyroid artery Hyoid artery Sternocleidomastoid artery Superior laryngeal artery Superior thyroid artery Thyrocervical trunk **V Thyroid Artery, Left** *See U Thyroid Artery, Right* **Y Upper Artery** Aortic intercostal artery Bronchial artery Esophageal artery Subcostal artery	**Ø Open** **3 Percutaneous** **4 Percutaneous Endoscopic**	**Z No Device**	**Z No Qualifier**

Ø Medical and Surgical
3 Upper Arteries
P Removal Definition: Taking out or off a device from a body part

Explanation: If a device is taken out and a similar device put in without cutting or puncturing the skin or mucous membrane, the procedure is coded to the root operation CHANGE. Otherwise, the procedure for taking out a device is coded to the root operation REMOVAL.

Body Part Character 4	Approach Character 5	Device Character 6	Qualifier Character 7
Y Upper Artery Aortic intercostal artery Bronchial artery Esophageal artery Subcostal artery	Ø Open 3 Percutaneous 4 Percutaneous Endoscopic	Ø Drainage Device 2 Monitoring Device 3 Infusion Device 7 Autologous Tissue Substitute C Extraluminal Device D Intraluminal Device J Synthetic Substitute K Nonautologous Tissue Substitute M Stimulator Lead Y Other Device	Z No Qualifier
Y Upper Artery Aortic intercostal artery Bronchial artery Esophageal artery Subcostal artery	X External	Ø Drainage Device 2 Monitoring Device 3 Infusion Device D Intraluminal Device M Stimulator Lead	Z No Qualifier

Non-OR Ø3PY3[Ø,2,3,D]Z
Non-OR Ø3PY[3,4]YZ
Non-OR Ø3PYX[Ø,2,3,D,M]Z

Ø Medical and Surgical
3 Upper Arteries
Q Repair Definition: Restoring, to the extent possible, a body part to its normal anatomic structure and function
Explanation: Used only when the method to accomplish the repair is not one of the other root operations

Body Part Character 4		Approach Character 5	Device Character 6	Qualifier Character 7
Ø Internal Mammary Artery, Right Anterior intercostal artery Internal thoracic artery Musculophrenic artery Pericardiophrenic artery Superior epigastric artery **1 Internal Mammary Artery, Left** *See Ø Internal Mammary Artery, Right* **2 Innominate Artery** Brachiocephalic artery Brachiocephalic trunk **3 Subclavian Artery, Right** Costocervical trunk Dorsal scapular artery Internal thoracic artery **4 Subclavian Artery, Left** *See 3 Subclavian Artery, Right* **5 Axillary Artery, Right** Anterior circumflex humeral artery Lateral thoracic artery Posterior circumflex humeral artery Subscapular artery Superior thoracic artery Thoracoacromial artery **6 Axillary Artery, Left** *See 5 Axillary Artery, Right* **7 Brachial Artery, Right** Inferior ulnar collateral artery Profunda brachii Superior ulnar collateral artery **8 Brachial Artery, Left** *See 7 Brachial Artery, Right* **9 Ulnar Artery, Right** Anterior ulnar recurrent artery Common interosseous artery Posterior ulnar recurrent artery **A Ulnar Artery, Left** *See 9 Ulnar Artery, Right* **B Radial Artery, Right** Radial recurrent artery **C Radial Artery, Left** *See B Radial Artery, Right* **D Hand Artery, Right** Deep palmar arch Princeps pollicis artery Radialis indicis Superficial palmar arch **F Hand Artery, Left** *See D Hand Artery, Right* **G Intracranial Artery** Anterior cerebral artery Anterior choroidal artery Anterior communicating artery Basilar artery Circle of Willis Internal carotid artery, intracranial portion Middle cerebral artery Ophthalmic artery Posterior cerebral artery Posterior communicating artery Posterior inferior cerebellar artery (PICA)	**H Common Carotid Artery, Right** **J Common Carotid Artery, Left** **K Internal Carotid Artery, Right** Caroticotympanic artery Carotid sinus **L Internal Carotid Artery, Left** *See K Internal Carotid Artery, Right* **M External Carotid Artery, Right** Ascending pharyngeal artery Internal maxillary artery Lingual artery Maxillary artery Occipital artery Posterior auricular artery Superior thyroid artery **N External Carotid Artery, Left** *See M External Carotid Artery, Right* **P Vertebral Artery, Right** Anterior spinal artery Posterior spinal artery **Q Vertebral Artery, Left** *See P Vertebral Artery, Right* **R Face Artery** Angular artery Ascending palatine artery External maxillary artery Facial artery Inferior labial artery Submental artery Superior labial artery **S Temporal Artery, Right** Middle temporal artery Superficial temporal artery Transverse facial artery **T Temporal Artery, Left** *See S Temporal Artery, Right* **U Thyroid Artery, Right** Cricothyroid artery Hyoid artery Sternocleidomastoid artery Superior laryngeal artery Superior thyroid artery Thyrocervical trunk **V Thyroid Artery, Left** *See U Thyroid Artery, Right* **Y Upper Artery** Aortic intercostal artery Bronchial artery Esophageal artery Subcostal artery	**Ø Open** **3 Percutaneous** **4 Percutaneous Endoscopic**	**Z No Device**	**Z No Qualifier**

Ø Medical and Surgical
3 Upper Arteries
R Replacement Definition: Putting in or on biological or synthetic material that physically takes the place and/or function of all or a portion of a body part

Explanation: The body part may have been taken out or replaced, or may be taken out, physically eradicated, or rendered nonfunctional during the REPLACEMENT procedure. A REMOVAL procedure is coded for taking out the device used in a previous replacement procedure.

Body Part Character 4		Approach Character 5	Device Character 6	Qualifier Character 7
Ø Internal Mammary Artery, Right Anterior intercostal artery Internal thoracic artery Musculophrenic artery Pericardiophrenic artery Superior epigastric artery **1 Internal Mammary Artery, Left** *See Ø Internal Mammary Artery, Right* **2 Innominate Artery** Brachiocephalic artery Brachiocephalic trunk **3 Subclavian Artery, Right** Costocervical trunk Dorsal scapular artery Internal thoracic artery **4 Subclavian Artery, Left** *See 3 Subclavian Artery, Right* **5 Axillary Artery, Right** Anterior circumflex humeral artery Lateral thoracic artery Posterior circumflex humeral artery Subscapular artery Superior thoracic artery Thoracoacromial artery **6 Axillary Artery, Left** *See 5 Axillary Artery, Right* **7 Brachial Artery, Right** Inferior ulnar collateral artery Profunda brachii Superior ulnar collateral artery **8 Brachial Artery, Left** *See 7 Brachial Artery, Right* **9 Ulnar Artery, Right** Anterior ulnar recurrent artery Common interosseous artery Posterior ulnar recurrent artery **A Ulnar Artery, Left** *See 9 Ulnar Artery, Right* **B Radial Artery, Right** Radial recurrent artery **C Radial Artery, Left** *See B Radial Artery, Right* **D Hand Artery, Right** Deep palmar arch Princeps pollicis artery Radialis indicis Superficial palmar arch **F Hand Artery, Left** *See D Hand Artery, Right* **G Intracranial Artery** Anterior cerebral artery Anterior choroidal artery Anterior communicating artery Basilar artery Circle of Willis Internal carotid artery, intracranial portion Middle cerebral artery Ophthalmic artery Posterior cerebral artery Posterior communicating artery Posterior inferior cerebellar artery (PICA)	**H Common Carotid Artery, Right** **J Common Carotid Artery, Left** **K Internal Carotid Artery, Right** Caroticotympanic artery Carotid sinus **L Internal Carotid Artery, Left** *See K Internal Carotid Artery, Right* **M External Carotid Artery, Right** Ascending pharyngeal artery Internal maxillary artery Lingual artery Maxillary artery Occipital artery Posterior auricular artery Superior thyroid artery **N External Carotid Artery, Left** *See M External Carotid Artery, Right* **P Vertebral Artery, Right** Anterior spinal artery Posterior spinal artery **Q Vertebral Artery, Left** *See P Vertebral Artery, Right* **R Face Artery** Angular artery Ascending palatine artery External maxillary artery Facial artery Inferior labial artery Submental artery Superior labial artery **S Temporal Artery, Right** Middle temporal artery Superficial temporal artery Transverse facial artery **T Temporal Artery, Left** *See S Temporal Artery, Right* **U Thyroid Artery, Right** Cricothyroid artery Hyoid artery Sternocleidomastoid artery Superior laryngeal artery Superior thyroid artery Thyrocervical trunk **V Thyroid Artery, Left** *See U Thyroid Artery, Right* **Y Upper Artery** Aortic intercostal artery Bronchial artery Esophageal artery Subcostal artery	**Ø Open** **4 Percutaneous Endoscopic**	**7 Autologous Tissue Substitute** **J Synthetic Substitute** **K Nonautologous Tissue Substitute**	**Z No Qualifier**

Ø Medical and Surgical
3 Upper Arteries
S Reposition Definition: Moving to its normal location, or other suitable location, all or a portion of a body part

Explanation: The body part is moved to a new location from an abnormal location, or from a normal location where it is not functioning correctly. The body part may or may not be cut out or off to be moved to the new location.

Body Part Character 4	Approach Character 5	Device Character 6	Qualifier Character 7
Ø Internal Mammary Artery, Right Anterior intercostal artery Internal thoracic artery Musculophrenic artery Pericardiophrenic artery Superior epigastric artery **1 Internal Mammary Artery, Left** *See Ø Internal Mammary Artery, Right* **2 Innominate Artery** Brachiocephalic artery Brachiocephalic trunk **3 Subclavian Artery, Right** Costocervical trunk Dorsal scapular artery Internal thoracic artery **4 Subclavian Artery, Left** *See 3 Subclavian Artery, Right* **5 Axillary Artery, Right** Anterior circumflex humeral artery Lateral thoracic artery Posterior circumflex humeral artery Subscapular artery Superior thoracic artery Thoracoacromial artery **6 Axillary Artery, Left** *See 5 Axillary Artery, Right* **7 Brachial Artery, Right** Inferior ulnar collateral artery Profunda brachii Superior ulnar collateral artery **8 Brachial Artery, Left** *See 7 Brachial Artery, Right* **9 Ulnar Artery, Right** Anterior ulnar recurrent artery Common interosseous artery Posterior ulnar recurrent artery **A Ulnar Artery, Left** *See 9 Ulnar Artery, Right* **B Radial Artery, Right** Radial recurrent artery **C Radial Artery, Left** *See B Radial Artery, Right* **D Hand Artery, Right** Deep palmar arch Princeps pollicis artery Radialis indicis Superficial palmar arch **F Hand Artery, Left** *See D Hand Artery, Right* **G Intracranial Artery** Anterior cerebral artery Anterior choroidal artery Anterior communicating artery Basilar artery Circle of Willis Internal carotid artery, intracranial portion Middle cerebral artery Ophthalmic artery Posterior cerebral artery Posterior communicating artery Posterior inferior cerebellar artery (PICA) **H Common Carotid Artery, Right** **J Common Carotid Artery, Left** **K Internal Carotid Artery, Right** Caroticotympanic artery Carotid sinus **L Internal Carotid Artery, Left** *See K Internal Carotid Artery, Right* **M External Carotid Artery, Right** Ascending pharyngeal artery Internal maxillary artery Lingual artery Maxillary artery Occipital artery Posterior auricular artery Superior thyroid artery **N External Carotid Artery, Left** *See M External Carotid Artery, Right* **P Vertebral Artery, Right** Anterior spinal artery Posterior spinal artery **Q Vertebral Artery, Left** *See P Vertebral Artery, Right* **R Face Artery** Angular artery Ascending palatine artery External maxillary artery Facial artery Inferior labial artery Submental artery Superior labial artery **S Temporal Artery, Right** Middle temporal artery Superficial temporal artery Transverse facial artery **T Temporal Artery, Left** *See S Temporal Artery, Right* **U Thyroid Artery, Right** Cricothyroid artery Hyoid artery Sternocleidomastoid artery Superior laryngeal artery Superior thyroid artery Thyrocervical trunk **V Thyroid Artery, Left** *See U Thyroid Artery, Right* **Y Upper Artery** Aortic intercostal artery Bronchial artery Esophageal artery Subcostal artery	**Ø Open** **3 Percutaneous** **4 Percutaneous Endoscopic**	**Z No Device**	**Z No Qualifier**

Ø Medical and Surgical
3 Upper Arteries
U Supplement Definition: Putting in or on biological or synthetic material that physically reinforces and/or augments the function of a portion of a body part

Explanation: The biological material is non-living, or is living and from the same individual. The body part may have been previously replaced, and the SUPPLEMENT procedure is performed to physically reinforce and/or augment the function of the replaced body part.

Body Part Character 4		Approach Character 5	Device Character 6	Qualifier Character 7
Ø Internal Mammary Artery, Right Anterior intercostal artery Internal thoracic artery Musculophrenic artery Pericardiophrenic artery Superior epigastric artery **1 Internal Mammary Artery, Left** ***See*** *Ø Internal Mammary Artery, Right* **2 Innominate Artery** Brachiocephalic artery Brachiocephalic trunk **3 Subclavian Artery, Right** Costocervical trunk Dorsal scapular artery Internal thoracic artery **4 Subclavian Artery, Left** ***See*** *3 Subclavian Artery, Right* **5 Axillary Artery, Right** Anterior circumflex humeral artery Lateral thoracic artery Posterior circumflex humeral artery Subscapular artery Superior thoracic artery Thoracoacromial artery **6 Axillary Artery, Left** ***See*** *5 Axillary Artery, Right* **7 Brachial Artery, Right** Inferior ulnar collateral artery Profunda brachii Superior ulnar collateral artery **8 Brachial Artery, Left** ***See*** *7 Brachial Artery, Right* **9 Ulnar Artery, Right** Anterior ulnar recurrent artery Common interosseous artery Posterior ulnar recurrent artery **A Ulnar Artery, Left** ***See*** *9 Ulnar Artery, Right* **B Radial Artery, Right** Radial recurrent artery **C Radial Artery, Left** ***See*** *B Radial Artery, Right* **D Hand Artery, Right** Deep palmar arch Princeps pollicis artery Radialis indicis Superficial palmar arch **F Hand Artery, Left** ***See*** *D Hand Artery, Right* **G Intracranial Artery** Anterior cerebral artery Anterior choroidal artery Anterior communicating artery Basilar artery Circle of Willis Internal carotid artery, intracranial portion Middle cerebral artery Ophthalmic artery Posterior cerebral artery Posterior communicating artery Posterior inferior cerebellar artery (PICA)	**H Common Carotid Artery, Right** **J Common Carotid Artery, Left** **K Internal Carotid Artery, Right** Caroticotympanic artery Carotid sinus **L Internal Carotid Artery, Left** ***See*** *K Internal Carotid Artery, Right* **M External Carotid Artery, Right** Ascending pharyngeal artery Internal maxillary artery Lingual artery Maxillary artery Occipital artery Posterior auricular artery Superior thyroid artery **N External Carotid Artery, Left** ***See*** *M External Carotid Artery, Right* **P Vertebral Artery, Right** Anterior spinal artery Posterior spinal artery **Q Vertebral Artery, Left** ***See*** *P Vertebral Artery, Right* **R Face Artery** Angular artery Ascending palatine artery External maxillary artery Facial artery Inferior labial artery Submental artery Superior labial artery **S Temporal Artery, Right** Middle temporal artery Superficial temporal artery Transverse facial artery **T Temporal Artery, Left** ***See*** *S Temporal Artery, Right* **U Thyroid Artery, Right** Cricothyroid artery Hyoid artery Sternocleidomastoid artery Superior laryngeal artery Superior thyroid artery Thyrocervical trunk **V Thyroid Artery, Left** ***See*** *U Thyroid Artery, Right* **Y Upper Artery** Aortic intercostal artery Bronchial artery Esophageal artery Subcostal artery	**Ø Open** **3 Percutaneous** **4 Percutaneous Endoscopic**	**7 Autologous Tissue Substitute** **J Synthetic Substitute** **K Nonautologous Tissue Substitute**	**Z No Qualifier**

Ø Medical and Surgical
3 Upper Arteries
V Restriction Definition: Partially closing an orifice or the lumen of a tubular body part
Explanation: The orifice can be a natural orifice or an artificially created orifice

Body Part Character 4		Approach Character 5	Device Character 6	Qualifier Character 7
Ø Internal Mammary Artery, Right Anterior intercostal artery Internal thoracic artery Musculophrenic artery Pericardiophrenic artery Superior epigastric artery **1 Internal Mammary Artery, Left** *See Ø Internal Mammary Artery, Right* **2 Innominate Artery** Brachiocephalic artery Brachiocephalic trunk **3 Subclavian Artery, Right** Costocervical trunk Dorsal scapular artery Internal thoracic artery **4 Subclavian Artery, Left** *See 3 Subclavian Artery, Right* **5 Axillary Artery, Right** Anterior circumflex humeral artery Lateral thoracic artery Posterior circumflex humeral artery Subscapular artery Superior thoracic artery Thoracoacromial artery **6 Axillary Artery, Left** *See 5 Axillary Artery, Right* **7 Brachial Artery, Right** Inferior ulnar collateral artery Profunda brachii Superior ulnar collateral artery **8 Brachial Artery, Left** *See 7 Brachial Artery, Right* **9 Ulnar Artery, Right** Anterior ulnar recurrent artery Common interosseous artery Posterior ulnar recurrent artery **A Ulnar Artery, Left** *See 9 Ulnar Artery, Right*	**B Radial Artery, Right** Radial recurrent artery **C Radial Artery, Left** *See B Radial Artery, Right* **D Hand Artery, Right** Deep palmar arch Princeps pollicis artery Radialis indicis Superficial palmar arch **F Hand Artery, Left** *See D Hand Artery, Right* **R Face Artery** Angular artery Ascending palatine artery External maxillary artery Facial artery Inferior labial artery Submental artery Superior labial artery **S Temporal Artery, Right** Middle temporal artery Superficial temporal artery Transverse facial artery **T Temporal Artery, Left** *See S Temporal Artery, Right* **U Thyroid Artery, Right** Cricothyroid artery Hyoid artery Sternocleidomastoid artery Superior laryngeal artery Superior thyroid artery Thyrocervical trunk **V Thyroid Artery, Left** *See U Thyroid Artery, Right* **Y Upper Artery** Aortic intercostal artery Bronchial artery Esophageal artery Subcostal artery	**Ø Open** **3 Percutaneous** **4 Percutaneous Endoscopic**	**C Extraluminal Device** **D Intraluminal Device** **Z No Device**	**Z No Qualifier**
G Intracranial Artery Anterior cerebral artery Anterior choroidal artery Anterior communicating artery Basilar artery Circle of Willis Internal carotid artery, intracranial portion Middle cerebral artery Ophthalmic artery Posterior cerebral artery Posterior communicating artery Posterior inferior cerebellar artery (PICA) **H Common Carotid Artery, Right** **J Common Carotid Artery, Left** **K Internal Carotid Artery, Right** Caroticotympanic artery Carotid sinus	**L Internal Carotid Artery, Left** *See K Internal Carotid Artery, Right* **M External Carotid Artery, Right** Ascending pharyngeal artery Internal maxillary artery Lingual artery Maxillary artery Occipital artery Posterior auricular artery Superior thyroid artery **N External Carotid Artery, Left** *See M External Carotid Artery, Right* **P Vertebral Artery, Right** Anterior spinal artery Posterior spinal artery **Q Vertebral Artery, Left** *See P Vertebral Artery, Right*	**Ø Open** **3 Percutaneous** **4 Percutaneous Endoscopic**	**B Intraluminal Device, Bioactive** **C Extraluminal Device** **D Intraluminal Device** **H Intraluminal Device, Flow Diverter** **Z No Device**	**Z No Qualifier**

Ø Medical and Surgical
3 Upper Arteries
W Revision

Definition: Correcting, to the extent possible, a portion of a malfunctioning device or the position of a displaced device

Explanation: Revision can include correcting a malfunctioning or displaced device by taking out or putting in components of the device such as a screw or pin

Body Part Character 4	Approach Character 5	Device Character 6	Qualifier Character 7
Y Upper Artery Aortic intercostal artery Bronchial artery Esophageal artery Subcostal artery	**Ø Open** **3 Percutaneous** **4 Percutaneous Endoscopic**	**Ø Drainage Device** **2 Monitoring Device** **3 Infusion Device** **7 Autologous Tissue Substitute** **C Extraluminal Device** **D Intraluminal Device** **J Synthetic Substitute** **K Nonautologous Tissue Substitute** **M Stimulator Lead** **Y Other Device**	**Z No Qualifier**
Y Upper Artery Aortic intercostal artery Bronchial artery Esophageal artery Subcostal artery	**X External**	**Ø Drainage Device** **2 Monitoring Device** **3 Infusion Device** **7 Autologous Tissue Substitute** **C Extraluminal Device** **D Intraluminal Device** **J Synthetic Substitute** **K Nonautologous Tissue Substitute** **M Stimulator Lead**	**Z No Qualifier**

Non-OR Ø3WY3[Ø,2,3,D]Z
Non-OR Ø3WY[3,4]YZ
Non-OR Ø3WYX[Ø,2,3,7,C,D,J,K,M]Z

Lower Arteries Ø41–Ø4W

Character Meanings

This Character Meaning table is provided as a guide to assist the user in the identification of character members that may be found in this section of code tables. It **SHOULD NOT** be used to build a PCS code.

Operation–Character 3	Body Part–Character 4	Approach–Character 5	Device–Character 6	Qualifier–Character 7
1 Bypass	Ø Abdominal Aorta	Ø Open	Ø Drainage Device	Ø Abdominal Aorta OR Ultrasonic
5 Destruction	1 Celiac Artery	3 Percutaneous	1 Radioactive Element	1 Celiac Artery OR Drug-Coated Balloon
7 Dilation	2 Gastric Artery	4 Percutaneous Endoscopic	2 Monitoring Device	2 Mesenteric Artery
9 Drainage	3 Hepatic Artery	X External	3 Infusion Device	3 Renal Artery, Right
B Excision	4 Splenic Artery		4 Intraluminal Device, Drug-eluting	4 Renal Artery, Left
C Extirpation	5 Superior Mesenteric Artery		5 Intraluminal Device, Drug-eluting, Two	5 Renal Artery, Bilateral
F Fragmentation	6 Colic Artery, Right		6 Intraluminal Device, Drug-eluting, Three	6 Common Iliac Artery, Right
H Insertion	7 Colic Artery, Left		7 Intraluminal Device, Drug-eluting, Four or More OR Autologous Tissue Substitute	7 Common Iliac Artery, Left
J Inspection	8 Colic Artery, Middle		9 Autologous Venous Tissue	8 Common Iliac Arteries, Bilateral
L Occlusion	9 Renal Artery, Right		A Autologous Arterial Tissue	9 Internal Iliac Artery, Right
N Release	A Renal Artery, Left		C Extraluminal Device	B Internal Iliac Artery, Left
P Removal	B Inferior Mesenteric Artery		D Intraluminal Device	C Internal Iliac Arteries, Bilateral
Q Repair	C Common Iliac Artery, Right		E Intraluminal Device, Two OR Intraluminal Device, Branched or Fenestrated, One or Two Arteries	D External Iliac Artery, Right
R Replacement	D Common Iliac Artery, Left		F Intraluminal Device, Three OR Intraluminal Device, Branched or Fenestrated, Three or More Arteries	F External Iliac Artery, Left
S Reposition	E Internal Iliac Artery, Right		G Intraluminal Device, Four or More	G External Iliac Arteries, Bilateral
U Supplement	F Internal Iliac Artery, Left		J Synthetic Substitute	H Femoral Artery, Right
V Restriction	H External Iliac Artery, Right		K Nonautologous Tissue Substitute	J Femoral Artery, Left OR Temporary
W Revision	J External Iliac Artery, Left		Y Other Device	K Femoral Arteries, Bilateral
	K Femoral Artery, Right		Z No Device	L Popliteal Artery
	L Femoral Artery, Left			M Peroneal Artery
	M Popliteal Artery, Right			N Posterior Tibial Artery
	N Popliteal Artery, Left			P Foot Artery
	P Anterior Tibial Artery, Right			Q Lower Extremity Artery
	Q Anterior Tibial Artery, Left			R Lower Artery
	R Posterior Tibial Artery, Right			S Lower Extremity Vein
	S Posterior Tibial Artery, Left			T Uterine Artery, Right
	T Peroneal Artery, Right			U Uterine Artery, Left
	U Peroneal Artery, Left			X Diagnostic
	V Foot Artery, Right			Z No Qualifier
	W Foot Artery, Left			
	Y Lower Artery			

AHA Coding Clinic for table Ø41

2019, 1Q, 23	Endovascular repair of shaggy aorta and deployment of chimney stent grafts
2018, 3Q, 25	Femoral artery to tibioperoneal trunk bypass
2017, 4Q, 46-47	New and revised body part values - Bypass hepatic artery to renal artery
2017, 3Q, 5	Femoral artery to posterior tibial artery bypass using autologous and synthetic grafts
2017, 3Q, 16	Abdominal aortic debranching with bypass of external iliac artery to bilateral renal arteries and superior mesenteric artery
2017, 1Q, 32	Peroneal artery to dorsalis pedis artery bypass using saphenous vein graft
2016, 2Q, 18	Femoral-tibial artery bypass and saphenous vein graft
2015, 3Q, 28	Bilateral renal artery bypass

AHA Coding Clinic for table Ø47

2020, 4Q, 50	Intravascular lithotripsy
2019, 4Q, 27	Bifurcation Qualifier
2019, 2Q, 14	Revision of occluded femoral-popliteal bypass graft
2018, 2Q, 24	Coronary artery bifurcation
2016, 4Q, 86	Peripheral artery, number of stents
2016, 4Q, 86-88	Coronary and peripheral artery bifurcation
2016, 3Q, 39	Infrarenal abdominal aortic aneurysm repair with iliac graft extension
2015, 4Q, 4-7, 15	Drug-coated balloon angioplasty in peripheral vessels
2015, 3Q, 9	Aborted endovascular stenting of superficial femoral artery

AHA Coding Clinic for table Ø4C

2021, 1Q, 15	Iliofemoral endarterectomy and furthest point of entry
2019, 4Q, 27	Bifurcation Qualifier
2019, 1Q, 23	Endovascular repair of shaggy aorta and deployment of chimney stent grafts
2018, 2Q, 24	Coronary artery bifurcation
2017, 2Q, 23	Thrombectomy via Fogarty catheter
2016, 4Q, 86-88	Coronary and peripheral artery bifurcation
2016, 1Q, 31	Iliofemoral endarterectomy with patch repair
2015, 1Q, 29	Discontinued carotid endarterectomy
2015, 1Q, 36	Percutaneous mechanical thrombectomy of femoropopliteal bypass graft

AHA Coding Clinic for table Ø4F

2020, 4Q, 45-49	New fragmentation tables
2020, 4Q, 49-50	Intravascular ultrasound assisted thrombolysis
2020, 4Q, 50-51	Intravascular lithotripsy

AHA Coding Clinic for table Ø4H

2019, 3Q, 20	Removal and revision of ECMO component
2019, 1Q, 23	Endovascular repair of shaggy aorta and deployment of chimney stent grafts
2017, 1Q, 30	Insertion of umbilical artery catheter

AHA Coding Clinic for table Ø4L

2020, 3Q, 43	Staged laparoscopic gastric conduit and placement of feeding tube
2018, 2Q, 18	Transverse rectus abdominis myocutaneous (TRAM) delay
2017, 4Q, 31	Resuscitative endovascular balloon occlusion of the aorta
2015, 2Q, 27	Uterine artery embolization using Gelfoam
2014, 3Q, 26	Coil embolization of gastroduodenal artery with chemoembolization of hepatic artery
2014, 1Q, 24	Endovascular embolization for gastrointestinal bleeding

AHA Coding Clinic for table Ø4N

2015, 2Q, 28	Release and replacement of celiac artery

AHA Coding Clinic for table Ø4P

2019, 3Q, 20	Removal and revision of ECMO component

AHA Coding Clinic for table Ø4Q

2014, 1Q, 21	Repair of femoral artery pseudoaneurysm

AHA Coding Clinic for table Ø4R

2019, 1Q, 22	Abdominal aortic aneurysm repair using tube graft
2015, 2Q, 28	Release and replacement of celiac artery

AHA Coding Clinic for table Ø4U

2019, 1Q, 22	Abdominal aortic aneurysm repair using tube graft
2016, 2Q, 18	Femoral-tibial artery bypass and saphenous vein graft
2016, 1Q, 31	Iliofemoral endarterectomy with patch repair
2014, 4Q, 37	Bovine patch arterioplasty
2014, 1Q, 22	Repair of pseudoaneurysm of femoral-popliteal bypass graft

AHA Coding Clinic for table Ø4V

2019, 4Q, 27	Bifurcation Qualifier
2019, 1Q, 22	Abdominal aortic aneurysm repair using tube graft
2018, 2Q, 24	Coronary artery bifurcation
2016, 4Q, 86-87	Coronary and peripheral artery bifurcation
2016, 4Q, 89-93	Branched and fenestrated endograft repair of aneurysms
2016, 3Q, 39	Infrarenal abdominal aortic aneurysm repair with iliac graft extension
2014, 1Q, 9	Endovascular repair of abdominal aortic aneurysm

AHA Coding Clinic for table Ø4W

2020, 3Q, 5	Types of endoleaks following endovascular aneurysm repair
2019, 2Q, 14	Revision of occluded femoral-popliteal bypass graft
2015, 1Q, 36	Revision of femoropopliteal bypass graft
2014, 1Q, 9	Endovascular repair of endoleak
2014, 1Q, 22	Repair of pseudoaneurysm of femoral-popliteal bypass graft

Lower Arteries

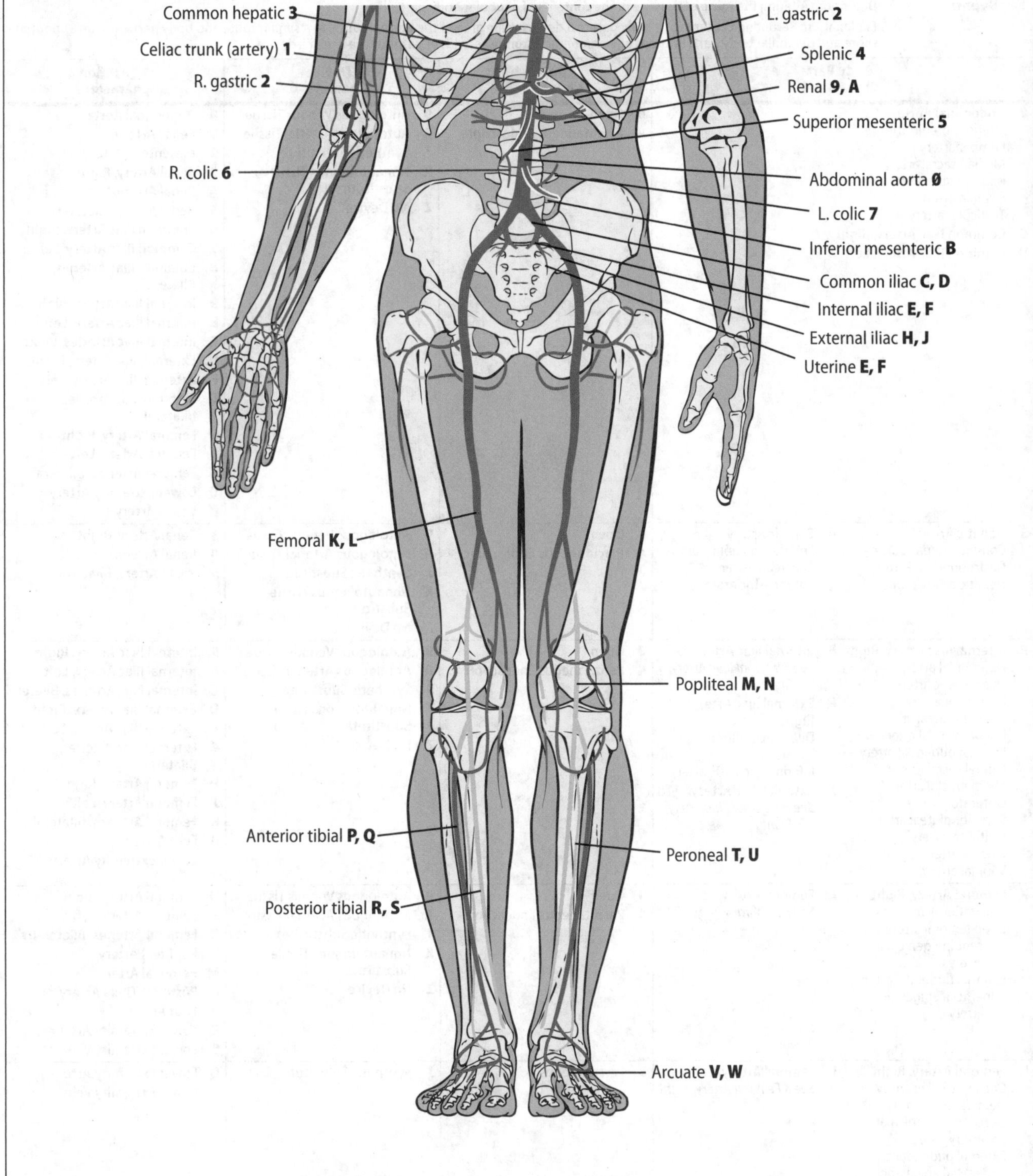

Ø Medical and Surgical
4 Lower Arteries
1 Bypass Definition: Altering the route of passage of the contents of a tubular body part

Explanation: Rerouting contents of a body part to a downstream area of the normal route, to a similar route and body part, or to an abnormal route and dissimilar body part. Includes one or more anastomoses, with or without the use of a device.

Body Part Character 4	Approach Character 5	Device Character 6	Qualifier Character 7
Ø Abdominal Aorta Inferior phrenic artery Lumbar artery Median sacral artery Middle suprarenal artery Ovarian artery Testicular artery **C Common Iliac Artery, Right** **D Common Iliac Artery, Left**	**Ø Open** **4 Percutaneous Endoscopic**	**9 Autologous Venous Tissue** **A Autologous Arterial Tissue** **J Synthetic Substitute** **K Nonautologous Tissue Substitute** **Z No Device**	**Ø Abdominal Aorta** **1 Celiac Artery** **2 Mesenteric Artery** **3 Renal Artery, Right** **4 Renal Artery, Left** **5 Renal Artery, Bilateral** **6 Common Iliac Artery, Right** **7 Common Iliac Artery, Left** **8 Common Iliac Arteries, Bilateral** **9 Internal Iliac Artery, Right** **B Internal Iliac Artery, Left** **C Internal Iliac Arteries, Bilateral** **D External Iliac Artery, Right** **F External Iliac Artery, Left** **G External Iliac Arteries, Bilateral** **H Femoral Artery, Right** **J Femoral Artery, Left** **K Femoral Arteries, Bilateral** **Q Lower Extremity Artery** **R Lower Artery**
3 Hepatic Artery Common hepatic artery Gastroduodenal artery Hepatic artery proper **4 Splenic Artery** Left gastroepiploic artery Pancreatic artery Short gastric artery	**Ø Open** **4 Percutaneous Endoscopic**	**9 Autologous Venous Tissue** **A Autologous Arterial Tissue** **J Synthetic Substitute** **K Nonautologous Tissue Substitute** **Z No Device**	**3 Renal Artery, Right** **4 Renal Artery, Left** **5 Renal Artery, Bilateral**
E Internal Iliac Artery, Right Deferential artery Hypogastric artery Iliolumbar artery Inferior gluteal artery Inferior vesical artery Internal pudendal artery Lateral sacral artery Middle rectal artery Obturator artery Superior gluteal artery Umbilical artery Uterine artery Vaginal artery **F Internal Iliac Artery, Left** *See E Internal Iliac Artery, Right* **H External Iliac Artery, Right** Deep circumflex iliac artery Inferior epigastric artery **J External Iliac Artery, Left** *See H External Iliac Artery, Right*	**Ø Open** **4 Percutaneous Endoscopic**	**9 Autologous Venous Tissue** **A Autologous Arterial Tissue** **J Synthetic Substitute** **K Nonautologous Tissue Substitute** **Z No Device**	**9 Internal Iliac Artery, Right** **B Internal Iliac Artery, Left** **C Internal Iliac Arteries, Bilateral** **D External Iliac Artery, Right** **F External Iliac Artery, Left** **G External Iliac Arteries, Bilateral** **H Femoral Artery, Right** **J Femoral Artery, Left** **K Femoral Arteries, Bilateral** **P Foot Artery** **Q Lower Extremity Artery**
K Femoral Artery, Right Circumflex iliac artery Deep femoral artery Descending genicular artery External pudendal artery Superficial epigastric artery **L Femoral Artery, Left** *See K Femoral Artery, Right*	**Ø Open** **4 Percutaneous Endoscopic**	**9 Autologous Venous Tissue** **A Autologous Arterial Tissue** **J Synthetic Substitute** **K Nonautologous Tissue Substitute** **Z No Device**	**H Femoral Artery, Right** **J Femoral Artery, Left** **K Femoral Arteries, Bilateral** **L Popliteal Artery** **M Peroneal Artery** **N Posterior Tibial Artery** **P Foot Artery** **Q Lower Extremity Artery** **S Lower Extremity Vein**
K Femoral Artery, Right Circumflex iliac artery Deep femoral artery Descending genicular artery External pudendal artery Superficial epigastric artery **L Femoral Artery, Left** *See K Femoral Artery, Right*	**3 Percutaneous**	**J Synthetic Substitute**	**Q Lower Extremity Artery** **S Lower Extremity Vein**
M Popliteal Artery, Right Inferior genicular artery Middle genicular artery Superior genicular artery Sural artery Tibioperoneal trunk **N Popliteal Artery, Left** *See M Popliteal Artery, Right*	**Ø Open** **4 Percutaneous Endoscopic**	**9 Autologous Venous Tissue** **A Autologous Arterial Tissue** **J Synthetic Substitute** **K Nonautologous Tissue Substitute** **Z No Device**	**L Popliteal Artery** **M Peroneal Artery** **P Foot Artery** **Q Lower Extremity Artery** **S Lower Extremity Vein**

Ø41 Continued on next page

Ø41 Continued

Ø Medical and Surgical
4 Lower Arteries
1 Bypass Definition: Altering the route of passage of the contents of a tubular body part

Explanation: Rerouting contents of a body part to a downstream area of the normal route, to a similar route and body part, or to an abnormal route and dissimilar body part. Includes one or more anastomoses, with or without the use of a device.

Body Part Character 4	Approach Character 5	Device Character 6	Qualifier Character 7
M Popliteal Artery, Right Inferior genicular artery Middle genicular artery Superior genicular artery Sural artery Tibioperoneal trunk **N Popliteal Artery, Left** *See M Popliteal Artery, Right*	**3 Percutaneous**	**J Synthetic Substitute**	**Q Lower Extremity Artery** **S Lower Extremity Vein**
P Anterior Tibial Artery, Right Anterior lateral malleolar artery Anterior medial malleolar artery Anterior tibial recurrent artery Dorsalis pedis artery Posterior tibial recurrent artery **Q Anterior Tibial Artery, Left** *See P Anterior Tibial Artery, Right* **R Posterior Tibial Artery, Right** **S Posterior Tibial Artery, Left**	**Ø Open** **3 Percutaneous** **4 Percutaneous Endoscopic**	**J Synthetic Substitute**	**Q Lower Extremity Artery** **S Lower Extremity Vein**
T Peroneal Artery, Right Fibular artery **U Peroneal Artery, Left** *See T Peroneal Artery, Right* **V Foot Artery, Right** Arcuate artery Dorsal metatarsal artery Lateral plantar artery Lateral tarsal artery Medial plantar artery **W Foot Artery, Left** *See V Foot Artery, Right*	**Ø Open** **4 Percutaneous Endoscopic**	**9 Autologous Venous Tissue** **A Autologous Arterial Tissue** **J Synthetic Substitute** **K Nonautologous Tissue Substitute** **Z No Device**	**P Foot Artery** **Q Lower Extremity Artery** **S Lower Extremity Vein**
T Peroneal Artery, Right Fibular artery **U Peroneal Artery, Left** *See T Peroneal Artery, Right* **V Foot Artery, Right** Arcuate artery Dorsal metatarsal artery Lateral plantar artery Lateral tarsal artery Medial plantar artery **W Foot Artery, Left** *See V Foot Artery, Right*	**3 Percutaneous**	**J Synthetic Substitute**	**Q Lower Extremity Artery** **S Lower Extremity Vein**

Ø Medical and Surgical
4 Lower Arteries
5 Destruction Definition: Physical eradication of all or a portion of a body part by the direct use of energy, force, or a destructive agent
Explanation: None of the body part is physically taken out

Body Part Character 4		Approach Character 5	Device Character 6	Qualifier Character 7
Ø Abdominal Aorta Inferior phrenic artery Lumbar artery Median sacral artery Middle suprarenal artery Ovarian artery Testicular artery **1 Celiac Artery** Celiac trunk **2 Gastric Artery** Left gastric artery Right gastric artery **3 Hepatic Artery** Common hepatic artery Gastroduodenal artery Hepatic artery proper **4 Splenic Artery** Left gastroepiploic artery Pancreatic artery Short gastric artery **5 Superior Mesenteric Artery** Ileal artery Ileocolic artery Inferior pancreaticoduodenal artery Jejunal artery **6 Colic Artery, Right** **7 Colic Artery, Left** **8 Colic Artery, Middle** **9 Renal Artery, Right** Inferior suprarenal artery Renal segmental artery **A Renal Artery, Left** *See 9 Renal Artery, Right* **B Inferior Mesenteric Artery** Sigmoid artery Superior rectal artery **C Common Iliac Artery, Right** **D Common Iliac Artery, Left** **E Internal Iliac Artery, Right** Deferential artery Hypogastric artery Iliolumbar artery Inferior gluteal artery Inferior vesical artery Internal pudendal artery Lateral sacral artery Middle rectal artery Obturator artery Superior gluteal artery Umbilical artery Uterine artery Vaginal artery	**F Internal Iliac Artery, Left** *See E Internal Iliac Artery, Right* **H External Iliac Artery, Right** Deep circumflex iliac artery Inferior epigastric artery **J External Iliac Artery, Left** *See H External Iliac Artery, Right* **K Femoral Artery, Right** Circumflex iliac artery Deep femoral artery Descending genicular artery External pudendal artery Superficial epigastric artery **L Femoral Artery, Left** *See K Femoral Artery, Right* **M Popliteal Artery, Right** Inferior genicular artery Middle genicular artery Superior genicular artery Sural artery Tibioperoneal trunk **N Popliteal Artery, Left** *See M Popliteal Artery, Right* **P Anterior Tibial Artery, Right** Anterior lateral malleolar artery Anterior medial malleolar artery Anterior tibial recurrent artery Dorsalis pedis artery Posterior tibial recurrent artery **Q Anterior Tibial Artery, Left** *See P Anterior Tibial Artery, Right* **R Posterior Tibial Artery, Right** **S Posterior Tibial Artery, Left** **T Peroneal Artery, Right** Fibular artery **U Peroneal Artery, Left** *See T Peroneal Artery, Right* **V Foot Artery, Right** Arcuate artery Dorsal metatarsal artery Lateral plantar artery Lateral tarsal artery Medial plantar artery **W Foot Artery, Left** *See V Foot Artery, Right* **Y Lower Artery** Umbilical artery	**Ø Open** **3 Percutaneous** **4 Percutaneous Endoscopic**	**Z No Device**	**Z No Qualifier**

Ø Medical and Surgical
4 Lower Arteries
7 Dilation

Definition: Expanding an orifice or the lumen of a tubular body part

Explanation: The orifice can be a natural orifice or an artificially created orifice. Accomplished by stretching a tubular body part using intraluminal pressure or by cutting part of the orifice or wall of the tubular body part.

Body Part Character 4		Approach Character 5	Device Character 6	Qualifier Character 7
Ø Abdominal Aorta Inferior phrenic artery Lumbar artery Median sacral artery Middle suprarenal artery Ovarian artery Testicular artery **1 Celiac Artery** Celiac trunk **2 Gastric Artery** Left gastric artery Right gastric artery **3 Hepatic Artery** Common hepatic artery Gastroduodenal artery Hepatic artery proper **4 Splenic Artery** Left gastroepiploic artery Pancreatic artery Short gastric artery **5 Superior Mesenteric Artery** Ileal artery Ileocolic artery Inferior pancreaticoduodenal artery Jejunal artery **6 Colic Artery, Right** **7 Colic Artery, Left** **8 Colic Artery, Middle** **9 Renal Artery, Right** Inferior suprarenal artery Renal segmental artery **A Renal Artery, Left** *See 9 Renal Artery, Right* **B Inferior Mesenteric Artery** Sigmoid artery Superior rectal artery **C Common Iliac Artery, Right** **D Common Iliac Artery, Left** **E Internal Iliac Artery, Right** Deferential artery Hypogastric artery Iliolumbar artery Inferior gluteal artery Inferior vesical artery Internal pudendal artery Lateral sacral artery Middle rectal artery Obturator artery Superior gluteal artery Umbilical artery Uterine artery Vaginal artery	**F Internal Iliac Artery, Left** *See E Internal Iliac Artery, Right* **H External Iliac Artery, Right** Deep circumflex iliac artery Inferior epigastric artery **J External Iliac Artery, Left** *See H External Iliac Artery, Right* **K Femoral Artery, Right** Circumflex iliac artery Deep femoral artery Descending genicular artery External pudendal artery Superficial epigastric artery **L Femoral Artery, Left** *See K Femoral Artery, Right* **M Popliteal Artery, Right** Inferior genicular artery Middle genicular artery Superior genicular artery Sural artery Tibioperoneal trunk **N Popliteal Artery, Left** *See M Popliteal Artery, Right* **P Anterior Tibial Artery, Right** Anterior lateral malleolar artery Anterior medial malleolar artery Anterior tibial recurrent artery Dorsalis pedis artery Posterior tibial recurrent artery **Q Anterior Tibial Artery, Left** *See P Anterior Tibial Artery, Right* **R Posterior Tibial Artery, Right** **S Posterior Tibial Artery, Left** **T Peroneal Artery, Right** Fibular artery **U Peroneal Artery, Left** *See T Peroneal Artery, Right* **V Foot Artery, Right** Arcuate artery Dorsal metatarsal artery Lateral plantar artery Lateral tarsal artery Medial plantar artery **W Foot Artery, Left** *See V Foot Artery, Right* **Y Lower Artery** Umbilical artery	**Ø Open** **3 Percutaneous** **4 Percutaneous Endoscopic**	**4 Intraluminal Device, Drug-eluting** **D Intraluminal Device** **Z No Device**	**1 Drug-Coated Balloon** **Z No Qualifier**

Ø47 Continued on next page

Ø Medical and Surgical
4 Lower Arteries
7 Dilation Definition: Expanding an orifice or the lumen of a tubular body part

Explanation: The orifice can be a natural orifice or an artificially created orifice. Accomplished by stretching a tubular body part using intraluminal pressure or by cutting part of the orifice or wall of the tubular body part.

Ø47 Continued

Body Part Character 4		Approach Character 5	Device Character 6	Qualifier Character 7
Ø Abdominal Aorta Inferior phrenic artery Lumbar artery Median sacral artery Middle suprarenal artery Ovarian artery Testicular artery **1 Celiac Artery** Celiac trunk **2 Gastric Artery** Left gastric artery Right gastric artery **3 Hepatic Artery** Common hepatic artery Gastroduodenal artery Hepatic artery proper **4 Splenic Artery** Left gastroepiploic artery Pancreatic artery Short gastric artery **5 Superior Mesenteric Artery** Ileal artery Ileocolic artery Inferior pancreaticoduodenal artery Jejunal artery **6 Colic Artery, Right** **7 Colic Artery, Left** **8 Colic Artery, Middle** **9 Renal Artery, Right** Inferior suprarenal artery Renal segmental artery **A Renal Artery, Left** ***See*** *9 Renal Artery, Right* **B Inferior Mesenteric Artery** Sigmoid artery Superior rectal artery **C Common Iliac Artery, Right** **D Common Iliac Artery, Left** **E Internal Iliac Artery, Right** Deferential artery Hypogastric artery Iliolumbar artery Inferior gluteal artery Inferior vesical artery Internal pudendal artery Lateral sacral artery Middle rectal artery Obturator artery Superior gluteal artery Umbilical artery Uterine artery Vaginal artery	**F Internal Iliac Artery, Left** ***See*** *E Internal Iliac Artery, Right* **H External Iliac Artery, Right** Deep circumflex iliac artery Inferior epigastric artery **J External Iliac Artery, Left** ***See*** *H External Iliac Artery, Right* **K Femoral Artery, Right** Circumflex iliac artery Deep femoral artery Descending genicular artery External pudendal artery Superficial epigastric artery **L Femoral Artery, Left** ***See*** *K Femoral Artery, Right* **M Popliteal Artery, Right** Inferior genicular artery Middle genicular artery Superior genicular artery Sural artery Tibioperoneal trunk **N Popliteal Artery, Left** ***See*** *M Popliteal Artery, Right* **P Anterior Tibial Artery, Right** Anterior lateral malleolar artery Anterior medial malleolar artery Anterior tibial recurrent artery Dorsalis pedis artery Posterior tibial recurrent artery **Q Anterior Tibial Artery, Left** ***See*** *P Anterior Tibial Artery, Right* **R Posterior Tibial Artery, Right** **S Posterior Tibial Artery, Left** **T Peroneal Artery, Right** Fibular artery **U Peroneal Artery, Left** ***See*** *T Peroneal Artery, Right* **V Foot Artery, Right** Arcuate artery Dorsal metatarsal artery Lateral plantar artery Lateral tarsal artery Medial plantar artery **W Foot Artery, Left** ***See*** *V Foot Artery, Right* **Y Lower Artery** Umbilical artery	**Ø Open** **3 Percutaneous** **4 Percutaneous Endoscopic**	**5 Intraluminal Device, Drug-eluting, Two** **6 Intraluminal Device, Drug-eluting, Three** **7 Intraluminal Device, Drug-eluting, Four or More** **E Intraluminal Device, Two** **F Intraluminal Device, Three** **G Intraluminal Device, Four or More**	**Z No Qualifier**

Ø Medical and Surgical
4 Lower Arteries
9 Drainage Definition: Taking or letting out fluids and/or gases from a body part
Explanation: The qualifier DIAGNOSTIC is used to identify drainage procedures that are biopsies

Body Part Character 4		Approach Character 5	Device Character 6	Qualifier Character 7
Ø Abdominal Aorta Inferior phrenic artery Lumbar artery Median sacral artery Middle suprarenal artery Ovarian artery Testicular artery **1 Celiac Artery** Celiac trunk **2 Gastric Artery** Left gastric artery Right gastric artery **3 Hepatic Artery** Common hepatic artery Gastroduodenal artery Hepatic artery proper **4 Splenic Artery** Left gastroepiploic artery Pancreatic artery Short gastric artery **5 Superior Mesenteric Artery** Ileal artery Ileocolic artery Inferior pancreaticoduodenal artery Jejunal artery **6 Colic Artery, Right** **7 Colic Artery, Left** **8 Colic Artery, Middle** **9 Renal Artery, Right** Inferior suprarenal artery Renal segmental artery **A Renal Artery, Left** ***See*** *9 Renal Artery, Right* **B Inferior Mesenteric Artery** Sigmoid artery Superior rectal artery **C Common Iliac Artery, Right** **D Common Iliac Artery, Left** **E Internal Iliac Artery, Right** Deferential artery Hypogastric artery Iliolumbar artery Inferior gluteal artery Inferior vesical artery Internal pudendal artery Lateral sacral artery Middle rectal artery Obturator artery Superior gluteal artery Umbilical artery Uterine artery Vaginal artery	**F Internal Iliac Artery, Left** ***See*** *E Internal Iliac Artery, Right* **H External Iliac Artery, Right** Deep circumflex iliac artery Inferior epigastric artery **J External Iliac Artery, Left** ***See*** *H External Iliac Artery, Right* **K Femoral Artery, Right** Circumflex iliac artery Deep femoral artery Descending genicular artery External pudendal artery Superficial epigastric artery **L Femoral Artery, Left** ***See*** *K Femoral Artery, Right* **M Popliteal Artery, Right** Inferior genicular artery Middle genicular artery Superior genicular artery Sural artery Tibioperoneal trunk **N Popliteal Artery, Left** ***See*** *M Popliteal Artery, Right* **P Anterior Tibial Artery, Right** Anterior lateral malleolar artery Anterior medial malleolar artery Anterior tibial recurrent artery Dorsalis pedis artery Posterior tibial recurrent artery **Q Anterior Tibial Artery, Left** ***See*** *P Anterior Tibial Artery, Right* **R Posterior Tibial Artery, Right** **S Posterior Tibial Artery, Left** **T Peroneal Artery, Right** Fibular artery **U Peroneal Artery, Left** ***See*** *T Peroneal Artery, Right* **V Foot Artery, Right** Arcuate artery Dorsal metatarsal artery Lateral plantar artery Lateral tarsal artery Medial plantar artery **W Foot Artery, Left** ***See*** *V Foot Artery, Right* **Y Lower Artery** Umbilical artery	**Ø Open** **3 Percutaneous** **4 Percutaneous Endoscopic**	**Ø Drainage Device**	**Z No Qualifier**

Non-OR Ø49[Ø,1,2,3,4,5,6,7,8,9,A,B,C,D,E,F,H,J,K,L,M,N,P,Q,R,S,T,U,V,W,Y][Ø,3,4]ØZ

Ø49 Continued on next page

Ø Medical and Surgical
4 Lower Arteries
9 Drainage Definition: Taking or letting out fluids and/or gases from a body part
Explanation: The qualifier DIAGNOSTIC is used to identify drainage procedures that are biopsies

Ø49 Continued

Body Part Character 4	Body Part Character 4 (cont.)	Approach Character 5	Device Character 6	Qualifier Character 7
Ø Abdominal Aorta Inferior phrenic artery Lumbar artery Median sacral artery Middle suprarenal artery Ovarian artery Testicular artery **1 Celiac Artery** Celiac trunk **2 Gastric Artery** Left gastric artery Right gastric artery **3 Hepatic Artery** Common hepatic artery Gastroduodenal artery Hepatic artery proper **4 Splenic Artery** Left gastroepiploic artery Pancreatic artery Short gastric artery **5 Superior Mesenteric Artery** Ileal artery Ileocolic artery Inferior pancreaticoduodenal artery Jejunal artery **6 Colic Artery, Right** **7 Colic Artery, Left** **8 Colic Artery, Middle** **9 Renal Artery, Right** Inferior suprarenal artery Renal segmental artery **A Renal Artery, Left** *See 9 Renal Artery, Right* **B Inferior Mesenteric Artery** Sigmoid artery Superior rectal artery **C Common Iliac Artery, Right** **D Common Iliac Artery, Left** **E Internal Iliac Artery, Right** Deferential artery Hypogastric artery Iliolumbar artery Inferior gluteal artery Inferior vesical artery Internal pudendal artery Lateral sacral artery Middle rectal artery Obturator artery Superior gluteal artery Umbilical artery Uterine artery Vaginal artery	**F Internal Iliac Artery, Left** *See E Internal Iliac Artery, Right* **H External Iliac Artery, Right** Deep circumflex iliac artery Inferior epigastric artery **J External Iliac Artery, Left** *See H External Iliac Artery, Right* **K Femoral Artery, Right** Circumflex iliac artery Deep femoral artery Descending genicular artery External pudendal artery Superficial epigastric artery **L Femoral Artery, Left** *See K Femoral Artery, Right* **M Popliteal Artery, Right** Inferior genicular artery Middle genicular artery Superior genicular artery Sural artery Tibioperoneal trunk **N Popliteal Artery, Left** *See M Popliteal Artery, Right* **P Anterior Tibial Artery, Right** Anterior lateral malleolar artery Anterior medial malleolar artery Anterior tibial recurrent artery Dorsalis pedis artery Posterior tibial recurrent artery **Q Anterior Tibial Artery, Left** *See P Anterior Tibial Artery, Right* **R Posterior Tibial Artery, Right** **S Posterior Tibial Artery, Left** **T Peroneal Artery, Right** Fibular artery **U Peroneal Artery, Left** *See T Peroneal Artery, Right* **V Foot Artery, Right** Arcuate artery Dorsal metatarsal artery Lateral plantar artery Lateral tarsal artery Medial plantar artery **W Foot Artery, Left** *See V Foot Artery, Right* **Y Lower Artery** Umbilical artery	**Ø Open** **3 Percutaneous** **4 Percutaneous Endoscopic**	**Z No Device**	**X Diagnostic** **Z No Qualifier**

Non-OR Ø49[Ø,1,2,3,4,5,6,7,8,9,A,B,C,D,E,F,H,J,K,L,M,N,P,Q,R,S,T,U,V,W,Y]3ZX
Non-OR Ø49[Ø,1,2,3,4,5,6,7,8,9,A,B,C,D,E,F,H,J,K,L,M,N,P,Q,R,S,T,U,V,W,Y][Ø,3,4]ZZ

Ø Medical and Surgical
4 Lower Arteries
B Excision Definition: Cutting out or off, without replacement, a portion of a body part
Explanation: The qualifier DIAGNOSTIC is used to identify excision procedures that are biopsies

Body Part Character 4	Approach Character 5	Device Character 6	Qualifier Character 7
Ø Abdominal Aorta Inferior phrenic artery Lumbar artery Median sacral artery Middle suprarenal artery Ovarian artery Testicular artery	**Ø Open**	**Z No Device**	**X Diagnostic**
1 Celiac Artery Celiac trunk	**3 Percutaneous**		**Z No Qualifier**
2 Gastric Artery Left gastric artery Right gastric artery	**4 Percutaneous Endoscopic**		
3 Hepatic Artery Common hepatic artery Gastroduodenal artery Hepatic artery proper			
4 Splenic Artery Left gastroepiploic artery Pancreatic artery Short gastric artery			
5 Superior Mesenteric Artery Ileal artery Ileocolic artery Inferior pancreaticoduodenal artery Jejunal artery			
6 Colic Artery, Right			
7 Colic Artery, Left			
8 Colic Artery, Middle			
9 Renal Artery, Right Inferior suprarenal artery Renal segmental artery			
A Renal Artery, Left *See 9 Renal Artery, Right*			
B Inferior Mesenteric Artery Sigmoid artery Superior rectal artery			
C Common Iliac Artery, Right			
D Common Iliac Artery, Left			
E Internal Iliac Artery, Right Deferential artery Hypogastric artery Iliolumbar artery Inferior gluteal artery Inferior vesical artery Internal pudendal artery Lateral sacral artery Middle rectal artery Obturator artery Superior gluteal artery Umbilical artery Uterine artery Vaginal artery			
F Internal Iliac Artery, Left *See E Internal Iliac Artery, Right*			
H External Iliac Artery, Right Deep circumflex iliac artery Inferior epigastric artery			
J External Iliac Artery, Left *See H External Iliac Artery, Right*			
K Femoral Artery, Right Circumflex iliac artery Deep femoral artery Descending genicular artery External pudendal artery Superficial epigastric artery			
L Femoral Artery, Left *See K Femoral Artery, Right*			
M Popliteal Artery, Right Inferior genicular artery Middle genicular artery Superior genicular artery Sural artery Tibioperoneal trunk			
N Popliteal Artery, Left *See M Popliteal Artery, Right*			
P Anterior Tibial Artery, Right Anterior lateral malleolar artery Anterior medial malleolar artery Anterior tibial recurrent artery Dorsalis pedis artery Posterior tibial recurrent artery			
Q Anterior Tibial Artery, Left *See P Anterior Tibial Artery, Right*			
R Posterior Tibial Artery, Right			
S Posterior Tibial Artery, Left			
T Peroneal Artery, Right Fibular artery			
U Peroneal Artery, Left *See T Peroneal Artery, Right*			
V Foot Artery, Right Arcuate artery Dorsal metatarsal artery Lateral plantar artery Lateral tarsal artery Medial plantar artery			
W Foot Artery, Left *See V Foot Artery, Right*			
Y Lower Artery Umbilical artery			

Ø Medical and Surgical
4 Lower Arteries
C Extirpation Definition: Taking or cutting out solid matter from a body part

Explanation: The solid matter may be an abnormal byproduct of a biological function or a foreign body; it may be imbedded in a body part or in the lumen of a tubular body part. The solid matter may or may not have been previously broken into pieces.

Body Part Character 4		Approach Character 5	Device Character 6	Qualifier Character 7
Ø Abdominal Aorta Inferior phrenic artery Lumbar artery Median sacral artery Middle suprarenal artery Ovarian artery Testicular artery **1 Celiac Artery** Celiac trunk **2 Gastric Artery** Left gastric artery Right gastric artery **3 Hepatic Artery** Common hepatic artery Gastroduodenal artery Hepatic artery proper **4 Splenic Artery** Left gastroepiploic artery Pancreatic artery Short gastric artery **5 Superior Mesenteric Artery** Ileal artery Ileocolic artery Inferior pancreaticoduodenal artery Jejunal artery **6 Colic Artery, Right** **7 Colic Artery, Left** **8 Colic Artery, Middle** **9 Renal Artery, Right** Inferior suprarenal artery Renal segmental artery **A Renal Artery, Left** *See 9 Renal Artery, Right* **B Inferior Mesenteric Artery** Sigmoid artery Superior rectal artery **C Common Iliac Artery, Right** **D Common Iliac Artery, Left** **E Internal Iliac Artery, Right** Deferential artery Hypogastric artery Iliolumbar artery Inferior gluteal artery Inferior vesical artery Internal pudendal artery Lateral sacral artery Middle rectal artery Obturator artery Superior gluteal artery Umbilical artery Uterine artery Vaginal artery	**F Internal Iliac Artery, Left** *See E Internal Iliac Artery, Right* **H External Iliac Artery, Right** Deep circumflex iliac artery Inferior epigastric artery **J External Iliac Artery, Left** *See H External Iliac Artery, Right* **K Femoral Artery, Right** Circumflex iliac artery Deep femoral artery Descending genicular artery External pudendal artery Superficial epigastric artery **L Femoral Artery, Left** *See K Femoral Artery, Right* **M Popliteal Artery, Right** Inferior genicular artery Middle genicular artery Superior genicular artery Sural artery Tibioperoneal trunk **N Popliteal Artery, Left** *See M Popliteal Artery, Right* **P Anterior Tibial Artery, Right** Anterior lateral malleolar artery Anterior medial malleolar artery Anterior tibial recurrent artery Dorsalis pedis artery Posterior tibial recurrent artery **Q Anterior Tibial Artery, Left** *See P Anterior Tibial Artery, Right* **R Posterior Tibial Artery, Right** **S Posterior Tibial Artery, Left** **T Peroneal Artery, Right** Fibular artery **U Peroneal Artery, Left** *See T Peroneal Artery, Right* **V Foot Artery, Right** Arcuate artery Dorsal metatarsal artery Lateral plantar artery Lateral tarsal artery Medial plantar artery **W Foot Artery, Left** *See V Foot Artery, Right* **Y Lower Artery** Umbilical artery	**Ø Open** **3 Percutaneous** **4 Percutaneous Endoscopic**	**Z No Device**	**Z No Qualifier**

Ø Medical and Surgical
4 Lower Arteries
F Fragmentation Definition: Breaking solid matter in a body part into pieces

Explanation: Physical force (e.g., manual, ultrasonic) applied directly or indirectly is used to break the solid matter into pieces. The solid matter may be an abnormal byproduct of a biological function or a foreign body. The pieces of solid matter are not taken out.

Body Part Character 4	Approach Character 5	Device Character 6	Qualifier Character 7
C Common Iliac Artery, Right **D Common Iliac Artery, Left** **E Internal Iliac Artery, Right** Deferential artery Hypogastric artery Iliolumbar artery Inferior gluteal artery Inferior vesical artery Internal pudendal artery Lateral sacral artery Middle rectal artery Obturator artery Superior gluteal artery Umbilical artery Uterine artery Vaginal artery **F Internal Iliac Artery, Left** *See E Internal Iliac Artery, Right* **H External Iliac Artery, Right** Deep circumflex iliac artery Inferior epigastric artery **J External Iliac Artery, Left** *See H External Iliac Artery, Right* **K Femoral Artery, Right** Circumflex iliac artery Deep femoral artery Descending genicular artery External pudendal artery Superficial epigastric artery **L Femoral Artery, Left** *See K Femoral Artery, Right* **M Popliteal Artery, Right** Inferior genicular artery Middle genicular artery Superior genicular artery Sural artery Tibioperoneal trunk **N Popliteal Artery, Left** *See M Popliteal Artery, Right* **P Anterior Tibial Artery, Right** Anterior lateral malleolar artery Anterior medial malleolar artery Anterior tibial recurrent artery Dorsalis pedis artery Posterior tibial recurrent artery **Q Anterior Tibial Artery, Left** *See P Anterior Tibial Artery, Right* **R Posterior Tibial Artery, Right** **S Posterior Tibial Artery, Left** **T Peroneal Artery, Right** Fibular artery **U Peroneal Artery, Left** *See T Peroneal Artery, Right* **Y Lower Artery** Umbilical artery	**3 Percutaneous**	**Z No Device**	**Ø Ultrasonic** **Z No Qualifier**

Ø Medical and Surgical
4 Lower Arteries
H Insertion Definition: Putting in a nonbiological appliance that monitors, assists, performs, or prevents a physiological function but does not physically take the place of a body part

Explanation: None

Body Part Character 4	Approach Character 5	Device Character 6	Qualifier Character 7
Ø Abdominal Aorta Inferior phrenic artery Lumbar artery Median sacral artery Middle suprarenal artery Ovarian artery Testicular artery	**Ø Open** **3 Percutaneous** **4 Percutaneous Endoscopic**	**2 Monitoring Device** **3 Infusion Device** **D Intraluminal Device**	**Z No Qualifier**
1 Celiac Artery Celiac trunk **2 Gastric Artery** Left gastric artery Right gastric artery **3 Hepatic Artery** Common hepatic artery Gastroduodenal artery Hepatic artery proper **4 Splenic Artery** Left gastroepiploic artery Pancreatic artery Short gastric artery **5 Superior Mesenteric Artery** Ileal artery Ileocolic artery Inferior pancreaticoduodenal artery Jejunal artery **6 Colic Artery, Right** **7 Colic Artery, Left** **8 Colic Artery, Middle** **9 Renal Artery, Right** Inferior suprarenal artery Renal segmental artery **A Renal Artery, Left** ***See*** *9 Renal Artery, Right* **B Inferior Mesenteric Artery** Sigmoid artery Superior rectal artery **C Common Iliac Artery, Right** **D Common Iliac Artery, Left** **E Internal Iliac Artery, Right** Deferential artery Hypogastric artery Iliolumbar artery Inferior gluteal artery Inferior vesical artery Internal pudendal artery Lateral sacral artery Middle rectal artery Obturator artery Superior gluteal artery Umbilical artery Uterine artery Vaginal artery **F Internal Iliac Artery, Left** ***See*** *E Internal Iliac Artery, Right* **H External Iliac Artery, Right** Deep circumflex iliac artery Inferior epigastric artery **J External Iliac Artery, Left** ***See*** *H External Iliac Artery, Right* **K Femoral Artery, Right** Circumflex iliac artery Deep femoral artery Descending genicular artery External pudendal artery Superficial epigastric artery **L Femoral Artery, Left** ***See*** *K Femoral Artery, Right* **M Popliteal Artery, Right** Inferior genicular artery Middle genicular artery Superior genicular artery Sural artery Tibioperoneal trunk **N Popliteal Artery, Left** ***See*** *M Popliteal Artery, Right* **P Anterior Tibial Artery, Right** Anterior lateral malleolar artery Anterior medial malleolar artery Anterior tibial recurrent artery Dorsalis pedis artery Posterior tibial recurrent artery **Q Anterior Tibial Artery, Left** ***See*** *P Anterior Tibial Artery, Right* **R Posterior Tibial Artery, Right** **S Posterior Tibial Artery, Left** **T Peroneal Artery, Right** Fibular artery **U Peroneal Artery, Left** ***See*** *T Peroneal Artery, Right* **V Foot Artery, Right** Arcuate artery Dorsal metatarsal artery Lateral plantar artery Lateral tarsal artery Medial plantar artery **W Foot Artery, Left** ***See*** *V Foot Artery, Right*	**Ø Open** **3 Percutaneous** **4 Percutaneous Endoscopic**	**3 Infusion Device** **D Intraluminal Device**	**Z No Qualifier**
Y Lower Artery Umbilical artery	**Ø Open** **3 Percutaneous** **4 Percutaneous Endoscopic**	**2 Monitoring Device** **3 Infusion Device** **D Intraluminal Device** **Y Other Device**	**Z No Qualifier**

Non-OR Ø4HØ[Ø,3,4][2,3]Z
Non-OR Ø4H[1,2,3,4,5,6,7,8,9,A,B,C,D,E,F,H,J,K,L,M,N,P,Q,R,S,T,U,V,W][Ø,3,4]3Z
Non-OR Ø4HY32Z
Non-OR Ø4HY[Ø,3,4]3Z
Non-OR Ø4HY[3,4]YZ

Ø Medical and Surgical
4 Lower Arteries
J Inspection Definition: Visually and/or manually exploring a body part

Explanation: Visual exploration may be performed with or without optical instrumentation. Manual exploration may be performed directly or through intervening body layers.

Body Part Character 4	Approach Character 5	Device Character 6	Qualifier Character 7
Y Lower Artery Umbilical artery	**Ø** Open **3** Percutaneous **4** Percutaneous Endoscopic **X** External	**Z** No Device	**Z** No Qualifier

Non-OR Ø4JY[3,4,X]ZZ

Ø Medical and Surgical
4 Lower Arteries
L Occlusion Definition: Completely closing an orifice or the lumen of a tubular body part

Explanation: The orifice can be a natural orifice or an artificially created orifice

Body Part Character 4	Approach Character 5	Device Character 6	Qualifier Character 7
Ø **Abdominal Aorta** Inferior phrenic artery Lumbar artery Median sacral artery Middle suprarenal artery Ovarian artery Testicular artery	**Ø** Open **4** Percutaneous Endoscopic	**C** Extraluminal Device **D** Intraluminal Device **Z** No Device	**Z** No Qualifier
Ø **Abdominal Aorta** Inferior phrenic artery Lumbar artery Median sacral artery Middle suprarenal artery Ovarian artery Testicular artery	**3** Percutaneous	**C** Extraluminal Device **Z** No Device	**Z** No Qualifier
Ø **Abdominal Aorta** Inferior phrenic artery Lumbar artery Median sacral artery Middle suprarenal artery Ovarian artery Testicular artery	**3** Percutaneous	**D** Intraluminal Device	**J** Temporary **Z** No Qualifier

Ø4L Continued on next page

Ø Medical and Surgical
4 Lower Arteries
L Occlusion Definition: Completely closing an orifice or the lumen of a tubular body part
Explanation: The orifice can be a natural orifice or an artificially created orifice

Ø4L Continued

Body Part Character 4	Approach Character 5	Device Character 6	Qualifier Character 7
1 Celiac Artery Celiac trunk **2 Gastric Artery** Left gastric artery, Right gastric artery **3 Hepatic Artery** Common hepatic artery, Gastroduodenal artery, Hepatic artery proper **4 Splenic Artery** Left gastroepiploic artery, Pancreatic artery, Short gastric artery **5 Superior Mesenteric Artery** Ileal artery, Ileocolic artery, Inferior pancreaticoduodenal artery, Jejunal artery **6 Colic Artery, Right** **7 Colic Artery, Left** **8 Colic Artery, Middle** **9 Renal Artery, Right** Inferior suprarenal artery, Renal segmental artery **A Renal Artery, Left** *See 9 Renal Artery, Right* **B Inferior Mesenteric Artery** Sigmoid artery, Superior rectal artery **C Common Iliac Artery, Right** **D Common Iliac Artery, Left** **H External Iliac Artery, Right** Deep circumflex iliac artery, Inferior epigastric artery **J External Iliac Artery, Left** *See H External Iliac Artery, Right* **K Femoral Artery, Right** Circumflex iliac artery, Deep femoral artery, Descending genicular artery, External pudendal artery, Superficial epigastric artery **L Femoral Artery, Left** *See K Femoral Artery, Right* **M Popliteal Artery, Right** Inferior genicular artery, Middle genicular artery, Superior genicular artery, Sural artery, Tibioperoneal trunk **N Popliteal Artery, Left** *See M Popliteal Artery, Right* **P Anterior Tibial Artery, Right** Anterior lateral malleolar artery, Anterior medial malleolar artery, Anterior tibial recurrent artery, Dorsalis pedis artery, Posterior tibial recurrent artery **Q Anterior Tibial Artery, Left** *See P Anterior Tibial Artery, Right* **R Posterior Tibial Artery, Right** **S Posterior Tibial Artery, Left** **T Peroneal Artery, Right** Fibular artery **U Peroneal Artery, Left** *See T Peroneal Artery, Right* **V Foot Artery, Right** Arcuate artery, Dorsal metatarsal artery, Lateral plantar artery, Lateral tarsal artery, Medial plantar artery **W Foot Artery, Left** *See V Foot Artery, Right* **Y Lower Artery** Umbilical artery	**Ø Open** **3 Percutaneous** **4 Percutaneous Endoscopic**	**C Extraluminal Device** **D Intraluminal Device** **Z No Device**	**Z No Qualifier**
E Internal Iliac Artery, Right Deferential artery, Hypogastric artery, Iliolumbar artery, Inferior gluteal artery, Inferior vesical artery, Internal pudendal artery, Lateral sacral artery, Middle rectal artery, Obturator artery, Superior gluteal artery, Umbilical artery, Uterine artery, Vaginal artery	**Ø Open** **3 Percutaneous** **4 Percutaneous Endoscopic**	**C Extraluminal Device** **D Intraluminal Device** **Z No Device**	**T Uterine Artery, Right** ♀ **Z No Qualifier**
F Internal Iliac Artery, Left Deferential artery, Hypogastric artery, Iliolumbar artery, Inferior gluteal artery, Inferior vesical artery, Internal pudendal artery, Lateral sacral artery, Middle rectal artery, Obturator artery, Superior gluteal artery, Umbilical artery, Uterine Artery, Vaginal artery	**Ø Open** **3 Percutaneous** **4 Percutaneous Endoscopic**	**C Extraluminal Device** **D Intraluminal Device** **Z No Device**	**U Uterine Artery, Left** ♀ **Z No Qualifier**

♀ Ø4LE[Ø,3,4][C,D,Z]T
♀ Ø4LF[Ø,3,4][C,D,Z]U

Ø Medical and Surgical
4 Lower Arteries
N Release Definition: Freeing a body part from an abnormal physical constraint by cutting or by the use of force
Explanation: Some of the restraining tissue may be taken out but none of the body part is taken out

Body Part Character 4	Approach Character 5	Device Character 6	Qualifier Character 7
Ø Abdominal Aorta Inferior phrenic artery Lumbar artery Median sacral artery Middle suprarenal artery Ovarian artery Testicular artery **1 Celiac Artery** Celiac trunk **2 Gastric Artery** Left gastric artery Right gastric artery **3 Hepatic Artery** Common hepatic artery Gastroduodenal artery Hepatic artery proper **4 Splenic Artery** Left gastroepiploic artery Pancreatic artery Short gastric artery **5 Superior Mesenteric Artery** Ileal artery Ileocolic artery Inferior pancreaticoduodenal artery Jejunal artery **6 Colic Artery, Right** **7 Colic Artery, Left** **8 Colic Artery, Middle** **9 Renal Artery, Right** Inferior suprarenal artery Renal segmental artery **A Renal Artery, Left** *See 9 Renal Artery, Right* **B Inferior Mesenteric Artery** Sigmoid artery Superior rectal artery **C Common Iliac Artery, Right** **D Common Iliac Artery, Left** **E Internal Iliac Artery, Right** Deferential artery Hypogastric artery Iliolumbar artery Inferior gluteal artery Inferior vesical artery Internal pudendal artery Lateral sacral artery Middle rectal artery Obturator artery Superior gluteal artery Umbilical artery Uterine artery Vaginal artery **F Internal Iliac Artery, Left** *See E Internal Iliac Artery, Right* **H External Iliac Artery, Right** Deep circumflex iliac artery Inferior epigastric artery **J External Iliac Artery, Left** *See H External Iliac Artery, Right* **K Femoral Artery, Right** Circumflex iliac artery Deep femoral artery Descending genicular artery External pudendal artery Superficial epigastric artery **L Femoral Artery, Left** *See K Femoral Artery, Right* **M Popliteal Artery, Right** Inferior genicular artery Middle genicular artery Superior genicular artery Sural artery Tibioperoneal trunk **N Popliteal Artery, Left** *See M Popliteal Artery, Right* **P Anterior Tibial Artery, Right** Anterior lateral malleolar artery Anterior medial malleolar artery Anterior tibial recurrent artery Dorsalis pedis artery Posterior tibial recurrent artery **Q Anterior Tibial Artery, Left** *See P Anterior Tibial Artery, Right* **R Posterior Tibial Artery, Right** **S Posterior Tibial Artery, Left** **T Peroneal Artery, Right** Fibular artery **U Peroneal Artery, Left** *See T Peroneal Artery, Right* **V Foot Artery, Right** Arcuate artery Dorsal metatarsal artery Lateral plantar artery Lateral tarsal artery Medial plantar artery **W Foot Artery, Left** *See V Foot Artery, Right* **Y Lower Artery** Umbilical artery	**Ø Open** **3 Percutaneous** **4 Percutaneous Endoscopic**	**Z No Device**	**Z No Qualifier**

Ø Medical and Surgical
4 Lower Arteries
P Removal Definition: Taking out or off a device from a body part

Explanation: If a device is taken out and a similar device put in without cutting or puncturing the skin or mucous membrane, the procedure is coded to the root operation CHANGE. Otherwise, the procedure for taking out a device is coded to the root operation REMOVAL.

Body Part Character 4	Approach Character 5	Device Character 6	Qualifier Character 7
Y Lower Artery Umbilical artery	Ø Open 3 Percutaneous 4 Percutaneous Endoscopic	Ø Drainage Device 2 Monitoring Device 3 Infusion Device 7 Autologous Tissue Substitute C Extraluminal Device D Intraluminal Device J Synthetic Substitute K Nonautologous Tissue Substitute Y Other Device	Z No Qualifier
Y Lower Artery Umbilical artery	X External	Ø Drainage Device 1 Radioactive Element 2 Monitoring Device 3 Infusion Device D Intraluminal Device	Z No Qualifier

Non-OR Ø4PY3[Ø,2,3,D]Z
Non-OR Ø4PY[3,4]YZ
Non-OR Ø4PYX[Ø,1,2,3,D]Z

Ø Medical and Surgical
4 Lower Arteries
Q Repair Definition: Restoring, to the extent possible, a body part to its normal anatomic structure and function
Explanation: Used only when the method to accomplish the repair is not one of the other root operations

Body Part Character 4	Approach Character 5	Device Character 6	Qualifier Character 7
Ø Abdominal Aorta Inferior phrenic artery Lumbar artery Median sacral artery Middle suprarenal artery Ovarian artery Testicular artery **1 Celiac Artery** Celiac trunk **2 Gastric Artery** Left gastric artery Right gastric artery **3 Hepatic Artery** Common hepatic artery Gastroduodenal artery Hepatic artery proper **4 Splenic Artery** Left gastroepiploic artery Pancreatic artery Short gastric artery **5 Superior Mesenteric Artery** Ileal artery Ileocolic artery Inferior pancreaticoduodenal artery Jejunal artery **6 Colic Artery, Right** **7 Colic Artery, Left** **8 Colic Artery, Middle** **9 Renal Artery, Right** Inferior suprarenal artery Renal segmental artery **A Renal Artery, Left** *See 9 Renal Artery, Right* **B Inferior Mesenteric Artery** Sigmoid artery Superior rectal artery **C Common Iliac Artery, Right** **D Common Iliac Artery, Left** **E Internal Iliac Artery, Right** Deferential artery Hypogastric artery Iliolumbar artery Inferior gluteal artery Inferior vesical artery Internal pudendal artery Lateral sacral artery Middle rectal artery Obturator artery Superior gluteal artery Umbilical artery Uterine artery Vaginal artery **F Internal Iliac Artery, Left** *See E Internal Iliac Artery, Right* **H External Iliac Artery, Right** Deep circumflex iliac artery Inferior epigastric artery **J External Iliac Artery, Left** *See H External Iliac Artery, Right* **K Femoral Artery, Right** Circumflex iliac artery Deep femoral artery Descending genicular artery External pudendal artery Superficial epigastric artery **L Femoral Artery, Left** *See K Femoral Artery, Right* **M Popliteal Artery, Right** Inferior genicular artery Middle genicular artery Superior genicular artery Sural artery Tibioperoneal trunk **N Popliteal Artery, Left** *See M Popliteal Artery, Right* **P Anterior Tibial Artery, Right** Anterior lateral malleolar artery Anterior medial malleolar artery Anterior tibial recurrent artery Dorsalis pedis artery Posterior tibial recurrent artery **Q Anterior Tibial Artery, Left** *See P Anterior Tibial Artery, Right* **R Posterior Tibial Artery, Right** **S Posterior Tibial Artery, Left** **T Peroneal Artery, Right** Fibular artery **U Peroneal Artery, Left** *See T Peroneal Artery, Right* **V Foot Artery, Right** Arcuate artery Dorsal metatarsal artery Lateral plantar artery Lateral tarsal artery Medial plantar artery **W Foot Artery, Left** *See V Foot Artery, Right* **Y Lower Artery** Umbilical artery	**Ø Open** **3 Percutaneous** **4 Percutaneous Endoscopic**	**Z No Device**	**Z No Qualifier**

Lower Arteries

Ø4Q–Ø4Q

Ø Medical and Surgical
4 Lower Arteries
R Replacement Definition: Putting in or on biological or synthetic material that physically takes the place and/or function of all or a portion of a body part

Explanation: The body part may have been taken out or replaced, or may be taken out, physically eradicated, or rendered nonfunctional during the REPLACEMENT procedure. A REMOVAL procedure is coded for taking out the device used in a previous replacement procedure.

Body Part Character 4		Approach Character 5	Device Character 6	Qualifier Character 7
Ø Abdominal Aorta Inferior phrenic artery Lumbar artery Median sacral artery Middle suprarenal artery Ovarian artery Testicular artery **1 Celiac Artery** Celiac trunk **2 Gastric Artery** Left gastric artery Right gastric artery **3 Hepatic Artery** Common hepatic artery Gastroduodenal artery Hepatic artery proper **4 Splenic Artery** Left gastroepiploic artery Pancreatic artery Short gastric artery **5 Superior Mesenteric Artery** Ileal artery Ileocolic artery Inferior pancreaticoduodenal artery Jejunal artery **6 Colic Artery, Right** **7 Colic Artery, Left** **8 Colic Artery, Middle** **9 Renal Artery, Right** Inferior suprarenal artery Renal segmental artery **A Renal Artery, Left** ***See*** *9 Renal Artery, Right* **B Inferior Mesenteric Artery** Sigmoid artery Superior rectal artery **C Common Iliac Artery, Right** **D Common Iliac Artery, Left** **E Internal Iliac Artery, Right** Deferential artery Hypogastric artery Iliolumbar artery Inferior gluteal artery Inferior vesical artery Internal pudendal artery Lateral sacral artery Middle rectal artery Obturator artery Superior gluteal artery Umbilical artery Uterine artery Vaginal artery	**F Internal Iliac Artery, Left** ***See*** *E Internal Iliac Artery, Right* **H External Iliac Artery, Right** Deep circumflex iliac artery Inferior epigastric artery **J External Iliac Artery, Left** ***See*** *H External Iliac Artery, Right* **K Femoral Artery, Right** Circumflex iliac artery Deep femoral artery Descending genicular artery External pudendal artery Superficial epigastric artery **L Femoral Artery, Left** ***See*** *K Femoral Artery, Right* **M Popliteal Artery, Right** Inferior genicular artery Middle genicular artery Superior genicular artery Sural artery Tibioperoneal trunk **N Popliteal Artery, Left** ***See*** *M Popliteal Artery, Right* **P Anterior Tibial Artery, Right** Anterior lateral malleolar artery Anterior medial malleolar artery Anterior tibial recurrent artery Dorsalis pedis artery Posterior tibial recurrent artery **Q Anterior Tibial Artery, Left** ***See*** *P Anterior Tibial Artery, Right* **R Posterior Tibial Artery, Right** **S Posterior Tibial Artery, Left** **T Peroneal Artery, Right** Fibular artery **U Peroneal Artery, Left** ***See*** *T Peroneal Artery, Right* **V Foot Artery, Right** Arcuate artery Dorsal metatarsal artery Lateral plantar artery Lateral tarsal artery Medial plantar artery **W Foot Artery, Left** ***See*** *V Foot Artery, Right* **Y Lower Artery** Umbilical artery	**Ø Open** **4 Percutaneous Endoscopic**	**7 Autologous Tissue Substitute** **J Synthetic Substitute** **K Nonautologous Tissue Substitute**	**Z No Qualifier**

Ø Medical and Surgical
4 Lower Arteries
S Reposition Definition: Moving to its normal location, or other suitable location, all or a portion of a body part

Explanation: The body part is moved to a new location from an abnormal location, or from a normal location where it is not functioning correctly. The body part may or may not be cut out or off to be moved to the new location.

Body Part Character 4		Approach Character 5	Device Character 6	Qualifier Character 7
Ø Abdominal Aorta Inferior phrenic artery Lumbar artery Median sacral artery Middle suprarenal artery Ovarian artery Testicular artery **1 Celiac Artery** Celiac trunk **2 Gastric Artery** Left gastric artery Right gastric artery **3 Hepatic Artery** Common hepatic artery Gastroduodenal artery Hepatic artery proper **4 Splenic Artery** Left gastroepiploic artery Pancreatic artery Short gastric artery **5 Superior Mesenteric Artery** Ileal artery Ileocolic artery Inferior pancreaticoduodenal artery Jejunal artery **6 Colic Artery, Right** **7 Colic Artery, Left** **8 Colic Artery, Middle** **9 Renal Artery, Right** Inferior suprarenal artery Renal segmental artery **A Renal Artery, Left** ***See*** *9 Renal Artery, Right* **B Inferior Mesenteric Artery** Sigmoid artery Superior rectal artery **C Common Iliac Artery, Right** **D Common Iliac Artery, Left** **E Internal Iliac Artery, Right** Deferential artery Hypogastric artery Iliolumbar artery Inferior gluteal artery Inferior vesical artery Internal pudendal artery Lateral sacral artery Middle rectal artery Obturator artery Superior gluteal artery Umbilical artery Uterine artery Vaginal artery	**F Internal Iliac Artery, Left** ***See*** *E Internal Iliac Artery, Right* **H External Iliac Artery, Right** Deep circumflex iliac artery Inferior epigastric artery **J External Iliac Artery, Left** ***See*** *H External Iliac Artery, Right* **K Femoral Artery, Right** Circumflex iliac artery Deep femoral artery Descending genicular artery External pudendal artery Superficial epigastric artery **L Femoral Artery, Left** ***See*** *K Femoral Artery, Right* **M Popliteal Artery, Right** Inferior genicular artery Middle genicular artery Superior genicular artery Sural artery Tibioperoneal trunk **N Popliteal Artery, Left** ***See*** *M Popliteal Artery, Right* **P Anterior Tibial Artery, Right** Anterior lateral malleolar artery Anterior medial malleolar artery Anterior tibial recurrent artery Dorsalis pedis artery Posterior tibial recurrent artery **Q Anterior Tibial Artery, Left** ***See*** *P Anterior Tibial Artery, Right* **R Posterior Tibial Artery, Right** **S Posterior Tibial Artery, Left** **T Peroneal Artery, Right** Fibular artery **U Peroneal Artery, Left** ***See*** *T Peroneal Artery, Right* **V Foot Artery, Right** Arcuate artery Dorsal metatarsal artery Lateral plantar artery Lateral tarsal artery Medial plantar artery **W Foot Artery, Left** ***See*** *V Foot Artery, Right* **Y Lower Artery** Umbilical artery	**Ø Open** **3 Percutaneous** **4 Percutaneous Endoscopic**	**Z No Device**	**Z No Qualifier**

Ø Medical and Surgical
4 Lower Arteries
U Supplement Definition: Putting in or on biological or synthetic material that physically reinforces and/or augments the function of a portion of a body part

Explanation: The biological material is non-living, or is living and from the same individual. The body part may have been previously replaced, and the SUPPLEMENT procedure is performed to physically reinforce and/or augment the function of the replaced body part.

Body Part Character 4		Approach Character 5	Device Character 6	Qualifier Character 7
Ø Abdominal Aorta Inferior phrenic artery Lumbar artery Median sacral artery Middle suprarenal artery Ovarian artery Testicular artery **1 Celiac Artery** Celiac trunk **2 Gastric Artery** Left gastric artery Right gastric artery **3 Hepatic Artery** Common hepatic artery Gastroduodenal artery Hepatic artery proper **4 Splenic Artery** Left gastroepiploic artery Pancreatic artery Short gastric artery **5 Superior Mesenteric Artery** Ileal artery Ileocolic artery Inferior pancreaticoduodenal artery Jejunal artery **6 Colic Artery, Right** **7 Colic Artery, Left** **8 Colic Artery, Middle** **9 Renal Artery, Right** Inferior suprarenal artery Renal segmental artery **A Renal Artery, Left** *See 9 Renal Artery, Right* **B Inferior Mesenteric Artery** Sigmoid artery Superior rectal artery **C Common Iliac Artery, Right** **D Common Iliac Artery, Left** **E Internal Iliac Artery, Right** Deferential artery Hypogastric artery Iliolumbar artery Inferior gluteal artery Inferior vesical artery Internal pudendal artery Lateral sacral artery Middle rectal artery Obturator artery Superior gluteal artery Umbilical artery Uterine artery Vaginal artery	**F Internal Iliac Artery, Left** *See E Internal Iliac Artery, Right* **H External Iliac Artery, Right** Deep circumflex iliac artery Inferior epigastric artery **J External Iliac Artery, Left** *See H External Iliac Artery, Right* **K Femoral Artery, Right** Circumflex iliac artery Deep femoral artery Descending genicular artery External pudendal artery Superficial epigastric artery **L Femoral Artery, Left** *See K Femoral Artery, Right* **M Popliteal Artery, Right** Inferior genicular artery Middle genicular artery Superior genicular artery Sural artery Tibioperoneal trunk **N Popliteal Artery, Left** *See M Popliteal Artery, Right* **P Anterior Tibial Artery, Right** Anterior lateral malleolar artery Anterior medial malleolar artery Anterior tibial recurrent artery Dorsalis pedis artery Posterior tibial recurrent artery **Q Anterior Tibial Artery, Left** *See P Anterior Tibial Artery, Right* **R Posterior Tibial Artery, Right** **S Posterior Tibial Artery, Left** **T Peroneal Artery, Right** Fibular artery **U Peroneal Artery, Left** *See T Peroneal Artery, Right* **V Foot Artery, Right** Arcuate artery Dorsal metatarsal artery Lateral plantar artery Lateral tarsal artery Medial plantar artery **W Foot Artery, Left** *See V Foot Artery, Right* **Y Lower Artery** Umbilical artery	**Ø Open** **3 Percutaneous** **4 Percutaneous Endoscopic**	**7 Autologous Tissue Substitute** **J Synthetic Substitute** **K Nonautologous Tissue Substitute**	**Z No Qualifier**

Ø Medical and Surgical
4 Lower Arteries
V Restriction Definition: Partially closing an orifice or the lumen of a tubular body part
Explanation: The orifice can be a natural orifice or an artificially created orifice

Body Part Character 4	Approach Character 5	Device Character 6	Qualifier Character 7
Ø Abdominal Aorta Inferior phrenic artery Lumbar artery Median sacral artery Middle suprarenal artery Ovarian artery Testicular artery	**Ø Open** **3 Percutaneous** **4 Percutaneous Endoscopic**	**C Extraluminal Device** **E Intraluminal Device, Branched or Fenestrated, One or Two Arteries** **F Intraluminal Device, Branched or Fenestrated, Three or More Arteries** **Z No Device**	**Z No Qualifier**
Ø Abdominal Aorta Inferior phrenic artery Lumbar artery Median sacral artery Middle suprarenal artery Ovarian artery Testicular artery	**Ø Open** **3 Percutaneous** **4 Percutaneous Endoscopic**	**D Intraluminal Device**	**J Temporary** **Z No Qualifier**
1 Celiac Artery Celiac trunk **2 Gastric Artery** Left gastric artery Right gastric artery **3 Hepatic Artery** Common hepatic artery Gastroduodenal artery Hepatic artery proper **4 Splenic Artery** Left gastroepiploic artery Pancreatic artery Short gastric artery **5 Superior Mesenteric Artery** Ileal artery Ileocolic artery Inferior pancreaticoduodenal artery Jejunal artery **6 Colic Artery, Right** **7 Colic Artery, Left** **8 Colic Artery, Middle** **9 Renal Artery, Right** Inferior suprarenal artery Renal segmental artery **A Renal Artery, Left** ***See*** *9 Renal Artery, Right* **B Inferior Mesenteric Artery** Sigmoid artery Superior rectal artery **E Internal Iliac Artery, Right** Deferential artery Hypogastric artery Iliolumbar artery Inferior gluteal artery Inferior vesical artery Internal pudendal artery Lateral sacral artery Middle rectal artery Obturator artery Superior gluteal artery Umbilical artery Uterine artery Vaginal artery **F Internal Iliac Artery, Left** ***See*** *E Internal Iliac Artery, Right* **H External Iliac Artery, Right** Deep circumflex iliac artery Inferior epigastric artery **J External Iliac Artery, Left** ***See*** *H External Iliac Artery, Right* **K Femoral Artery, Right** Circumflex iliac artery Deep femoral artery Descending genicular artery External pudendal artery Superficial epigastric artery **L Femoral Artery, Left** ***See*** *K Femoral Artery, Right* **M Popliteal Artery, Right** Inferior genicular artery Middle genicular artery Superior genicular artery Sural artery Tibioperoneal trunk **N Popliteal Artery, Left** ***See*** *M Popliteal Artery, Right* **P Anterior Tibial Artery, Right** Anterior lateral malleolar artery Anterior medial malleolar artery Anterior tibial recurrent artery Dorsalis pedis artery Posterior tibial recurrent artery **Q Anterior Tibial Artery, Left** ***See*** *P Anterior Tibial Artery, Right* **R Posterior Tibial Artery, Right** **S Posterior Tibial Artery, Left** **T Peroneal Artery, Right** Fibular artery **U Peroneal Artery, Left** ***See*** *T Peroneal Artery, Right* **V Foot Artery, Right** Arcuate artery Dorsal metatarsal artery Lateral plantar artery Lateral tarsal artery Medial plantar artery **W Foot Artery, Left** ***See*** *V Foot Artery, Right* **Y Lower Artery** Umbilical artery	**Ø Open** **3 Percutaneous** **4 Percutaneous Endoscopic**	**C Extraluminal Device** **D Intraluminal Device** **Z No Device**	**Z No Qualifier**
C Common Iliac Artery, Right **D Common Iliac Artery, Left**	**Ø Open** **3 Percutaneous** **4 Percutaneous Endoscopic**	**C Extraluminal Device** **D Intraluminal Device** **E Intraluminal Device, Branched or Fenestrated, One or Two Arteries** **Z No Device**	**Z No Qualifier**

Ø Medical and Surgical
4 Lower Arteries
W Revision

Definition: Correcting, to the extent possible, a portion of a malfunctioning device or the position of a displaced device

Explanation: Revision can include correcting a malfunctioning or displaced device by taking out or putting in components of the device such as a screw or pin

Body Part Character 4	Approach Character 5	Device Character 6	Qualifier Character 7
Y Lower Artery Umbilical artery	Ø Open 3 Percutaneous 4 Percutaneous Endoscopic	Ø Drainage Device 2 Monitoring Device 3 Infusion Device 7 Autologous Tissue Substitute C Extraluminal Device D Intraluminal Device J Synthetic Substitute K Nonautologous Tissue Substitute Y Other Device	Z No Qualifier
Y Lower Artery Umbilical artery	X External	Ø Drainage Device 2 Monitoring Device 3 Infusion Device 7 Autologous Tissue Substitute C Extraluminal Device D Intraluminal Device J Synthetic Substitute K Nonautologous Tissue Substitute	Z No Qualifier

Non-OR Ø4WY3[Ø,2,3,D]Z
Non-OR Ø4WY[3,4]YZ
Non-OR Ø4WYX[Ø,2,3,7,C,D,J,K]Z

Upper Veins Ø51–Ø5W

Character Meanings

This Character Meaning table is provided as a guide to assist the user in the identification of character members that may be found in this section of code tables. It **SHOULD NOT** be used to build a PCS code.

Operation–Character 3	Body Part–Character 4	Approach–Character 5	Device–Character 6	Qualifier–Character 7
1 Bypass	Ø Azygos Vein	Ø Open	Ø Drainage Device	Ø Ultrasonic
5 Destruction	1 Hemiazygos Vein	3 Percutaneous	2 Monitoring Device	1 Drug-Coated Balloon
7 Dilation	3 Innominate Vein, Right	4 Percutaneous Endoscopic	3 Infusion Device	X Diagnostic
9 Drainage	4 Innominate Vein, Left	X External	7 Autologous Tissue Substitute	Y Upper Vein
B Excision	5 Subclavian Vein, Right		9 Autologous Venous Tissue	Z No Qualifier
C Extirpation	6 Subclavian Vein, Left		A Autologous Arterial Tissue	
D Extraction	7 Axillary Vein, Right		C Extraluminal Device	
F Fragmentation	8 Axillary Vein, Left		D Intraluminal Device	
H Insertion	9 Brachial Vein, Right		J Synthetic Substitute	
J Inspection	A Brachial Vein, Left		K Nonautologous Tissue Substitute	
L Occlusion	B Basilic Vein, Right		M Neurostimulator Lead	
N Release	C Basilic Vein, Left		Y Other Device	
P Removal	D Cephalic Vein, Right		Z No Device	
Q Repair	F Cephalic Vein, Left			
R Replacement	G Hand Vein, Right			
S Reposition	H Hand Vein, Left			
U Supplement	L Intracranial Vein			
V Restriction	M Internal Jugular Vein, Right			
W Revision	N Internal Jugular Vein, Left			
	P External Jugular Vein, Right			
	Q External Jugular Vein, Left			
	R Vertebral Vein, Right			
	S Vertebral Vein, Left			
	T Face Vein, Right			
	V Face Vein, Left			
	Y Upper Vein			

AHA Coding Clinic for table Ø51
2020, 1Q, 28 Free flap microvascular breast reconstruction
2017, 3Q, 15 Bypass of innominate vein to atrial appendage

AHA Coding Clinic for table Ø57
2020, 3Q, 38 Thrombectomy of arteriovenous fistula with angioplasty and stent placement

AHA Coding Clinic for table Ø59
2018, 3Q, 7 Catheter placement for treatment of congestive heart failure

AHA Coding Clinic for table Ø5B
2021, 2Q, 15 Excision of pituitary macroadenoma within cavernous sinus
2020, 3Q, 40 Excision of ulceration of arteriovenous fistula
2020, 1Q, 24 Resection of vascular malformation, likely cavernoma
2016, 2Q, 12 Resection of malignant neoplasm of infratemporal fossa

AHA Coding Clinic for table Ø5C
2020, 3Q, 37 Repair of aneurysm of arteriovenous fistula with endovenectomy
2020, 3Q, 38 Thrombectomy of arteriovenous fistula with angioplasty and stent placement

AHA Coding Clinic for table Ø5F
2020, 4Q, 45-49 New fragmentation tables
2020, 4Q, 49-50 Intravascular ultrasound assisted thrombolysis
2020, 4Q, 50 Intravascular lithotripsy

AHA Coding Clinic for table Ø5H
2016, 4Q, 97-98 Phrenic neurostimulator

AHA Coding Clinic for table Ø5P
2016, 4Q, 97-98 Phrenic neurostimulator

AHA Coding Clinic for table Ø5Q
2017, 3Q, 15 Bypass of innominate vein to atrial appendage

AHA Coding Clinic for table Ø5S
2013, 4Q, 125 Stage II cephalic vein transposition (superficialization) of arteriovenous fistula

AHA Coding Clinic for table Ø5V
2020, 3Q, 37 Repair of aneurysm of arteriovenous fistula with endovenectomy

AHA Coding Clinic for table Ø5W
2016, 4Q, 97-98 Phrenic neurostimulator

Head and Neck Veins

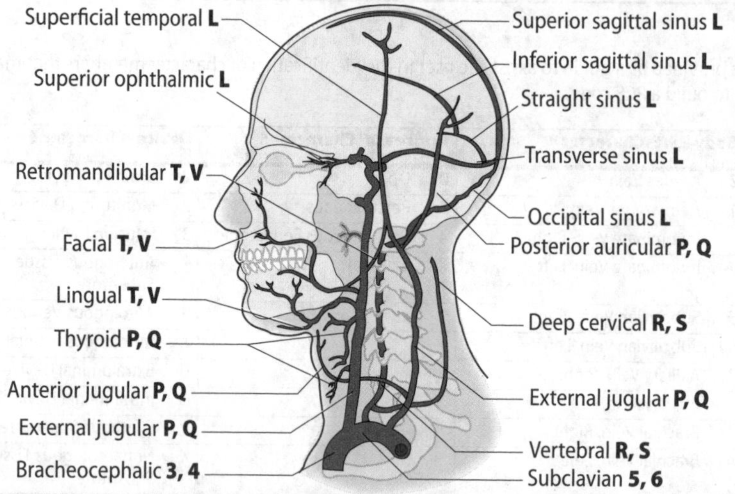

Upper Veins

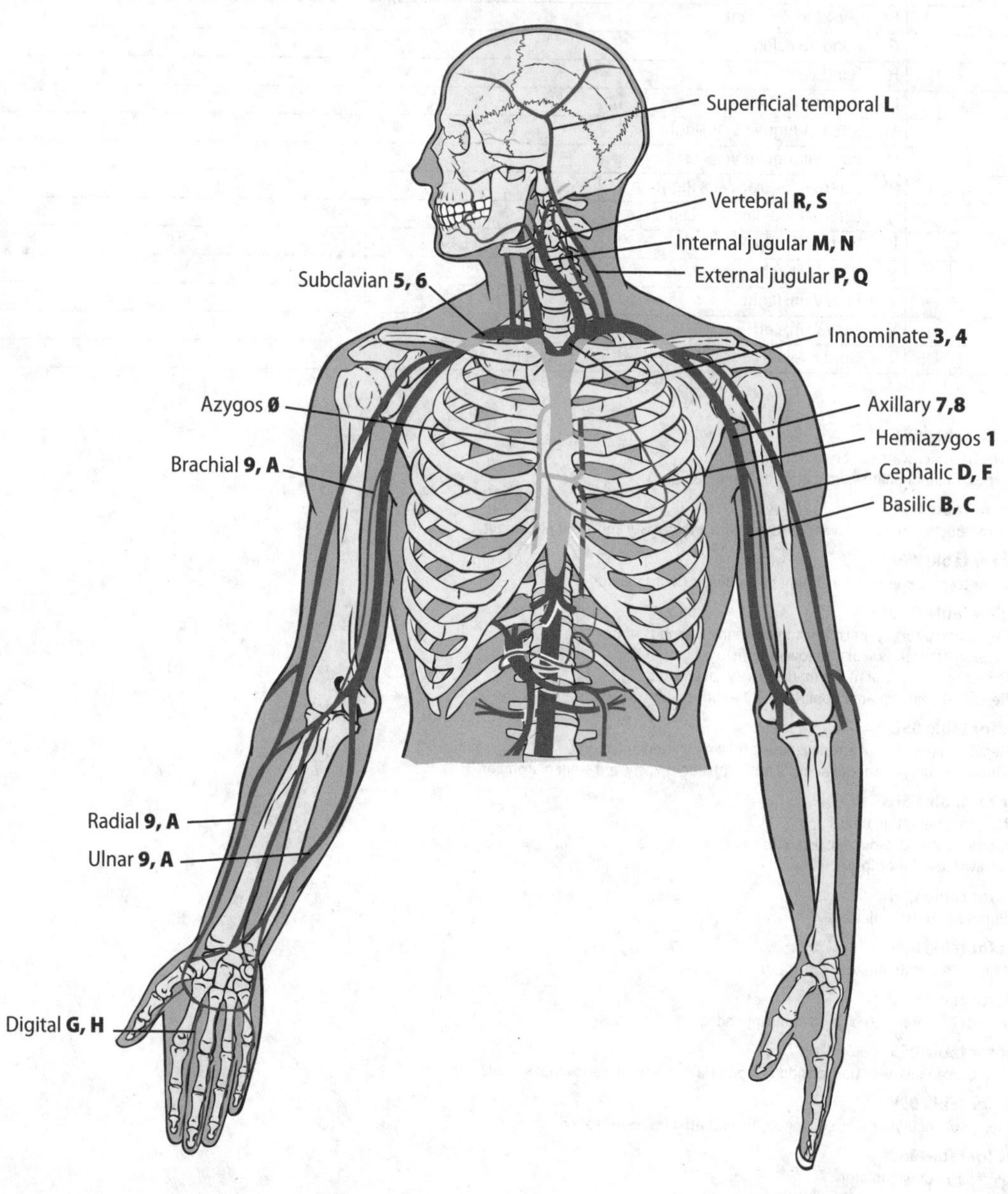

Ø Medical and Surgical
5 Upper Veins
1 Bypass Definition: Altering the route of passage of the contents of a tubular body part

Explanation: Rerouting contents of a body part to a downstream area of the normal route, to a similar route and body part, or to an abnormal route and dissimilar body part. Includes one or more anastomoses, with or without the use of a device.

Body Part Character 4	Approach Character 5	Device Character 6	Qualifier Character 7
Ø Azygos Vein Right ascending lumbar vein Right subcostal vein **1 Hemiazygos Vein** Left ascending lumbar vein Left subcostal vein **3 Innominate Vein, Right** Brachiocephalic vein Inferior thyroid vein **4 Innominate Vein, Left** ***See*** *3 Innominate Vein, Right* **5 Subclavian Vein, Right** **6 Subclavian Vein, Left** **7 Axillary Vein, Right** **8 Axillary Vein, Left** **9 Brachial Vein, Right** Radial vein Ulnar vein **A Brachial Vein, Left** ***See*** *9 Brachial Vein, Right* **B Basilic Vein, Right** Median antebrachial vein Median cubital vein **C Basilic Vein, Left** ***See*** *B Basilic Vein, Right* **D Cephalic Vein, Right** Accessory cephalic vein **F Cephalic Vein, Left** ***See*** *D Cephalic Vein, Right* **G Hand Vein, Right** Dorsal metacarpal vein Palmar (volar) digital vein Palmar (volar) metacarpal vein Superficial palmar venous arch Volar (palmar) digital vein Volar (palmar) metacarpal vein **H Hand Vein, Left** ***See*** *G Hand Vein, Right* **L Intracranial Vein** Anterior cerebral vein Basal (internal) cerebral vein Dural venous sinus Great cerebral vein Inferior cerebellar vein Inferior cerebral vein Internal (basal) cerebral vein Middle cerebral vein Ophthalmic vein Superior cerebellar vein Superior cerebral vein **M Internal Jugular Vein, Right** **N Internal Jugular Vein, Left** **P External Jugular Vein, Right** Posterior auricular vein **Q External Jugular Vein, Left** ***See*** *P External Jugular Vein, Right* **R Vertebral Vein, Right** Deep cervical vein Suboccipital venous plexus **S Vertebral Vein, Left** ***See*** *R Vertebral Vein, Right* **T Face Vein, Right** Angular vein Anterior facial vein Common facial vein Deep facial vein Frontal vein Posterior facial (retromandibular) vein Supraorbital vein **V Face Vein, Left** ***See*** *T Face Vein, Right*	**Ø Open** **4 Percutaneous Endoscopic**	**7 Autologous Tissue Substitute** **9 Autologous Venous Tissue** **A Autologous Arterial Tissue** **J Synthetic Substitute** **K Nonautologous Tissue Substitute** **Z No Device**	**Y Upper Vein**

Ø Medical and Surgical
5 Upper Veins
5 Destruction Definition: Physical eradication of all or a portion of a body part by the direct use of energy, force, or a destructive agent
Explanation: None of the body part is physically taken out

Body Part Character 4	Approach Character 5	Device Character 6	Qualifier Character 7
Ø Azygos Vein Right ascending lumbar vein Right subcostal vein **1 Hemiazygos Vein** Left ascending lumbar vein Left subcostal vein **3 Innominate Vein, Right** Brachiocephalic vein Inferior thyroid vein **4 Innominate Vein, Left** *See 3 Innominate Vein, Right* **5 Subclavian Vein, Right** **6 Subclavian Vein, Left** **7 Axillary Vein, Right** **8 Axillary Vein, Left** **9 Brachial Vein, Right** Radial vein Ulnar vein **A Brachial Vein, Left** *See 9 Brachial Vein, Right* **B Basilic Vein, Right** Median antebrachial vein Median cubital vein **C Basilic Vein, Left** *See B Basilic Vein, Right* **D Cephalic Vein, Right** Accessory cephalic vein **F Cephalic Vein, Left** *See D Cephalic Vein, Right* **G Hand Vein, Right** Dorsal metacarpal vein Palmar (volar) digital vein Palmar (volar) metacarpal vein Superficial palmar venous arch Volar (palmar) digital vein Volar (palmar) metacarpal vein **H Hand Vein, Left** *See G Hand Vein, Right* **L Intracranial Vein** Anterior cerebral vein Basal (internal) cerebral vein Dural venous sinus Great cerebral vein Inferior cerebellar vein Inferior cerebral vein Internal (basal) cerebral vein Middle cerebral vein Ophthalmic vein Superior cerebellar vein Superior cerebral vein **M Internal Jugular Vein, Right** **N Internal Jugular Vein, Left** **P External Jugular Vein, Right** Posterior auricular vein **Q External Jugular Vein, Left** *See P External Jugular Vein, Right* **R Vertebral Vein, Right** Deep cervical vein Suboccipital venous plexus **S Vertebral Vein, Left** *See R Vertebral Vein, Right* **T Face Vein, Right** Angular vein Anterior facial vein Common facial vein Deep facial vein Frontal vein Posterior facial (retromandibular) vein Supraorbital vein **V Face Vein, Left** *See T Face Vein, Right* **Y Upper Vein**	**Ø Open** **3 Percutaneous** **4 Percutaneous Endoscopic**	**Z No Device**	**Z No Qualifier**

Ø Medical and Surgical
5 Upper Veins
7 Dilation Definition: Expanding an orifice or the lumen of a tubular body part

Explanation: The orifice can be a natural orifice or an artificially created orifice. Accomplished by stretching a tubular body part using intraluminal pressure or by cutting part of the orifice or wall of the tubular body part.

Body Part Character 4	Approach Character 5	Device Character 6	Qualifier Character 7
Ø Azygos Vein Right ascending lumbar vein Right subcostal vein **1 Hemiazygos Vein** Left ascending lumbar vein Left subcostal vein **G Hand Vein, Right** Dorsal metacarpal vein Palmar (volar) digital vein Palmar (volar) metacarpal vein Superficial palmar venous arch Volar (palmar) digital vein Volar (palmar) metacarpal vein **H Hand Vein, Left** *See G Hand Vein, Right* **L Intracranial Vein** NC Anterior cerebral vein Basal (internal) cerebral vein Dural venous sinus Great cerebral vein Inferior cerebellar vein Inferior cerebral vein Internal (basal) cerebral vein Middle cerebral vein Ophthalmic vein Superior cerebellar vein Superior cerebral vein **M Internal Jugular Vein, Right** **N Internal Jugular Vein, Left** **P External Jugular Vein, Right** Posterior auricular vein **Q External Jugular Vein, Left** *See P External Jugular Vein, Right* **R Vertebral Vein, Right** Deep cervical vein Suboccipital venous plexus **S Vertebral Vein, Left** *See R Vertebral Vein, Right* **T Face Vein, Right** Angular vein Anterior facial vein Common facial vein Deep facial vein Frontal vein Posterior facial (retromandibular) vein Supraorbital vein **V Face Vein, Left** *See T Face Vein, Right* **Y Upper Vein**	**Ø Open** **3 Percutaneous** **4 Percutaneous Endoscopic**	**D Intraluminal Device** **Z No Device**	**Z No Qualifier**
3 Innominate Vein, Right Brachiocephalic vein Inferior thyroid vein **4 Innominate Vein, Left** *See 3 Innominate Vein, Right* **5 Subclavian Vein, Right** **6 Subclavian Vein, Left** **7 Axillary Vein, Right** **8 Axillary Vein, Left** **9 Brachial Vein, Right** Radial vein Ulnar vein **A Brachial Vein, Left** *See 9 Brachial Vein, Right* **B Basilic Vein, Right** Median antebrachial vein Median cubital vein **C Basilic Vein, Left** *See B Basilic Vein, Right* **D Cephalic Vein, Right** Accessory cephalic vein **F Cephalic Vein, Left** *See D Cephalic Vein, Right*	**Ø Open** **3 Percutaneous** **4 Percutaneous Endoscopic**	**D Intraluminal Device** **Z No Device**	**1 Drug-Coated Balloon** **Z No Qualifier**

NC Ø57L[3,4]ZZ

Ø Medical and Surgical
5 Upper Veins
9 Drainage Definition: Taking or letting out fluids and/or gases from a body part
Explanation: The qualifier DIAGNOSTIC is used to identify drainage procedures that are biopsies

Body Part Character 4		Approach Character 5	Device Character 6	Qualifier Character 7
Ø Azygos Vein Right ascending lumbar vein Right subcostal vein **1 Hemiazygos Vein** Left ascending lumbar vein Left subcostal vein **3 Innominate Vein, Right** Brachiocephalic vein Inferior thyroid vein **4 Innominate Vein, Left** ***See*** *3 Innominate Vein, Right* **5 Subclavian Vein, Right** **6 Subclavian Vein, Left** **7 Axillary Vein, Right** **8 Axillary Vein, Left** **9 Brachial Vein, Right** Radial vein Ulnar vein **A Brachial Vein, Left** ***See*** *9 Brachial Vein, Right* **B Basilic Vein, Right** Median antebrachial vein Median cubital vein **C Basilic Vein, Left** ***See*** *B Basilic Vein, Right* **D Cephalic Vein, Right** Accessory cephalic vein **F Cephalic Vein, Left** ***See*** *D Cephalic Vein, Right* **G Hand Vein, Right** Dorsal metacarpal vein Palmar (volar) digital vein Palmar (volar) metacarpal vein Superficial palmar venous arch Volar (palmar) digital vein Volar (palmar) metacarpal vein	**H Hand Vein, Left** ***See*** *G Hand Vein, Right* **L Intracranial Vein** Anterior cerebral vein Basal (internal) cerebral vein Dural venous sinus Great cerebral vein Inferior cerebellar vein Inferior cerebral vein Internal (basal) cerebral vein Middle cerebral vein Ophthalmic vein Superior cerebellar vein Superior cerebral vein **M Internal Jugular Vein, Right** **N Internal Jugular Vein, Left** **P External Jugular Vein, Right** Posterior auricular vein **Q External Jugular Vein, Left** ***See*** *P External Jugular Vein, Right* **R Vertebral Vein, Right** Deep cervical vein Suboccipital venous plexus **S Vertebral Vein, Left** ***See*** *R Vertebral Vein, Right* **T Face Vein, Right** Angular vein Anterior facial vein Common facial vein Deep facial vein Frontal vein Posterior facial (retromandibular) vein Supraorbital vein **V Face Vein, Left** ***See*** *T Face Vein, Right* **Y Upper Vein**	**Ø Open** **3 Percutaneous** **4 Percutaneous Endoscopic**	**Ø Drainage Device**	**Z No Qualifier**
Ø Azygos Vein Right ascending lumbar vein Right subcostal vein **1 Hemiazygos Vein** Left ascending lumbar vein Left subcostal vein **3 Innominate Vein, Right** Brachiocephalic vein Inferior thyroid vein **4 Innominate Vein, Left** ***See*** *3 Innominate Vein, Right* **5 Subclavian Vein, Right** **6 Subclavian Vein, Left** **7 Axillary Vein, Right** **8 Axillary Vein, Left** **9 Brachial Vein, Right** Radial vein Ulnar vein **A Brachial Vein, Left** ***See*** *9 Brachial Vein, Right* **B Basilic Vein, Right** Median antebrachial vein Median cubital vein **C Basilic Vein, Left** ***See*** *B Basilic Vein, Right* **D Cephalic Vein, Right** Accessory cephalic vein **F Cephalic Vein, Left** ***See*** *D Cephalic Vein, Right* **G Hand Vein, Right** Dorsal metacarpal vein Palmar (volar) digital vein Palmar (volar) metacarpal vein Superficial palmar venous arch Volar (palmar) digital vein Volar (palmar) metacarpal vein	**H Hand Vein, Left** ***See*** *G Hand Vein, Right* **L Intracranial Vein** Anterior cerebral vein Basal (internal) cerebral vein Dural venous sinus Great cerebral vein Inferior cerebellar vein Inferior cerebral vein Internal (basal) cerebral vein Middle cerebral vein Ophthalmic vein Superior cerebellar vein Superior cerebral vein **M Internal Jugular Vein, Right** **N Internal Jugular Vein, Left** **P External Jugular Vein, Right** Posterior auricular vein **Q External Jugular Vein, Left** ***See*** *P External Jugular Vein, Right* **R Vertebral Vein, Right** Deep cervical vein Suboccipital venous plexus **S Vertebral Vein, Left** ***See*** *R Vertebral Vein, Right* **T Face Vein, Right** Angular vein Anterior facial vein Common facial vein Deep facial vein Frontal vein Posterior facial (retromandibular) vein Supraorbital vein **V Face Vein, Left** ***See*** *T Face Vein, Right* **Y Upper Vein**	**Ø Open** **3 Percutaneous** **4 Percutaneous Endoscopic**	**Z No Device**	**X Diagnostic** **Z No Qualifier**

Non-OR Ø59[Ø,1,3,4,5,6,7,8,9,A,B,C,D,F,G,H,L,M,N,P,Q,R,S,T,V,Y][Ø,3,4]ØZ
Non-OR Ø59[Ø,1,3,4,5,6,7,8,9,A,B,C,D,F,G,H,L,M,N,P,Q,R,S,T,V,Y]3ZX
Non-OR Ø59[Ø,1,3,4,5,6,7,8,9,A,B,C,D,F,G,H,L,M,N,P,Q,R,S,T,V,Y][Ø,3,4]ZZ

Ø Medical and Surgical
5 Upper Veins
B Excision Definition: Cutting out or off, without replacement, a portion of a body part
Explanation: The qualifier DIAGNOSTIC is used to identify excision procedures that are biopsies

Body Part Character 4	Approach Character 5	Device Character 6	Qualifier Character 7
Ø Azygos Vein Right ascending lumbar vein Right subcostal vein **1 Hemiazygos Vein** Left ascending lumbar vein Left subcostal vein **3 Innominate Vein, Right** Brachiocephalic vein Inferior thyroid vein **4 Innominate Vein, Left** *See 3 Innominate Vein, Right* **5 Subclavian Vein, Right** **6 Subclavian Vein, Left** **7 Axillary Vein, Right** **8 Axillary Vein, Left** **9 Brachial Vein, Right** Radial vein Ulnar vein **A Brachial Vein, Left** *See 9 Brachial Vein, Right* **B Basilic Vein, Right** Median antebrachial vein Median cubital vein **C Basilic Vein, Left** *See B Basilic Vein, Right* **D Cephalic Vein, Right** Accessory cephalic vein **F Cephalic Vein, Left** *See D Cephalic Vein, Right* **G Hand Vein, Right** Dorsal metacarpal vein Palmar (volar) digital vein Palmar (volar) metacarpal vein Superficial palmar venous arch Volar (palmar) digital vein Volar (palmar) metacarpal vein **H Hand Vein, Left** *See G Hand Vein, Right* **L Intracranial Vein** Anterior cerebral vein Basal (internal) cerebral vein Dural venous sinus Great cerebral vein Inferior cerebellar vein Inferior cerebral vein Internal (basal) cerebral vein Middle cerebral vein Ophthalmic vein Superior cerebellar vein Superior cerebral vein **M Internal Jugular Vein, Right** **N Internal Jugular Vein, Left** **P External Jugular Vein, Right** Posterior auricular vein **Q External Jugular Vein, Left** *See P External Jugular Vein, Right* **R Vertebral Vein, Right** Deep cervical vein Suboccipital venous plexus **S Vertebral Vein, Left** *See R Vertebral Vein, Right* **T Face Vein, Right** Angular vein Anterior facial vein Common facial vein Deep facial vein Frontal vein Posterior facial (retromandibular) vein Supraorbital vein **V Face Vein, Left** *See T Face Vein, Right* **Y Upper Vein**	**Ø Open** **3 Percutaneous** **4 Percutaneous Endoscopic**	**Z No Device**	**X Diagnostic** **Z No Qualifier**

Ø Medical and Surgical
5 Upper Veins
C Extirpation Definition: Taking or cutting out solid matter from a body part

Explanation: The solid matter may be an abnormal byproduct of a biological function or a foreign body; it may be imbedded in a body part or in the lumen of a tubular body part. The solid matter may or may not have been previously broken into pieces.

Body Part Character 4	Approach Character 5	Device Character 6	Qualifier Character 7
Ø Azygos Vein Right ascending lumbar vein Right subcostal vein **1 Hemiazygos Vein** Left ascending lumbar vein Left subcostal vein **3 Innominate Vein, Right** Brachiocephalic vein Inferior thyroid vein **4 Innominate Vein, Left** *See 3 Innominate Vein, Right* **5 Subclavian Vein, Right** **6 Subclavian Vein, Left** **7 Axillary Vein, Right** **8 Axillary Vein, Left** **9 Brachial Vein, Right** Radial vein Ulnar vein **A Brachial Vein, Left** *See 9 Brachial Vein, Right* **B Basilic Vein, Right** Median antebrachial vein Median cubital vein **C Basilic Vein, Left** *See B Basilic Vein, Right* **D Cephalic Vein, Right** Accessory cephalic vein **F Cephalic Vein, Left** *See D Cephalic Vein, Right* **G Hand Vein, Right** Dorsal metacarpal vein Palmar (volar) digital vein Palmar (volar) metacarpal vein Superficial palmar venous arch Volar (palmar) digital vein Volar (palmar) metacarpal vein **H Hand Vein, Left** *See G Hand Vein, Right* **L Intracranial Vein** Anterior cerebral vein Basal (internal) cerebral vein Dural venous sinus Great cerebral vein Inferior cerebellar vein Inferior cerebral vein Internal (basal) cerebral vein Middle cerebral vein Ophthalmic vein Superior cerebellar vein Superior cerebral vein **M Internal Jugular Vein, Right** **N Internal Jugular Vein, Left** **P External Jugular Vein, Right** Posterior auricular vein **Q External Jugular Vein, Left** *See P External Jugular Vein, Right* **R Vertebral Vein, Right** Deep cervical vein Suboccipital venous plexus **S Vertebral Vein, Left** *See R Vertebral Vein, Right* **T Face Vein, Right** Angular vein Anterior facial vein Common facial vein Deep facial vein Frontal vein Posterior facial (retromandibular) vein Supraorbital vein **V Face Vein, Left** *See T Face Vein, Right* **Y Upper Vein**	**Ø Open** **3 Percutaneous** **4 Percutaneous Endoscopic**	**Z No Device**	**Z No Qualifier**

Ø Medical and Surgical
5 Upper Veins
D Extraction Definition: Pulling or stripping out or off all or a portion of a body part by the use of force

Explanation: The qualifier DIAGNOSTIC is used to identify extraction procedures that are biopsies

Body Part Character 4	Approach Character 5	Device Character 6	Qualifier Character 7
9 Brachial Vein, Right Radial vein Ulnar vein **A Brachial Vein, Left** *See 9 Brachial Vein, Right* **B Basilic Vein, Right** Median antebrachial vein Median cubital vein **C Basilic Vein, Left** *See B Basilic Vein, Right* **D Cephalic Vein, Right** Accessory cephalic vein **F Cephalic Vein, Left** *See D Cephalic Vein, Right* **G Hand Vein, Right** Dorsal metacarpal vein Palmar (volar) digital vein Palmar (volar) metacarpal vein Superficial palmar venous arch Volar (palmar) digital vein Volar (palmar) metacarpal vein **H Hand Vein, Left** *See G Hand Vein, Right* **Y Upper Vein**	**Ø Open** **3 Percutaneous**	**Z No Device**	**Z No Qualifier**

Ø Medical and Surgical
5 Upper Veins
F Fragmentation Definition: Breaking solid matter in a body part into pieces

Explanation: Physical force (e.g., manual, ultrasonic) applied directly or indirectly is used to break the solid matter into pieces. The solid matter may be an abnormal byproduct of a biological function or a foreign body. The pieces of solid matter are not taken out.

Body Part Character 4	Approach Character 5	Device Character 6	Qualifier Character 7
3 Innominate Vein, Right Brachiocephalic vein Inferior thyroid vein **4 Innominate Vein, Left** *See 3 Innominate Vein, Right* **5 Subclavian Vein, Right** **6 Subclavian Vein, Left** **7 Axillary Vein, Right** **8 Axillary Vein, Left** **9 Brachial Vein, Right** Radial vein Ulnar vein **A Brachial Vein, Left** *See 9 Brachial Vein, Right* **B Basilic Vein, Right** Median antebrachial vein Median cubital vein **C Basilic Vein, Left** *See B Basilic Vein, Right* **D Cephalic Vein, Right** Accessory cephalic vein **F Cephalic Vein, Left** *See D Cephalic Vein, Right* **Y Upper Vein**	**3 Percutaneous**	**Z No Device**	**Ø Ultrasonic** **Z No Qualifier**

Ø Medical and Surgical
5 Upper Veins
H Insertion

Definition: Putting in a nonbiological appliance that monitors, assists, performs, or prevents a physiological function but does not physically take the place of a body part

Explanation: None

Body Part Character 4	Approach Character 5	Device Character 6	Qualifier Character 7
Ø Azygos Vein ⊞ Right ascending lumbar vein Right subcostal vein	**Ø** Open **3** Percutaneous **4** Percutaneous Endoscopic	**2** Monitoring Device **3** Infusion Device **D** Intraluminal Device **M** Neurostimulator Lead	**Z** No Qualifier
1 Hemiazygos Vein Left ascending lumbar vein Left subcostal vein **5 Subclavian Vein, Right** **6 Subclavian Vein, Left** **7 Axillary Vein, Right** **8 Axillary Vein, Left** **9 Brachial Vein, Right** Radial vein Ulnar vein **A Brachial Vein, Left** *See 9 Brachial Vein, Right* **B Basilic Vein, Right** Median antebrachial vein Median cubital vein **C Basilic Vein, Left** *See B Basilic Vein, Right* **D Cephalic Vein, Right** Accessory cephalic vein **F Cephalic Vein, Left** *See D Cephalic Vein, Right* **G Hand Vein, Right** Dorsal metacarpal vein Palmar (volar) digital vein Palmar (volar) metacarpal vein Superficial palmar venous arch Volar (palmar) digital vein Volar (palmar) metacarpal vein **H Hand Vein, Left** *See G Hand Vein, Right* **L Intracranial Vein** Anterior cerebral vein Basal (internal) cerebral vein Dural venous sinus Great cerebral vein Inferior cerebellar vein Inferior cerebral vein Internal (basal) cerebral vein Middle cerebral vein Ophthalmic vein Superior cerebellar vein Superior cerebral vein **M Internal Jugular Vein, Right** **N Internal Jugular Vein, Left** **P External Jugular Vein, Right** Posterior auricular vein **Q External Jugular Vein, Left** *See P External Jugular Vein, Right* **R Vertebral Vein, Right** Deep cervical vein Suboccipital venous plexus **S Vertebral Vein, Left** *See R Vertebral Vein, Right* **T Face Vein, Right** Angular vein Anterior facial vein Common facial vein Deep facial vein Frontal vein Posterior facial (retromandibular) vein Supraorbital vein **V Face Vein, Left** *See T Face Vein, Right*	**Ø** Open **3** Percutaneous **4** Percutaneous Endoscopic	**3** Infusion Device **D** Intraluminal Device	**Z** No Qualifier
3 Innominate Vein, Right ⊞ Brachiocephalic vein Inferior thyroid vein **4 Innominate Vein, Left** ⊞ *See 3 Innominate Vein, Right*	**Ø** Open **3** Percutaneous **4** Percutaneous Endoscopic	**3** Infusion Device **D** Intraluminal Device **M** Neurostimulator Lead	**Z** No Qualifier
Y Upper Vein	**Ø** Open **3** Percutaneous **4** Percutaneous Endoscopic	**2** Monitoring Device **3** Infusion Device **D** Intraluminal Device **Y** Other Device	**Z** No Qualifier

Non-OR Ø5HØ[Ø,3,4]3Z
Non-OR Ø5H[1,5,6,7,8,9,A,B,C,D,F,G,H,L,M,N,P,Q,R,S,T,V][Ø,3,4]3Z
Non-OR Ø5H[3,4][Ø,3,4]3Z
Non-OR Ø5HY[Ø,3,4]3Z
Non-OR Ø5HY32Z
Non-OR Ø5HY[3,4]YZ
HAC Ø5HØ[3,4]3Z when reported with SDx J95.811
HAC Ø5H[1,5,6][3,4]3Z when reported with SDx J95.811
HAC Ø5H[M,N,P,Q]33Z when reported with SDx J95.811
HAC Ø5H[3,4][3,4]3Z when reported with SDx J95.811

See Appendix L for Procedure Combinations
⊞ Ø5HØ[Ø,3,4]MZ
⊞ Ø5H[3,4][Ø,3,4]MZ

Ø Medical and Surgical
5 Upper Veins
J Inspection

Definition: Visually and/or manually exploring a body part

Explanation: Visual exploration may be performed with or without optical instrumentation. Manual exploration may be performed directly or through intervening body layers.

Body Part Character 4	Approach Character 5	Device Character 6	Qualifier Character 7
Y Upper Vein	**Ø** Open **3** Percutaneous **4** Percutaneous Endoscopic **X** External	**Z** No Device	**Z** No Qualifier

Non-OR Ø5JY[3,X]ZZ

Ø Medical and Surgical
5 Upper Veins
L Occlusion Definition: Completely closing an orifice or the lumen of a tubular body part
Explanation: The orifice can be a natural orifice or an artificially created orifice

Body Part Character 4	Approach Character 5	Device Character 6	Qualifier Character 7
Ø Azygos Vein Right ascending lumbar vein Right subcostal vein **1 Hemiazygos Vein** Left ascending lumbar vein Left subcostal vein **3 Innominate Vein, Right** Brachiocephalic vein Inferior thyroid vein **4 Innominate Vein, Left** *See 3 Innominate Vein, Right* **5 Subclavian Vein, Right** **6 Subclavian Vein, Left** **7 Axillary Vein, Right** **8 Axillary Vein, Left** **9 Brachial Vein, Right** Radial vein Ulnar vein **A Brachial Vein, Left** *See 9 Brachial Vein, Right* **B Basilic Vein, Right** Median antebrachial vein Median cubital vein **C Basilic Vein, Left** *See B Basilic Vein, Right* **D Cephalic Vein, Right** Accessory cephalic vein **F Cephalic Vein, Left** *See D Cephalic Vein, Right* **G Hand Vein, Right** Dorsal metacarpal vein Palmar (volar) digital vein Palmar (volar) metacarpal vein Superficial palmar venous arch Volar (palmar) digital vein Volar (palmar) metacarpal vein **H Hand Vein, Left** *See G Hand Vein, Right* **L Intracranial Vein** Anterior cerebral vein Basal (internal) cerebral vein Dural venous sinus Great cerebral vein Inferior cerebellar vein Inferior cerebral vein Internal (basal) cerebral vein Middle cerebral vein Ophthalmic vein Superior cerebellar vein Superior cerebral vein **M Internal Jugular Vein, Right** **N Internal Jugular Vein, Left** **P External Jugular Vein, Right** Posterior auricular vein **Q External Jugular Vein, Left** *See P External Jugular Vein, Right* **R Vertebral Vein, Right** Deep cervical vein Suboccipital venous plexus **S Vertebral Vein, Left** *See R Vertebral Vein, Right* **T Face Vein, Right** Angular vein Anterior facial vein Common facial vein Deep facial vein Frontal vein Posterior facial (retromandibular) vein Supraorbital vein **V Face Vein, Left** *See T Face Vein, Right* **Y Upper Vein**	**Ø Open** **3 Percutaneous** **4 Percutaneous Endoscopic**	**C Extraluminal Device** **D Intraluminal Device** **Z No Device**	**Z No Qualifier**

Ø Medical and Surgical
5 Upper Veins
N Release Definition: Freeing a body part from an abnormal physical constraint by cutting or by the use of force
Explanation: Some of the restraining tissue may be taken out but none of the body part is taken out

Body Part Character 4	Approach Character 5	Device Character 6	Qualifier Character 7
Ø Azygos Vein Right ascending lumbar vein Right subcostal vein **1 Hemiazygos Vein** Left ascending lumbar vein Left subcostal vein **3 Innominate Vein, Right** Brachiocephalic vein Inferior thyroid vein **4 Innominate Vein, Left** *See 3 Innominate Vein, Right* **5 Subclavian Vein, Right** **6 Subclavian Vein, Left** **7 Axillary Vein, Right** **8 Axillary Vein, Left** **9 Brachial Vein, Right** Radial vein Ulnar vein **A Brachial Vein, Left** *See 9 Brachial Vein, Right* **B Basilic Vein, Right** Median antebrachial vein Median cubital vein **C Basilic Vein, Left** *See B Basilic Vein, Right* **D Cephalic Vein, Right** Accessory cephalic vein **F Cephalic Vein, Left** *See D Cephalic Vein, Right* **G Hand Vein, Right** Dorsal metacarpal vein Palmar (volar) digital vein Palmar (volar) metacarpal vein Superficial palmar venous arch Volar (palmar) digital vein Volar (palmar) metacarpal vein **H Hand Vein, Left** *See G Hand Vein, Right* **L Intracranial Vein** Anterior cerebral vein Basal (internal) cerebral vein Dural venous sinus Great cerebral vein Inferior cerebellar vein Inferior cerebral vein Internal (basal) cerebral vein Middle cerebral vein Ophthalmic vein Superior cerebellar vein Superior cerebral vein **M Internal Jugular Vein, Right** **N Internal Jugular Vein, Left** **P External Jugular Vein, Right** Posterior auricular vein **Q External Jugular Vein, Left** *See P External Jugular Vein, Right* **R Vertebral Vein, Right** Deep cervical vein Suboccipital venous plexus **S Vertebral Vein, Left** *See R Vertebral Vein, Right* **T Face Vein, Right** Angular vein Anterior facial vein Common facial vein Deep facial vein Frontal vein Posterior facial (retromandibular) vein Supraorbital vein **V Face Vein, Left** *See T Face Vein, Right* **Y Upper Vein**	**Ø Open** **3 Percutaneous** **4 Percutaneous Endoscopic**	**Z No Device**	**Z No Qualifier**

Ø Medical and Surgical
5 Upper Veins
P Removal Definition: Taking out or off a device from a body part

Explanation: If a device is taken out and a similar device put in without cutting or puncturing the skin or mucous membrane, the procedure is coded to the root operation CHANGE. Otherwise, the procedure for taking out a device is coded to the root operation REMOVAL.

Body Part Character 4	Approach Character 5	Device Character 6	Qualifier Character 7
Ø Azygos Vein Right ascending lumbar vein Right subcostal vein	**Ø Open** **3 Percutaneous** **4 Percutaneous Endoscopic** **X External**	**2 Monitoring Device** **M Neurostimulator Lead**	**Z No Qualifier**
3 Innominate Vein, Right Brachiocephalic vein Inferior thyroid vein **4 Innominate Vein, Left** *See 3 Innominate Vein, Right*	**Ø Open** **3 Percutaneous** **4 Percutaneous Endoscopic** **X External**	**M Neurostimulator Lead**	**Z No Qualifier**
Y Upper Vein	**Ø Open** **3 Percutaneous** **4 Percutaneous Endoscopic**	**Ø Drainage Device** **2 Monitoring Device** **3 Infusion Device** **7 Autologous Tissue Substitute** **C Extraluminal Device** **D Intraluminal Device** **J Synthetic Substitute** **K Nonautologous Tissue Substitute** **Y Other Device**	**Z No Qualifier**
Y Upper Vein	**X External**	**Ø Drainage Device** **2 Monitoring Device** **3 Infusion Device** **D Intraluminal Device**	**Z No Qualifier**

Non-OR Ø5PØ[Ø,3,4,X]2Z
Non-OR Ø5PY3[Ø,2,3]Z
Non-OR Ø5PY[3,4]YZ
Non-OR Ø5PYX[Ø,2,3,D]Z

Ø Medical and Surgical
5 Upper Veins
Q Repair Definition: Restoring, to the extent possible, a body part to its normal anatomic structure and function
Explanation: Used only when the method to accomplish the repair is not one of the other root operations

Body Part Character 4	Approach Character 5	Device Character 6	Qualifier Character 7
Ø Azygos Vein Right ascending lumbar vein Right subcostal vein **1 Hemiazygos Vein** Left ascending lumbar vein Left subcostal vein **3 Innominate Vein, Right** Brachiocephalic vein Inferior thyroid vein **4 Innominate Vein, Left** *See 3 Innominate Vein, Right* **5 Subclavian Vein, Right** **6 Subclavian Vein, Left** **7 Axillary Vein, Right** **8 Axillary Vein, Left** **9 Brachial Vein, Right** Radial vein Ulnar vein **A Brachial Vein, Left** *See 9 Brachial Vein, Right* **B Basilic Vein, Right** Median antebrachial vein Median cubital vein **C Basilic Vein, Left** *See B Basilic Vein, Right* **D Cephalic Vein, Right** Accessory cephalic vein **F Cephalic Vein, Left** *See D Cephalic Vein, Right* **G Hand Vein, Right** Dorsal metacarpal vein Palmar (volar) digital vein Palmar (volar) metacarpal vein Superficial palmar venous arch Volar (palmar) digital vein Volar (palmar) metacarpal vein **H Hand Vein, Left** *See G Hand Vein, Right* **L Intracranial Vein** Anterior cerebral vein Basal (internal) cerebral vein Dural venous sinus Great cerebral vein Inferior cerebellar vein Inferior cerebral vein Internal (basal) cerebral vein Middle cerebral vein Ophthalmic vein Superior cerebellar vein Superior cerebral vein **M Internal Jugular Vein, Right** **N Internal Jugular Vein, Left** **P External Jugular Vein, Right** Posterior auricular vein **Q External Jugular Vein, Left** *See P External Jugular Vein, Right* **R Vertebral Vein, Right** Deep cervical vein Suboccipital venous plexus **S Vertebral Vein, Left** *See R Vertebral Vein, Right* **T Face Vein, Right** Angular vein Anterior facial vein Common facial vein Deep facial vein Frontal vein Posterior facial (retromandibular) vein Supraorbital vein **V Face Vein, Left** *See T Face Vein, Right* **Y Upper Vein**	**Ø Open** **3 Percutaneous** **4 Percutaneous Endoscopic**	**Z No Device**	**Z No Qualifier**

Ø Medical and Surgical
5 Upper Veins
R Replacement Definition: Putting in or on biological or synthetic material that physically takes the place and/or function of all or a portion of a body part

Explanation: The body part may have been taken out or replaced, or may be taken out, physically eradicated, or rendered nonfunctional during the REPLACEMENT procedure. A REMOVAL procedure is coded for taking out the device used in a previous replacement procedure.

Body Part Character 4	Approach Character 5	Device Character 6	Qualifier Character 7
Ø Azygos Vein Right ascending lumbar vein Right subcostal vein **1 Hemiazygos Vein** Left ascending lumbar vein Left subcostal vein **3 Innominate Vein, Right** Brachiocephalic vein Inferior thyroid vein **4 Innominate Vein, Left** *See 3 Innominate Vein, Right* **5 Subclavian Vein, Right** **6 Subclavian Vein, Left** **7 Axillary Vein, Right** **8 Axillary Vein, Left** **9 Brachial Vein, Right** Radial vein Ulnar vein **A Brachial Vein, Left** *See 9 Brachial Vein, Right* **B Basilic Vein, Right** Median antebrachial vein Median cubital vein **C Basilic Vein, Left** *See B Basilic Vein, Right* **D Cephalic Vein, Right** Accessory cephalic vein **F Cephalic Vein, Left** *See D Cephalic Vein, Right* **G Hand Vein, Right** Dorsal metacarpal vein Palmar (volar) digital vein Palmar (volar) metacarpal vein Superficial palmar venous arch Volar (palmar) digital vein Volar (palmar) metacarpal vein **H Hand Vein, Left** *See G Hand Vein, Right* **L Intracranial Vein** Anterior cerebral vein Basal (internal) cerebral vein Dural venous sinus Great cerebral vein Inferior cerebellar vein Inferior cerebral vein Internal (basal) cerebral vein Middle cerebral vein Ophthalmic vein Superior cerebellar vein Superior cerebral vein **M Internal Jugular Vein, Right** **N Internal Jugular Vein, Left** **P External Jugular Vein, Right** Posterior auricular vein **Q External Jugular Vein, Left** *See P External Jugular Vein, Right* **R Vertebral Vein, Right** Deep cervical vein Suboccipital venous plexus **S Vertebral Vein, Left** *See R Vertebral Vein, Right* **T Face Vein, Right** Angular vein Anterior facial vein Common facial vein Deep facial vein Frontal vein Posterior facial (retromandibular) vein Supraorbital vein **V Face Vein, Left** *See T Face Vein, Right* **Y Upper Vein**	**Ø Open** **4 Percutaneous Endoscopic**	**7 Autologous Tissue Substitute** **J Synthetic Substitute** **K Nonautologous Tissue Substitute**	**Z No Qualifier**

Ø Medical and Surgical
5 Upper Veins
S Reposition Definition: Moving to its normal location, or other suitable location, all or a portion of a body part

Explanation: The body part is moved to a new location from an abnormal location, or from a normal location where it is not functioning correctly. The body part may or may not be cut out or off to be moved to the new location.

Body Part Character 4	Approach Character 5	Device Character 6	Qualifier Character 7
Ø Azygos Vein Right ascending lumbar vein Right subcostal vein **1 Hemiazygos Vein** Left ascending lumbar vein Left subcostal vein **3 Innominate Vein, Right** Brachiocephalic vein Inferior thyroid vein **4 Innominate Vein, Left** *See 3 Innominate Vein, Right* **5 Subclavian Vein, Right** **6 Subclavian Vein, Left** **7 Axillary Vein, Right** **8 Axillary Vein, Left** **9 Brachial Vein, Right** Radial vein Ulnar vein **A Brachial Vein, Left** *See 9 Brachial Vein, Right* **B Basilic Vein, Right** Median antebrachial vein Median cubital vein **C Basilic Vein, Left** *See B Basilic Vein, Right* **D Cephalic Vein, Right** Accessory cephalic vein **F Cephalic Vein, Left** *See D Cephalic Vein, Right* **G Hand Vein, Right** Dorsal metacarpal vein Palmar (volar) digital vein Palmar (volar) metacarpal vein Superficial palmar venous arch Volar (palmar) digital vein Volar (palmar) metacarpal vein **H Hand Vein, Left** *See G Hand Vein, Right* **L Intracranial Vein** Anterior cerebral vein Basal (internal) cerebral vein Dural venous sinus Great cerebral vein Inferior cerebellar vein Inferior cerebral vein Internal (basal) cerebral vein Middle cerebral vein Ophthalmic vein Superior cerebellar vein Superior cerebral vein **M Internal Jugular Vein, Right** **N Internal Jugular Vein, Left** **P External Jugular Vein, Right** Posterior auricular vein **Q External Jugular Vein, Left** *See P External Jugular Vein, Right* **R Vertebral Vein, Right** Deep cervical vein Suboccipital venous plexus **S Vertebral Vein, Left** *See R Vertebral Vein, Right* **T Face Vein, Right** Angular vein Anterior facial vein Common facial vein Deep facial vein Frontal vein Posterior facial (retromandibular) vein Supraorbital vein **V Face Vein, Left** *See T Face Vein, Right* **Y Upper Vein**	**Ø Open** **3 Percutaneous** **4 Percutaneous Endoscopic**	**Z No Device**	**Z No Qualifier**

Ø Medical and Surgical
5 Upper Veins
U Supplement Definition: Putting in or on biological or synthetic material that physically reinforces and/or augments the function of a portion of a body part

Explanation: The biological material is non-living, or is living and from the same individual. The body part may have been previously replaced, and the SUPPLEMENT procedure is performed to physically reinforce and/or augment the function of the replaced body part.

Body Part Character 4	Approach Character 5	Device Character 6	Qualifier Character 7
Ø Azygos Vein Right ascending lumbar vein Right subcostal vein **1 Hemiazygos Vein** Left ascending lumbar vein Left subcostal vein **3 Innominate Vein, Right** Brachiocephalic vein Inferior thyroid vein **4 Innominate Vein, Left** *See 3 Innominate Vein, Right* **5 Subclavian Vein, Right** **6 Subclavian Vein, Left** **7 Axillary Vein, Right** **8 Axillary Vein, Left** **9 Brachial Vein, Right** Radial vein Ulnar vein **A Brachial Vein, Left** *See 9 Brachial Vein, Right* **B Basilic Vein, Right** Median antebrachial vein Median cubital vein **C Basilic Vein, Left** *See B Basilic Vein, Right* **D Cephalic Vein, Right** Accessory cephalic vein **F Cephalic Vein, Left** *See D Cephalic Vein, Right* **G Hand Vein, Right** Dorsal metacarpal vein Palmar (volar) digital vein Palmar (volar) metacarpal vein Superficial palmar venous arch Volar (palmar) digital vein Volar (palmar) metacarpal vein **H Hand Vein, Left** *See G Hand Vein, Right* **L Intracranial Vein** Anterior cerebral vein Basal (internal) cerebral vein Dural venous sinus Great cerebral vein Inferior cerebellar vein Inferior cerebral vein Internal (basal) cerebral vein Middle cerebral vein Ophthalmic vein Superior cerebellar vein Superior cerebral vein **M Internal Jugular Vein, Right** **N Internal Jugular Vein, Left** **P External Jugular Vein, Right** Posterior auricular vein **Q External Jugular Vein, Left** *See P External Jugular Vein, Right* **R Vertebral Vein, Right** Deep cervical vein Suboccipital venous plexus **S Vertebral Vein, Left** *See R Vertebral Vein, Right* **T Face Vein, Right** Angular vein Anterior facial vein Common facial vein Deep facial vein Frontal vein Posterior facial (retromandibular) vein Supraorbital vein **V Face Vein, Left** *See T Face Vein, Right* **Y Upper Vein**	**Ø Open** **3 Percutaneous** **4 Percutaneous Endoscopic**	**7 Autologous Tissue Substitute** **J Synthetic Substitute** **K Nonautologous Tissue Substitute**	**Z No Qualifier**

Ø Medical and Surgical
5 Upper Veins
V Restriction Definition: Partially closing an orifice or the lumen of a tubular body part
Explanation: The orifice can be a natural orifice or an artificially created orifice

Body Part Character 4	Approach Character 5	Device Character 6	Qualifier Character 7
Ø Azygos Vein Right ascending lumbar vein Right subcostal vein **1 Hemiazygos Vein** Left ascending lumbar vein Left subcostal vein **3 Innominate Vein, Right** Brachiocephalic vein Inferior thyroid vein **4 Innominate Vein, Left** *See 3 Innominate Vein, Right* **5 Subclavian Vein, Right** **6 Subclavian Vein, Left** **7 Axillary Vein, Right** **8 Axillary Vein, Left** **9 Brachial Vein, Right** Radial vein Ulnar vein **A Brachial Vein, Left** *See 9 Brachial Vein, Right* **B Basilic Vein, Right** Median antebrachial vein Median cubital vein **C Basilic Vein, Left** *See B Basilic Vein, Right* **D Cephalic Vein, Right** Accessory cephalic vein **F Cephalic Vein, Left** *See D Cephalic Vein, Right* **G Hand Vein, Right** Dorsal metacarpal vein Palmar (volar) digital vein Palmar (volar) metacarpal vein Superficial palmar venous arch Volar (palmar) digital vein Volar (palmar) metacarpal vein **H Hand Vein, Left** *See G Hand Vein, Right* **L Intracranial Vein** Anterior cerebral vein Basal (internal) cerebral vein Dural venous sinus Great cerebral vein Inferior cerebellar vein Inferior cerebral vein Internal (basal) cerebral vein Middle cerebral vein Ophthalmic vein Superior cerebellar vein Superior cerebral vein **M Internal Jugular Vein, Right** **N Internal Jugular Vein, Left** **P External Jugular Vein, Right** Posterior auricular vein **Q External Jugular Vein, Left** *See P External Jugular Vein, Right* **R Vertebral Vein, Right** Deep cervical vein Suboccipital venous plexus **S Vertebral Vein, Left** *See R Vertebral Vein, Right* **T Face Vein, Right** Angular vein Anterior facial vein Common facial vein Deep facial vein Frontal vein Posterior facial (retromandibular) vein Supraorbital vein **V Face Vein, Left** *See T Face Vein, Right* **Y Upper Vein**	**Ø Open** **3 Percutaneous** **4 Percutaneous Endoscopic**	**C Extraluminal Device** **D Intraluminal Device** **Z No Device**	**Z No Qualifier**

Ø Medical and Surgical
5 Upper Veins
W Revision

Definition: Correcting, to the extent possible, a portion of a malfunctioning device or the position of a displaced device

Explanation: Revision can include correcting a malfunctioning or displaced device by taking out or putting in components of the device such as a screw or pin

Body Part Character 4	Approach Character 5	Device Character 6	Qualifier Character 7
Ø Azygos Vein Right ascending lumbar vein Right subcostal vein	**Ø** Open **3** Percutaneous **4** Percutaneous Endoscopic **X** External	**2** Monitoring Device **M** Neurostimulator Lead	**Z** No Qualifier
3 Innominate Vein, Right Brachiocephalic vein Inferior thyroid vein **4** Innominate Vein, Left *See 3 Innominate Vein, Right*	**Ø** Open **3** Percutaneous **4** Percutaneous Endoscopic **X** External	**M** Neurostimulator Lead	**Z** No Qualifier
Y Upper Vein	**Ø** Open **3** Percutaneous **4** Percutaneous Endoscopic	**Ø** Drainage Device **2** Monitoring Device **3** Infusion Device **7** Autologous Tissue Substitute **C** Extraluminal Device **D** Intraluminal Device **J** Synthetic Substitute **K** Nonautologous Tissue Substitute **Y** Other Device	**Z** No Qualifier
Y Upper Vein	**X** External	**Ø** Drainage Device **2** Monitoring Device **3** Infusion Device **7** Autologous Tissue Substitute **C** Extraluminal Device **D** Intraluminal Device **J** Synthetic Substitute **K** Nonautologous Tissue Substitute	**Z** No Qualifier

Non-OR Ø5WØXMZ
Non-OR Ø5W[3,4]XMZ
Non-OR Ø5WY3[Ø,2,3,D]Z
Non-OR Ø5WY[3,4]YZ
Non-OR Ø5WYX[Ø,2,3,7,C,D,J,K]Z

Lower Veins Ø61–Ø6W

Character Meanings

This Character Meaning table is provided as a guide to assist the user in the identification of character members that may be found in this section of code tables. It **SHOULD NOT** be used to build a PCS code.

Operation–Character 3	Body Part–Character 4	Approach–Character 5	Device–Character 6	Qualifier–Character 7
1 Bypass	Ø Inferior Vena Cava	Ø Open	Ø Drainage Device	Ø Ultrasonic
5 Destruction	1 Splenic Vein	3 Percutaneous	2 Monitoring Device	4 Hepatic Vein
7 Dilation	2 Gastric Vein	4 Percutaneous Endoscopic	3 Infusion Device	5 Superior Mesenteric Vein
9 Drainage	3 Esophageal Vein	7 Via Natural or Artificial Opening	7 Autologous Tissue Substitute	6 Inferior Mesenteric Vein
B Excision	4 Hepatic Vein	8 Via Natural or Artificial Opening Endoscopic	9 Autologous Venous Tissue	9 Renal Vein, Right
C Extirpation	5 Superior Mesenteric Vein	X External	A Autologous Arterial Tissue	B Renal Vein, Left
D Extraction	6 Inferior Mesenteric Vein		C Extraluminal Device	C Hemorrhoidal Plexus
F Fragmentation	7 Colic Vein		D Intraluminal Device	P Pulmonary Trunk
H Insertion	8 Portal Vein		J Synthetic Substitute	Q Pulmonary Artery, Right
J Inspection	9 Renal Vein, Right		K Nonautologous Tissue Substitute	R Pulmonary Artery, Left
L Occlusion	B Renal Vein, Left		Y Other Device	T Via Umbilical Vein
N Release	C Common Iliac Vein, Right		Z No Device	X Diagnostic
P Removal	D Common Iliac Vein, Left			Y Lower Vein
Q Repair	F External Iliac Vein, Right			Z No Qualifier
R Replacement	G External Iliac Vein, Left			
S Reposition	H Hypogastric Vein, Right			
U Supplement	J Hypogastric Vein, Left			
V Restriction	M Femoral Vein, Right			
W Revision	N Femoral Vein, Left			
	P Saphenous Vein, Right			
	Q Saphenous Vein, Left			
	T Foot Vein, Right			
	V Foot Vein, Left			
	Y Lower Vein			

AHA Coding Clinic for table Ø61

2017, 4Q, 36-38	Fontan completion procedure
2017, 4Q, 66-67	New qualifier values - Portal to hepatic shunt

AHA Coding Clinic for table Ø6B

2020, 1Q, 28	Free flap microvascular breast reconstruction
2017, 3Q, 5	Femoral artery to posterior tibial artery bypass using autologous and synthetic grafts
2017, 1Q, 31	Left to right common carotid artery bypass
2017, 1Q, 32	Peroneal artery to dorsalis pedis artery bypass using saphenous vein graft
2016, 3Q, 31	Femoral to peroneal artery bypass with in-situ saphenous vein graft and lysis of valves
2016, 2Q, 18	Femoral-tibial artery bypass and saphenous vein graft
2016, 1Q, 27	Aortocoronary bypass graft utilizing Y-graft
2014, 3Q, 8	Excision of saphenous vein for coronary artery bypass graft
2014, 3Q, 20	MAZE procedure performed with coronary artery bypass graft
2014, 1Q, 10	Repair of thoracic aortic aneurysm & coronary artery bypass graft

AHA Coding Clinic for table Ø6F

2020, 4Q, 45-49	New fragmentation tables
2020, 4Q, 49-50	Intravascular ultrasound assisted thrombolysis
2020, 4Q, 50	Intravascular lithotripsy

AHA Coding Clinic for table Ø6H

2017, 3Q, 11	Placement of peripherally inserted central catheter using 3CG ECG technology
2017, 1Q, 31	Umbilical vein catheterization
2017, 1Q, 31	Central catheter placement in femoral vein
2013, 3Q, 18	Heart transplant surgery

AHA Coding Clinic for table Ø6L

2020, 3Q, 44	Cardiophrenic vein embolization
2019, 4Q, 28	Transorifice occlusion of gastric varices
2018, 2Q, 18	Transverse rectus abdominis myocutaneous (TRAM) delay
2017, 4Q, 57-58	Added approach values - Transorifice esophageal vein banding
2013, 4Q, 112	Endoscopic banding of esophageal varices

AHA Coding Clinic for table Ø6V

2018, 3Q, 11	Transvenous transcatheter placement of valve in inferior vena cava
2018, 1Q, 10	Revision of transjugular intrahepatic portosystemic shunt

AHA Coding Clinic for table Ø6W

2019, 2Q, 39	Transjugular intrahepatic portosystemic shunt revision
2018, 1Q, 10	Revision of transjugular intrahepatic portosystemic shunt
2014, 3Q, 25	Revision of transjugular intrahepatic portosystemic shunt (TIPS)

Lower Veins

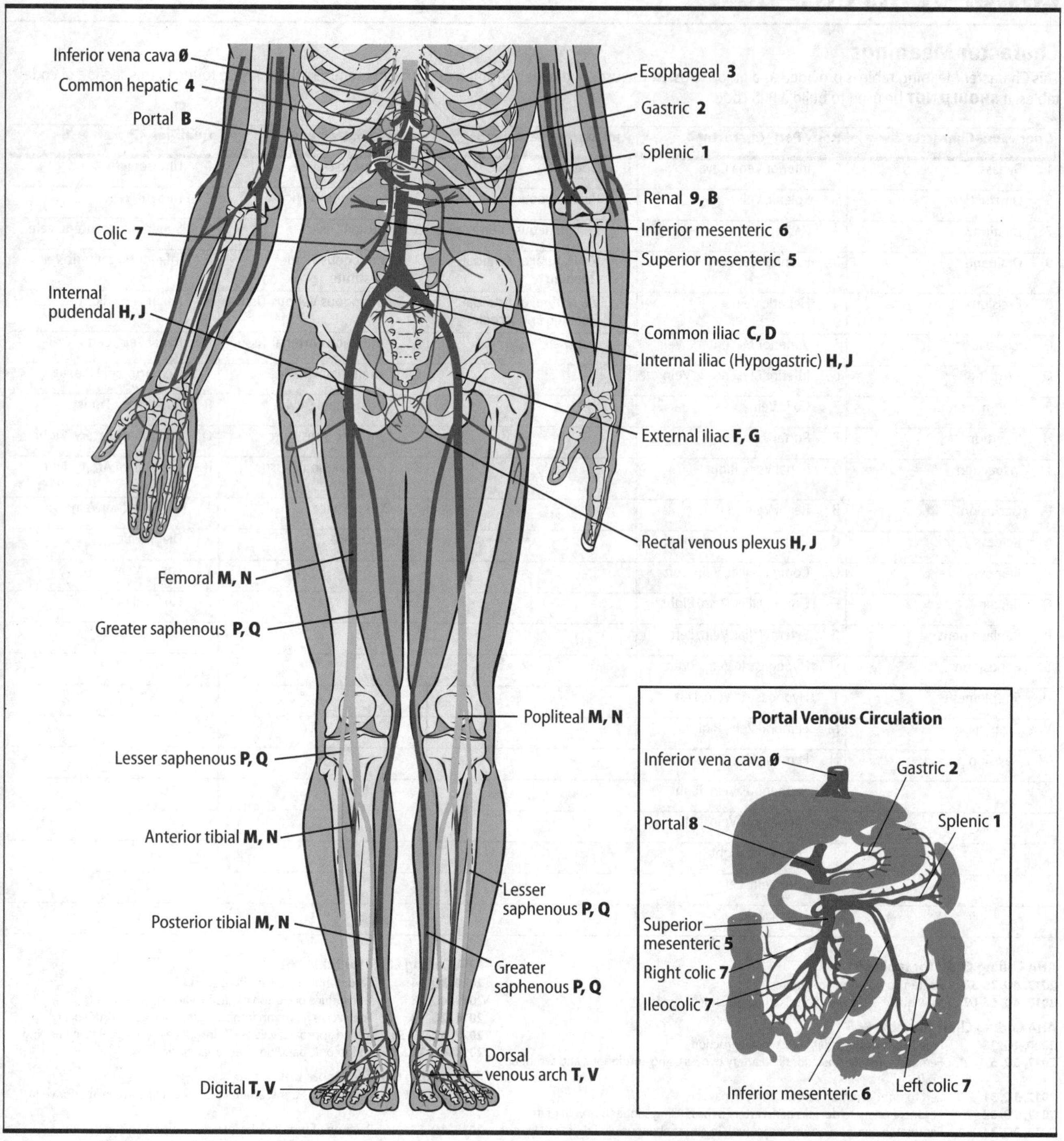
Inferior vena cava Ø
Common hepatic 4
Portal B
Colic 7
Internal pudendal H, J
Esophageal 3
Gastric 2
Splenic 1
Renal 9, B
Inferior mesenteric 6
Superior mesenteric 5
Common iliac C, D
Internal iliac (Hypogastric) H, J
External iliac F, G
Rectal venous plexus H, J
Femoral M, N
Greater saphenous P, Q
Popliteal M, N
Lesser saphenous P, Q
Anterior tibial M, N
Lesser saphenous P, Q
Posterior tibial M, N
Greater saphenous P, Q
Dorsal venous arch T, V
Digital T, V
Portal Venous Circulation
Inferior vena cava Ø
Gastric 2
Portal 8
Splenic 1
Superior mesenteric 5
Right colic 7
Ileocolic 7
Inferior mesenteric 6
Left colic 7

Ø Medical and Surgical
6 Lower Veins
1 Bypass Definition: Altering the route of passage of the contents of a tubular body part

Explanation: Rerouting contents of a body part to a downstream area of the normal route, to a similar route and body part, or to an abnormal route and dissimilar body part. Includes one or more anastomoses, with or without the use of a device.

Body Part Character 4	Approach Character 5	Device Character 6	Qualifier Character 7
Ø Inferior Vena Cava Postcava Right inferior phrenic vein Right ovarian vein Right second lumbar vein Right suprarenal vein Right testicular vein	**Ø Open** **4 Percutaneous Endoscopic**	**7 Autologous Tissue Substitute** **9 Autologous Venous Tissue** **A Autologous Arterial Tissue** **J Synthetic Substitute** **K Nonautologous Tissue Substitute** **Z No Device**	**5 Superior Mesenteric Vein** **6 Inferior Mesenteric Vein** **P Pulmonary Trunk** **Q Pulmonary Artery, Right** **R Pulmonary Artery, Left** **Y Lower Vein**
1 Splenic Vein Left gastroepiploic vein Pancreatic vein	**Ø Open** **4 Percutaneous Endoscopic**	**7 Autologous Tissue Substitute** **9 Autologous Venous Tissue** **A Autologous Arterial Tissue** **J Synthetic Substitute** **K Nonautologous Tissue Substitute** **Z No Device**	**9 Renal Vein, Right** **B Renal Vein, Left** **Y Lower Vein**
2 Gastric Vein **3 Esophageal Vein** **4 Hepatic Vein** **5 Superior Mesenteric Vein** Right gastroepiploic vein **6 Inferior Mesenteric Vein** Sigmoid vein Superior rectal vein **7 Colic Vein** Ileocolic vein Left colic vein Middle colic vein Right colic vein **9 Renal Vein, Right** **B Renal Vein, Left** Left inferior phrenic vein Left ovarian vein Left second lumbar vein Left suprarenal vein Left testicular vein **C Common Iliac Vein, Right** **D Common Iliac Vein, Left** **F External Iliac Vein, Right** **G External Iliac Vein, Left** **H Hypogastric Vein, Right** Gluteal vein Internal iliac vein Internal pudendal vein Lateral sacral vein Middle hemorrhoidal vein Obturator vein Uterine vein Vaginal vein Vesical vein **J Hypogastric Vein, Left** *See H Hypogastric Vein, Right* **M Femoral Vein, Right** Deep femoral (profunda femoris) vein Popliteal vein Profunda femoris (deep femoral) vein **N Femoral Vein, Left** *See M Femoral Vein, Right* **P Saphenous Vein, Right** External pudendal vein Great(er) saphenous vein Lesser saphenous vein Small saphenous vein Superficial circumflex iliac vein Superficial epigastric vein **Q Saphenous Vein, Left** *See P Saphenous Vein, Right* **T Foot Vein, Right** Common digital vein Dorsal metatarsal vein Dorsal venous arch Plantar digital vein Plantar metatarsal vein Plantar venous arch **V Foot Vein, Left** *See T Foot Vein, Right*	**Ø Open** **4 Percutaneous Endoscopic**	**7 Autologous Tissue Substitute** **9 Autologous Venous Tissue** **A Autologous Arterial Tissue** **J Synthetic Substitute** **K Nonautologous Tissue Substitute** **Z No Device**	**Y Lower Vein**
8 Portal Vein Hepatic portal vein	**Ø Open**	**7 Autologous Tissue Substitute** **9 Autologous Venous Tissue** **A Autologous Arterial Tissue** **J Synthetic Substitute** **K Nonautologous Tissue Substitute** **Z No Device**	**9 Renal Vein, Right** **B Renal Vein, Left** **Y Lower Vein**
8 Portal Vein Hepatic portal vein	**3 Percutaneous**	**J Synthetic Substitute**	**4 Hepatic Vein** **Y Lower Vein**
8 Portal Vein Hepatic portal vein	**4 Percutaneous Endoscopic**	**7 Autologous Tissue Substitute** **9 Autologous Venous Tissue** **A Autologous Arterial Tissue** **K Nonautologous Tissue Substitute** **Z No Device**	**9 Renal Vein, Right** **B Renal Vein, Left** **Y Lower Vein**
8 Portal Vein Hepatic portal vein	**4 Percutaneous Endoscopic**	**J Synthetic Substitute**	**4 Hepatic Vein** **9 Renal Vein, Right** **B Renal Vein, Left** **Y Lower Vein**

Ø Medical and Surgical
6 Lower Veins
5 Destruction Definition: Physical eradication of all or a portion of a body part by the direct use of energy, force, or a destructive agent

Explanation: None of the body part is physically taken out

Body Part Character 4	Approach Character 5	Device Character 6	Qualifier Character 7
Ø Inferior Vena Cava Postcava Right inferior phrenic vein Right ovarian vein Right second lumbar vein Right suprarenal vein Right testicular vein **1 Splenic Vein** Left gastroepiploic vein Pancreatic vein **2 Gastric Vein** **3 Esophageal Vein** **4 Hepatic Vein** **5 Superior Mesenteric Vein** Right gastroepiploic vein **6 Inferior Mesenteric Vein** Sigmoid vein Superior rectal vein **7 Colic Vein** Ileocolic vein Left colic vein Middle colic vein Right colic vein **8 Portal Vein** Hepatic portal vein **9 Renal Vein, Right** **B Renal Vein, Left** Left inferior phrenic vein Left ovarian vein Left second lumbar vein Left suprarenal vein Left testicular vein **C Common Iliac Vein, Right** **D Common Iliac Vein, Left** **F External Iliac Vein, Right** **G External Iliac Vein, Left** **H Hypogastric Vein, Right** Gluteal vein Internal iliac vein Internal pudendal vein Lateral sacral vein Middle hemorrhoidal vein Obturator vein Uterine vein Vaginal vein Vesical vein **J Hypogastric Vein, Left** *See H Hypogastric Vein, Right* **M Femoral Vein, Right** Deep femoral (profunda femoris) vein Popliteal vein Profunda femoris (deep femoral) vein **N Femoral Vein, Left** *See M Femoral Vein, Right* **P Saphenous Vein, Right** External pudendal vein Great(er) saphenous vein Lesser saphenous vein Small saphenous vein Superficial circumflex iliac vein Superficial epigastric vein **Q Saphenous Vein, Left** *See P Saphenous Vein, Right* **T Foot Vein, Right** Common digital vein Dorsal metatarsal vein Dorsal venous arch Plantar digital vein Plantar metatarsal vein Plantar venous arch **V Foot Vein, Left** *See T Foot Vein, Right*	**Ø Open** **3 Percutaneous** **4 Percutaneous Endoscopic**	**Z No Device**	**Z No Qualifier**
Y Lower Vein	**Ø Open** **3 Percutaneous** **4 Percutaneous Endoscopic**	**Z No Device**	**C Hemorrhoidal Plexus** **Z No Qualifier**

Ø Medical and Surgical
6 Lower Veins
7 Dilation Definition: Expanding an orifice or the lumen of a tubular body part

Explanation: The orifice can be a natural orifice or an artificially created orifice. Accomplished by stretching a tubular body part using intraluminal pressure or by cutting part of the orifice or wall of the tubular body part.

Body Part Character 4	Approach Character 5	Device Character 6	Qualifier Character 7
Ø Inferior Vena Cava Postcava Right inferior phrenic vein Right ovarian vein Right second lumbar vein Right suprarenal vein Right testicular vein **1 Splenic Vein** Left gastroepiploic vein Pancreatic vein **2 Gastric Vein** **3 Esophageal Vein** **4 Hepatic Vein** **5 Superior Mesenteric Vein** Right gastroepiploic vein **6 Inferior Mesenteric Vein** Sigmoid vein Superior rectal vein **7 Colic Vein** Ileocolic vein Left colic vein Middle colic vein Right colic vein **8 Portal Vein** Hepatic portal vein **9 Renal Vein, Right** **B Renal Vein, Left** Left inferior phrenic vein Left ovarian vein Left second lumbar vein Left suprarenal vein Left testicular vein **C Common Iliac Vein, Right** **D Common Iliac Vein, Left** **F External Iliac Vein, Right** **G External Iliac Vein, Left** **H Hypogastric Vein, Right** Gluteal vein Internal iliac vein Internal pudendal vein Lateral sacral vein Middle hemorrhoidal vein Obturator vein Uterine vein Vaginal vein Vesical vein **J Hypogastric Vein, Left** ***See** H Hypogastric Vein, Right* **M Femoral Vein, Right** Deep femoral (profunda femoris) vein Popliteal vein Profunda femoris (deep femoral) vein **N Femoral Vein, Left** ***See** M Femoral Vein, Right* **P Saphenous Vein, Right** External pudendal vein Great(er) saphenous vein Lesser saphenous vein Small saphenous vein Superficial circumflex iliac vein Superficial epigastric vein **Q Saphenous Vein, Left** ***See** P Saphenous Vein, Right* **T Foot Vein, Right** Common digital vein Dorsal metatarsal vein Dorsal venous arch Plantar digital vein Plantar metatarsal vein Plantar venous arch **V Foot Vein, Left** ***See** T Foot Vein, Right* **Y Lower Vein**	**Ø Open** **3 Percutaneous** **4 Percutaneous Endoscopic**	**D Intraluminal Device** **Z No Device**	**Z No Qualifier**

Ø Medical and Surgical
6 Lower Veins
9 Drainage Definition: Taking or letting out fluids and/or gases from a body part
Explanation: The qualifier DIAGNOSTIC is used to identify drainage procedures that are biopsies

Body Part Character 4	Approach Character 5	Device Character 6	Qualifier Character 7
Ø Inferior Vena Cava Postcava Right inferior phrenic vein Right ovarian vein Right second lumbar vein Right suprarenal vein Right testicular vein **1 Splenic Vein** Left gastroepiploic vein Pancreatic vein **2 Gastric Vein** **3 Esophageal Vein** **4 Hepatic Vein** **5 Superior Mesenteric Vein** Right gastroepiploic vein **6 Inferior Mesenteric Vein** Sigmoid vein Superior rectal vein **7 Colic Vein** Ileocolic vein Left colic vein Middle colic vein Right colic vein **8 Portal Vein** Hepatic portal vein **9 Renal Vein, Right** **B Renal Vein, Left** Left inferior phrenic vein Left ovarian vein Left second lumbar vein Left suprarenal vein Left testicular vein **C Common Iliac Vein, Right** **D Common Iliac Vein, Left** **F External Iliac Vein, Right** **G External Iliac Vein, Left** **H Hypogastric Vein, Right** Gluteal vein Internal iliac vein Internal pudendal vein Lateral sacral vein Middle hemorrhoidal vein Obturator vein Uterine vein Vaginal vein Vesical vein **J Hypogastric Vein, Left** *See H Hypogastric Vein, Right* **M Femoral Vein, Right** Deep femoral (profunda femoris) vein Popliteal vein Profunda femoris (deep femoral) vein **N Femoral Vein, Left** *See M Femoral Vein, Right* **P Saphenous Vein, Right** External pudendal vein Great(er) saphenous vein Lesser saphenous vein Small saphenous vein Superficial circumflex iliac vein Superficial epigastric vein **Q Saphenous Vein, Left** *See P Saphenous Vein, Right* **T Foot Vein, Right** Common digital vein Dorsal metatarsal vein Dorsal venous arch Plantar digital vein Plantar metatarsal vein Plantar venous arch **V Foot Vein, Left** *See T Foot Vein, Right* **Y Lower Vein**	**Ø Open** **3 Percutaneous** **4 Percutaneous Endoscopic**	**Ø Drainage Device**	**Z No Qualifier**

Non-OR Ø69[Ø,1,2,4,5,6,7,8,9,B,C,D,F,G,H,J,M,N,P,Q,T,V,Y][Ø,3,4]ØZ
Non-OR Ø6933ØZ

Ø69 Continued on next page

Ø69 Continued

Ø Medical and Surgical
6 Lower Veins
9 Drainage Definition: Taking or letting out fluids and/or gases from a body part
Explanation: The qualifier DIAGNOSTIC is used to identify drainage procedures that are biopsies

Body Part Character 4	Approach Character 5	Device Character 6	Qualifier Character 7
Ø Inferior Vena Cava Postcava Right inferior phrenic vein Right ovarian vein Right second lumbar vein Right suprarenal vein Right testicular vein **1 Splenic Vein** Left gastroepiploic vein Pancreatic vein **2 Gastric Vein** **3 Esophageal Vein** **4 Hepatic Vein** **5 Superior Mesenteric Vein** Right gastroepiploic vein **6 Inferior Mesenteric Vein** Sigmoid vein Superior rectal vein **7 Colic Vein** Ileocolic vein Left colic vein Middle colic vein Right colic vein **8 Portal Vein** Hepatic portal vein **9 Renal Vein, Right** **B Renal Vein, Left** Left inferior phrenic vein Left ovarian vein Left second lumbar vein Left suprarenal vein Left testicular vein **C Common Iliac Vein, Right** **D Common Iliac Vein, Left** **F External Iliac Vein, Right** **G External Iliac Vein, Left** **H Hypogastric Vein, Right** Gluteal vein Internal iliac vein Internal pudendal vein Lateral sacral vein Middle hemorrhoidal vein Obturator vein Uterine vein Vaginal vein Vesical vein **J Hypogastric Vein, Left** *See H Hypogastric Vein, Right* **M Femoral Vein, Right** Deep femoral (profunda femoris) vein Popliteal vein Profunda femoris (deep femoral) vein **N Femoral Vein, Left** *See M Femoral Vein, Right* **P Saphenous Vein, Right** External pudendal vein Great(er) saphenous vein Lesser saphenous vein Small saphenous vein Superficial circumflex iliac vein Superficial epigastric vein **Q Saphenous Vein, Left** *See P Saphenous Vein, Right* **T Foot Vein, Right** Common digital vein Dorsal metatarsal vein Dorsal venous arch Plantar digital vein Plantar metatarsal vein Plantar venous arch **V Foot Vein, Left** *See T Foot Vein, Right* **Y Lower Vein**	**Ø Open** **3 Percutaneous** **4 Percutaneous Endoscopic**	**Z No Device**	**X Diagnostic** **Z No Qualifier**

Non-OR Ø69[Ø,1,2,3,4,5,6,7,8,9,B,C,D,F,G,H,J,M,N,P,Q,T,V,Y]3ZX
Non-OR Ø69[Ø,1,2,4,5,6,7,8,9,B,C,D,F,G,H,J,M,N,P,Q,T,V,Y][Ø,3,4]ZZ
Non-OR Ø6933ZZ

Ø Medical and Surgical
6 Lower Veins
B Excision Definition: Cutting out or off, without replacement, a portion of a body part
Explanation: The qualifier DIAGNOSTIC is used to identify excision procedures that are biopsies

Body Part Character 4	Approach Character 5	Device Character 6	Qualifier Character 7
Ø Inferior Vena Cava Postcava Right inferior phrenic vein Right ovarian vein Right second lumbar vein Right suprarenal vein Right testicular vein **1 Splenic Vein** Left gastroepiploic vein Pancreatic vein **2 Gastric Vein** **3 Esophageal Vein** **4 Hepatic Vein** **5 Superior Mesenteric Vein** Right gastroepiploic vein **6 Inferior Mesenteric Vein** Sigmoid vein Superior rectal vein **7 Colic Vein** Ileocolic vein Left colic vein Middle colic vein Right colic vein **8 Portal Vein** Hepatic portal vein **9 Renal Vein, Right** **B Renal Vein, Left** Left inferior phrenic vein Left ovarian vein Left second lumbar vein Left suprarenal vein Left testicular vein **C Common Iliac Vein, Right** **D Common Iliac Vein, Left** **F External Iliac Vein, Right** **G External Iliac Vein, Left** **H Hypogastric Vein, Right** Gluteal vein Internal iliac vein Internal pudendal vein Lateral sacral vein Middle hemorrhoidal vein Obturator vein Uterine vein Vaginal vein Vesical vein **J Hypogastric Vein, Left** *See H Hypogastric Vein, Right* **M Femoral Vein, Right** Deep femoral (profunda femoris) vein Popliteal vein Profunda femoris (deep femoral) vein **N Femoral Vein, Left** *See M Femoral Vein, Right* **P Saphenous Vein, Right** External pudendal vein Great(er) saphenous vein Lesser saphenous vein Small saphenous vein Superficial circumflex iliac vein Superficial epigastric vein **Q Saphenous Vein, Left** *See P Saphenous Vein, Right* **T Foot Vein, Right** Common digital vein Dorsal metatarsal vein Dorsal venous arch Plantar digital vein Plantar metatarsal vein Plantar venous arch **V Foot Vein, Left** *See T Foot Vein, Right*	**Ø Open** **3 Percutaneous** **4 Percutaneous Endoscopic**	**Z No Device**	**X Diagnostic** **Z No Qualifier**
Y Lower Vein	**Ø Open** **3 Percutaneous** **4 Percutaneous Endoscopic**	**Z No Device**	**C Hemorrhoidal Plexus** **X Diagnostic** **Z No Qualifier**

Ø Medical and Surgical
6 Lower Veins
C Extirpation Definition: Taking or cutting out solid matter from a body part

Explanation: The solid matter may be an abnormal byproduct of a biological function or a foreign body; it may be imbedded in a body part or in the lumen of a tubular body part. The solid matter may or may not have been previously broken into pieces.

Body Part Character 4	Approach Character 5	Device Character 6	Qualifier Character 7
Ø Inferior Vena Cava Postcava Right inferior phrenic vein Right ovarian vein Right second lumbar vein Right suprarenal vein Right testicular vein **1 Splenic Vein** Left gastroepiploic vein Pancreatic vein **2 Gastric Vein** **3 Esophageal Vein** **4 Hepatic Vein** **5 Superior Mesenteric Vein** Right gastroepiploic vein **6 Inferior Mesenteric Vein** Sigmoid vein Superior rectal vein **7 Colic Vein** Ileocolic vein Left colic vein Middle colic vein Right colic vein **8 Portal Vein** Hepatic portal vein **9 Renal Vein, Right** **B Renal Vein, Left** Left inferior phrenic vein Left ovarian vein Left second lumbar vein Left suprarenal vein Left testicular vein **C Common Iliac Vein, Right** **D Common Iliac Vein, Left** **F External Iliac Vein, Right** **G External Iliac Vein, Left** **H Hypogastric Vein, Right** Gluteal vein Internal iliac vein Internal pudendal vein Lateral sacral vein Middle hemorrhoidal vein Obturator vein Uterine vein Vaginal vein Vesical vein **J Hypogastric Vein, Left** *See H Hypogastric Vein, Right* **M Femoral Vein, Right** Deep femoral (profunda femoris) vein Popliteal vein Profunda femoris (deep femoral) vein **N Femoral Vein, Left** *See M Femoral Vein, Right* **P Saphenous Vein, Right** External pudendal vein Great(er) saphenous vein Lesser saphenous vein Small saphenous vein Superficial circumflex iliac vein Superficial epigastric vein **Q Saphenous Vein, Left** *See P Saphenous Vein, Right* **T Foot Vein, Right** Common digital vein Dorsal metatarsal vein Dorsal venous arch Plantar digital vein Plantar metatarsal vein Plantar venous arch **V Foot Vein, Left** *See T Foot Vein, Right* **Y Lower Vein**	**Ø Open** **3 Percutaneous** **4 Percutaneous Endoscopic**	**Z No Device**	**Z No Qualifier**

Ø Medical and Surgical
6 Lower Veins
D Extraction Definition: Pulling or stripping out or off all or a portion of a body part by the use of force

Explanation: The qualifier DIAGNOSTIC is used to identify extraction procedures that are biopsies

Body Part Character 4	Approach Character 5	Device Character 6	Qualifier Character 7
M Femoral Vein, Right Deep femoral (profunda femoris) vein Popliteal vein Profunda femoris (deep femoral) vein **N Femoral Vein, Left** *See M Femoral Vein, Right* **P Saphenous Vein, Right** External pudendal vein Great(er) saphenous vein Lesser saphenous vein Small saphenous vein Superficial circumflex iliac vein Superficial epigastric vein **Q Saphenous Vein, Left** *See P Saphenous Vein, Right* **T Foot Vein, Right** Common digital vein Dorsal metatarsal vein Dorsal venous arch Plantar digital vein Plantar metatarsal vein Plantar venous arch **V Foot Vein, Left** *See T Foot Vein, Right* **Y Lower Vein**	**Ø Open** **3 Percutaneous** **4 Percutaneous Endoscopic**	**Z No Device**	**Z No Qualifier**

Ø Medical and Surgical
6 Lower Veins
F Fragmentation Definition: Breaking solid matter in a body part into pieces

Explanation: Physical force (e.g., manual, ultrasonic) applied directly or indirectly is used to break the solid matter into pieces. The solid matter may be an abnormal byproduct of a biological function or a foreign body. The pieces of solid matter are not taken out.

Body Part Character 4	Approach Character 5	Device Character 6	Qualifier Character 7
C Common Iliac Vein, Right **D Common Iliac Vein, Left** **F External Iliac Vein, Right** **G External Iliac Vein, Left** **H Hypogastric Vein, Right** Gluteal vein Internal iliac vein Internal pudendal vein Lateral sacral vein Middle hemorrhoidal vein Obturator vein Uterine vein Vaginal vein Vesical vein **J Hypogastric Vein, Left** *See H Hypogastric Vein, Right* **M Femoral Vein, Right** Deep femoral (profunda femoris) vein Popliteal vein Profunda femoris (deep femoral) vein **N Femoral Vein, Left** *See M Femoral Vein, Right* **P Saphenous Vein, Right** External pudendal vein Great(er) saphenous vein Lesser saphenous vein Small saphenous vein Superficial circumflex iliac vein Superficial epigastric vein **Q Saphenous Vein, Left** *See P Saphenous Vein, Right* **Y Lower Vein**	**3 Percutaneous**	**Z No Device**	**Ø Ultrasonic** **Z No Qualifier**

Ø Medical and Surgical
6 Lower Veins
H Insertion Definition: Putting in a nonbiological appliance that monitors, assists, performs, or prevents a physiological function but does not physically take the place of a body part

Explanation: None

Body Part Character 4	Approach Character 5	Device Character 6	Qualifier Character 7
Ø Inferior Vena Cava Postcava Right inferior phrenic vein Right ovarian vein Right second lumbar vein Right suprarenal vein Right testicular vein	**Ø Open** **3 Percutaneous**	**3 Infusion Device**	**T Via Umbilical Vein** **Z No Qualifier**
Ø Inferior Vena Cava Postcava Right inferior phrenic vein Right ovarian vein Right second lumbar vein Right suprarenal vein Right testicular vein	**Ø Open** **3 Percutaneous**	**D Intraluminal Device**	**Z No Qualifier**
Ø Inferior Vena Cava Postcava Right inferior phrenic vein Right ovarian vein Right second lumbar vein Right suprarenal vein Right testicular vein	**4 Percutaneous Endoscopic**	**3 Infusion Device** **D Intraluminal Device**	**Z No Qualifier**
1 Splenic Vein Left gastroepiploic vein Pancreatic vein **2 Gastric Vein** **3 Esophageal Vein** **4 Hepatic Vein** **5 Superior Mesenteric Vein** Right gastroepiploic vein **6 Inferior Mesenteric Vein** Sigmoid vein Superior rectal vein **7 Colic Vein** Ileocolic vein Left colic vein Middle colic vein Right colic vein **8 Portal Vein** Hepatic portal vein **9 Renal Vein, Right** **B Renal Vein, Left** Left inferior phrenic vein Left ovarian vein Left second lumbar vein Left suprarenal vein Left testicular vein **C Common Iliac Vein, Right** **D Common Iliac Vein, Left** **F External Iliac Vein, Right** **G External Iliac Vein, Left** **H Hypogastric Vein, Right** Gluteal vein Internal iliac vein Internal pudendal vein Lateral sacral vein Middle hemorrhoidal vein Obturator vein Uterine vein Vaginal vein Vesical vein **J Hypogastric Vein, Left** ***See** H Hypogastric Vein, Right* **M Femoral Vein, Right** Deep femoral (profunda femoris) vein Popliteal vein Profunda femoris (deep femoral) vein **N Femoral Vein, Left** ***See** M Femoral Vein, Right* **P Saphenous Vein, Right** External pudendal vein Great(er) saphenous vein Lesser saphenous vein Small saphenous vein Superficial circumflex iliac vein Superficial epigastric vein **Q Saphenous Vein, Left** ***See** P Saphenous Vein, Right* **T Foot Vein, Right** Common digital vein Dorsal metatarsal vein Dorsal venous arch Plantar digital vein Plantar metatarsal vein Plantar venous arch **V Foot Vein, Left** ***See** T Foot Vein, Right*	**Ø Open** **3 Percutaneous** **4 Percutaneous Endoscopic**	**3 Infusion Device** **D Intraluminal Device**	**Z No Qualifier**
Y Lower Vein	**Ø Open** **3 Percutaneous** **4 Percutaneous Endoscopic**	**2 Monitoring Device** **3 Infusion Device** **D Intraluminal Device** **Y Other Device**	**Z No Qualifier**

Non-OR Ø6HØ[Ø,3]3[T,Z]
Non-OR Ø6HØ3DZ
Non-OR Ø6HØ43Z
Non-OR Ø6H[1,2,3,4,5,6,7,8,9,B,C,D,F,G,H,J,M,N,P,Q,T,V][Ø,3,4]3Z
Non-OR Ø6HY[Ø,3,4]3Z
Non-OR Ø6HY32Z
Non-OR Ø6HY[3,4]YZ

Ø Medical and Surgical
6 Lower Veins
J Inspection Definition: Visually and/or manually exploring a body part

Explanation: Visual exploration may be performed with or without optical instrumentation. Manual exploration may be performed directly or through intervening body layers.

Body Part Character 4	Approach Character 5	Device Character 6	Qualifier Character 7
Y Lower Vein	**Ø** Open **3** Percutaneous **4** Percutaneous Endoscopic **X** External	**Z** No Device	**Z** No Qualifier

Non-OR Ø6JY[3,X]ZZ

Ø Medical and Surgical
6 Lower Veins
L Occlusion Definition: Completely closing an orifice or the lumen of a tubular body part

Explanation: The orifice can be a natural orifice or an artificially created orifice

Body Part Character 4		Approach Character 5	Device Character 6	Qualifier Character 7
Ø **Inferior Vena Cava** Postcava Right inferior phrenic vein Right ovarian vein Right second lumbar vein Right suprarenal vein Right testicular vein **1** **Splenic Vein** Left gastroepiploic vein Pancreatic vein **4** **Hepatic Vein** **5** **Superior Mesenteric Vein** Right gastroepiploic vein **6** **Inferior Mesenteric Vein** Sigmoid vein Superior rectal vein **7** **Colic Vein** Ileocolic vein Left colic vein Middle colic vein Right colic vein **8** **Portal Vein** Hepatic portal vein **9** **Renal Vein, Right** **B** **Renal Vein, Left** Left inferior phrenic vein Left ovarian vein Left second lumbar vein Left suprarenal vein Left testicular vein **C** **Common Iliac Vein, Right** **D** **Common Iliac Vein, Left** **F** **External Iliac Vein, Right** **G** **External Iliac Vein, Left**	**H** **Hypogastric Vein, Right** Gluteal vein Internal iliac vein Internal pudendal vein Lateral sacral vein Middle hemorrhoidal vein Obturator vein Uterine vein Vaginal vein Vesical vein **J** **Hypogastric Vein, Left** *See H Hypogastric Vein, Right* **M** **Femoral Vein, Right** Deep femoral (profunda femoris) vein Popliteal vein Profunda femoris (deep femoral) vein **N** **Femoral Vein, Left** *See M Femoral Vein, Right* **P** **Saphenous Vein, Right** External pudendal vein Great(er) saphenous vein Lesser saphenous vein Small saphenous vein Superficial circumflex iliac vein Superficial epigastric vein **Q** **Saphenous Vein, Left** *See P Saphenous Vein, Right* **T** **Foot Vein, Right** Common digital vein Dorsal metatarsal vein Dorsal venous arch Plantar digital vein Plantar metatarsal vein Plantar venous arch **V** **Foot Vein, Left** *See T Foot Vein, Right*	**Ø** Open **3** Percutaneous **4** Percutaneous Endoscopic	**C** Extraluminal Device **D** Intraluminal Device **Z** No Device	**Z** No Qualifier
2 Gastric Vein **3** Esophageal Vein		**Ø** Open **3** Percutaneous **4** Percutaneous Endoscopic **7** Via Natural or Artificial Opening **8** Via Natural or Artificial Opening Endoscopic	**C** Extraluminal Device **D** Intraluminal Device **Z** No Device	**Z** No Qualifier
Y Lower Vein		**Ø** Open **3** Percutaneous **4** Percutaneous Endoscopic **7** Via Natural or Artificial Opening **8** Via Natural or Artificial Opening Endoscopic	**C** Extraluminal Device **D** Intraluminal Device **Z** No Device	**C** Hemorrhoidal Plexus **Z** No Qualifier

Non-OR Ø6L2[7,8][C,D,Z]Z
Non-OR Ø6L3[3,4,7,8][C,D,Z]Z

Ø Medical and Surgical
6 Lower Veins
N Release Definition: Freeing a body part from an abnormal physical constraint by cutting or by the use of force
Explanation: Some of the restraining tissue may be taken out but none of the body part is taken out

Body Part Character 4		Approach Character 5	Device Character 6	Qualifier Character 7
Ø Inferior Vena Cava Postcava Right inferior phrenic vein Right ovarian vein Right second lumbar vein Right suprarenal vein Right testicular vein **1 Splenic Vein** Left gastroepiploic vein Pancreatic vein **2 Gastric Vein** **3 Esophageal Vein** **4 Hepatic Vein** **5 Superior Mesenteric Vein** Right gastroepiploic vein **6 Inferior Mesenteric Vein** Sigmoid vein Superior rectal vein **7 Colic Vein** Ileocolic vein Left colic vein Middle colic vein Right colic vein **8 Portal Vein** Hepatic portal vein **9 Renal Vein, Right** **B Renal Vein, Left** Left inferior phrenic vein Left ovarian vein Left second lumbar vein Left suprarenal vein Left testicular vein **C Common Iliac Vein, Right** **D Common Iliac Vein, Left** **F External Iliac Vein, Right** **G External Iliac Vein, Left**	**H Hypogastric Vein, Right** Gluteal vein Internal iliac vein Internal pudendal vein Lateral sacral vein Middle hemorrhoidal vein Obturator vein Uterine vein Vaginal vein Vesical vein **J Hypogastric Vein, Left** *See H Hypogastric Vein, Right* **M Femoral Vein, Right** Deep femoral (profunda femoris) vein Popliteal vein Profunda femoris (deep femoral) vein **N Femoral Vein, Left** *See M Femoral Vein, Right* **P Saphenous Vein, Right** External pudendal vein Great(er) saphenous vein Lesser saphenous vein Small saphenous vein Superficial circumflex iliac vein Superficial epigastric vein **Q Saphenous Vein, Left** *See P Saphenous Vein, Right* **T Foot Vein, Right** Common digital vein Dorsal metatarsal vein Dorsal venous arch Plantar digital vein Plantar metatarsal vein Plantar venous arch **V Foot Vein, Left** *See T Foot Vein, Right* **Y Lower Vein**	**Ø Open** **3 Percutaneous** **4 Percutaneous Endoscopic**	**Z No Device**	**Z No Qualifier**

Ø Medical and Surgical
6 Lower Veins
P Removal Definition: Taking out or off a device from a body part
Explanation: If a device is taken out and a similar device put in without cutting or puncturing the skin or mucous membrane, the procedure is coded to the root operation CHANGE. Otherwise, the procedure for taking out a device is coded to the root operation REMOVAL.

Body Part Character 4	Approach Character 5	Device Character 6	Qualifier Character 7
Y Lower Vein	**Ø Open** **3 Percutaneous** **4 Percutaneous Endoscopic**	**Ø Drainage Device** **2 Monitoring Device** **3 Infusion Device** **7 Autologous Tissue Substitute** **C Extraluminal Device** **D Intraluminal Device** **J Synthetic Substitute** **K Nonautologous Tissue Substitute** **Y Other Device**	**Z No Qualifier**
Y Lower Vein	**X External**	**Ø Drainage Device** **2 Monitoring Device** **3 Infusion Device** **D Intraluminal Device**	**Z No Qualifier**

Non-OR Ø6PY3[Ø,2,3]Z
Non-OR Ø6PY[3,4]YZ
Non-OR Ø6PYX[Ø,2,3,D]Z

Ø Medical and Surgical
6 Lower Veins
Q Repair Definition: Restoring, to the extent possible, a body part to its normal anatomic structure and function
Explanation: Used only when the method to accomplish the repair is not one of the other root operations

Body Part Character 4	Approach Character 5	Device Character 6	Qualifier Character 7
Ø Inferior Vena Cava Postcava Right inferior phrenic vein Right ovarian vein Right second lumbar vein Right suprarenal vein Right testicular vein **1 Splenic Vein** Left gastroepiploic vein Pancreatic vein **2 Gastric Vein** **3 Esophageal Vein** **4 Hepatic Vein** **5 Superior Mesenteric Vein** Right gastroepiploic vein **6 Inferior Mesenteric Vein** Sigmoid vein Superior rectal vein **7 Colic Vein** Ileocolic vein Left colic vein Middle colic vein Right colic vein **8 Portal Vein** Hepatic portal vein **9 Renal Vein, Right** **B Renal Vein, Left** Left inferior phrenic vein Left ovarian vein Left second lumbar vein Left suprarenal vein Left testicular vein **C Common Iliac Vein, Right** **D Common Iliac Vein, Left** **F External Iliac Vein, Right** **G External Iliac Vein, Left** **H Hypogastric Vein, Right** Gluteal vein Internal iliac vein Internal pudendal vein Lateral sacral vein Middle hemorrhoidal vein Obturator vein Uterine vein Vaginal vein Vesical vein **J Hypogastric Vein, Left** *See H Hypogastric Vein, Right* **M Femoral Vein, Right** Deep femoral (profunda femoris) vein Popliteal vein Profunda femoris (deep femoral) vein **N Femoral Vein, Left** *See M Femoral Vein, Right* **P Saphenous Vein, Right** External pudendal vein Great(er) saphenous vein Lesser saphenous vein Small saphenous vein Superficial circumflex iliac vein Superficial epigastric vein **Q Saphenous Vein, Left** *See P Saphenous Vein, Right* **T Foot Vein, Right** Common digital vein Dorsal metatarsal vein Dorsal venous arch Plantar digital vein Plantar metatarsal vein Plantar venous arch **V Foot Vein, Left** *See T Foot Vein, Right* **Y Lower Vein**	**Ø Open** **3 Percutaneous** **4 Percutaneous Endoscopic**	**Z No Device**	**Z No Qualifier**

Ø Medical and Surgical
6 Lower Veins
R Replacement Definition: Putting in or on biological or synthetic material that physically takes the place and/or function of all or a portion of a body part

Explanation: The body part may have been taken out or replaced, or may be taken out, physically eradicated, or rendered nonfunctional during the REPLACEMENT procedure. A REMOVAL procedure is coded for taking out the device used in a previous replacement procedure.

Body Part Character 4	Approach Character 5	Device Character 6	Qualifier Character 7
Ø Inferior Vena Cava Postcava Right inferior phrenic vein Right ovarian vein Right second lumbar vein Right suprarenal vein Right testicular vein **1 Splenic Vein** Left gastroepiploic vein Pancreatic vein **2 Gastric Vein** **3 Esophageal Vein** **4 Hepatic Vein** **5 Superior Mesenteric Vein** Right gastroepiploic vein **6 Inferior Mesenteric Vein** Sigmoid vein Superior rectal vein **7 Colic Vein** Ileocolic vein Left colic vein Middle colic vein Right colic vein **8 Portal Vein** Hepatic portal vein **9 Renal Vein, Right** **B Renal Vein, Left** Left inferior phrenic vein Left ovarian vein Left second lumbar vein Left suprarenal vein Left testicular vein **C Common Iliac Vein, Right** **D Common Iliac Vein, Left** **F External Iliac Vein, Right** **G External Iliac Vein, Left** **H Hypogastric Vein, Right** Gluteal vein Internal iliac vein Internal pudendal vein Lateral sacral vein Middle hemorrhoidal vein Obturator vein Uterine vein Vaginal vein Vesical vein **J Hypogastric Vein, Left** *See H Hypogastric Vein, Right* **M Femoral Vein, Right** Deep femoral (profunda femoris) vein Popliteal vein Profunda femoris (deep femoral) vein **N Femoral Vein, Left** *See M Femoral Vein, Right* **P Saphenous Vein, Right** External pudendal vein Great(er) saphenous vein Lesser saphenous vein Small saphenous vein Superficial circumflex iliac vein Superficial epigastric vein **Q Saphenous Vein, Left** *See P Saphenous Vein, Right* **T Foot Vein, Right** Common digital vein Dorsal metatarsal vein Dorsal venous arch Plantar digital vein Plantar metatarsal vein Plantar venous arch **V Foot Vein, Left** *See T Foot Vein, Right* **Y Lower Vein**	**Ø Open** **4 Percutaneous Endoscopic**	**7 Autologous Tissue Substitute** **J Synthetic Substitute** **K Nonautologous Tissue Substitute**	**Z No Qualifier**

Ø Medical and Surgical
6 Lower Veins
S Reposition Definition: Moving to its normal location, or other suitable location, all or a portion of a body part

Explanation: The body part is moved to a new location from an abnormal location, or from a normal location where it is not functioning correctly. The body part may or may not be cut out or off to be moved to the new location.

Body Part Character 4	Approach Character 5	Device Character 6	Qualifier Character 7
Ø Inferior Vena Cava Postcava Right inferior phrenic vein Right ovarian vein Right second lumbar vein Right suprarenal vein Right testicular vein **1 Splenic Vein** Left gastroepiploic vein Pancreatic vein **2 Gastric Vein** **3 Esophageal Vein** **4 Hepatic Vein** **5 Superior Mesenteric Vein** Right gastroepiploic vein **6 Inferior Mesenteric Vein** Sigmoid vein Superior rectal vein **7 Colic Vein** Ileocolic vein Left colic vein Middle colic vein Right colic vein **8 Portal Vein** Hepatic portal vein **9 Renal Vein, Right** **B Renal Vein, Left** Left inferior phrenic vein Left ovarian vein Left second lumbar vein Left suprarenal vein Left testicular vein **C Common Iliac Vein, Right** **D Common Iliac Vein, Left** **F External Iliac Vein, Right** **G External Iliac Vein, Left** **H Hypogastric Vein, Right** Gluteal vein Internal iliac vein Internal pudendal vein Lateral sacral vein Middle hemorrhoidal vein Obturator vein Uterine vein Vaginal vein Vesical vein **J Hypogastric Vein, Left** *See H Hypogastric Vein, Right* **M Femoral Vein, Right** Deep femoral (profunda femoris) vein Popliteal vein Profunda femoris (deep femoral) vein **N Femoral Vein, Left** *See M Femoral Vein, Right* **P Saphenous Vein, Right** External pudendal vein Great(er) saphenous vein Lesser saphenous vein Small saphenous vein Superficial circumflex iliac vein Superficial epigastric vein **Q Saphenous Vein, Left** *See P Saphenous Vein, Right* **T Foot Vein, Right** Common digital vein Dorsal metatarsal vein Dorsal venous arch Plantar digital vein Plantar metatarsal vein Plantar venous arch **V Foot Vein, Left** *See T Foot Vein, Right* **Y Lower Vein**	**Ø Open** **3 Percutaneous** **4 Percutaneous Endoscopic**	**Z No Device**	**Z No Qualifier**

Ø Medical and Surgical
6 Lower Veins
U Supplement Definition: Putting in or on biological or synthetic material that physically reinforces and/or augments the function of a portion of a body part

Explanation: The biological material is non-living, or is living and from the same individual. The body part may have been previously replaced, and the SUPPLEMENT procedure is performed to physically reinforce and/or augment the function of the replaced body part.

Body Part Character 4	Approach Character 5	Device Character 6	Qualifier Character 7
Ø Inferior Vena Cava Postcava Right inferior phrenic vein Right ovarian vein Right second lumbar vein Right suprarenal vein Right testicular vein **1 Splenic Vein** Left gastroepiploic vein Pancreatic vein **2 Gastric Vein** **3 Esophageal Vein** **4 Hepatic Vein** **5 Superior Mesenteric Vein** Right gastroepiploic vein **6 Inferior Mesenteric Vein** Sigmoid vein Superior rectal vein **7 Colic Vein** Ileocolic vein Left colic vein Middle colic vein Right colic vein **8 Portal Vein** Hepatic portal vein **9 Renal Vein, Right** **B Renal Vein, Left** Left inferior phrenic vein Left ovarian vein Left second lumbar vein Left suprarenal vein Left testicular vein **C Common Iliac Vein, Right** **D Common Iliac Vein, Left** **F External Iliac Vein, Right** **G External Iliac Vein, Left** **H Hypogastric Vein, Right** Gluteal vein Internal iliac vein Internal pudendal vein Lateral sacral vein Middle hemorrhoidal vein Obturator vein Uterine vein Vaginal vein Vesical vein **J Hypogastric Vein, Left** *See H Hypogastric Vein, Right* **M Femoral Vein, Right** Deep femoral (profunda femoris) vein Popliteal vein Profunda femoris (deep femoral) vein **N Femoral Vein, Left** *See M Femoral Vein, Right* **P Saphenous Vein, Right** External pudendal vein Great(er) saphenous vein Lesser saphenous vein Small saphenous vein Superficial circumflex iliac vein Superficial epigastric vein **Q Saphenous Vein, Left** *See P Saphenous Vein, Right* **T Foot Vein, Right** Common digital vein Dorsal metatarsal vein Dorsal venous arch Plantar digital vein Plantar metatarsal vein Plantar venous arch **V Foot Vein, Left** *See T Foot Vein, Right* **Y Lower Vein**	**Ø Open** **3 Percutaneous** **4 Percutaneous Endoscopic**	**7 Autologous Tissue Substitute** **J Synthetic Substitute** **K Nonautologous Tissue Substitute**	**Z No Qualifier**

Ø Medical and Surgical
6 Lower Veins
V Restriction Definition: Partially closing an orifice or the lumen of a tubular body part
Explanation: The orifice can be a natural orifice or an artificially created orifice

Body Part Character 4	Approach Character 5	Device Character 6	Qualifier Character 7
Ø Inferior Vena Cava Postcava Right inferior phrenic vein Right ovarian vein Right second lumbar vein Right suprarenal vein Right testicular vein **1 Splenic Vein** Left gastroepiploic vein Pancreatic vein **2 Gastric Vein** **3 Esophageal Vein** **4 Hepatic Vein** **5 Superior Mesenteric Vein** Right gastroepiploic vein **6 Inferior Mesenteric Vein** Sigmoid vein Superior rectal vein **7 Colic Vein** Ileocolic vein Left colic vein Middle colic vein Right colic vein **8 Portal Vein** Hepatic portal vein **9 Renal Vein, Right** **B Renal Vein, Left** Left inferior phrenic vein Left ovarian vein Left second lumbar vein Left suprarenal vein Left testicular vein **C Common Iliac Vein, Right** **D Common Iliac Vein, Left** **F External Iliac Vein, Right** **G External Iliac Vein, Left** **H Hypogastric Vein, Right** Gluteal vein Internal iliac vein Internal pudendal vein Lateral sacral vein Middle hemorrhoidal vein Obturator vein Uterine vein Vaginal vein Vesical vein **J Hypogastric Vein, Left** *See H Hypogastric Vein, Right* **M Femoral Vein, Right** Deep femoral (profunda femoris) vein Popliteal vein Profunda femoris (deep femoral) vein **N Femoral Vein, Left** *See M Femoral Vein, Right* **P Saphenous Vein, Right** External pudendal vein Great(er) saphenous vein Lesser saphenous vein Small saphenous vein Superficial circumflex iliac vein Superficial epigastric vein **Q Saphenous Vein, Left** *See P Saphenous Vein, Right* **T Foot Vein, Right** Common digital vein Dorsal metatarsal vein Dorsal venous arch Plantar digital vein Plantar metatarsal vein Plantar venous arch **V Foot Vein, Left** *See T Foot Vein, Right* **Y Lower Vein**	**Ø Open** **3 Percutaneous** **4 Percutaneous Endoscopic**	**C Extraluminal Device** **D Intraluminal Device** **Z No Device**	**Z No Qualifier**

Ø Medical and Surgical
6 Lower Veins
W Revision

Definition: Correcting, to the extent possible, a portion of a malfunctioning device or the position of a displaced device

Explanation: Revision can include correcting a malfunctioning or displaced device by taking out or putting in components of the device such as a screw or pin

Body Part Character 4	Approach Character 5	Device Character 6	Qualifier Character 7
Y Lower Vein	Ø Open 3 Percutaneous 4 Percutaneous Endoscopic	Ø Drainage Device 2 Monitoring Device 3 Infusion Device 7 Autologous Tissue Substitute C Extraluminal Device D Intraluminal Device J Synthetic Substitute K Nonautologous Tissue Substitute Y Other Device	Z No Qualifier
Y Lower Vein	X External	Ø Drainage Device 2 Monitoring Device 3 Infusion Device 7 Autologous Tissue Substitute C Extraluminal Device D Intraluminal Device J Synthetic Substitute K Nonautologous Tissue Substitute	Z No Qualifier

Non-OR Ø6WY3[Ø,2,3,D]Z
Non-OR Ø6WY[3,4]YZ
Non-OR Ø6WYX[Ø,2,3,7,C,D,J,K]Z

Lymphatic and Hemic Systems Ø72–Ø7Y

Character Meanings*

This Character Meaning table is provided as a guide to assist the user in the identification of character members that may be found in this section of code tables. It **SHOULD NOT** be used to build a PCS code.

Operation–Character 3	Body Part–Character 4	Approach–Character 5	Device–Character 6	Qualifier–Character 7
2 Change	Ø Lymphatic, Head	Ø Open	Ø Drainage Device	Ø Allogeneic
5 Destruction	1 Lymphatic, Right Neck	3 Percutaneous	1 Radioactive Element	1 Syngeneic
9 Drainage	2 Lymphatic, Left Neck	4 Percutaneous Endoscopic	3 Infusion Device	2 Zooplastic
B Excision	3 Lymphatic, Right Upper Extremity	8 Via Natural or Artificial Opening Endoscopic	7 Autologous Tissue Substitute	X Diagnostic
C Extirpation	4 Lymphatic, Left Upper Extremity	X External	C Extraluminal Device	Z No Qualifier
D Extraction	5 Lymphatic, Right Axillary		D Intraluminal Device	
H Insertion	6 Lymphatic, Left Axillary		J Synthetic Substitute	
J Inspection	7 Lymphatic, Thorax		K Nonautologous Tissue Substitute	
L Occlusion	8 Lymphatic, Internal Mammary, Right		Y Other Device	
N Release	9 Lymphatic, Internal Mammary, Left		Z No Device	
P Removal	B Lymphatic, Mesenteric			
Q Repair	C Lymphatic, Pelvis			
S Reposition	D Lymphatic, Aortic			
T Resection	F Lymphatic, Right Lower Extremity			
U Supplement	G Lymphatic, Left Lower Extremity			
V Restriction	H Lymphatic, Right Inguinal			
W Revision	J Lymphatic, Left Inguinal			
Y Transplantation	K Thoracic Duct			
	L Cisterna Chyli			
	M Thymus			
	N Lymphatic			
	P Spleen			
	Q Bone Marrow, Sternum			
	R Bone Marrow, Iliac			
	S Bone Marrow, Vertebral			
	T Bone Marrow			

* Includes lymph vessels and lymph nodes.

AHA Coding Clinic for table Ø79
2018, 4Q, 84 Fine needle aspiration biopsy of lymphatic tissue
2017, 1Q, 34 Lymphovenous bypass following mastectomy
2014, 1Q, 26 Transbronchial needle aspiration lymph node biopsy
2013, 4Q, 111 Transbronchial needle aspiration lymph node biopsy

AHA Coding Clinic for table Ø7B
2019, 1Q, 3-8 Whipple procedure
2018, 4Q, 84 Fine needle aspiration biopsy of lymphatic tissue
2018, 1Q, 22 Resection of lymph node chains
2016, 1Q, 30 Axillary lymph node resection with modified radical mastectomy
2014, 3Q, 10 Selective excision of paratracheal lymph nodes
2014, 1Q, 20 Fiducial marker placement
2014, 1Q, 26 Transbronchial endoscopic lymph node aspiration biopsy

AHA Coding Clinic for table Ø7D
2018, 4Q, 84 Fine needle aspiration biopsy of lymphatic tissue
2013, 4Q, 111 Root operation for bone marrow biopsy

AHA Coding Clinic for table Ø7H
2020, 4Q, 43-44 Insertion of radioactive element
2020, 4Q, 53 Bone marrow body part

AHA Coding Clinic for table Ø7Q
2017, 1Q, 34 Lymphovenous bypass following mastectomy

AHA Coding Clinic for table Ø7S
2019, 3Q, 29 Thymus transplant for T-Cell production

AHA Coding Clinic for table Ø7T
2018, 1Q, 22 Resection of lymph node chains
2016, 2Q, 12 Resection of malignant neoplasm of infratemporal fossa
2016, 1Q, 30 Axillary lymph node resection with modified radical mastectomy
2015, 4Q, 13 New Section X codes—New Technology procedures
2014, 3Q, 9 Radical resection of level I lymph nodes
2014, 3Q, 16 Repair of Tetralogy of Fallot

AHA Coding Clinic for table Ø7Y
2019, 3Q, 29 Thymus transplant for T-Cell production

Lymphatic System

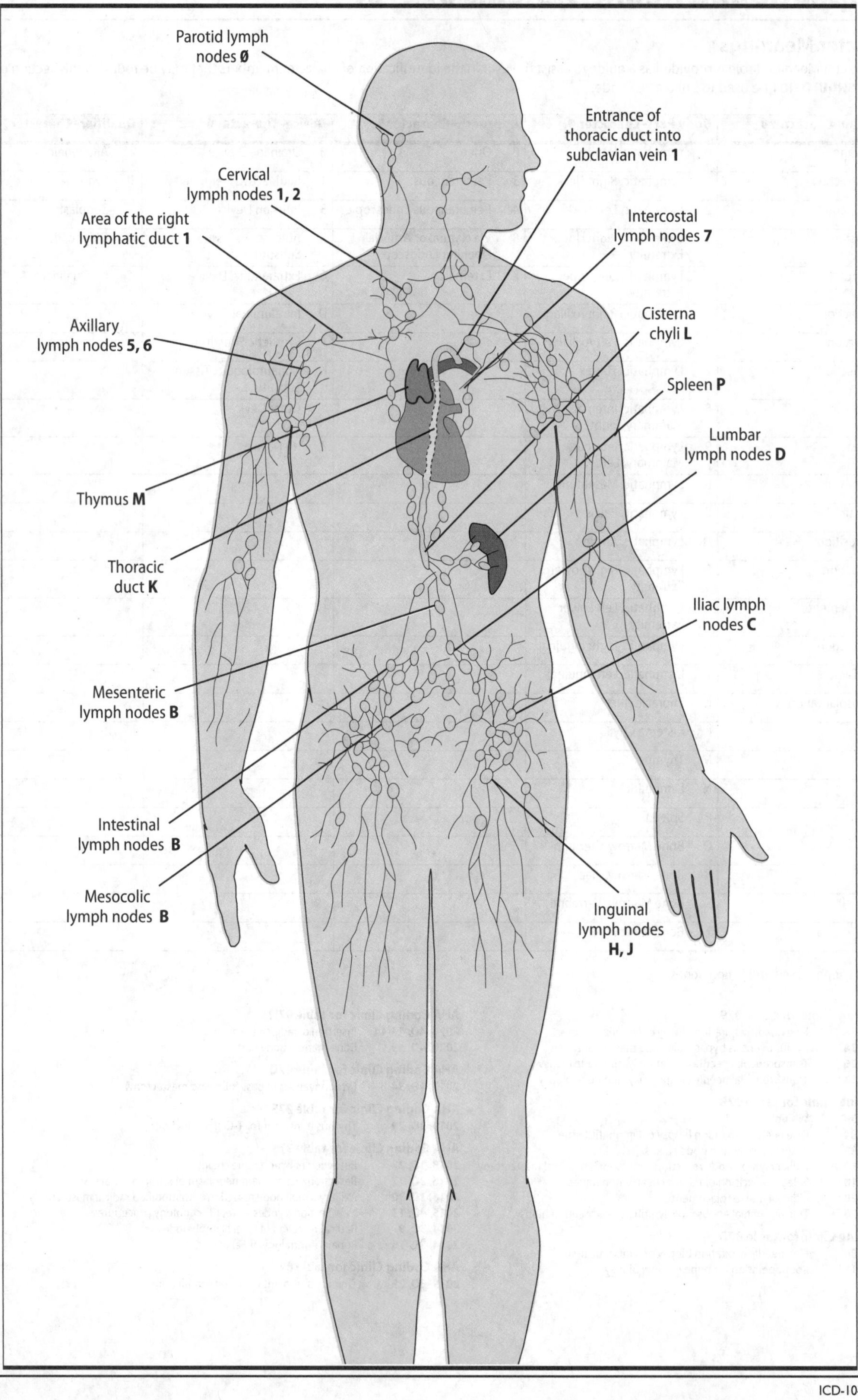

Ø Medical and Surgical
7 Lymphatic and Hemic Systems
2 Change Definition: Taking out or off a device from a body part and putting back an identical or similar device in or on the same body part without cutting or puncturing the skin or a mucous membrane

Explanation: All CHANGE procedures are coded using the approach EXTERNAL

Body Part Character 4		Approach Character 5	Device Character 6	Qualifier Character 7
K Thoracic Duct Left jugular trunk Left subclavian trunk **L Cisterna Chyli** Intestinal lymphatic trunk Lumbar lymphatic trunk	**M Thymus** Thymus gland **N Lymphatic** **P Spleen** Accessory spleen **T Bone Marrow**	**X External**	**Ø Drainage Device** **Y Other Device**	**Z No Qualifier**

Non-OR All body part, approach, device, and qualifier values

Ø Medical and Surgical
7 Lymphatic and Hemic Systems
5 Destruction Definition: Physical eradication of all or a portion of a body part by the direct use of energy, force, or a destructive agent

Explanation: None of the body part is physically taken out

Body Part Character 4		Approach Character 5	Device Character 6	Qualifier Character 7
Ø Lymphatic, Head Buccinator lymph node Infraauricular lymph node Infraparotid lymph node Parotid lymph node Preauricular lymph node Submandibular lymph node Submaxillary lymph node Submental lymph node Subparotid lymph node Suprahyoid lymph node **1 Lymphatic, Right Neck** Cervical lymph node Jugular lymph node Mastoid (postauricular) lymph node Occipital lymph node Postauricular (mastoid) lymph node Retropharyngeal lymph node Right jugular trunk Right lymphatic duct Right subclavian trunk Supraclavicular (Virchow's) lymph node Virchow's (supraclavicular) lymph node **2 Lymphatic, Left Neck** Cervical lymph node Jugular lymph node Mastoid (postauricular) lymph node Occipital lymph node Postauricular (mastoid) lymph node Retropharyngeal lymph node Supraclavicular (Virchow's) lymph node Virchow's (supraclavicular) lymph node **3 Lymphatic, Right Upper Extremity** Cubital lymph node Deltopectoral (infraclavicular) lymph node Epitrochlear lymph node Infraclavicular (deltopectoral) lymph node Supratrochlear lymph node **4 Lymphatic, Left Upper Extremity** *See 3 Lymphatic, Right Upper Extremity* **5 Lymphatic, Right Axillary** Anterior (pectoral) lymph node Apical (subclavicular) lymph node Brachial (lateral) lymph node Central axillary lymph node Lateral (brachial) lymph node Pectoral (anterior) lymph node Posterior (subscapular) lymph node Subclavicular (apical) lymph node Subscapular (posterior) lymph node	**6 Lymphatic, Left Axillary** *See 5 Lymphatic, Right Axillary* **7 Lymphatic, Thorax** Intercostal lymph node Mediastinal lymph node Parasternal lymph node Paratracheal lymph node Tracheobronchial lymph node **8 Lymphatic, Internal Mammary, Right** **9 Lymphatic, Internal Mammary, Left** **B Lymphatic, Mesenteric** Inferior mesenteric lymph node Pararectal lymph node Superior mesenteric lymph node **C Lymphatic, Pelvis** Common iliac (subaortic) lymph node Gluteal lymph node Iliac lymph node Inferior epigastric lymph node Obturator lymph node Sacral lymph node Subaortic (common iliac) lymph node Suprainguinal lymph node **D Lymphatic, Aortic** Celiac lymph node Gastric lymph node Hepatic lymph node Lumbar lymph node Pancreaticosplenic lymph node Paraaortic lymph node Retroperitoneal lymph node **F Lymphatic, Right Lower Extremity** Femoral lymph node Popliteal lymph node **G Lymphatic, Left Lower Extremity** *See F Lymphatic, Right Lower Extremity* **H Lymphatic, Right Inguinal** **J Lymphatic, Left Inguinal** **K Thoracic Duct** Left jugular trunk Left subclavian trunk **L Cisterna Chyli** Intestinal lymphatic trunk Lumbar lymphatic trunk **M Thymus** Thymus gland **P Spleen** Accessory spleen	**Ø Open** **3 Percutaneous** **4 Percutaneous Endoscopic**	**Z No Device**	**Z No Qualifier**

Ø Medical and Surgical
7 Lymphatic and Hemic Systems
9 Drainage Definition: Taking or letting out fluids and/or gases from a body part
Explanation: The qualifier DIAGNOSTIC is used to identify drainage procedures that are biopsies

Body Part Character 4	Approach Character 5	Device Character 6	Qualifier Character 7
Ø Lymphatic, Head Buccinator lymph node Infraauricular lymph node Infraparotid lymph node Parotid lymph node Preauricular lymph node Submandibular lymph node Submaxillary lymph node Submental lymph node Subparotid lymph node Suprahyoid lymph node **1 Lymphatic, Right Neck** Cervical lymph node Jugular lymph node Mastoid (postauricular) lymph node Occipital lymph node Postauricular (mastoid) lymph node Retropharyngeal lymph node Right jugular trunk Right lymphatic duct Right subclavian trunk Supraclavicular (Virchow's) lymph node Virchow's (supraclavicular) lymph node **2 Lymphatic, Left Neck** Cervical lymph node Jugular lymph node Mastoid (postauricular) lymph node Occipital lymph node Postauricular (mastoid) lymph node Retropharyngeal lymph node Supraclavicular (Virchow's) lymph node Virchow's (supraclavicular) lymph node **3 Lymphatic, Right Upper Extremity** Cubital lymph node Deltopectoral (infraclavicular) lymph node Epitrochlear lymph node Infraclavicular (deltopectoral) lymph node Supratrochlear lymph node **4 Lymphatic, Left Upper Extremity** *See 3 Lymphatic, Right Upper Extremity* **5 Lymphatic, Right Axillary** Anterior (pectoral) lymph node Apical (subclavicular) lymph node Brachial (lateral) lymph node Central axillary lymph node Lateral (brachial) lymph node Pectoral (anterior) lymph node Posterior (subscapular) lymph node Subclavicular (apical) lymph node Subscapular (posterior) lymph node **6 Lymphatic, Left Axillary** *See 5 Lymphatic, Right Axillary* **7 Lymphatic, Thorax** Intercostal lymph node Mediastinal lymph node Parasternal lymph node Paratracheal lymph node Tracheobronchial lymph node **8 Lymphatic, Internal Mammary, Right** **9 Lymphatic, Internal Mammary, Left** **B Lymphatic, Mesenteric** Inferior mesenteric lymph node Pararectal lymph node Superior mesenteric lymph node **C Lymphatic, Pelvis** Common iliac (subaortic) lymph node Gluteal lymph node Iliac lymph node Inferior epigastric lymph node Obturator lymph node Sacral lymph node Subaortic (common iliac) lymph node Suprainguinal lymph node **D Lymphatic, Aortic** Celiac lymph node Gastric lymph node Hepatic lymph node Lumbar lymph node Pancreaticosplenic lymph node Paraaortic lymph node Retroperitoneal lymph node **F Lymphatic, Right Lower Extremity** Femoral lymph node Popliteal lymph node **G Lymphatic, Left Lower Extremity** *See F Lymphatic, Right Lower Extremity* **H Lymphatic, Right Inguinal** **J Lymphatic, Left Inguinal** **K Thoracic Duct** Left jugular trunk Left subclavian trunk **L Cisterna Chyli** Intestinal lymphatic trunk Lumbar lymphatic trunk	**Ø Open** **3 Percutaneous** **4 Percutaneous Endoscopic** **8 Via Natural or Artificial Opening Endoscopic**	**Ø Drainage Device**	**Z No Qualifier**

Non-OR Ø79[Ø,1,2,3,4,5,6,7,8,9,B,C,D,F,G,H,J,K,L][3,8]ØZ

Ø79 Continued on next page

Ø Medical and Surgical
7 Lymphatic and Hemic Systems
9 Drainage Definition: Taking or letting out fluids and/or gases from a body part
Explanation: The qualifier DIAGNOSTIC is used to identify drainage procedures that are biopsies

Ø79 Continued

Body Part Character 4	Approach Character 5	Device Character 6	Qualifier Character 7
Ø Lymphatic, Head Buccinator lymph node Infraauricular lymph node Infraparotid lymph node Parotid lymph node Preauricular lymph node Submandibular lymph node Submaxillary lymph node Submental lymph node Subparotid lymph node Suprahyoid lymph node **1 Lymphatic, Right Neck** Cervical lymph node Jugular lymph node Mastoid (postauricular) lymph node Occipital lymph node Postauricular (mastoid) lymph node Retropharyngeal lymph node Right jugular trunk Right lymphatic duct Right subclavian trunk Supraclavicular (Virchow's) lymph node Virchow's (supraclavicular) lymph node **2 Lymphatic, Left Neck** Cervical lymph node Jugular lymph node Mastoid (postauricular) lymph node Occipital lymph node Postauricular (mastoid) lymph node Retropharyngeal lymph node Supraclavicular (Virchow's) lymph node Virchow's (supraclavicular) lymph node **3 Lymphatic, Right Upper Extremity** Cubital lymph node Deltopectoral (infraclavicular) lymph node Epitrochlear lymph node Infraclavicular (deltopectoral) lymph node Supratrochlear lymph node **4 Lymphatic, Left Upper Extremity** *See 3 Lymphatic, Right Upper Extremity* **5 Lymphatic, Right Axillary** Anterior (pectoral) lymph node Apical (subclavicular) lymph node Brachial (lateral) lymph node Central axillary lymph node Lateral (brachial) lymph node Pectoral (anterior) lymph node Posterior (subscapular) lymph node Subclavicular (apical) lymph node Subscapular (posterior) lymph node **6 Lymphatic, Left Axillary** *See 5 Lymphatic, Right Axillary* **7 Lymphatic, Thorax** Intercostal lymph node Mediastinal lymph node Parasternal lymph node Paratracheal lymph node Tracheobronchial lymph node **8 Lymphatic, Internal Mammary, Right** **9 Lymphatic, Internal Mammary, Left** **B Lymphatic, Mesenteric** Inferior mesenteric lymph node Pararectal lymph node Superior mesenteric lymph node **C Lymphatic, Pelvis** Common iliac (subaortic) lymph node Gluteal lymph node Iliac lymph node Inferior epigastric lymph node Obturator lymph node Sacral lymph node Subaortic (common iliac) lymph node Suprainguinal lymph node **D Lymphatic, Aortic** Celiac lymph node Gastric lymph node Hepatic lymph node Lumbar lymph node Pancreaticosplenic lymph node Paraaortic lymph node Retroperitoneal lymph node **F Lymphatic, Right Lower Extremity** Femoral lymph node Popliteal lymph node **G Lymphatic, Left Lower Extremity** *See F Lymphatic, Right Lower Extremity* **H Lymphatic, Right Inguinal** **J Lymphatic, Left Inguinal** **K Thoracic Duct** Left jugular trunk Left subclavian trunk **L Cisterna Chyli** Intestinal lymphatic trunk Lumbar lymphatic trunk	**Ø Open** **3 Percutaneous** **4 Percutaneous Endoscopic** **8 Via Natural or Artificial Opening Endoscopic**	**Z No Device**	**X Diagnostic** **Z No Qualifier**
M Thymus Thymus gland **P Spleen** Accessory spleen **T Bone Marrow**	**Ø Open** **3 Percutaneous** **4 Percutaneous Endoscopic**	**Ø Drainage Device**	**Z No Qualifier**
M Thymus Thymus gland **P Spleen** Accessory spleen **T Bone Marrow**	**Ø Open** **3 Percutaneous** **4 Percutaneous Endoscopic**	**Z No Device**	**X Diagnostic** **Z No Qualifier**

Non-OR Ø79[Ø,1,2,3,4,5,6,7,8,9,B,C,D,F,G,H,J,K,L]8ZX
Non-OR Ø79[Ø,1,2,3,4,5,6,7,8,9,B,C,D,F,G,H,J,K,L][3,8]ZZ
Non-OR Ø79M3ØZ
Non-OR Ø79P[3,4]ØZ
Non-OR Ø79T[Ø,3,4]ØZ
Non-OR Ø79M3ZZ
Non-OR Ø79P[3,4]Z[X,Z]
Non-OR Ø79T[Ø,3,4]Z[X,Z]

Ø Medical and Surgical
7 Lymphatic and Hemic Systems
B Excision Definition: Cutting out or off, without replacement, a portion of a body part
Explanation: The qualifier DIAGNOSTIC is used to identify excision procedures that are biopsies

Body Part Character 4	Approach Character 5	Device Character 6	Qualifier Character 7
Ø Lymphatic, Head Buccinator lymph node Infraauricular lymph node Infraparotid lymph node Parotid lymph node Preauricular lymph node Submandibular lymph node Submaxillary lymph node Submental lymph node Subparotid lymph node Suprahyoid lymph node **1 Lymphatic, Right Neck** Cervical lymph node Jugular lymph node Mastoid (postauricular) lymph node Occipital lymph node Postauricular (mastoid) lymph node Retropharyngeal lymph node Right jugular trunk Right lymphatic duct Right subclavian trunk Supraclavicular (Virchow's) lymph node Virchow's (supraclavicular) lymph node **2 Lymphatic, Left Neck** Cervical lymph node Jugular lymph node Mastoid (postauricular) lymph node Occipital lymph node Postauricular (mastoid) lymph node Retropharyngeal lymph node Supraclavicular (Virchow's) lymph node Virchow's (supraclavicular) lymph node **3 Lymphatic, Right Upper Extremity** Cubital lymph node Deltopectoral (infraclavicular) lymph node Epitrochlear lymph node Infraclavicular (deltopectoral) lymph node Supratrochlear lymph node **4 Lymphatic, Left Upper Extremity** ***See*** *3 Lymphatic, Right Upper Extremity* **5 Lymphatic, Right Axillary** Anterior (pectoral) lymph node Apical (subclavicular) lymph node Brachial (lateral) lymph node Central axillary lymph node Lateral (brachial) lymph node Pectoral (anterior) lymph node Posterior (subscapular) lymph node Subclavicular (apical) lymph node Subscapular (posterior) lymph node **6 Lymphatic, Left Axillary** ***See*** *5 Lymphatic, Right Axillary* **7 Lymphatic, Thorax** Intercostal lymph node Mediastinal lymph node Parasternal lymph node Paratracheal lymph node Tracheobronchial lymph node **8 Lymphatic, Internal Mammary, Right** **9 Lymphatic, Internal Mammary, Left** **B Lymphatic, Mesenteric** Inferior mesenteric lymph node Pararectal lymph node Superior mesenteric lymph node **C Lymphatic, Pelvis** Common iliac (subaortic) lymph node Gluteal lymph node Iliac lymph node Inferior epigastric lymph node Obturator lymph node Sacral lymph node Subaortic (common iliac) lymph node Suprainguinal lymph node **D Lymphatic, Aortic** Celiac lymph node Gastric lymph node Hepatic lymph node Lumbar lymph node Pancreaticosplenic lymph node Paraaortic lymph node Retroperitoneal lymph node **F Lymphatic, Right Lower Extremity** Femoral lymph node Popliteal lymph node **G Lymphatic, Left Lower Extremity** ***See*** *F Lymphatic, Right Lower Extremity* **H Lymphatic, Right Inguinal** ⊞ **J Lymphatic, Left Inguinal** ⊞ **K Thoracic Duct** Left jugular trunk Left subclavian trunk **L Cisterna Chyli** Intestinal lymphatic trunk Lumbar lymphatic trunk **M Thymus** Thymus gland **P Spleen** Accessory spleen	**Ø Open** **3 Percutaneous** **4 Percutaneous Endoscopic**	**Z No Device**	**X Diagnostic** **Z No Qualifier**

Non-OR Ø7BP[3,4]ZX

See Appendix L for Procedure Combinations
⊞ Ø7B[H,J][Ø,4]ZZ

Ø Medical and Surgical
7 Lymphatic and Hemic Systems
C Extirpation Definition: Taking or cutting out solid matter from a body part

Explanation: The solid matter may be an abnormal byproduct of a biological function or a foreign body; it may be imbedded in a body part or in the lumen of a tubular body part. The solid matter may or may not have been previously broken into pieces.

Body Part Character 4		Approach Character 5	Device Character 6	Qualifier Character 7
Ø Lymphatic, Head Buccinator lymph node Infraauricular lymph node Infraparotid lymph node Parotid lymph node Preauricular lymph node Submandibular lymph node Submaxillary lymph node Submental lymph node Subparotid lymph node Suprahyoid lymph node **1 Lymphatic, Right Neck** Cervical lymph node Jugular lymph node Mastoid (postauricular) lymph node Occipital lymph node Postauricular (mastoid) lymph node Retropharyngeal lymph node Right jugular trunk Right lymphatic duct Right subclavian trunk Supraclavicular (Virchow's) lymph node Virchow's (supraclavicular) lymph node **2 Lymphatic, Left Neck** Cervical lymph node Jugular lymph node Mastoid (postauricular) lymph node Occipital lymph node Postauricular (mastoid) lymph node Retropharyngeal lymph node Supraclavicular (Virchow's) lymph node Virchow's (supraclavicular) lymph node **3 Lymphatic, Right Upper Extremity** Cubital lymph node Deltopectoral (infraclavicular) lymph node Epitrochlear lymph node Infraclavicular (deltopectoral) lymph node Supratrochlear lymph node **4 Lymphatic, Left Upper Extremity** *See 3 Lymphatic, Right Upper Extremity* **5 Lymphatic, Right Axillary** Anterior (pectoral) lymph node Apical (subclavicular) lymph node Brachial (lateral) lymph node Central axillary lymph node Lateral (brachial) lymph node Pectoral (anterior) lymph node Posterior (subscapular) lymph node Subclavicular (apical) lymph node Subscapular (posterior) lymph node	**6 Lymphatic, Left Axillary** *See 5 Lymphatic, Right Axillary* **7 Lymphatic, Thorax** Intercostal lymph node Mediastinal lymph node Parasternal lymph node Paratracheal lymph node Tracheobronchial lymph node **8 Lymphatic, Internal Mammary, Right** **9 Lymphatic, Internal Mammary, Left** **B Lymphatic, Mesenteric** Inferior mesenteric lymph node Pararectal lymph node Superior mesenteric lymph node **C Lymphatic, Pelvis** Common iliac (subaortic) lymph node Gluteal lymph node Iliac lymph node Inferior epigastric lymph node Obturator lymph node Sacral lymph node Subaortic (common iliac) lymph node Suprainguinal lymph node **D Lymphatic, Aortic** Celiac lymph node Gastric lymph node Hepatic lymph node Lumbar lymph node Pancreaticosplenic lymph node Paraaortic lymph node Retroperitoneal lymph node **F Lymphatic, Right Lower Extremity** Femoral lymph node Popliteal lymph node **G Lymphatic, Left Lower Extremity** *See F Lymphatic, Right Lower Extremity* **H Lymphatic, Right Inguinal** **J Lymphatic, Left Inguinal** **K Thoracic Duct** Left jugular trunk Left subclavian trunk **L Cisterna Chyli** Intestinal lymphatic trunk Lumbar lymphatic trunk **M Thymus** Thymus gland **P Spleen** Accessory spleen	**Ø Open** **3 Percutaneous** **4 Percutaneous Endoscopic**	**Z No Device**	**Z No Qualifier**

Non-OR Ø7CP[3,4]ZZ

Ø Medical and Surgical
7 Lymphatic and Hemic Systems
D Extraction Definition: Pulling or stripping out or off all or a portion of a body part by the use of force

Explanation: The qualifier DIAGNOSTIC is used to identify extraction procedures that are biopsies

Body Part Character 4	Approach Character 5	Device Character 6	Qualifier Character 7
Ø Lymphatic, Head Buccinator lymph node Infraauricular lymph node Infraparotid lymph node Parotid lymph node Preauricular lymph node Submandibular lymph node Submaxillary lymph node Submental lymph node Subparotid lymph node Suprahyoid lymph node **1 Lymphatic, Right Neck** Cervical lymph node Jugular lymph node Mastoid (postauricular) lymph node Occipital lymph node Postauricular (mastoid) lymph node Retropharyngeal lymph node Right jugular trunk Right lymphatic duct Right subclavian trunk Supraclavicular (Virchow's) lymph node Virchow's (supraclavicular) lymph node **2 Lymphatic, Left Neck** Cervical lymph node Jugular lymph node Mastoid (postauricular) lymph node Occipital lymph node Postauricular (mastoid) lymph node Retropharyngeal lymph node Supraclavicular (Virchow's) lymph node Virchow's (supraclavicular) lymph node **3 Lymphatic, Right Upper Extremity** Cubital lymph node Deltopectoral (infraclavicular) lymph node Epitrochlear lymph node Infraclavicular (deltopectoral) lymph node Supratrochlear lymph node **4 Lymphatic, Left Upper Extremity** ***See*** *3 Lymphatic, Right Upper Extremity* **5 Lymphatic, Right Axillary** Anterior (pectoral) lymph node Apical (subclavicular) lymph node Brachial (lateral) lymph node Central axillary lymph node Lateral (brachial) lymph node Pectoral (anterior) lymph node Posterior (subscapular) lymph node Subclavicular (apical) lymph node Subscapular (posterior) lymph node **6 Lymphatic, Left Axillary** ***See*** *5 Lymphatic, Right Axillary* **7 Lymphatic, Thorax** Intercostal lymph node Mediastinal lymph node Parasternal lymph node Paratracheal lymph node Tracheobronchial lymph node **8 Lymphatic, Internal Mammary, Right** **9 Lymphatic, Internal Mammary, Left** **B Lymphatic, Mesenteric** Inferior mesenteric lymph node Pararectal lymph node Superior mesenteric lymph node **C Lymphatic, Pelvis** Common iliac (subaortic) lymph node Gluteal lymph node Iliac lymph node Inferior epigastric lymph node Obturator lymph node Sacral lymph node Subaortic (common iliac) lymph node Suprainguinal lymph node **D Lymphatic, Aortic** Celiac lymph node Gastric lymph node Hepatic lymph node Lumbar lymph node Pancreaticosplenic lymph node Paraaortic lymph node Retroperitoneal lymph node **F Lymphatic, Right Lower Extremity** Femoral lymph node Popliteal lymph node **G Lymphatic, Left Lower Extremity** ***See*** *F Lymphatic, Right Lower Extremity* **H Lymphatic, Right Inguinal** **J Lymphatic, Left Inguinal** **K Thoracic Duct** Left jugular trunk Left subclavian trunk **L Cisterna Chyli** Intestinal lymphatic trunk Lumbar lymphatic trunk	**3** Percutaneous **4** Percutaneous Endoscopic **8** Via Natural or Artificial Opening Endoscopic	**Z** No Device	**X** Diagnostic
M Thymus Thymus gland **P Spleen** Accessory spleen	**3** Percutaneous **4** Percutaneous Endoscopic	**Z** No Device	**X** Diagnostic
Q Bone Marrow, Sternum **R Bone Marrow, Iliac** **S Bone Marrow, Vertebral** **T Bone Marrow**	**Ø** Open **3** Percutaneous	**Z** No Device	**X** Diagnostic **Z** No Qualifier

Non-OR All body part, approach, device, and qualifier values

Ø Medical and Surgical
7 Lymphatic and Hemic Systems
H Insertion Definition: Putting in a nonbiological appliance that monitors, assists, performs, or prevents a physiological function but does not physically take the place of a body part

Explanation: None

Body Part Character 4	Approach Character 5	Device Character 6	Qualifier Character 7
K Thoracic Duct Left jugular trunk Left subclavian trunk **L** Cisterna Chyli Intestinal lymphatic trunk Lumbar lymphatic trunk **M** Thymus Thymus gland **N** Lymphatic **P** Spleen Accessory spleen **T** Bone Marrow	**Ø** Open **3** Percutaneous **4** Percutaneous Endoscopic	**1** Radioactive Element **3** Infusion Device **Y** Other Device	**Z** No Qualifier

Non-OR Ø7H[K,L,M,N,P][Ø,4]3Z
Non-OR Ø7H[K,L,M,N,P,T]3[1,3,Y]Z
Non-OR Ø7H[N,P]4YZ
Non-OR Ø7HT[Ø,4][1,3,Y]Z

Ø Medical and Surgical
7 Lymphatic and Hemic Systems
J Inspection Definition: Visually and/or manually exploring a body part

Explanation: Visual exploration may be performed with or without optical instrumentation. Manual exploration may be performed directly or through intervening body layers.

Body Part Character 4	Approach Character 5	Device Character 6	Qualifier Character 7
K Thoracic Duct Left jugular trunk Left subclavian trunk **L** Cisterna Chyli Intestinal lymphatic trunk Lumbar lymphatic trunk **M** Thymus Thymus gland **T** Bone Marrow	**Ø** Open **3** Percutaneous **4** Percutaneous Endoscopic	**Z** No Device	**Z** No Qualifier
N Lymphatic	**Ø** Open **3** Percutaneous **4** Percutaneous Endoscopic **8** Via Natural or Artificial Opening Endoscopic **X** External	**Z** No Device	**Z** No Qualifier
P Spleen Accessory spleen	**Ø** Open **3** Percutaneous **4** Percutaneous Endoscopic **X** External	**Z** No Device	**Z** No Qualifier

Non-OR Ø7J[K,L,M]3ZZ
Non-OR Ø7JT[Ø,3,4]ZZ
Non-OR Ø7JN[3,8,X]ZZ
Non-OR Ø7JP[3,4,X]ZZ

Ø Medical and Surgical
7 Lymphatic and Hemic Systems
L Occlusion Definition: Completely closing an orifice or the lumen of a tubular body part
Explanation: The orifice can be a natural orifice or an artificially created orifice

Body Part Character 4		Approach Character 5	Device Character 6	Qualifier Character 7
Ø Lymphatic, Head Buccinator lymph node Infraauricular lymph node Infraparotid lymph node Parotid lymph node Preauricular lymph node Submandibular lymph node Submaxillary lymph node Submental lymph node Subparotid lymph node Suprahyoid lymph node **1 Lymphatic, Right Neck** Cervical lymph node Jugular lymph node Mastoid (postauricular) lymph node Occipital lymph node Postauricular (mastoid) lymph node Retropharyngeal lymph node Right jugular trunk Right lymphatic duct Right subclavian trunk Supraclavicular (Virchow's) lymph node Virchow's (supraclavicular) lymph node **2 Lymphatic, Left Neck** Cervical lymph node Jugular lymph node Mastoid (postauricular) lymph node Occipital lymph node Postauricular (mastoid) lymph node Retropharyngeal lymph node Supraclavicular (Virchow's) lymph node Virchow's (supraclavicular) lymph node **3 Lymphatic, Right Upper Extremity** Cubital lymph node Deltopectoral (infraclavicular) lymph node Epitrochlear lymph node Infraclavicular (deltopectoral) lymph node Supratrochlear lymph node **4 Lymphatic, Left Upper Extremity** *See 3 Lymphatic, Right Upper Extremity* **5 Lymphatic, Right Axillary** Anterior (pectoral) lymph node Apical (subclavicular) lymph node Brachial (lateral) lymph node Central axillary lymph node Lateral (brachial) lymph node Pectoral (anterior) lymph node Posterior (subscapular) lymph node Subclavicular (apical) lymph node Subscapular (posterior) lymph node	**6 Lymphatic, Left Axillary** *See 5 Lymphatic, Right Axillary* **7 Lymphatic, Thorax** Intercostal lymph node Mediastinal lymph node Parasternal lymph node Paratracheal lymph node Tracheobronchial lymph node **8 Lymphatic, Internal Mammary, Right** **9 Lymphatic, Internal Mammary, Left** **B Lymphatic, Mesenteric** Inferior mesenteric lymph node Pararectal lymph node Superior mesenteric lymph node **C Lymphatic, Pelvis** Common iliac (subaortic) lymph node Gluteal lymph node Iliac lymph node Inferior epigastric lymph node Obturator lymph node Sacral lymph node Subaortic (common iliac) lymph node Suprainguinal lymph node **D Lymphatic, Aortic** Celiac lymph node Gastric lymph node Hepatic lymph node Lumbar lymph node Pancreaticosplenic lymph node Paraaortic lymph node Retroperitoneal lymph node **F Lymphatic, Right Lower Extremity** Femoral lymph node Popliteal lymph node **G Lymphatic, Left Lower Extremity** *See F Lymphatic, Right Lower Extremity* **H Lymphatic, Right Inguinal** **J Lymphatic, Left Inguinal** **K Thoracic Duct** Left jugular trunk Left subclavian trunk **L Cisterna Chyli** Intestinal lymphatic trunk Lumbar lymphatic trunk	**Ø Open** **3 Percutaneous** **4 Percutaneous Endoscopic**	**C Extraluminal Device** **D Intraluminal Device** **Z No Device**	**Z No Qualifier**

Ø Medical and Surgical
7 Lymphatic and Hemic Systems
N Release Definition: Freeing a body part from an abnormal physical constraint by cutting or by the use of force

Explanation: Some of the restraining tissue may be taken out but none of the body part is taken out

Body Part Character 4	Approach Character 5	Device Character 6	Qualifier Character 7
Ø Lymphatic, Head Buccinator lymph node Infraauricular lymph node Infraparotid lymph node Parotid lymph node Preauricular lymph node Submandibular lymph node Submaxillary lymph node Submental lymph node Subparotid lymph node Suprahyoid lymph node **1 Lymphatic, Right Neck** Cervical lymph node Jugular lymph node Mastoid (postauricular) lymph node Occipital lymph node Postauricular (mastoid) lymph node Retropharyngeal lymph node Right jugular trunk Right lymphatic duct Right subclavian trunk Supraclavicular (Virchow's) lymph node Virchow's (supraclavicular) lymph node **2 Lymphatic, Left Neck** Cervical lymph node Jugular lymph node Mastoid (postauricular) lymph node Occipital lymph node Postauricular (mastoid) lymph node Retropharyngeal lymph node Supraclavicular (Virchow's) lymph node Virchow's (supraclavicular) lymph node **3 Lymphatic, Right Upper Extremity** Cubital lymph node Deltopectoral (infraclavicular) lymph node Epitrochlear lymph node Infraclavicular (deltopectoral) lymph node Supratrochlear lymph node **4 Lymphatic, Left Upper Extremity** *See 3 Lymphatic, Right Upper Extremity* **5 Lymphatic, Right Axillary** Anterior (pectoral) lymph node Apical (subclavicular) lymph node Brachial (lateral) lymph node Central axillary lymph node Lateral (brachial) lymph node Pectoral (anterior) lymph node Posterior (subscapular) lymph node Subclavicular (apical) lymph node Subscapular (posterior) lymph node **6 Lymphatic, Left Axillary** *See 5 Lymphatic, Right Axillary* **7 Lymphatic, Thorax** Intercostal lymph node Mediastinal lymph node Parasternal lymph node Paratracheal lymph node Tracheobronchial lymph node **8 Lymphatic, Internal Mammary, Right** **9 Lymphatic, Internal Mammary, Left** **B Lymphatic, Mesenteric** Inferior mesenteric lymph node Pararectal lymph node Superior mesenteric lymph node **C Lymphatic, Pelvis** Common iliac (subaortic) lymph node Gluteal lymph node Iliac lymph node Inferior epigastric lymph node Obturator lymph node Sacral lymph node Subaortic (common iliac) lymph node Suprainguinal lymph node **D Lymphatic, Aortic** Celiac lymph node Gastric lymph node Hepatic lymph node Lumbar lymph node Pancreaticosplenic lymph node Paraaortic lymph node Retroperitoneal lymph node **F Lymphatic, Right Lower Extremity** Femoral lymph node Popliteal lymph node **G Lymphatic, Left Lower Extremity** *See F Lymphatic, Right Lower Extremity* **H Lymphatic, Right Inguinal** **J Lymphatic, Left Inguinal** **K Thoracic Duct** Left jugular trunk Left subclavian trunk **L Cisterna Chyli** Intestinal lymphatic trunk Lumbar lymphatic trunk **M Thymus** Thymus gland **P Spleen** Accessory spleen	**Ø Open** **3 Percutaneous** **4 Percutaneous Endoscopic**	**Z** No Device	**Z** No Qualifier

Ø Medical and Surgical
7 Lymphatic and Hemic Systems
P Removal Definition: Taking out or off a device from a body part

Explanation: If a device is taken out and a similar device put in without cutting or puncturing the skin or mucous membrane, the procedure is coded to the root operation CHANGE. Otherwise, the procedure for taking out a device is coded to the root operation REMOVAL.

Body Part Character 4	Approach Character 5	Device Character 6	Qualifier Character 7
K Thoracic Duct Left jugular trunk Left subclavian trunk L Cisterna Chyli Intestinal lymphatic trunk Lumbar lymphatic trunk N Lymphatic	Ø Open 3 Percutaneous 4 Percutaneous Endoscopic	Ø Drainage Device 3 Infusion Device 7 Autologous Tissue Substitute C Extraluminal Device D Intraluminal Device J Synthetic Substitute K Nonautologous Tissue Substitute Y Other Device	Z No Qualifier
K Thoracic Duct Left jugular trunk Left subclavian trunk L Cisterna Chyli Intestinal lymphatic trunk Lumbar lymphatic trunk N Lymphatic	X External	Ø Drainage Device 3 Infusion Device D Intraluminal Device	Z No Qualifier
M Thymus Thymus gland P Spleen Accessory spleen	Ø Open 3 Percutaneous 4 Percutaneous Endoscopic	Ø Drainage Device 3 Infusion Device Y Other Device	Z No Qualifier
M Thymus Thymus gland P Spleen Accessory spleen	X External	Ø Drainage Device 3 Infusion Device	Z No Qualifier
T Bone Marrow	Ø Open 3 Percutaneous 4 Percutaneous Endoscopic X External	Ø Drainage Device	Z No Qualifier

Non-OR Ø7P[K,L,N][3,4]YZ
Non-OR Ø7P[K,L,N]X[Ø,3,D]Z
Non-OR Ø7P[M,P][3,4]YZ
Non-OR Ø7P[M,P]X[Ø,3]Z
Non-OR Ø7PT[Ø,3,4,X]ØZ

Ø Medical and Surgical
7 Lymphatic and Hemic Systems
Q Repair Definition: Restoring, to the extent possible, a body part to its normal anatomic structure and function
Explanation: Used only when the method to accomplish the repair is not one of the other root operations

Body Part Character 4		Approach Character 5	Device Character 6	Qualifier Character 7
Ø Lymphatic, Head Buccinator lymph node Infraauricular lymph node Infraparotid lymph node Parotid lymph node Preauricular lymph node Submandibular lymph node Submaxillary lymph node Submental lymph node Subparotid lymph node Suprahyoid lymph node **1 Lymphatic, Right Neck** Cervical lymph node Jugular lymph node Mastoid (postauricular) lymph node Occipital lymph node Postauricular (mastoid) lymph node Retropharyngeal lymph node Right jugular trunk Right lymphatic duct Right subclavian trunk Supraclavicular (Virchow's) lymph node Virchow's (supraclavicular) lymph node **2 Lymphatic, Left Neck** Cervical lymph node Jugular lymph node Mastoid (postauricular) lymph node Occipital lymph node Postauricular (mastoid) lymph node Retropharyngeal lymph node Supraclavicular (Virchow's) lymph node Virchow's (supraclavicular) lymph node **3 Lymphatic, Right Upper Extremity** Cubital lymph node Deltopectoral (infraclavicular) lymph node Epitrochlear lymph node Infraclavicular (deltopectoral) lymph node Supratrochlear lymph node **4 Lymphatic, Left Upper Extremity** ***See*** *3 Lymphatic, Right Upper Extremity* **5 Lymphatic, Right Axillary** Anterior (pectoral) lymph node Apical (subclavicular) lymph node Brachial (lateral) lymph node Central axillary lymph node Lateral (brachial) lymph node Pectoral (anterior) lymph node Posterior (subscapular) lymph node Subclavicular (apical) lymph node Subscapular (posterior) lymph node	**6 Lymphatic, Left Axillary** ***See*** *5 Lymphatic, Right Axillary* **7 Lymphatic, Thorax** Intercostal lymph node Mediastinal lymph node Parasternal lymph node Paratracheal lymph node Tracheobronchial lymph node **8 Lymphatic, Internal Mammary, Right** **9 Lymphatic, Internal Mammary, Left** **B Lymphatic, Mesenteric** Inferior mesenteric lymph node Pararectal lymph node Superior mesenteric lymph node **C Lymphatic, Pelvis** Common iliac (subaortic) lymph node Gluteal lymph node Iliac lymph node Inferior epigastric lymph node Obturator lymph node Sacral lymph node Subaortic (common iliac) lymph node Suprainguinal lymph node **D Lymphatic, Aortic** Celiac lymph node Gastric lymph node Hepatic lymph node Lumbar lymph node Pancreaticosplenic lymph node Paraaortic lymph node Retroperitoneal lymph node **F Lymphatic, Right Lower Extremity** Femoral lymph node Popliteal lymph node **G Lymphatic, Left Lower Extremity** ***See*** *F Lymphatic, Right Lower Extremity* **H Lymphatic, Right Inguinal** **J Lymphatic, Left Inguinal** **K Thoracic Duct** Left jugular trunk Left subclavian trunk **L Cisterna Chyli** Intestinal lymphatic trunk Lumbar lymphatic trunk	**Ø Open** **3 Percutaneous** **4 Percutaneous Endoscopic** **8 Via Natural or Artificial Opening Endoscopic**	**Z No Device**	**Z No Qualifier**
M Thymus Thymus gland **P Spleen** Accessory spleen		**Ø Open** **3 Percutaneous** **4 Percutaneous Endoscopic**	**Z No Device**	**Z No Qualifier**

0 Medical and Surgical
7 Lymphatic and Hemic Systems
S Reposition Definition: Moving to its normal location, or other suitable location, all or a portion of a body part

Explanation: The body part is moved to a new location from an abnormal location, or from a normal location where it is not functioning correctly. The body part may or may not be cut out or off to be moved to the new location.

Body Part Character 4	Approach Character 5	Device Character 6	Qualifier Character 7
M Thymus Thymus gland **P Spleen** Accessory spleen	**0 Open**	**Z No Device**	**Z No Qualifier**

0 Medical and Surgical
7 Lymphatic and Hemic Systems
T Resection Definition: Cutting out or off, without replacement, all of a body part

Explanation: None

Body Part Character 4		Approach Character 5	Device Character 6	Qualifier Character 7
0 Lymphatic, Head Buccinator lymph node Infraauricular lymph node Infraparotid lymph node Parotid lymph node Preauricular lymph node Submandibular lymph node Submaxillary lymph node Submental lymph node Subparotid lymph node Suprahyoid lymph node **1 Lymphatic, Right Neck** Cervical lymph node Jugular lymph node Mastoid (postauricular) lymph node Occipital lymph node Postauricular (mastoid) lymph node Retropharyngeal lymph node Right jugular trunk Right lymphatic duct Right subclavian trunk Supraclavicular (Virchow's) lymph node Virchow's (supraclavicular) lymph node **2 Lymphatic, Left Neck** Cervical lymph node Jugular lymph node Mastoid (postauricular) lymph node Occipital lymph node Postauricular (mastoid) lymph node Retropharyngeal lymph node Supraclavicular (Virchow's) lymph node Virchow's (supraclavicular) lymph node **3 Lymphatic, Right Upper Extremity** Cubital lymph node Deltopectoral (infraclavicular) lymph node Epitrochlear lymph node Infraclavicular (deltopectoral) lymph node Supratrochlear lymph node **4 Lymphatic, Left Upper Extremity** ***See** 3 Lymphatic, Right Upper Extremity* **5 Lymphatic, Right Axillary** ⊞ Anterior (pectoral) lymph node Apical (subclavicular) lymph node Brachial (lateral) lymph node Central axillary lymph node Lateral (brachial) lymph node Pectoral (anterior) lymph node Posterior (subscapular) lymph node Subclavicular (apical) lymph node Subscapular (posterior) lymph node	**6 Lymphatic, Left Axillary** ⊞ ***See** 5 Lymphatic, Right Axillary* **7 Lymphatic, Thorax** ⊞ Intercostal lymph node Mediastinal lymph node Parasternal lymph node Paratracheal lymph node Tracheobronchial lymph node **8 Lymphatic, Internal Mammary, Right** ⊞ **9 Lymphatic, Internal Mammary, Left** ⊞ **B Lymphatic, Mesenteric** Inferior mesenteric lymph node Pararectal lymph node Superior mesenteric lymph node **C Lymphatic, Pelvis** Common iliac (subaortic) lymph node Gluteal lymph node Iliac lymph node Inferior epigastric lymph node Obturator lymph node Sacral lymph node Subaortic (common iliac) lymph node Suprainguinal lymph node **D Lymphatic, Aortic** Celiac lymph node Gastric lymph node Hepatic lymph node Lumbar lymph node Pancreaticosplenic lymph node Paraaortic lymph node Retroperitoneal lymph node **F Lymphatic, Right Lower Extremity** Femoral lymph node Popliteal lymph node **G Lymphatic, Left Lower Extremity** ***See** F Lymphatic, Right Lower Extremity* **H Lymphatic, Right Inguinal** **J Lymphatic, Left Inguinal** **K Thoracic Duct** Left jugular trunk Left subclavian trunk **L Cisterna Chyli** Intestinal lymphatic trunk Lumbar lymphatic trunk **M Thymus** Thymus gland **P Spleen** Accessory spleen	**0 Open** **4 Percutaneous Endoscopic**	**Z No Device**	**Z No Qualifier**

See Appendix L for Procedure Combinations
⊞ 07T[5,6,7,8,9]0ZZ

Ø Medical and Surgical
7 Lymphatic and Hemic Systems
U Supplement Definition: Putting in or on biological or synthetic material that physically reinforces and/or augments the function of a portion of a body part

Explanation: The biological material is non-living, or is living and from the same individual. The body part may have been previously replaced, and the SUPPLEMENT procedure is performed to physically reinforce and/or augment the function of the replaced body part.

Body Part Character 4	Approach Character 5	Device Character 6	Qualifier Character 7
Ø Lymphatic, Head Buccinator lymph node Infraauricular lymph node Infraparotid lymph node Parotid lymph node Preauricular lymph node Submandibular lymph node Submaxillary lymph node Submental lymph node Subparotid lymph node Suprahyoid lymph node **1 Lymphatic, Right Neck** Cervical lymph node Jugular lymph node Mastoid (postauricular) lymph node Occipital lymph node Postauricular (mastoid) lymph node Retropharyngeal lymph node Right jugular trunk Right lymphatic duct Right subclavian trunk Supraclavicular (Virchow's) lymph node Virchow's (supraclavicular) lymph node **2 Lymphatic, Left Neck** Cervical lymph node Jugular lymph node Mastoid (postauricular) lymph node Occipital lymph node Postauricular (mastoid) lymph node Retropharyngeal lymph node Supraclavicular (Virchow's) lymph node Virchow's (supraclavicular) lymph node **3 Lymphatic, Right Upper Extremity** Cubital lymph node Deltopectoral (infraclavicular) lymph node Epitrochlear lymph node Infraclavicular (deltopectoral) lymph node Supratrochlear lymph node **4 Lymphatic, Left Upper Extremity** ***See** 3 Lymphatic, Right Upper Extremity* **5 Lymphatic, Right Axillary** Anterior (pectoral) lymph node Apical (subclavicular) lymph node Brachial (lateral) lymph node Central axillary lymph node Lateral (brachial) lymph node Pectoral (anterior) lymph node Posterior (subscapular) lymph node Subclavicular (apical) lymph node Subscapular (posterior) lymph node **6 Lymphatic, Left Axillary** ***See** 5 Lymphatic, Right Axillary* **7 Lymphatic, Thorax** Intercostal lymph node Mediastinal lymph node Parasternal lymph node Paratracheal lymph node Tracheobronchial lymph node **8 Lymphatic, Internal Mammary, Right** **9 Lymphatic, Internal Mammary, Left** **B Lymphatic, Mesenteric** Inferior mesenteric lymph node Pararectal lymph node Superior mesenteric lymph node **C Lymphatic, Pelvis** Common iliac (subaortic) lymph node Gluteal lymph node Iliac lymph node Inferior epigastric lymph node Obturator lymph node Sacral lymph node Subaortic (common iliac) lymph node Suprainguinal lymph node **D Lymphatic, Aortic** Celiac lymph node Gastric lymph node Hepatic lymph node Lumbar lymph node Pancreaticosplenic lymph node Paraaortic lymph node Retroperitoneal lymph node **F Lymphatic, Right Lower Extremity** Femoral lymph node Popliteal lymph node **G Lymphatic, Left Lower Extremity** ***See** F Lymphatic, Right Lower Extremity* **H Lymphatic, Right Inguinal** **J Lymphatic, Left Inguinal** **K Thoracic Duct** Left jugular trunk Left subclavian trunk **L Cisterna Chyli** Intestinal lymphatic trunk Lumbar lymphatic trunk	**Ø Open** **4 Percutaneous Endoscopic**	**7 Autologous Tissue Substitute** **J Synthetic Substitute** **K Nonautologous Tissue Substitute**	**Z No Qualifier**

Ø Medical and Surgical
7 Lymphatic and Hemic Systems
V Restriction Definition: Partially closing an orifice or the lumen of a tubular body part
Explanation: The orifice can be a natural orifice or an artificially created orifice

Body Part Character 4	Approach Character 5	Device Character 6	Qualifier Character 7
Ø Lymphatic, Head Buccinator lymph node Infraauricular lymph node Infraparotid lymph node Parotid lymph node Preauricular lymph node Submandibular lymph node Submaxillary lymph node Submental lymph node Subparotid lymph node Suprahyoid lymph node **1 Lymphatic, Right Neck** Cervical lymph node Jugular lymph node Mastoid (postauricular) lymph node Occipital lymph node Postauricular (mastoid) lymph node Retropharyngeal lymph node Right jugular trunk Right lymphatic duct Right subclavian trunk Supraclavicular (Virchow's) lymph node Virchow's (supraclavicular) lymph node **2 Lymphatic, Left Neck** Cervical lymph node Jugular lymph node Mastoid (postauricular) lymph node Occipital lymph node Postauricular (mastoid) lymph node Retropharyngeal lymph node Supraclavicular (Virchow's) lymph node Virchow's (supraclavicular) lymph node **3 Lymphatic, Right Upper Extremity** Cubital lymph node Deltopectoral (infraclavicular) lymph node Epitrochlear lymph node Infraclavicular (deltopectoral) lymph node Supratrochlear lymph node **4 Lymphatic, Left Upper Extremity** *See 3 Lymphatic, Right Upper Extremity* **5 Lymphatic, Right Axillary** Anterior (pectoral) lymph node Apical (subclavicular) lymph node Brachial (lateral) lymph node Central axillary lymph node Lateral (brachial) lymph node Pectoral (anterior) lymph node Posterior (subscapular) lymph node Subclavicular (apical) lymph node Subscapular (posterior) lymph node **6 Lymphatic, Left Axillary** *See 5 Lymphatic, Right Axillary* **7 Lymphatic, Thorax** Intercostal lymph node Mediastinal lymph node Parasternal lymph node Paratracheal lymph node Tracheobronchial lymph node **8 Lymphatic, Internal Mammary, Right** **9 Lymphatic, Internal Mammary, Left** **B Lymphatic, Mesenteric** Inferior mesenteric lymph node Pararectal lymph node Superior mesenteric lymph node **C Lymphatic, Pelvis** Common iliac (subaortic) lymph node Gluteal lymph node Iliac lymph node Inferior epigastric lymph node Obturator lymph node Sacral lymph node Subaortic (common iliac) lymph node Suprainguinal lymph node **D Lymphatic, Aortic** Celiac lymph node Gastric lymph node Hepatic lymph node Lumbar lymph node Pancreaticosplenic lymph node Paraaortic lymph node Retroperitoneal lymph node **F Lymphatic, Right Lower Extremity** Femoral lymph node Popliteal lymph node **G Lymphatic, Left Lower Extremity** *See F Lymphatic, Right Lower Extremity* **H Lymphatic, Right Inguinal** **J Lymphatic, Left Inguinal** **K Thoracic Duct** Left jugular trunk Left subclavian trunk **L Cisterna Chyli** Intestinal lymphatic trunk Lumbar lymphatic trunk	**Ø Open** **3 Percutaneous** **4 Percutaneous Endoscopic**	**C Extraluminal Device** **D Intraluminal Device** **Z No Device**	**Z No Qualifier**

Ø Medical and Surgical
7 Lymphatic and Hemic Systems
W Revision Definition: Correcting, to the extent possible, a portion of a malfunctioning device or the position of a displaced device

Explanation: Revision can include correcting a malfunctioning or displaced device by taking out or putting in components of the device such as a screw or pin

Body Part Character 4	Approach Character 5	Device Character 6	Qualifier Character 7
K Thoracic Duct Left jugular trunk Left subclavian trunk L Cisterna Chyli Intestinal lymphatic trunk Lumbar lymphatic trunk N Lymphatic	Ø Open 3 Percutaneous 4 Percutaneous Endoscopic	Ø Drainage Device 3 Infusion Device 7 Autologous Tissue Substitute C Extraluminal Device D Intraluminal Device J Synthetic Substitute K Nonautologous Tissue Substitute Y Other Device	Z No Qualifier
K Thoracic Duct Left jugular trunk Left subclavian trunk L Cisterna Chyli Intestinal lymphatic trunk Lumbar lymphatic trunk N Lymphatic	X External	Ø Drainage Device 3 Infusion Device 7 Autologous Tissue Substitute C Extraluminal Device D Intraluminal Device J Synthetic Substitute K Nonautologous Tissue Substitute	Z No Qualifier
M Thymus Thymus gland P Spleen Accessory spleen	Ø Open 3 Percutaneous 4 Percutaneous Endoscopic	Ø Drainage Device 3 Infusion Device Y Other Device	Z No Qualifier
M Thymus Thymus gland P Spleen Accessory spleen	X External	Ø Drainage Device 3 Infusion Device	Z No Qualifier
T Bone Marrow	Ø Open 3 Percutaneous 4 Percutaneous Endoscopic X External	Ø Drainage Device	Z No Qualifier

Non-OR Ø7W[K,L,N][3,4]YZ
Non-OR Ø7W[K,L,N]X[Ø,3,7,C,D,J,K]Z
Non-OR Ø7W[M,P][3,4]YZ
Non-OR Ø7W[M,P]X[Ø,3]Z
Non-OR Ø7WT[Ø,3,4,X]ØZ

Ø Medical and Surgical
7 Lymphatic and Hemic Systems
Y Transplantation Definition: Putting in or on all or a portion of a living body part taken from another individual or animal to physically take the place and/or function of all or a portion of a similar body part

Explanation: The native body part may or may not be taken out, and the transplanted body part may take over all or a portion of its function

Body Part Character 4	Approach Character 5	Device Character 6	Qualifier Character 7
M Thymus Thymus gland P Spleen Accessory spleen	Ø Open	Z No Device	Ø Allogeneic 1 Syngeneic 2 Zooplastic

Eye Ø8Ø–Ø8X

Character Meanings

This Character Meaning table is provided as a guide to assist the user in the identification of character members that may be found in this section of code tables. It **SHOULD NOT** be used to build a PCS code.

Operation–Character 3	Body Part–Character 4	Approach–Character 5	Device–Character 6	Qualifier–Character 7
Ø Alteration	Ø Eye, Right	Ø Open	Ø Drainage Device OR Synthetic Substitute, Intraocular Telescope	3 Nasal Cavity
1 Bypass	1 Eye, Left	3 Percutaneous	1 Radioactive Element	4 Sclera
2 Change	2 Anterior Chamber, Right	7 Via Natural or Artificial Opening	3 Infusion Device	X Diagnostic
5 Destruction	3 Anterior Chamber, Left	8 Via Natural or Artificial Opening Endoscopic	5 Epiretinal Visual Prosthesis	Z No Qualifier
7 Dilation	4 Vitreous, Right	X External	7 Autologous Tissue Substitute	
9 Drainage	5 Vitreous, Left		C Extraluminal Device	
B Excision	6 Sclera, Right		D Intraluminal Device	
C Extirpation	7 Sclera, Left		J Synthetic Substitute	
D Extraction	8 Cornea, Right		K Nonautologous Tissue Substitute	
F Fragmentation	9 Cornea, Left		Y Other Device	
H Insertion	A Choroid, Right		Z No Device	
J Inspection	B Choroid, Left			
L Occlusion	C Iris, Right			
M Reattachment	D Iris, Left			
N Release	E Retina, Right			
P Removal	F Retina, Left			
Q Repair	G Retinal Vessel, Right			
R Replacement	H Retinal Vessel, Left			
S Reposition	J Lens, Right			
T Resection	K Lens, Left			
U Supplement	L Extraocular Muscle, Right			
V Restriction	M Extraocular Muscle, Left			
W Revision	N Upper Eyelid, Right			
X Transfer	P Upper Eyelid, Left			
	Q Lower Eyelid, Right			
	R Lower Eyelid, Left			
	S Conjunctiva, Right			
	T Conjunctiva, Left			
	V Lacrimal Gland, Right			
	W Lacrimal Gland, Left			
	X Lacrimal Duct, Right			
	Y Lacrimal Duct, Left			

AHA Coding Clinic for table Ø81
2019, 1Q, 27 Glaucoma tube shunt

AHA Coding Clinic for table Ø89
2016, 2Q, 21 Laser trabeculoplasty

AHA Coding Clinic for table Ø8B
2014, 4Q, 35 Vitrectomy with air/fluid exchange
2014, 4Q, 36 Pars plans vitrectomy without mention of instillation of oil, air or fluid

AHA Coding Clinic for table Ø8J
2015, 1Q, 35 Attempted removal of foreign body from cornea

AHA Coding Clinic for table Ø8N
2015, 2Q, 24 Penetrating keratoplasty and anterior segment reconstruction

AHA Coding Clinic for table Ø8Q
2018, 3Q, 13 Repair of ruptured globe

AHA Coding Clinic for table Ø8R
2015, 2Q, 24 Penetrating keratoplasty and anterior segment reconstruction
2015, 2Q, 25 Penetrating keratoplasty and placement of viscoelastic eye with paracentesis

AHA Coding Clinic for table Ø8T
2015, 2Q, 12 Orbital exenteration

AHA Coding Clinic for table Ø8U
2014, 3Q, 31 Corneal amniotic membrane transplantation

Eye

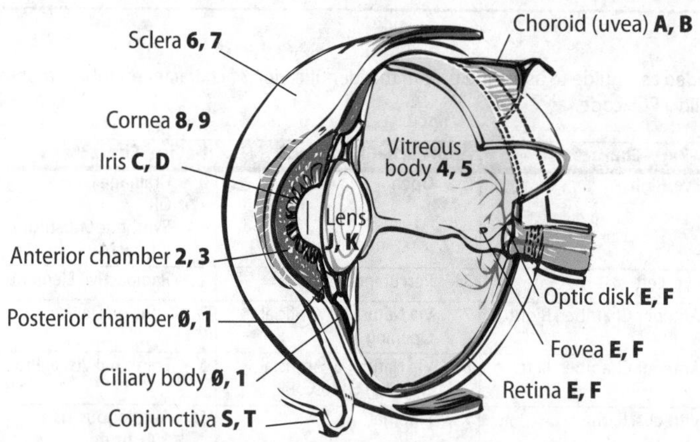

Eye Musculature

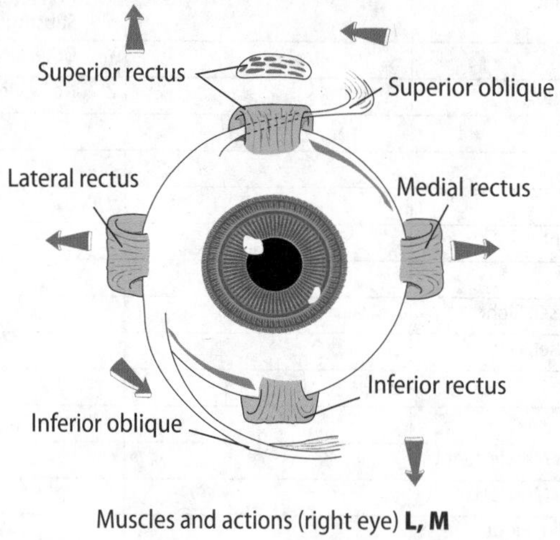

Lacrimal System

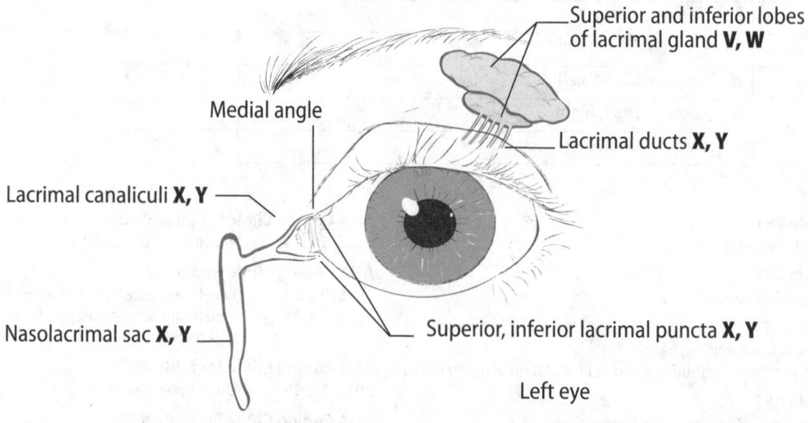

0 Medical and Surgical
8 Eye
0 Alteration Definition: Modifying the anatomic structure of a body part without affecting the function of the body part
Explanation: Principal purpose is to improve appearance

Body Part Character 4	Approach Character 5	Device Character 6	Qualifier Character 7
N Upper Eyelid, Right Lateral canthus Levator palpebrae superioris muscle Orbicularis oculi muscle Superior tarsal plate P Upper Eyelid, Left *See N Upper Eyelid, Right* Q Lower Eyelid, Right Inferior tarsal plate Medial canthus R Lower Eyelid, Left *See Q Lower Eyelid, Right*	0 Open 3 Percutaneous X External	7 Autologous Tissue Substitute J Synthetic Substitute K Nonautologous Tissue Substitute Z No Device	Z No Qualifier

Non-OR All body part, approach, device, and qualifier values

0 Medical and Surgical
8 Eye
1 Bypass Definition: Altering the route of passage of the contents of a tubular body part
Explanation: Rerouting contents of a body part to a downstream area of the normal route, to a similar route and body part, or to an abnormal route and dissimilar body part. Includes one or more anastomoses, with or without the use of a device.

Body Part Character 4	Approach Character 5	Device Character 6	Qualifier Character 7
2 Anterior Chamber, Right Aqueous humour 3 Anterior Chamber, Left *See 2 Anterior Chamber, Right*	3 Percutaneous	J Synthetic Substitute K Nonautologous Tissue Substitute Z No Device	4 Sclera
X Lacrimal Duct, Right Lacrimal canaliculus Lacrimal punctum Lacrimal sac Nasolacrimal duct Y Lacrimal Duct, Left *See X Lacrimal Duct, Right*	0 Open 3 Percutaneous	J Synthetic Substitute K Nonautologous Tissue Substitute Z No Device	3 Nasal Cavity

0 Medical and Surgical
8 Eye
2 Change Definition: Taking out or off a device from a body part and putting back an identical or similar device in or on the same body part without cutting or puncturing the skin or a mucous membrane
Explanation: All CHANGE procedures are coded using the approach EXTERNAL

Body Part Character 4	Approach Character 5	Device Character 6	Qualifier Character 7
0 Eye, Right Ciliary body Posterior chamber 1 Eye, Left *See 0 Eye, Right*	X External	0 Drainage Device Y Other Device	Z No Qualifier

Non-OR All body part, approach, device, and qualifier values

Ø Medical and Surgical
8 Eye
5 Destruction Definition: Physical eradication of all or a portion of a body part by the direct use of energy, force, or a destructive agent
Explanation: None of the body part is physically taken out

Body Part Character 4		Approach Character 5	Device Character 6	Qualifier Character 7
Ø Eye, Right Ciliary body Posterior chamber **1 Eye, Left** *See Ø Eye, Right* **6 Sclera, Right** **7 Sclera, Left**	**8 Cornea, Right** **9 Cornea, Left** **S Conjunctiva, Right** Plica semilunaris **T Conjunctiva, Left** *See S Conjunctiva, Right*	**X External**	**Z No Device**	**Z No Qualifier**
2 Anterior Chamber, Right Aqueous humour **3 Anterior Chamber, Left** *See 2 Anterior Chamber, Right* **4 Vitreous, Right** Vitreous body **5 Vitreous, Left** *See 4 Vitreous, Right* **C Iris, Right** **D Iris, Left**	**E Retina, Right** Fovea Macula Optic disc **F Retina, Left** *See E Retina, Right* **G Retinal Vessel, Right** **H Retinal Vessel, Left** **J Lens, Right** Zonule of Zinn **K Lens, Left** *See J Lens, Right*	**3 Percutaneous**	**Z No Device**	**Z No Qualifier**
A Choroid, Right **B Choroid, Left** **L Extraocular Muscle, Right** Inferior oblique muscle Inferior rectus muscle Lateral rectus muscle Medial rectus muscle Superior oblique muscle Superior rectus muscle	**M Extraocular Muscle, Left** *See L Extraocular Muscle, Right* **V Lacrimal Gland, Right** **W Lacrimal Gland, Left**	**Ø Open** **3 Percutaneous**	**Z No Device**	**Z No Qualifier**
N Upper Eyelid, Right Lateral canthus Levator palpebrae superioris muscle Orbicularis oculi muscle Superior tarsal plate **P Upper Eyelid, Left** *See N Upper Eyelid, Right*	**Q Lower Eyelid, Right** Inferior tarsal plate Medial canthus **R Lower Eyelid, Left** *See Q Lower Eyelid, Right*	**Ø Open** **3 Percutaneous** **X External**	**Z No Device**	**Z No Qualifier**
X Lacrimal Duct, Right Lacrimal canaliculus Lacrimal punctum Lacrimal sac Nasolacrimal duct	**Y Lacrimal Duct, Left** *See X Lacrimal Duct, Right*	**Ø Open** **3 Percutaneous** **7 Via Natural or Artificial Opening** **8 Via Natural or Artificial Opening Endoscopic**	**Z No Device**	**Z No Qualifier**

Non-OR Ø85[E,F]3ZZ

Ø Medical and Surgical
8 Eye
7 Dilation Definition: Expanding an orifice or the lumen of a tubular body part
Explanation: The orifice can be a natural orifice or an artificially created orifice. Accomplished by stretching a tubular body part using intraluminal pressure or by cutting part of the orifice or wall of the tubular body part.

Body Part Character 4	Approach Character 5	Device Character 6	Qualifier Character 7
X Lacrimal Duct, Right Lacrimal canaliculus Lacrimal punctum Lacrimal sac Nasolacrimal duct **Y Lacrimal Duct, Left** *See X Lacrimal Duct, Right*	**Ø Open** **3 Percutaneous** **7 Via Natural or Artificial Opening** **8 Via Natural or Artificial Opening Endoscopic**	**D Intraluminal Device** **Z No Device**	**Z No Qualifier**

Ø Medical and Surgical
8 Eye
9 Drainage Definition: Taking or letting out fluids and/or gases from a body part
Explanation: The qualifier DIAGNOSTIC is used to identify drainage procedures that are biopsies

Body Part Character 4		Approach Character 5	Device Character 6	Qualifier Character 7
Ø Eye, Right Ciliary body Posterior chamber **1 Eye, Left** *See Ø Eye, Right* **6 Sclera, Right** **7 Sclera, Left**	**8 Cornea, Right** **9 Cornea, Left** **S Conjunctiva, Right** Plica semilunaris **T Conjunctiva, Left** *See S Conjunctiva, Right*	**X** External	**Ø** Drainage Device	**Z** No Qualifier
Ø Eye, Right Ciliary body Posterior chamber **1 Eye, Left** *See Ø Eye, Right* **6 Sclera, Right** **7 Sclera, Left**	**8 Cornea, Right** **9 Cornea, Left** **S Conjunctiva, Right** Plica semilunaris **T Conjunctiva, Left** *See S Conjunctiva, Right*	**X** External	**Z** No Device	**X** Diagnostic **Z** No Qualifier
2 Anterior Chamber, Right Aqueous humour **3 Anterior Chamber, Left** *See 2 Anterior Chamber, Right* **4 Vitreous, Right** Vitreous body **5 Vitreous, Left** *See 4 Vitreous, Right* **C Iris, Right** **D Iris, Left**	**E Retina, Right** Fovea Macula Optic disc **F Retina, Left** *See E Retina, Right* **G Retinal Vessel, Right** **H Retinal Vessel, Left** **J Lens, Right** Zonule of Zinn **K Lens, Left** *See J Lens, Right*	**3** Percutaneous	**Ø** Drainage Device	**Z** No Qualifier
2 Anterior Chamber, Right Aqueous humour **3 Anterior Chamber, Left** *See 2 Anterior Chamber, Right* **4 Vitreous, Right** Vitreous body **5 Vitreous, Left** *See 4 Vitreous, Right* **C Iris, Right** **D Iris, Left**	**E Retina, Right** Fovea Macula Optic disc **F Retina, Left** *See E Retina, Right* **G Retinal Vessel, Right** **H Retinal Vessel, Left** **J Lens, Right** Zonule of Zinn **K Lens, Left** *See J Lens, Right*	**3** Percutaneous	**Z** No Device	**X** Diagnostic **Z** No Qualifier
A Choroid, Right **B Choroid, Left** **L Extraocular Muscle, Right** Inferior oblique muscle Inferior rectus muscle Lateral rectus muscle Medial rectus muscle Superior oblique muscle Superior rectus muscle	**M Extraocular Muscle, Left** *See L Extraocular Muscle, Right* **V Lacrimal Gland, Right** **W Lacrimal Gland, Left**	**Ø** Open **3** Percutaneous	**Ø** Drainage Device	**Z** No Qualifier
A Choroid, Right **B Choroid, Left** **L Extraocular Muscle, Right** Inferior oblique muscle Inferior rectus muscle Lateral rectus muscle Medial rectus muscle Superior oblique muscle Superior rectus muscle	**M Extraocular Muscle, Left** *See L Extraocular Muscle, Right* **V Lacrimal Gland, Right** **W Lacrimal Gland, Left**	**Ø** Open **3** Percutaneous	**Z** No Device	**X** Diagnostic **Z** No Qualifier
N Upper Eyelid, Right Lateral canthus Levator palpebrae superioris muscle Orbicularis oculi muscle Superior tarsal plate **P Upper Eyelid, Left** *See N Upper Eyelid, Right*	**Q Lower Eyelid, Right** Inferior tarsal plate Medial canthus **R Lower Eyelid, Left** *See Q Lower Eyelid, Right*	**Ø** Open **3** Percutaneous **X** External	**Ø** Drainage Device	**Z** No Qualifier

Non-OR Ø89[Ø,1,6,7,8,9,S,T]XZ[X,Z]
Non-OR Ø89[N,P,Q,R][Ø,3,X]ØZ

Ø89 Continued on next page

Ø Medical and Surgical
8 Eye
9 Drainage

Ø89 Continued

Definition: Taking or letting out fluids and/or gases from a body part
Explanation: The qualifier DIAGNOSTIC is used to identify drainage procedures that are biopsies

Body Part Character 4		Approach Character 5	Device Character 6	Qualifier Character 7
N Upper Eyelid, Right Lateral canthus Levator palpebrae superioris muscle Orbicularis oculi muscle Superior tarsal plate **P Upper Eyelid, Left** *See N Upper Eyelid, Right*	**Q Lower Eyelid, Right** Inferior tarsal plate Medial canthus **R Lower Eyelid, Left** *See Q Lower Eyelid, Right*	**Ø Open** **3 Percutaneous** **X External**	**Z No Device**	**X Diagnostic** **Z No Qualifier**
X Lacrimal Duct, Right Lacrimal canaliculus Lacrimal punctum Lacrimal sac Nasolacrimal duct	**Y Lacrimal Duct, Left** *See X Lacrimal Duct, Right*	**Ø Open** **3 Percutaneous** **7 Via Natural or Artificial Opening** **8 Via Natural or Artificial Opening Endoscopic**	**Ø Drainage Device**	**Z No Qualifier**
X Lacrimal Duct, Right Lacrimal canaliculus Lacrimal punctum Lacrimal sac Nasolacrimal duct	**Y Lacrimal Duct, Left** *See X Lacrimal Duct, Right*	**Ø Open** **3 Percutaneous** **7 Via Natural or Artificial Opening** **8 Via Natural or Artificial Opening Endoscopic**	**Z No Device**	**X Diagnostic** **Z No Qualifier**

Non-OR Ø89[N,P,Q,R]ØZZ
Non-OR Ø89[N,P,Q,R][3,X]Z[X,Z]

Ø Medical and Surgical
8 Eye
B Excision

Definition: Cutting out or off, without replacement, a portion of a body part
Explanation: The qualifier DIAGNOSTIC is used to identify excision procedures that are biopsies

Body Part Character 4		Approach Character 5	Device Character 6	Qualifier Character 7
Ø Eye, Right Ciliary body Posterior chamber **1 Eye, Left** *See Ø Eye, Right* **N Upper Eyelid, Right** Lateral canthus Levator palpebrae superioris muscle Orbicularis oculi muscle Superior tarsal plate	**P Upper Eyelid, Left** *See N Upper Eyelid, Right* **Q Lower Eyelid, Right** Inferior tarsal plate Medial canthus **R Lower Eyelid, Left** *See Q Lower Eyelid, Right*	**Ø Open** **3 Percutaneous** **X External**	**Z No Device**	**X Diagnostic** **Z No Qualifier**
4 Vitreous, Right Vitreous body **5 Vitreous, Left** *See 4 Vitreous, Right* **C Iris, Right** **D Iris, Left** **E Retina, Right** Fovea Macula Optic disc	**F Retina, Left** *See E Retina, Right* **J Lens, Right** Zonule of Zinn **K Lens, Left** *See J Lens, Right*	**3 Percutaneous**	**Z No Device**	**X Diagnostic** **Z No Qualifier**
6 Sclera, Right **7 Sclera, Left** **8 Cornea, Right** **9 Cornea, Left**	**S Conjunctiva, Right** Plica semilunaris **T Conjunctiva, Left** *See S Conjunctiva, Right*	**X External**	**Z No Device**	**X Diagnostic** **Z No Qualifier**
A Choroid, Right **B Choroid, Left** **L Extraocular Muscle, Right** Inferior oblique muscle Inferior rectus muscle Lateral rectus muscle Medial rectus muscle Superior oblique muscle Superior rectus muscle	**M Extraocular Muscle, Left** *See L Extraocular Muscle, Right* **V Lacrimal Gland, Right** **W Lacrimal Gland, Left**	**Ø Open** **3 Percutaneous**	**Z No Device**	**X Diagnostic** **Z No Qualifier**
X Lacrimal Duct, Right Lacrimal canaliculus Lacrimal punctum Lacrimal sac Nasolacrimal duct	**Y Lacrimal Duct, Left** *See X Lacrimal Duct, Right*	**Ø Open** **3 Percutaneous** **7 Via Natural or Artificial Opening** **8 Via Natural or Artificial Opening Endoscopic**	**Z No Device**	**X Diagnostic** **Z No Qualifier**

Ø Medical and Surgical
8 Eye
C Extirpation Definition: Taking or cutting out solid matter from a body part

Explanation: The solid matter may be an abnormal byproduct of a biological function or a foreign body; it may be imbedded in a body part or in the lumen of a tubular body part. The solid matter may or may not have been previously broken into pieces.

Body Part Character 4	Approach Character 5	Device Character 6	Qualifier Character 7
Ø Eye, Right Ciliary body Posterior chamber **1 Eye, Left** *See Ø Eye, Right* **6 Sclera, Right** **7 Sclera, Left** **8 Cornea, Right** **9 Cornea, Left** **S Conjunctiva, Right** Plica semilunaris **T Conjunctiva, Left** *See S Conjunctiva, Right*	**X External**	**Z No Device**	**Z No Qualifier**
2 Anterior Chamber, Right Aqueous humour **3 Anterior Chamber, Left** *See 2 Anterior Chamber, Right* **4 Vitreous, Right** Vitreous body **5 Vitreous, Left** *See 4 Vitreous, Right* **C Iris, Right** **D Iris, Left** **E Retina, Right** Fovea Macula Optic disc **F Retina, Left** *See* E Retina, Right **G Retinal Vessel, Right** **H Retinal Vessel, Left** **J Lens, Right** Zonule of Zinn **K Lens, Left** *See J Lens, Right*	**3 Percutaneous** **X External**	**Z No Device**	**Z No Qualifier**
A Choroid, Right **B Choroid, Left** **L Extraocular Muscle, Right** Inferior oblique muscle Inferior rectus muscle Lateral rectus muscle Medial rectus muscle Superior oblique muscle Superior rectus muscle **M Extraocular Muscle, Left** *See L Extraocular Muscle, Right* **N Upper Eyelid, Right** Lateral canthus Levator palpebrae superioris muscle Orbicularis oculi muscle Superior tarsal plate **P Upper Eyelid, Left** *See N Upper Eyelid, Right* **Q Lower Eyelid, Right** Inferior tarsal plate Medial canthus **R Lower Eyelid, Left** *See Q Lower Eyelid, Right* **V Lacrimal Gland, Right** **W Lacrimal Gland, Left**	**Ø Open** **3 Percutaneous** **X External**	**Z No Device**	**Z No Qualifier**
X Lacrimal Duct, Right Lacrimal canaliculus Lacrimal punctum Lacrimal sac Nasolacrimal duct **Y Lacrimal Duct, Left** *See X Lacrimal Duct, Right*	**Ø Open** **3 Percutaneous** **7 Via Natural or Artificial Opening** **8 Via Natural or Artificial Opening Endoscopic**	**Z No Device**	**Z No Qualifier**

Non-OR Ø8C[Ø,1,6,7,S,T]XZZ
Non-OR Ø8C[2,3]XZZ
Non-OR Ø8C[N,P,Q,R][Ø,3,X]ZZ

Ø Medical and Surgical
8 Eye
D Extraction Definition: Pulling or stripping out or off all or a portion of a body part by the use of force
Explanation: The qualifier DIAGNOSTIC is used to identify extraction procedures that are biopsies

Body Part Character 4	Approach Character 5	Device Character 6	Qualifier Character 7
8 Cornea, Right 9 Cornea, Left	X External	Z No Device	X Diagnostic Z No Qualifier
J Lens, Right Zonule of Zinn K Lens, Left *See J Lens, Right*	3 Percutaneous	Z No Device	Z No Qualifier

Ø Medical and Surgical
8 Eye
F Fragmentation Definition: Breaking solid matter in a body part into pieces
Explanation: Physical force (e.g., manual, ultrasonic) applied directly or indirectly is used to break the solid matter into pieces. The solid matter may be an abnormal byproduct of a biological function or a foreign body. The pieces of solid matter are not taken out.

Body Part Character 4	Approach Character 5	Device Character 6	Qualifier Character 7
4 Vitreous, Right NC Vitreous body 5 Vitreous, Left NC *See 4 Vitreous, Right*	3 Percutaneous X External	Z No Device	Z No Qualifier

Non-OR Ø8F[4,5]XZZ
NC Ø8F[4,5]XZZ

Ø Medical and Surgical
8 Eye
H Insertion Definition: Putting in a nonbiological appliance that monitors, assists, performs, or prevents a physiological function but does not physically take the place of a body part
Explanation: None

Body Part Character 4	Approach Character 5	Device Character 6	Qualifier Character 7
Ø Eye, Right Ciliary body Posterior chamber 1 Eye, Left *See Ø Eye, Right*	Ø Open	5 Epiretinal Visual Prosthesis Y Other Device	Z No Qualifier
Ø Eye, Right Ciliary body Posterior chamber 1 Eye, Left *See Ø Eye, Right*	3 Percutaneous	1 Radioactive Element 3 Infusion Device Y Other Device	Z No Qualifier
Ø Eye, Right Ciliary body Posterior chamber 1 Eye, Left *See Ø Eye, Right*	7 Via Natural or Artificial Opening 8 Via Natural or Artificial Opening Endoscopic	Y Other Device	Z No Qualifier
Ø Eye, Right Ciliary body Posterior chamber 1 Eye, Left *See Ø Eye, Right*	X External	1 Radioactive Element 3 Infusion Device	Z No Qualifier

Non-OR Ø8H[Ø,1]3YZ
Non-OR Ø8H[Ø,1][7,8]YZ

Ø Medical and Surgical
8 Eye
J Inspection Definition: Visually and/or manually exploring a body part

Explanation: Visual exploration may be performed with or without optical instrumentation. Manual exploration may be performed directly or through intervening body layers.

Body Part Character 4	Approach Character 5	Device Character 6	Qualifier Character 7
Ø Eye, Right Ciliary body Posterior chamber **1 Eye, Left** *See Ø Eye, Right* **J Lens, Right** Zonule of Zinn **K Lens, Left** *See J Lens, Right*	X External	Z No Device	Z No Qualifier
L Extraocular Muscle, Right Inferior oblique muscle Inferior rectus muscle Lateral rectus muscle Medial rectus muscle Superior oblique muscle Superior rectus muscle **M Extraocular Muscle, Left** *See L Extraocular Muscle, Right*	Ø Open X External	Z No Device	Z No Qualifier

Non-OR Ø8J[Ø,1,J,K]XZZ
Non-OR Ø8J[L,M]XZZ

Ø Medical and Surgical
8 Eye
L Occlusion Definition: Completely closing an orifice or the lumen of a tubular body part

Explanation: The orifice can be a natural orifice or an artificially created orifice

Body Part Character 4	Approach Character 5	Device Character 6	Qualifier Character 7
X Lacrimal Duct, Right Lacrimal canaliculus Lacrimal punctum Lacrimal sac Nasolacrimal duct **Y Lacrimal Duct, Left** *See X Lacrimal Duct, Right*	Ø Open 3 Percutaneous	C Extraluminal Device D Intraluminal Device Z No Device	Z No Qualifier
X Lacrimal Duct, Right Lacrimal canaliculus Lacrimal punctum Lacrimal sac Nasolacrimal duct **Y Lacrimal Duct, Left** *See X Lacrimal Duct, Right*	7 Via Natural or Artificial Opening 8 Via Natural or Artificial Opening Endoscopic	D Intraluminal Device Z No Device	Z No Qualifier

Ø Medical and Surgical
8 Eye
M Reattachment Definition: Putting back in or on all or a portion of a separated body part to its normal location or other suitable location

Explanation: Vascular circulation and nervous pathways may or may not be reestablished

Body Part Character 4	Approach Character 5	Device Character 6	Qualifier Character 7
N Upper Eyelid, Right Lateral canthus Levator palpebrae superioris muscle Orbicularis oculi muscle Superior tarsal plate **P Upper Eyelid, Left** *See N Upper Eyelid, Right* **Q Lower Eyelid, Right** Inferior tarsal plate Medial canthus **R Lower Eyelid, Left** *See Q Lower Eyelid, Right*	X External	Z No Device	Z No Qualifier

Ø Medical and Surgical
8 Eye
N Release Definition: Freeing a body part from an abnormal physical constraint by cutting or by the use of force
Explanation: Some of the restraining tissue may be taken out but none of the body part is taken out

Body Part Character 4	Approach Character 5	Device Character 6	Qualifier Character 7
Ø Eye, Right Ciliary body Posterior chamber **1 Eye, Left** *See Ø Eye, Right* **6 Sclera, Right** **7 Sclera, Left** **8 Cornea, Right** **9 Cornea, Left** **S Conjunctiva, Right** Plica semilunaris **T Conjunctiva, Left** *See S Conjunctiva, Right*	**X External**	**Z No Device**	**Z No Qualifier**
2 Anterior Chamber, Right Aqueous humour **3 Anterior Chamber, Left** *See 2 Anterior Chamber, Right* **4 Vitreous, Right** Vitreous body **5 Vitreous, Left** *See 4 Vitreous, Right* **C Iris, Right** **D Iris, Left** **E Retina, Right** Fovea Macula Optic disc **F Retina, Left** *See E Retina, Right* **G Retinal Vessel, Right** **H Retinal Vessel, Left** **J Lens, Right** Zonule of Zinn **K Lens, Left** *See J Lens, Right*	**3 Percutaneous**	**Z No Device**	**Z No Qualifier**
A Choroid, Right **B Choroid, Left** **L Extraocular Muscle, Right** Inferior oblique muscle Inferior rectus muscle Lateral rectus muscle Medial rectus muscle Superior oblique muscle Superior rectus muscle **M Extraocular Muscle, Left** *See L Extraocular Muscle, Right* **V Lacrimal Gland, Right** **W Lacrimal Gland, Left**	**Ø Open** **3 Percutaneous**	**Z No Device**	**Z No Qualifier**
N Upper Eyelid, Right Lateral canthus Levator palpebrae superioris muscle Orbicularis oculi muscle Superior tarsal plate **P Upper Eyelid, Left** *See N Upper Eyelid, Right* **Q Lower Eyelid, Right** Inferior tarsal plate Medial canthus **R Lower Eyelid, Left** *See Q Lower Eyelid, Right*	**Ø Open** **3 Percutaneous** **X External**	**Z No Device**	**Z No Qualifier**
X Lacrimal Duct, Right Lacrimal canaliculus Lacrimal punctum Lacrimal sac Nasolacrimal duct **Y Lacrimal Duct, Left** *See X Lacrimal Duct, Right*	**Ø Open** **3 Percutaneous** **7 Via Natural or Artificial Opening** **8 Via Natural or Artificial Opening Endoscopic**	**Z No Device**	**Z No Qualifier**

Ø Medical and Surgical
8 Eye
P Removal Definition: Taking out or off a device from a body part

Explanation: If a device is taken out and a similar device put in without cutting or puncturing the skin or mucous membrane, the procedure is coded to the root operation CHANGE. Otherwise, the procedure for taking out a device is coded to the root operation REMOVAL.

Body Part Character 4	Approach Character 5	Device Character 6	Qualifier Character 7
Ø Eye, Right Ciliary body Posterior chamber 1 Eye, Left *See Ø Eye, Right*	Ø Open 3 Percutaneous 7 Via Natural or Artificial Opening 8 Via Natural or Artificial Opening Endoscopic	Ø Drainage Device 1 Radioactive Element 3 Infusion Device 7 Autologous Tissue Substitute C Extraluminal Device D Intraluminal Device J Synthetic Substitute K Nonautologous Tissue Substitute Y Other Device	Z No Qualifier
Ø Eye, Right Ciliary body Posterior chamber 1 Eye, Left *See Ø Eye, Right*	X External	Ø Drainage Device 1 Radioactive Element 3 Infusion Device 7 Autologous Tissue Substitute C Extraluminal Device D Intraluminal Device J Synthetic Substitute K Nonautologous Tissue Substitute	Z No Qualifier
J Lens, Right Zonule of Zinn K Lens, Left *See J Lens, Right*	3 Percutaneous	J Synthetic Substitute Y Other Device	Z No Qualifier
L Extraocular Muscle, Right Inferior oblique muscle Inferior rectus muscle Lateral rectus muscle Medial rectus muscle Superior oblique muscle Superior rectus muscle M Extraocular Muscle, Left *See L Extraocular Muscle, Right*	Ø Open 3 Percutaneous	Ø Drainage Device 7 Autologous Tissue Substitute J Synthetic Substitute K Nonautologous Tissue Substitute Y Other Device	Z No Qualifier

Non-OR Ø8P[Ø,1]3YZ
Non-OR Ø8P[Ø,1][7,8][Ø,3,D,Y]Z
Non-OR Ø8P[Ø,1]X[Ø,1,3,C,D,J]Z
Non-OR Ø8P[J,K]3YZ
Non-OR Ø8P[L,M]3YZ

Ø Medical and Surgical
8 Eye
Q Repair Definition: Restoring, to the extent possible, a body part to its normal anatomic structure and function
Explanation: Used only when the method to accomplish the repair is not one of the other root operations

Body Part Character 4	Approach Character 5	Device Character 6	Qualifier Character 7
Ø Eye, Right Ciliary body Posterior chamber **1 Eye, Left** *See Ø Eye, Right* **6 Sclera, Right** **7 Sclera, Left** **8 Cornea, Right** NC **9 Cornea, Left** NC **S Conjunctiva, Right** Plica semilunaris **T Conjunctiva, Left** *See S Conjunctiva, Right*	**X External**	**Z No Device**	**Z No Qualifier**
2 Anterior Chamber, Right Aqueous humour **3 Anterior Chamber, Left** *See 2 Anterior Chamber, Right* **4 Vitreous, Right** Vitreous body **5 Vitreous, Left** *See 4 Vitreous, Right* **C Iris, Right** **D Iris, Left** **E Retina, Right** Fovea Macula Optic disc **F Retina, Left** *See E Retina, Right* **G Retinal Vessel, Right** **H Retinal Vessel, Left** **J Lens, Right** Zonule of Zinn **K Lens, Left** *See J Lens, Right*	**3 Percutaneous**	**Z No Device**	**Z No Qualifier**
A Choroid, Right **B Choroid, Left** **L Extraocular Muscle, Right** Inferior oblique muscle Inferior rectus muscle Lateral rectus muscle Medial rectus muscle Superior oblique muscle Superior rectus muscle **M Extraocular Muscle, Left** *See L Extraocular Muscle, Right* **V Lacrimal Gland, Right** **W Lacrimal Gland, Left**	**Ø Open** **3 Percutaneous**	**Z No Device**	**Z No Qualifier**
N Upper Eyelid, Right Lateral canthus Levator palpebrae superioris muscle Orbicularis oculi muscle Superior tarsal plate **P Upper Eyelid, Left** *See N Upper Eyelid, Right* **Q Lower Eyelid, Right** Inferior tarsal plate Medial canthus **R Lower Eyelid, Left** *See Q Lower Eyelid, Right*	**Ø Open** **3 Percutaneous** **X External**	**Z No Device**	**Z No Qualifier**
X Lacrimal Duct, Right Lacrimal canaliculus Lacrimal punctum Lacrimal sac Nasolacrimal duct **Y Lacrimal Duct, Left** *See X Lacrimal Duct, Right*	**Ø Open** **3 Percutaneous** **7 Via Natural or Artificial Opening** **8 Via Natural or Artificial Opening Endoscopic**	**Z No Device**	**Z No Qualifier**

Non-OR Ø8Q[N,P,Q,R][Ø,3,X]ZZ
NC Ø8Q[8,9]XZZ

Ø Medical and Surgical
8 Eye
R Replacement Definition: Putting in or on biological or synthetic material that physically takes the place and/or function of all or a portion of a body part

Explanation: The body part may have been taken out or replaced, or may be taken out, physically eradicated, or rendered nonfunctional during the REPLACEMENT procedure. A REMOVAL procedure is coded for taking out the device used in a previous replacement procedure.

Body Part Character 4	Approach Character 5	Device Character 6	Qualifier Character 7
Ø Eye, Right Ciliary body Posterior chamber **1 Eye, Left** *See Ø Eye, Right* **A Choroid, Right** **B Choroid, Left**	**Ø Open** **3 Percutaneous**	**7 Autologous Tissue Substitute** **J Synthetic Substitute** **K Nonautologous Tissue Substitute**	**Z No Qualifier**
4 Vitreous, Right Vitreous body **5 Vitreous, Left** *See 4 Vitreous, Right* **C Iris, Right** **D Iris, Left** **G Retinal Vessel, Right** **H Retinal Vessel, Left**	**3 Percutaneous**	**7 Autologous Tissue Substitute** **J Synthetic Substitute** **K Nonautologous Tissue Substitute**	**Z No Qualifier**
6 Sclera, Right **7 Sclera, Left** **S Conjunctiva, Right** Plica semilunaris **T Conjunctiva, Left** *See S Conjunctiva, Right*	**X External**	**7 Autologous Tissue Substitute** **J Synthetic Substitute** **K Nonautologous Tissue Substitute**	**Z No Qualifier**
8 Cornea, Right **9 Cornea, Left**	**3 Percutaneous** **X External**	**7 Autologous Tissue Substitute** **J Synthetic Substitute** **K Nonautologous Tissue Substitute**	**Z No Qualifier**
J Lens, Right Zonule of Zinn **K Lens, Left** *See J Lens, Right*	**3 Percutaneous**	**Ø Synthetic Substitute, Intraocular Telescope** **7 Autologous Tissue Substitute** **J Synthetic Substitute** **K Nonautologous Tissue Substitute**	**Z No Qualifier**
N Upper Eyelid, Right Lateral canthus Levator palpebrae superioris muscle Orbicularis oculi muscle Superior tarsal plate **P Upper Eyelid, Left** *See N Upper Eyelid, Right* **Q Lower Eyelid, Right** Inferior tarsal plate Medial canthus **R Lower Eyelid, Left** *See Q Lower Eyelid, Right*	**Ø Open** **3 Percutaneous** **X External**	**7 Autologous Tissue Substitute** **J Synthetic Substitute** **K Nonautologous Tissue Substitute**	**Z No Qualifier**
X Lacrimal Duct, Right Lacrimal canaliculus Lacrimal punctum Lacrimal sac Nasolacrimal duct **Y Lacrimal Duct, Left** *See X Lacrimal Duct, Right*	**Ø Open** **3 Percutaneous** **7 Via Natural or Artificial Opening** **8 Via Natural or Artificial Opening Endoscopic**	**7 Autologous Tissue Substitute** **J Synthetic Substitute** **K Nonautologous Tissue Substitute**	**Z No Qualifier**

Ø Medical and Surgical
8 Eye
S Reposition Definition: Moving to its normal location, or other suitable location, all or a portion of a body part

Explanation: The body part is moved to a new location from an abnormal location, or from a normal location where it is not functioning correctly. The body part may or may not be cut out or off to be moved to the new location.

Body Part Character 4	Approach Character 5	Device Character 6	Qualifier Character 7
C Iris, Right **D Iris, Left** **G Retinal Vessel, Right** **H Retinal Vessel, Left** **J Lens, Right** Zonule of Zinn **K Lens, Left** *See J Lens, Right*	**3 Percutaneous**	**Z No Device**	**Z No Qualifier**
L Extraocular Muscle, Right Inferior oblique muscle Inferior rectus muscle Lateral rectus muscle Medial rectus muscle Superior oblique muscle Superior rectus muscle **M Extraocular Muscle, Left** *See L Extraocular Muscle, Right* **V Lacrimal Gland, Right** **W Lacrimal Gland, Left**	**Ø Open** **3 Percutaneous**	**Z No Device**	**Z No Qualifier**
N Upper Eyelid, Right Lateral canthus Levator palpebrae superioris muscle Orbicularis oculi muscle Superior tarsal plate **P Upper Eyelid, Left** *See N Upper Eyelid, Right* **Q Lower Eyelid, Right** Inferior tarsal plate Medial canthus **R Lower Eyelid, Left** *See Q Lower Eyelid, Right*	**Ø Open** **3 Percutaneous** **X External**	**Z No Device**	**Z No Qualifier**
X Lacrimal Duct, Right Lacrimal canaliculus Lacrimal punctum Lacrimal sac Nasolacrimal duct **Y Lacrimal Duct, Left** *See X Lacrimal Duct, Right*	**Ø Open** **3 Percutaneous** **7 Via Natural or Artificial Opening** **8 Via Natural or Artificial Opening Endoscopic**	**Z No Device**	**Z No Qualifier**

Ø Medical and Surgical
8 Eye
T Resection Definition: Cutting out or off, without replacement, all of a body part

Explanation: None

Body Part Character 4	Approach Character 5	Device Character 6	Qualifier Character 7
Ø Eye, Right Ciliary body Posterior chamber **1 Eye, Left** *See Ø Eye, Right* **8 Cornea, Right** **9 Cornea, Left**	**X External**	**Z No Device**	**Z No Qualifier**
4 Vitreous, Right Vitreous body **5 Vitreous, Left** *See 4 Vitreous, Right* **C Iris, Right** **D Iris, Left** **J Lens, Right** Zonule of Zinn **K Lens, Left** *See J Lens, Right*	**3 Percutaneous**	**Z No Device**	**Z No Qualifier**
L Extraocular Muscle, Right Inferior oblique muscle Inferior rectus muscle Lateral rectus muscle Medial rectus muscle Superior oblique muscle Superior rectus muscle **M Extraocular Muscle, Left** *See L Extraocular Muscle, Right* **V Lacrimal Gland, Right** **W Lacrimal Gland, Left**	**Ø Open** **3 Percutaneous**	**Z No Device**	**Z No Qualifier**
N Upper Eyelid, Right Lateral canthus Levator palpebrae superioris muscle Orbicularis oculi muscle Superior tarsal plate **P Upper Eyelid, Left** *See N Upper Eyelid, Right* **Q Lower Eyelid, Right** Inferior tarsal plate Medial canthus **R Lower Eyelid, Left** *See Q Lower Eyelid, Right*	**Ø Open** **X External**	**Z No Device**	**Z No Qualifier**
X Lacrimal Duct, Right Lacrimal canaliculus Lacrimal punctum Lacrimal sac Nasolacrimal duct **Y Lacrimal Duct, Left** *See X Lacrimal Duct, Right*	**Ø Open** **3 Percutaneous** **7 Via Natural or Artificial Opening** **8 Via Natural or Artificial Opening Endoscopic**	**Z No Device**	**Z No Qualifier**

Ø Medical and Surgical
8 Eye
U Supplement Definition: Putting in or on biological or synthetic material that physically reinforces and/or augments the function of a portion of a body part

Explanation: The biological material is non-living, or is living and from the same individual. The body part may have been previously replaced, and the SUPPLEMENT procedure is performed to physically reinforce and/or augment the function of the replaced body part.

Body Part Character 4	Approach Character 5	Device Character 6	Qualifier Character 7
Ø Eye, Right Ciliary body Posterior chamber **1 Eye, Left** *See Ø Eye, Right* **C Iris, Right** **D Iris, Left** **E Retina, Right** Fovea Macula Optic disc **F Retina, Left** *See E Retina, Right* **G Retinal Vessel, Right** **H Retinal Vessel, Left** **L Extraocular Muscle, Right** Inferior oblique muscle Inferior rectus muscle Lateral rectus muscle Medial rectus muscle Superior oblique muscle Superior rectus muscle **M Extraocular Muscle, Left** *See L Extraocular Muscle, Right*	**Ø Open** **3 Percutaneous**	**7 Autologous Tissue Substitute** **J Synthetic Substitute** **K Nonautologous Tissue Substitute**	**Z No Qualifier**
8 Cornea, Right NC **9 Cornea, Left** NC **N Upper Eyelid, Right** Lateral canthus Levator palpebrae superioris muscle Orbicularis oculi muscle Superior tarsal plate **P Upper Eyelid, Left** *See N Upper Eyelid, Right* **Q Lower Eyelid, Right** Inferior tarsal plate Medial canthus **R Lower Eyelid, Left** *See Q Lower Eyelid, Right*	**Ø Open** **3 Percutaneous** **X External**	**7 Autologous Tissue Substitute** **J Synthetic Substitute** **K Nonautologous Tissue Substitute**	**Z No Qualifier**
X Lacrimal Duct, Right Lacrimal canaliculus Lacrimal punctum Lacrimal sac Nasolacrimal duct **Y Lacrimal Duct, Left** *See X Lacrimal Duct, Right*	**Ø Open** **3 Percutaneous** **7 Via Natural or Artificial Opening** **8 Via Natural or Artificial Opening Endoscopic**	**7 Autologous Tissue Substitute** **J Synthetic Substitute** **K Nonautologous Tissue Substitute**	**Z No Qualifier**

NC Ø8U[8,9][Ø,3,X]KZ

Ø Medical and Surgical
8 Eye
V Restriction Definition: Partially closing an orifice or the lumen of a tubular body part

Explanation: The orifice can be a natural orifice or an artificially created orifice

Body Part Character 4	Approach Character 5	Device Character 6	Qualifier Character 7
X Lacrimal Duct, Right Lacrimal canaliculus Lacrimal punctum Lacrimal sac Nasolacrimal duct **Y Lacrimal Duct, Left** *See X Lacrimal Duct, Right*	**Ø Open** **3 Percutaneous**	**C Extraluminal Device** **D Intraluminal Device** **Z No Device**	**Z No Qualifier**
X Lacrimal Duct, Right Lacrimal canaliculus Lacrimal punctum Lacrimal sac Nasolacrimal duct **Y Lacrimal Duct, Left** *See X Lacrimal Duct, Right*	**7 Via Natural or Artificial Opening** **8 Via Natural or Artificial Opening Endoscopic**	**D Intraluminal Device** **Z No Device**	**Z No Qualifier**

Ø Medical and Surgical
8 Eye
W Revision Definition: Correcting, to the extent possible, a portion of a malfunctioning device or the position of a displaced device

Explanation: Revision can include correcting a malfunctioning or displaced device by taking out or putting in components of the device such as a screw or pin

Body Part Character 4	Approach Character 5	Device Character 6	Qualifier Character 7
Ø Eye, Right Ciliary body Posterior chamber **1 Eye, Left** *See Ø Eye, Right*	**Ø Open** **3 Percutaneous** **7 Via Natural or Artificial Opening** **8 Via Natural or Artificial Opening Endoscopic**	**Ø Drainage Device** **3 Infusion Device** **7 Autologous Tissue Substitute** **C Extraluminal Device** **D Intraluminal Device** **J Synthetic Substitute** **K Nonautologous Tissue Substitute** **Y Other Device**	**Z No Qualifier**
Ø Eye, Right Ciliary body Posterior chamber **1 Eye, Left** *See Ø Eye, Right*	**X External**	**Ø Drainage Device** **3 Infusion Device** **7 Autologous Tissue Substitute** **C Extraluminal Device** **D Intraluminal Device** **J Synthetic Substitute** **K Nonautologous Tissue Substitute**	**Z No Qualifier**
J Lens, Right Zonule of Zinn **K Lens, Left** *See J Lens, Right*	**3 Percutaneous**	**J Synthetic Substitute** **Y Other Device**	**Z No Qualifier**
J Lens, Right Zonule of Zinn **K Lens, Left** *See J Lens, Right*	**X External**	**J Synthetic Substitute**	**Z No Qualifier**
L Extraocular Muscle, Right Inferior oblique muscle Inferior rectus muscle Lateral rectus muscle Medial rectus muscle Superior oblique muscle Superior rectus muscle **M Extraocular Muscle, Left** *See L Extraocular Muscle, Right*	**Ø Open** **3 Percutaneous**	**Ø Drainage Device** **7 Autologous Tissue Substitute** **J Synthetic Substitute** **K Nonautologous Tissue Substitute** **Y Other Device**	**Z No Qualifier**

Non-OR Ø8W[Ø,1][3,7,8]YZ
Non-OR Ø8W[Ø,1]X[Ø,3,7,C,D,J,K]Z
Non-OR Ø8W[J,K]3YZ
Non-OR Ø8W[J,K]XJZ
Non-OR Ø8W[L,M]3YZ

Ø Medical and Surgical
8 Eye
X Transfer Definition: Moving, without taking out, all or a portion of a body part to another location to take over the function of all or a portion of a body part

Explanation: The body part transferred remains connected to its vascular and nervous supply

Body Part Character 4	Approach Character 5	Device Character 6	Qualifier Character 7
L Extraocular Muscle, Right Inferior oblique muscle Inferior rectus muscle Lateral rectus muscle Medial rectus muscle Superior oblique muscle Superior rectus muscle **M Extraocular Muscle, Left** *See L Extraocular Muscle, Right*	**Ø Open** **3 Percutaneous**	**Z No Device**	**Z No Qualifier**

Ear, Nose, Sinus 090–09W

Character Meanings*

This Character Meaning table is provided as a guide to assist the user in the identification of character members that may be found in this section of code tables. It **SHOULD NOT** be used to build a PCS code.

Operation–Character 3	Body Part–Character 4	Approach–Character 5	Device–Character 6	Qualifier–Character 7
0 Alteration	0 External Ear, Right	0 Open	0 Drainage Device	0 Endolymphatic
1 Bypass	1 External Ear, Left	3 Percutaneous	1 Radioactive Element	X Diagnostic
2 Change	2 External Ear, Bilateral	4 Percutaneous Endoscopic	4 Hearing Device, Bone Conduction	Z No Qualifier
3 Control	3 External Auditory Canal, Right	7 Via Natural or Artificial Opening	5 Hearing Device, Single Channel Cochlear Prosthesis	
5 Destruction	4 External Auditory Canal, Left	8 Via Natural or Artificial Opening Endoscopic	6 Hearing Device, Multiple Channel Cochlear Prosthesis	
7 Dilation	5 Middle Ear, Right	X External	7 Autologous Tissue Substitute	
8 Division	6 Middle Ear, Left		B Intraluminal Device, Airway	
9 Drainage	7 Tympanic Membrane, Right		D Intraluminal Device	
B Excision	8 Tympanic Membrane, Left		J Synthetic Substitute	
C Extirpation	9 Auditory Ossicle, Right		K Nonautologous Tissue Substitute	
D Extraction	A Auditory Ossicle, Left		S Hearing Device	
H Insertion	B Mastoid Sinus, Right		Y Other Device	
J Inspection	C Mastoid Sinus, Left		Z No Device	
M Reattachment	D Inner Ear, Right			
N Release	E Inner Ear, Left			
P Removal	F Eustachian Tube, Right			
Q Repair	G Eustachian Tube, Left			
R Replacement	H Ear, Right			
S Reposition	J Ear, Left			
T Resection	K Nasal Mucosa and Soft Tissue			
U Supplement	L Nasal Turbinate			
W Revision	M Nasal Septum			
	N Nasopharynx			
	P Accessory Sinus			
	Q Maxillary Sinus, Right			
	R Maxillary Sinus, Left			
	S Frontal Sinus, Right			
	T Frontal Sinus, Left			
	U Ethmoid Sinus, Right			
	V Ethmoid Sinus, Left			
	W Sphenoid Sinus, Right			
	X Sphenoid Sinus, Left			
	Y Sinus			

* Includes sinus ducts.

AHA Coding Clinic for table 093
2018, 4Q, 38 Control of epistaxis

AHA Coding Clinic for table 095
2018, 1Q, 19 Control of epistaxis via silver nitrate cauterization

AHA Coding Clinic for table 09H
2020, 4Q, 43-44 Insertion of radioactive element

AHA Coding Clinic for table 09Q
2018, 1Q, 19 Control of epistaxis via silver nitrate cauterization
2017, 4Q, 106 Control of bleeding of external naris using suture
2014, 4Q, 20 Control of epistaxis
2014, 3Q, 22 Transsphenoidal removal of pituitary tumor and fat graft placement
2013, 4Q, 114 Balloon sinuplasty

AHA Coding Clinic for table 09U
2019, 4Q, 28-29 Sinus supplement

Ear Anatomy

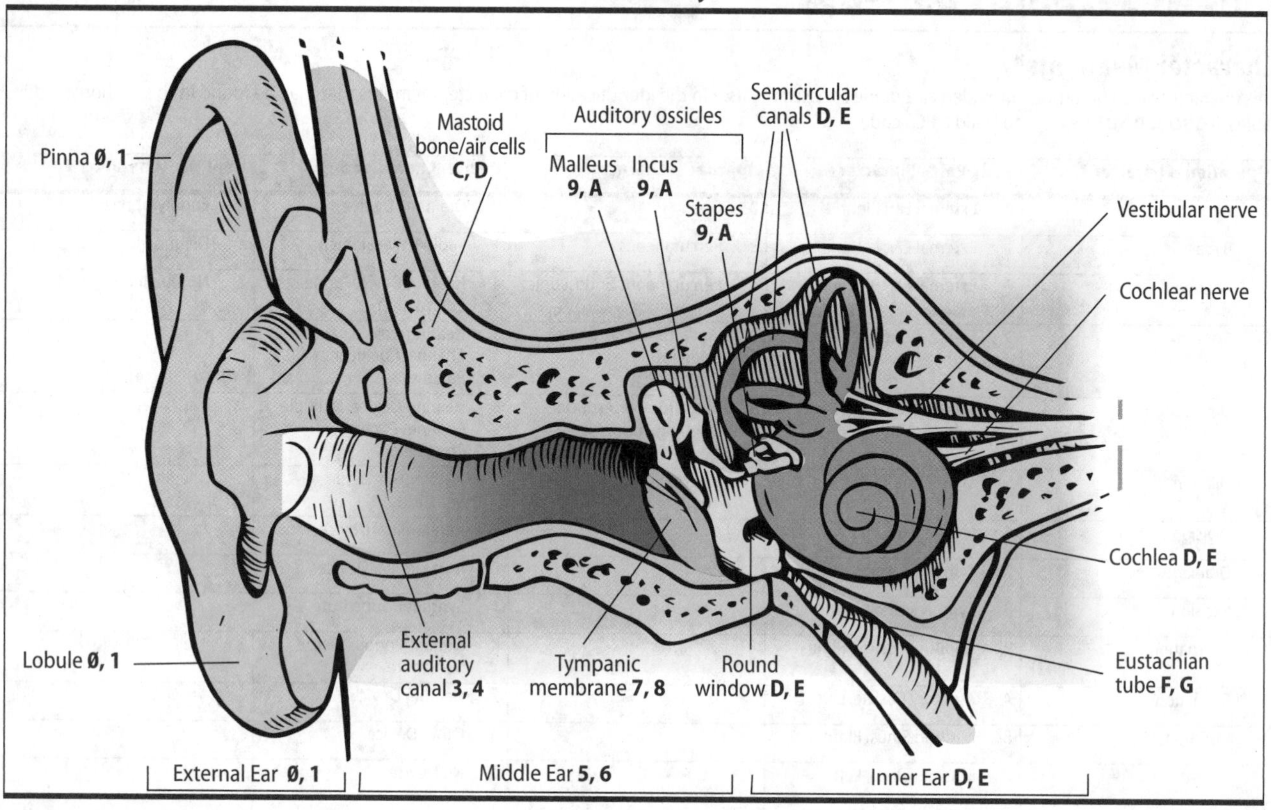

Nasal Turbinates

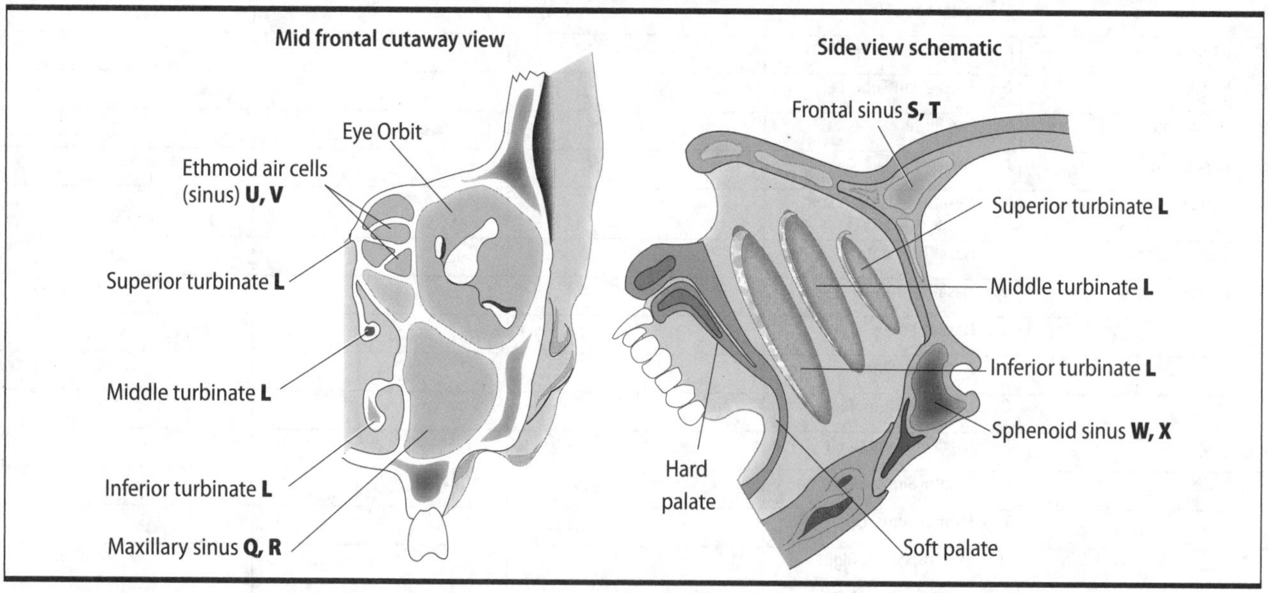

Paranasal Sinuses

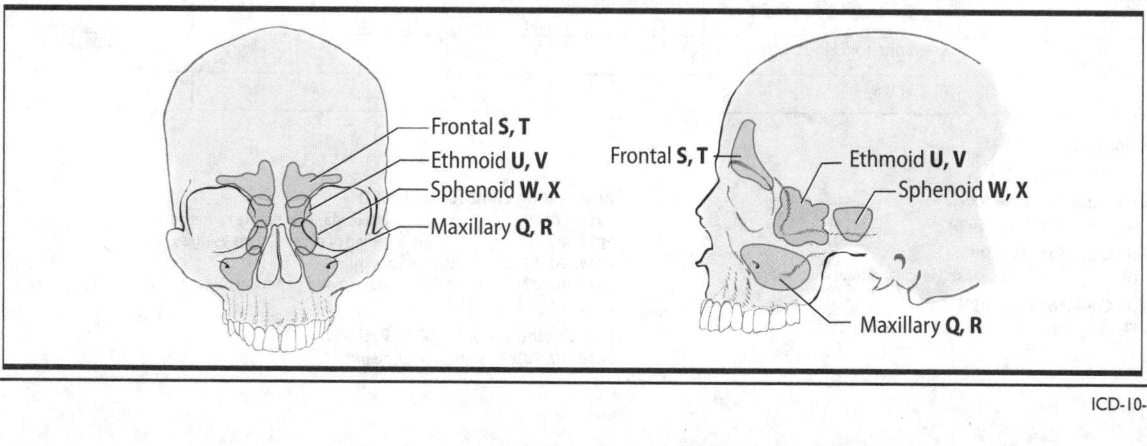

Ø Medical and Surgical
9 Ear, Nose, Sinus
Ø Alteration Definition: Modifying the anatomic structure of a body part without affecting the function of the body part
Explanation: Principal purpose is to improve appearance

Body Part Character 4		Approach Character 5	Device Character 6	Qualifier Character 7
Ø External Ear, Right Antihelix Antitragus Auricle Earlobe Helix Pinna Tragus **1 External Ear, Left** *See Ø External Ear, Right*	**2 External Ear, Bilateral** *See Ø External Ear, Right* **K Nasal Mucosa and Soft Tissue** Columella External naris Greater alar cartilage Internal naris Lateral nasal cartilage Lesser alar cartilage Nasal cavity Nostril	**Ø Open** **3 Percutaneous** **4 Percutaneous Endoscopic** **X External**	**7 Autologous Tissue Substitute** **J Synthetic Substitute** **K Nonautologous Tissue Substitute** **Z No Device**	**Z No Qualifier**

Ø Medical and Surgical
9 Ear, Nose, Sinus
1 Bypass Definition: Altering the route of passage of the contents of a tubular body part
Explanation: Rerouting contents of a body part to a downstream area of the normal route, to a similar route and body part, or to an abnormal route and dissimilar body part. Includes one or more anastomoses, with or without the use of a device.

Body Part Character 4	Approach Character 5	Device Character 6	Qualifier Character 7
D Inner Ear, Right Bony labyrinth Bony vestibule Cochlea Round window Semicircular canal **E Inner Ear, Left** *See D Inner Ear, Right*	**Ø Open**	**7 Autologous Tissue Substitute** **J Synthetic Substitute** **K Nonautologous Tissue Substitute** **Z No Device**	**Ø Endolymphatic**

Ø Medical and Surgical
9 Ear, Nose, Sinus
2 Change Definition: Taking out or off a device from a body part and putting back an identical or similar device in or on the same body part without cutting or puncturing the skin or a mucous membrane
Explanation: All CHANGE procedures are coded using the approach EXTERNAL

Body Part Character 4	Approach Character 5	Device Character 6	Qualifier Character 7
H Ear, Right **J Ear, Left** **K Nasal Mucosa and Soft Tissue** Columella External naris Greater alar cartilage Internal naris Lateral nasal cartilage Lesser alar cartilage Nasal cavity Nostril **Y Sinus**	**X External**	**Ø Drainage Device** **Y Other Device**	**Z No Qualifier**

Non-OR All body part, approach, device, and qualifier values

Ø Medical and Surgical
9 Ear, Nose, Sinus
3 Control Definition: Stopping, or attempting to stop, postprocedural or other acute bleeding
Explanation: None

Body Part Character 4	Approach Character 5	Device Character 6	Qualifier Character 7
K Nasal Mucosa and Soft Tissue Columella External naris Greater alar cartilage Internal naris Lateral nasal cartilage Lesser alar cartilage Nasal cavity Nostril	**7 Via Natural or Artificial Opening** **8 Via Natural or Artificial Opening Endoscopic**	**Z No Device**	**Z No Qualifier**

Non-OR Ø93K[7,8]ZZ

Ø Medical and Surgical
9 Ear, Nose, Sinus
5 Destruction Definition: Physical eradication of all or a portion of a body part by the direct use of energy, force, or a destructive agent
Explanation: None of the body part is physically taken out

Body Part Character 4		Approach Character 5	Device Character 6	Qualifier Character 7
Ø External Ear, Right Antihelix Antitragus Auricle Earlobe Helix Pinna Tragus	**1 External Ear, Left** *See Ø External Ear, Right*	**Ø Open** **3 Percutaneous** **4 Percutaneous Endoscopic** **X External**	**Z No Device**	**Z No Qualifier**
3 External Auditory Canal, Right External auditory meatus	**4 External Auditory Canal, Left** *See 3 External Auditory Canal, Right*	**Ø Open** **3 Percutaneous** **4 Percutaneous Endoscopic** **7 Via Natural or Artificial Opening** **8 Via Natural or Artificial Opening Endoscopic** **X External**	**Z No Device**	**Z No Qualifier**
5 Middle Ear, Right Oval window Tympanic cavity **6 Middle Ear, Left** *See 5 Middle Ear, Right* **9 Auditory Ossicle, Right** Incus Malleus Stapes **A Auditory Ossicle, Left** *See 9 Auditory Ossicle, Right*	**D Inner Ear, Right** Bony labyrinth Bony vestibule Cochlea Round window Semicircular canal **E Inner Ear, Left** *See D Inner Ear, Right*	**Ø Open** **8 Via Natural or Artificial Opening Endoscopic**	**Z No Device**	**Z No Qualifier**
7 Tympanic Membrane, Right Pars flaccida **8 Tympanic Membrane, Left** *See 7 Tympanic Membrane, Right* **F Eustachian Tube, Right** Auditory tube Pharyngotympanic tube **G Eustachian Tube, Left** *See F Eustachian Tube, Right*	**L Nasal Turbinate** Inferior turbinate Middle turbinate Nasal concha Superior turbinate **N Nasopharynx** Choana Fossa of Rosenmuller Pharyngeal recess Rhinopharynx	**Ø Open** **3 Percutaneous** **4 Percutaneous Endoscopic** **7 Via Natural or Artificial Opening** **8 Via Natural or Artificial Opening Endoscopic**	**Z No Device**	**Z No Qualifier**
B Mastoid Sinus, Right Mastoid air cells **C Mastoid Sinus, Left** *See B Mastoid Sinus, Right* **M Nasal Septum** Quadrangular cartilage Septal cartilage Vomer bone **P Accessory Sinus** **Q Maxillary Sinus, Right** Antrum of Highmore	**R Maxillary Sinus, Left** *See Q Maxillary Sinus, Right* **S Frontal Sinus, Right** **T Frontal Sinus, Left** **U Ethmoid Sinus, Right** Ethmoidal air cell **V Ethmoid Sinus, Left** *See U Ethmoid Sinus, Right* **W Sphenoid Sinus, Right** **X Sphenoid Sinus, Left**	**Ø Open** **3 Percutaneous** **4 Percutaneous Endoscopic** **8 Via Natural or Artificial Opening Endoscopic**	**Z No Device**	**Z No Qualifier**
K Nasal Mucosa and Soft Tissue Columella External naris Greater alar cartilage Internal naris Lateral nasal cartilage Lesser alar cartilage Nasal cavity Nostril		**Ø Open** **3 Percutaneous** **4 Percutaneous Endoscopic** **8 Via Natural or Artificial Opening Endoscopic** **X External**	**Z No Device**	**Z No Qualifier**

Non-OR Ø95[Ø,1][Ø,3,4,X]ZZ
Non-OR Ø95[3,4][Ø,3,4,7,8,X]ZZ
Non-OR Ø95[F,G][Ø,3,4,7,8]ZZ
Non-OR Ø95M[Ø,3,4,8]ZZ
Non-OR Ø95K[Ø,3,4,8,X]ZZ

Ø Medical and Surgical
9 Ear, Nose, Sinus
7 Dilation Definition: Expanding an orifice or the lumen of a tubular body part

Explanation: The orifice can be a natural orifice or an artificially created orifice. Accomplished by stretching a tubular body part using intraluminal pressure or by cutting part of the orifice or wall of the tubular body part.

Body Part Character 4	Approach Character 5	Device Character 6	Qualifier Character 7
F Eustachian Tube, Right Auditory tube Pharyngotympanic tube **G Eustachian Tube, Left** *See F Eustachian Tube, Right*	**Ø Open** **7 Via Natural or Artificial Opening** **8 Via Natural or Artificial Opening Endoscopic**	**D Intraluminal Device** **Z No Device**	**Z No Qualifier**
F Eustachian Tube, Right Auditory tube Pharyngotympanic tube **G Eustachian Tube, Left** *See F Eustachian Tube, Right*	**3 Percutaneous** **4 Percutaneous Endoscopic**	**Z No Device**	**Z No Qualifier**

Non-OR All body part, approach, device, and qualifier values

Ø Medical and Surgical
9 Ear, Nose, Sinus
8 Division Definition: Cutting into a body part, without draining fluids and/or gases from the body part, in order to separate or transect a body part

Explanation: All or a portion of the body part is separated into two or more portions

Body Part Character 4	Approach Character 5	Device Character 6	Qualifier Character 7
L Nasal Turbinate Inferior turbinate Middle turbinate Nasal concha Superior turbinate	**Ø Open** **3 Percutaneous** **4 Percutaneous Endoscopic** **7 Via Natural or Artificial Opening** **8 Via Natural or Artificial Opening Endoscopic**	**Z No Device**	**Z No Qualifier**

Ø Medical and Surgical
9 Ear, Nose, Sinus
9 Drainage Definition: Taking or letting out fluids and/or gases from a body part
Explanation: The qualifier DIAGNOSTIC is used to identify drainage procedures that are biopsies

Body Part Character 4		Approach Character 5	Device Character 6	Qualifier Character 7
Ø External Ear, Right Antihelix Antitragus Auricle Earlobe Helix Pinna Tragus	**1 External Ear, Left** *See Ø External Ear, Right*	**Ø Open** **3 Percutaneous** **4 Percutaneous Endoscopic** **X External**	**Ø Drainage Device**	**Z No Qualifier**
Ø External Ear, Right Antihelix Antitragus Auricle Earlobe Helix Pinna Tragus	**1 External Ear, Left** *See Ø External Ear, Right*	**Ø Open** **3 Percutaneous** **4 Percutaneous Endoscopic** **X External**	**Z No Device**	**X Diagnostic** **Z No Qualifier**
3 External Auditory Canal, Right External auditory meatus **4 External Auditory Canal, Left** *See 3 External Auditory Canal, Right*	**K Nasal Mucosa and Soft Tissue** Columella External naris Greater alar cartilage Internal naris Lateral nasal cartilage Lesser alar cartilage Nasal cavity Nostril	**Ø Open** **3 Percutaneous** **4 Percutaneous Endoscopic** **7 Via Natural or Artificial Opening** **8 Via Natural or Artificial Opening Endoscopic** **X External**	**Ø Drainage Device**	**Z No Qualifier**
3 External Auditory Canal, Right External auditory meatus **4 External Auditory Canal, Left** *See 3 External Auditory Canal, Right*	**K Nasal Mucosa and Soft Tissue** Columella External naris Greater alar cartilage Internal naris Lateral nasal cartilage Lesser alar cartilage Nasal cavity Nostril	**Ø Open** **3 Percutaneous** **4 Percutaneous Endoscopic** **7 Via Natural or Artificial Opening** **8 Via Natural or Artificial Opening Endoscopic** **X External**	**Z No Device**	**X Diagnostic** **Z No Qualifier**
5 Middle Ear, Right Oval window Tympanic cavity **6 Middle Ear, Left** *See 5 Middle Ear, Right* **9 Auditory Ossicle, Right** Incus Malleus Stapes	**A Auditory Ossicle, Left** *See 9 Auditory Ossicle, Right* **D Inner Ear, Right** Bony labyrinth Bony vestibule Cochlea Round window Semicircular canal **E Inner Ear, Left** *See D Inner Ear, Right*	**Ø Open** **7 Via Natural or Artificial Opening** **8 Via Natural or Artificial Opening Endoscopic**	**Ø Drainage Device**	**Z No Qualifier**
5 Middle Ear, Right Oval window Tympanic cavity **6 Middle Ear, Left** *See 5 Middle Ear, Right* **9 Auditory Ossicle, Right** Incus Malleus Stapes	**A Auditory Ossicle, Left** *See 9 Auditory Ossicle, Right* **D Inner Ear, Right** Bony labyrinth Bony vestibule Cochlea Round window Semicircular canal **E Inner Ear, Left** *See D Inner Ear, Right*	**Ø Open** **7 Via Natural or Artificial Opening** **8 Via Natural or Artificial Opening Endoscopic**	**Z No Device**	**X Diagnostic** **Z No Qualifier**

Non-OR Ø99[Ø,1][Ø,3,4,X]ØZ
Non-OR Ø99[Ø,1][Ø,3,4,X]Z[X,Z]
Non-OR Ø99[3,4,K][Ø,3,4,7,8,X]ØZ
Non-OR Ø99[3,4,K][Ø,3,4,7,8,X]Z[X,Z]
Non-OR Ø99[5,6]8ØZ
Non-OR Ø99[9,A,D,E][7,8]ØZ
Non-OR Ø99[5,6]ØZZ
Non-OR Ø99[5,6,9,A,D,E][7,8]Z[X,Z]

Ø99 Continued on next page

Ø99 Continued

Ø Medical and Surgical
9 Ear, Nose, Sinus
9 Drainage Definition: Taking or letting out fluids and/or gases from a body part
Explanation: The qualifier DIAGNOSTIC is used to identify drainage procedures that are biopsies

Body Part Character 4		Approach Character 5	Device Character 6	Qualifier Character 7
7 Tympanic Membrane, Right Pars flaccida **8 Tympanic Membrane, Left** *See 7 Tympanic Membrane, Right* **B Mastoid Sinus, Right** Mastoid air cells **C Mastoid Sinus, Left** *See B Mastoid Sinus, Right* **F Eustachian Tube, Right** Auditory tube Pharyngotympanic tube **G Eustachian Tube, Left** *See F Eustachian Tube, Right* **L Nasal Turbinate** Inferior turbinate Middle turbinate Nasal concha Superior turbinate **M Nasal Septum** Quadrangular cartilage Septal cartilage Vomer bone	**N Nasopharynx** Choana Fossa of Rosenmuller Pharyngeal recess Rhinopharynx **P Accessory Sinus** **Q Maxillary Sinus, Right** Antrum of Highmore **R Maxillary Sinus, Left** *See Q Maxillary Sinus, Right* **S Frontal Sinus, Right** **T Frontal Sinus, Left** **U Ethmoid Sinus, Right** Ethmoidal air cell **V Ethmoid Sinus, Left** *See U Ethmoid Sinus, Right* **W Sphenoid Sinus, Right** **X Sphenoid Sinus, Left**	**Ø Open** **3 Percutaneous** **4 Percutaneous Endoscopic** **7 Via Natural or Artificial Opening** **8 Via Natural or Artificial Opening Endoscopic**	**Ø Drainage Device**	**Z No Qualifier**
7 Tympanic Membrane, Right Pars flaccida **8 Tympanic Membrane, Left** *See 7 Tympanic Membrane, Right* **B Mastoid Sinus, Right** Mastoid air cells **C Mastoid Sinus, Left** *See B Mastoid Sinus, Right* **F Eustachian Tube, Right** Auditory tube Pharyngotympanic tube **G Eustachian Tube, Left** *See F Eustachian Tube, Right* **L Nasal Turbinate** Inferior turbinate Middle turbinate Nasal concha Superior turbinate **M Nasal Septum** Quadrangular cartilage Septal cartilage Vomer bone	**N Nasopharynx** Choana Fossa of Rosenmuller Pharyngeal recess Rhinopharynx **P Accessory Sinus** **Q Maxillary Sinus, Right** Antrum of Highmore **R Maxillary Sinus, Left** *See Q Maxillary Sinus, Right* **S Frontal Sinus, Right** **T Frontal Sinus, Left** **U Ethmoid Sinus, Right** Ethmoidal air cell **V Ethmoid Sinus, Left** *See U Ethmoid Sinus, Right* **W Sphenoid Sinus, Right** **X Sphenoid Sinus, Left**	**Ø Open** **3 Percutaneous** **4 Percutaneous Endoscopic** **7 Via Natural or Artificial Opening** **8 Via Natural or Artificial Opening Endoscopic**	**Z No Device**	**X Diagnostic** **Z No Qualifier**

Non-OR Ø99[B,C][3,7,8]ØZ
Non-OR Ø99[F,G,L,M][Ø,3,4,7,8]ØZ
Non-OR Ø99N3ØZ
Non-OR Ø99[P,Q,R,S,T,U,V,W,X][3,4,7,8]ØZ
Non-OR Ø99[7,8][Ø,3,4,7,8]ZZ
Non-OR Ø99[7,8][7,8]ZX
Non-OR Ø99[B,C]3ZZ
Non-OR Ø99[B,C][7,8]Z[X,Z]
Non-OR Ø99[F,G][Ø,3,4,7,8]ZZ
Non-OR Ø99[F,G][7,8]ZX
Non-OR Ø99[L,M][Ø,3,4,7,8]Z[X,Z]
Non-OR Ø99N[Ø,3,4,7,8]ZX
Non-OR Ø99N3ZZ
Non-OR Ø99[P,Q,R,S,T,U,V,W,X][3,4,7,8]Z[X,Z]

Ø Medical and Surgical
9 Ear, Nose, Sinus
B Excision Definition: Cutting out or off, without replacement, a portion of a body part
Explanation: The qualifier DIAGNOSTIC is used to identify excision procedures that are biopsies

Body Part Character 4		Approach Character 5	Device Character 6	Qualifier Character 7
Ø External Ear, Right Antihelix Antitragus Auricle Earlobe Helix Pinna Tragus	**1 External Ear, Left** *See Ø External Ear, Right*	**Ø Open** **3 Percutaneous** **4 Percutaneous Endoscopic** **X External**	**Z No Device**	**X Diagnostic** **Z No Qualifier**
3 External Auditory Canal, Right External auditory meatus	**4 External Auditory Canal, Left** *See 3 External Auditory Canal, Right*	**Ø Open** **3 Percutaneous** **4 Percutaneous Endoscopic** **7 Via Natural or Artificial Opening** **8 Via Natural or Artificial Opening Endoscopic** **X External**	**Z No Device**	**X Diagnostic** **Z No Qualifier**
5 Middle Ear, Right Oval window Tympanic cavity **6 Middle Ear, Left** *See 5 Middle Ear, Right* **9 Auditory Ossicle, Right** Incus Malleus Stapes	**A Auditory Ossicle, Left** *See 9 Auditory Ossicle, Right* **D Inner Ear, Right** Bony labyrinth Bony vestibule Cochlea Round window Semicircular canal **E Inner Ear, Left** *See D Inner Ear, Right*	**Ø Open** **8 Via Natural or Artificial Opening Endoscopic**	**Z No Device**	**X Diagnostic** **Z No Qualifier**
7 Tympanic Membrane, Right Pars flaccida **8 Tympanic Membrane, Left** *See 7 Tympanic Membrane, Right* **F Eustachian Tube, Right** Auditory tube Pharyngotympanic tube **G Eustachian Tube, Left** *See F Eustachian Tube, Right*	**L Nasal Turbinate** Inferior turbinate Middle turbinate Nasal concha Superior turbinate **N Nasopharynx** Choana Fossa of Rosenmuller Pharyngeal recess Rhinopharynx	**Ø Open** **3 Percutaneous** **4 Percutaneous Endoscopic** **7 Via Natural or Artificial Opening** **8 Via Natural or Artificial Opening Endoscopic**	**Z No Device**	**X Diagnostic** **Z No Qualifier**
B Mastoid Sinus, Right Mastoid air cells **C Mastoid Sinus, Left** *See B Mastoid Sinus, Right* **M Nasal Septum** Quadrangular cartilage Septal cartilage Vomer bone **P Accessory Sinus** **Q Maxillary Sinus, Right** Antrum of Highmore	**R Maxillary Sinus, Left** *See Q Maxillary Sinus, Right* **S Frontal Sinus, Right** **T Frontal Sinus, Left** **U Ethmoid Sinus, Right** Ethmoidal air cell **V Ethmoid Sinus, Left** *See U Ethmoid Sinus, Right* **W Sphenoid Sinus, Right** **X Sphenoid Sinus, Left**	**Ø Open** **3 Percutaneous** **4 Percutaneous Endoscopic** **8 Via Natural or Artificial Opening Endoscopic**	**Z No Device**	**X Diagnostic** **Z No Qualifier**
K Nasal Mucosa and Soft Tissue Columella External naris Greater alar cartilage Internal naris Lateral nasal cartilage Lesser alar cartilage Nasal cavity Nostril		**Ø Open** **3 Percutaneous** **4 Percutaneous Endoscopic** **8 Via Natural or Artificial Opening Endoscopic** **X External**	**Z No Device**	**X Diagnostic** **Z No Qualifier**

Non-OR Ø9B[Ø,1][Ø,3,4,X]Z[X,Z]
Non-OR Ø9B[3,4][Ø,3,4,7,8,X]Z[X,Z]
Non-OR Ø9B[F,G,L,N][Ø,3,4,7,8]Z[X,Z]
Non-OR Ø9BM[Ø,3,4,8]ZX
Non-OR Ø9B[P,Q,R,S,T,U,V,W,X][3,4,8]ZX
Non-OR Ø9BK8Z[X,Z]

Ø Medical and Surgical
9 Ear, Nose, Sinus
C Extirpation Definition: Taking or cutting out solid matter from a body part

Explanation: The solid matter may be an abnormal byproduct of a biological function or a foreign body; it may be imbedded in a body part or in the lumen of a tubular body part. The solid matter may or may not have been previously broken into pieces.

Body Part Character 4		Approach Character 5	Device Character 6	Qualifier Character 7
Ø External Ear, Right Antihelix Antitragus Auricle Earlobe Helix Pinna Tragus	**1 External Ear, Left** *See Ø External Ear, Right*	**Ø Open** **3 Percutaneous** **4 Percutaneous Endoscopic** **X External**	**Z No Device**	**Z No Qualifier**
3 External Auditory Canal, Right External auditory meatus	**4 External Auditory Canal, Left** *See 3 External Auditory Canal, Right*	**Ø Open** **3 Percutaneous** **4 Percutaneous Endoscopic** **7 Via Natural or Artificial Opening** **8 Via Natural or Artificial Opening Endoscopic** **X External**	**Z No Device**	**Z No Qualifier**
5 Middle Ear, Right Oval window Tympanic cavity **6 Middle Ear, Left** *See 5 Middle Ear, Right* **9 Auditory Ossicle, Right** Incus Malleus Stapes	**A Auditory Ossicle, Left** *See 9 Auditory Ossicle, Right* **D Inner Ear, Right** Bony labyrinth Bony vestibule Cochlea Round window Semicircular canal **E Inner Ear, Left** *See D Inner Ear, Right*	**Ø Open** **8 Via Natural or Artificial Opening Endoscopic**	**Z No Device**	**Z No Qualifier**
7 Tympanic Membrane, Right Pars flaccida **8 Tympanic Membrane, Left** *See 7 Tympanic Membrane, Right* **F Eustachian Tube, Right** Auditory tube Pharyngotympanic tube **G Eustachian Tube, Left** *See F Eustachian Tube, Right*	**L Nasal Turbinate** Inferior turbinate Middle turbinate Nasal concha Superior turbinate **N Nasopharynx** Choana Fossa of Rosenmuller Pharyngeal recess Rhinopharynx	**Ø Open** **3 Percutaneous** **4 Percutaneous Endoscopic** **7 Via Natural or Artificial Opening** **8 Via Natural or Artificial Opening Endoscopic**	**Z No Device**	**Z No Qualifier**
B Mastoid Sinus, Right Mastoid air cells **C Mastoid Sinus, Left** *See B Mastoid Sinus, Right* **M Nasal Septum** Quadrangular cartilage Septal cartilage Vomer bone **P Accessory Sinus** **Q Maxillary Sinus, Right** Antrum of Highmore	**R Maxillary Sinus, Left** *See Q Maxillary Sinus, Right* **S Frontal Sinus, Right** **T Frontal Sinus, Left** **U Ethmoid Sinus, Right** Ethmoidal air cell **V Ethmoid Sinus, Left** *See U Ethmoid Sinus, Right* **W Sphenoid Sinus, Right** **X Sphenoid Sinus, Left**	**Ø Open** **3 Percutaneous** **4 Percutaneous Endoscopic** **8 Via Natural or Artificial Opening Endoscopic**	**Z No Device**	**Z No Qualifier**
K Nasal Mucosa and Soft Tissue Columella External naris Greater alar cartilage Internal naris Lateral nasal cartilage Lesser alar cartilage Nasal cavity Nostril		**Ø Open** **3 Percutaneous** **4 Percutaneous Endoscopic** **8 Via Natural or Artificial Opening Endoscopic** **X External**	**Z No Device**	**Z No Qualifier**

Non-OR Ø9C[Ø,1][Ø,3,4,X]ZZ
Non-OR Ø9C[3,4][Ø,3,4,7,8,X]ZZ
Non-OR Ø9C[7,8,F,G,L][Ø,3,4,7,8]ZZ
Non-OR Ø9CM[Ø,3,4,8]ZZ
Non-OR Ø9CK8ZZ

Ø Medical and Surgical
9 Ear, Nose, Sinus
D Extraction Definition: Pulling or stripping out or off all or a portion of a body part by the use of force
Explanation: The qualifier DIAGNOSTIC is used to identify extraction procedures that are biopsies

Body Part Character 4	Approach Character 5	Device Character 6	Qualifier Character 7
7 Tympanic Membrane, Right Pars flaccida **8 Tympanic Membrane, Left** *See 7 Tympanic Membrane, Right* **L Nasal Turbinate** Inferior turbinate Middle turbinate Nasal concha Superior turbinate	**Ø Open** **3 Percutaneous** **4 Percutaneous Endoscopic** **7 Via Natural or Artificial Opening** **8 Via Natural or Artificial Opening Endoscopic**	**Z No Device**	**Z No Qualifier**
9 Auditory Ossicle, Right Incus Malleus Stapes **A Auditory Ossicle, Left** *See 9 Auditory Ossicle, Right*	**Ø Open**	**Z No Device**	**Z No Qualifier**
B Mastoid Sinus, Right Mastoid air cells **C Mastoid Sinus, Left** *See B Mastoid Sinus, Right* **M Nasal Septum** Quadrangular cartilage Septal cartilage Vomer bone **P Accessory Sinus** **Q Maxillary Sinus, Right** Antrum of Highmore **R Maxillary Sinus, Left** *See Q Maxillary Sinus, Right* **S Frontal Sinus, Right** **T Frontal Sinus, Left** **U Ethmoid Sinus, Right** Ethmoidal air cell **V Ethmoid Sinus, Left** *See U Ethmoid Sinus, Right* **W Sphenoid Sinus, Right** **X Sphenoid Sinus, Left**	**Ø Open** **3 Percutaneous** **4 Percutaneous Endoscopic**	**Z No Device**	**Z No Qualifier**

Ø Medical and Surgical
9 Ear, Nose, Sinus
H Insertion Definition: Putting in a nonbiological appliance that monitors, assists, performs, or prevents a physiological function but does not physically take the place of a body part
Explanation: None

Body Part Character 4	Approach Character 5	Device Character 6	Qualifier Character 7
D Inner Ear, Right Bony labyrinth Bony vestibule Cochlea Round window Semicircular canal **E Inner Ear, Left** *See D Inner Ear, Right*	**Ø Open** **3 Percutaneous** **4 Percutaneous Endoscopic**	**1 Radioactive Element** **4 Hearing Device, Bone Conduction** **5 Hearing Device, Single Channel Cochlear Prosthesis** **6 Hearing Device, Multiple Channel Cochlear Prosthesis** **S Hearing Device**	**Z No Qualifier**
H Ear, Right **J Ear, Left** **K Nasal Mucosa and Soft Tissue** Columella External naris Greater alar cartilage Internal naris Lateral nasal cartilage Lesser alar cartilage Nasal cavity Nostril **Y Sinus**	**Ø Open** **3 Percutaneous** **4 Percutaneous Endoscopic** **7 Via Natural or Artificial Opening** **8 Via Natural or Artificial Opening Endoscopic**	**1 Radioactive Element** **Y Other Device**	**Z No Qualifier**
N Nasopharynx Choana Fossa of Rosenmuller Pharyngeal recess Rhinopharynx	**7 Via Natural or Artificial Opening** **8 Via Natural or Artificial Opening Endoscopic**	**1 Radioactive Element** **B Intraluminal Device, Airway**	**Z No Qualifier**

Non-OR Ø9H[H,J,K]Ø1Z
Non-OR Ø9HKØYZ
Non-OR Ø9H[H,J,K,Y][3,4,7,8][1,Y]Z
Non-OR Ø9HN[7,8][1,B]Z

Ø Medical and Surgical
9 Ear, Nose, Sinus
J Inspection Definition: Visually and/or manually exploring a body part

Explanation: Visual exploration may be performed with or without optical instrumentation. Manual exploration may be performed directly or through intervening body layers.

Body Part Character 4	Approach Character 5	Device Character 6	Qualifier Character 7
7 Tympanic Membrane, Right Pars flaccida **8 Tympanic Membrane, Left** *See 7 Tympanic Membrane, Right* **H Ear, Right** **J Ear, Left**	**Ø Open** **3 Percutaneous** **4 Percutaneous Endoscopic** **7 Via Natural or Artificial Opening** **8 Via Natural or Artificial Opening Endoscopic** **X External**	**Z No Device**	**Z No Qualifier**
D Inner Ear, Right Bony labyrinth Bony vestibule Cochlea Round window Semicircular canal **E Inner Ear, Left** *See D Inner Ear, Right* **K Nasal Mucosa and Soft Tissue** Columella External naris Greater alar cartilage Internal naris Lateral nasal cartilage Lesser alar cartilage Nasal cavity Nostril **Y Sinus**	**Ø Open** **3 Percutaneous** **4 Percutaneous Endoscopic** **8 Via Natural or Artificial Opening Endoscopic** **X External**	**Z No Device**	**Z No Qualifier**

Non-OR Ø9J[7,8][3,7,8,X]ZZ
Non-OR Ø9J[H,J][Ø,3,4,7,8,X]ZZ
Non-OR Ø9J[D,E][3,8,X]ZZ
Non-OR Ø9J[K,Y][Ø,3,4,8,X]ZZ

Ø Medical and Surgical
9 Ear, Nose, Sinus
M Reattachment Definition: Putting back in or on all or a portion of a separated body part to its normal location or other suitable location

Explanation: Vascular circulation and nervous pathways may or may not be reestablished

Body Part Character 4	Approach Character 5	Device Character 6	Qualifier Character 7
Ø External Ear, Right Antihelix Antitragus Auricle Earlobe Helix Pinna Tragus **1 External Ear, Left** *See Ø External Ear, Right* **K Nasal Mucosa and Soft Tissue** Columella External naris Greater alar cartilage Internal naris Lateral nasal cartilage Lesser alar cartilage Nasal cavity Nostril	**X External**	**Z No Device**	**Z No Qualifier**

Ø Medical and Surgical
9 Ear, Nose, Sinus
N Release Definition: Freeing a body part from an abnormal physical constraint by cutting or by the use of force
Explanation: Some of the restraining tissue may be taken out but none of the body part is taken out

Body Part Character 4		Approach Character 5	Device Character 6	Qualifier Character 7
Ø External Ear, Right Antihelix Antitragus Auricle Earlobe Helix Pinna Tragus	**1 External Ear, Left** *See Ø External Ear, Right*	**Ø Open** **3 Percutaneous** **4 Percutaneous Endoscopic** **X External**	**Z No Device**	**Z No Qualifier**
3 External Auditory Canal, Right External auditory meatus	**4 External Auditory Canal, Left** *See 3 External Auditory Canal, Right*	**Ø Open** **3 Percutaneous** **4 Percutaneous Endoscopic** **7 Via Natural or Artificial Opening** **8 Via Natural or Artificial Opening Endoscopic** **X External**	**Z No Device**	**Z No Qualifier**
5 Middle Ear, Right Oval window Tympanic cavity **6 Middle Ear, Left** *See 5 Middle Ear, Right* **9 Auditory Ossicle, Right** Incus Malleus Stapes	**A Auditory Ossicle, Left** *See 9 Auditory Ossicle, Right* **D Inner Ear, Right** Bony labyrinth Bony vestibule Cochlea Round window Semicircular canal **E Inner Ear, Left** *See D Inner Ear, Right*	**Ø Open** **8 Via Natural or Artificial Opening Endoscopic**	**Z No Device**	**Z No Qualifier**
7 Tympanic Membrane, Right Pars flaccida **8 Tympanic Membrane, Left** *See 7 Tympanic Membrane, Right* **F Eustachian Tube, Right** Auditory tube Pharyngotympanic tube **G Eustachian Tube, Left** *See F Eustachian Tube, Right*	**L Nasal Turbinate** Inferior turbinate Middle turbinate Nasal concha Superior turbinate **N Nasopharynx** Choana Fossa of Rosenmuller Pharyngeal recess Rhinopharynx	**Ø Open** **3 Percutaneous** **4 Percutaneous Endoscopic** **7 Via Natural or Artificial Opening** **8 Via Natural or Artificial Opening Endoscopic**	**Z No Device**	**Z No Qualifier**
B Mastoid Sinus, Right Mastoid air cells **C Mastoid Sinus, Left** *See B Mastoid Sinus, Right* **M Nasal Septum** Quadrangular cartilage Septal cartilage Vomer bone **P Accessory Sinus** **Q Maxillary Sinus, Right** Antrum of Highmore	**R Maxillary Sinus, Left** *See Q Maxillary Sinus, Right* **S Frontal Sinus, Right** **T Frontal Sinus, Left** **U Ethmoid Sinus, Right** Ethmoidal air cell **V Ethmoid Sinus, Left** *See U Ethmoid Sinus, Right* **W Sphenoid Sinus, Right** **X Sphenoid Sinus, Left**	**Ø Open** **3 Percutaneous** **4 Percutaneous Endoscopic** **8 Via Natural or Artificial Opening Endoscopic**	**Z No Device**	**Z No Qualifier**
K Nasal Mucosa and Soft Tissue Columella External naris Greater alar cartilage Internal naris Lateral nasal cartilage Lesser alar cartilage Nasal cavity Nostril		**Ø Open** **3 Percutaneous** **4 Percutaneous Endoscopic** **8 Via Natural or Artificial Opening Endoscopic** **X External**	**Z No Device**	**Z No Qualifier**

Non-OR Ø9N[Ø,1]XZZ
Non-OR Ø9N[3,4]XZZ
Non-OR Ø9N[F,G,L][Ø,3,4,7,8]ZZ
Non-OR Ø9NM[Ø,3,4,8]ZZ
Non-OR Ø9NK[Ø,3,4,8,X]ZZ

Ø Medical and Surgical
9 Ear, Nose, Sinus
P Removal Definition: Taking out or off a device from a body part

Explanation: If a device is taken out and a similar device put in without cutting or puncturing the skin or mucous membrane, the procedure is coded to the root operation CHANGE. Otherwise, the procedure for taking out a device is coded to the root operation REMOVAL.

Body Part Character 4	Approach Character 5	Device Character 6	Qualifier Character 7
7 Tympanic Membrane, Right Pars flaccida **8 Tympanic Membrane, Left** *See 7 Tympanic Membrane, Right*	**Ø Open** **7 Via Natural or Artificial Opening** **8 Via Natural or Artificial Opening Endoscopic** **X External**	**Ø Drainage Device**	**Z No Qualifier**
D Inner Ear, Right Bony labyrinth Bony vestibule Cochlea Round window Semicircular canal **E Inner Ear, Left** *See D Inner Ear, Right*	**Ø Open** **7 Via Natural or Artificial Opening** **8 Via Natural or Artificial Opening Endoscopic**	**S Hearing Device**	**Z No Qualifier**
H Ear, Right **J Ear, Left** **K Nasal Mucosa and Soft Tissue** Columella External naris Greater alar cartilage Internal naris Lateral nasal cartilage Lesser alar cartilage Nasal cavity Nostril	**Ø Open** **3 Percutaneous** **4 Percutaneous Endoscopic** **7 Via Natural or Artificial Opening** **8 Via Natural or Artificial Opening Endoscopic**	**Ø Drainage Device** **7 Autologous Tissue Substitute** **D Intraluminal Device** **J Synthetic Substitute** **K Nonautologous Tissue Substitute** **Y Other Device**	**Z No Qualifier**
H Ear, Right **J Ear, Left** **K Nasal Mucosa and Soft Tissue** Columella External naris Greater alar cartilage Internal naris Lateral nasal cartilage Lesser alar cartilage Nasal cavity Nostril	**X External**	**Ø Drainage Device** **7 Autologous Tissue Substitute** **D Intraluminal Device** **J Synthetic Substitute** **K Nonautologous Tissue Substitute**	**Z No Qualifier**
Y Sinus	**Ø Open** **3 Percutaneous** **4 Percutaneous Endoscopic**	**Ø Drainage Device** **Y Other Device**	**Z No Qualifier**
Y Sinus	**7 Via Natural or Artificial Opening** **8 Via Natural or Artificial Opening Endoscopic**	**Y Other Device**	**Z No Qualifier**
Y Sinus	**X External**	**Ø Drainage Device**	**Z No Qualifier**

Non-OR Ø9P[7,8][Ø,7,8,X]ØZ
Non-OR Ø9P[H,J][3,4][Ø,J,K,Y]Z
Non-OR Ø9P[H,J][7,8][Ø,D,Y]Z
Non-OR Ø9PK[Ø,3,4,7,8][Ø,7,D,J,K,Y]Z
Non-OR Ø9P[H,J]X[Ø,7,D,J,K]Z
Non-OR Ø9PKX[Ø,7,D,J,K]Z
Non-OR Ø9PY[3,4]YZ
Non-OR Ø9PY[7,8]YZ
Non-OR Ø9PYXØZ

Ø Medical and Surgical
9 Ear, Nose, Sinus
Q Repair Definition: Restoring, to the extent possible, a body part to its normal anatomic structure and function
Explanation: Used only when the method to accomplish the repair is not one of the other root operations

Body Part Character 4	Approach Character 5	Device Character 6	Qualifier Character 7
Ø External Ear, Right Antihelix Antitragus Auricle Earlobe Helix Pinna Tragus **1 External Ear, Left** *See Ø External Ear, Right* **2 External Ear, Bilateral** *See Ø External Ear, Right*	**Ø Open** **3 Percutaneous** **4 Percutaneous Endoscopic** **X External**	**Z No Device**	**Z No Qualifier**
3 External Auditory Canal, Right External auditory meatus **4 External Auditory Canal, Left** *See 3 External Auditory Canal, Right* **F Eustachian Tube, Right** Auditory tube Pharyngotympanic tube **G Eustachian Tube, Left** *See F Eustachian Tube, Right*	**Ø Open** **3 Percutaneous** **4 Percutaneous Endoscopic** **7 Via Natural or Artificial Opening** **8 Via Natural or Artificial Opening Endoscopic** **X External**	**Z No Device**	**Z No Qualifier**
5 Middle Ear, Right Oval window Tympanic cavity **6 Middle Ear, Left** *See 5 Middle Ear, Right* **9 Auditory Ossicle, Right** Incus Malleus Stapes **A Auditory Ossicle, Left** *See 9 Auditory Ossicle, Right* **D Inner Ear, Right** Bony labyrinth Bony vestibule Cochlea Round window Semicircular canal **E Inner Ear, Left** *See D Inner Ear, Right*	**Ø Open** **8 Via Natural or Artificial Opening Endoscopic**	**Z No Device**	**Z No Qualifier**
7 Tympanic Membrane, Right Pars flaccida **8 Tympanic Membrane, Left** *See 7 Tympanic Membrane, Right* **L Nasal Turbinate** Inferior turbinate Middle turbinate Nasal concha Superior turbinate **N Nasopharynx** Choana Fossa of Rosenmuller Pharyngeal recess Rhinopharynx	**Ø Open** **3 Percutaneous** **4 Percutaneous Endoscopic** **7 Via Natural or Artificial Opening** **8 Via Natural or Artificial Opening Endoscopic**	**Z No Device**	**Z No Qualifier**
B Mastoid Sinus, Right Mastoid air cells **C Mastoid Sinus, Left** *See B Mastoid Sinus, Right* **M Nasal Septum** Quadrangular cartilage Septal cartilage Vomer bone **P Accessory Sinus** **Q Maxillary Sinus, Right** Antrum of Highmore **R Maxillary Sinus, Left** *See Q Maxillary Sinus, Right* **S Frontal Sinus, Right** **T Frontal Sinus, Left** **U Ethmoid Sinus, Right** Ethmoidal air cell **V Ethmoid Sinus, Left** *See U Ethmoid Sinus, Right* **W Sphenoid Sinus, Right** **X Sphenoid Sinus, Left**	**Ø Open** **3 Percutaneous** **4 Percutaneous Endoscopic** **8 Via Natural or Artificial Opening Endoscopic**	**Z No Device**	**Z No Qualifier**
K Nasal Mucosa and Soft Tissue Columella External naris Greater alar cartilage Internal naris Lateral nasal cartilage Lesser alar cartilage Nasal cavity Nostril	**Ø Open** **3 Percutaneous** **4 Percutaneous Endoscopic** **8 Via Natural or Artificial Opening Endoscopic** **X External**	**Z No Device**	**Z No Qualifier**

Non-OR Ø9Q[Ø,1,2]XZZ
Non-OR Ø9Q[3,4]XZZ
Non-OR Ø9Q[F,G][Ø,3,4,7,8,X]ZZ
Non-OR Ø9QKXZZ

Ø **Medical and Surgical**
9 **Ear, Nose, Sinus**
R **Replacement** Definition: Putting in or on biological or synthetic material that physically takes the place and/or function of all or a portion of a body part

Explanation: The body part may have been taken out or replaced, or may be taken out, physically eradicated, or rendered nonfunctional during the REPLACEMENT procedure. A REMOVAL procedure is coded for taking out the device used in a previous replacement procedure.

Body Part Character 4	Approach Character 5	Device Character 6	Qualifier Character 7
Ø External Ear, Right Antihelix Antitragus Auricle Earlobe Helix Pinna Tragus **1 External Ear, Left** *See Ø External Ear, Right* **2 External Ear, Bilateral** *See Ø External Ear, Right* **K Nasal Mucosa and Soft Tissue** Columella External naris Greater alar cartilage Internal naris Lateral nasal cartilage Lesser alar cartilage Nasal cavity Nostril	**Ø Open** **X External**	**7 Autologous Tissue Substitute** **J Synthetic Substitute** **K Nonautologous Tissue Substitute**	**Z No Qualifier**
5 Middle Ear, Right Oval window Tympanic cavity **6 Middle Ear, Left** *See 5 Middle Ear, Right* **9 Auditory Ossicle, Right** Incus Malleus Stapes **A Auditory Ossicle, Left** *See 9 Auditory Ossicle, Right* **D Inner Ear, Right** Bony labyrinth Bony vestibule Cochlea Round window Semicircular canal **E Inner Ear, Left** *See D Inner Ear, Right*	**Ø Open**	**7 Autologous Tissue Substitute** **J Synthetic Substitute** **K Nonautologous Tissue Substitute**	**Z No Qualifier**
7 Tympanic Membrane, Right Pars flaccida **8 Tympanic Membrane, Left** *See 7 Tympanic Membrane, Right* **N Nasopharynx** Choana Fossa of Rosenmuller Pharyngeal recess Rhinopharynx	**Ø Open** **7 Via Natural or Artificial Opening** **8 Via Natural or Artificial Opening Endoscopic**	**7 Autologous Tissue Substitute** **J Synthetic Substitute** **K Nonautologous Tissue Substitute**	**Z No Qualifier**
L Nasal Turbinate Inferior turbinate Middle turbinate Nasal concha Superior turbinate	**Ø Open** **3 Percutaneous** **4 Percutaneous Endoscopic** **7 Via Natural or Artificial Opening** **8 Via Natural or Artificial Opening Endoscopic**	**7 Autologous Tissue Substitute** **J Synthetic Substitute** **K Nonautologous Tissue Substitute**	**Z No Qualifier**
M Nasal Septum Quadrangular cartilage Septal cartilage Vomer bone	**Ø Open** **3 Percutaneous** **4 Percutaneous Endoscopic**	**7 Autologous Tissue Substitute** **J Synthetic Substitute** **K Nonautologous Tissue Substitute**	**Z No Qualifier**

Ø Medical and Surgical
9 Ear, Nose, Sinus
S Reposition Definition: Moving to its normal location, or other suitable location, all or a portion of a body part

Explanation: The body part is moved to a new location from an abnormal location, or from a normal location where it is not functioning correctly. The body part may or may not be cut out or off to be moved to the new location.

Body Part Character 4	Approach Character 5	Device Character 6	Qualifier Character 7
Ø External Ear, Right Antihelix Antitragus Auricle Earlobe Helix Pinna Tragus **1 External Ear, Left** *See Ø External Ear, Right* **2 External Ear, Bilateral** *See Ø External Ear, Right* **K Nasal Mucosa and Soft Tissue** Columella External naris Greater alar cartilage Internal naris Lateral nasal cartilage Lesser alar cartilage Nasal cavity Nostril	**Ø Open** **4 Percutaneous Endoscopic** **X External**	**Z No Device**	**Z No Qualifier**
7 Tympanic Membrane, Right Pars flaccida **8 Tympanic Membrane, Left** *See 7 Tympanic Membrane, Right* **F Eustachian Tube, Right** Auditory tube Pharyngotympanic tube **G Eustachian Tube, Left** *See F Eustachian Tube, Right* **L Nasal Turbinate** Inferior turbinate Middle turbinate Nasal concha Superior turbinate	**Ø Open** **4 Percutaneous Endoscopic** **7 Via Natural or Artificial Opening** **8 Via Natural or Artificial Opening Endoscopic**	**Z No Device**	**Z No Qualifier**
9 Auditory Ossicle, Right Incus Malleus Stapes **A Auditory Ossicle, Left** *See 9 Auditory Ossicle, Right* **M Nasal Septum** Quadrangular cartilage Septal cartilage Vomer bone	**Ø Open** **4 Percutaneous Endoscopic**	**Z No Device**	**Z No Qualifier**

Non-OR Ø9S[F,G][Ø,4,7,8]ZZ

Ø Medical and Surgical
9 Ear, Nose, Sinus
T Resection Definition: Cutting out or off, without replacement, all of a body part

Explanation: None

Body Part Character 4		Approach Character 5	Device Character 6	Qualifier Character 7
Ø External Ear, Right Antihelix Antitragus Auricle Earlobe Helix Pinna Tragus	**1 External Ear, Left** *See Ø External Ear, Right*	**Ø Open** **4 Percutaneous Endoscopic** **X External**	**Z No Device**	**Z No Qualifier**
5 Middle Ear, Right Oval window Tympanic cavity **6 Middle Ear, Left** *See 5 Middle Ear, Right* **9 Auditory Ossicle, Right** Incus Malleus Stapes	**A Auditory Ossicle, Left** *See 9 Auditory Ossicle, Right* **D Inner Ear, Right** Bony labyrinth Bony vestibule Cochlea Round window Semicircular canal **E Inner Ear, Left** *See D Inner Ear, Right*	**Ø Open** **8 Via Natural or Artificial Opening Endoscopic**	**Z No Device**	**Z No Qualifier**
7 Tympanic Membrane, Right Pars flaccida **8 Tympanic Membrane, Left** *See 7 Tympanic Membrane, Right* **F Eustachian Tube, Right** Auditory tube Pharyngotympanic tube **G Eustachian Tube, Left** *See F Eustachian Tube, Right*	**L Nasal Turbinate** Inferior turbinate Middle turbinate Nasal concha Superior turbinate **N Nasopharynx** Choana Fossa of Rosenmuller Pharyngeal recess Rhinopharynx	**Ø Open** **4 Percutaneous Endoscopic** **7 Via Natural or Artificial Opening** **8 Via Natural or Artificial Opening Endoscopic**	**Z No Device**	**Z No Qualifier**
B Mastoid Sinus, Right Mastoid air cells **C Mastoid Sinus, Left** *See B Mastoid Sinus, Right* **M Nasal Septum** Quadrangular cartilage Septal cartilage Vomer bone **P Accessory Sinus** **Q Maxillary Sinus, Right** Antrum of Highmore	**R Maxillary Sinus, Left** *See Q Maxillary Sinus, Right* **S Frontal Sinus, Right** **T Frontal Sinus, Left** **U Ethmoid Sinus, Right** Ethmoidal air cell **V Ethmoid Sinus, Left** *See U Ethmoid Sinus, Right* **W Sphenoid Sinus, Right** **X Sphenoid Sinus, Left**	**Ø Open** **4 Percutaneous Endoscopic** **8 Via Natural or Artificial Opening Endoscopic**	**Z No Device**	**Z No Qualifier**
K Nasal Mucosa and Soft Tissue Columella External naris Greater alar cartilage Internal naris Lateral nasal cartilage Lesser alar cartilage Nasal cavity Nostril		**Ø Open** **4 Percutaneous Endoscopic** **8 Via Natural or Artificial Opening Endoscopic** **X External**	**Z No Device**	**Z No Qualifier**

Non-OR Ø9T[F,G][Ø,4,7,8]ZZ

Ø Medical and Surgical
9 Ear, Nose, Sinus
U Supplement Definition: Putting in or on biological or synthetic material that physically reinforces and/or augments the function of a portion of a body part

Explanation: The biological material is non-living, or is living and from the same individual. The body part may have been previously replaced, and the SUPPLEMENT procedure is performed to physically reinforce and/or augment the function of the replaced body part.

Body Part Character 4		Approach Character 5	Device Character 6	Qualifier Character 7
Ø External Ear, Right Antihelix Antitragus Auricle Earlobe Helix Pinna Tragus	**1 External Ear, Left** *See Ø External Ear, Right* **2 External Ear, Bilateral** *See Ø External Ear, Right*	**Ø Open** **X External**	**7 Autologous Tissue Substitute** **J Synthetic Substitute** **K Nonautologous Tissue Substitute**	**Z No Qualifier**
5 Middle Ear, Right Oval window Tympanic cavity **6 Middle Ear, Left** *See 5 Middle Ear, Right* **9 Auditory Ossicle, Right** Incus Malleus Stapes **A Auditory Ossicle, Left** *See 9 Auditory Ossicle, Right*	**D Inner Ear, Right** Bony labyrinth Bony vestibule Cochlea Round window Semicircular canal **E Inner Ear, Left** *See D Inner Ear, Right*	**Ø Open** **8 Via Natural or Artificial Opening Endoscopic**	**7 Autologous Tissue Substitute** **J Synthetic Substitute** **K Nonautologous Tissue Substitute**	**Z No Qualifier**
7 Tympanic Membrane, Right Pars flaccida **8 Tympanic Membrane, Left** *See 7 Tympanic Membrane, Right*	**N Nasopharynx** Choana Fossa of Rosenmuller Pharyngeal recess Rhinopharynx	**Ø Open** **7 Via Natural or Artificial Opening** **8 Via Natural or Artificial Opening Endoscopic**	**7 Autologous Tissue Substitute** **J Synthetic Substitute** **K Nonautologous Tissue Substitute**	**Z No Qualifier**
B Mastoid Sinus, Right Mastoid air cells **C Mastoid Sinus, Left** *See B Mastoid Sinus, Right* **L Nasal Turbinate** Inferior turbinate Middle turbinate Nasal concha Superior turbinate **P Accessory Sinus** **Q Maxillary Sinus, Right** Antrum of Highmore	**R Maxillary Sinus, Left** *See Q Maxillary Sinus, Right* **S Frontal Sinus, Right** **T Frontal Sinus, Left** **U Ethmoid Sinus, Right** Ethmoidal air cell **V Ethmoid Sinus, Left** *See U Ethmoid Sinus, Right* **W Sphenoid Sinus, Right** **X Sphenoid Sinus, Left**	**Ø Open** **3 Percutaneous** **4 Percutaneous Endoscopic** **7 Via Natural or Artificial Opening** **8 Via Natural or Artificial Opening Endoscopic**	**7 Autologous Tissue Substitute** **J Synthetic Substitute** **K Nonautologous Tissue Substitute**	**Z No Qualifier**
K Nasal Mucosa and Soft Tissue Columella External naris Greater alar cartilage Internal naris Lateral nasal cartilage Lesser alar cartilage Nasal cavity Nostril		**Ø Open** **8 Via Natural or Artificial Opening Endoscopic** **X External**	**7 Autologous Tissue Substitute** **J Synthetic Substitute** **K Nonautologous Tissue Substitute**	**Z No Qualifier**
M Nasal Septum Quadrangular cartilage Septal cartilage Vomer bone		**Ø Open** **3 Percutaneous** **4 Percutaneous Endoscopic** **8 Via Natural or Artificial Opening Endoscopic**	**7 Autologous Tissue Substitute** **J Synthetic Substitute** **K Nonautologous Tissue Substitute**	**Z No Qualifier**

Ø Medical and Surgical
9 Ear, Nose, Sinus
W Revision Definition: Correcting, to the extent possible, a portion of a malfunctioning device or the position of a displaced device

Explanation: Revision can include correcting a malfunctioning or displaced device by taking out or putting in components of the device such as a screw or pin

Body Part Character 4	Approach Character 5	Device Character 6	Qualifier Character 7
7 Tympanic Membrane, Right Pars flaccida **8 Tympanic Membrane, Left** *See 7 Tympanic Membrane, Right* **9 Auditory Ossicle, Right** Incus Malleus Stapes **A Auditory Ossicle, Left** *See 9 Auditory Ossicle, Right*	**Ø Open** **7 Via Natural or Artificial Opening** **8 Via Natural or Artificial Opening Endoscopic**	**7 Autologous Tissue Substitute** **J Synthetic Substitute** **K Nonautologous Tissue Substitute**	**Z No Qualifier**
D Inner Ear, Right Bony labyrinth Bony vestibule Cochlea Round window Semicircular canal **E Inner Ear, Left** *See D Inner Ear, Right*	**Ø Open** **7 Via Natural or Artificial Opening** **8 Via Natural or Artificial Opening Endoscopic**	**S Hearing Device**	**Z No Qualifier**
H Ear, Right **J Ear, Left** **K Nasal Mucosa and Soft Tissue** Columella External naris Greater alar cartilage Internal naris Lateral nasal cartilage Lesser alar cartilage Nasal cavity Nostril	**Ø Open** **3 Percutaneous** **4 Percutaneous Endoscopic** **7 Via Natural or Artificial Opening** **8 Via Natural or Artificial Opening Endoscopic**	**Ø Drainage Device** **7 Autologous Tissue Substitute** **D Intraluminal Device** **J Synthetic Substitute** **K Nonautologous Tissue Substitute** **Y Other Device**	**Z No Qualifier**
H Ear, Right **J Ear, Left** **K Nasal Mucosa and Soft Tissue** Columella External naris Greater alar cartilage Internal naris Lateral nasal cartilage Lesser alar cartilage Nasal cavity Nostril	**X External**	**Ø Drainage Device** **7 Autologous Tissue Substitute** **D Intraluminal Device** **J Synthetic Substitute** **K Nonautologous Tissue Substitute**	**Z No Qualifier**
Y Sinus	**Ø Open** **3 Percutaneous** **4 Percutaneous Endoscopic**	**Ø Drainage Device** **Y Other Device**	**Z No Qualifier**
Y Sinus	**7 Via Natural or Artificial Opening** **8 Via Natural or Artificial Opening Endoscopic**	**Y Other Device**	**Z No Qualifier**
Y Sinus	**X External**	**Ø Drainage Device**	**Z No Qualifier**

Non-OR Ø9W[H,J][3,4][J,K,Y]Z
Non-OR Ø9W[H,J][7,8][D,Y]Z
Non-OR Ø9WK[Ø,3,4,7,8][Ø,7,D,J,K,Y]Z
Non-OR Ø9W[H,J,K]X[Ø,7,D,J,K]Z
Non-OR Ø9WY[3,4]YZ
Non-OR Ø9WY[7,8]YZ
Non-OR Ø9WYXØZ

Respiratory System ØB1–ØBY

Character Meanings

This Character Meaning table is provided as a guide to assist the user in the identification of character members that may be found in this section of code tables. It **SHOULD NOT** be used to build a PCS code.

Operation–Character 3	Body Part–Character 4	Approach–Character 5	Device–Character 6	Qualifier–Character 7
1 Bypass	Ø Tracheobronchial Tree	Ø Open	Ø Drainage Device	Ø Allogeneic
2 Change	1 Trachea	3 Percutaneous	1 Radioactive Element	1 Syngeneic
5 Destruction	2 Carina	4 Percutaneous Endoscopic	2 Monitoring Device	2 Zooplastic
7 Dilation	3 Main Bronchus, Right	7 Via Natural or Artificial Opening	3 Infusion Device	4 Cutaneous
9 Drainage	4 Upper Lobe Bronchus, Right	8 Via Natural or Artificial Opening Endoscopic	7 Autologous Tissue Substitute	6 Esophagus
B Excision	5 Middle Lobe Bronchus, Right	X External	C Extraluminal Device	X Diagnostic
C Extirpation	6 Lower Lobe Bronchus, Right		D Intraluminal Device	Z No Qualifier
D Extraction	7 Main Bronchus, Left		E Intraluminal Device, Endotracheal Airway	
F Fragmentation	8 Upper Lobe Bronchus, Left		F Tracheostomy Device	
H Insertion	9 Lingula Bronchus		G Intraluminal Device, Endobronchial Valve	
J Inspection	B Lower Lobe Bronchus, Left		J Synthetic Substitute	
L Occlusion	C Upper Lung Lobe, Right		K Nonautologous Tissue Substitute	
M Reattachment	D Middle Lung Lobe, Right		M Diaphragmatic Pacemaker Lead	
N Release	F Lower Lung Lobe, Right		Y Other Device	
P Removal	G Upper Lung Lobe, Left		Z No Device	
Q Repair	H Lung Lingula			
R Replacement	J Lower Lung Lobe, Left			
S Reposition	K Lung, Right			
T Resection	L Lung, Left			
U Supplement	M Lungs, Bilateral			
V Restriction	N Pleura, Right			
W Revision	P Pleura, Left			
Y Transplantation	Q Pleura			
	T Diaphragm			

AHA Coding Clinic for table ØB5
2016, 2Q, 17 Photodynamic therapy for treatment of malignant mesothelioma
2015, 2Q, 31 Thoracoscopic talc pleurodesis

AHA Coding Clinic for table ØB7
2020, 3Q, 43 Tracheobronchomalacia with placement of tracheobronchial stent

AHA Coding Clinic for table ØB9
2017, 3Q, 15 Bronchoscopy with suctioning for removal of retained secretions
2017, 1Q, 51 Bronchoalveolar lavage
2016, 1Q, 26 Bronchoalveolar lavage, endobronchial biopsy and transbronchial biopsy
2016, 1Q, 27 Fiberoptic bronchoscopy with brushings and bronchoalveolar lavage

AHA Coding Clinic for table ØBB
2016, 1Q, 26 Bronchoalveolar lavage, endobronchial biopsy and transbronchial biopsy
2016, 1Q, 27 Fiberoptic bronchoscopy with brushings and bronchoalveolar lavage
2014, 1Q, 20 Fiducial marker placement

AHA Coding Clinic for table ØBC
2017, 3Q, 14 Bronchoscopy with suctioning and washings for removal of mucus plug

AHA Coding Clinic for table ØBD
2020, 3Q, 40 Transbronchial cryobiopsy of upper, middle and lower lobes of lung
2018, 3Q, 28 Lung decortication for empyema

AHA Coding Clinic for table ØBH
2019, 3Q, 33 Insertion of endobronchial valve
2014, 4Q, 3-10 Mechanical ventilation

AHA Coding Clinic for table ØBJ
2015, 2Q, 31 Thoracoscopic talc pleurodesis
2014, 1Q, 20 Fiducial marker placement

AHA Coding Clinic for table ØBL
2019, 3Q, 33 Insertion of endobronchial valve

AHA Coding Clinic for table ØBN
2019, 2Q, 20 Pericardiectomy for constrictive pericarditis
2018, 3Q, 28 Lung decortication
2018, 3Q, 28 Lung decortication for empyema
2015, 3Q, 15 Vascular ring surgery with release of esophagus and trachea

AHA Coding Clinic for table ØBQ
2020, 3Q, 41 Plication of diaphragm
2016, 2Q, 22 Esophageal lengthening Collis gastroplasty with Nissen fundoplication and hiatal hernia
2014, 3Q, 28 Laparoscopic Nissen fundoplication and diaphragmatic hernia repair

AHA Coding Clinic for table ØBU
2020, 3Q, 43 Tracheobronchomalacia with placement of tracheobronchial stent
2015, 1Q, 28 Repair of bronchopleural fistula using omental pedicle graft

AHA Coding Clinic for table ØBV
2020, 3Q, 41 Plication of diaphragm

Respiratory System

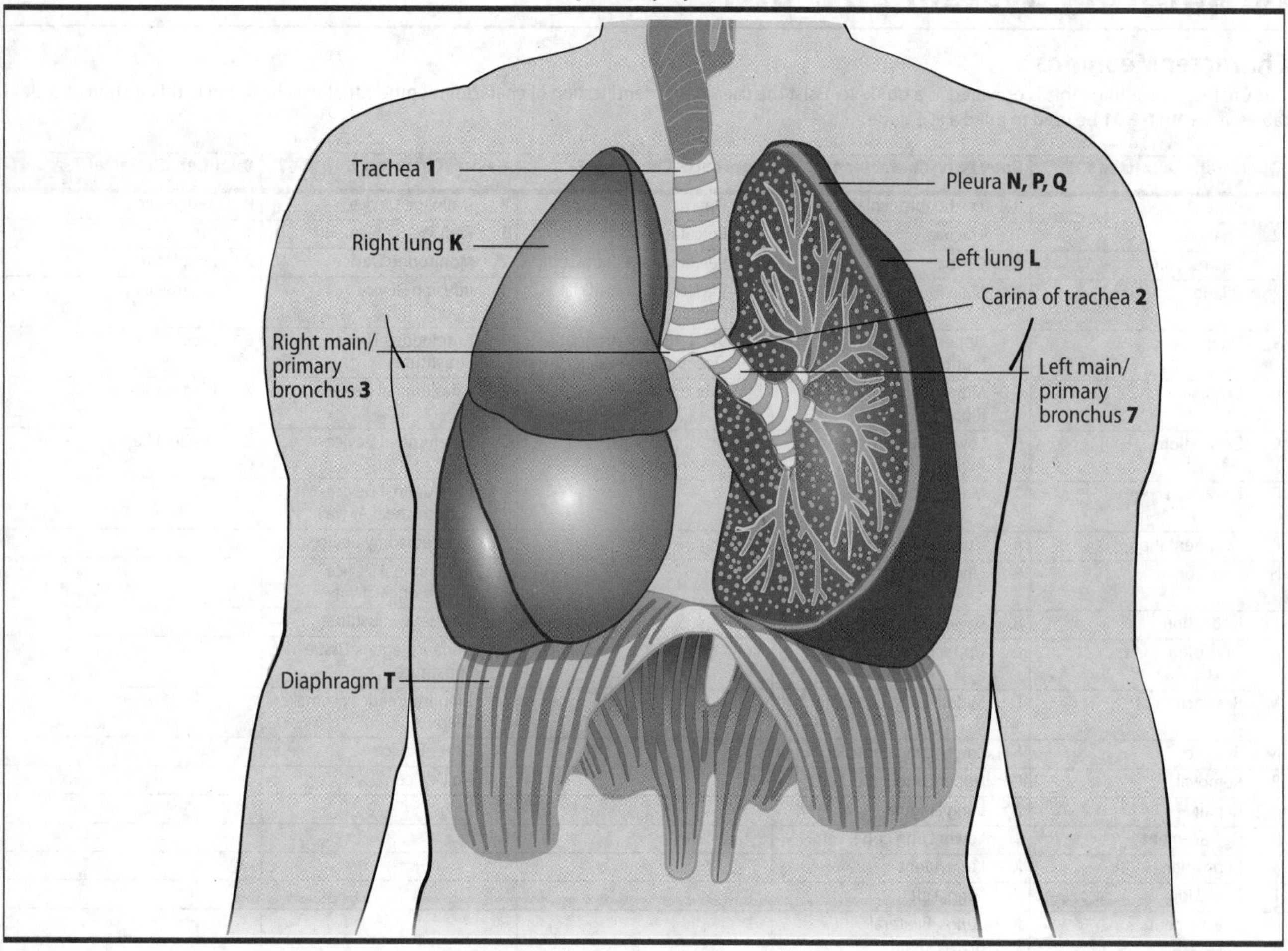

Right Lung Bronchi

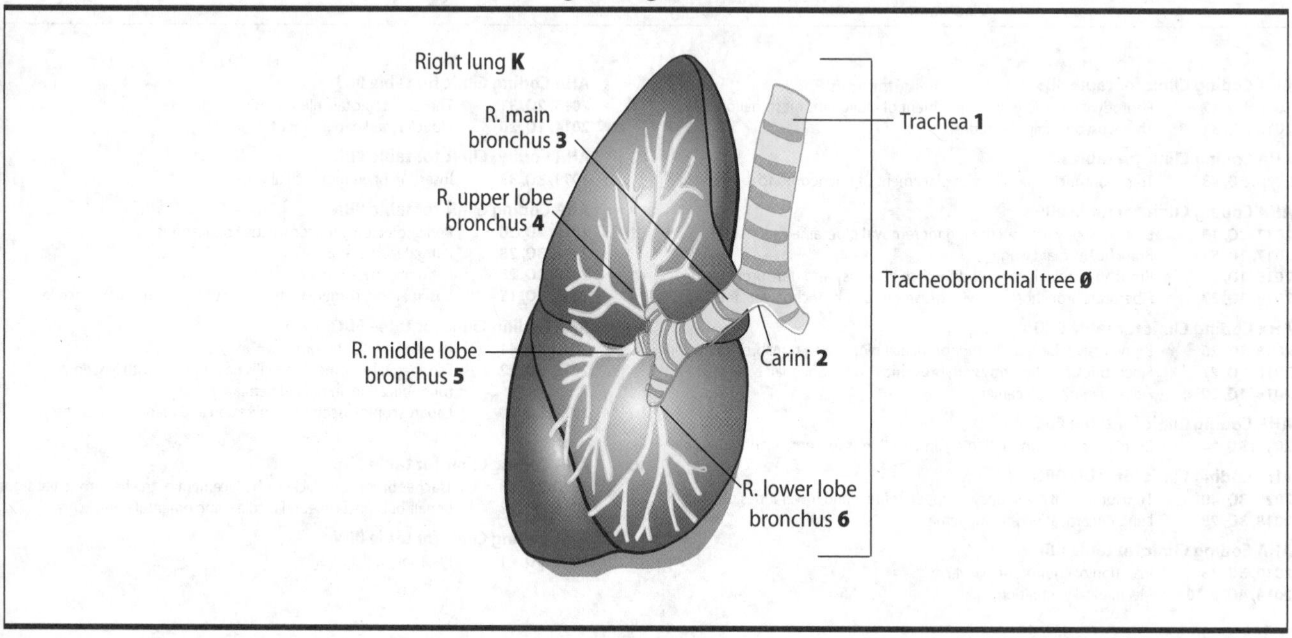

Ø Medical and Surgical
B Respiratory System
1 Bypass Definition: Altering the route of passage of the contents of a tubular body part

Explanation: Rerouting contents of a body part to a downstream area of the normal route, to a similar route and body part, or to an abnormal route and dissimilar body part. Includes one or more anastomoses, with or without the use of a device.

Body Part Character 4	Approach Character 5	Device Character 6	Qualifier Character 7
1 Trachea Cricoid cartilage	Ø Open	D Intraluminal Device	6 Esophagus
1 Trachea Cricoid cartilage	Ø Open	F Tracheostomy Device Z No Device	4 Cutaneous
1 Trachea Cricoid cartilage	3 Percutaneous 4 Percutaneous Endoscopic	F Tracheostomy Device Z No Device	4 Cutaneous

DRG Non-OR ØB113[F,Z]4
Non-OR ØB11ØD6

Ø Medical and Surgical
B Respiratory System
2 Change Definition: Taking out or off a device from a body part and putting back an identical or similar device in or on the same body part without cutting or puncturing the skin or a mucous membrane

Explanation: All CHANGE procedures are coded using the approach EXTERNAL

Body Part Character 4	Approach Character 5	Device Character 6	Qualifier Character 7
Ø Tracheobronchial Tree K Lung, Right L Lung, Left Q Pleura T Diaphragm	X External	Ø Drainage Device Y Other Device	Z No Qualifier
1 Trachea Cricoid cartilage	X External	Ø Drainage Device E Intraluminal Device, Endotracheal Airway F Tracheostomy Device Y Other Device	Z No Qualifier

Non-OR All body part, approach, device, and qualifier values

Ø Medical and Surgical
B Respiratory System
5 Destruction Definition: Physical eradication of all or a portion of a body part by the direct use of energy, force, or a destructive agent

Explanation: None of the body part is physically taken out

Body Part Character 4	Approach Character 5	Device Character 6	Qualifier Character 7
1 Trachea Cricoid cartilage 2 Carina 3 Main Bronchus, Right Bronchus intermedius Intermediate bronchus 4 Upper Lobe Bronchus, Right 5 Middle Lobe Bronchus, Right 6 Lower Lobe Bronchus, Right 7 Main Bronchus, Left 8 Upper Lobe Bronchus, Left 9 Lingula Bronchus B Lower Lobe Bronchus, Left C Upper Lung Lobe, Right D Middle Lung Lobe, Right F Lower Lung Lobe, Right G Upper Lung Lobe, Left H Lung Lingula J Lower Lung Lobe, Left K Lung, Right L Lung, Left M Lungs, Bilateral	Ø Open 3 Percutaneous 4 Percutaneous Endoscopic 7 Via Natural or Artificial Opening 8 Via Natural or Artificial Opening Endoscopic	Z No Device	Z No Qualifier
N Pleura, Right P Pleura, Left T Diaphragm	Ø Open 3 Percutaneous 4 Percutaneous Endoscopic	Z No Device	Z No Qualifier

Non-OR ØB5[3,4,5,6,7,8,9,B][4,8]ZZ
Non-OR ØB5[C,D,F,G,H,J,K,L,M]8ZZ

Ø Medical and Surgical
B Respiratory System
7 Dilation Definition: Expanding an orifice or the lumen of a tubular body part

Explanation: The orifice can be a natural orifice or an artificially created orifice. Accomplished by stretching a tubular body part using intraluminal pressure or by cutting part of the orifice or wall of the tubular body part.

Body Part Character 4	Approach Character 5	Device Character 6	Qualifier Character 7
1 Trachea Cricoid cartilage **2 Carina** **3 Main Bronchus, Right** Bronchus intermedius Intermediate bronchus **4 Upper Lobe Bronchus, Right** **5 Middle Lobe Bronchus, Right** **6 Lower Lobe Bronchus, Right** **7 Main Bronchus, Left** **8 Upper Lobe Bronchus, Left** **9 Lingula Bronchus** **B Lower Lobe Bronchus, Left**	**Ø Open** **3 Percutaneous** **4 Percutaneous Endoscopic** **7 Via Natural or Artificial Opening** **8 Via Natural or Artificial Opening Endoscopic**	**D Intraluminal Device** **Z No Device**	**Z No Qualifier**

Non-OR ØB7[3,4,5,6,7,8,9,B][Ø,3,4,7,8][D,Z]Z

Ø Medical and Surgical
B Respiratory System
9 Drainage Definition: Taking or letting out fluids and/or gases from a body part

Explanation: The qualifier DIAGNOSTIC is used to identify drainage procedures that are biopsies

Body Part Character 4	Body Part Character 4 (cont.)	Approach Character 5	Device Character 6	Qualifier Character 7
1 Trachea Cricoid cartilage **2 Carina** **3 Main Bronchus, Right** Bronchus intermedius Intermediate bronchus **4 Upper Lobe Bronchus, Right** **5 Middle Lobe Bronchus, Right** **6 Lower Lobe Bronchus, Right** **7 Main Bronchus, Left**	**8 Upper Lobe Bronchus, Left** **9 Lingula Bronchus** **B Lower Lobe Bronchus, Left** **C Upper Lung Lobe, Right** **D Middle Lung Lobe, Right** **F Lower Lung Lobe, Right** **G Upper Lung Lobe, Left** **H Lung Lingula** **J Lower Lung Lobe, Left** **K Lung, Right** **L Lung, Left** **M Lungs, Bilateral**	**Ø Open** **3 Percutaneous** **4 Percutaneous Endoscopic** **7 Via Natural or Artificial Opening** **8 Via Natural or Artificial Opening Endoscopic**	**Ø Drainage Device**	**Z No Qualifier**
1 Trachea Cricoid cartilage **2 Carina** **3 Main Bronchus, Right** Bronchus intermedius Intermediate bronchus **4 Upper Lobe Bronchus, Right** **5 Middle Lobe Bronchus, Right** **6 Lower Lobe Bronchus, Right** **7 Main Bronchus, Left**	**8 Upper Lobe Bronchus, Left** **9 Lingula Bronchus** **B Lower Lobe Bronchus, Left** **C Upper Lung Lobe, Right** **D Middle Lung Lobe, Right** **F Lower Lung Lobe, Right** **G Upper Lung Lobe, Left** **H Lung Lingula** **J Lower Lung Lobe, Left** **K Lung, Right** **L Lung, Left** **M Lungs, Bilateral**	**Ø Open** **3 Percutaneous** **4 Percutaneous Endoscopic** **7 Via Natural or Artificial Opening** **8 Via Natural or Artificial Opening Endoscopic**	**Z No Device**	**X Diagnostic** **Z No Qualifier**
N Pleura, Right **P Pleura, Left**		**Ø Open** **3 Percutaneous** **4 Percutaneous Endoscopic** **8 Via Natural or Artificial Opening Endoscopic**	**Ø Drainage Device**	**Z No Qualifier**
N Pleura, Right **P Pleura, Left**		**Ø Open** **3 Percutaneous** **4 Percutaneous Endoscopic** **8 Via Natural or Artificial Opening Endoscopic**	**Z No Device**	**X Diagnostic** **Z No Qualifier**
T Diaphragm		**Ø Open** **3 Percutaneous** **4 Percutaneous Endoscopic**	**Ø Drainage Device**	**Z No Qualifier**
T Diaphragm		**Ø Open** **3 Percutaneous** **4 Percutaneous Endoscopic**	**Z No Device**	**X Diagnostic** **Z No Qualifier**

Non-OR ØB9[1,2,3,4,5,6,7,8,9,B][7,8]ØZ
Non-OR ØB9[1,2,3,4,5,6,7,8,9,B][3,4]ZX
Non-OR ØB9[1,2,3,4,5,6,7,8,9,B][7,8]Z[X,Z]
Non-OR ØB9[C,D,F,G,H,J,K,L,M][3,4,7]ZX
Non-OR ØB9[C,D,F,G,H,J,K,L,M]8Z[X,Z]
Non-OR ØB9[N,P][Ø,3,8]ØZ
Non-OR ØB9[N,P][Ø,3,8]Z[X,Z]
Non-OR ØB9[N,P]4ZX
Non-OR ØB9T[3,4]ØZ
Non-OR ØB9T[3,4]Z[X,Z]

Ø Medical and Surgical
B Respiratory System
B Excision Definition: Cutting out or off, without replacement, a portion of a body part

Explanation: The qualifier DIAGNOSTIC is used to identify excision procedures that are biopsies

Body Part Character 4	Approach Character 5	Device Character 6	Qualifier Character 7
1 Trachea Cricoid cartilage 2 Carina 3 Main Bronchus, Right Bronchus intermedius Intermediate bronchus 4 Upper Lobe Bronchus, Right 5 Middle Lobe Bronchus, Right 6 Lower Lobe Bronchus, Right 7 Main Bronchus, Left 8 Upper Lobe Bronchus, Left 9 Lingula Bronchus B Lower Lobe Bronchus, Left C Upper Lung Lobe, Right D Middle Lung Lobe, Right F Lower Lung Lobe, Right G Upper Lung Lobe, Left H Lung Lingula J Lower Lung Lobe, Left K Lung, Right L Lung, Left M Lungs, Bilateral	Ø Open 3 Percutaneous 4 Percutaneous Endoscopic 7 Via Natural or Artificial Opening 8 Via Natural or Artificial Opening Endoscopic	Z No Device	X Diagnostic Z No Qualifier
N Pleura, Right P Pleura, Left	Ø Open 3 Percutaneous 4 Percutaneous Endoscopic 8 Via Natural or Artificial Opening Endoscopic	Z No Device	X Diagnostic Z No Qualifier
T Diaphragm	Ø Open 3 Percutaneous 4 Percutaneous Endoscopic	Z No Device	X Diagnostic Z No Qualifier

Non-OR ØBB[1,2,3,4,5,6,7,8,9,B][3,4,7,8]ZX
Non-OR ØBB[3,4,5,6,7,8,9,B,M][4,8]ZZ
Non-OR ØBB[C,D,F,G,H,J,K,L,M]3ZX
Non-OR ØBB[C,D,F,G,H,J,K,L]8ZZ
Non-OR ØBB[N,P][Ø,3]ZX

Ø Medical and Surgical
B Respiratory System
C Extirpation Definition: Taking or cutting out solid matter from a body part

Explanation: The solid matter may be an abnormal byproduct of a biological function or a foreign body; it may be imbedded in a body part or in the lumen of a tubular body part. The solid matter may or may not have been previously broken into pieces.

Body Part Character 4	Approach Character 5	Device Character 6	Qualifier Character 7
1 Trachea Cricoid cartilage 2 Carina 3 Main Bronchus, Right Bronchus intermedius Intermediate bronchus 4 Upper Lobe Bronchus, Right 5 Middle Lobe Bronchus, Right 6 Lower Lobe Bronchus, Right 7 Main Bronchus, Left 8 Upper Lobe Bronchus, Left 9 Lingula Bronchus B Lower Lobe Bronchus, Left C Upper Lung Lobe, Right D Middle Lung Lobe, Right F Lower Lung Lobe, Right G Upper Lung Lobe, Left H Lung Lingula J Lower Lung Lobe, Left K Lung, Right L Lung, Left M Lungs, Bilateral	Ø Open 3 Percutaneous 4 Percutaneous Endoscopic 7 Via Natural or Artificial Opening 8 Via Natural or Artificial Opening Endoscopic	Z No Device	Z No Qualifier
N Pleura, Right P Pleura, Left T Diaphragm	Ø Open 3 Percutaneous 4 Percutaneous Endoscopic	Z No Device	Z No Qualifier

Non-OR ØBC[1,2,3,4,5,6,7,8,9,B][7,8]ZZ
Non-OR ØBC[N,P]3ZZ

Ø Medical and Surgical
B Respiratory System
D Extraction Definition: Pulling or stripping out or off all or a portion of a body part by the use of force

Explanation: The qualifier DIAGNOSTIC is used to identify extraction procedures that are biopsies

Body Part Character 4	Approach Character 5	Device Character 6	Qualifier Character 7
1 Trachea Cricoid cartilage 2 Carina 3 Main Bronchus, Right Bronchus intermedius Intermediate bronchus 4 Upper Lobe Bronchus, Right 5 Middle Lobe Bronchus, Right 6 Lower Lobe Bronchus, Right 7 Main Bronchus, Left 8 Upper Lobe Bronchus, Left 9 Lingula Bronchus B Lower Lobe Bronchus, Left C Upper Lung Lobe, Right D Middle Lung Lobe, Right F Lower Lung Lobe, Right G Upper Lung Lobe, Left H Lung Lingula J Lower Lung Lobe, Left K Lung, Right L Lung, Left M Lungs, Bilateral	4 Percutaneous Endoscopic 8 Via Natural or Artificial Opening Endoscopic	Z No Device	X Diagnostic
N Pleura, Right P Pleura, Left	Ø Open 3 Percutaneous 4 Percutaneous Endoscopic	Z No Device	X Diagnostic Z No Qualifier

Non-OR ØBD[1,2,3,4,5,6,7,8,9,B,C,D,F,G,H,J,K,L,M][4,8]ZX

Ø Medical and Surgical
B Respiratory System
F Fragmentation Definition: Breaking solid matter in a body part into pieces

Explanation: Physical force (e.g., manual, ultrasonic) applied directly or indirectly is used to break the solid matter into pieces. The solid matter may be an abnormal byproduct of a biological function or a foreign body. The pieces of solid matter are not taken out.

Body Part Character 4	Approach Character 5	Device Character 6	Qualifier Character 7
1 Trachea NC Cricoid cartilage 2 Carina NC 3 Main Bronchus, Right NC Bronchus intermedius Intermediate bronchus 4 Upper Lobe Bronchus, Right NC 5 Middle Lobe Bronchus, Right NC 6 Lower Lobe Bronchus, Right NC 7 Main Bronchus, Left NC 8 Upper Lobe Bronchus, Left NC 9 Lingula Bronchus NC B Lower Lobe Bronchus, Left NC	Ø Open 3 Percutaneous 4 Percutaneous Endoscopic 7 Via Natural or Artificial Opening 8 Via Natural or Artificial Opening Endoscopic X External	Z No Device	Z No Qualifier

Non-OR ØBF[1,2,3,4,5,6,7,8,9,B]XZZ
Non-OR ØBF[3,4,5,6,7,8,9,B][7,8]ZZ
NC ØBF[1,2,3,4,5,6,7,8,9,B]XZZ

Ø Medical and Surgical
B Respiratory System
H Insertion Definition: Putting in a nonbiological appliance that monitors, assists, performs, or prevents a physiological function but does not physically take the place of a body part

Explanation: None

Body Part Character 4	Approach Character 5	Device Character 6	Qualifier Character 7
Ø Tracheobronchial Tree	Ø Open 3 Percutaneous 4 Percutaneous Endoscopic 7 Via Natural or Artificial Opening 8 Via Natural or Artificial Opening Endoscopic	1 Radioactive Element 2 Monitoring Device 3 Infusion Device D Intraluminal Device Y Other Device	Z No Qualifier
1 Trachea Cricoid cartilage	Ø Open	2 Monitoring Device D Intraluminal Device Y Other Device	Z No Qualifier
1 Trachea Cricoid cartilage	3 Percutaneous	D Intraluminal Device E Intraluminal Device, Endotracheal Airway Y Other Device	Z No Qualifier
1 Trachea Cricoid cartilage	4 Percutaneous Endoscopic	D Intraluminal Device Y Other Device	Z No Qualifier
1 Trachea Cricoid cartilage	7 Via Natural or Artificial Opening 8 Via Natural or Artificial Opening Endoscopic	2 Monitoring Device D Intraluminal Device E Intraluminal Device, Endotracheal Airway Y Other Device	Z No Qualifier
3 Main Bronchus, Right Bronchus intermedius Intermediate bronchus 4 Upper Lobe Bronchus, Right 5 Middle Lobe Bronchus, Right 6 Lower Lobe Bronchus, Right 7 Main Bronchus, Left 8 Upper Lobe Bronchus, Left 9 Lingula Bronchus B Lower Lobe Bronchus, Left	Ø Open 3 Percutaneous 4 Percutaneous Endoscopic 7 Via Natural or Artificial Opening 8 Via Natural or Artificial Opening Endoscopic	G Intraluminal Device, Endobronchial Valve	Z No Qualifier
K Lung, Right L Lung, Left	Ø Open 3 Percutaneous 4 Percutaneous Endoscopic 7 Via Natural or Artificial Opening 8 Via Natural or Artificial Opening Endoscopic	1 Radioactive Element 2 Monitoring Device 3 Infusion Device Y Other Device	Z No Qualifier
Q Pleura	Ø Open 3 Percutaneous 4 Percutaneous Endoscopic 7 Via Natural or Artificial Opening 8 Via Natural or Artificial Opening Endoscopic	Y Other Device	Z No Qualifier
T Diaphragm	Ø Open 3 Percutaneous 4 Percutaneous Endoscopic	2 Monitoring Device M Diaphragmatic Pacemaker Lead Y Other Device	Z No Qualifier
T Diaphragm	7 Via Natural or Artificial Opening 8 Via Natural or Artificial Opening Endoscopic	Y Other Device	Z No Qualifier

DRG Non-OR ØBH[3,4,5,6,7,8,9,B]8GZ
Non-OR ØBHØ3YZ
Non-OR ØBHØ[7,8][2,3,D,Y]Z
Non-OR ØBH13[E,Y]Z
Non-OR ØBH1[7,8][2,D,E,Y]Z
Non-OR ØBH[K,L]3YZ
Non-OR ØBH[K,L]7[2,3,Y]Z
Non-OR ØBH[K,L]8[2,3]Z
Non-OR ØBHQ[3,7]YZ
Non-OR ØBHT3YZ
Non-OR ØBHT[7,8]YZ

Ø Medical and Surgical
B Respiratory System
J Inspection Definition: Visually and/or manually exploring a body part

Explanation: Visual exploration may be performed with or without optical instrumentation. Manual exploration may be performed directly or through intervening body layers.

Body Part Character 4	Approach Character 5	Device Character 6	Qualifier Character 7
Ø Tracheobronchial Tree **1** Trachea Cricoid cartilage **K** Lung, Right **L** Lung, Left **Q** Pleura **T** Diaphragm	**Ø** Open **3** Percutaneous **4** Percutaneous Endoscopic **7** Via Natural or Artificial Opening **8** Via Natural or Artificial Opening Endoscopic **X** External	**Z** No Device	**Z** No Qualifier

Non-OR ØBJ[Ø,K,L,Q,T][3,7,8,X]ZZ
Non-OR ØBJ1[3,4,7,8,X]ZZ

Ø Medical and Surgical
B Respiratory System
L Occlusion Definition: Completely closing an orifice or the lumen of a tubular body part

Explanation: The orifice can be a natural orifice or an artificially created orifice

Body Part Character 4	Approach Character 5	Device Character 6	Qualifier Character 7
1 Trachea Cricoid cartilage **2** Carina **3** Main Bronchus, Right Bronchus intermedius Intermediate bronchus **4** Upper Lobe Bronchus, Right **5** Middle Lobe Bronchus, Right **6** Lower Lobe Bronchus, Right **7** Main Bronchus, Left **8** Upper Lobe Bronchus, Left **9** Lingula Bronchus **B** Lower Lobe Bronchus, Left	**Ø** Open **3** Percutaneous **4** Percutaneous Endoscopic	**C** Extraluminal Device **D** Intraluminal Device **Z** No Device	**Z** No Qualifier
1 Trachea Cricoid cartilage **2** Carina **3** Main Bronchus, Right Bronchus intermedius Intermediate bronchus **4** Upper Lobe Bronchus, Right **5** Middle Lobe Bronchus, Right **6** Lower Lobe Bronchus, Right **7** Main Bronchus, Left **8** Upper Lobe Bronchus, Left **9** Lingula Bronchus **B** Lower Lobe Bronchus, Left	**7** Via Natural or Artificial Opening **8** Via Natural or Artificial Opening Endoscopic	**D** Intraluminal Device **Z** No Device	**Z** No Qualifier

Ø Medical and Surgical
B Respiratory System
M Reattachment Definition: Putting back in or on all or a portion of a separated body part to its normal location or other suitable location
Explanation: Vascular circulation and nervous pathways may or may not be reestablished

Body Part Character 4	Approach Character 5	Device Character 6	Qualifier Character 7
1 Trachea Cricoid cartilage **2 Carina** **3 Main Bronchus, Right** Bronchus intermedius Intermediate bronchus **4 Upper Lobe Bronchus, Right** **5 Middle Lobe Bronchus, Right** **6 Lower Lobe Bronchus, Right** **7 Main Bronchus, Left** **8 Upper Lobe Bronchus, Left** **9 Lingula Bronchus** **B Lower Lobe Bronchus, Left** **C Upper Lung Lobe, Right** **D Middle Lung Lobe, Right** **F Lower Lung Lobe, Right** **G Upper Lung Lobe, Left** **H Lung Lingula** **J Lower Lung Lobe, Left** **K Lung, Right** **L Lung, Left** **T Diaphragm**	**Ø Open**	**Z No Device**	**Z No Qualifier**

Ø Medical and Surgical
B Respiratory System
N Release Definition: Freeing a body part from an abnormal physical constraint by cutting or by the use of force
Explanation: Some of the restraining tissue may be taken out but none of the body part is taken out

Body Part Character 4	Approach Character 5	Device Character 6	Qualifier Character 7
1 Trachea Cricoid cartilage **2 Carina** **3 Main Bronchus, Right** Bronchus intermedius Intermediate bronchus **4 Upper Lobe Bronchus, Right** **5 Middle Lobe Bronchus, Right** **6 Lower Lobe Bronchus, Right** **7 Main Bronchus, Left** **8 Upper Lobe Bronchus, Left** **9 Lingula Bronchus** **B Lower Lobe Bronchus, Left** **C Upper Lung Lobe, Right** **D Middle Lung Lobe, Right** **F Lower Lung Lobe, Right** **G Upper Lung Lobe, Left** **H Lung Lingula** **J Lower Lung Lobe, Left** **K Lung, Right** **L Lung, Left** **M Lungs, Bilateral**	**Ø Open** **3 Percutaneous** **4 Percutaneous Endoscopic** **7 Via Natural or Artificial Opening** **8 Via Natural or Artificial Opening Endoscopic**	**Z No Device**	**Z No Qualifier**
N Pleura, Right **P Pleura, Left** **T Diaphragm**	**Ø Open** **3 Percutaneous** **4 Percutaneous Endoscopic**	**Z No Device**	**Z No Qualifier**

Ø Medical and Surgical
B Respiratory System
P Removal Definition: Taking out or off a device from a body part

Explanation: If a device is taken out and a similar device put in without cutting or puncturing the skin or mucous membrane, the procedure is coded to the root operation CHANGE. Otherwise, the procedure for taking out a device is coded to the root operation REMOVAL.

Body Part Character 4	Approach Character 5	Device Character 6	Qualifier Character 7
Ø Tracheobronchial Tree	Ø Open 3 Percutaneous 4 Percutaneous Endoscopic 7 Via Natural or Artificial Opening 8 Via Natural or Artificial Opening Endoscopic	Ø Drainage Device 1 Radioactive Element 2 Monitoring Device 3 Infusion Device 7 Autologous Tissue Substitute C Extraluminal Device D Intraluminal Device J Synthetic Substitute K Nonautologous Tissue Substitute Y Other Device	Z No Qualifier
Ø Tracheobronchial Tree	X External	Ø Drainage Device 1 Radioactive Element 2 Monitoring Device 3 Infusion Device D Intraluminal Device	Z No Qualifier
1 Trachea Cricoid cartilage	Ø Open 3 Percutaneous 4 Percutaneous Endoscopic 7 Via Natural or Artificial Opening 8 Via Natural or Artificial Opening Endoscopic	Ø Drainage Device 2 Monitoring Device 7 Autologous Tissue Substitute C Extraluminal Device D Intraluminal Device F Tracheostomy Device J Synthetic Substitute K Nonautologous Tissue Substitute	Z No Qualifier
1 Trachea Cricoid cartilage	X External	Ø Drainage Device 2 Monitoring Device D Intraluminal Device F Tracheostomy Device	Z No Qualifier
K Lung, Right L Lung, Left	Ø Open 3 Percutaneous 4 Percutaneous Endoscopic 7 Via Natural or Artificial Opening 8 Via Natural or Artificial Opening Endoscopic	Ø Drainage Device 1 Radioactive Element 2 Monitoring Device 3 Infusion Device Y Other Device	Z No Qualifier
K Lung, Right L Lung, Left	X External	Ø Drainage Device 1 Radioactive Element 2 Monitoring Device 3 Infusion Device	Z No Qualifier
Q Pleura	Ø Open 3 Percutaneous 4 Percutaneous Endoscopic 7 Via Natural or Artificial Opening 8 Via Natural or Artificial Opening Endoscopic	Ø Drainage Device 1 Radioactive Element 2 Monitoring Device Y Other Device	Z No Qualifier
Q Pleura	X External	Ø Drainage Device 1 Radioactive Element 2 Monitoring Device	Z No Qualifier
T Diaphragm	Ø Open 3 Percutaneous 4 Percutaneous Endoscopic 7 Via Natural or Artificial Opening 8 Via Natural or Artificial Opening Endoscopic	Ø Drainage Device 2 Monitoring Device 7 Autologous Tissue Substitute J Synthetic Substitute K Nonautologous Tissue Substitute M Diaphragmatic Pacemaker Lead Y Other Device	Z No Qualifier
T Diaphragm	X External	Ø Drainage Device 2 Monitoring Device M Diaphragmatic Pacemaker Lead	Z No Qualifier

Non-OR ØBPØ[3,4]YZ
Non-OR ØBPØ[7,8][Ø,2,3,D,Y]Z
Non-OR ØBPØX[Ø,1,2,3,D]Z
Non-OR ØBP1[Ø,3,4]FZ
Non-OR ØBP1[7,8][Ø,2,D,F]Z
Non-OR ØBP1X[Ø,2,D,F]Z
Non-OR ØBP[K,L]3YZ
Non-OR ØBPK7[Ø,1,2,3,Y]Z
Non-OR ØBPK8[Ø,1,2,3]Z
Non-OR ØBPL7[Ø,2,3,Y]Z
Non-OR ØBPL8[Ø,2,3]Z
Non-OR ØBP[K,L]X[Ø,1,2,3]Z
Non-OR ØBPQ[Ø,3,4,7,8][Ø,1,2,]Z
Non-OR ØBPQ[3,7]YZ
Non-OR ØBPQX[Ø,1,2]Z
Non-OR ØBPT3YZ
Non-OR ØBPT[7,8][Ø,2,Y]Z
Non-OR ØBPTX[Ø,2,M]Z

Ø Medical and Surgical
B Respiratory System
Q Repair Definition: Restoring, to the extent possible, a body part to its normal anatomic structure and function
Explanation: Used only when the method to accomplish the repair is not one of the other root operations

Body Part Character 4	Approach Character 5	Device Character 6	Qualifier Character 7
1 Trachea Cricoid cartilage **2 Carina** **3 Main Bronchus, Right** Bronchus intermedius Intermediate bronchus **4 Upper Lobe Bronchus, Right** **5 Middle Lobe Bronchus, Right** **6 Lower Lobe Bronchus, Right** **7 Main Bronchus, Left** **8 Upper Lobe Bronchus, Left** **9 Lingula Bronchus** **B Lower Lobe Bronchus, Left** **C Upper Lung Lobe, Right** **D Middle Lung Lobe, Right** **F Lower Lung Lobe, Right** **G Upper Lung Lobe, Left** **H Lung Lingula** **J Lower Lung Lobe, Left** **K Lung, Right** **L Lung, Left** **M Lungs, Bilateral**	**Ø Open** **3 Percutaneous** **4 Percutaneous Endoscopic** **7 Via Natural or Artificial Opening** **8 Via Natural or Artificial Opening Endoscopic**	**Z No Device**	**Z No Qualifier**
N Pleura, Right **P Pleura, Left** **T Diaphragm**	**Ø Open** **3 Percutaneous** **4 Percutaneous Endoscopic**	**Z No Device**	**Z No Qualifier**

Ø Medical and Surgical
B Respiratory System
R Replacement Definition: Putting in or on biological or synthetic material that physically takes the place and/or function of all or a portion of a body part

Explanation: The body part may have been taken out or replaced, or may be taken out, physically eradicated, or rendered nonfunctional during the REPLACEMENT procedure. A REMOVAL procedure is coded for taking out the device used in a previous replacement procedure.

Body Part Character 4	Approach Character 5	Device Character 6	Qualifier Character 7
1 Trachea Cricoid cartilage **2 Carina** **3 Main Bronchus, Right** Bronchus intermedius Intermediate bronchus **4 Upper Lobe Bronchus, Right** **5 Middle Lobe Bronchus, Right** **6 Lower Lobe Bronchus, Right** **7 Main Bronchus, Left** **8 Upper Lobe Bronchus, Left** **9 Lingula Bronchus** **B Lower Lobe Bronchus, Left** **T Diaphragm**	**Ø Open** **4 Percutaneous Endoscopic**	**7 Autologous Tissue Substitute** **J Synthetic Substitute** **K Nonautologous Tissue Substitute**	**Z No Qualifier**

Ø Medical and Surgical
B Respiratory System
S Reposition Definition: Moving to its normal location, or other suitable location, all or a portion of a body part

Explanation: The body part is moved to a new location from an abnormal location, or from a normal location where it is not functioning correctly. The body part may or may not be cut out or off to be moved to the new location.

Body Part Character 4	Approach Character 5	Device Character 6	Qualifier Character 7
1 Trachea Cricoid cartilage **2 Carina** **3 Main Bronchus, Right** Bronchus intermedius Intermediate bronchus **4 Upper Lobe Bronchus, Right** **5 Middle Lobe Bronchus, Right** **6 Lower Lobe Bronchus, Right** **7 Main Bronchus, Left** **8 Upper Lobe Bronchus, Left** **9 Lingula Bronchus** **B Lower Lobe Bronchus, Left** **C Upper Lung Lobe, Right** **D Middle Lung Lobe, Right** **F Lower Lung Lobe, Right** **G Upper Lung Lobe, Left** **H Lung Lingula** **J Lower Lung Lobe, Left** **K Lung, Right** **L Lung, Left** **T Diaphragm**	**Ø Open**	**Z No Device**	**Z No Qualifier**

Ø Medical and Surgical
B Respiratory System
T Resection Definition: Cutting out or off, without replacement, all of a body part
Explanation: None

Body Part Character 4	Approach Character 5	Device Character 6	Qualifier Character 7
1 Trachea Cricoid cartilage **2 Carina** **3 Main Bronchus, Right** Bronchus intermedius Intermediate bronchus **4 Upper Lobe Bronchus, Right** **5 Middle Lobe Bronchus, Right** **6 Lower Lobe Bronchus, Right** **7 Main Bronchus, Left** **8 Upper Lobe Bronchus, Left** **9 Lingula Bronchus** **B Lower Lobe Bronchus, Left** **C Upper Lung Lobe, Right** **D Middle Lung Lobe, Right** **F Lower Lung Lobe, Right** **G Upper Lung Lobe, Left** **H Lung Lingula** **J Lower Lung Lobe, Left** **K Lung, Right** **L Lung, Left** **M Lungs, Bilateral** **T Diaphragm**	**Ø Open** **4 Percutaneous Endoscopic**	**Z No Device**	**Z No Qualifier**

Ø Medical and Surgical
B Respiratory System
U Supplement Definition: Putting in or on biological or synthetic material that physically reinforces and/or augments the function of a portion of a body part
Explanation: The biological material is non-living, or is living and from the same individual. The body part may have been previously replaced, and the SUPPLEMENT procedure is performed to physically reinforce and/or augment the function of the replaced body part.

Body Part Character 4	Approach Character 5	Device Character 6	Qualifier Character 7
1 Trachea Cricoid cartilage **2 Carina** **3 Main Bronchus, Right** Bronchus intermedius Intermediate bronchus **4 Upper Lobe Bronchus, Right** **5 Middle Lobe Bronchus, Right** **6 Lower Lobe Bronchus, Right** **7 Main Bronchus, Left** **8 Upper Lobe Bronchus, Left** **9 Lingula Bronchus** **B Lower Lobe Bronchus, Left**	**Ø Open** **4 Percutaneous Endoscopic** **8 Via Natural or Artificial Opening Endoscopic**	**7 Autologous Tissue Substitute** **J Synthetic Substitute** **K Nonautologous Tissue Substitute**	**Z No Qualifier**
T Diaphragm	**Ø Open** **4 Percutaneous Endoscopic**	**7 Autologous Tissue Substitute** **J Synthetic Substitute** **K Nonautologous Tissue Substitute**	**Z No Qualifier**

Ø Medical and Surgical
B Respiratory System
V Restriction Definition: Partially closing an orifice or the lumen of a tubular body part
Explanation: The orifice can be a natural orifice or an artificially created orifice

Body Part Character 4	Approach Character 5	Device Character 6	Qualifier Character 7
1 Trachea Cricoid cartilage **2 Carina** **3 Main Bronchus, Right** Bronchus intermedius Intermediate bronchus **4 Upper Lobe Bronchus, Right** **5 Middle Lobe Bronchus, Right** **6 Lower Lobe Bronchus, Right** **7 Main Bronchus, Left** **8 Upper Lobe Bronchus, Left** **9 Lingula Bronchus** **B Lower Lobe Bronchus, Left**	**Ø Open** **3 Percutaneous** **4 Percutaneous Endoscopic**	**C Extraluminal Device** **D Intraluminal Device** **Z No Device**	**Z No Qualifier**
1 Trachea Cricoid cartilage **2 Carina** **3 Main Bronchus, Right** Bronchus intermedius Intermediate bronchus **4 Upper Lobe Bronchus, Right** **5 Middle Lobe Bronchus, Right** **6 Lower Lobe Bronchus, Right** **7 Main Bronchus, Left** **8 Upper Lobe Bronchus, Left** **9 Lingula Bronchus** **B Lower Lobe Bronchus, Left**	**7 Via Natural or Artificial Opening** **8 Via Natural or Artificial Opening Endoscopic**	**D Intraluminal Device** **Z No Device**	**Z No Qualifier**

Ø Medical and Surgical
B Respiratory System
W Revision

Definition: Correcting, to the extent possible, a portion of a malfunctioning device or the position of a displaced device

Explanation: Revision can include correcting a malfunctioning or displaced device by taking out or putting in components of the device such as a screw or pin

Body Part Character 4	Approach Character 5	Device Character 6	Qualifier Character 7
Ø Tracheobronchial Tree	**Ø** Open **3** Percutaneous **4** Percutaneous Endoscopic **7** Via Natural or Artificial Opening **8** Via Natural or Artificial Opening Endoscopic	**Ø** Drainage Device **2** Monitoring Device **3** Infusion Device **7** Autologous Tissue Substitute **C** Extraluminal Device **D** Intraluminal Device **J** Synthetic Substitute **K** Nonautologous Tissue Substitute **Y** Other Device	**Z** No Qualifier
Ø Tracheobronchial Tree	**X** External	**Ø** Drainage Device **2** Monitoring Device **3** Infusion Device **7** Autologous Tissue Substitute **C** Extraluminal Device **D** Intraluminal Device **J** Synthetic Substitute **K** Nonautologous Tissue Substitute	**Z** No Qualifier
1 Trachea Cricoid cartilage	**Ø** Open **3** Percutaneous **4** Percutaneous Endoscopic **7** Via Natural or Artificial Opening **8** Via Natural or Artificial Opening Endoscopic **X** External	**Ø** Drainage Device **2** Monitoring Device **7** Autologous Tissue Substitute **C** Extraluminal Device **D** Intraluminal Device **F** Tracheostomy Device **J** Synthetic Substitute **K** Nonautologous Tissue Substitute	**Z** No Qualifier
K Lung, Right **L** Lung, Left	**Ø** Open **3** Percutaneous **4** Percutaneous Endoscopic **7** Via Natural or Artificial Opening **8** Via Natural or Artificial Opening Endoscopic	**Ø** Drainage Device **2** Monitoring Device **3** Infusion Device **Y** Other Device	**Z** No Qualifier
K Lung, Right **L** Lung, Left	**X** External	**Ø** Drainage Device **2** Monitoring Device **3** Infusion Device	**Z** No Qualifier
Q Pleura	**Ø** Open **3** Percutaneous **4** Percutaneous Endoscopic **7** Via Natural or Artificial Opening **8** Via Natural or Artificial Opening Endoscopic	**Ø** Drainage Device **2** Monitoring Device **Y** Other Device	**Z** No Qualifier
Q Pleura	**X** External	**Ø** Drainage Device **2** Monitoring Device	**Z** No Qualifier
T Diaphragm	**Ø** Open **3** Percutaneous **4** Percutaneous Endoscopic **7** Via Natural or Artificial Opening **8** Via Natural or Artificial Opening Endoscopic	**Ø** Drainage Device **2** Monitoring Device **7** Autologous Tissue Substitute **J** Synthetic Substitute **K** Nonautologous Tissue Substitute **M** Diaphragmatic Pacemaker Lead **Y** Other Device	**Z** No Qualifier
T Diaphragm	**X** External	**Ø** Drainage Device **2** Monitoring Device **7** Autologous Tissue Substitute **J** Synthetic Substitute **K** Nonautologous Tissue Substitute **M** Diaphragmatic Pacemaker Lead	**Z** No Qualifier

Non-OR ØBWØ[3,4]YZ
Non-OR ØBWØ[7,8][2,3,D,Y]Z
Non-OR ØBWØX[Ø,2,3,7,C,D,J,K]Z
Non-OR ØBW1X[Ø,2,7,C,D,F,J,K]Z
Non-OR ØBW[K,L]3YZ
Non-OR ØBW[K,L]7[Ø,2,3,Y]Z
Non-OR ØBW[K,L]8[Ø,2,3]Z
Non-OR ØBW[K,L]X[Ø,2,3]Z
Non-OR ØBWQ[Ø,3,4,7,8][Ø,2]Z
Non-OR ØBWQ[Ø,3,7]YZ
Non-OR ØBWQX[Ø,2]Z
Non-OR ØBWT[3,7,8]YZ
Non-OR ØBWTX[Ø,2,7,J,K,M]Z

Respiratory System

Ø Medical and Surgical
B Respiratory System
Y Transplantation Definition: Putting in or on all or a portion of a living body part taken from another individual or animal to physically take the place and/or function of all or a portion of a similar body part

Explanation: The native body part may or may not be taken out, and the transplanted body part may take over all or a portion of its function

Body Part Character 4	Approach Character 5	Device Character 6	Qualifier Character 7
C Upper Lung Lobe, Right LC D Middle Lung Lobe, Right LC F Lower Lung Lobe, Right LC G Upper Lung Lobe, Left LC H Lung Lingula LC J Lower Lung Lobe, Left LC K Lung, Right LC L Lung, Left LC M Lungs, Bilateral LC	Ø Open	Z No Device	Ø Allogeneic 1 Syngeneic 2 Zooplastic

LC ØBY[C,D,F,G,H,J,K,L,M]ØZ[Ø,1,2]

ØBY–ØBY

Mouth and Throat ØCØ–ØCX

Character Meanings

This Character Meaning table is provided as a guide to assist the user in the identification of character members that may be found in this section of code tables. It **SHOULD NOT** be used to build a PCS code.

Operation–Character 3		Body Part–Character 4		Approach–Character 5		Device–Character 6		Qualifier–Character 7	
Ø	Alteration	Ø	Upper Lip	Ø	Open	Ø	Drainage Device	Ø	Single
2	Change	1	Lower Lip	3	Percutaneous	1	Radioactive Element	1	Multiple
5	Destruction	2	Hard Palate	4	Percutaneous Endoscopic	5	External Fixation Device	2	All
7	Dilation	3	Soft Palate	7	Via Natural or Artificial Opening	7	Autologous Tissue Substitute	X	Diagnostic
9	Drainage	4	Buccal Mucosa	8	Via Natural or Artificial Opening Endoscopic	B	Intraluminal Device, Airway	Z	No Qualifier
B	Excision	5	Upper Gingiva	X	External	C	Extraluminal Device		
C	Extirpation	6	Lower Gingiva			D	Intraluminal Device		
D	Extraction	7	Tongue			J	Synthetic Substitute		
F	Fragmentation	8	Parotid Gland, Right			K	Nonautologous Tissue Substitute		
H	Insertion	9	Parotid Gland, Left			Y	Other Device		
J	Inspection	A	Salivary Gland			Z	No Device		
L	Occlusion	B	Parotid Duct, Right						
M	Reattachment	C	Parotid Duct, Left						
N	Release	D	Sublingual Gland, Right						
P	Removal	F	Sublingual Gland, Left						
Q	Repair	G	Submaxillary Gland, Right						
R	Replacement	H	Submaxillary Gland, Left						
S	Reposition	J	Minor Salivary Gland						
T	Resection	M	Pharynx						
U	Supplement	N	Uvula						
V	Restriction	P	Tonsils						
W	Revision	Q	Adenoids						
X	Transfer	R	Epiglottis						
		S	Larynx						
		T	Vocal Cord, Right						
		V	Vocal Cord, Left						
		W	Upper Tooth						
		X	Lower Tooth						
		Y	Mouth and Throat						

AHA Coding Clinic for table ØC9
2017, 2Q, 16 Incision and drainage of floor of mouth

AHA Coding Clinic for table ØCB
2017, 2Q, 16 Excision of floor of mouth
2016, 3Q, 28 Lingual tonsillectomy, tongue base excision and epiglottopexy
2016, 2Q, 19 Biopsy of the base of tongue
2014, 3Q, 21 Superficial parotidectomy

AHA Coding Clinic for table ØCC
2016, 2Q, 20 Sialendoscopy with stone removal

AHA Coding Clinic for table ØCH
2020, 4Q, 43-44 Insertion of radioactive element

AHA Coding Clinic for table ØCQ
2017, 1Q, 20 Preparatory nasal adhesion repair before definitive cleft palate repair

AHA Coding Clinic for table ØCR
2014, 3Q, 25 Excision of soft palate with placement of surgical obturator
2014, 2Q, 5 Oasis acellular matrix graft
2014, 2Q, 6 Composite grafting (synthetic versus nonautologous tissue substitute)

AHA Coding Clinic for table ØCS
2016, 3Q, 28 Lingual tonsillectomy, tongue base excision and epiglottopexy

AHA Coding Clinic for table ØCT
2016, 2Q, 12 Resection of malignant neoplasm of infratemporal fossa
2014, 3Q, 21 Superficial parotidectomy
2014, 3Q, 23 Le Fort I osteotomy

Salivary Glands

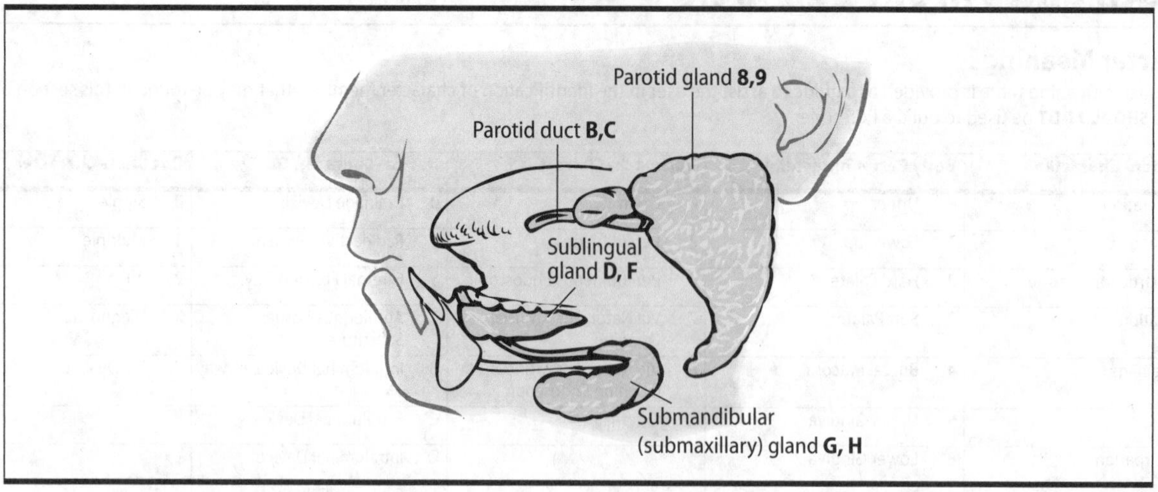

Oral Anatomy

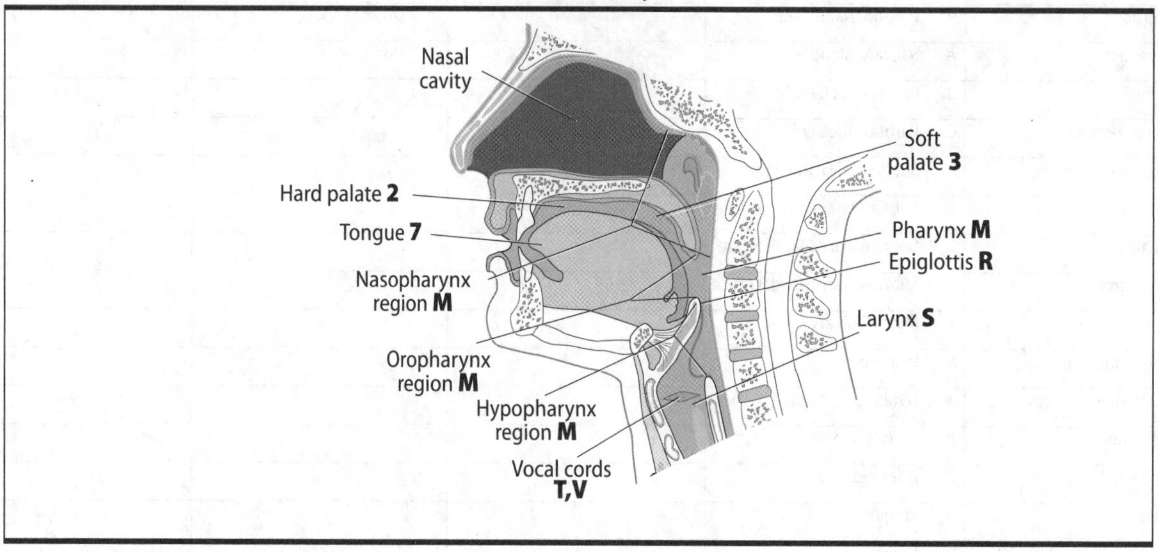

Mouth Frontal View (Upper)

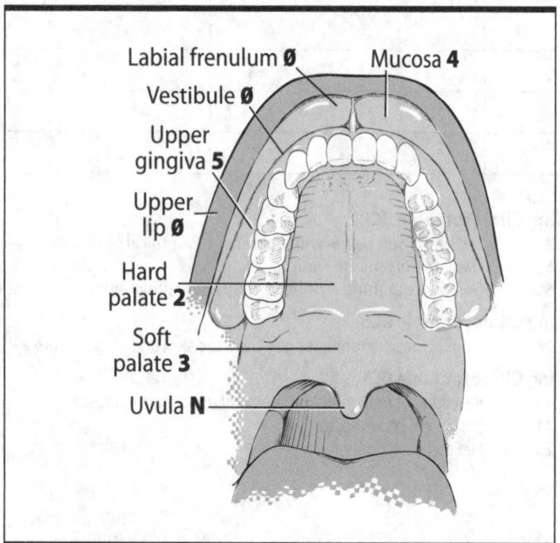

Mouth Frontal View (Lower)

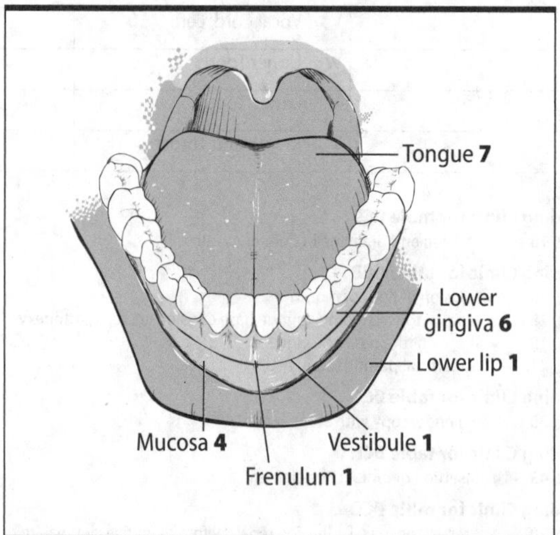

Ø Medical and Surgical
C Mouth and Throat
Ø Alteration Definition: Modifying the anatomic structure of a body part without affecting the function of the body part
Explanation: Principal purpose is to improve appearance

Body Part Character 4	Approach Character 5	Device Character 6	Qualifier Character 7
Ø Upper Lip Frenulum labii superioris Labial gland Vermilion border **1 Lower Lip** Frenulum labii inferioris Labial gland Vermilion border	**X External**	**7 Autologous Tissue Substitute** **J Synthetic Substitute** **K Nonautologous Tissue Substitute** **Z No Device**	**Z No Qualifier**

Ø Medical and Surgical
C Mouth and Throat
2 Change Definition: Taking out or off a device from a body part and putting back an identical or similar device in or on the same body part without cutting or puncturing the skin or a mucous membrane
Explanation: All CHANGE procedures are coded using the approach EXTERNAL

Body Part Character 4	Approach Character 5	Device Character 6	Qualifier Character 7
A Salivary Gland **S Larynx** Aryepiglottic fold Arytenoid cartilage Corniculate cartilage Cuneiform cartilage False vocal cord Glottis Rima glottidis Thyroid cartilage Ventricular fold **Y Mouth and Throat**	**X External**	**Ø Drainage Device** **Y Other Device**	**Z No Qualifier**

Non-OR All body part, approach, device, and qualifier values

Ø Medical and Surgical
C Mouth and Throat
5 Destruction Definition: Physical eradication of all or a portion of a body part by the direct use of energy, force, or a destructive agent

Explanation: None of the body part is physically taken out

Body Part Character 4		Approach Character 5	Device Character 6	Qualifier Character 7
Ø Upper Lip Frenulum labii superioris Labial gland Vermilion border **1 Lower Lip** Frenulum labii inferioris Labial gland Vermilion border **2 Hard Palate** **3 Soft Palate** **4 Buccal Mucosa** Buccal gland Molar gland Palatine gland	**5 Upper Gingiva** **6 Lower Gingiva** **7 Tongue** Frenulum linguae **N Uvula** Palatine uvula **P Tonsils** Palatine tonsil **Q Adenoids** Pharyngeal tonsil	**Ø Open** **3 Percutaneous** **X External**	**Z No Device**	**Z No Qualifier**
8 Parotid Gland, Right **9 Parotid Gland, Left** **B Parotid Duct, Right** Stensen's duct **C Parotid Duct, Left** *See B Parotid Duct, Right* **D Sublingual Gland, Right**	**F Sublingual Gland, Left** **G Submaxillary Gland, Right** Submandibular gland **H Submaxillary Gland, Left** *See G Submaxillary Gland, Right* **J Minor Salivary Gland** Anterior lingual gland	**Ø Open** **3 Percutaneous**	**Z No Device**	**Z No Qualifier**
M Pharynx Base of tongue Hypopharynx Laryngopharynx Lingual tonsil Oropharynx Piriform recess (sinus) Tongue, base of **R Epiglottis** Glossoepiglottic fold	**S Larynx** Aryepiglottic fold Arytenoid cartilage Corniculate cartilage Cuneiform cartilage False vocal cord Glottis Rima glottidis Thyroid cartilage Ventricular fold **T Vocal Cord, Right** Vocal fold **V Vocal Cord, Left** *See T Vocal Cord, Right*	**Ø Open** **3 Percutaneous** **4 Percutaneous Endoscopic** **7 Via Natural or Artificial Opening** **8 Via Natural or Artificial Opening Endoscopic**	**Z No Device**	**Z No Qualifier**
W Upper Tooth **X Lower Tooth**		**Ø Open** **X External**	**Z No Device**	**Ø Single** **1 Multiple** **2 All**

Non-OR ØC5[5,6][Ø,3,X]ZZ
Non-OR ØC5[W,X][Ø,X]Z[Ø,1,2]

Ø Medical and Surgical
C Mouth and Throat
7 Dilation Definition: Expanding an orifice or the lumen of a tubular body part

Explanation: The orifice can be a natural orifice or an artificially created orifice. Accomplished by stretching a tubular body part using intraluminal pressure or by cutting part of the orifice or wall of the tubular body part.

Body Part Character 4	Approach Character 5	Device Character 6	Qualifier Character 7
B Parotid Duct, Right Stensen's duct **C Parotid Duct, Left** *See B Parotid Duct, Right*	**Ø Open** **3 Percutaneous** **7 Via Natural or Artificial Opening**	**D Intraluminal Device** **Z No Device**	**Z No Qualifier**
M Pharynx Base of tongue Hypopharynx Laryngopharynx Lingual tonsil Oropharynx Piriform recess (sinus) Tongue, base of	**7 Via Natural or Artificial Opening** **8 Via Natural or Artificial Opening Endoscopic**	**D Intraluminal Device** **Z No Device**	**Z No Qualifier**
S Larynx Aryepiglottic fold Arytenoid cartilage Corniculate cartilage Cuneiform cartilage False vocal cord Glottis Rima glottidis Thyroid cartilage Ventricular fold	**Ø Open** **3 Percutaneous** **4 Percutaneous Endoscopic** **7 Via Natural or Artificial Opening** **8 Via Natural or Artificial Opening Endoscopic**	**D Intraluminal Device** **Z No Device**	**Z No Qualifier**

Non-OR ØC7[B,C][Ø,3,7][D,Z]Z
Non-OR ØC7M[7,8][D,Z]Z

Ø Medical and Surgical
C Mouth and Throat
9 Drainage Definition: Taking or letting out fluids and/or gases from a body part
Explanation: The qualifier DIAGNOSTIC is used to identify drainage procedures that are biopsies

Body Part Character 4		Approach Character 5	Device Character 6	Qualifier Character 7
Ø Upper Lip Frenulum labii superioris Labial gland Vermilion border **1 Lower Lip** Frenulum labii inferioris Labial gland Vermilion border **2 Hard Palate** **3 Soft Palate** **4 Buccal Mucosa** Buccal gland Molar gland Palatine gland	**5 Upper Gingiva** **6 Lower Gingiva** **7 Tongue** Frenulum linguae **N Uvula** Palatine uvula **P Tonsils** Palatine tonsil **Q Adenoids** Pharyngeal tonsil	**Ø Open** **3 Percutaneous** **X External**	**Ø Drainage Device**	**Z No Qualifier**
Ø Upper Lip Frenulum labii superioris Labial gland Vermilion border **1 Lower Lip** Frenulum labii inferioris Labial gland Vermilion border **2 Hard Palate** **3 Soft Palate** **4 Buccal Mucosa** Buccal gland Molar gland Palatine gland	**5 Upper Gingiva** **6 Lower Gingiva** **7 Tongue** Frenulum linguae **N Uvula** Palatine uvula **P Tonsils** Palatine tonsil **Q Adenoids** Pharyngeal tonsil	**Ø Open** **3 Percutaneous** **X External**	**Z No Device**	**X Diagnostic** **Z No Qualifier**
8 Parotid Gland, Right **9 Parotid Gland, Left** **B Parotid Duct, Right** Stensen's duct **C Parotid Duct, Left** *See B Parotid Duct, Right* **D Sublingual Gland, Right**	**F Sublingual Gland, Left** **G Submaxillary Gland, Right** Submandibular gland **H Submaxillary Gland, Left** *See G Submaxillary Gland, Right* **J Minor Salivary Gland** Anterior lingual gland	**Ø Open** **3 Percutaneous**	**Ø Drainage Device**	**Z No Qualifier**
8 Parotid Gland, Right **9 Parotid Gland, Left** **B Parotid Duct, Right** Stensen's duct **C Parotid Duct, Left** *See B Parotid Duct, Right*	**D Sublingual Gland, Right** **F Sublingual Gland, Left** **G Submaxillary Gland, Right** Submandibular gland **H Submaxillary Gland, Left** *See G Submaxillary Gland, Right* **J Minor Salivary Gland** Anterior lingual gland	**Ø Open** **3 Percutaneous**	**Z No Device**	**X Diagnostic** **Z No Qualifier**
M Pharynx Base of tongue Hypopharynx Laryngopharynx Lingual tonsil Oropharynx Piriform recess (sinus) Tongue, base of **R Epiglottis** Glossoepiglottic fold	**S Larynx** Aryepiglottic fold Arytenoid cartilage Corniculate cartilage Cuneiform cartilage False vocal cord Glottis Rima glottidis Thyroid cartilage Ventricular fold **T Vocal Cord, Right** Vocal fold **V Vocal Cord, Left** *See T Vocal Cord, Right*	**Ø Open** **3 Percutaneous** **4 Percutaneous Endoscopic** **7 Via Natural or Artificial Opening** **8 Via Natural or Artificial Opening Endoscopic**	**Ø Drainage Device**	**Z No Qualifier**

Non-OR ØC9[Ø,1,2,3,4,7,N,P,Q]3ØZ
Non-OR ØC9[5,6][Ø,3,X]ØZ
Non-OR ØC9[Ø,1,4][Ø,3,X]ZX
Non-OR ØC9[Ø,1,2,3,4,7,N,P,Q]3ZZ
Non-OR ØC9[5,6][Ø,3,X]Z[X,Z]
Non-OR ØC97[3,X]ZX
Non-OR ØC9[8,9,B,C,D,F,G,H,J][Ø,3]ØZ
Non-OR ØC9[8,9,B,C,D,F,G,H,J]3ZX
Non-OR ØC9[8,9,G,H]3ZZ
Non-OR ØC9[B,C,D, F,J][Ø,3]ZZ
Non-OR ØC9[M,R,S,T,V]3ØZ

ØC9 Continued on next page

ØC9 Continued

Ø Medical and Surgical
C Mouth and Throat
9 Drainage Definition: Taking or letting out fluids and/or gases from a body part
Explanation: The qualifier DIAGNOSTIC is used to identify drainage procedures that are biopsies

Body Part Character 4		Approach Character 5	Device Character 6	Qualifier Character 7
M Pharynx Base of tongue Hypopharynx Laryngopharynx Lingual tonsil Oropharynx Piriform recess (sinus) Tongue, base of **R Epiglottis** Glossoepiglottic fold	**S Larynx** Aryepiglottic fold Arytenoid cartilage Corniculate cartilage Cuneiform cartilage False vocal cord Glottis Rima glottidis Thyroid cartilage Ventricular fold **T Vocal Cord, Right** Vocal fold **V Vocal Cord, Left** *See T Vocal Cord, Right*	**Ø Open** **3 Percutaneous** **4 Percutaneous Endoscopic** **7 Via Natural or Artificial Opening** **8 Via Natural or Artificial Opening Endoscopic**	**Z No Device**	**X Diagnostic** **Z No Qualifier**
W Upper Tooth **X Lower Tooth**		**Ø Open** **X External**	**Ø Drainage Device** **Z No Device**	**Ø Single** **1 Multiple** **2 All**

Non-OR ØC9M[Ø,3,4,7,8]ZX
Non-OR ØC9[M,R,S,T,V]3ZZ
Non-OR ØC9[R,S,T,V][3,4,7,8]ZX
Non-OR ØC9[W,X][Ø,X][Ø,Z][Ø,1,2]

Ø Medical and Surgical
C Mouth and Throat
B Excision Definition: Cutting out or off, without replacement, a portion of a body part
Explanation: The qualifier DIAGNOSTIC is used to identify excision procedures that are biopsies

Body Part Character 4		Approach Character 5	Device Character 6	Qualifier Character 7
Ø Upper Lip Frenulum labii superioris Labial gland Vermilion border **1 Lower Lip** Frenulum labii inferioris Labial gland Vermilion border **2 Hard Palate** **3 Soft Palate** **4 Buccal Mucosa** Buccal gland Molar gland Palatine gland	**5 Upper Gingiva** **6 Lower Gingiva** **7 Tongue** Frenulum linguae **N Uvula** Palatine uvula **P Tonsils** Palatine tonsil **Q Adenoids** Pharyngeal tonsil	**Ø Open** **3 Percutaneous** **X External**	**Z No Device**	**X Diagnostic** **Z No Qualifier**
8 Parotid Gland, Right **9 Parotid Gland, Left** **B Parotid Duct, Right** Stensen's duct **C Parotid Duct, Left** *See B Parotid Duct, Right* **D Sublingual Gland, Right**	**F Sublingual Gland, Left** **G Submaxillary Gland, Right** Submandibular gland **H Submaxillary Gland, Left** *See G Submaxillary Gland, Right* **J Minor Salivary Gland** Anterior lingual gland	**Ø Open** **3 Percutaneous**	**Z No Device**	**X Diagnostic** **Z No Qualifier**
M Pharynx Base of tongue Hypopharynx Laryngopharynx Lingual tonsil Oropharynx Piriform recess (sinus) Tongue, base of **R Epiglottis** Glossoepiglottic fold	**S Larynx** Aryepiglottic fold Arytenoid cartilage Corniculate cartilage Cuneiform cartilage False vocal cord Glottis Rima glottidis Thyroid cartilage Ventricular fold **T Vocal Cord, Right** Vocal fold **V Vocal Cord, Left** *See T Vocal Cord, Right*	**Ø Open** **3 Percutaneous** **4 Percutaneous Endoscopic** **7 Via Natural or Artificial Opening** **8 Via Natural or Artificial Opening Endoscopic**	**Z No Device**	**X Diagnostic** **Z No Qualifier**
W Upper Tooth **X Lower Tooth**		**Ø Open** **X External**	**Z No Device**	**Ø Single** **1 Multiple** **2 All**

Non-OR ØCB[Ø,1,4][Ø,3,X]ZX
Non-OR ØCB[5,6][Ø,3,X]Z[X,Z]
Non-OR ØCB7[3,X]ZX
Non-OR ØCB[8,9,B,C,D,F,G,H,J]3ZX
Non-OR ØCBM[Ø,3,4,7,8]ZX
Non-OR ØCB[R,S,T,V][3,4,7,8]ZX
Non-OR ØCB[W,X][Ø,X]Z[Ø,1,2]

Ø Medical and Surgical
C Mouth and Throat
C Extirpation Definition: Taking or cutting out solid matter from a body part

Explanation: The solid matter may be an abnormal byproduct of a biological function or a foreign body; it may be imbedded in a body part or in the lumen of a tubular body part. The solid matter may or may not have been previously broken into pieces.

Body Part Character 4		Approach Character 5	Device Character 6	Qualifier Character 7
Ø Upper Lip Frenulum labii superioris Labial gland Vermilion border **1 Lower Lip** Frenulum labii inferioris Labial gland Vermilion border **2 Hard Palate** **3 Soft Palate** **4 Buccal Mucosa** Buccal gland Molar gland Palatine gland	**5 Upper Gingiva** **6 Lower Gingiva** **7 Tongue** Frenulum linguae **N Uvula** Palatine uvula **P Tonsils** Palatine tonsil **Q Adenoids** Pharyngeal tonsil	**Ø Open** **3 Percutaneous** **X External**	**Z No Device**	**Z No Qualifier**
8 Parotid Gland, Right **9 Parotid Gland, Left** **B Parotid Duct, Right** Stensen's duct **C Parotid Duct, Left** *See B Parotid Duct, Right* **D Sublingual Gland, Right**	**F Sublingual Gland, Left** **G Submaxillary Gland, Right** Submandibular gland **H Submaxillary Gland, Left** *See G Submaxillary Gland, Right* **J Minor Salivary Gland** Anterior lingual gland	**Ø Open** **3 Percutaneous**	**Z No Device**	**Z No Qualifier**
M Pharynx Base of tongue Hypopharynx Laryngopharynx Lingual tonsil Oropharynx Piriform recess (sinus) Tongue, base of **R Epiglottis** Glossoepiglottic fold	**S Larynx** Aryepiglottic fold Arytenoid cartilage Corniculate cartilage Cuneiform cartilage False vocal cord Glottis Rima glottidis Thyroid cartilage Ventricular fold **T Vocal Cord, Right** Vocal fold **V Vocal Cord, Left** *See T Vocal Cord, Right*	**Ø Open** **3 Percutaneous** **4 Percutaneous Endoscopic** **7 Via Natural or Artificial Opening** **8 Via Natural or Artificial Opening Endoscopic**	**Z No Device**	**Z No Qualifier**
W Upper Tooth **X Lower Tooth**		**Ø Open** **X External**	**Z No Device**	**Ø Single** **1 Multiple** **2 All**

Non-OR ØCC[Ø,1,2,3,4,7,N,P,Q]XZZ
Non-OR ØCC[5,6][Ø,3,X]ZZ
Non-OR ØCC[8,9,G,H]3ZZ
Non-OR ØCC[B,C,D, F,J][Ø,3]ZZ
Non-OR ØCC[M,S][7,8]ZZ
Non-OR ØCC[W,X][Ø,X]Z[Ø,1,2]

Ø Medical and Surgical
C Mouth and Throat
D Extraction Definition: Pulling or stripping out or off all or a portion of a body part by the use of force

Explanation: The qualifier DIAGNOSTIC is used to identify extraction procedures that are biopsies

Body Part Character 4	Approach Character 5	Device Character 6	Qualifier Character 7
T Vocal Cord, Right Vocal fold **V Vocal Cord, Left** *See T Vocal Cord, Right*	**Ø Open** **3 Percutaneous** **4 Percutaneous Endoscopic** **7 Via Natural or Artificial Opening** **8 Via Natural or Artificial Opening Endoscopic**	**Z No Device**	**Z No Qualifier**
W Upper Tooth **X Lower Tooth**	**X External**	**Z No Device**	**Ø Single** **1 Multiple** **2 All**

Non-OR ØCD[W,X]XZ[Ø,1,2]

Ø Medical and Surgical
C Mouth and Throat
F Fragmentation Definition: Breaking solid matter in a body part into pieces

Explanation: Physical force (e.g., manual, ultrasonic) applied directly or indirectly is used to break the solid matter into pieces. The solid matter may be an abnormal byproduct of a biological function or a foreign body. The pieces of solid matter are not taken out.

Body Part Character 4	Approach Character 5	Device Character 6	Qualifier Character 7
B Parotid Duct, Right NC Stensen's duct **C** Parotid Duct, Left NC *See B Parotid Duct, Right*	**Ø** Open **3** Percutaneous **7** Via Natural or Artificial Opening **X** External	**Z** No Device	**Z** No Qualifier

Non-OR All body part, approach, device, and qualifier values
NC ØCF[B,C]XZZ

Ø Medical and Surgical
C Mouth and Throat
H Insertion Definition: Putting in a nonbiological appliance that monitors, assists, performs, or prevents a physiological function but does not physically take the place of a body part

Explanation: None

Body Part Character 4	Approach Character 5	Device Character 6	Qualifier Character 7
7 Tongue Frenulum linguae	**Ø** Open **3** Percutaneous **X** External	**1** Radioactive Element	**Z** No Qualifier
A Salivary Gland **S** Larynx Aryepiglottic fold Arytenoid cartilage Corniculate cartilage Cuneiform cartilage False vocal cord Glottis Rima glottidis Thyroid cartilage Ventricular fold	**Ø** Open **3** Percutaneous **7** Via Natural or Artificial Opening **8** Via Natural or Artificial Opening Endoscopic	**1** Radioactive Element **Y** Other Device	**Z** No Qualifier
Y Mouth and Throat	**Ø** Open **3** Percutaneous	**1** Radioactive Element **Y** Other Device	**Z** No Qualifier
Y Mouth and Throat	**7** Via Natural or Artificial Opening **8** Via Natural or Artificial Opening Endoscopic	**1** Radioactive Element **B** Intraluminal Device, Airway **Y** Other Device	**Z** No Qualifier

Non-OR ØCH[A,S]Ø1Z
Non-OR ØCHSØYZ
Non-OR ØCH[A,S][3,7,8][1,Y]Z
Non-OR ØCHY[Ø,3][1,Y]Z
Non-OR ØCHY[7,8][1,B,Y]Z

Ø Medical and Surgical
C Mouth and Throat
J Inspection Definition: Visually and/or manually exploring a body part

Explanation: Visual exploration may be performed with or without optical instrumentation. Manual exploration may be performed directly or through intervening body layers.

Body Part Character 4	Approach Character 5	Device Character 6	Qualifier Character 7
A Salivary Gland	**Ø** Open **3** Percutaneous **X** External	**Z** No Device	**Z** No Qualifier
S Larynx Aryepiglottic fold Arytenoid cartilage Corniculate cartilage Cuneiform cartilage False vocal cord Glottis Rima glottidis Thyroid cartilage Ventricular fold **Y** Mouth and Throat	**Ø** Open **3** Percutaneous **4** Percutaneous Endoscopic **7** Via Natural or Artificial Opening **8** Via Natural or Artificial Opening Endoscopic **X** External	**Z** No Device	**Z** No Qualifier

Non-OR All body part, approach, device, and qualifier values

Ø Medical and Surgical
C Mouth and Throat
L Occlusion Definition: Completely closing an orifice or the lumen of a tubular body part
Explanation: The orifice can be a natural orifice or an artificially created orifice

Body Part Character 4	Approach Character 5	Device Character 6	Qualifier Character 7
B Parotid Duct, Right Stensen's duct **C Parotid Duct, Left** *See B Parotid Duct, Right*	**Ø Open** **3 Percutaneous** **4 Percutaneous Endoscopic**	**C Extraluminal Device** **D Intraluminal Device** **Z No Device**	**Z No Qualifier**
B Parotid Duct, Right Stensen's duct **C Parotid Duct, Left** *See B Parotid Duct, Right*	**7 Via Natural or Artificial Opening** **8 Via Natural or Artificial Opening Endoscopic**	**D Intraluminal Device** **Z No Device**	**Z No Qualifier**

Ø Medical and Surgical
C Mouth and Throat
M Reattachment Definition: Putting back in or on all or a portion of a separated body part to its normal location or other suitable location
Explanation: Vascular circulation and nervous pathways may or may not be reestablished

Body Part Character 4	Approach Character 5	Device Character 6	Qualifier Character 7
Ø Upper Lip Frenulum labii superioris Labial gland Vermilion border **1 Lower Lip** Frenulum labii inferioris Labial gland Vermilion border **3 Soft Palate** **7 Tongue** Frenulum linguae **N Uvula** Palatine uvula	**Ø Open**	**Z No Device**	**Z No Qualifier**
W Upper Tooth **X Lower Tooth**	**Ø Open** **X External**	**Z No Device**	**Ø Single** **1 Multiple** **2 All**

Non-OR ØCM[W,X][Ø,X]Z[Ø,1,2]

Ø Medical and Surgical
C Mouth and Throat
N Release Definition: Freeing a body part from an abnormal physical constraint by cutting or by the use of force
Explanation: Some of the restraining tissue may be taken out but none of the body part is taken out

Body Part Character 4	Approach Character 5	Device Character 6	Qualifier Character 7
Ø Upper Lip Frenulum labii superioris Labial gland Vermilion border **1 Lower Lip** Frenulum labii inferioris Labial gland Vermilion border **2 Hard Palate** **3 Soft Palate** **4 Buccal Mucosa** Buccal gland Molar gland Palatine gland **5 Upper Gingiva** **6 Lower Gingiva** **7 Tongue** Frenulum linguae **N Uvula** Palatine uvula **P Tonsils** Palatine tonsil **Q Adenoids** Pharyngeal tonsil	**Ø Open** **3 Percutaneous** **X External**	**Z No Device**	**Z No Qualifier**
8 Parotid Gland, Right **9 Parotid Gland, Left** **B Parotid Duct, Right** Stensen's duct **C Parotid Duct, Left** *See B Parotid Duct, Right* **D Sublingual Gland, Right** **F Sublingual Gland, Left** **G Submaxillary Gland, Right** Submandibular gland **H Submaxillary Gland, Left** *See G Submaxillary Gland, Right* **J Minor Salivary Gland** Anterior lingual gland	**Ø Open** **3 Percutaneous**	**Z No Device**	**Z No Qualifier**
M Pharynx Base of tongue Hypopharynx Laryngopharynx Lingual tonsil Oropharynx Piriform recess (sinus) Tongue, base of **R Epiglottis** Glossoepiglottic fold **S Larynx** Aryepiglottic fold Arytenoid cartilage Corniculate cartilage Cuneiform cartilage False vocal cord Glottis Rima glottidis Thyroid cartilage Ventricular fold **T Vocal Cord, Right** Vocal fold **V Vocal Cord, Left** *See T Vocal Cord, Right*	**Ø Open** **3 Percutaneous** **4 Percutaneous Endoscopic** **7 Via Natural or Artificial Opening** **8 Via Natural or Artificial Opening Endoscopic**	**Z No Device**	**Z No Qualifier**
W Upper Tooth **X Lower Tooth**	**Ø Open** **X External**	**Z No Device**	**Ø Single** **1 Multiple** **2 All**

Non-OR ØCN[Ø,1,5,6,7][Ø,3,X]ZZ
Non-OR ØCN[W,X][Ø,X]Z[Ø,1,2]

Ø Medical and Surgical
C Mouth and Throat
P Removal Definition: Taking out or off a device from a body part

Explanation: If a device is taken out and a similar device put in without cutting or puncturing the skin or mucous membrane, the procedure is coded to the root operation CHANGE. Otherwise, the procedure for taking out a device is coded to the root operation REMOVAL.

Body Part Character 4	Approach Character 5	Device Character 6	Qualifier Character 7
A Salivary Gland	Ø Open 3 Percutaneous	Ø Drainage Device C Extraluminal Device Y Other Device	Z No Qualifier
A Salivary Gland	7 Via Natural or Artificial Opening 8 Via Natural or Artificial Opening Endoscopic	Y Other Device	Z No Qualifier
S Larynx Aryepiglottic fold Arytenoid cartilage Corniculate cartilage Cuneiform cartilage False vocal cord Glottis Rima glottidis Thyroid cartilage Ventricular fold	Ø Open 3 Percutaneous 7 Via Natural or Artificial Opening 8 Via Natural or Artificial Opening Endoscopic	Ø Drainage Device 7 Autologous Tissue Substitute D Intraluminal Device J Synthetic Substitute K Nonautologous Tissue Substitute Y Other Device	Z No Qualifier
S Larynx Aryepiglottic fold Arytenoid cartilage Corniculate cartilage Cuneiform cartilage False vocal cord Glottis Rima glottidis Thyroid cartilage Ventricular fold	X External	Ø Drainage Device 7 Autologous Tissue Substitute D Intraluminal Device J Synthetic Substitute K Nonautologous Tissue Substitute	Z No Qualifier
Y Mouth and Throat	Ø Open 3 Percutaneous 7 Via Natural or Artificial Opening 8 Via Natural or Artificial Opening Endoscopic	Ø Drainage Device 1 Radioactive Element 7 Autologous Tissue Substitute D Intraluminal Device J Synthetic Substitute K Nonautologous Tissue Substitute Y Other Device	Z No Qualifier
Y Mouth and Throat	X External	Ø Drainage Device 1 Radioactive Element 7 Autologous Tissue Substitute D Intraluminal Device J Synthetic Substitute K Nonautologous Tissue Substitute	Z No Qualifier

Non-OR ØCPA[Ø,3][Ø,C,Y]Z
Non-OR ØCPA[7,8]YZ
Non-OR ØCPS3YZ
Non-OR ØCPS[7,8][Ø,D,Y]Z
Non-OR ØCPSX[Ø,7,D,J,K]Z
Non-OR ØCPY3YZ
Non-OR ØCPY[7,8][Ø,D,Y]Z
Non-OR ØCPYX[Ø,1,7,D,J,K]Z

Ø Medical and Surgical
C Mouth and Throat
Q Repair Definition: Restoring, to the extent possible, a body part to its normal anatomic structure and function
Explanation: Used only when the method to accomplish the repair is not one of the other root operations

Body Part Character 4	Approach Character 5	Device Character 6	Qualifier Character 7
Ø Upper Lip Frenulum labii superioris Labial gland Vermilion border **1 Lower Lip** Frenulum labii inferioris Labial gland Vermilion border **2 Hard Palate** **3 Soft Palate** **4 Buccal Mucosa** Buccal gland Molar gland Palatine gland **5 Upper Gingiva** **6 Lower Gingiva** **7 Tongue** Frenulum linguae **N Uvula** Palatine uvula **P Tonsils** Palatine tonsil **Q Adenoids** Pharyngeal tonsil	**Ø Open** **3 Percutaneous** **X External**	**Z No Device**	**Z No Qualifier**
8 Parotid Gland, Right **9 Parotid Gland, Left** **B Parotid Duct, Right** Stensen's duct **C Parotid Duct, Left** *See B Parotid Duct, Right* **D Sublingual Gland, Right** **F Sublingual Gland, Left** **G Submaxillary Gland, Right** Submandibular gland **H Submaxillary Gland, Left** *See G Submaxillary Gland, Right* **J Minor Salivary Gland** Anterior lingual gland	**Ø Open** **3 Percutaneous**	**Z No Device**	**Z No Qualifier**
M Pharynx Base of tongue Hypopharynx Laryngopharynx Lingual tonsil Oropharynx Piriform recess (sinus) Tongue, base of **R Epiglottis** Glossoepiglottic fold **S Larynx** Aryepiglottic fold Arytenoid cartilage Corniculate cartilage Cuneiform cartilage False vocal cord Glottis Rima glottidis Thyroid cartilage Ventricular fold **T Vocal Cord, Right** Vocal fold **V Vocal Cord, Left** *See T Vocal Cord, Right*	**Ø Open** **3 Percutaneous** **4 Percutaneous Endoscopic** **7 Via Natural or Artificial Opening** **8 Via Natural or Artificial Opening Endoscopic**	**Z No Device**	**Z No Qualifier**
W Upper Tooth **X Lower Tooth**	**Ø Open** **X External**	**Z No Device**	**Ø Single** **1 Multiple** **2 All**

Non-OR ØCQ[Ø,1,4,7]XZZ
Non-OR ØCQ[5,6][Ø,3,X]ZZ
Non-OR ØCQ[W,X][Ø,X]Z[Ø,1,2]

Ø Medical and Surgical
C Mouth and Throat
R Replacement Definition: Putting in or on biological or synthetic material that physically takes the place and/or function of all or a portion of a body part

Explanation: The body part may have been taken out or replaced, or may be taken out, physically eradicated, or rendered nonfunctional during the REPLACEMENT procedure. A REMOVAL procedure is coded for taking out the device used in a previous replacement procedure.

Body Part Character 4	Approach Character 5	Device Character 6	Qualifier Character 7
Ø Upper Lip Frenulum labii superioris Labial gland Vermilion border **1 Lower Lip** Frenulum labii inferioris Labial gland Vermilion border **2 Hard Palate** **3 Soft Palate** **4 Buccal Mucosa** Buccal gland Molar gland Palatine gland **5 Upper Gingiva** **6 Lower Gingiva** **7 Tongue** Frenulum linguae **N Uvula** Palatine uvula	**Ø Open** **3 Percutaneous** **X External**	**7 Autologous Tissue Substitute** **J Synthetic Substitute** **K Nonautologous Tissue Substitute**	**Z No Qualifier**
B Parotid Duct, Right Stensen's duct **C Parotid Duct, Left** *See B Parotid Duct, Right*	**Ø Open** **3 Percutaneous**	**7 Autologous Tissue Substitute** **J Synthetic Substitute** **K Nonautologous Tissue Substitute**	**Z No Qualifier**
M Pharynx Base of tongue Hypopharynx Laryngopharynx Lingual tonsil Oropharynx Piriform recess (sinus) Tongue, base of **R Epiglottis** Glossoepiglottic fold **S Larynx** Aryepiglottic fold Arytenoid cartilage Corniculate cartilage Cuneiform cartilage False vocal cord Glottis Rima glottidis Thyroid cartilage Ventricular fold **T Vocal Cord, Right** Vocal fold **V Vocal Cord, Left** *See T Vocal Cord, Right*	**Ø Open** **7 Via Natural or Artificial Opening** **8 Via Natural or Artificial Opening Endoscopic**	**7 Autologous Tissue Substitute** **J Synthetic Substitute** **K Nonautologous Tissue Substitute**	**Z No Qualifier**
W Upper Tooth **X Lower Tooth**	**Ø Open** **X External**	**7 Autologous Tissue Substitute** **J Synthetic Substitute** **K Nonautologous Tissue Substitute**	**Ø Single** **1 Multiple** **2 All**

Non-OR ØCR[W,X][Ø,X][7,J,K][Ø,1,2]

Ø Medical and Surgical
C Mouth and Throat
S Reposition Definition: Moving to its normal location, or other suitable location, all or a portion of a body part

Explanation: The body part is moved to a new location from an abnormal location, or from a normal location where it is not functioning correctly. The body part may or may not be cut out or off to be moved to the new location.

Body Part Character 4	Approach Character 5	Device Character 6	Qualifier Character 7
Ø Upper Lip Frenulum labii superioris Labial gland Vermilion border **1 Lower Lip** Frenulum labii inferioris Labial gland Vermilion border **2 Hard Palate** **3 Soft Palate** **7 Tongue** Frenulum linguae **N Uvula** Palatine uvula	**Ø Open** **X External**	**Z No Device**	**Z No Qualifier**
B Parotid Duct, Right Stensen's duct **C Parotid Duct, Left** *See B Parotid Duct, Right*	**Ø Open** **3 Percutaneous**	**Z No Device**	**Z No Qualifier**
R Epiglottis Glossoepiglottic fold **T Vocal Cord, Right** Vocal fold **V Vocal Cord, Left** *See T Vocal Cord, Right*	**Ø Open** **7 Via Natural or Artificial Opening** **8 Via Natural or Artificial Opening Endoscopic**	**Z No Device**	**Z No Qualifier**
W Upper Tooth **X Lower Tooth**	**Ø Open** **X External**	**5 External Fixation Device** **Z No Device**	**Ø Single** **1 Multiple** **2 All**

Non-OR ØCS[W,X][Ø,X][5,Z][Ø,1,2]

Ø Medical and Surgical
C Mouth and Throat
T Resection Definition: Cutting out or off, without replacement, all of a body part
Explanation: None

Body Part Character 4	Approach Character 5	Device Character 6	Qualifier Character 7
Ø Upper Lip Frenulum labii superioris Labial gland Vermilion border **1 Lower Lip** Frenulum labii inferioris Labial gland Vermilion border **2 Hard Palate** **3 Soft Palate** **7 Tongue** Frenulum linguae **N Uvula** Palatine uvula **P Tonsils** Palatine tonsil **Q Adenoids** Pharyngeal tonsil	**Ø Open** **X External**	**Z No Device**	**Z No Qualifier**
8 Parotid Gland, Right **9 Parotid Gland, Left** **B Parotid Duct, Right** Stensen's duct **C Parotid Duct, Left** *See B Parotid Duct, Right* **D Sublingual Gland, Right** **F Sublingual Gland, Left** **G Submaxillary Gland, Right** Submandibular gland **H Submaxillary Gland, Left** *See G Submaxillary Gland, Right* **J Minor Salivary Gland** Anterior lingual gland	**Ø Open**	**Z No Device**	**Z No Qualifier**
M Pharynx Base of tongue Hypopharynx Laryngopharynx Lingual tonsil Oropharynx Piriform recess (sinus) Tongue, base of **R Epiglottis** Glossoepiglottic fold **S Larynx** Aryepiglottic fold Arytenoid cartilage Corniculate cartilage Cuneiform cartilage False vocal cord Glottis Rima glottidis Thyroid cartilage Ventricular fold **T Vocal Cord, Right** Vocal fold **V Vocal Cord, Left** *See T Vocal Cord, Right*	**Ø Open** **4 Percutaneous Endoscopic** **7 Via Natural or Artificial Opening** **8 Via Natural or Artificial Opening Endoscopic**	**Z No Device**	**Z No Qualifier**
W Upper Tooth **X Lower Tooth**	**Ø Open**	**Z No Device**	**Ø Single** **1 Multiple** **2 All**

Non-OR ØCT[W,X]ØZ[Ø,1,2]

Ø Medical and Surgical
C Mouth and Throat
U Supplement Definition: Putting in or on biological or synthetic material that physically reinforces and/or augments the function of a portion of a body part

Explanation: The biological material is non-living, or is living and from the same individual. The body part may have been previously replaced, and the SUPPLEMENT procedure is performed to physically reinforce and/or augment the function of the replaced body part.

Body Part Character 4	Approach Character 5	Device Character 6	Qualifier Character 7
Ø Upper Lip Frenulum labii superioris Labial gland Vermilion border **1 Lower Lip** Frenulum labii inferioris Labial gland Vermilion border **2 Hard Palate** **3 Soft Palate** **4 Buccal Mucosa** Buccal gland Molar gland Palatine gland **5 Upper Gingiva** **6 Lower Gingiva** **7 Tongue** Frenulum linguae **N Uvula** Palatine uvula	**Ø Open** **3 Percutaneous** **X External**	**7 Autologous Tissue Substitute** **J Synthetic Substitute** **K Nonautologous Tissue Substitute**	**Z No Qualifier**
M Pharynx Base of tongue Hypopharynx Laryngopharynx Lingual tonsil Oropharynx Piriform recess (sinus) Tongue, base of **R Epiglottis** Glossoepiglottic fold **S Larynx** Aryepiglottic fold Arytenoid cartilage Corniculate cartilage Cuneiform cartilage False vocal cord Glottis Rima glottidis Thyroid cartilage Ventricular fold **T Vocal Cord, Right** Vocal fold **V Vocal Cord, Left** *See T Vocal Cord, Right*	**Ø Open** **7 Via Natural or Artificial Opening** **8 Via Natural or Artificial Opening Endoscopic**	**7 Autologous Tissue Substitute** **J Synthetic Substitute** **K Nonautologous Tissue Substitute**	**Z No Qualifier**

Non-OR ØCU2[Ø,3]JZ

Ø Medical and Surgical
C Mouth and Throat
V Restriction Definition: Partially closing an orifice or the lumen of a tubular body part

Explanation: The orifice can be a natural orifice or an artificially created orifice

Body Part Character 4	Approach Character 5	Device Character 6	Qualifier Character 7
B Parotid Duct, Right Stensen's duct **C Parotid Duct, Left** *See B Parotid Duct, Right*	**Ø Open** **3 Percutaneous**	**C Extraluminal Device** **D Intraluminal Device** **Z No Device**	**Z No Qualifier**
B Parotid Duct, Right Stensen's duct **C Parotid Duct, Left** *See B Parotid Duct, Right*	**7 Via Natural or Artificial Opening** **8 Via Natural or Artificial Opening Endoscopic**	**D Intraluminal Device** **Z No Device**	**Z No Qualifier**

Ø Medical and Surgical
C Mouth and Throat
W Revision

Definition: Correcting, to the extent possible, a portion of a malfunctioning device or the position of a displaced device

Explanation: Revision can include correcting a malfunctioning or displaced device by taking out or putting in components of the device such as a screw or pin

Body Part Character 4	Approach Character 5	Device Character 6	Qualifier Character 7
A Salivary Gland	Ø Open 3 Percutaneous	Ø Drainage Device C Extraluminal Device Y Other Device	Z No Qualifier
A Salivary Gland	7 Via Natural or Artificial Opening 8 Via Natural or Artificial Opening Endoscopic	Y Other Device	Z No Qualifier
A Salivary Gland	X External	Ø Drainage Device C Extraluminal Device	Z No Qualifier
S Larynx Aryepiglottic fold Arytenoid cartilage Corniculate cartilage Cuneiform cartilage False vocal cord Glottis Rima glottidis Thyroid cartilage Ventricular fold	Ø Open 3 Percutaneous 7 Via Natural or Artificial Opening 8 Via Natural or Artificial Opening Endoscopic	Ø Drainage Device 7 Autologous Tissue Substitute D Intraluminal Device J Synthetic Substitute K Nonautologous Tissue Substitute Y Other Device	Z No Qualifier
S Larynx Aryepiglottic fold Arytenoid cartilage Corniculate cartilage Cuneiform cartilage False vocal cord Glottis Rima glottidis Thyroid cartilage Ventricular fold	X External	Ø Drainage Device 7 Autologous Tissue Substitute D Intraluminal Device J Synthetic Substitute K Nonautologous Tissue Substitute	Z No Qualifier
Y Mouth and Throat	Ø Open 3 Percutaneous 7 Via Natural or Artificial Opening 8 Via Natural or Artificial Opening Endoscopic	Ø Drainage Device 1 Radioactive Element 7 Autologous Tissue Substitute D Intraluminal Device J Synthetic Substitute K Nonautologous Tissue Substitute Y Other Device	Z No Qualifier
Y Mouth and Throat	X External	Ø Drainage Device 1 Radioactive Element 7 Autologous Tissue Substitute D Intraluminal Device J Synthetic Substitute K Nonautologous Tissue Substitute	Z No Qualifier

Non-OR ØCWA[Ø,3][Ø,C,Y]Z
Non-OR ØCWA[7,8]YZ
Non-OR ØCWAX[Ø,C]Z
Non-OR ØCWS[3,7,8]YZ
Non-OR ØCWSX[Ø,7,D,J,K]Z
Non-OR ØCWYØ7Z
Non-OR ØCWY[3,7,8]YZ
Non-OR ØCWYX[Ø,1,7,D,J,K]Z

Ø Medical and Surgical
C Mouth and Throat
X Transfer Definition: Moving, without taking out, all or a portion of a body part to another location to take over the function of all or a portion of a body part

Explanation: The body part transferred remains connected to its vascular and nervous supply

Body Part Character 4	Approach Character 5	Device Character 6	Qualifier Character 7
Ø Upper Lip Frenulum labii superioris Labial gland Vermilion border **1 Lower Lip** Frenulum labii inferioris Labial gland Vermilion border **3 Soft Palate** **4 Buccal Mucosa** Buccal gland Molar gland Palatine gland **5 Upper Gingiva** **6 Lower Gingiva** **7 Tongue** Frenulum linguae	**Ø Open** **X External**	**Z No Device**	**Z No Qualifier**

Gastrointestinal System ØD1–ØDY

Character Meanings

This Character Meaning table is provided as a guide to assist the user in the identification of character members that may be found in this section of code tables. It **SHOULD NOT** be used to build a PCS code.

Operation–Character 3		Body Part–Character 4		Approach–Character 5		Device–Character 6		Qualifier–Character 7	
1	Bypass	Ø	Upper Intestinal Tract	Ø	Open	Ø	Drainage Device	Ø	Allogeneic
2	Change	1	Esophagus, Upper	3	Percutaneous	1	Radioactive Element	1	Syngeneic
5	Destruction	2	Esophagus, Middle	4	Percutaneous Endoscopic	2	Monitoring Device	2	Zooplastic
7	Dilation	3	Esophagus, Lower	7	Via Natural or Artificial Opening	3	Infusion Device	3	Vertical
8	Division	4	Esophagogastric Junction	8	Via Natural or Artificial Opening Endoscopic	7	Autologous Tissue Substitute	4	Cutaneous
9	Drainage	5	Esophagus	F	Via Natural or Artificial Opening with Percutaneous Endoscopic Assistance	B	Intraluminal Device, Airway	5	Esophagus
B	Excision	6	Stomach	X	External	C	Extraluminal Device	6	Stomach
C	Extirpation	7	Stomach, Pylorus			D	Intraluminal Device	7	Vagina
D	Extraction	8	Small Intestine			J	Synthetic Substitute	8	Small Intestine
F	Fragmentation	9	Duodenum			K	Nonautologous Tissue Substitute	9	Duodenum
H	Insertion	A	Jejunum			L	Artificial Sphincter	A	Jejunum
J	Inspection	B	Ileum			M	Stimulator Lead	B	Ileum
L	Occlusion	C	Ileocecal Valve			U	Feeding Device	E	Large Intestine
M	Reattachment	D	Lower Intestinal Tract			Y	Other Device	H	Cecum
N	Release	E	Large Intestine			Z	No Device	K	Ascending Colon
P	Removal	F	Large Intestine, Right					L	Transverse Colon
Q	Repair	G	Large Intestine, Left					M	Descending Colon
R	Replacement	H	Cecum					N	Sigmoid Colon
S	Reposition	J	Appendix					P	Rectum
T	Resection	K	Ascending Colon					Q	Anus
U	Supplement	L	Transverse Colon					X	Diagnostic
V	Restriction	M	Descending Colon					Z	No Qualifier
W	Revision	N	Sigmoid Colon						
X	Transfer	P	Rectum						
Y	Transplantation	Q	Anus						
		R	Anal Sphincter						
		U	Omentum						
		V	Mesentery						
		W	Peritoneum						

AHA Coding Clinic for table ØD1

2021, 1Q, 19	Kock pouch revision surgery
2019, 4Q, 29	Intestinal bypass
2017, 2Q, 17	Billroth II (distal gastrectomy and gastrojejunostomy)
2016, 2Q, 31	Laparoscopic biliopancreatic diversion with duodenal switch
2014, 4Q, 41	Abdominoperineal resection (APR) with flap closure of perineum and colostomy

AHA Coding Clinic for table ØD2

2019, 1Q, 26	Exchange of clogged gastrojejunostomy tube

AHA Coding Clinic for table ØD5

2017, 1Q, 34	Debulking of tumor and peritoneum ablation

AHA Coding Clinic for table ØD7

2020, 3Q, 45	Dilation versus drainage of perirectal cyst
2017, 3Q, 23	Laparoscopic pyloromyotomy
2014, 4Q, 40	Dilation of gastrojejunostomy anastomosis stricture

AHA Coding Clinic for table ØD8

2019, 2Q, 15	Reversal of Roux-en-Y bypass
2017, 3Q, 22	Laparoscopic esophagomyotomy (Heller type) and Toupet fundoplication
2017, 3Q, 23	Laparoscopic pyloromyotomy

AHA Coding Clinic for table ØD9

2020, 3Q, 45	Dilation versus drainage of perirectal cyst
2015, 2Q, 29	Insertion of nasogastric tube for drainage and feeding

AHA Coding Clinic for table ØDB

2021, 2Q, 11	Serosal injury with excision of small intestine
2021, 1Q, 20	Rectal suction biopsy
2021, 1Q, 22	Total proctocolectomy with creation of J-pouch
2019, 2Q, 15	Reversal of Roux-en-Y bypass
2019, 1Q, 3-8	Whipple procedure
2019, 1Q, 27	Excision of pelvic sidewall mass
2017, 2Q, 17	Billroth II (distal gastrectomy and gastrojejunostomy)
2017, 1Q, 16	Hepatic flexure versus transverse colon
2016, 3Q, 3-7	Stoma creation & takedown procedures
2016, 2Q, 31	Laparoscopic biliopancreatic diversion with duodenal switch
2016, 1Q, 22	Perineal proctectomy
2016, 1Q, 24	Endoscopic brush biopsy of esophagus
2014, 4Q, 40	Abdominoperineal resection (APR) with flap closure of perineum and colostomy
2014, 3Q, 28	Ileostomy takedown and parastomal hernia repair
2014, 3Q, 32	Pyloric-sparing Whipple procedure

AHA Coding Clinic for table ØDD

2021, 1Q, 20	Rectal suction biopsy
2017, 4Q, 41-42	Extraction procedures

AHA Coding Clinic for table ØDH

2020, 4Q, 43-44	Insertion of radioactive element
2020, 3Q, 43	Staged laparoscopic gastric conduit and placement of feeding tube
2019, 2Q, 18	Endoscopic wound VAC placement
2016, 3Q, 26	Insertion of gastrostomy tube
2013, 4Q,117	Percutaneous endoscopic placement of gastrostomy tube

AHA Coding Clinic for table ØDJ

2019, 1Q, 25	Laparoscopic appendectomy converted to open procedure
2019, 1Q, 25	Milking of inspissated material from ileum to colon
2017, 2Q, 15	Low anterior resection with sigmoidoscopy
2016, 2Q, 20	Capsule endoscopy of small intestine
2015, 3Q, 24	Esophagogastroduodenoscopy with epinephrine injection for control of bleeding

AHA Coding Clinic for table ØDL

2013, 4Q, 112	Endoscopic banding of esophageal varices

AHA Coding Clinic for table ØDN

2017, 4Q, 49-50	New and revised body part values - Repositioning of the intestine
2017, 1Q, 35	Lysis of omental and peritoneal adhesions
2015, 3Q, 15	Vascular ring surgery with release of esophagus and trachea
2015, 3Q, 16	Vascular ring surgery and double aortic arch

AHA Coding Clinic for table ØDP

2019, 2Q, 18	Removal of wound VAC

AHA Coding Clinic for table ØDQ

2019, 2Q, 15	Reversal of Roux-en-Y bypass
2018, 2Q, 25	Third and fourth degree obstetric lacerations
2018, 1Q, 11	Repair of internal hernia at Petersen space
2017, 3Q, 17	Posterior sagittal anorectoplasty
2016, 3Q, 3-7	Stoma creation & takedown procedures
2016, 3Q, 26	Insertion of gastrostomy tube
2016, 1Q, 7	Obstetrical perineal laceration repair
2016, 1Q, 8	Obstetrical perineal laceration repair
2014, 4Q, 20	Control of bleeding duodenal ulcer

AHA Coding Clinic for table ØDS

2019, 1Q, 30	Laparoscopic-assisted rectopexy with manual reduction of prolapse
2017, 4Q, 49-50	New and revised body part values - Repositioning of the intestine
2017, 3Q, 9	Ileocolic intussusception reduction via air enema
2017, 3Q, 17	Posterior sagittal anorectoplasty
2016, 3Q, 3-5	Stoma creation & takedown procedures

AHA Coding Clinic for table ØDT

2021, 1Q, 22	Total proctocolectomy with creation of J-pouch
2020, 4Q, 100	Robotic-assisted sigmoid colectomy with extension of incision for specimen removal
2019, 1Q, 3-8	Whipple procedure
2019, 1Q, 14	Esophagectomy with colon interposition
2017, 4Q, 49-50	New and revised body part values - Repositioning of the intestine
2014, 4Q, 40	Abdominoperineal resection (APR) with flap closure of perineum and colostomy
2014, 4Q, 42	Right colectomy with side-to-side functional end-to-end anastomosis
2014, 3Q, 6	Ileocecectomy including cecum, terminal ileum and appendix
2014, 3Q, 6	Right colectomy

AHA Coding Clinic for table ØDU

2021, 2Q, 20	Malone antegrade continence enema procedure
2021, 1Q, 22	Total proctocolectomy with creation of J-pouch
2019, 1Q, 30	Laparoscopic-assisted rectopexy with manual reduction of prolapse

AHA Coding Clinic for table ØDV

2017, 3Q, 22	Laparoscopic esophagomyotomy (Heller type) and Toupet fundoplication
2016, 2Q, 22	Esophageal lengthening Collis gastroplasty with Nissen fundoplication and hiatal hernia
2014, 3Q, 28	Laparoscopic Nissen fundoplication and diaphragmatic hernia repair

AHA Coding Clinic for table ØDW

2021, 1Q, 19	Kock pouch revision surgery
2018, 1Q, 20	Adjustment of gastric band

AHA Coding Clinic for table ØDX

2019, 4Q, 29-30	Transfer large intestine to vagina
2019, 1Q, 14	Esophagectomy with colon interposition
2017, 2Q, 18	Esophagectomy and esophagogastrectomy with cervical esophagogastrostomy
2016, 2Q, 22	Esophageal lengthening Collis gastroplasty with Nissen fundoplication and hiatal hernia
2015, 1Q, 28	Repair of bronchopleural fistula using omental pedicle graft

Upper Intestinal Tract (Ø) and Lower Intestinal Tract (D)

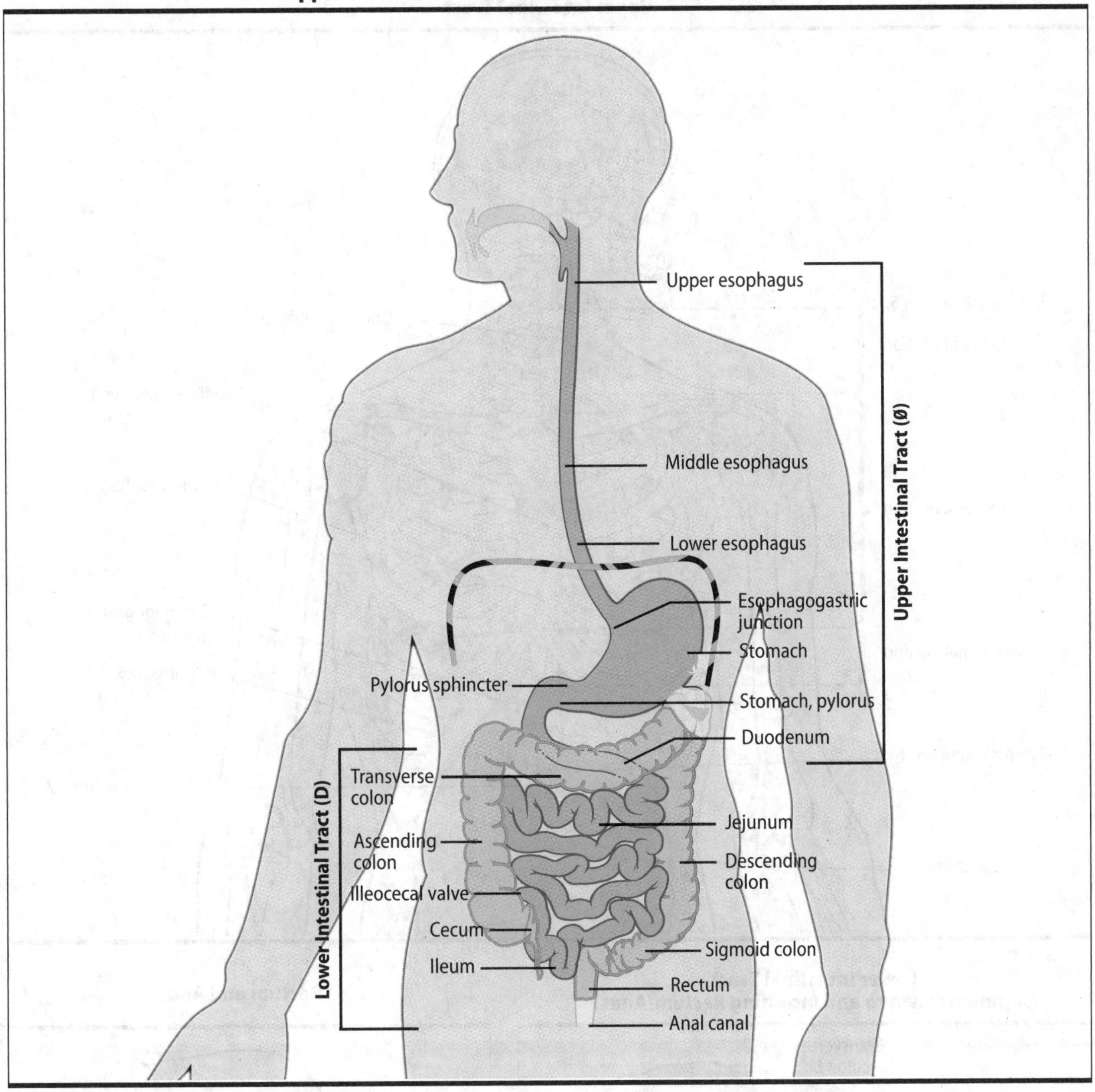

Upper Intestinal Tract

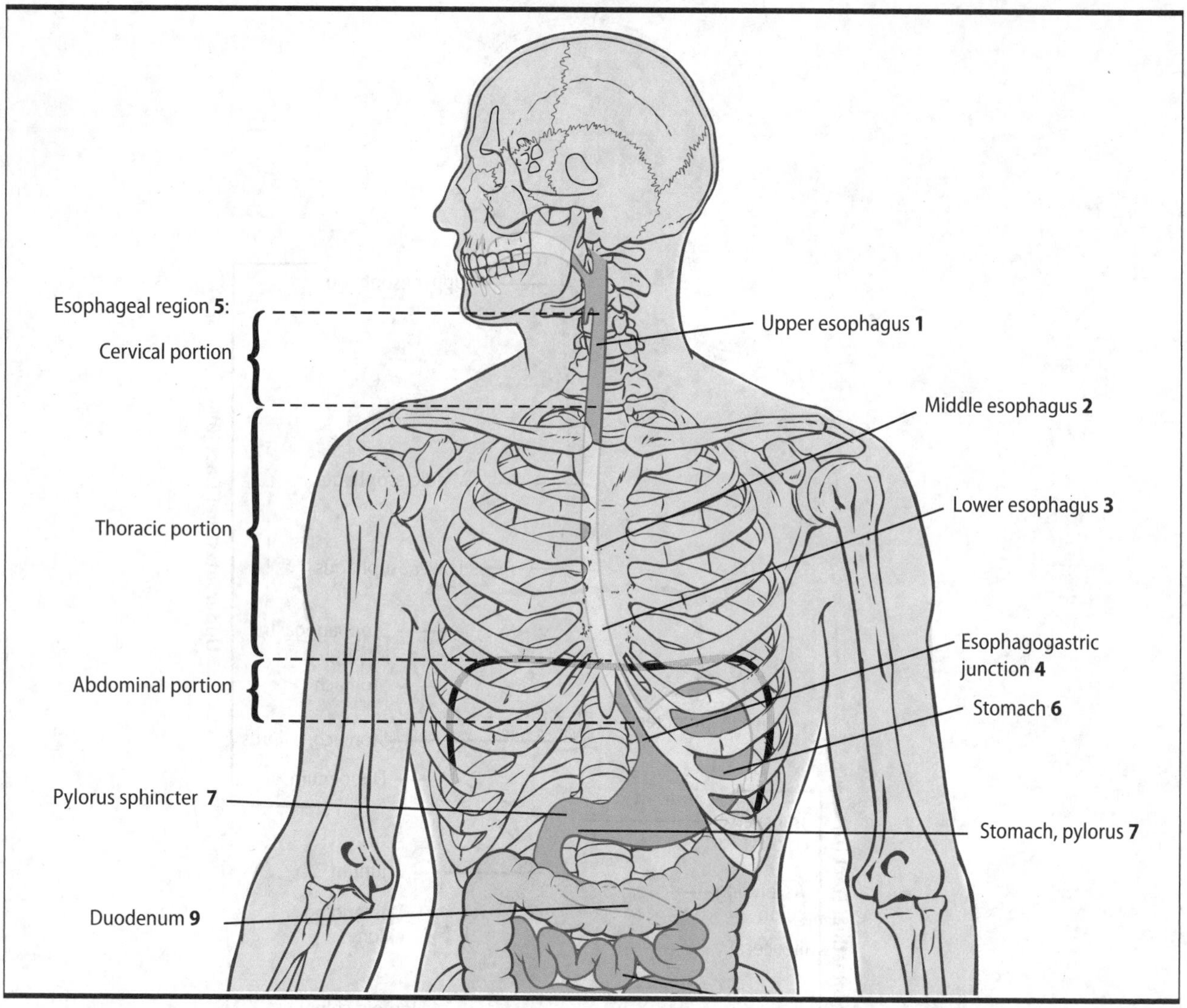

Lower Intestinal Tract (Jejunum Down to and Including Rectum/Anus)

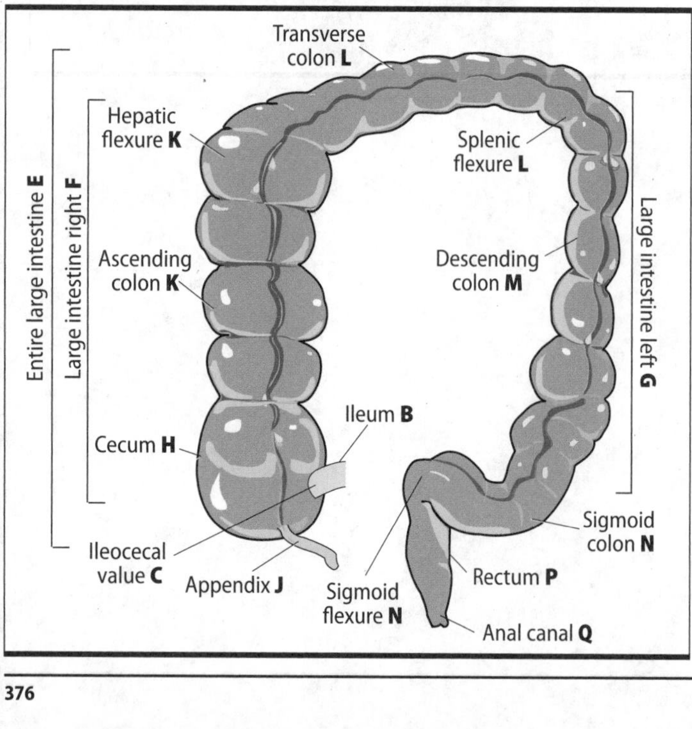

Rectum and Anus

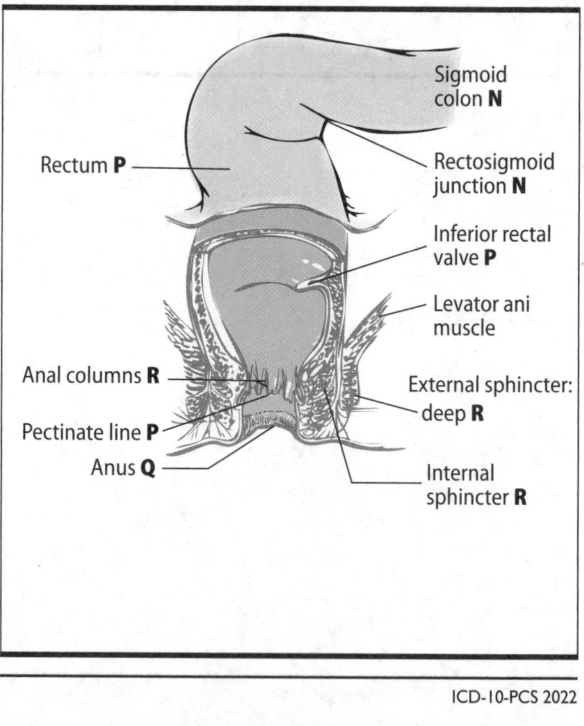

Ø Medical and Surgical
D Gastrointestinal System
1 Bypass Definition: Altering the route of passage of the contents of a tubular body part

Explanation: Rerouting contents of a body part to a downstream area of the normal route, to a similar route and body part, or to an abnormal route and dissimilar body part. Includes one or more anastomoses, with or without the use of a device.

Body Part Character 4	Approach Character 5	Device Character 6	Qualifier Character 7
1 Esophagus, Upper Cervical esophagus **2 Esophagus, Middle** Thoracic esophagus **3 Esophagus, Lower** Abdominal esophagus **5 Esophagus**	**Ø Open** **4 Percutaneous Endoscopic** **8 Via Natural or Artificial Opening Endoscopic**	**7 Autologous Tissue Substitute** **J Synthetic Substitute** **K Nonautologous Tissue Substitute** **Z No Device**	**4 Cutaneous** **6 Stomach** **9 Duodenum** **A Jejunum** **B Ileum**
1 Esophagus, Upper Cervical esophagus **2 Esophagus, Middle** Thoracic esophagus **3 Esophagus, Lower** Abdominal esophagus **5 Esophagus**	**3 Percutaneous**	**J Synthetic Substitute**	**4 Cutaneous**
6 Stomach **9 Duodenum**	**Ø Open** **4 Percutaneous Endoscopic** **8 Via Natural or Artificial Opening Endoscopic**	**7 Autologous Tissue Substitute** **J Synthetic Substitute** **K Nonautologous Tissue Substitute** **Z No Device**	**4 Cutaneous** **9 Duodenum** **A Jejunum** **B Ileum** **L Transverse Colon**
6 Stomach **9 Duodenum**	**3 Percutaneous**	**J Synthetic Substitute**	**4 Cutaneous**
8 Small Intestine	**Ø Open** **4 Percutaneous Endoscopic** **8 Via Natural or Artificial Opening Endoscopic**	**7 Autologous Tissue Substitute** **J Synthetic Substitute** **K Nonautologous Tissue Substitute** **Z No Device**	**4 Cutaneous** **8 Small Intestine** **H Cecum** **K Ascending Colon** **L Transverse Colon** **M Descending Colon** **N Sigmoid Colon** **P Rectum** **Q Anus**
A Jejunum Duodenojejunal flexure	**Ø Open** **4 Percutaneous Endoscopic** **8 Via Natural or Artificial Opening Endoscopic**	**7 Autologous Tissue Substitute** **J Synthetic Substitute** **K Nonautologous Tissue Substitute** **Z No Device**	**4 Cutaneous** **A Jejunum** **B Ileum** **H Cecum** **K Ascending Colon** **L Transverse Colon** **M Descending Colon** **N Sigmoid Colon** **P Rectum** **Q Anus**
A Jejunum Duodenojejunal flexure	**3 Percutaneous**	**J Synthetic Substitute**	**4 Cutaneous**
B Ileum	**Ø Open** **4 Percutaneous Endoscopic** **8 Via Natural or Artificial Opening Endoscopic**	**7 Autologous Tissue Substitute** **J Synthetic Substitute** **K Nonautologous Tissue Substitute** **Z No Device**	**4 Cutaneous** **B Ileum** **H Cecum** **K Ascending Colon** **L Transverse Colon** **M Descending Colon** **N Sigmoid Colon** **P Rectum** **Q Anus**
B Ileum	**3 Percutaneous**	**J Synthetic Substitute**	**4 Cutaneous**
E Large Intestine	**Ø Open** **4 Percutaneous Endoscopic** **8 Via Natural or Artificial Opening Endoscopic**	**7 Autologous Tissue Substitute** **J Synthetic Substitute** **K Nonautologous Tissue Substitute** **Z No Device**	**4 Cutaneous** **E Large Intestine** **P Rectum**
H Cecum	**Ø Open** **4 Percutaneous Endoscopic** **8 Via Natural or Artificial Opening Endoscopic**	**7 Autologous Tissue Substitute** **J Synthetic Substitute** **K Nonautologous Tissue Substitute** **Z No Device**	**4 Cutaneous** **H Cecum** **K Ascending Colon** **L Transverse Colon** **M Descending Colon** **N Sigmoid Colon** **P Rectum**
H Cecum	**3 Percutaneous**	**J Synthetic Substitute**	**4 Cutaneous**

Non-OR ØD16[Ø,4,8][7,J,K,Z]4
Non-OR ØD163J4
HAC ØD16[Ø,4,8][7,J,K,Z][9,A,B,L] when reported with PDx E66.Ø1 and SDx K68.11, K95.Ø1, K95.81 or T81.4Ø–T81.49 with 7th character A

ØD1 Continued on next page

Ø Medical and Surgical
D Gastrointestinal System
1 Bypass Definition: Altering the route of passage of the contents of a tubular body part

Explanation: Rerouting contents of a body part to a downstream area of the normal route, to a similar route and body part, or to an abnormal route and dissimilar body part. Includes one or more anastomoses, with or without the use of a device.

ØD1 Continued

Body Part Character 4	Approach Character 5	Device Character 6	Qualifier Character 7
K Ascending Colon	Ø Open 4 Percutaneous Endoscopic 8 Via Natural or Artificial Opening Endoscopic	7 Autologous Tissue Substitute J Synthetic Substitute K Nonautologous Tissue Substitute Z No Device	4 Cutaneous K Ascending Colon L Transverse Colon M Descending Colon N Sigmoid Colon P Rectum
K Ascending Colon	3 Percutaneous	J Synthetic Substitute	4 Cutaneous
L Transverse Colon Hepatic flexure Splenic flexure	Ø Open 4 Percutaneous Endoscopic 8 Via Natural or Artificial Opening Endoscopic	7 Autologous Tissue Substitute J Synthetic Substitute K Nonautologous Tissue Substitute Z No Device	4 Cutaneous L Transverse Colon M Descending Colon N Sigmoid Colon P Rectum
L Transverse Colon Hepatic flexure Splenic flexure	3 Percutaneous	J Synthetic Substitute	4 Cutaneous
M Descending Colon	Ø Open 4 Percutaneous Endoscopic 8 Via Natural or Artificial Opening Endoscopic	7 Autologous Tissue Substitute J Synthetic Substitute K Nonautologous Tissue Substitute Z No Device	4 Cutaneous M Descending Colon N Sigmoid Colon P Rectum
M Descending Colon	3 Percutaneous	J Synthetic Substitute	4 Cutaneous
N Sigmoid Colon Rectosigmoid junction Sigmoid flexure	Ø Open 4 Percutaneous Endoscopic 8 Via Natural or Artificial Opening Endoscopic	7 Autologous Tissue Substitute J Synthetic Substitute K Nonautologous Tissue Substitute Z No Device	4 Cutaneous N Sigmoid Colon P Rectum
N Sigmoid Colon Rectosigmoid junction Sigmoid flexure	3 Percutaneous	J Synthetic Substitute	4 Cutaneous

Ø Medical and Surgical
D Gastrointestinal System
2 Change Definition: Taking out or off a device from a body part and putting back an identical or similar device in or on the same body part without cutting or puncturing the skin or a mucous membrane

Explanation: All CHANGE procedures are coded using the approach EXTERNAL

Body Part Character 4	Approach Character 5	Device Character 6	Qualifier Character 7
Ø Upper Intestinal Tract D Lower Intestinal Tract	X External	Ø Drainage Device U Feeding Device Y Other Device	Z No Qualifier
U Omentum Gastrocolic ligament Gastrocolic omentum Gastrohepatic omentum Gastrophrenic ligament Gastrosplenic ligament Greater Omentum Hepatogastric ligament Lesser Omentum V Mesentery Mesoappendix Mesocolon W Peritoneum Epiploic foramen	X External	Ø Drainage Device Y Other Device	Z No Qualifier

Non-OR All body part, approach, device, and qualifier values

Ø Medical and Surgical
D Gastrointestinal System
5 Destruction Definition: Physical eradication of all or a portion of a body part by the direct use of energy, force, or a destructive agent

Explanation: None of the body part is physically taken out

Body Part Character 4	Approach Character 5	Device Character 6	Qualifier Character 7
1 Esophagus, Upper Cervical esophagus **2 Esophagus, Middle** Thoracic esophagus **3 Esophagus, Lower** Abdominal esophagus **4 Esophagogastric Junction** Cardia Cardioesophageal junction Gastroesophageal (GE) junction **5 Esophagus** **6 Stomach** **7 Stomach, Pylorus** Pyloric antrum Pyloric canal Pyloric sphincter **8 Small Intestine** **9 Duodenum** **A Jejunum** Duodenojejunal flexure **B Ileum** **C Ileocecal Valve** **E Large Intestine** **F Large Intestine, Right** **G Large Intestine, Left** **H Cecum** **J Appendix** Vermiform appendix **K Ascending Colon** **L Transverse Colon** Hepatic flexure Splenic flexure **M Descending Colon** **N Sigmoid Colon** Rectosigmoid junction Sigmoid flexure **P Rectum** Anorectal junction	**Ø Open** **3 Percutaneous** **4 Percutaneous Endoscopic** **7 Via Natural or Artificial Opening** **8 Via Natural or Artificial Opening Endoscopic**	**Z No Device**	**Z No Qualifier**
Q Anus Anal orifice	**Ø Open** **3 Percutaneous** **4 Percutaneous Endoscopic** **7 Via Natural or Artificial Opening** **8 Via Natural or Artificial Opening Endoscopic** **X External**	**Z No Device**	**Z No Qualifier**
R Anal Sphincter External anal sphincter Internal anal sphincter **U Omentum** Gastrocolic ligament Gastrocolic omentum Gastrohepatic omentum Gastrophrenic ligament Gastrosplenic ligament Greater Omentum Hepatogastric ligament Lesser Omentum **V Mesentery** Mesoappendix Mesocolon **W Peritoneum** Epiploic foramen	**Ø Open** **3 Percutaneous** **4 Percutaneous Endoscopic**	**Z No Device**	**Z No Qualifier**

Non-OR ØD5[1,2,3,4,5,6,7,9,E,F,G,H,K,L,M,N][4,8]ZZ
Non-OR ØD5[8,A,B,C]8ZZ
Non-OR ØD5P[Ø,3,4,7,8]ZZ
Non-OR ØD5Q[4,8]ZZ
Non-OR ØD5R4ZZ

Ø Medical and Surgical
D Gastrointestinal System
7 Dilation Definition: Expanding an orifice or the lumen of a tubular body part

Explanation: The orifice can be a natural orifice or an artificially created orifice. Accomplished by stretching a tubular body part using intraluminal pressure or by cutting part of the orifice or wall of the tubular body part.

Body Part Character 4	Approach Character 5	Device Character 6	Qualifier Character 7
1 Esophagus, Upper Cervical esophagus **2 Esophagus, Middle** Thoracic esophagus **3 Esophagus, Lower** Abdominal esophagus **4 Esophagogastric Junction** Cardia Cardioesophageal junction Gastroesophageal (GE) junction **5 Esophagus** **6 Stomach** **7 Stomach, Pylorus** Pyloric antrum Pyloric canal Pyloric sphincter **8 Small Intestine** **9 Duodenum** **A Jejunum** Duodenojejunal flexure **B Ileum** **C Ileocecal Valve** **E Large Intestine** **F Large Intestine, Right** **G Large Intestine, Left** **H Cecum** **K Ascending Colon** **L Transverse Colon** Hepatic flexure Splenic flexure **M Descending Colon** **N Sigmoid Colon** Rectosigmoid junction Sigmoid flexure **P Rectum** Anorectal junction **Q Anus** Anal orifice	**Ø Open** **3 Percutaneous** **4 Percutaneous Endoscopic** **7 Via Natural or Artificial Opening** **8 Via Natural or Artificial Opening Endoscopic**	**D Intraluminal Device** **Z No Device**	**Z No Qualifier**

Non-OR ØD7[1,2,3,4,5,6,8,9,A,B,C,E,F,G,H,K,L,M,N,P,Q][7,8][D,Z]Z
Non-OR ØD77[4,8]DZ
Non-OR ØD777[D,Z]Z
Non-OR ØD7[8,9,A,B,C,E,F,G,H,K,L,M,N][Ø,3,4]DZ

Ø Medical and Surgical
D Gastrointestinal System
8 Division Definition: Cutting into a body part, without draining fluids and/or gases from the body part, in order to separate or transect a body part

Explanation: All or a portion of the body part is separated into two or more portions

Body Part Character 4	Approach Character 5	Device Character 6	Qualifier Character 7
4 Esophagogastric Junction Cardia Cardioesophageal junction Gastroesophageal (GE) junction **7 Stomach, Pylorus** Pyloric antrum Pyloric canal Pyloric sphincter	**Ø Open** **3 Percutaneous** **4 Percutaneous Endoscopic** **7 Via Natural or Artificial Opening** **8 Via Natural or Artificial Opening Endoscopic**	**Z No Device**	**Z No Qualifier**
R Anal Sphincter External anal sphincter Internal anal sphincter	**Ø Open** **3 Percutaneous**	**Z No Device**	**Z No Qualifier**

Ø Medical and Surgical
D Gastrointestinal System
9 Drainage Definition: Taking or letting out fluids and/or gases from a body part
Explanation: The qualifier DIAGNOSTIC is used to identify drainage procedures that are biopsies

Body Part Character 4	Approach Character 5	Device Character 6	Qualifier Character 7
1 Esophagus, Upper Cervical esophagus **2 Esophagus, Middle** Thoracic esophagus **3 Esophagus, Lower** Abdominal esophagus **4 Esophagogastric Junction** Cardia Cardioesophageal junction Gastroesophageal (GE) junction **5 Esophagus** **6 Stomach** **7 Stomach, Pylorus** Pyloric antrum Pyloric canal Pyloric sphincter **8 Small Intestine** **9Duodenum** **A Jejunum** Duodenojejunal flexure **B Ileum** **C Ileocecal Valve** **E Large Intestine** **F Large Intestine, Right** **G Large Intestine, Left** **H Cecum** **J Appendix** Vermiform appendix **K Ascending Colon** **L Transverse Colon** Hepatic flexure Splenic flexure **M Descending Colon** **N Sigmoid Colon** Rectosigmoid junction Sigmoid flexure **P Rectum** Anorectal junction	**Ø Open** **3 Percutaneous** **4 Percutaneous Endoscopic** **7 Via Natural or Artificial Opening** **8 Via Natural or Artificial Opening Endoscopic**	**Ø Drainage Device**	**Z No Qualifier**
1 Esophagus, Upper Cervical esophagus **2 Esophagus, Middle** Thoracic esophagus **3 Esophagus, Lower** Abdominal esophagus **4 Esophagogastric Junction** Cardia Cardioesophageal junction Gastroesophageal (GE) junction **5 Esophagus** **6 Stomach** **7 Stomach, Pylorus** Pyloric antrum Pyloric canal Pyloric sphincter **8 Small Intestine** **9Duodenum** **A Jejunum** Duodenojejunal flexure **B Ileum** **C Ileocecal Valve** **E Large Intestine** **F Large Intestine, Right** **G Large Intestine, Left** **H Cecum** **J Appendix** Vermiform appendix **K Ascending Colon** **L Transverse Colon** Hepatic flexure Splenic flexure **M Descending Colon** **N Sigmoid Colon** Rectosigmoid junction Sigmoid flexure **P Rectum** Anorectal junction	**Ø Open** **3 Percutaneous** **4 Percutaneous Endoscopic** **7 Via Natural or Artificial Opening** **8 Via Natural or Artificial Opening Endoscopic**	**Z No Device**	**X Diagnostic** **Z No Qualifier**
Q Anus Anal orifice	**Ø Open** **3 Percutaneous** **4 Percutaneous Endoscopic** **7 Via Natural or Artificial Opening** **8 Via Natural or Artificial Opening Endoscopic** **X External**	**Ø Drainage Device**	**Z No Qualifier**
Q Anus Anal orifice	**Ø Open** **3 Percutaneous** **4 Percutaneous Endoscopic** **7 Via Natural or Artificial Opening** **8 Via Natural or Artificial Opening Endoscopic** **X External**	**Z No Device**	**X Diagnostic** **Z No Qualifier**

Non-OR ØD9[1,2,3,4,5,C,J]3ØZ
Non-OR ØD9[6,7,8,9,A,B,E,F,G,H,K,L,M,N,P][3,7,8]ØZ
Non-OR ØD9[1,2,3,4,5,6,7,8,9,A,B,C,E,F,G,H,K,L,M,N,P][3,4,7,8]ZX
Non-OR ØD9[1,2,3,4,5,6,7,8,9,A,B,C,E,F,G,H,J,K,L,M,N,P]3ZZ
Non-OR ØD9Q3ØZ
Non-OR ØD9Q[Ø,3,4,7,8,X]ZX
Non-OR ØD9Q3ZZ

ØD9 Continued on next page

ØD9 Continued

Ø Medical and Surgical
D Gastrointestinal System
9 Drainage Definition: Taking or letting out fluids and/or gases from a body part
Explanation: The qualifier DIAGNOSTIC is used to identify drainage procedures that are biopsies

Body Part Character 4	Approach Character 5	Device Character 6	Qualifier Character 7
R Anal Sphincter External anal sphincter Internal anal sphincter **U Omentum** Gastrocolic ligament Gastrocolic omentum Gastrohepatic omentum Gastrophrenic ligament Gastrosplenic ligament Greater Omentum Hepatogastric ligament Lesser Omentum **V Mesentery** Mesoappendix Mesocolon **W Peritoneum** Epiploic foramen	**Ø Open** **3 Percutaneous** **4 Percutaneous Endoscopic**	**Ø Drainage Device**	**Z No Qualifier**
R Anal Sphincter External anal sphincter Internal anal sphincter **U Omentum** Gastrocolic ligament Gastrocolic omentum Gastrohepatic omentum Gastrophrenic ligament Gastrosplenic ligament Greater Omentum Hepatogastric ligament Lesser Omentum **V Mesentery** Mesoappendix Mesocolon **W Peritoneum** Epiploic foramen	**Ø Open** **3 Percutaneous** **4 Percutaneous Endoscopic**	**Z No Device**	**X Diagnostic** **Z No Qualifier**

Non-OR ØD9[R,W]3ØZ
Non-OR ØD9[U,V][3,4]ØZ
Non-OR ØD9[R,U,V,W]3Z[X,Z]
Non-OR ØD9R[Ø,4]ZX
Non-OR ØD9[U,V]4ZZ

Ø Medical and Surgical
D Gastrointestinal System
B Excision Definition: Cutting out or off, without replacement, a portion of a body part
Explanation: The qualifier DIAGNOSTIC is used to identify excision procedures that are biopsies

Body Part Character 4	Approach Character 5	Device Character 6	Qualifier Character 7
1 Esophagus, Upper Cervical esophagus **2 Esophagus, Middle** Thoracic esophagus **3 Esophagus, Lower** Abdominal esophagus **4 Esophagogastric Junction** Cardia, Cardioesophageal junction, Gastroesophageal (GE) junction **5 Esophagus** **7 Stomach, Pylorus** Pyloric antrum, Pyloric canal, Pyloric sphincter **8 Small Intestine** **9 Duodenum** **A Jejunum** Duodenojejunal flexure **B Ileum** **C Ileocecal Valve** **E Large Intestine** **F Large Intestine, Right** **H Cecum** **J Appendix** Vermiform appendix **K Ascending Colon** **P Rectum** Anorectal junction	**Ø Open** **3 Percutaneous** **4 Percutaneous Endoscopic** **7 Via Natural or Artificial Opening** **8 Via Natural or Artificial Opening Endoscopic**	**Z No Device**	**X Diagnostic** **Z No Qualifier**
6 Stomach	**Ø Open** **3 Percutaneous** **4 Percutaneous Endoscopic** **7 Via Natural or Artificial Opening** **8 Via Natural or Artificial Opening Endoscopic**	**Z No Device**	**3 Vertical** **X Diagnostic** **Z No Qualifier**
G Large Intestine, Left **L Transverse Colon** Hepatic flexure, Splenic flexure **M Descending Colon** **N Sigmoid Colon** Rectosigmoid junction, Sigmoid flexure	**Ø Open** **3 Percutaneous** **4 Percutaneous Endoscopic** **7 Via Natural or Artificial Opening** **8 Via Natural or Artificial Opening Endoscopic**	**Z No Device**	**X Diagnostic** **Z No Qualifier**
G Large Intestine, Left **L Transverse Colon** Hepatic flexure, Splenic flexure **M Descending Colon** **N Sigmoid Colon** Rectosigmoid junction, Sigmoid flexure	**F Via Natural or Artificial Opening with Percutaneous Endoscopic Assistance**	**Z No Device**	**Z No Qualifier**
Q Anus Anal orifi	**Ø Open** **3 Percutaneous** **4 Percutaneous Endoscopic** **7 Via Natural or Artificial Opening** **8 Via Natural or Artificial Opening Endoscopic** **X External**	**Z No Device**	**X Diagnostic** **Z No Qualifier**
R Anal Sphincter External anal sphincter, Internal anal sphincter **U Omentum** Gastrocolic ligament, Gastrocolic omentum, Gastrohepatic omentum, Gastrophrenic ligament, Gastrosplenic ligament, Greater Omentum, Hepatogastric ligament, Lesser Omentum **V Mesentery** Mesoappendix, Mesocolon **W Peritoneum** Epiploic foramen	**Ø Open** **3 Percutaneous** **4 Percutaneous Endoscopic**	**Z No Device**	**X Diagnostic** **Z No Qualifier**

Non-OR ØDB[1,2,3,4,5,7,8,9,A,B,C,E,F,H,K,P][3,4,7,8]ZX
Non-OR ØDB[1,2,3,5,7,9][4,8]ZZ
Non-OR ØDB[4,E,F,H,K,P]8ZZ
Non-OR ØDB6[3,7]ZX
Non-OR ØDB68Z[X,Z]
Non-OR ØDB[G,L,M,N][3,4,7,8]ZX
Non-OR ØDB[G,L,M,N]8ZZ
Non-OR ØDBQ[Ø,3,4,7,8,X]ZX
Non-OR ØDBQ8ZZ
Non-OR ØDBR[Ø,3,4]ZX
Non-OR ØDB[U,V,W][3,4]ZX

Ø Medical and Surgical
D Gastrointestinal System
C Extirpation Definition: Taking or cutting out solid matter from a body part

Explanation: The solid matter may be an abnormal byproduct of a biological function or a foreign body; it may be imbedded in a body part or in the lumen of a tubular body part. The solid matter may or may not have been previously broken into pieces.

Body Part Character 4	Approach Character 5	Device Character 6	Qualifier Character 7
1 Esophagus, Upper Cervical esophagus **2 Esophagus, Middle** Thoracic esophagus **3 Esophagus, Lower** Abdominal esophagus **4 Esophagogastric Junction** Cardia Cardioesophageal junction Gastroesophageal (GE) junction **5 Esophagus** **6 Stomach** **7 Stomach, Pylorus** Pyloric antrum Pyloric canal Pyloric sphincter **8 Small Intestine** **9 Duodenum** **A Jejunum** Duodenojejunal flexure **B Ileum** **C Ileocecal Valve** **E Large Intestine** **F Large Intestine, Right** **G Large Intestine, Left** **H Cecum** **J Appendix** Vermiform appendix **K Ascending Colon** **L Transverse Colon** Hepatic flexure Splenic flexure **M Descending Colon** **N Sigmoid Colon** Rectosigmoid junction Sigmoid flexure **P Rectum** Anorectal junction	**Ø Open** **3 Percutaneous** **4 Percutaneous Endoscopic** **7 Via Natural or Artificial Opening** **8 Via Natural or Artificial Opening Endoscopic**	**Z No Device**	**Z No Qualifier**
Q Anus Anal orifice	**Ø Open** **3 Percutaneous** **4 Percutaneous Endoscopic** **7 Via Natural or Artificial Opening** **8 Via Natural or Artificial Opening Endoscopic** **X External**	**Z No Device**	**Z No Qualifier**
R Anal Sphincter External anal sphincter Internal anal sphincter **U Omentum** Gastrocolic ligament Gastrocolic omentum Gastrohepatic omentum Gastrophrenic ligament Gastrosplenic ligament Greater Omentum Hepatogastric ligament Lesser Omentum **V Mesentery** Mesoappendix Mesocolon **W Peritoneum** Epiploic foramen	**Ø Open** **3 Percutaneous** **4 Percutaneous Endoscopic**	**Z No Device**	**Z No Qualifier**

Non-OR ØDC[1,2,3,4,5,6,7,8,9,A,B,C,E,F,G,H,K,L,M,N,P][7,8]ZZ
Non-OR ØDCQ[7,8,X]ZZ

Ø Medical and Surgical
D Gastrointestinal System
D Extraction Definition: Pulling or stripping out or off all or a portion of a body part by the use of force
Explanation: The qualifier DIAGNOSTIC is used to identify extraction procedures that are biopsies

Body Part Character 4	Approach Character 5	Device Character 6	Qualifier Character 7
1 Esophagus, Upper Cervical esophagus 2 Esophagus, Middle Thoracic esophagus 3 Esophagus, Lower Abdominal esophagus 4 Esophagogastric Junction Cardia Cardioesophageal junction Gastroesophageal (GE) junction 5 Esophagus 6 Stomach 7 Stomach, Pylorus Pyloric antrum Pyloric canal Pyloric sphincter 8 Small Intestine 9 Duodenum A Jejunum Duodenojejunal flexure B Ileum C Ileocecal Valve E Large Intestine F Large Intestine, Right G Large Intestine, Left H Cecum J Appendix Vermiform appendix K Ascending Colon L Transverse Colon Hepatic flexure Splenic flexure M Descending Colon N Sigmoid Colon Rectosigmoid junction Sigmoid flexure P Rectum Anorectal junction	3 Percutaneous 4 Percutaneous Endoscopic 8 Via Natural or Artificial Opening Endoscopic	Z No Device	X Diagnostic
Q Anus Anal orifice	3 Percutaneous 4 Percutaneous Endoscopic 8 Via Natural or Artificial Opening Endoscopic X External	Z No Device	X Diagnostic

Non-OR ØDD[1,2,3,4,5,6,7,8,9,A,B,C,E,F,G,H,K,L,M,N,P][3,4,8]ZX
Non-OR ØDDQ[3,4,8,X]ZX

Ø Medical and Surgical
D Gastrointestinal System
F Fragmentation Definition: Breaking solid matter in a body part into pieces

Explanation: Physical force (e.g., manual, ultrasonic) applied directly or indirectly is used to break the solid matter into pieces. The solid matter may be an abnormal byproduct of a biological function or a foreign body. The pieces of solid matter are not taken out.

Body Part Character 4	Approach Character 5	Device Character 6	Qualifier Character 7
5 Esophagus NC 6 Stomach NC 8 Small Intestine NC 9 Duodenum NC A Jejunum NC Duodenojejunal flexure B Ileum NC E Large Intestine NC F Large Intestine, Right NC G Large Intestine, Left NC H Cecum NC J Appendix NC Vermiform appendix K Ascending Colon NC L Transverse Colon NC Hepatic flexure Splenic flexure M Descending Colon NC N Sigmoid Colon NC Rectosigmoid junction Sigmoid flexure P Rectum NC Anorectal junction Q Anus NC Anal orifice	Ø Open 3 Percutaneous 4 Percutaneous Endoscopic 7 Via Natural or Artificial Opening 8 Via Natural or Artificial Opening Endoscopic X External	Z No Device	Z No Qualifier

Non-OR ØDF[5,6,8,9,A,B,E,F,G,H,J,K,L,M,N,P,Q]XZZ
NC ØDF[5,6,8,9,A,B,E,F,G,H,J,K,L,M,N,P,Q]XZZ

Ø Medical and Surgical
D Gastrointestinal System
H Insertion Definition: Putting in a nonbiological appliance that monitors, assists, performs, or prevents a physiological function but does not physically take the place of a body part

Explanation: None

Body Part Character 4	Approach Character 5	Device Character 6	Qualifier Character 7
Ø Upper Intestinal Tract **D Lower Intestinal Tract**	**Ø Open** **3 Percutaneous** **4 Percutaneous Endoscopic** **7 Via Natural or Artificial Opening** **8 Via Natural or Artificial Opening Endoscopic**	**Y Other Device**	**Z No Qualifier**
5 Esophagus	**Ø Open** **3 Percutaneous** **4 Percutaneous Endoscopic**	**1 Radioactive Element** **2 Monitoring Device** **3 Infusion Device** **D Intraluminal Device** **U Feeding Device** **Y Other Device**	**Z No Qualifier**
5 Esophagus	**7 Via Natural or Artificial Opening** **8 Via Natural or Artificial Opening Endoscopic**	**1 Radioactive Element** **2 Monitoring Device** **3 Infusion Device** **B Intraluminal Device, Airway** **D Intraluminal Device** **U Feeding Device** **Y Other Device**	**Z No Qualifier**
6 Stomach ⊞	**Ø Open** **3 Percutaneous** **4 Percutaneous Endoscopic**	**1 Radioactive Element** **2 Monitoring Device** **3 Infusion Device** **D Intraluminal Device** **M Stimulator Lead** **U Feeding Device** **Y Other Device**	**Z No Qualifier**
6 Stomach	**7 Via Natural or Artificial Opening** **8 Via Natural or Artificial Opening Endoscopic**	**1 Radioactive Element** **2 Monitoring Device** **3 Infusion Device** **D Intraluminal Device** **U Feeding Device** **Y Other Device**	**Z No Qualifier**
8 Small Intestine **9 Duodenum** **A Jejunum** Duodenojejunal flexure **B Ileum**	**Ø Open** **3 Percutaneous** **4 Percutaneous Endoscopic** **7 Via Natural or Artificial Opening** **8 Via Natural or Artificial Opening Endoscopic**	**1 Radioactive Element** **2 Monitoring Device** **3 Infusion Device** **D Intraluminal Device** **U Feeding Device**	**Z No Qualifier**
E Large Intestine **P Rectum** Anorectal junction	**Ø Open** **3 Percutaneous** **4 Percutaneous Endoscopic** **7 Via Natural or Artificial Opening** **8 Via Natural or Artificial Opening Endoscopic**	**1 Radioactive Element** **D Intraluminal Device**	**Z No Qualifier**
Q Anus Anal orifice	**Ø Open** **3 Percutaneous** **4 Percutaneous Endoscopic**	**D Intraluminal Device** **L Artificial Sphincter**	**Z No Qualifier**
Q Anus Anal orifice	**7 Via Natural or Artificial Opening** **8 Via Natural or Artificial Opening Endoscopic**	**D Intraluminal Device**	**Z No Qualifier**
R Anal Sphincter External anal sphincter Internal anal sphincter	**Ø Open** **3 Percutaneous** **4 Percutaneous Endoscopic**	**M Stimulator Lead**	**Z No Qualifier**

Non-OR ØDH[Ø,D][Ø,3,4,7,8]YZ
Non-OR ØDH5[Ø,3,4][D,U]Z
Non-OR ØDH5[3,4]YZ
Non-OR ØDH5[7,8][2,3,B,D,U,Y]Z
Non-OR ØDH631Z
Non-OR ØDH6[3,4][U,Y]Z
Non-OR ØDH6[7,8][1,2,3,D,U,Y]Z
Non-OR ØDH[8,9,A,B][Ø,3,4,7,8][1,D,U]Z
Non-OR ØDH[8,9,A,B][7,8][2,3]Z
Non-OR ØDHE[Ø,3,4,7,8][1,D]Z
Non-OR ØDHP[Ø,3,4,7,8]DZ

See Appendix L for Procedure Combinations
⊞ ØDH6[Ø,3,4]MZ

Ø Medical and Surgical
D Gastrointestinal System
J Inspection Definition: Visually and/or manually exploring a body part

Explanation: Visual exploration may be performed with or without optical instrumentation. Manual exploration may be performed directly or through intervening body layers.

Body Part Character 4	Approach Character 5	Device Character 6	Qualifier Character 7
Ø Upper Intestinal Tract **6 Stomach** **D Lower Intestinal Tract**	**Ø Open** **3 Percutaneous** **4 Percutaneous Endoscopic** **7 Via Natural or Artificial Opening** **8 Via Natural or Artificial Opening Endoscopic** **X External**	**Z No Device**	**Z No Qualifier**
U Omentum Gastrocolic ligament Gastrocolic omentum Gastrohepatic omentum Gastrophrenic ligament Gastrosplenic ligament Greater Omentum Hepatogastric ligament Lesser Omentum **V Mesentery** Mesoappendix Mesocolon **W Peritoneum** Epiploic foramen	**Ø Open** **3 Percutaneous** **4 Percutaneous Endoscopic** **X External**	**Z No Device**	**Z No Qualifier**

Non-OR ØDJ[Ø,6,D][3,7,8,X]ZZ
Non-OR ØDJ[U,V,W][3,X]ZZ

Ø Medical and Surgical
D Gastrointestinal System
L Occlusion Definition: Completely closing an orifice or the lumen of a tubular body part
Explanation: The orifice can be a natural orifice or an artificially created orifice

Body Part Character 4		Approach Character 5	Device Character 6	Qualifier Character 7
1 Esophagus, Upper Cervical esophagus **2 Esophagus, Middle** Thoracic esophagus **3 Esophagus, Lower** Abdominal esophagus **4 Esophagogastric Junction** Cardia; Cardioesophageal junction; Gastroesophageal (GE) junction **5 Esophagus** **6 Stomach** **7 Stomach, Pylorus** Pyloric antrum; Pyloric canal; Pyloric sphincter **8 Small Intestine**	**9 Duodenum** **A Jejunum** Duodenojejunal flexure **B Ileum** **C Ileocecal Valve** **E Large Intestine** **F Large Intestine, Right** **G Large Intestine, Left** **H Cecum** **K Ascending Colon** **L Transverse Colon** Hepatic flexure; Splenic flexure **M Descending Colon** **N Sigmoid Colon** Rectosigmoid junction; Sigmoid flexure **P Rectum** Anorectal junction	**Ø Open** **3 Percutaneous** **4 Percutaneous Endoscopic**	**C Extraluminal Device** **D Intraluminal Device** **Z No Device**	**Z No Qualifier**
1 Esophagus, Upper Cervical esophagus **2 Esophagus, Middle** Thoracic esophagus **3 Esophagus, Lower** Abdominal esophagus **4 Esophagogastric Junction** Cardia; Cardioesophageal junction; Gastroesophageal (GE) junction **5 Esophagus** **6 Stomach** **7 Stomach, Pylorus** Pyloric antrum; Pyloric canal; Pyloric sphincter **8 Small Intestine**	**9 Duodenum** **A Jejunum** Duodenojejunal flexure **B Ileum** **C Ileocecal Valve** **E Large Intestine** **F Large Intestine, Right** **G Large Intestine, Left** **H Cecum** **K Ascending Colon** **L Transverse Colon** Hepatic flexure; Splenic flexure **M Descending Colon** **N Sigmoid Colon** Rectosigmoid junction; Sigmoid flexure **P Rectum** Anorectal junction	**7 Via Natural or Artificial Opening** **8 Via Natural or Artificial Opening Endoscopic**	**D Intraluminal Device** **Z No Device**	**Z No Qualifier**
Q Anus Anal orifice		**Ø Open** **3 Percutaneous** **4 Percutaneous Endoscopic** **X External**	**C Extraluminal Device** **D Intraluminal Device** **Z No Device**	**Z No Qualifier**
Q Anus Anal orifice		**7 Via Natural or Artificial Opening** **8 Via Natural or Artificial Opening Endoscopic**	**D Intraluminal Device** **Z No Device**	**Z No Qualifier**

Non-OR ØDL[1,2,3,4,5][Ø,3,4][C,D,Z]Z
Non-OR ØDL[1,2,3,4,5][7,8][D,Z]Z

Gastrointestinal System

Ø Medical and Surgical
D Gastrointestinal System
M Reattachment Definition: Putting back in or on all or a portion of a separated body part to its normal location or other suitable location
Explanation: Vascular circulation and nervous pathways may or may not be reestablished

Body Part Character 4	Approach Character 5	Device Character 6	Qualifier Character 7
5 Esophagus **6 Stomach** **8 Small Intestine** **9 Duodenum** **A Jejunum** Duodenojejunal flexure **B Ileum** **E Large Intestine** **F Large Intestine, Right** **G Large Intestine, Left** **H Cecum** **K Ascending Colon** **L Transverse Colon** Hepatic flexure Splenic flexure **M Descending Colon** **N Sigmoid Colon** Rectosigmoid junction Sigmoid flexure **P Rectum** Anorectal junction	**Ø Open** **4 Percutaneous Endoscopic**	**Z No Device**	**Z No Qualifier**

Ø Medical and Surgical
D Gastrointestinal System
N Release Definition: Freeing a body part from an abnormal physical constraint by cutting or by the use of force
Explanation: Some of the restraining tissue may be taken out but none of the body part is taken out

Body Part Character 4	Approach Character 5	Device Character 6	Qualifier Character 7
1 Esophagus, Upper Cervical esophagus **2 Esophagus, Middle** Thoracic esophagus **3 Esophagus, Lower** Abdominal esophagus **4 Esophagogastric Junction** Cardia Cardioesophageal junction Gastroesophageal (GE) junction **5 Esophagus** **6 Stomach** **7 Stomach, Pylorus** Pyloric antrum Pyloric canal Pyloric sphincter **8 Small Intestine** **9 Duodenum** **A Jejunum** Duodenojejunal flexure **B Ileum** **C Ileocecal Valve** **E Large Intestine** **F Large Intestine, Right** **G Large Intestine, Left** **H Cecum** **J Appendix** Vermiform appendix **K Ascending Colon** **L Transverse Colon** Hepatic flexure Splenic flexure **M Descending Colon** **N Sigmoid Colon** Rectosigmoid junction Sigmoid flexure **P Rectum** Anorectal junction	**Ø Open** **3 Percutaneous** **4 Percutaneous Endoscopic** **7 Via Natural or Artificial Opening** **8 Via Natural or Artificial Opening Endoscopic**	**Z No Device**	**Z No Qualifier**
Q Anus Anal orifice	**Ø Open** **3 Percutaneous** **4 Percutaneous Endoscopic** **7 Via Natural or Artificial Opening** **8 Via Natural or Artificial Opening Endoscopic** **X External**	**Z No Device**	**Z No Qualifier**
R Anal Sphincter External anal sphincter Internal anal sphincter **U Omentum** Gastrocolic ligament Gastrocolic omentum Gastrohepatic omentum Gastrophrenic ligament Gastrosplenic ligament Greater Omentum Hepatogastric ligament Lesser Omentum **V Mesentery** Mesoappendix Mesocolon **W Peritoneum** Epiploic foramen	**Ø Open** **3 Percutaneous** **4 Percutaneous Endoscopic**	**Z No Device**	**Z No Qualifier**

Non-OR ØDN[8,9,A,B,E,F,G,H,K,L,M,N][7,8]ZZ

Ø Medical and Surgical
D Gastrointestinal System
P Removal Definition: Taking out or off a device from a body part

Explanation: If a device is taken out and a similar device put in without cutting or puncturing the skin or mucous membrane, the procedure is coded to the root operation CHANGE. Otherwise, the procedure for taking out a device is coded to the root operation REMOVAL.

Body Part Character 4	Approach Character 5	Device Character 6	Qualifier Character 7
Ø Upper Intestinal Tract **D** Lower Intestinal Tract	**Ø** Open **3** Percutaneous **4** Percutaneous Endoscopic **7** Via Natural or Artificial Opening **8** Via Natural or Artificial Opening Endoscopic	**Ø** Drainage Device **2** Monitoring Device **3** Infusion Device **7** Autologous Tissue Substitute **C** Extraluminal Device **D** Intraluminal Device **J** Synthetic Substitute **K** Nonautologous Tissue Substitute **U** Feeding Device **Y** Other Device	**Z** No Qualifier
Ø Upper Intestinal Tract **D** Lower Intestinal Tract	**X** External	**Ø** Drainage Device **2** Monitoring Device **3** Infusion Device **D** Intraluminal Device **U** Feeding Device	**Z** No Qualifier
5 Esophagus	**Ø** Open **3** Percutaneous **4** Percutaneous Endoscopic	**1** Radioactive Element **2** Monitoring Device **3** Infusion Device **U** Feeding Device **Y** Other Device	**Z** No Qualifier
5 Esophagus	**7** Via Natural or Artificial Opening **8** Via Natural or Artificial Opening Endoscopic	**1** Radioactive Element **D** Intraluminal Device **Y** Other Device	**Z** No Qualifier
5 Esophagus	**X** External	**1** Radioactive Element **2** Monitoring Device **3** Infusion Device **D** Intraluminal Device **U** Feeding Device	**Z** No Qualifier
6 Stomach	**Ø** Open **3** Percutaneous **4** Percutaneous Endoscopic	**Ø** Drainage Device **2** Monitoring Device **3** Infusion Device **7** Autologous Tissue Substitute **C** Extraluminal Device **D** Intraluminal Device **J** Synthetic Substitute **K** Nonautologous Tissue Substitute **M** Stimulator Lead **U** Feeding Device **Y** Other Device	**Z** No Qualifier
6 Stomach	**7** Via Natural or Artificial Opening **8** Via Natural or Artificial Opening Endoscopic	**Ø** Drainage Device **2** Monitoring Device **3** Infusion Device **7** Autologous Tissue Substitute **C** Extraluminal Device **D** Intraluminal Device **J** Synthetic Substitute **K** Nonautologous Tissue Substitute **U** Feeding Device **Y** Other Device	**Z** No Qualifier
6 Stomach	**X** External	**Ø** Drainage Device **2** Monitoring Device **3** Infusion Device **D** Intraluminal Device **U** Feeding Device	**Z** No Qualifier

Non-OR ØDP[Ø,D][3,4]YZ
Non-OR ØDP[Ø,D][7,8][Ø,2,3,D,U,Y]Z
Non-OR ØDP[Ø,D]X[Ø,2,3,D,U]Z
Non-OR ØDP5[3,4]YZ
Non-OR ØDP5[7,8][1,D,Y]Z
Non-OR ØDP5X[1,2,3,D,U]Z
Non-OR ØDP6[3,4]YZ
Non-OR ØDP6[7,8][Ø,2,3,D,U,Y]Z
Non-OR ØDP6X[Ø,2,3,D,U]Z

ØDP Continued on next page

Ø Medical and Surgical
D Gastrointestinal System
P Removal Definition: Taking out or off a device from a body part

Explanation: If a device is taken out and a similar device put in without cutting or puncturing the skin or mucous membrane, the procedure is coded to the root operation CHANGE. Otherwise, the procedure for taking out a device is coded to the root operation REMOVAL.

ØDP Continued

Body Part Character 4	Approach Character 5	Device Character 6	Qualifier Character 7
P Rectum Anorectal junction	**Ø Open** **3 Percutaneous** **4 Percutaneous Endoscopic** **7 Via Natural or Artificial Opening** **8 Via Natural or Artificial Opening Endoscopic** **X External**	**1 Radioactive Element**	**Z No Qualifier**
Q Anus Anal orifice	**Ø Open** **3 Percutaneous** **4 Percutaneous Endoscopic** **7 Via Natural or Artificial Opening** **8 Via Natural or Artificial Opening Endoscopic**	**L Artificial Sphincter**	**Z No Qualifier**
R Anal Sphincter External anal sphincter Internal anal sphincter	**Ø Open** **3 Percutaneous** **4 Percutaneous Endoscopic**	**M Stimulator Lead**	**Z No Qualifier**
U Omentum Gastrocolic ligament Gastrocolic omentum Gastrohepatic omentum Gastrophrenic ligament Gastrosplenic ligament Greater Omentum Hepatogastric ligament Lesser Omentum **V Mesentery** Mesoappendix Mesocolon **W Peritoneum** Epiploic foramen	**Ø Open** **3 Percutaneous** **4 Percutaneous Endoscopic**	**Ø Drainage Device** **1 Radioactive Element** **7 Autologous Tissue Substitute** **J Synthetic Substitute** **K Nonautologous Tissue Substitute**	**Z No Qualifier**

Non-OR ØDPP[7,8,X]1Z

Ø Medical and Surgical
D Gastrointestinal System
Q Repair Definition: Restoring, to the extent possible, a body part to its normal anatomic structure and function
Explanation: Used only when the method to accomplish the repair is not one of the other root operations

Body Part Character 4	Approach Character 5	Device Character 6	Qualifier Character 7
1 Esophagus, Upper Cervical esophagus **2 Esophagus, Middle** Thoracic esophagus **3 Esophagus, Lower** Abdominal esophagus **4 Esophagogastric Junction** Cardia, Cardioesophageal junction, Gastroesophageal (GE) junction **5 Esophagus** **6 Stomach** **7 Stomach, Pylorus** Pyloric antrum, Pyloric canal, Pyloric sphincter **8 Small Intestine** ⊞ **9 Duodenum** ⊞ **A Jejunum** ⊞ Duodenojejunal flexure **B Ileum** ⊞ **C Ileocecal Valve** **E Large Intestine** ⊞ **F Large Intestine, Right** ⊞ **G Large Intestine, Left** ⊞ **H Cecum** ⊞ **J Appendix** Vermiform appendix **K Ascending Colon** ⊞ **L Transverse Colon** ⊞ Hepatic flexure, Splenic flexure **M Descending Colon** ⊞ **N Sigmoid Colon** ⊞ Rectosigmoid junction, Sigmoid flexure **P Rectum** Anorectal junction	**Ø Open** **3 Percutaneous** **4 Percutaneous Endoscopic** **7 Via Natural or Artificial Opening** **8 Via Natural or Artificial Opening Endoscopic**	**Z No Device**	**Z No Qualifier**
Q Anus Anal orifice	**Ø Open** **3 Percutaneous** **4 Percutaneous Endoscopic** **7 Via Natural or Artificial Opening** **8 Via Natural or Artificial Opening Endoscopic** **X External**	**Z No Device**	**Z No Qualifier**
R Anal Sphincter External anal sphincter, Internal anal sphincter **U Omentum** Gastrocolic ligament, Gastrocolic omentum, Gastrohepatic omentum, Gastrophrenic ligament, Gastrosplenic ligament, Greater Omentum, Hepatogastric ligament, Lesser Omentum **V Mesentery** Mesoappendix, Mesocolon **W Peritoneum** Epiploic foramen	**Ø Open** **3 Percutaneous** **4 Percutaneous Endoscopic**	**Z No Device**	**Z No Qualifier**

Non-OR ØDQU[Ø,3,4]ZZ

See Appendix L for Procedure Combinations
⊞ ØDQ[8,9,A,B,E,F,G,H,K,L,M,N]ØZZ

Ø Medical and Surgical
D Gastrointestinal System
R Replacement Definition: Putting in or on biological or synthetic material that physically takes the place and/or function of all or a portion of a body part

Explanation: The body part may have been taken out or replaced, or may be taken out, physically eradicated, or rendered nonfunctional during the REPLACEMENT procedure. A REMOVAL procedure is coded for taking out the device used in a previous replacement procedure.

Body Part Character 4	Approach Character 5	Device Character 6	Qualifier Character 7
5 Esophagus	**Ø Open** **4 Percutaneous Endoscopic** **7 Via Natural or Artificial Opening** **8 Via Natural or Artificial Opening Endoscopic**	**7 Autologous Tissue Substitute** **J Synthetic Substitute** **K Nonautologous Tissue Substitute**	**Z No Qualifier**
R Anal Sphincter External anal sphincter Internal anal sphincter **U Omentum** Gastrocolic ligament Gastrocolic omentum Gastrohepatic omentum Gastrophrenic ligament Gastrosplenic ligament Greater Omentum Hepatogastric ligament Lesser Omentum **V Mesentery** Mesoappendix Mesocolon **W Peritoneum** Epiploic foramen	**Ø Open** **4 Percutaneous Endoscopic**	**7 Autologous Tissue Substitute** **J Synthetic Substitute** **K Nonautologous Tissue Substitute**	**Z No Qualifier**

Ø Medical and Surgical
D Gastrointestinal System
S Reposition Definition: Moving to its normal location, or other suitable location, all or a portion of a body part

Explanation: The body part is moved to a new location from an abnormal location, or from a normal location where it is not functioning correctly. The body part may or may not be cut out or off to be moved to the new location.

Body Part Character 4	Approach Character 5	Device Character 6	Qualifier Character 7
5 Esophagus **6 Stomach** **9 Duodenum** **A Jejunum** Duodenojejunal flexure **B Ileum** **H Cecum** **K Ascending Colon** **L Transverse Colon** Hepatic flexure Splenic flexure **M Descending Colon** **N Sigmoid Colon** Rectosigmoid junction Sigmoid flexure **P Rectum** Anorectal junction **Q Anus** Anal orifice	**Ø Open** **4 Percutaneous Endoscopic** **7 Via Natural or Artificial Opening** **8 Via Natural or Artificial Opening Endoscopic** **X External**	**Z No Device**	**Z No Qualifier**
8 Small Intestine **E Large Intestine**	**Ø Open** **4 Percutaneous Endoscopic** **7 Via Natural or Artificial Opening** **8 Via Natural or Artificial Opening Endoscopic**	**Z No Device**	**Z No Qualifier**

Non-OR ØDS[5,6,9,A,B,H,K,L,M,N,P,Q]XZZ

Ø Medical and Surgical
D Gastrointestinal System
T Resection Definition: Cutting out or off, without replacement, all of a body part

Explanation: None

Body Part Character 4	Approach Character 5	Device Character 6	Qualifier Character 7
1 Esophagus, Upper Cervical esophagus **2 Esophagus, Middle** Thoracic esophagus **3 Esophagus, Lower** Abdominal esophagus **4 Esophagogastric Junction** Cardia Cardioesophageal junction Gastroesophageal (GE) junction **5 Esophagus** **6 Stomach** **7 Stomach, Pylorus** Pyloric antrum Pyloric canal Pyloric sphincter **8 Small Intestine** **9 Duodenum** ⊞ **A Jejunum** Duodenojejunal flexure **B Ileum** **C Ileocecal Valve** **E Large Intestine** **F Large Intestine, Right** **H Cecum** **J Appendix** Vermiform appendix **K Ascending Colon** **P Rectum** Anorectal junction **Q Anus** Anal orifice	**Ø Open** **4 Percutaneous Endoscopic** **7 Via Natural or Artificial Opening** **8 Via Natural or Artificial Opening Endoscopic**	**Z No Device**	**Z No Qualifier**
G Large Intestine, Left **L Transverse Colon** Hepatic flexure Splenic flexure **M Descending Colon** **N Sigmoid Colon** Rectosigmoid junction Sigmoid flexure	**Ø Open** **4 Percutaneous Endoscopic** **7 Via Natural or Artificial Opening** **8 Via Natural or Artificial Opening Endoscopic** **F Via Natural or Artificial Opening with Percutaneous Endoscopic Assistance**	**Z No Device**	**Z No Qualifier**
R Anal Sphincter External anal sphincter Internal anal sphincter **U Omentum** Gastrocolic ligament Gastrocolic omentum Gastrohepatic omentum Gastrophrenic ligament Gastrosplenic ligament Greater Omentum Hepatogastric ligament Lesser Omentum	**Ø Open** **4 Percutaneous Endoscopic**	**Z No Device**	**Z No Qualifier**

See Appendix L for Procedure Combinations
⊞ ØDT9ØZZ

Ø Medical and Surgical
D Gastrointestinal System
U Supplement Definition: Putting in or on biological or synthetic material that physically reinforces and/or augments the function of a portion of a body part

Explanation: The biological material is non-living, or is living and from the same individual. The body part may have been previously replaced, and the SUPPLEMENT procedure is performed to physically reinforce and/or augment the function of the replaced body part.

Body Part Character 4	Approach Character 5	Device Character 6	Qualifier Character 7
1 Esophagus, Upper Cervical esophagus **2 Esophagus, Middle** Thoracic esophagus **3 Esophagus, Lower** Abdominal esophagus **4 Esophagogastric Junction** Cardia, Cardioesophageal junction, Gastroesophageal (GE) junction **5 Esophagus** **6 Stomach** **7 Stomach, Pylorus** Pyloric antrum, Pyloric canal, Pyloric sphincter **8 Small Intestine** **9 Duodenum** **A Jejunum** Duodenojejunal flexure **B Ileum** **C Ileocecal Valve** **E Large Intestine** **F Large Intestine, Right** **G Large Intestine, Left** **H Cecum** **K Ascending Colon** **L Transverse Colon** Hepatic flexure, Splenic flexure **M Descending Colon** **N Sigmoid Colon** Rectosigmoid junction, Sigmoid flexure **P Rectum** Anorectal junction	**Ø Open** **4 Percutaneous Endoscopic** **7 Via Natural or Artificial Opening** **8 Via Natural or Artificial Opening Endoscopic**	**7 Autologous Tissue Substitute** **J Synthetic Substitute** **K Nonautologous Tissue Substitute**	**Z No Qualifier**
Q Anus Anal orifice	**Ø Open** **4 Percutaneous Endoscopic** **7 Via Natural or Artificial Opening** **8 Via Natural or Artificial Opening Endoscopic** **X External**	**7 Autologous Tissue Substitute** **J Synthetic Substitute** **K Nonautologous Tissue Substitute**	**Z No Qualifier**
R Anal Sphincter External anal sphincter, Internal anal sphincter **U Omentum** Gastrocolic ligament, Gastrocolic omentum, Gastrohepatic omentum, Gastrophrenic ligament, Gastrosplenic ligament, Greater Omentum, Hepatogastric ligament, Lesser Omentum **V Mesentery** Mesoappendix, Mesocolon **W Peritoneum** Epiploic foramen	**Ø Open** **4 Percutaneous Endoscopic**	**7 Autologous Tissue Substitute** **J Synthetic Substitute** **K Nonautologous Tissue Substitute**	**Z No Qualifier**

Ø Medical and Surgical
D Gastrointestinal System
V Restriction Definition: Partially closing an orifice or the lumen of a tubular body part
Explanation: The orifice can be a natural orifice or an artificially created orifice

Body Part Character 4	Approach Character 5	Device Character 6	Qualifier Character 7
1 Esophagus, Upper Cervical esophagus **2 Esophagus, Middle** Thoracic esophagus **3 Esophagus, Lower** Abdominal esophagus **4 Esophagogastric Junction** Cardia Cardioesophageal junction Gastroesophageal (GE) junction **5 Esophagus** **6 Stomach** **7 Stomach, Pylorus** Pyloric antrum Pyloric canal Pyloric sphincter **8 Small Intestine** **9 Duodenum** **A Jejunum** Duodenojejunal flexure **B Ileum** **C Ileocecal Valve** **E Large Intestine** **F Large Intestine, Right** **G Large Intestine, Left** **H Cecum** **K Ascending Colon** **L Transverse Colon** Hepatic flexure Splenic flexure **M Descending Colon** **N Sigmoid Colon** Rectosigmoid junction Sigmoid flexure **P Rectum** Anorectal junction	**Ø Open** **3 Percutaneous** **4 Percutaneous Endoscopic**	**C Extraluminal Device** **D Intraluminal Device** **Z No Device**	**Z No Qualifier**
1 Esophagus, Upper Cervical esophagus **2 Esophagus, Middle** Thoracic esophagus **3 Esophagus, Lower** Abdominal esophagus **4 Esophagogastric Junction** Cardia Cardioesophageal junction Gastroesophageal (GE) junction **5 Esophagus** **6 Stomach** NC **7 Stomach, Pylorus** Pyloric antrum Pyloric canal Pyloric sphincter **8 Small Intestine** **9 Duodenum** **A Jejunum** Duodenojejunal flexure **B Ileum** **C Ileocecal Valve** **E Large Intestine** **F Large Intestine, Right** **G Large Intestine, Left** **H Cecum** **K Ascending Colon** **L Transverse Colon** Hepatic flexure Splenic flexure **M Descending Colon** **N Sigmoid Colon** Rectosigmoid junction Sigmoid flexure **P Rectum** Anorectal junction	**7 Via Natural or Artificial Opening** **8 Via Natural or Artificial Opening Endoscopic**	**D Intraluminal Device** **Z No Device**	**Z No Qualifier**
Q Anus Anal orifice	**Ø Open** **3 Percutaneous** **4 Percutaneous Endoscopic** **X External**	**C Extraluminal Device** **D Intraluminal Device** **Z No Device**	**Z No Qualifier**
Q Anus Anal orifice	**7 Via Natural or Artificial Opening** **8 Via Natural or Artificial Opening Endoscopic**	**D Intraluminal Device** **Z No Device**	**Z No Qualifier**

Non-OR ØDV6[7,8]DZ
HAC ØDV64CZ when reported with PDx E66.Ø1 and SDx K68.11, K95.Ø1, K95.81, or T81.4Ø–T81.49 with 7th character A
NC ØDV6[7,8]DZ

Ø Medical and Surgical
D Gastrointestinal System
W Revision Definition: Correcting, to the extent possible, a portion of a malfunctioning device or the position of a displaced device

Explanation: Revision can include correcting a malfunctioning or displaced device by taking out or putting in components of the device such as a screw or pin

Body Part Character 4	Approach Character 5	Device Character 6	Qualifier Character 7
Ø Upper Intestinal Tract D Lower Intestinal Tract	Ø Open 3 Percutaneous 4 Percutaneous Endoscopic 7 Via Natural or Artificial Opening 8 Via Natural or Artificial Opening Endoscopic	Ø Drainage Device 2 Monitoring Device 3 Infusion Device 7 Autologous Tissue Substitute C Extraluminal Device D Intraluminal Device J Synthetic Substitute K Nonautologous Tissue Substitute U Feeding Device Y Other Device	Z No Qualifier
Ø Upper Intestinal Tract D Lower Intestinal Tract	X External	Ø Drainage Device 2 Monitoring Device 3 Infusion Device 7 Autologous Tissue Substitute C Extraluminal Device D Intraluminal Device J Synthetic Substitute K Nonautologous Tissue Substitute U Feeding Device	Z No Qualifier
5 Esophagus	Ø Open 3 Percutaneous 4 Percutaneous Endoscopic	Y Other Device	Z No Qualifier
5 Esophagus	7 Via Natural or Artificial Opening 8 Via Natural or Artificial Opening Endoscopic	D Intraluminal Device Y Other Device	Z No Qualifier
5 Esophagus	X External	D Intraluminal Device	Z No Qualifier
6 Stomach	Ø Open 3 Percutaneous 4 Percutaneous Endoscopic	Ø Drainage Device 2 Monitoring Device 3 Infusion Device 7 Autologous Tissue Substitute C Extraluminal Device D Intraluminal Device J Synthetic Substitute K Nonautologous Tissue Substitute M Stimulator Lead U Feeding Device Y Other Device	Z No Qualifier
6 Stomach	7 Via Natural or Artificial Opening 8 Via Natural or Artificial Opening Endoscopic	Ø Drainage Device 2 Monitoring Device 3 Infusion Device 7 Autologous Tissue Substitute C Extraluminal Device D Intraluminal Device J Synthetic Substitute K Nonautologous Tissue Substitute U Feeding Device Y Other Device	Z No Qualifier
6 Stomach	X External	Ø Drainage Device 2 Monitoring Device 3 Infusion Device 7 Autologous Tissue Substitute C Extraluminal Device D Intraluminal Device J Synthetic Substitute K Nonautologous Tissue Substitute U Feeding Device	Z No Qualifier

Non-OR ØDW[Ø,D][3,4,7,8]YZ
Non-OR ØDW[Ø,D]8UZ
Non-OR ØDW[Ø,D]X[Ø,2,3,7,C,D,J,K,U]Z
Non-OR ØDW5[Ø,3,4]YZ
Non-OR ØDW5[7,8]YZ
Non-OR ØDW5XDZ
Non-OR ØDW6[3,4]YZ
Non-OR ØDW68UZ
Non-OR ØDW6[7,8]YZ
Non-OR ØDW6X[Ø,2,3,7,C,D,J,K,U]Z

ØDW Continued on next page

ØDW Continued

Ø Medical and Surgical
D Gastrointestinal System
W Revision Definition: Correcting, to the extent possible, a portion of a malfunctioning device or the position of a displaced device

Explanation: Revision can include correcting a malfunctioning or displaced device by taking out or putting in components of the device such as a screw or pin

Body Part Character 4	Approach Character 5	Device Character 6	Qualifier Character 7
8 Small Intestine E Large Intestine	Ø Open 4 Percutaneous Endoscopic 7 Via Natural or Artificial Opening 8 Via Natural or Artificial Opening Endoscopic	7 Autologous Tissue Substitute J Synthetic Substitute K Nonautologous Tissue Substitute	Z No Qualifier
Q Anus Anal orifice	Ø Open 3 Percutaneous 4 Percutaneous Endoscopic 7 Via Natural or Artificial Opening 8 Via Natural or Artificial Opening Endoscopic	L Artificial Sphincter	Z No Qualifier
R Anal Sphincter External anal sphincter Internal anal sphincter	Ø Open 3 Percutaneous 4 Percutaneous Endoscopic	M Stimulator Lead	Z No Qualifier
U Omentum Gastrocolic ligament Gastrocolic omentum Gastrohepatic omentum Gastrophrenic ligament Gastrosplenic ligament Greater Omentum Hepatogastric ligament Lesser Omentum V Mesentery Mesoappendix Mesocolon W Peritoneum Epiploic foramen	Ø Open 3 Percutaneous 4 Percutaneous Endoscopic	Ø Drainage Device 7 Autologous Tissue Substitute J Synthetic Substitute K Nonautologous Tissue Substitute	Z No Qualifier

Non-OR ØDW[U,V,W][Ø,3,4]ØZ

Ø Medical and Surgical
D Gastrointestinal System
X Transfer Definition: Moving, without taking out, all or a portion of a body part to another location to take over the function of all or a portion of a body part

Explanation: The body part transferred remains connected to its vascular and nervous supply

Body Part Character 4	Approach Character 5	Device Character 6	Qualifier Character 7
6 Stomach 8 Small Intestine	Ø Open 4 Percutaneous Endoscopic	Z No Device	5 Esophagus
E Large Intestine	Ø Open 4 Percutaneous Endoscopic	Z No Device	5 Esophagus 7 Vagina ♀

♀ ØDXE[Ø,4]Z7

Ø Medical and Surgical
D Gastrointestinal System
Y Transplantation Definition: Putting in or on all or a portion of a living body part taken from another individual or animal to physically take the place and/or function of all or a portion of a similar body part

Explanation: The native body part may or may not be taken out, and the transplanted body part may take over all or a portion of its function

Body Part Character 4	Approach Character 5	Device Character 6	Qualifier Character 7
5 Esophagus 6 Stomach 8 Small Intestine LC E Large Intestine LC	Ø Open	Z No Device	Ø Allogeneic 1 Syngeneic 2 Zooplastic

Non-OR ØDY5ØZ[Ø,1,2]
LC ØDY[8,E]ØZ[Ø,1,2]

Hepatobiliary System and Pancreas ØF1–ØFY

Character Meanings

This Character Meaning table is provided as a guide to assist the user in the identification of character members that may be found in this section of code tables. It **SHOULD NOT** be used to build a PCS code.

Operation–Character 3	Body Part–Character 4	Approach–Character 5	Device–Character 6	Qualifier–Character 7
1 Bypass	Ø Liver	Ø Open	Ø Drainage Device	Ø Allogeneic
2 Change	1 Liver, Right Lobe	3 Percutaneous	1 Radioactive Element	1 Syngeneic
5 Destruction	2 Liver, Left Lobe	4 Percutaneous Endoscopic	2 Monitoring Device	2 Zooplastic
7 Dilation	4 Gallbladder	7 Via Natural or Artificial Opening	3 Infusion Device	3 Duodenum
8 Division	5 Hepatic Duct, Right	8 Via Natural or Artificial Opening Endoscopic	7 Autologous Tissue Substitute	4 Stomach
9 Drainage	6 Hepatic Duct, Left	X External	C Extraluminal Device	5 Hepatic Duct, Right
B Excision	7 Hepatic Duct, Common		D Intraluminal Device	6 Hepatic Duct, Left
C Extirpation	8 Cystic Duct		J Synthetic Substitute	7 Hepatic Duct, Caudate
D Extraction	9 Common Bile Duct		K Nonautologous Tissue Substitute	8 Cystic Duct
F Fragmentation	B Hepatobiliary Duct		Y Other Device	9 Common Bile Duct
H Insertion	C Ampulla of Vater		Z No Device	B Small Intestine
J Inspection	D Pancreatic Duct			C Large Intestine
L Occlusion	F Pancreatic Duct, Accessory			F Irreversible Electroporation
M Reattachment	G Pancreas			X Diagnostic
N Release				Z No Qualifier
P Removal				
Q Repair				
R Replacement				
S Reposition				
T Resection				
U Supplement				
V Restriction				
W Revision				
Y Transplantation				

AHA Coding Clinic for table ØF1
2020, 4Q, 53 Bypass pancreatic duct to stomach

AHA Coding Clinic for table ØF5
2018, 4Q, 39 Irreversible electroporation

AHA Coding Clinic for table ØF7
2016, 3Q, 27 Endoscopic retrograde cholangiopancreatography with sphincterotomy and insertion of pancreatic stent
2016, 1Q, 25 Endoscopic retrograde cholangiopancreatography with brush biopsy of pancreatic and common bile ducts
2015, 1Q, 32 Percutaneous transhepatic biliary drainage catheter placement
2014, 3Q, 15 Drainage of pancreatic pseudocyst

AHA Coding Clinic for table ØF9
2020, 3Q, 34 Cystogastrostomy with stent insertion
2015, 1Q, 32 Percutaneous transhepatic biliary drainage catheter placement
2014, 3Q, 15 Drainage of pancreatic pseudocyst

AHA Coding Clinic for table ØFB
2019, 1Q, 3-8 Whipple procedure
2016, 3Q, 41 Open cholecystectomy with needle biopsy of liver
2016, 1Q, 23 Endoscopic ultrasound with aspiration biopsy of common hepatic duct
2016, 1Q, 25 Endoscopic retrograde cholangiopancreatography with brush biopsy of pancreatic and common bile ducts
2014, 3Q, 32 Pyloric-sparing Whipple procedure

AHA Coding Clinic for table ØFC
2016, 3Q, 27 Endoscopic retrograde cholangiopancreatography with sphincterotomy and insertion of pancreatic stent

AHA Coding Clinic for table ØFH
2020, 4Q, 43-44 Insertion of radioactive element

AHA Coding Clinic for table ØFQ
2016, 3Q, 27 Revision of common bile duct anastomosis
2013, 4Q, 109 Separating conjoined twins

AHA Coding Clinic for table ØFT
2019, 1Q, 3-8 Whipple Procedure
2012, 4Q, 99 Domino liver transplant

AHA Coding Clinic for table ØFY
2014, 3Q, 13 Orthotopic liver transplant with end to side cavoplasty
2012, 4Q, 99 Domino liver transplant

Liver

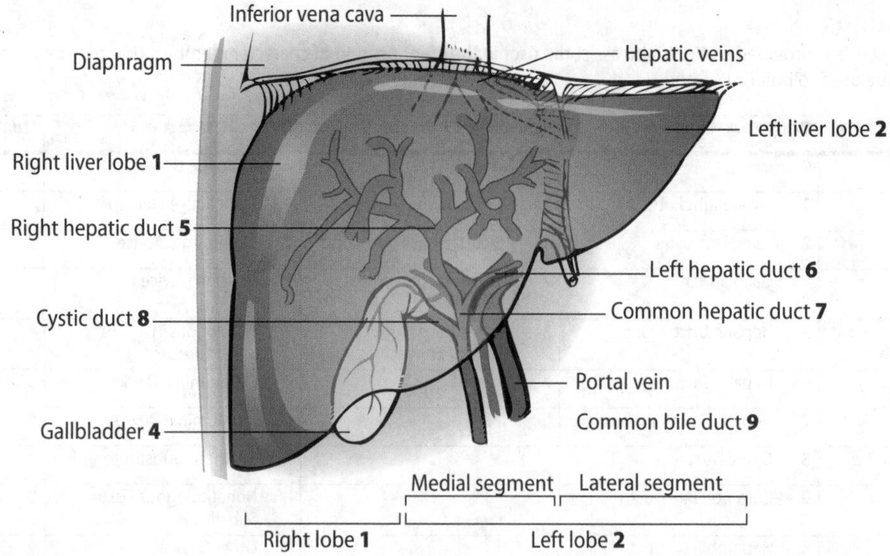

Pancreas

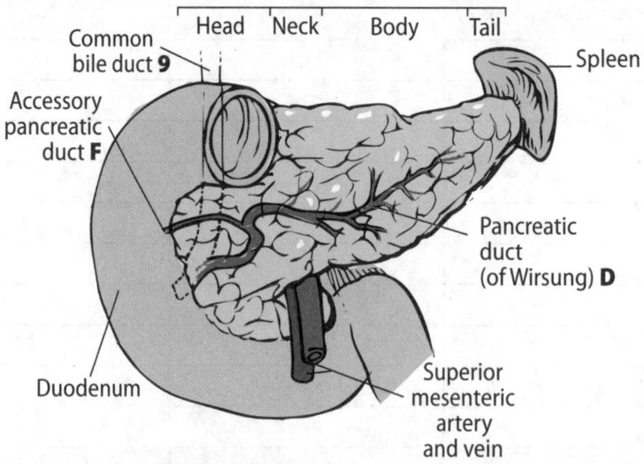

Gallbladder and Ducts

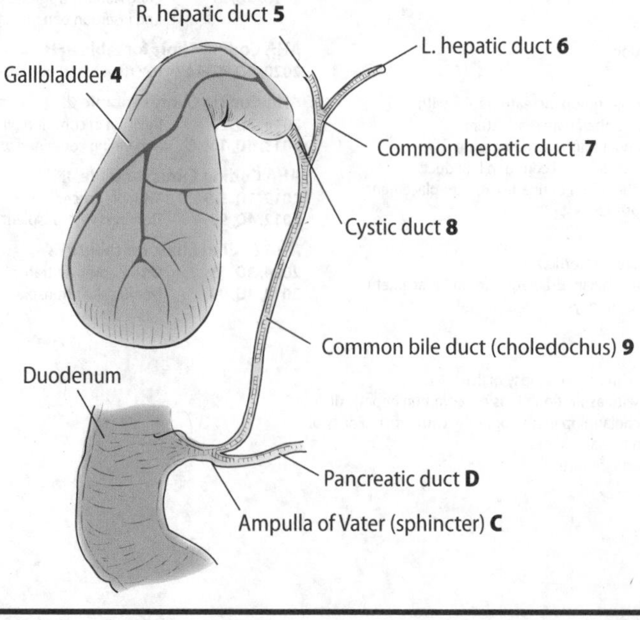

Ø Medical and Surgical
F Hepatobiliary System and Pancreas
1 Bypass Definition: Altering the route of passage of the contents of a tubular body part

Explanation: Rerouting contents of a body part to a downstream area of the normal route, to a similar route and body part, or to an abnormal route and dissimilar body part. Includes one or more anastomoses, with or without the use of a device.

Body Part Character 4	Approach Character 5	Device Character 6	Qualifier Character 7
4 Gallbladder 5 Hepatic Duct, Right 6 Hepatic Duct, Left 7 Hepatic Duct, Common 8 Cystic Duct 9 Common Bile Duct	Ø Open 4 Percutaneous Endoscopic	D Intraluminal Device Z No Device	3 Duodenum 4 Stomach 5 Hepatic Duct, Right 6 Hepatic Duct, Left 7 Hepatic Duct, Caudate 8 Cystic Duct 9 Common Bile Duct B Small Intestine
D Pancreatic Duct Duct of Wirsung	Ø Open 4 Percutaneous Endoscopic	D Intraluminal Device Z No Device	3 Duodenum 4 Stomach B Small Intestine C Large Intestine
F Pancreatic Duct, Accessory Duct of Santorini G Pancreas	Ø Open 4 Percutaneous Endoscopic	D Intraluminal Device Z No Device	3 Duodenum B Small Intestine C Large Intestine

Ø Medical and Surgical
F Hepatobiliary System and Pancreas
2 Change Definition: Taking out or off a device from a body part and putting back an identical or similar device in or on the same body part without cutting or puncturing the skin or a mucous membrane

Explanation: All CHANGE procedures are coded using the approach EXTERNAL

Body Part Character 4	Approach Character 5	Device Character 6	Qualifier Character 7
Ø Liver Quadrate lobe 4 Gallbladder B Hepatobiliary Duct D Pancreatic Duct Duct of Wirsung G Pancreas	X External	Ø Drainage Device Y Other Device	Z No Qualifier

Non-OR All body part, approach, device, and qualifier values

Ø Medical and Surgical
F Hepatobiliary System and Pancreas
5 Destruction Definition: Physical eradication of all or a portion of a body part by the direct use of energy, force, or a destructive agent

Explanation: None of the body part is physically taken out

Body Part Character 4	Approach Character 5	Device Character 6	Qualifier Character 7
Ø Liver Quadrate lobe 1 Liver, Right Lobe 2 Liver, Left Lobe	Ø Open 3 Percutaneous 4 Percutaneous Endoscopic	Z No Device	F Irreversible Electroporation Z No Qualifier
4 Gallbladder	Ø Open 3 Percutaneous 4 Percutaneous Endoscopic 8 Via Natural or Artificial Opening Endoscopic	Z No Device	Z No Qualifier
5 Hepatic Duct, Right 6 Hepatic Duct, Left 7 Hepatic Duct, Common 8 Cystic Duct 9 Common Bile Duct C Ampulla of Vater Duodenal ampulla Hepatopancreatic ampulla D Pancreatic Duct Duct of Wirsung F Pancreatic Duct, Accessory Duct of Santorini	Ø Open 3 Percutaneous 4 Percutaneous Endoscopic 7 Via Natural or Artificial Opening 8 Via Natural or Artificial Opening Endoscopic	Z No Device	Z No Qualifier
G Pancreas	Ø Open 3 Percutaneous 4 Percutaneous Endoscopic	Z No Device	F Irreversible Electroporation Z No Qualifier
G Pancreas	8 Via Natural or Artificial Opening Endoscopic	Z No Device	Z No Qualifier

Non-OR ØF5[5,6,7,8,9,C,D,F][4,8]ZZ
Non-OR ØF5G4Z[F,Z]
Non-OR ØF5G8ZZ

NC Noncovered Procedure LC Limited Coverage QA Questionable OB Admit NT New Tech Add-on ⊞ Combination Member ♂ Male ♀ Female

Ø Medical and Surgical
F Hepatobiliary System and Pancreas
7 Dilation Definition: Expanding an orifice or the lumen of a tubular body part

Explanation: The orifice can be a natural orifice or an artificially created orifice. Accomplished by stretching a tubular body part using intraluminal pressure or by cutting part of the orifice or wall of the tubular body part.

Body Part Character 4	Approach Character 5	Device Character 6	Qualifier Character 7
5 Hepatic Duct, Right 6 Hepatic Duct, Left 7 Hepatic Duct, Common 8 Cystic Duct 9 Common Bile Duct C Ampulla of Vater Duodenal ampulla Hepatopancreatic ampulla D Pancreatic Duct Duct of Wirsung F Pancreatic Duct, Accessory Duct of Santorini	Ø Open 3 Percutaneous 4 Percutaneous Endoscopic 7 Via Natural or Artificial Opening 8 Via Natural or Artificial Opening Endoscopic	D Intraluminal Device Z No Device	Z No Qualifier

Non-OR ØF7[5,6,7,8,9][3,4,8][D,Z]Z
Non-OR ØF7[5,6,7,8,9,D]]7DZ
Non-OR ØF7C8[D,Z]Z
Non-OR ØF7[D,F][4,8][D,Z]Z

Ø Medical and Surgical
F Hepatobiliary System and Pancreas
8 Division Definition: Cutting into a body part, without draining fluids and/or gases from the body part, in order to separate or transect a body part

Explanation: All or a portion of the body part is separated into two or more portions

Body Part Character 4	Approach Character 5	Device Character 6	Qualifier Character 7
Ø Liver 1 Liver, Right Lobe 2 Liver, Left Lobe G Pancreas	Ø Open 3 Percutaneous 4 Percutaneous Endoscopic	Z No Device	Z No Qualifier

Non-OR ØF8[Ø,1,2]3ZZ

Ø Medical and Surgical
F Hepatobiliary System and Pancreas
9 Drainage Definition: Taking or letting out fluids and/or gases from a body part

Explanation: The qualifier DIAGNOSTIC is used to identify drainage procedures that are biopsies

Body Part Character 4	Approach Character 5	Device Character 6	Qualifier Character 7
Ø Liver Quadrate lobe **1 Liver, Right Lobe** **2 Liver, Left Lobe**	**Ø Open** **3 Percutaneous** **4 Percutaneous Endoscopic**	**Ø Drainage Device**	**Z No Qualifier**
Ø Liver Quadrate lobe **1 Liver, Right Lobe** **2 Liver, Left Lobe**	**Ø Open** **3 Percutaneous** **4 Percutaneous Endoscopic**	**Z No Device**	**X Diagnostic** **Z No Qualifier**
4 Gallbladder **G Pancreas**	**Ø Open** **3 Percutaneous** **4 Percutaneous Endoscopic** **8 Via Natural or Artificial Opening Endoscopic**	**Ø Drainage Device**	**Z No Qualifier**
4 Gallbladder **G Pancreas**	**Ø Open** **3 Percutaneous** **4 Percutaneous Endoscopic** **8 Via Natural or Artificial Opening Endoscopic**	**Z No Device**	**X Diagnostic** **Z No Qualifier**
5 Hepatic Duct, Right **6 Hepatic Duct, Left** **7 Hepatic Duct, Common** **8 Cystic Duct** **9 Common Bile Duct** **C Ampulla of Vater** Duodenal ampulla Hepatopancreatic ampulla **D Pancreatic Duct** Duct of Wirsung **F Pancreatic Duct, Accessory** Duct of Santorini	**Ø Open** **3 Percutaneous** **4 Percutaneous Endoscopic** **7 Via Natural or Artificial Opening** **8 Via Natural or Artificial Opening Endoscopic**	**Ø Drainage Device**	**Z No Qualifier**
5 Hepatic Duct, Right **6 Hepatic Duct, Left** **7 Hepatic Duct, Common** **8 Cystic Duct** **9 Common Bile Duct** **C Ampulla of Vater** Duodenal ampulla Hepatopancreatic ampulla **D Pancreatic Duct** Duct of Wirsung **F Pancreatic Duct, Accessory** Duct of Santorini	**Ø Open** **3 Percutaneous** **4 Percutaneous Endoscopic** **7 Via Natural or Artificial Opening** **8 Via Natural or Artificial Opening Endoscopic**	**Z No Device**	**X Diagnostic** **Z No Qualifier**

Non-OR ØF9[Ø,1,2][3,4]ØZ
Non-OR ØF9[Ø,1,2][3,4]Z[X,Z]
Non-OR ØF9[4,G]8ØZ
Non-OR ØF9G3ØZ
Non-OR ØF9[4,G]8Z[X,Z]
Non-OR ØF9G3Z[XZ]
Non-OR ØF9G4ZX
Non-OR ØF9[5,6,8][3,8]ØZ
Non-OR ØF97[3,4,7,8]ØZ
Non-OR ØF99[3,8]ØZ
Non-OR ØF9C[3,4,8]ØZ
Non-OR ØF9[D,F][3,8]ØZ
Non-OR ØF9[5,6,8,9,C,D,F]3Z[X,Z]
Non-OR ØF9[5,6,8,9,C,D,F][4,7,8]ZX
Non-OR ØF9[5,6,8,D,F]8ZZ
Non-OR ØF97[3,4,7,8]Z[X,Z]
Non-OR ØF99[4,7,8]ZZ
Non-OR ØF9C[4,8]ZZ

Ø Medical and Surgical
F Hepatobiliary System and Pancreas
B Excision Definition: Cutting out or off, without replacement, a portion of a body part
Explanation: The qualifier DIAGNOSTIC is used to identify excision procedures that are biopsies

Body Part Character 4	Approach Character 5	Device Character 6	Qualifier Character 7
Ø Liver Quadrate lobe 1 Liver, Right Lobe 2 Liver, Left Lobe	Ø Open 3 Percutaneous 4 Percutaneous Endoscopic	Z No Device	X Diagnostic Z No Qualifier
4 Gallbladder G Pancreas	Ø Open 3 Percutaneous 4 Percutaneous Endoscopic 8 Via Natural or Artificial Opening Endoscopic	Z No Device	X Diagnostic Z No Qualifier
5 Hepatic Duct, Right 6 Hepatic Duct, Left 7 Hepatic Duct, Common 8 Cystic Duct 9 Common Bile Duct C Ampulla of Vater Duodenal ampulla Hepatopancreatic ampulla D Pancreatic Duct Duct of Wirsung F Pancreatic Duct, Accessory Duct of Santorini	Ø Open 3 Percutaneous 4 Percutaneous Endoscopic 7 Via Natural or Artificial Opening 8 Via Natural or Artificial Opening Endoscopic	Z No Device	X Diagnostic Z No Qualifier

Non-OR ØFB[Ø,1,2]3ZX
Non-OR ØFB[4,G][3,4,8]ZX
Non-OR ØFB[5,6,7,8,9,C,D,F][3,4,7,8]ZX
Non-OR ØFB[5,6,7,8,9,C,D,F][4,8]ZZ

Ø Medical and Surgical
F Hepatobiliary System and Pancreas
C Extirpation Definition: Taking or cutting out solid matter from a body part
Explanation: The solid matter may be an abnormal byproduct of a biological function or a foreign body; it may be imbedded in a body part or in the lumen of a tubular body part. The solid matter may or may not have been previously broken into pieces.

Body Part Character 4	Approach Character 5	Device Character 6	Qualifier Character 7
Ø Liver Quadrate lobe 1 Liver, Right Lobe 2 Liver, Left Lobe	Ø Open 3 Percutaneous 4 Percutaneous Endoscopic	Z No Device	Z No Qualifier
4 Gallbladder G Pancreas	Ø Open 3 Percutaneous 4 Percutaneous Endoscopic 8 Via Natural or Artificial Opening Endoscopic	Z No Device	Z No Qualifier
5 Hepatic Duct, Right 6 Hepatic Duct, Left 7 Hepatic Duct, Common 8 Cystic Duct 9 Common Bile Duct C Ampulla of Vater Duodenal ampulla Hepatopancreatic ampulla D Pancreatic Duct Duct of Wirsung F Pancreatic Duct, Accessory Duct of Santorini	Ø Open 3 Percutaneous 4 Percutaneous Endoscopic 7 Via Natural or Artificial Opening 8 Via Natural or Artificial Opening Endoscopic	Z No Device	Z No Qualifier

Non-OR ØFC[5,6,7,8,9][3,4,7,8]ZZ
Non-OR ØFCC[4,8]ZZ
Non-OR ØFC[D,F][3,4,8]ZZ

Ø Medical and Surgical
F Hepatobiliary System and Pancreas
D Extraction Definition: Pulling or stripping out or off all or a portion of a body part by the use of force

Explanation: The qualifier DIAGNOSTIC is used to identify extraction procedures that are biopsies

Body Part Character 4	Approach Character 5	Device Character 6	Qualifier Character 7
Ø Liver Quadrate lobe 1 Liver, Right Lobe 2 Liver, Left Lobe	3 Percutaneous 4 Percutaneous Endoscopic	Z No Device	X Diagnostic
4 Gallbladder 5 Hepatic Duct, Right 6 Hepatic Duct, Left 7 Hepatic Duct, Common 8 Cystic Duct 9 Common Bile Duct C Ampulla of Vater Duodenal ampulla Hepatopancreatic ampulla D Pancreatic Duct Duct of Wirsung F Pancreatic Duct, Accessory Duct of Santorini G Pancreas	3 Percutaneous 4 Percutaneous Endoscopic 8 Via Natural or Artificial Opening Endoscopic	Z No Device	X Diagnostic

Non-OR ØFD[Ø,1,2]3ZX
Non-OR ØFD[4,5,6,7,8,9,C,D,F,G][3,4,8]ZX

Ø Medical and Surgical
F Hepatobiliary System and Pancreas
F Fragmentation Definition: Breaking solid matter in a body part into pieces

Explanation: Physical force (e.g., manual, ultrasonic) applied directly or indirectly is used to break the solid matter into pieces. The solid matter may be an abnormal byproduct of a biological function or a foreign body. The pieces of solid matter are not taken out.

Body Part Character 4	Approach Character 5	Device Character 6	Qualifier Character 7
4 Gallbladder NC 5 Hepatic Duct, Right NC 6 Hepatic Duct, Left NC 7 Hepatic Duct, Common 8 Cystic Duct NC 9 Common Bile Duct NC C Ampulla of Vater NC Duodenal ampulla Hepatopancreatic ampulla D Pancreatic Duct NC Duct of Wirsung F Pancreatic Duct, Accessory NC Duct of Santorini	Ø Open 3 Percutaneous 4 Percutaneous Endoscopic 7 Via Natural or Artificial Opening 8 Via Natural or Artificial Opening Endoscopic X External	Z No Device	Z No Qualifier

Non-OR ØFF[4,5,6,7,8,9,C,D,F][8,X]ZZ
NC ØFF[4,5,6,8,9,C,D,F]XZZ

Ø Medical and Surgical
F Hepatobiliary System and Pancreas
H Insertion Definition: Putting in a nonbiological appliance that monitors, assists, performs, or prevents a physiological function but does not physically take the place of a body part

Explanation: None

Body Part Character 4	Approach Character 5	Device Character 6	Qualifier Character 7
Ø Liver Quadrate lobe 4 Gallbladder G Pancreas	Ø Open 3 Percutaneous 4 Percutaneous Endoscopic	1 Radioactive Element 2 Monitoring Device 3 Infusion Device Y Other Device	Z No Qualifier
1 Liver, Right Lobe 2 Liver, Left Lobe	Ø Open 3 Percutaneous 4 Percutaneous Endoscopic	2 Monitoring Device 3 Infusion Device	Z No Qualifier
B Hepatobiliary Duct ⊞ D Pancreatic Duct Duct of Wirsung	Ø Open 3 Percutaneous 4 Percutaneous Endoscopic 7 Via Natural or Artificial Opening 8 Via Natural or Artificial Opening Endoscopic	1 Radioactive Element 2 Monitoring Device 3 Infusion Device D Intraluminal Device Y Other Device	Z No Qualifier

Non-OR ØFH[Ø,4,G]31Z
Non-OR ØFH[Ø,4,G][Ø,3,4]3Z
Non-OR ØFH[Ø,4,G][3,4]YZ
Non-OR ØFH[1,2][Ø,3,4]3Z
Non-OR ØFH[B,D][Ø,3,4]3Z
Non-OR ØFH[B,D][4,8]DZ
Non-OR ØFH[B,D][7,8][2,3]Z
Non-OR ØFH[B,D][3,4,7,8]YZ

See Appendix L for Procedure Combinations
⊞ ØFHB7DZ

NC Noncovered Procedure LC Limited Coverage QA Questionable OB Admit NT New Tech Add-on ⊞ Combination Member ♂ Male ♀ Female

Ø Medical and Surgical
F Hepatobiliary System and Pancreas
J Inspection Definition: Visually and/or manually exploring a body part

Explanation: Visual exploration may be performed with or without optical instrumentation. Manual exploration may be performed directly or through intervening body layers.

Body Part Character 4	Approach Character 5	Device Character 6	Qualifier Character 7
Ø Liver Quadrate lobe	**Ø Open** **3 Percutaneous** **4 Percutaneous Endoscopic** **X External**	**Z No Device**	**Z No Qualifier**
4 Gallbladder **G Pancreas**	**Ø Open** **3 Percutaneous** **4 Percutaneous Endoscopic** **8 Via Natural or Artificial Opening Endoscopic** **X External**	**Z No Device**	**Z No Qualifier**
B Hepatobiliary Duct **D Pancreatic Duct** Duct of Wirsung	**Ø Open** **3 Percutaneous** **4 Percutaneous Endoscopic** **7 Via Natural or Artificial Opening** **8 Via Natural or Artificial Opening Endoscopic**	**Z No Device**	**Z No Qualifier**

Non-OR ØFJØ[3,X]ZZ
Non-OR ØFJ[4,G][3,8,X]ZZ
Non-OR ØFJ[B,D][3,7,8]ZZ

Ø Medical and Surgical
F Hepatobiliary System and Pancreas
L Occlusion Definition: Completely closing an orifice or the lumen of a tubular body part

Explanation: The orifice can be a natural orifice or an artificially created orifice

Body Part Character 4	Approach Character 5	Device Character 6	Qualifier Character 7
5 Hepatic Duct, Right **6 Hepatic Duct, Left** **7 Hepatic Duct, Common** **8 Cystic Duct** **9 Common Bile Duct** **C Ampulla of Vater** Duodenal ampulla Hepatopancreatic ampulla **D Pancreatic Duct** Duct of Wirsung **F Pancreatic Duct, Accessory** Duct of Santorini	**Ø Open** **3 Percutaneous** **4 Percutaneous Endoscopic**	**C Extraluminal Device** **D Intraluminal Device** **Z No Device**	**Z No Qualifier**
5 Hepatic Duct, Right **6 Hepatic Duct, Left** **7 Hepatic Duct, Common** **8 Cystic Duct** **9 Common Bile Duct** **C Ampulla of Vater** Duodenal ampulla Hepatopancreatic ampulla **D Pancreatic Duct** Duct of Wirsung **F Pancreatic Duct, Accessory** Duct of Santorini	**7 Via Natural or Artificial Opening** **8 Via Natural or Artificial Opening Endoscopic**	**D Intraluminal Device** **Z No Device**	**Z No Qualifier**

Non-OR ØFL[5,6,7,8,9][3,4][C,D,Z]Z
Non-OR ØFL[5,6,7,8,9][7,8][D,Z]Z

Ø Medical and Surgical
F Hepatobiliary System and Pancreas
M Reattachment Definition: Putting back in or on all or a portion of a separated body part to its normal location or other suitable location
Explanation: Vascular circulation and nervous pathways may or may not be reestablished

Body Part Character 4	Approach Character 5	Device Character 6	Qualifier Character 7
Ø Liver Quadrate lobe **1 Liver, Right Lobe** **2 Liver, Left Lobe** **4 Gallbladder** **5 Hepatic Duct, Right** **6 Hepatic Duct, Left** **7 Hepatic Duct, Common** **8 Cystic Duct** **9 Common Bile Duct** **C Ampulla of Vater** Duodenal ampulla Hepatopancreatic ampulla **D Pancreatic Duct** Duct of Wirsung **F Pancreatic Duct, Accessory** Duct of Santorini **G Pancreas**	**Ø Open** **4 Percutaneous Endoscopic**	**Z No Device**	**Z No Qualifier**

Non-OR ØFM[4,5,6,7,8,9]4ZZ

Ø Medical and Surgical
F Hepatobiliary System and Pancreas
N Release Definition: Freeing a body part from an abnormal physical constraint by cutting or by the use of force
Explanation: Some of the restraining tissue may be taken out but none of the body part is taken out

Body Part Character 4	Approach Character 5	Device Character 6	Qualifier Character 7
Ø Liver Quadrate lobe **1 Liver, Right Lobe** **2 Liver, Left Lobe**	**Ø Open** **3 Percutaneous** **4 Percutaneous Endoscopic**	**Z No Device**	**Z No Qualifier**
4 Gallbladder **G Pancreas**	**Ø Open** **3 Percutaneous** **4 Percutaneous Endoscopic** **8 Via Natural or Artificial Opening Endoscopic**	**Z No Device**	**Z No Qualifier**
5 Hepatic Duct, Right **6 Hepatic Duct, Left** **7 Hepatic Duct, Common** **8 Cystic Duct** **9 Common Bile Duct** **C Ampulla of Vater** Duodenal ampulla Hepatopancreatic ampulla **D Pancreatic Duct** Duct of Wirsung **F Pancreatic Duct, Accessory** Duct of Santorini	**Ø Open** **3 Percutaneous** **4 Percutaneous Endoscopic** **7 Via Natural or Artificial Opening** **8 Via Natural or Artificial Opening Endoscopic**	**Z No Device**	**Z No Qualifier**

Ø Medical and Surgical
F Hepatobiliary System and Pancreas
P Removal Definition: Taking out or off a device from a body part

Explanation: If a device is taken out and a similar device put in without cutting or puncturing the skin or mucous membrane, the procedure is coded to the root operation CHANGE. Otherwise, the procedure for taking out a device is coded to the root operation REMOVAL.

Body Part Character 4	Approach Character 5	Device Character 6	Qualifier Character 7
Ø Liver Quadrate lobe	**Ø Open** **3 Percutaneous** **4 Percutaneous Endoscopic**	**Ø Drainage Device** **2 Monitoring Device** **3 Infusion Device** **Y Other Device**	**Z No Qualifier**
Ø Liver Quadrate lobe	**X External**	**Ø Drainage Device** **2 Monitoring Device** **3 Infusion Device**	**Z No Qualifier**
4 Gallbladder **G Pancreas**	**Ø Open** **3 Percutaneous** **4 Percutaneous Endoscopic**	**Ø Drainage Device** **2 Monitoring Device** **3 Infusion Device** **D Intraluminal Device** **Y Other Device**	**Z No Qualifier**
4 Gallbladder **G Pancreas**	**X External**	**Ø Drainage Device** **2 Monitoring Device** **3 Infusion Device** **D Intraluminal Device**	**Z No Qualifier**
B Hepatobiliary Duct **D Pancreatic Duct** Duct of Wirsung	**Ø Open** **3 Percutaneous** **4 Percutaneous Endoscopic** **7 Via Natural or Artificial Opening** **8 Via Natural or Artificial Opening Endoscopic**	**Ø Drainage Device** **1 Radioactive Element** **2 Monitoring Device** **3 Infusion Device** **7 Autologous Tissue Substitute** **C Extraluminal Device** **D Intraluminal Device** **J Synthetic Substitute** **K Nonautologous Tissue Substitute** **Y Other Device**	**Z No Qualifier**
B Hepatobiliary Duct **D Pancreatic Duct** Duct of Wirsung	**X External**	**Ø Drainage Device** **1 Radioactive Element** **2 Monitoring Device** **3 Infusion Device** **D Intraluminal Device**	**Z No Qualifier**

Non-OR ØFPØ[3,4]YZ
Non-OR ØFPØX[Ø,2,3]Z
Non-OR ØFPG3ØZ
Non-OR ØFP[4,G][3,4]YZ
Non-OR ØFP4X[Ø,2,3,D]Z
Non-OR ØFPGX[Ø,2,3]Z
Non-OR ØFP[B,D][3,4]YZ
Non-OR ØFP[B,D][7,8][Ø,2,3,D,Y]Z
Non-OR ØFP[B,D]X[Ø,1,2,3,D]Z

See Appendix L for Procedure Combinations
Combo-only ØFP[B,D][7,8]DZ
Combo-only ØFP[B,D]XDZ

Ø Medical and Surgical
F Hepatobiliary System and Pancreas
Q Repair Definition: Restoring, to the extent possible, a body part to its normal anatomic structure and function

Explanation: Used only when the method to accomplish the repair is not one of the other root operations

Body Part Character 4	Approach Character 5	Device Character 6	Qualifier Character 7
Ø Liver Quadrate lobe **1 Liver, Right Lobe** **2 Liver, Left Lobe**	**Ø Open** **3 Percutaneous** **4 Percutaneous Endoscopic**	**Z No Device**	**Z No Qualifier**
4 Gallbladder **G Pancreas**	**Ø Open** **3 Percutaneous** **4 Percutaneous Endoscopic** **8 Via Natural or Artificial Opening Endoscopic**	**Z No Device**	**Z No Qualifier**
5 Hepatic Duct, Right **6 Hepatic Duct, Left** **7 Hepatic Duct, Common** **8 Cystic Duct** **9 Common Bile Duct** **C Ampulla of Vater** Duodenal ampulla Hepatopancreatic ampulla **D Pancreatic Duct** Duct of Wirsung **F Pancreatic Duct, Accessory** Duct of Santorini	**Ø Open** **3 Percutaneous** **4 Percutaneous Endoscopic** **7 Via Natural or Artificial Opening** **8 Via Natural or Artificial Opening Endoscopic**	**Z No Device**	**Z No Qualifier**

Ø Medical and Surgical
F Hepatobiliary System and Pancreas
R Replacement Definition: Putting in or on biological or synthetic material that physically takes the place and/or function of all or a portion of a body part

Explanation: The body part may have been taken out or replaced, or may be taken out, physically eradicated, or rendered nonfunctional during the REPLACEMENT procedure. A REMOVAL procedure is coded for taking out the device used in a previous replacement procedure.

Body Part Character 4	Approach Character 5	Device Character 6	Qualifier Character 7
5 Hepatic Duct, Right **6 Hepatic Duct, Left** **7 Hepatic Duct, Common** **8 Cystic Duct** **9 Common Bile Duct** **C Ampulla of Vater** Duodenal ampulla Hepatopancreatic ampulla **D Pancreatic Duct** Duct of Wirsung **F Pancreatic Duct, Accessory** Duct of Santorini	**Ø Open** **4 Percutaneous Endoscopic** **8 Via Natural or Artificial Opening Endoscopic**	**7 Autologous Tissue Substitute** **J Synthetic Substitute** **K Nonautologous Tissue Substitute**	**Z No Qualifier**

Ø Medical and Surgical
F Hepatobiliary System and Pancreas
S Reposition Definition: Moving to its normal location, or other suitable location, all or a portion of a body part

Explanation: The body part is moved to a new location from an abnormal location, or from a normal location where it is not functioning correctly. The body part may or may not be cut out or off to be moved to the new location.

Body Part Character 4	Approach Character 5	Device Character 6	Qualifier Character 7
Ø Liver Quadrate lobe **4 Gallbladder** **5 Hepatic Duct, Right** **6 Hepatic Duct, Left** **7 Hepatic Duct, Common** **8 Cystic Duct** **9 Common Bile Duct** **C Ampulla of Vater** Duodenal ampulla Hepatopancreatic ampulla **D Pancreatic Duct** Duct of Wirsung **F Pancreatic Duct, Accessory** Duct of Santorini **G Pancreas**	**Ø Open** **4 Percutaneous Endoscopic**	**Z No Device**	**Z No Qualifier**

Ø Medical and Surgical
F Hepatobiliary System and Pancreas
T Resection Definition: Cutting out or off, without replacement, all of a body part
Explanation: None

Body Part Character 4	Approach Character 5	Device Character 6	Qualifier Character 7
Ø Liver Quadrate lobe **1 Liver, Right Lobe** **2 Liver, Left Lobe** **4 Gallbladder** **G Pancreas**	**Ø Open** **4 Percutaneous Endoscopic**	**Z No Device**	**Z No Qualifier**
5 Hepatic Duct, Right **6 Hepatic Duct, Left** **7 Hepatic Duct, Common** **8 Cystic Duct** **9 Common Bile Duct** **C Ampulla of Vater** Duodenal ampulla Hepatopancreatic ampulla **D Pancreatic Duct** Duct of Wirsung **F Pancreatic Duct, Accessory** Duct of Santorini	**Ø Open** **4 Percutaneous Endoscopic** **7 Via Natural or Artificial Opening** **8 Via Natural or Artificial Opening Endoscopic**	**Z No Device**	**Z No Qualifier**

Non-OR ØFT[D,F][4,8]ZZ

See Appendix L for Procedure Combinations
ØFTGØZZ

Ø Medical and Surgical
F Hepatobiliary System and Pancreas
U Supplement Definition: Putting in or on biological or synthetic material that physically reinforces and/or augments the function of a portion of a body part
Explanation: The biological material is non-living, or is living and from the same individual. The body part may have been previously replaced, and the SUPPLEMENT procedure is performed to physically reinforce and/or augment the function of the replaced body part.

Body Part Character 4	Approach Character 5	Device Character 6	Qualifier Character 7
5 Hepatic Duct, Right **6 Hepatic Duct, Left** **7 Hepatic Duct, Common** **8 Cystic Duct** **9 Common Bile Duct** **C Ampulla of Vater** Duodenal ampulla Hepatopancreatic ampulla **D Pancreatic Duct** Duct of Wirsung **F Pancreatic Duct, Accessory** Duct of Santorini	**Ø Open** **3 Percutaneous** **4 Percutaneous Endoscopic** **8 Via Natural or Artificial Opening Endoscopic**	**7 Autologous Tissue Substitute** **J Synthetic Substitute** **K Nonautologous Tissue Substitute**	**Z No Qualifier**

Ø Medical and Surgical
F Hepatobiliary System and Pancreas
V Restriction Definition: Partially closing an orifice or the lumen of a tubular body part
Explanation: The orifice can be a natural orifice or an artificially created orifice

Body Part Character 4	Approach Character 5	Device Character 6	Qualifier Character 7
5 Hepatic Duct, Right **6 Hepatic Duct, Left** **7 Hepatic Duct, Common** **8 Cystic Duct** **9 Common Bile Duct** **C Ampulla of Vater** Duodenal ampulla Hepatopancreatic ampulla **D Pancreatic Duct** Duct of Wirsung **F Pancreatic Duct, Accessory** Duct of Santorini	**Ø Open** **3 Percutaneous** **4 Percutaneous Endoscopic**	**C Extraluminal Device** **D Intraluminal Device** **Z No Device**	**Z No Qualifier**
5 Hepatic Duct, Right **6 Hepatic Duct, Left** **7 Hepatic Duct, Common** **8 Cystic Duct** **9 Common Bile Duct** **C Ampulla of Vater** Duodenal ampulla Hepatopancreatic ampulla **D Pancreatic Duct** Duct of Wirsung **F Pancreatic Duct, Accessory** Duct of Santorini	**7 Via Natural or Artificial Opening** **8 Via Natural or Artificial Opening Endoscopic**	**D Intraluminal Device** **Z No Device**	**Z No Qualifier**

Non-OR ØFV[5,6,7,8,9][3,4][C,D,Z]Z
Non-OR ØFV[5,6,7,8,9][7,8][D,Z]Z

Ø Medical and Surgical
F Hepatobiliary System and Pancreas
W Revision Definition: Correcting, to the extent possible, a portion of a malfunctioning device or the position of a displaced device

Explanation: Revision can include correcting a malfunctioning or displaced device by taking out or putting in components of the device such as a screw or pin

Body Part Character 4	Approach Character 5	Device Character 6	Qualifier Character 7
Ø Liver Quadrate lobe	Ø Open 3 Percutaneous 4 Percutaneous Endoscopic	Ø Drainage Device 2 Monitoring Device 3 Infusion Device Y Other Device	Z No Qualifier
Ø Liver Quadrate lobe	X External	Ø Drainage Device 2 Monitoring Device 3 Infusion Device	Z No Qualifier
4 Gallbladder G Pancreas	Ø Open 3 Percutaneous 4 Percutaneous Endoscopic	Ø Drainage Device 2 Monitoring Device 3 Infusion Device D Intraluminal Device Y Other Device	Z No Qualifier
4 Gallbladder G Pancreas	X External	Ø Drainage Device 2 Monitoring Device 3 Infusion Device D Intraluminal Device	Z No Qualifier
B Hepatobiliary Duct D Pancreatic Duct Duct of Wirsung	Ø Open 3 Percutaneous 4 Percutaneous Endoscopic 7 Via Natural or Artificial Opening 8 Via Natural or Artificial Opening Endoscopic	Ø Drainage Device 2 Monitoring Device 3 Infusion Device 7 Autologous Tissue Substitute C Extraluminal Device D Intraluminal Device J Synthetic Substitute K Nonautologous Tissue Substitute Y Other Device	Z No Qualifier
B Hepatobiliary Duct D Pancreatic Duct Duct of Wirsung	X External	Ø Drainage Device 2 Monitoring Device 3 Infusion Device 7 Autologous Tissue Substitute C Extraluminal Device D Intraluminal Device J Synthetic Substitute K Nonautologous Tissue Substitute	Z No Qualifier

Non-OR ØFWØ[3,4]YZ
Non-OR ØFWØX[Ø,2,3]Z
Non-OR ØFW[4,G][3,4]YZ
Non-OR ØFW[4,G]X[Ø,2,3,D]Z
Non-OR ØFW[B,D][3,4,7,8]YZ
Non-OR ØFW[B,D]X[Ø,2,3,7,C,D,J,K]Z

Ø Medical and Surgical
F Hepatobiliary System and Pancreas
Y Transplantation Definition: Putting in or on all or a portion of a living body part taken from another individual or animal to physically take the place and/or function of all or a portion of a similar body part

Explanation: The native body part may or may not be taken out, and the transplanted body part may take over all or a portion of its function

Body Part Character 4	Approach Character 5	Device Character 6	Qualifier Character 7
Ø Liver LC Quadrate lobe G Pancreas LC NC ⊞	Ø Open	Z No Device	Ø Allogeneic 1 Syngeneic 2 Zooplastic

LC ØFYØØZ[Ø,1,2]
LC ØFYGØZ[Ø,1]
NC ØFYGØZ2
NC ØFYGØZ[Ø,1] If reported alone without one of the following procedures ØTYØØZ[Ø,1,2], ØTY1ØZ[Ø,1,2] and without one of the following diagnoses E1Ø.1Ø-E1Ø.9, E89.1

See Appendix L for Procedure Combinations
⊞ ØFYGØZ[Ø,1,2]

Endocrine System ØG2–ØGW

Character Meanings

This Character Meaning table is provided as a guide to assist the user in the identification of character members that may be found in this section of code tables. It **SHOULD NOT** be used to build a PCS code.

Operation–Character 3	Body Part–Character 4	Approach–Character 5	Device–Character 6	Qualifier–Character 7
2 Change	Ø Pituitary Gland	Ø Open	Ø Drainage Device	X Diagnostic
5 Destruction	1 Pineal Body	3 Percutaneous	1 Radioactive Element	Z No Qualifier
8 Division	2 Adrenal Gland, Left	4 Percutaneous Endoscopic	2 Monitoring Device	
9 Drainage	3 Adrenal Gland, Right	X External	3 Infusion Device	
B Excision	4 Adrenal Glands, Bilateral		Y Other Device	
C Extirpation	5 Adrenal Gland		Z No Device	
H Insertion	6 Carotid Body, Left			
J Inspection	7 Carotid Body, Right			
M Reattachment	8 Carotid Bodies, Bilateral			
N Release	9 Para-aortic Body			
P Removal	B Coccygeal Glomus			
Q Repair	C Glomus Jugulare			
S Reposition	D Aortic Body			
T Resection	F Paraganglion Extremity			
W Revision	G Thyroid Gland Lobe, Left			
	H Thyroid Gland Lobe, Right			
	J Thyroid Gland Isthmus			
	K Thyroid Gland			
	L Superior Parathyroid Gland, Right			
	M Superior Parathyroid Gland, Left			
	N Inferior Parathyroid Gland, Right			
	P Inferior Parathyroid Gland, Left			
	Q Parathyroid Glands, Multiple			
	R Parathyroid Gland			
	S Endocrine Gland			

AHA Coding Clinic for table ØGB
2021, 2Q, 7 Infrarenal para-aortic paraganglioma with excision
2017, 2Q, 20 Near total thyroidectomy
2014, 3Q, 22 Transsphenoidal removal of pituitary tumor and fat graft placement

AHA Coding Clinic for table ØGH
2020, 4Q, 43-44 Insertion of radioactive element

AHA Coding Clinic for table ØGT
2017, 2Q, 20 Near total thyroidectomy

Endocrine System

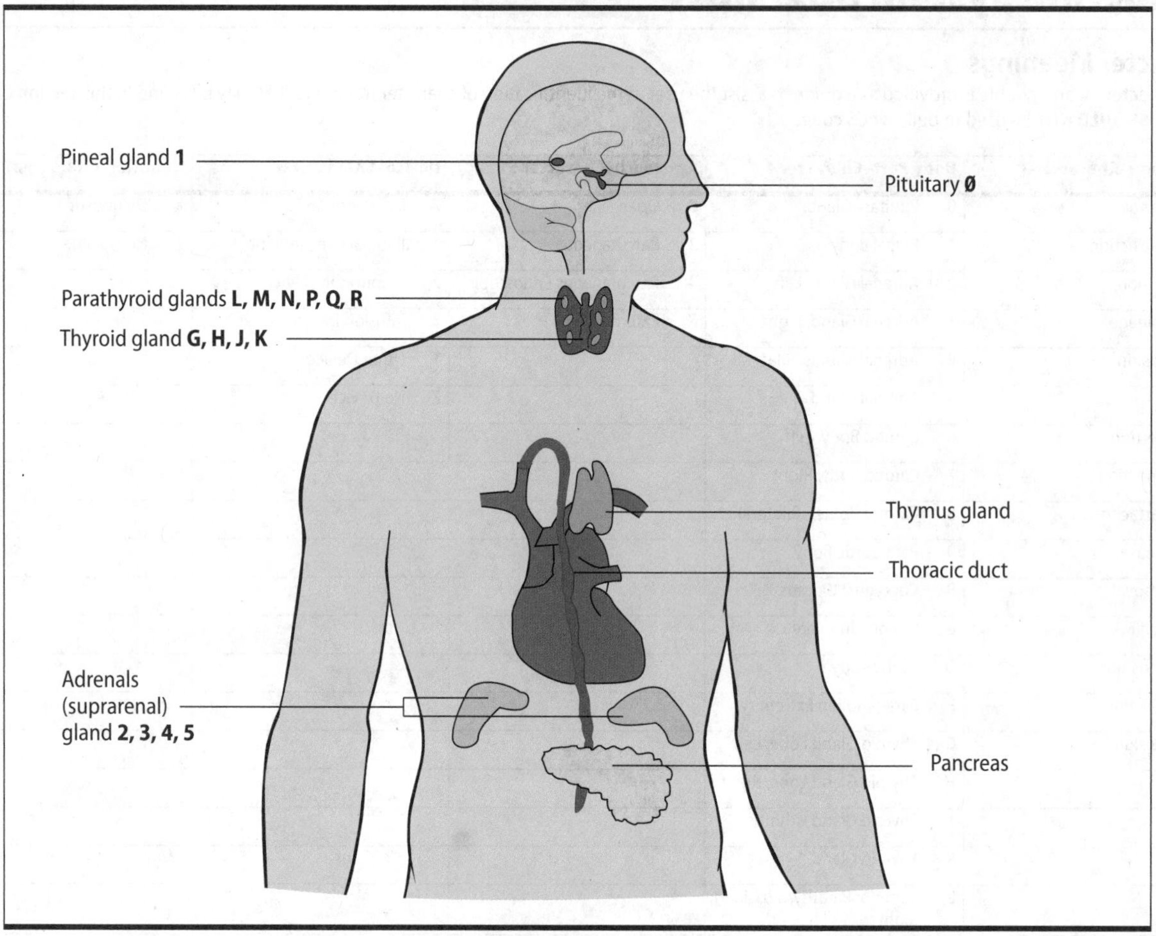

Left Adrenal Gland

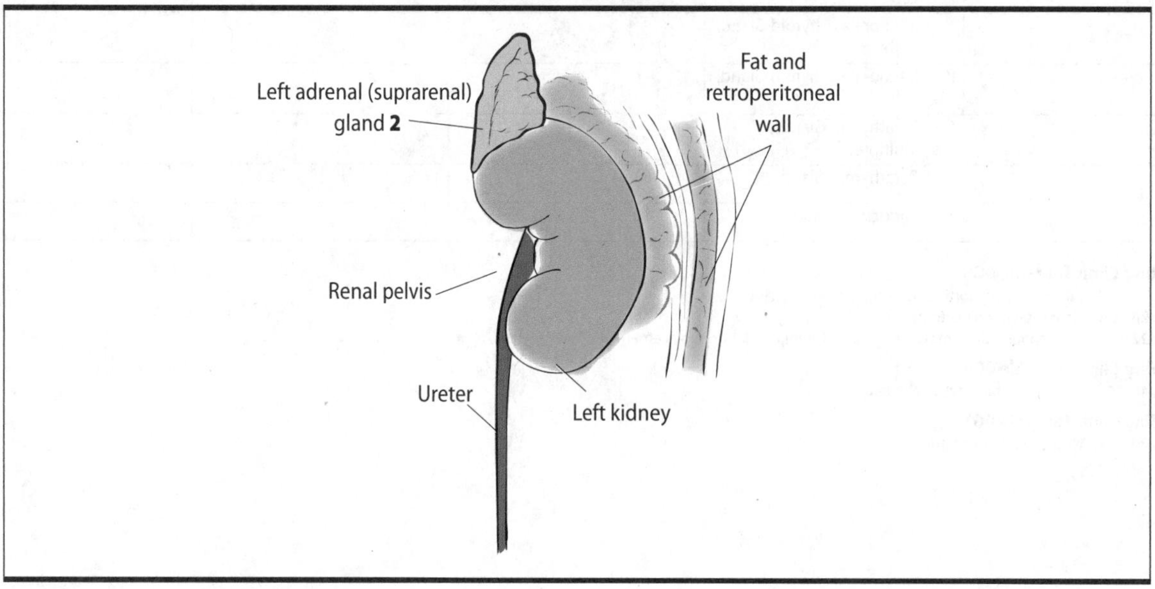

Thyroid

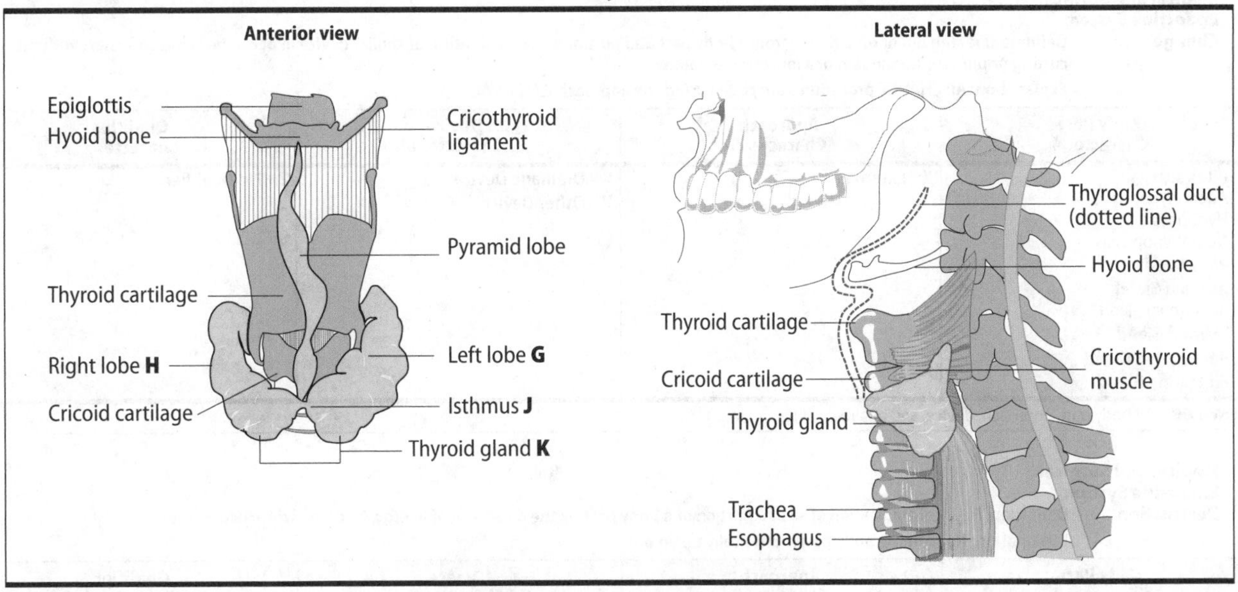

Thyroid and Parathyroid Glands

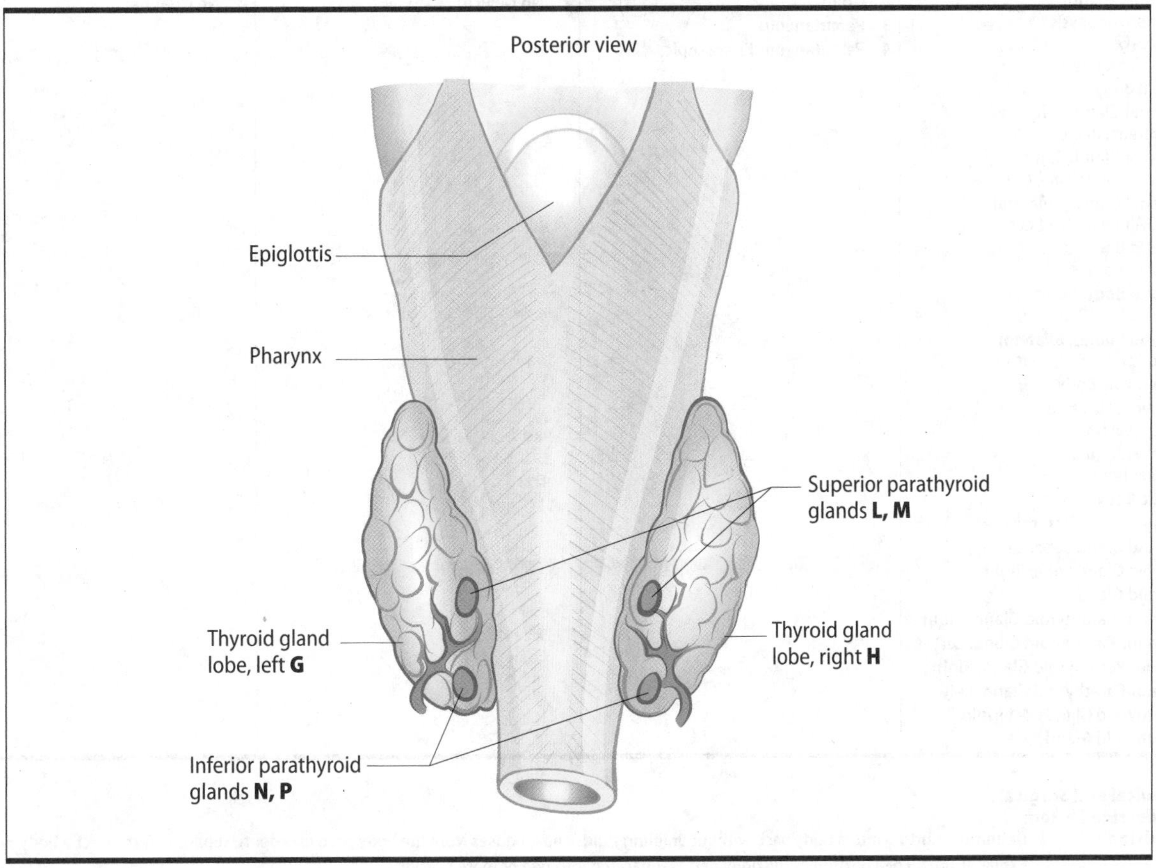

Ø Medical and Surgical
G Endocrine System
2 Change Definition: Taking out or off a device from a body part and putting back an identical or similar device in or on the same body part without cutting or puncturing the skin or a mucous membrane

Explanation: All CHANGE procedures are coded using the approach EXTERNAL

Body Part Character 4	Approach Character 5	Device Character 6	Qualifier Character 7
Ø Pituitary Gland Adenohypophysis Hypophysis Neurohypophysis **1 Pineal Body** **5 Adrenal Gland** Suprarenal gland **K Thyroid Gland** **R Parathyroid Gland** **S Endocrine Gland**	**X External**	**Ø Drainage Device** **Y Other Device**	**Z No Qualifier**

Non-OR All body part, approach, device, and qualifier values

Ø Medical and Surgical
G Endocrine System
5 Destruction Definition: Physical eradication of all or a portion of a body part by the direct use of energy, force, or a destructive agent

Explanation: None of the body part is physically taken out

Body Part Character 4	Approach Character 5	Device Character 6	Qualifier Character 7
Ø Pituitary Gland Adenohypophysis Hypophysis Neurohypophysis **1 Pineal Body** **2 Adrenal Gland, Left** Suprarenal gland **3 Adrenal Gland, Right** *See 2 Adrenal Gland, Left* **4 Adrenal Glands, Bilateral** *See 2 Adrenal Gland, Left* **6 Carotid Body, Left** Carotid glomus **7 Carotid Body, Right** *See 6 Carotid Body, Left* **8 Carotid Bodies, Bilateral** *See 6 Carotid Body, Left* **9 Para-aortic Body** **B Coccygeal Glomus** Coccygeal body **C Glomus Jugulare** Jugular body **D Aortic Body** **F Paraganglion Extremity** **G Thyroid Gland Lobe, Left** **H Thyroid Gland Lobe, Right** **K Thyroid Gland** **L Superior Parathyroid Gland, Right** **M Superior Parathyroid Gland, Left** **N Inferior Parathyroid Gland, Right** **P Inferior Parathyroid Gland, Left** **Q Parathyroid Glands, Multiple** **R Parathyroid Gland**	**Ø Open** **3 Percutaneous** **4 Percutaneous Endoscopic**	**Z No Device**	**Z No Qualifier**

Ø Medical and Surgical
G Endocrine System
8 Division Definition: Cutting into a body part, without draining fluids and/or gases from the body part, in order to separate or transect a body part

Explanation: All or a portion of the body part is separated into two or more portions

Body Part Character 4	Approach Character 5	Device Character 6	Qualifier Character 7
Ø Pituitary Gland Adenohypophysis Hypophysis Neurohypophysis **J Thyroid Gland Isthmus**	**Ø Open** **3 Percutaneous** **4 Percutaneous Endoscopic**	**Z No Device**	**Z No Qualifier**

Ø Medical and Surgical
G Endocrine System
9 Drainage Definition: Taking or letting out fluids and/or gases from a body part

Explanation: The qualifier DIAGNOSTIC is used to identify drainage procedures that are biopsies

Body Part Character 4	Approach Character 5	Device Character 6	Qualifier Character 7
Ø Pituitary Gland Adenohypophysis Hypophysis Neurohypophysis **1 Pineal Body** **2 Adrenal Gland, Left** Suprarenal gland **3 Adrenal Gland, Right** *See 2 Adrenal Gland, Left* **4 Adrenal Glands, Bilateral** *See 2 Adrenal Gland, Left* **6 Carotid Body, Left** Carotid glomus **7 Carotid Body, Right** *See 6 Carotid Body, Left* **8 Carotid Bodies, Bilateral** *See 6 Carotid Body, Left* **9 Para-aortic Body** **B Coccygeal Glomus** Coccygeal body **C Glomus Jugulare** Jugular body **D Aortic Body** **F Paraganglion Extremity** **G Thyroid Gland Lobe, Left** **H Thyroid Gland Lobe, Right** **K Thyroid Gland** **L Superior Parathyroid Gland, Right** **M Superior Parathyroid Gland, Left** **N Inferior Parathyroid Gland, Right** **P Inferior Parathyroid Gland, Left** **Q Parathyroid Glands, Multiple** **R Parathyroid Gland**	**Ø Open** **3 Percutaneous** **4 Percutaneous Endoscopic**	**Ø Drainage Device**	**Z No Qualifier**
Ø Pituitary Gland Adenohypophysis Hypophysis Neurohypophysis **1 Pineal Body** **2 Adrenal Gland, Left** Suprarenal gland **3 Adrenal Gland, Right** *See 2 Adrenal Gland, Left* **4 Adrenal Glands, Bilateral** *See 2 Adrenal Gland, Left* **6 Carotid Body, Left** Carotid glomus **7 Carotid Body, Right** *See 6 Carotid Body, Left* **8 Carotid Bodies, Bilateral** *See 6 Carotid Body, Left* **9 Para-aortic Body** **B Coccygeal Glomus** Coccygeal body **C Glomus Jugulare** Jugular body **D Aortic Body** **F Paraganglion Extremity** **G Thyroid Gland Lobe, Left** **H Thyroid Gland Lobe, Right** **K Thyroid Gland** **L Superior Parathyroid Gland, Right** **M Superior Parathyroid Gland, Left** **N Inferior Parathyroid Gland, Right** **P Inferior Parathyroid Gland, Left** **Q Parathyroid Glands, Multiple** **R Parathyroid Gland**	**Ø Open** **3 Percutaneous** **4 Percutaneous Endoscopic**	**Z No Device**	**X Diagnostic** **Z No Qualifier**

Non-OR ØG9[Ø,1,2,3,4,6,7,8,9,B,C,D,F,G,H,K,L,M,N,P,Q,R]3ØZ
Non-OR ØG9[G,H,K,L,M,N,P,Q,R]4ØZ
Non-OR ØG9[2,3,4,G,H,K][3,4]ZX
Non-OR ØG9[Ø,1,2,3,4,6,7,8,9,B,C,D,F,G,H,K,L,M,N,P,Q,R]3ZZ
Non-OR ØG9[G,H,K,L,M,N,P,Q,R]4ZZ

Ø Medical and Surgical
G Endocrine System
B Excision Definition: Cutting out or off, without replacement, a portion of a body part

Explanation: The qualifier DIAGNOSTIC is used to identify excision procedures that are biopsies

Body Part Character 4	Approach Character 5	Device Character 6	Qualifier Character 7
Ø Pituitary Gland Adenohypophysis Hypophysis Neurohypophysis **1 Pineal Body** **2 Adrenal Gland, Left** Suprarenal gland **3 Adrenal Gland, Right** *See 2 Adrenal Gland, Left* **4 Adrenal Glands, Bilateral** *See 2 Adrenal Gland, Left* **6 Carotid Body, Left** Carotid glomus **7 Carotid Body, Right** *See 6 Carotid Body, Left* **8 Carotid Bodies, Bilateral** *See 6 Carotid Body, Left* **9 Para-aortic Body** **B Coccygeal Glomus** Coccygeal body **C Glomus Jugulare** Jugular body **D Aortic Body** **F Paraganglion Extremity** **G Thyroid Gland Lobe, Left** **H Thyroid Gland Lobe, Right** **J Thyroid Gland Isthmus** **L Superior Parathyroid Gland, Right** **M Superior Parathyroid Gland, Left** **N Inferior Parathyroid Gland, Right** **P Inferior Parathyroid Gland, Left** **Q Parathyroid Glands, Multiple** **R Parathyroid Gland**	**Ø Open** **3 Percutaneous** **4 Percutaneous Endoscopic**	**Z No Device**	**X Diagnostic** **Z No Qualifier**

Non-OR ØGB[2,3,4,G,H,J][3,4]ZX

Ø Medical and Surgical
G Endocrine System
C Extirpation Definition: Taking or cutting out solid matter from a body part

Explanation: The solid matter may be an abnormal byproduct of a biological function or a foreign body; it may be imbedded in a body part or in the lumen of a tubular body part. The solid matter may or may not have been previously broken into pieces.

Body Part Character 4	Approach Character 5	Device Character 6	Qualifier Character 7
Ø Pituitary Gland Adenohypophysis Hypophysis Neurohypophysis **1 Pineal Body** **2 Adrenal Gland, Left** Suprarenal gland **3 Adrenal Gland, Right** *See 2 Adrenal Gland, Left* **4 Adrenal Glands, Bilateral** *See 2 Adrenal Gland, Left* **6 Carotid Body, Left** Carotid glomus **7 Carotid Body, Right** *See 6 Carotid Body, Left* **8 Carotid Bodies, Bilateral** *See 6 Carotid Body, Left* **9 Para-aortic Body** **B Coccygeal Glomus** Coccygeal body **C Glomus Jugulare** Jugular body **D Aortic Body** **F Paraganglion Extremity** **G Thyroid Gland Lobe, Left** **H Thyroid Gland Lobe, Right** **K Thyroid Gland** **L Superior Parathyroid Gland, Right** **M Superior Parathyroid Gland, Left** **N Inferior Parathyroid Gland, Right** **P Inferior Parathyroid Gland, Left** **Q Parathyroid Glands, Multiple** **R Parathyroid Gland**	**Ø Open** **3 Percutaneous** **4 Percutaneous Endoscopic**	**Z No Device**	**Z No Qualifier**

Ø Medical and Surgical
G Endocrine System
H Insertion Definition: Putting in a nonbiological appliance that monitors, assists, performs, or prevents a physiological function but does not physically take the place of a body part

Explanation: None

Body Part Character 4	Approach Character 5	Device Character 6	Qualifier Character 7
S Endocrine Gland	Ø Open 3 Percutaneous 4 Percutaneous Endoscopic	1 Radioactive Element 2 Monitoring Device 3 Infusion Device Y Other Device	Z No Qualifier

Non-OR ØGHS31Z
Non-OR ØGHS[3,4]YZ

Ø Medical and Surgical
G Endocrine System
J Inspection Definition: Visually and/or manually exploring a body part

Explanation: Visual exploration may be performed with or without optical instrumentation. Manual exploration may be performed directly or through intervening body layers.

Body Part Character 4	Approach Character 5	Device Character 6	Qualifier Character 7
Ø Pituitary Gland Adenohypophysis Hypophysis Neurohypophysis 1 Pineal Body 5 Adrenal Gland Suprarenal gland K Thyroid Gland R Parathyroid Gland S Endocrine Gland	Ø Open 3 Percutaneous 4 Percutaneous Endoscopic	Z No Device	Z No Qualifier

Non-OR ØGJ[Ø,1,5,K,R,S]3ZZ

Ø Medical and Surgical
G Endocrine System
M Reattachment Definition: Putting back in or on all or a portion of a separated body part to its normal location or other suitable location

Explanation: Vascular circulation and nervous pathways may or may not be reestablished

Body Part Character 4	Approach Character 5	Device Character 6	Qualifier Character 7
2 Adrenal Gland, Left Suprarenal gland 3 Adrenal Gland, Right *See 2 Adrenal Gland, Left* G Thyroid Gland Lobe, Left H Thyroid Gland Lobe, Right L Superior Parathyroid Gland, Right M Superior Parathyroid Gland, Left N Inferior Parathyroid Gland, Right P Inferior Parathyroid Gland, Left Q Parathyroid Glands, Multiple R Parathyroid Gland	Ø Open 4 Percutaneous Endoscopic	Z No Device	Z No Qualifier

Ø Medical and Surgical
G Endocrine System
N Release Definition: Freeing a body part from an abnormal physical constraint by cutting or by the use of force

Explanation: Some of the restraining tissue may be taken out but none of the body part is taken out

Body Part Character 4	Approach Character 5	Device Character 6	Qualifier Character 7
Ø Pituitary Gland Adenohypophysis Hypophysis Neurohypophysis **1 Pineal Body** **2 Adrenal Gland, Left** Suprarenal gland **3 Adrenal Gland, Right** *See 2 Adrenal Gland, Left* **4 Adrenal Glands, Bilateral** *See 2 Adrenal Gland, Left* **6 Carotid Body, Left** Carotid glomus **7 Carotid Body, Right** *See 6 Carotid Body, Left* **8 Carotid Bodies, Bilateral** *See 6 Carotid Body, Left* **9 Para-aortic Body** **B Coccygeal Glomus** Coccygeal body **C Glomus Jugulare** Jugular body **D Aortic Body** **F Paraganglion Extremity** **G Thyroid Gland Lobe, Left** **H Thyroid Gland Lobe, Right** **K Thyroid Gland** **L Superior Parathyroid Gland, Right** **M Superior Parathyroid Gland, Left** **N Inferior Parathyroid Gland, Right** **P Inferior Parathyroid Gland, Left** **Q Parathyroid Glands, Multiple** **R Parathyroid Gland**	**Ø Open** **3 Percutaneous** **4 Percutaneous Endoscopic**	**Z No Device**	**Z No Qualifier**

Non-OR ØGN[6,7,8,9,B,C,D,F][Ø,3,4]ZZ

Ø Medical and Surgical
G Endocrine System
P Removal Definition: Taking out or off a device from a body part

Explanation: If a device is taken out and a similar device put in without cutting or puncturing the skin or mucous membrane, the procedure is coded to the root operation CHANGE. Otherwise, the procedure for taking out a device is coded to the root operation REMOVAL.

Body Part Character 4	Approach Character 5	Device Character 6	Qualifier Character 7
Ø Pituitary Gland Adenohypophysis Hypophysis Neurohypophysis **1 Pineal Body** **5 Adrenal Gland** Suprarenal gland **K Thyroid Gland** **R Parathyroid Gland**	**Ø Open** **3 Percutaneous** **4 Percutaneous Endoscopic** **X External**	**Ø Drainage Device**	**Z No Qualifier**
S Endocrine Gland	**Ø Open** **3 Percutaneous** **4 Percutaneous Endoscopic**	**Ø Drainage Device** **2 Monitoring Device** **3 Infusion Device** **Y Other Device**	**Z No Qualifier**
S Endocrine Gland	**X External**	**Ø Drainage Device** **2 Monitoring Device** **3 Infusion Device**	**Z No Qualifier**

Non-OR ØGP[Ø,1,5,K,R]XØZ
Non-OR ØGPS[3,4]YZ
Non-OR ØGPSX[Ø,2,3]Z

Ø Medical and Surgical
G Endocrine System
Q Repair Definition: Restoring, to the extent possible, a body part to its normal anatomic structure and function

Explanation: Used only when the method to accomplish the repair is not one of the other root operations

Body Part Character 4	Approach Character 5	Device Character 6	Qualifier Character 7
Ø Pituitary Gland Adenohypophysis Hypophysis Neurohypophysis **1 Pineal Body** **2 Adrenal Gland, Left** Suprarenal gland **3 Adrenal Gland, Right** *See 2 Adrenal Gland, Left* **4 Adrenal Glands, Bilateral** *See 2 Adrenal Gland, Left* **6 Carotid Body, Left** Carotid glomus **7 Carotid Body, Right** *See 6 Carotid Body, Left* **8 Carotid Bodies, Bilateral** *See 6 Carotid Body, Left* **9 Para-aortic Body** **B Coccygeal Glomus** Coccygeal body **C Glomus Jugulare** Jugular body **D Aortic Body** **F Paraganglion Extremity** **G Thyroid Gland Lobe, Left** **H Thyroid Gland Lobe, Right** **J Thyroid Gland Isthmus** **K Thyroid Gland** **L Superior Parathyroid Gland, Right** **M Superior Parathyroid Gland, Left** **N Inferior Parathyroid Gland, Right** **P Inferior Parathyroid Gland, Left** **Q Parathyroid Glands, Multiple** **R Parathyroid Gland**	**Ø Open** **3 Percutaneous** **4 Percutaneous Endoscopic**	**Z No Device**	**Z No Qualifier**

Ø Medical and Surgical
G Endocrine System
S Reposition Definition: Moving to its normal location, or other suitable location, all or a portion of a body part

Explanation: The body part is moved to a new location from an abnormal location, or from a normal location where it is not functioning correctly. The body part may or may not be cut out or off to be moved to the new location.

Body Part Character 4	Approach Character 5	Device Character 6	Qualifier Character 7
2 Adrenal Gland, Left Suprarenal gland **3 Adrenal Gland, Right** *See 2 Adrenal Gland, Left* **G Thyroid Gland Lobe, Left** **H Thyroid Gland Lobe, Right** **L Superior Parathyroid Gland, Right** **M Superior Parathyroid Gland, Left** **N Inferior Parathyroid Gland, Right** **P Inferior Parathyroid Gland, Left** **Q Parathyroid Glands, Multiple** **R Parathyroid Gland**	**Ø Open** **4 Percutaneous Endoscopic**	**Z No Device**	**Z No Qualifier**

Ø Medical and Surgical
G Endocrine System
T Resection Definition: Cutting out or off, without replacement, all of a body part

Explanation: None

Body Part Character 4	Approach Character 5	Device Character 6	Qualifier Character 7
Ø Pituitary Gland Adenohypophysis Hypophysis Neurohypophysis 1 Pineal Body 2 Adrenal Gland, Left Suprarenal gland 3 Adrenal Gland, Right *See 2 Adrenal Gland, Left* 4 Adrenal Glands, Bilateral *See 2 Adrenal Gland, Left* 6 Carotid Body, Left Carotid glomus 7 Carotid Body, Right *See 6 Carotid Body, Left* 8 Carotid Bodies, Bilateral *See 6 Carotid Body, Left* 9 Para-aortic Body B Coccygeal Glomus Coccygeal body C Glomus Jugulare Jugular body D Aortic Body F Paraganglion Extremity G Thyroid Gland Lobe, Left H Thyroid Gland Lobe, Right J Thyroid Gland Isthmus K Thyroid Gland L Superior Parathyroid Gland, Right M Superior Parathyroid Gland, Left N Inferior Parathyroid Gland, Right P Inferior Parathyroid Gland, Left Q Parathyroid Glands, Multiple R Parathyroid Gland	Ø Open 4 Percutaneous Endoscopic	Z No Device	Z No Qualifier

Non-OR ØGT[6,7,8,9,B,C,D,F][Ø,4]ZZ

Ø Medical and Surgical
G Endocrine System
W Revision Definition: Correcting, to the extent possible, a portion of a malfunctioning device or the position of a displaced device

Explanation: Revision can include correcting a malfunctioning or displaced device by taking out or putting in components of the device such as a screw or pin

Body Part Character 4	Approach Character 5	Device Character 6	Qualifier Character 7
Ø Pituitary Gland Adenohypophysis Hypophysis Neurohypophysis 1 Pineal Body 5 Adrenal Gland Suprarenal gland K Thyroid Gland R Parathyroid Gland	Ø Open 3 Percutaneous 4 Percutaneous Endoscopic X External	Ø Drainage Device	Z No Qualifier
S Endocrine Gland	Ø Open 3 Percutaneous 4 Percutaneous Endoscopic	Ø Drainage Device 2 Monitoring Device 3 Infusion Device Y Other Device	Z No Qualifier
S Endocrine Gland	X External	Ø Drainage Device 2 Monitoring Device 3 Infusion Device	Z No Qualifier

Non-OR ØGW[Ø,1,5,K,R]XØZ
Non-OR ØGWS[3,4]YZ
Non-OR ØGWSX[Ø,2,3]Z

Skin and Breast ØHØ–ØHX

Character Meanings*

This Character Meaning table is provided as a guide to assist the user in the identification of character members that may be found in this section of code tables. It **SHOULD NOT** be used to build a PCS code.

Operation–Character 3	Body Part–Character 4	Approach–Character 5	Device–Character 6	Qualifier–Character 7
Ø Alteration	Ø Skin, Scalp	Ø Open	Ø Drainage Device	2 Cell Suspension Technique
2 Change	1 Skin, Face	3 Percutaneous	1 Radioactive Element	3 Full Thickness
5 Destruction	2 Skin, Right Ear	7 Via Natural or Artificial Opening	7 Autologous Tissue Substitute	4 Partial Thickness
8 Division	3 Skin, Left Ear	8 Via Natural or Artificial Opening Endoscopic	J Synthetic Substitute	5 Latissimus Dorsi Myocutaneous Flap
9 Drainage	4 Skin, Neck	X External	K Nonautologous Tissue Substitute	6 Transverse Rectus Abdominis Myocutaneous Flap
B Excision	5 Skin, Chest		N Tissue Expander	7 Deep Inferior Epigastric Artery Perforator Flap
C Extirpation	6 Skin, Back		Y Other Device	8 Superficial Inferior Epigastric Artery Flap
D Extraction	7 Skin, Abdomen		Z No Device	9 Gluteal Artery Perforator Flap
H Insertion	8 Skin, Buttock			D Multiple
J Inspection	9 Skin, Perineum			X Diagnostic
M Reattachment	A Skin, Inguinal			Z No Qualifier
N Release	B Skin, Right Upper Arm			
P Removal	C Skin, Left Upper Arm			
Q Repair	D Skin, Right Lower Arm			
R Replacement	E Skin, Left Lower Arm			
S Reposition	F Skin, Right Hand			
T Resection	G Skin, Left Hand			
U Supplement	H Skin, Right Upper Leg			
W Revision	J Skin, Left Upper Leg			
X Transfer	K Skin, Right Lower Leg			
	L Skin, Left Lower Leg			
	M Skin, Right Foot			
	N Skin, Left Foot			
	P Skin			
	Q Finger Nail			
	R Toe Nail			
	S Hair			
	T Breast, Right			
	U Breast, Left			
	V Breast, Bilateral			
	W Nipple, Right			
	X Nipple, Left			
	Y Supernumerary Breast			

* Includes skin and breast glands and ducts.

AHA Coding Clinic for table ØHØ

2019, 4Q, 30-31 Breast procedures

AHA Coding Clinic for table ØH5

2019, 4Q, 30-31 Breast procedures

AHA Coding Clinic for table ØH9

2019, 4Q, 30-31 Breast procedures

AHA Coding Clinic for table ØHB

2020, 1Q, 31 Repair of buried penis
2019, 4Q, 30-31 Breast procedures
2018, 1Q, 14 Excisional debridement of breast tissue and skin
2016, 3Q, 29 Closure of bilateral alveolar clefts
2015, 3Q, 3-8 Excisional and nonexcisional debridement

AHA Coding Clinic for table ØHC

2019, 4Q, 30-31 Breast procedures

AHA Coding Clinic for table ØHD

2019, 4Q, 30-31 Breast procedures
2016, 1Q, 40 Nonexcisional debridement of skin and subcutaneous tissue
2015, 3Q, 3-8 Excisional and nonexcisional debridement

AHA Coding Clinic for table ØHH

2019, 4Q, 30-31 Breast procedures
2017, 4Q, 67 New qualifier values - Pedicle flap procedures
2014, 2Q, 12 Pedicle latissimus myocutaneous flap with placement of breast tissue expanders
2013, 4Q, 107 Breast tissue expander placement using acellular dermal matrix

AHA Coding Clinic for table ØHJ

2019, 4Q, 30-31 Breast procedures

AHA Coding Clinic for table ØHN

2019, 4Q, 30-31 Breast procedures

AHA Coding Clinic for table ØHP

2019, 4Q, 30-31 Breast procedures
2018, 3Q, 13 Deep inferior epigastric artery perforator flap breast reconstruction
2016, 2Q, 27 Removal of nonviable transverse rectus abdominis myocutaneous (TRAM) flaps

AHA Coding Clinic for table ØHQ

2019, 4Q, 30-31 Breast procedures
2018, 2Q, 25 Third and fourth degree obstetric lacerations
2016, 1Q, 7 Obstetrical perineal laceration repair
2014, 4Q, 31 Delayed wound closure following fracture treatment

AHA Coding Clinic for table ØHR

2020, 1Q, 27 Delayed reconstruction following mastectomy using gracilis musculocutaneous free flap
2020, 1Q, 28 Free flap microvascular breast reconstruction
2020, 1Q, 30 Polarity Skin TE™ application
2019, 4Q, 30-31 Breast procedures
2019, 4Q, 32 Cell suspension epithelial autograft
2019, 3Q, 32 Breast reconstruction with neurotization
2018, 3Q, 13 Deep inferior epigastric artery perforator flap breast reconstruction
2017, 1Q, 35 Epifix® allograft
2014, 3Q, 14 Application of TheraSkin® and excisional debridement

AHA Coding Clinic for table ØHT

2021, 2Q, 16 Goldilocks breast reconstruction
2018, 3Q, 13 Deep inferior epigastric artery perforator flap breast reconstruction
2014, 4Q, 34 Skin-sparing mastectomy

AHA Coding Clinic for table ØHU

2019, 4Q, 30-31 Breast procedures

AHA Coding Clinic for table ØHW

2019, 4Q, 30-31 Breast procedures

Integumentary Anatomy

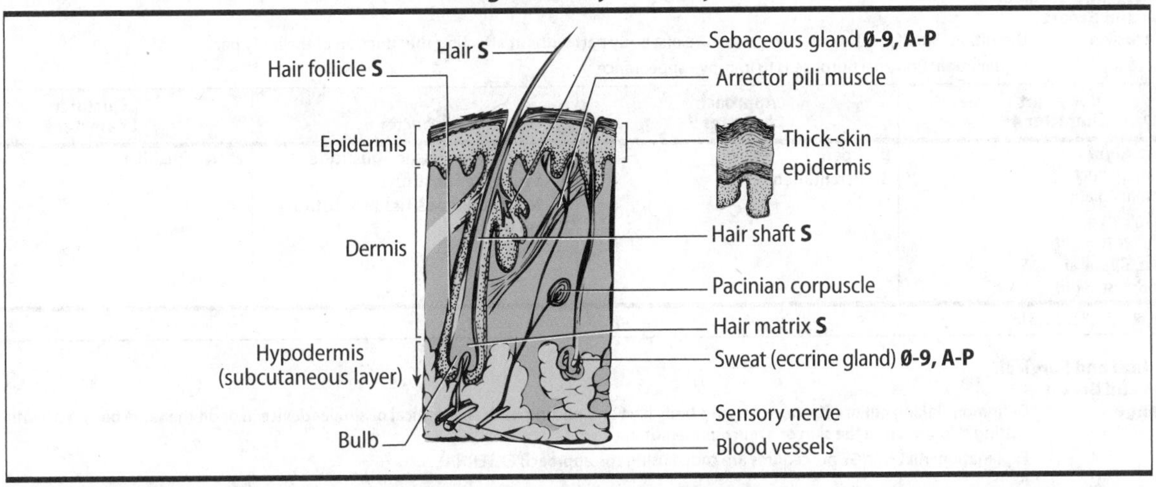

Nail Anatomy

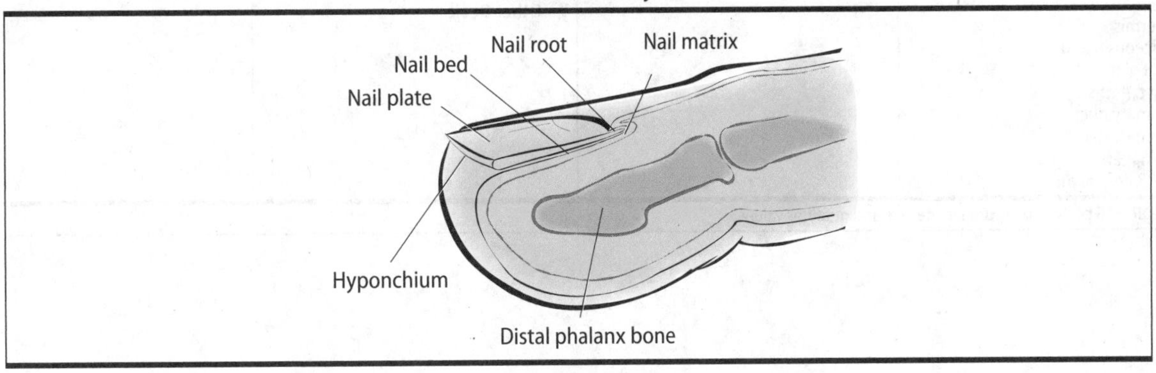

Breast

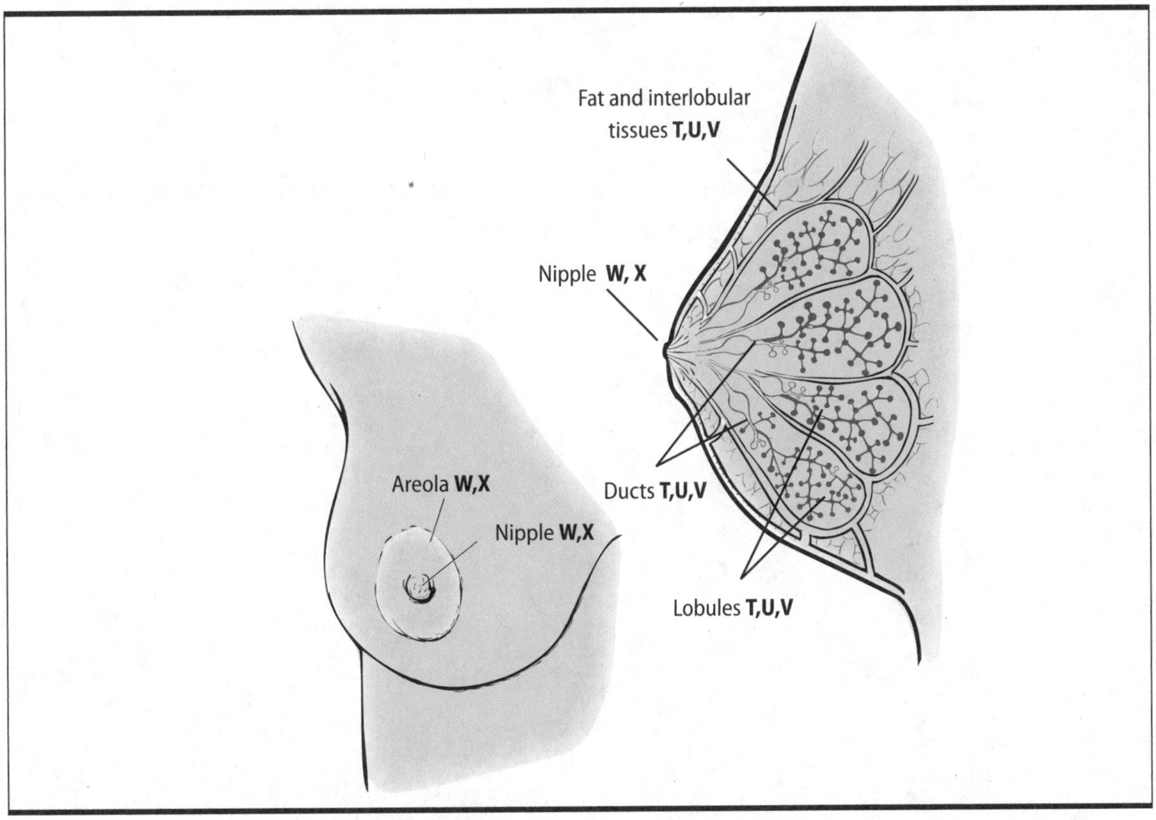

Ø Medical and Surgical
H Skin and Breast
Ø Alteration Definition: Modifying the anatomic structure of a body part without affecting the function of the body part

Explanation: Principal purpose is to improve appearance

Body Part Character 4	Approach Character 5	Device Character 6	Qualifier Character 7
T Breast, Right Mammary duct Mammary gland U Breast, Left *See T Breast, Right* V Breast, Bilateral *See T Breast, Right*	Ø Open 3 Percutaneous	7 Autologous Tissue Substitute J Synthetic Substitute K Nonautologous Tissue Substitute Z No Device	Z No Qualifier

Non-OR ØHØ[T,U,V]3JZ

Ø Medical and Surgical
H Skin and Breast
2 Change Definition: Taking out or off a device from a body part and putting back an identical or similar device in or on the same body part without cutting or puncturing the skin or a mucous membrane

Explanation: All CHANGE procedures are coded using the approach EXTERNAL

Body Part Character 4	Approach Character 5	Device Character 6	Qualifier Character 7
P Skin Dermis Epidermis Sebaceous gland Sweat gland T Breast, Right Mammary duct Mammary gland U Breast, Left *See T Breast, Right*	X External	Ø Drainage Device Y Other Device	Z No Qualifier

Non-OR All body part, approach, device, and qualifier values

Ø Medical and Surgical
H Skin and Breast
5 Destruction Definition: Physical eradication of all or a portion of a body part by the direct use of energy, force, or a destructive agent
Explanation: None of the body part is physically taken out

Body Part Character 4	Approach Character 5	Device Character 6	Qualifier Character 7
Ø Skin, Scalp **1 Skin, Face** **2 Skin, Right Ear** **3 Skin, Left Ear** **4 Skin, Neck** **5 Skin, Chest** Breast procedures, skin only **6 Skin, Back** **7 Skin, Abdomen** **8 Skin, Buttock** **9 Skin, Perineum** **A Skin, Inguinal** **B Skin, Right Upper Arm** **C Skin, Left Upper Arm** **D Skin, Right Lower Arm** **E Skin, Left Lower Arm** **F Skin, Right Hand** **G Skin, Left Hand** **H Skin, Right Upper Leg** **J Skin, Left Upper Leg** **K Skin, Right Lower Leg** **L Skin, Left Lower Leg** **M Skin, Right Foot** **N Skin, Left Foot**	**X External**	**Z No Device**	**D Multiple** **Z No Qualifier**
Q Finger Nail Nail bed Nail plate **R Toe Nail** *See Q Finger Nail*	**X External**	**Z No Device**	**Z No Qualifier**
T Breast, Right Mammary duct Mammary gland **U Breast, Left** *See T Breast, Right* **V Breast, Bilateral** *See T Breast, Right*	**Ø Open** **3 Percutaneous** **7 Via Natural or Artificial Opening** **8 Via Natural or Artificial Opening Endoscopic**	**Z No Device**	**Z No Qualifier**
W Nipple, Right Areola **X Nipple, Left** *See W Nipple, Right*	**Ø Open** **3 Percutaneous** **7 Via Natural or Artificial Opening** **8 Via Natural or Artificial Opening Endoscopic** **X External**	**Z No Device**	**Z No Qualifier**

DRG Non-OR ØH5[Ø,1,4,5,6,7,8,9,A,B,C,D,E,F,G,H,J,K,L,M,N]XZ[D,Z]
DRG Non-OR ØH5[Q,R]XZZ
Non-OR ØH5[2,3]XZ[D,Z]

Ø Medical and Surgical
H Skin and Breast
8 Division

Definition: Cutting into a body part, without draining fluids and/or gases from the body part, in order to separate or transect a body part

Explanation: All or a portion of the body part is separated into two or more portions

Body Part Character 4	Approach Character 5	Device Character 6	Qualifier Character 7
Ø Skin, Scalp 1 Skin, Face 2 Skin, Right Ear 3 Skin, Left Ear 4 Skin, Neck 5 Skin, Chest Breast procedures, skin only 6 Skin, Back 7 Skin, Abdomen 8 Skin, Buttock 9 Skin, Perineum A Skin, Inguinal B Skin, Right Upper Arm C Skin, Left Upper Arm D Skin, Right Lower Arm E Skin, Left Lower Arm F Skin, Right Hand G Skin, Left Hand H Skin, Right Upper Leg J Skin, Left Upper Leg K Skin, Right Lower Leg L Skin, Left Lower Leg M Skin, Right Foot N Skin, Left Foot	X External	Z No Device	Z No Qualifier

Non-OR All body part, approach, device, and qualifier values

Ø Medical and Surgical
H Skin and Breast
9 Drainage Definition: Taking or letting out fluids and/or gases from a body part
Explanation: The qualifier DIAGNOSTIC is used to identify drainage procedures that are biopsies

Body Part Character 4	Approach Character 5	Device Character 6	Qualifier Character 7
Ø Skin, Scalp **1** Skin, Face **2** Skin, Right Ear **3** Skin, Left Ear **4** Skin, Neck **5** Skin, Chest Breast procedures, skin only **6** Skin, Back **7** Skin, Abdomen **8** Skin, Buttock **9** Skin, Perineum **A** Skin, Inguinal **B** Skin, Right Upper Arm **C** Skin, Left Upper Arm **D** Skin, Right Lower Arm **E** Skin, Left Lower Arm **F** Skin, Right Hand **G** Skin, Left Hand **H** Skin, Right Upper Leg **J** Skin, Left Upper Leg **K** Skin, Right Lower Leg **L** Skin, Left Lower Leg **M** Skin, Right Foot **N** Skin, Left Foot **Q** Finger Nail Nail bed Nail plate **R** Toe Nail *See Q Finger Nail*	**X** External	**Ø** Drainage Device	**Z** No Qualifier
Ø Skin, Scalp **1** Skin, Face **2** Skin, Right Ear **3** Skin, Left Ear **4** Skin, Neck **5** Skin, Chest Breast procedures, skin only **6** Skin, Back **7** Skin, Abdomen **8** Skin, Buttock **9** Skin, Perineum **A** Skin, Inguinal **B** Skin, Right Upper Arm **C** Skin, Left Upper Arm **D** Skin, Right Lower Arm **E** Skin, Left Lower Arm **F** Skin, Right Hand **G** Skin, Left Hand **H** Skin, Right Upper Leg **J** Skin, Left Upper Leg **K** Skin, Right Lower Leg **L** Skin, Left Lower Leg **M** Skin, Right Foot **N** Skin, Left Foot **Q** Finger Nail Nail bed Nail plate **R** Toe Nail *See Q Finger Nail*	**X** External	**Z** No Device	**X** Diagnostic **Z** No Qualifier
T Breast, Right Mammary duct Mammary gland **U** Breast, Left *See T Breast, Right* **V** Breast, Bilateral *See T Breast, Right*	**Ø** Open **3** Percutaneous **7** Via Natural or Artificial Opening **8** Via Natural or Artificial Opening Endoscopic	**Ø** Drainage Device	**Z** No Qualifier
T Breast, Right Mammary duct Mammary gland **U** Breast, Left *See T Breast, Right* **V** Breast, Bilateral *See T Breast, Right*	**Ø** Open **3** Percutaneous **7** Via Natural or Artificial Opening **8** Via Natural or Artificial Opening Endoscopic	**Z** No Device	**X** Diagnostic **Z** No Qualifier
W Nipple, Right Areola **X** Nipple, Left *See W Nipple, Right*	**Ø** Open **3** Percutaneous **7** Via Natural or Artificial Opening **8** Via Natural or Artificial Opening Endoscopic **X** External	**Ø** Drainage Device	**Z** No Qualifier
W Nipple, Right Areola **X** Nipple, Left *See W Nipple, Right*	**Ø** Open **3** Percutaneous **7** Via Natural or Artificial Opening **8** Via Natural or Artificial Opening Endoscopic **X** External	**Z** No Device	**X** Diagnostic **Z** No Qualifier

Non-OR ØH9[Ø,1,2,3,4,5,6,7,8,A,B,C,D,E,F,G,H,J,K,L,M,N,Q,R]XØZ
Non-OR ØH9[Ø,1,2,3,4,5,6,7,8,A,B,C,D,E,F,G,H,J,K,L,M,N,Q,R]XZ[X,Z]
Non-OR ØH99XZX
Non-OR ØH9[T,U,V][Ø,3,7,8]ØZ
Non-OR ØH9[T,U,V][3,7,8]Z[X,Z]
Non-OR ØH9[W,X][Ø,3,7,8,X]ØZ
Non-OR ØH9[W,X][3,7,8,X]Z[X,Z]

Ø Medical and Surgical
H Skin and Breast
B Excision Definition: Cutting out or off, without replacement, a portion of a body part
Explanation: The qualifier DIAGNOSTIC is used to identify excision procedures that are biopsies

Body Part Character 4	Approach Character 5	Device Character 6	Qualifier Character 7
Ø Skin, Scalp **1** Skin, Face **2** Skin, Right Ear **3** Skin, Left Ear **4** Skin, Neck **5** Skin, Chest Breast procedures, skin only **6** Skin, Back **7** Skin, Abdomen **8** Skin, Buttock **9** Skin, Perineum **A** Skin, Inguinal **B** Skin, Right Upper Arm **C** Skin, Left Upper Arm **D** Skin, Right Lower Arm **E** Skin, Left Lower Arm **F** Skin, Right Hand **G** Skin, Left Hand **H** Skin, Right Upper Leg **J** Skin, Left Upper Leg **K** Skin, Right Lower Leg **L** Skin, Left Lower Leg **M** Skin, Right Foot **N** Skin, Left Foot **Q** Finger Nail Nail bed Nail plate **R** Toe Nail *See Q Finger Nail*	**X** External	**Z** No Device	**X** Diagnostic **Z** No Qualifier
T Breast, Right Mammary duct Mammary gland **U** Breast, Left *See T Breast, Right* **V** Breast, Bilateral *See T Breast, Right* **Y** Supernumerary Breast	**Ø** Open **3** Percutaneous **7** Via Natural or Artificial Opening **8** Via Natural or Artificial Opening Endoscopic	**Z** No Device	**X** Diagnostic **Z** No Qualifier
W Nipple, Right Areola **X** Nipple, Left *See W Nipple, Right*	**Ø** Open **3** Percutaneous **7** Via Natural or Artificial Opening **8** Via Natural or Artificial Opening Endoscopic **X** External	**Z** No Device	**X** Diagnostic **Z** No Qualifier

DRG Non-OR ØHB9XZZ
Non-OR ØHB[Ø,1,2,3,4,5,6,7,8,A,B,C,D,E,F,G,H,J,K,L,M,N,Q,R]XZ[X,Z]
Non-OR ØHB9XZX
Non-OR ØHB[T,U,V,Y][3,7,8]ZX
Non-OR ØHB[W,X][3,7,8,X]ZX

Ø Medical and Surgical
H Skin and Breast
C Extirpation Definition: Taking or cutting out solid matter from a body part

Explanation: The solid matter may be an abnormal byproduct of a biological function or a foreign body; it may be imbedded in a body part or in the lumen of a tubular body part. The solid matter may or may not have been previously broken into pieces.

Body Part Character 4	Approach Character 5	Device Character 6	Qualifier Character 7
Ø Skin, Scalp **1** Skin, Face **2** Skin, Right Ear **3** Skin, Left Ear **4** Skin, Neck **5** Skin, Chest Breast procedures, skin only **6** Skin, Back **7** Skin, Abdomen **8** Skin, Buttock **9** Skin, Perineum **A** Skin, Inguinal **B** Skin, Right Upper Arm **C** Skin, Left Upper Arm **D** Skin, Right Lower Arm **E** Skin, Left Lower Arm **F** Skin, Right Hand **G** Skin, Left Hand **H** Skin, Right Upper Leg **J** Skin, Left Upper Leg **K** Skin, Right Lower Leg **L** Skin, Left Lower Leg **M** Skin, Right Foot **N** Skin, Left Foot **Q** Finger Nail Nail bed Nail plate **R** Toe Nail *See Q Finger Nail*	**X** External	**Z** No Device	**Z** No Qualifier
T Breast, Right Mammary duct Mammary gland **U** Breast, Left *See T Breast, Right* **V** Breast, Bilateral *See T Breast, Right*	**Ø** Open **3** Percutaneous **7** Via Natural or Artificial Opening **8** Via Natural or Artificial Opening Endoscopic	**Z** No Device	**Z** No Qualifier
W Nipple, Right Areola **X** Nipple, Left *See W Nipple, Right*	**Ø** Open **3** Percutaneous **7** Via Natural or Artificial Opening **8** Via Natural or Artificial Opening Endoscopic **X** External	**Z** No Device	**Z** No Qualifier

Non-OR ØHC[Ø,1,2,3,4,5,6,7,8,9,A,B,C,D,E,F,G,H,J,K,L,M,N,Q,R]XZZ
Non-OR ØHC[T,U,V][3,7,8]ZZ
Non-OR ØHC[W,X][3,7,8,X]ZZ

Ø Medical and Surgical
H Skin and Breast
D Extraction Definition: Pulling or stripping out or off all or a portion of a body part by the use of force
Explanation: The qualifier DIAGNOSTIC is used to identify extraction procedures that are biopsies

Body Part Character 4	Approach Character 5	Device Character 6	Qualifier Character 7
Ø Skin, Scalp **1 Skin, Face** **2 Skin, Right Ear** **3 Skin, Left Ear** **4 Skin, Neck** **5 Skin, Chest** Breast procedures, skin only **6 Skin, Back** **7 Skin, Abdomen** **8 Skin, Buttock** **9 Skin, Perineum** **A Skin, Inguinal** **B Skin, Right Upper Arm** **C Skin, Left Upper Arm** **D Skin, Right Lower Arm** **E Skin, Left Lower Arm** **F Skin, Right Hand** **G Skin, Left Hand** **H Skin, Right Upper Leg** **J Skin, Left Upper Leg** **K Skin, Right Lower Leg** **L Skin, Left Lower Leg** **M Skin, Right Foot** **N Skin, Left Foot** **Q Finger Nail** Nail bed Nail plate **R Toe Nail** *See Q Finger Nail* **S Hair**	**X External**	**Z No Device**	**Z No Qualifier**
T Breast, Right Mammary duct Mammary gland **U Breast, Left** *See T Breast, Right* **V Breast, Bilateral** *See T Breast, Right* **Y Supernumerary Breast**	**Ø Open**	**Z No Device**	**Z No Qualifier**

Non-OR All body part, approach, device, and qualifier values

Ø Medical and Surgical
H Skin and Breast
H Insertion Definition: Putting in a nonbiological appliance that monitors, assists, performs, or prevents a physiological function but does not physically take the place of a body part

Explanation: None

Body Part Character 4	Approach Character 5	Device Character 6	Qualifier Character 7
P Skin	**X External**	**Y Other Device**	**Z No Qualifier**
T Breast, Right Mammary duct Mammary gland **U Breast, Left** *See T Breast, Right*	**Ø Open** **3 Percutaneous** **7 Via Natural or Artificial Opening** **8 Via Natural or Artificial Opening Endoscopic**	**1 Radioactive Element** **N Tissue Expander** **Y Other Device**	**Z No Qualifier**
V Breast, Bilateral Mammary duct Mammary gland	**Ø Open** **3 Percutaneous** **7 Via Natural or Artificial Opening** **8 Via Natural or Artificial Opening Endoscopic**	**1 Radioactive Element** **N Tissue Expander**	**Z No Qualifier**
W Nipple, Right Areola **X Nipple, Left** *See W Nipple, Right*	**Ø Open** **3 Percutaneous** **7 Via Natural or Artificial Opening** **8 Via Natural or Artificial Opening Endoscopic**	**1 Radioactive Element** **N Tissue Expander**	**Z No Qualifier**
W Nipple, Right Areola **X Nipple, Left** *See W Nipple, Right*	**X External**	**1 Radioactive Element**	**Z No Qualifier**

Non-OR ØHHPXYZ
Non-OR ØHH[T,U][3,7,8]YZ

Ø Medical and Surgical
H Skin and Breast
J Inspection Definition: Visually and/or manually exploring a body part

Explanation: Visual exploration may be performed with or without optical instrumentation. Manual exploration may be performed directly or through intervening body layers.

Body Part Character 4	Approach Character 5	Device Character 6	Qualifier Character 7
P Skin Dermis Epidermis Sebaceous gland Sweat gland **Q Finger Nail** Nail bed Nail plate **R Toe Nail** *See Q Finger Nail*	**X External**	**Z No Device**	**Z No Qualifier**
T Breast, Right Mammary duct Mammary gland **U Breast, Left** *See T Breast, Right*	**Ø Open** **3 Percutaneous** **7 Via Natural or Artificial Opening** **8 Via Natural or Artificial Opening Endoscopic**	**Z No Device**	**Z No Qualifier**

Non-OR All body part, approach, device and qualifier values

Ø Medical and Surgical
H Skin and Breast
M Reattachment Definition: Putting back in or on all or a portion of a separated body part to its normal location or other suitable location
Explanation: Vascular circulation and nervous pathways may or may not be reestablished

Body Part Character 4	Approach Character 5	Device Character 6	Qualifier Character 7
Ø Skin, Scalp **1 Skin, Face** **2 Skin, Right Ear** **3 Skin, Left Ear** **4 Skin, Neck** **5 Skin, Chest** Breast procedures, skin only **6 Skin, Back** **7 Skin, Abdomen** **8 Skin, Buttock** **9 Skin, Perineum** **A Skin, Inguinal** **B Skin, Right Upper Arm** **C Skin, Left Upper Arm** **D Skin, Right Lower Arm** **E Skin, Left Lower Arm** **F Skin, Right Hand** **G Skin, Left Hand** **H Skin, Right Upper Leg** **J Skin, Left Upper Leg** **K Skin, Right Lower Leg** **L Skin, Left Lower Leg** **M Skin, Right Foot** **N Skin, Left Foot** **T Breast, Right** Mammary duct Mammary gland **U Breast, Left** *See T Breast, Right* **V Breast, Bilateral** *See T Breast, Right* **W Nipple, Right** Areola **X Nipple, Left** *See W Nipple, Right*	**X External**	**Z No Device**	**Z No Qualifier**

Non-OR ØHMØXZZ

Ø Medical and Surgical
H Skin and Breast
N Release Definition: Freeing a body part from an abnormal physical constraint by cutting or by the use of force
Explanation: Some of the restraining tissue may be taken out but none of the body part is taken out

Body Part Character 4	Approach Character 5	Device Character 6	Qualifier Character 7
Ø Skin, Scalp **1 Skin, Face** **2 Skin, Right Ear** **3 Skin, Left Ear** **4 Skin, Neck** **5 Skin, Chest** Breast procedures, skin only **6 Skin, Back** **7 Skin, Abdomen** **8 Skin, Buttock** **9 Skin, Perineum** **A Skin, Inguinal** **B Skin, Right Upper Arm** **C Skin, Left Upper Arm** **D Skin, Right Lower Arm** **E Skin, Left Lower Arm** **F Skin, Right Hand** **G Skin, Left Hand** **H Skin, Right Upper Leg** **J Skin, Left Upper Leg** **K Skin, Right Lower Leg** **L Skin, Left Lower Leg** **M Skin, Right Foot** **N Skin, Left Foot** **Q Finger Nail** Nail bed Nail plate **R Toe Nail** *See Q Finger Nail*	**X External**	**Z No Device**	**Z No Qualifier**
T Breast, Right Mammary duct Mammary gland **U Breast, Left** *See T Breast, Right* **V Breast, Bilateral** *See T Breast, Right*	**Ø Open** **3 Percutaneous** **7 Via Natural or Artificial Opening** **8 Via Natural or Artificial Opening Endoscopic**	**Z No Device**	**Z No Qualifier**
W Nipple, Right Areola **X Nipple, Left** *See W Nipple, Right*	**Ø Open** **3 Percutaneous** **7 Via Natural or Artificial Opening** **8 Via Natural or Artificial Opening Endoscopic** **X External**	**Z No Device**	**Z No Qualifier**

Ø Medical and Surgical
H Skin and Breast
P Removal Definition: Taking out or off a device from a body part

Explanation: If a device is taken out and a similar device put in without cutting or puncturing the skin or mucous membrane, the procedure is coded to the root operation CHANGE. Otherwise, the procedure for taking out a device is coded to the root operation REMOVAL.

Body Part Character 4	Approach Character 5	Device Character 6	Qualifier Character 7
P Skin Dermis Epidermis Sebaceous gland Sweat gland	X External	Ø Drainage Device 7 Autologous Tissue Substitute J Synthetic Substitute K Nonautologous Tissue Substitute Y Other Device	Z No Qualifier
Q Finger Nail Nail bed Nail plate R Toe Nail *See Q Finger Nail*	X External	Ø Drainage Device 7 Autologous Tissue Substitute J Synthetic Substitute K Nonautologous Tissue Substitute	Z No Qualifier
S Hair	X External	7 Autologous Tissue Substitute J Synthetic Substitute K Nonautologous Tissue Substitute	Z No Qualifier
T Breast, Right Mammary duct Mammary gland U Breast, Left *See T Breast, Right*	Ø Open 3 Percutaneous 7 Via Natural or Artificial Opening 8 Via Natural or Artificial Opening Endoscopic	Ø Drainage Device 1 Radioactive Element 7 Autologous Tissue Substitute J Synthetic Substitute K Nonautologous Tissue Substitute N Tissue Expander Y Other Device	Z No Qualifier

Non-OR ØHPPX[Ø,7,J,K,Y]Z
Non-OR ØHP[Q,R]X[Ø,7,J,K]Z
Non-OR ØHPSX[7,J,K]Z
Non-OR ØHP[T,U]Ø[Ø,1,7,K]Z
Non-OR ØHP[T,U]3[Ø,1,7,K,Y]Z
Non-OR ØHP[T,U][7,8][Ø,1,7,J,K,N,Y]Z

Ø Medical and Surgical
H Skin and Breast
Q Repair Definition: Restoring, to the extent possible, a body part to its normal anatomic structure and function
Explanation: Used only when the method to accomplish the repair is not one of the other root operations

Body Part Character 4	Approach Character 5	Device Character 6	Qualifier Character 7
Ø Skin, Scalp **1 Skin, Face** **2 Skin, Right Ear** **3 Skin, Left Ear** **4 Skin, Neck** **5 Skin, Chest** Breast procedures, skin only **6 Skin, Back** **7 Skin, Abdomen** **8 Skin, Buttock** **9 Skin, Perineum** **A Skin, Inguinal** **B Skin, Right Upper Arm** **C Skin, Left Upper Arm** **D Skin, Right Lower Arm** **E Skin, Left Lower Arm** **F Skin, Right Hand** **G Skin, Left Hand** **H Skin, Right Upper Leg** **J Skin, Left Upper Leg** **K Skin, Right Lower Leg** **L Skin, Left Lower Leg** **M Skin, Right Foot** **N Skin, Left Foot** **Q Finger Nail** Nail bed Nail plate **R Toe Nail** *See Q Finger Nail*	**X External**	**Z No Device**	**Z No Qualifier**
T Breast, Right Mammary duct Mammary gland **U Breast, Left** *See T Breast, Right* **V Breast, Bilateral** *See T Breast, Right* **Y Supernumerary Breast**	**Ø Open** **3 Percutaneous** **7 Via Natural or Artificial Opening** **8 Via Natural or Artificial Opening Endoscopic**	**Z No Device**	**Z No Qualifier**
W Nipple, Right Areola **X Nipple, Left** *See W Nipple, Right*	**Ø Open** **3 Percutaneous** **7 Via Natural or Artificial Opening** **8 Via Natural or Artificial Opening Endoscopic** **X External**	**Z No Device**	**Z No Qualifier**

DRG Non-OR ØHQ9XZZ
Non-OR ØHQ[Ø,1,2,3,4,5,6,7,8,A,B,C,D,E,F,G,H,J,K,L,M,N]XZZ

Ø Medical and Surgical
H Skin and Breast
R Replacement Definition: Putting in or on biological or synthetic material that physically takes the place and/or function of all or a portion of a body part

Explanation: The body part may have been taken out or replaced, or may be taken out, physically eradicated, or rendered nonfunctional during the REPLACEMENT procedure. A REMOVAL procedure is coded for taking out the device used in a previous replacement procedure.

Body Part Character 4	Approach Character 5	Device Character 6	Qualifier Character 7
Ø Skin, Scalp **1** Skin, Face **2** Skin, Right Ear **3** Skin, Left Ear **4** Skin, Neck **5** Skin, Chest Breast procedures, skin only **6** Skin, Back **7** Skin, Abdomen **8** Skin, Buttock **9** Skin, Perineum **A** Skin, Inguinal **B** Skin, Right Upper Arm **C** Skin, Left Upper Arm **D** Skin, Right Lower Arm **E** Skin, Left Lower Arm **F** Skin, Right Hand **G** Skin, Left Hand **H** Skin, Right Upper Leg **J** Skin, Left Upper Leg **K** Skin, Right Lower Leg **L** Skin, Left Lower Leg **M** Skin, Right Foot **N** Skin, Left Foot	**X** External	**7** Autologous Tissue Substitute	**2** Cell Suspension Technique **3** Full Thickness **4** Partial Thickness
Ø Skin, Scalp **1** Skin, Face **2** Skin, Right Ear **3** Skin, Left Ear **4** Skin, Neck **5** Skin, Chest Breast procedures, skin only **6** Skin, Back **7** Skin, Abdomen **8** Skin, Buttock **9** Skin, Perineum **A** Skin, Inguinal **B** Skin, Right Upper Arm **C** Skin, Left Upper Arm **D** Skin, Right Lower Arm **E** Skin, Left Lower Arm **F** Skin, Right Hand **G** Skin, Left Hand **H** Skin, Right Upper Leg **J** Skin, Left Upper Leg **K** Skin, Right Lower Leg **L** Skin, Left Lower Leg **M** Skin, Right Foot **N** Skin, Left Foot	**X** External	**J** Synthetic Substitute	**3** Full Thickness **4** Partial Thickness **Z** No Qualifier
Ø Skin, Scalp **1** Skin, Face **2** Skin, Right Ear **3** Skin, Left Ear **4** Skin, Neck **5** Skin, Chest Breast procedures, skin only **6** Skin, Back **7** Skin, Abdomen **8** Skin Buttock **9** Skin, Perineum **A** Skin, Inguinal **B** Skin, Right Upper Arm **C** Skin, Left Upper Arm **D** Skin, Right Lower Arm **E** Skin, Left Lower Arm **F** Skin, Right Hand **G** Skin, Left Hand **H** Skin, Right Upper Leg **J** Skin, Left Upper Leg **K** Skin, Right Lower Leg **L** Skin, Left Lower Leg **M** Skin, Right Foot **N** Skin, Left Foot	**X** External	**K** Nonautologous Tissue Substitute	**3** Full Thickness **4** Partial Thickness
Q Finger Nail Nail bed Nail plate **R** Toe Nail *See Q Finger Nail* **S** Hair	**X** External	**7** Autologous Tissue Substitute **J** Synthetic Substitute **K** Nonautologous Tissue Substitute	**Z** No Qualifier
T Breast, Right Mammary duct Mammary gland **U** Breast, Left *See T Breast, Right* **V** Breast, Bilateral *See T Breast, Right*	**Ø** Open	**7** Autologous Tissue Substitute	**5** Latissimus Dorsi Myocutaneous Flap **6** Transverse Rectus Abdominis Myocutaneous Flap **7** Deep Inferior Epigastric Artery Perforator Flap **8** Superficial Inferior Epigastric Artery Flap **9** Gluteal Artery Perforator Flap **Z** No Qualifier
T Breast, Right Mammary duct Mammary gland **U** Breast, Left *See T Breast, Right* **V** Breast, Bilateral *See T Breast, Right*	**Ø** Open	**J** Synthetic Substitute **K** Nonautologous Tissue Substitute	**Z** No Qualifier
T Breast, Right ⊞ Mammary duct Mammary gland **U** Breast, Left ⊞ *See T Breast, Right* **V** Breast, Bilateral ⊞ *See T Breast, Right*	**3** Percutaneous	**7** Autologous Tissue Substitute **J** Synthetic Substitute **K** Nonautologous Tissue Substitute	**Z** No Qualifier
W Nipple, Right Areola **X** Nipple, Left *See W Nipple, Right*	**Ø** Open **3** Percutaneous **X** External	**7** Autologous Tissue Substitute **J** Synthetic Substitute **K** Nonautologous Tissue Substitute	**Z** No Qualifier

Non-OR ØHRSX7Z

See Appendix L for Procedure Combinations
⊞ ØHR[T,U,V]37Z

Ø Medical and Surgical
H Skin and Breast
S Reposition Definition: Moving to its normal location, or other suitable location, all or a portion of a body part

Explanation: The body part is moved to a new location from an abnormal location, or from a normal location where it is not functioning correctly. The body part may or may not be cut out or off to be moved to the new location.

Body Part Character 4	Approach Character 5	Device Character 6	Qualifier Character 7
S Hair **W Nipple, Right** Areola **X Nipple, Left** *See W Nipple, Right*	**X External**	**Z No Device**	**Z No Qualifier**
T Breast, Right Mammary duct Mammary gland **U Breast, Left** *See T Breast, Right* **V Breast, Bilateral** *See T Breast, Right*	**Ø Open**	**Z No Device**	**Z No Qualifier**

Non-OR ØHSSXZZ

Ø Medical and Surgical
H Skin and Breast
T Resection Definition: Cutting out or off, without replacement, all of a body part

Explanation: None

Body Part Character 4	Approach Character 5	Device Character 6	Qualifier Character 7
Q Finger Nail Nail bed Nail plate **R Toe Nail** *See Q Finger Nail* **W Nipple, Right** Areola **X Nipple, Left** *See W Nipple, Right*	**X External**	**Z No Device**	**Z No Qualifier**
T Breast, Right ⊞ Mammary duct Mammary gland **U Breast, Left** ⊞ *See T Breast, Right* **V Breast, Bilateral** ⊞ *See T Breast, Right* **Y Supernumerary Breast**	**Ø Open**	**Z No Device**	**Z No Qualifier**

Non-OR ØHT[Q,R]XZZ

See Appendix L for Procedure Combinations
⊞ ØHT[T,U,V]ØZZ

Ø Medical and Surgical
H Skin and Breast
U Supplement Definition: Putting in or on biological or synthetic material that physically reinforces and/or augments the function of a portion of a body part

Explanation: The biological material is non-living, or is living and from the same individual. The body part may have been previously replaced, and the SUPPLEMENT procedure is performed to physically reinforce and/or augment the function of the replaced body part.

Body Part Character 4	Approach Character 5	Device Character 6	Qualifier Character 7
T Breast, Right Mammary duct Mammary gland **U Breast, Left** *See T Breast, Right* **V Breast, Bilateral** *See T Breast, Right*	**Ø Open** **3 Percutaneous** **7 Via Natural or Artificial Opening** **8 Via Natural or Artificial Opening Endoscopic**	**7 Autologous Tissue Substitute** **J Synthetic Substitute** **K Nonautologous Tissue Substitute**	**Z No Qualifier**
W Nipple, Right Areola **X Nipple, Left** *See W Nipple, Right*	**Ø Open** **3 Percutaneous** **7 Via Natural or Artificial Opening** **8 Via Natural or Artificial Opening Endoscopic** **X External**	**7 Autologous Tissue Substitute** **J Synthetic Substitute** **K Nonautologous Tissue Substitute**	**Z No Qualifier**

Non-OR ØHU[T,U,V]3JZ

Ø Medical and Surgical
H Skin and Breast
W Revision

Definition: Correcting, to the extent possible, a portion of a malfunctioning device or the position of a displaced device

Explanation: Revision can include correcting a malfunctioning or displaced device by taking out or putting in components of the device such as a screw or pin

Body Part Character 4	Approach Character 5	Device Character 6	Qualifier Character 7
P Skin Dermis Epidermis Sebaceous gland Sweat gland	**X External**	**Ø Drainage Device** **7 Autologous Tissue Substitute** **J Synthetic Substitute** **K Nonautologous Tissue Substitute** **Y Other Device**	**Z No Qualifier**
Q Finger Nail Nail bed Nail plate **R Toe Nail** *See Q Finger Nail*	**X External**	**Ø Drainage Device** **7 Autologous Tissue Substitute** **J Synthetic Substitute** **K Nonautologous Tissue Substitute**	**Z No Qualifier**
S Hair	**X External**	**7 Autologous Tissue Substitute** **J Synthetic Substitute** **K Nonautologous Tissue Substitute**	**Z No Qualifier**
T Breast, Right Mammary duct Mammary gland **U Breast, Left** *See T Breast, Right*	**Ø Open** **3 Percutaneous** **7 Via Natural or Artificial Opening** **8 Via Natural or Artificial Opening Endoscopic**	**Ø Drainage Device** **7 Autologous Tissue Substitute** **J Synthetic Substitute** **K Nonautologous Tissue Substitute** **N Tissue Expander** **Y Other Device**	**Z No Qualifier**

Non-OR ØHWPX[Ø,7,J,K,Y]Z
Non-OR ØHW[Q,R]X[Ø,7,J,K]Z
Non-OR ØHWSX[7,J,K]Z
Non-OR ØHW[T,U]Ø[Ø,7,K,N]Z
Non-OR ØHW[T,U]3[Ø,7,K,N,Y]Z
Non-OR ØHW[T,U][7,8][Ø,7,J,K,N,Y]Z

Ø Medical and Surgical
H Skin and Breast
X Transfer

Definition: Moving, without taking out, all or a portion of a body part to another location to take over the function of all or a portion of a body part

Explanation: The body part transferred remains connected to its vascular and nervous supply

Body Part Character 4	Approach Character 5	Device Character 6	Qualifier Character 7
Ø Skin, Scalp **1 Skin, Face** **2 Skin, Right Ear** **3 Skin, Left Ear** **4 Skin, Neck** **5 Skin, Chest** Breast procedures, skin only **6 Skin, Back** **7 Skin, Abdomen** **8 Skin, Buttock** **9 Skin, Perineum** **A Skin, Inguinal** **B Skin, Right Upper Arm** **C Skin, Left Upper Arm** **D Skin, Right Lower Arm** **E Skin, Left Lower Arm** **F Skin, Right Hand** **G Skin, Left Hand** **H Skin, Right Upper Leg** **J Skin, Left Upper Leg** **K Skin, Right Lower Leg** **L Skin, Left Lower Leg** **M Skin, Right Foot** **N Skin, Left Foot**	**X External**	**Z No Device**	**Z No Qualifier**

Subcutaneous Tissue and Fascia ØJØ–ØJX

Character Meanings

This Character Meaning table is provided as a guide to assist the user in the identification of character members that may be found in this section of code tables. It **SHOULD NOT** be used to build a PCS code.

Operation–Character 3	Body Part–Character 4	Approach–Character 5	Device–Character 6	Qualifier–Character 7
Ø Alteration	Ø Subcutaneous Tissue and Fascia, Scalp	Ø Open	Ø Drainage Device OR Monitoring Device, Hemodynamic	B Skin and Subcutaneous Tissue
2 Change	1 Subcutaneous Tissue and Fascia, Face	3 Percutaneous	1 Radioactive Element	C Skin, Subcutaneous Tissue and Fascia
5 Destruction	4 Subcutaneous Tissue and Fascia, Right Neck	X External	2 Monitoring Device	X Diagnostic
8 Division	5 Subcutaneous Tissue and Fascia, Left Neck		3 Infusion Device	Z No Qualifier
9 Drainage	6 Subcutaneous Tissue and Fascia, Chest		4 Pacemaker, Single Chamber	
B Excision	7 Subcutaneous Tissue and Fascia, Back		5 Pacemaker, Single Chamber Rate Responsive	
C Extirpation	8 Subcutaneous Tissue and Fascia, Abdomen		6 Pacemaker, Dual Chamber	
D Extraction	9 Subcutaneous Tissue and Fascia, Buttock		7 Autologous Tissue Substitute OR Cardiac Resynchronization Pacemaker Pulse Generator	
H Insertion	B Subcutaneous Tissue and Fascia, Perineum		8 Defibrillator Generator	
J Inspection	C Subcutaneous Tissue and Fascia, Pelvic Region		9 Cardiac Resynchronization Defibrillator Pulse Generator	
N Release	D Subcutaneous Tissue and Fascia, Right Upper Arm		A Contractility Modulation Device	
P Removal	F Subcutaneous Tissue and Fascia, Left Upper Arm		B Stimulator Generator, Single Array	
Q Repair	G Subcutaneous Tissue and Fascia, Right Lower Arm		C Stimulator Generator, Single Array Rechargeable	
R Replacement	H Subcutaneous Tissue and Fascia, Left Lower Arm		D Stimulator Generator, Multiple Array	
U Supplement	J Subcutaneous Tissue and Fascia, Right Hand		E Stimulator Generator, Multiple Array Rechargeable	
W Revision	K Subcutaneous Tissue and Fascia, Left Hand		F Subcutaneous Defibrillator Lead	
X Transfer	L Subcutaneous Tissue and Fascia, Right Upper Leg		H Contraceptive Device	
	M Subcutaneous Tissue and Fascia, Left Upper Leg		J Synthetic Substitute	
	N Subcutaneous Tissue and Fascia, Right Lower Leg		K Nonautologous Tissue Substitute	
	P Subcutaneous Tissue and Fascia, Left Lower Leg		M Stimulator Generator	
	Q Subcutaneous Tissue and Fascia, Right Foot		N Tissue Expander	
	R Subcutaneous Tissue and Fascia, Left Foot		P Cardiac Rhythm Related Device	
	S Subcutaneous Tissue and Fascia, Head and Neck		V Infusion Device, Pump	
	T Subcutaneous Tissue and Fascia, Trunk		W Vascular Access Device, Totally Implantable	
	V Subcutaneous Tissue and Fascia, Upper Extremity		X Vascular Access Device, Tunneled	
	W Subcutaneous Tissue and Fascia, Lower Extremity		Y Other Device	
			Z No Device	

AHA Coding Clinic for table ØJ2

2018, 3Q, 10	Disruption of perma-catheter fibrin sheath via angioplasty of superior vena cava
2017, 2Q, 26	Exchange of tunneled catheter

AHA Coding Clinic for table ØJ5

2019, 3Q, 25	Endoscopic removal of pilonidal sinus and cyst

AHA Coding Clinic for table ØJ8

2017, 3Q, 11	Bilateral escharotomy of leg, thigh and foot

AHA Coding Clinic for table ØJ9

2018, 3Q, 16	Incision and drainage of submandibular space
2018, 3Q, 16	Incision and drainage of neck abscess
2015, 3Q, 23	Incision and drainage of multiple abscess cavities using vessel loop

AHA Coding Clinic for table ØJB

2020, 1Q, 31	Repair of buried penis
2019, 3Q, 25	Endoscopic removal of pilonidal sinus and cyst
2018, 3Q, 17	Excisional debridement of periosteum
2018, 1Q, 7	Placement of fat graft following lumbar decompression surgery
2015, 3Q, 3-8	Excisional and nonexcisional debridement
2015, 2Q, 13	Transfer of free flap to reconstruct orbital defect
2015, 1Q, 29	Fistulectomy with placement of seton
2014, 4Q, 38	Abdominoplasty and abdominal wall plication for hernia repair
2014, 3Q, 22	Transsphenoidal removal of pituitary tumor and fat graft placement

AHA Coding Clinic for table ØJC

2017, 3Q, 22	Replacement of native skull bone flap

AHA Coding Clinic for table ØJD

2016, 3Q, 20	VersaJet™ nonexcisional debridement of leg muscle
2016, 3Q, 21	Nonexcisional debridement of infected lumbar wound
2016, 3Q, 21	Nonexcisional pulsed lavage debridement
2016, 3Q, 22	Debridement of bone and tendon using Tenex ultrasound device
2016, 1Q, 40	Nonexcisional debridement of skin and subcutaneous tissue
2015, 3Q, 3-8	Excisional and nonexcisional debridement
2015, 1Q, 23	Non-Excisional debridement with lavage of wound

AHA Coding Clinic for table ØJH

2020, 4Q, 54	Insertion of other device into subcutaneous tissue and fascia
2020, 4Q, 55	Insertion of subcutaneous pump system for ascites drainage
2020, 2Q, 15	Ommaya Reservoir with Ventricular Catheter Placement
2020, 2Q, 16	Ommaya Reservoir Placement for Cerebrospinal Fluid Infusion Therapy
2019, 4Q, 33	Subcutaneous implantable cardioverter defibrillator lead
2017, 4Q, 63-64	Added and revised device values - Vascular access reservoir
2017, 2Q, 24	Tunneled catheter versus totally implantable catheter
2017, 2Q, 26	Exchange of tunneled catheter
2016, 4Q, 97-98	Phrenic neurostimulator
2016, 2Q, 14	Insertion of peritoneal totally implantable venous access device
2016, 2Q, 15	Removal and replacement of tunneled internal jugular catheter
2015, 4Q, 14	New Section X codes—New Technology procedures
2015, 4Q, 30-31	Vascular access devices
2015, 2Q, 33	Totally implantable central venous access device (Port-a-Cath)
2014, 3Q, 19	End of life replacement of Baclofen pump
2013, 4Q, 116	Device character for Port-A-Cath placement
2012, 4Q, 104	Placement of subcutaneous implantable cardioverter defibrillator

AHA Coding Clinic for table ØJN

2017, 3Q, 11	Bilateral escharotomy of leg, thigh and foot

AHA Coding Clinic for table ØJP

2019, 4Q, 33	Subcutaneous implantable cardioverter defibrillator lead
2018, 4Q, 86	Placement of lumboatrial shunt
2018, 3Q, 29	Decommissioning of left ventricular assist device with exploration of mediastinum
2016, 2Q, 15	Removal and replacement of tunneled internal jugular catheter
2015, 4Q, 31	Vascular access devices
2014, 3Q, 19	End of life replacement of Baclofen pump
2013, 4Q, 109	Separating conjoined twins
2012, 4Q, 104	Placement of subcutaneous implantable cardioverter defibrillator

AHA Coding Clinic for table ØJQ

2017, 3Q, 19	Anterior repair of cystocele
2014, 4Q, 44	Posterior colporrhaphy/rectocele repair

AHA Coding Clinic for table ØJR

2015, 2Q, 13	Transfer of free flap to reconstruct orbital defect

AHA Coding Clinic for table ØJU

2018, 2Q, 20	Prelaminated free flap graft using Alloderm™
2018, 1Q, 7	Placement of fat graft following lumbar decompression surgery

AHA Coding Clinic for table ØJW

2019, 4Q, 33	Subcutaneous implantable cardioverter defibrillator lead
2018, 1Q, 8	Ventricular peritoneal shunt ligation
2015, 4Q, 33	Externalization of peritoneal dialysis catheter
2015, 2Q, 9	Revision of ventriculoperitoneal (VP) shunt
2012, 4Q, 104	Placement of subcutaneous implantable cardioverter defibrillator

AHA Coding Clinic for table ØJX

2021, 2Q, 16	Goldilocks breast reconstruction
2018, 1Q, 10	Complex wound closure using pericranial flap
2014, 3Q, 18	Placement of reverse sural fasciocutaneous pedicle flap
2013, 4Q, 109	Separating conjoined twins

Ø Medical and Surgical
J Subcutaneous Tissue and Fascia
Ø Alteration Definition: Modifying the anatomic structure of a body part without affecting the function of the body part
Explanation: Principal purpose is to improve appearance

Body Part Character 4	Approach Character 5	Device Character 6	Qualifier Character 7
1 Subcutaneous Tissue and Fascia, Face Masseteric fascia Orbital fascia Submandibular space **4 Subcutaneous Tissue and Fascia, Right Neck** Deep cervical fascia Pretracheal fascia Prevertebral fascia **5 Subcutaneous Tissue and Fascia, Left Neck** *See 4 Subcutaneous Tissue and Fascia, Right Neck* **6 Subcutaneous Tissue and Fascia, Chest** Pectoral fascia **7 Subcutaneous Tissue and Fascia, Back** **8 Subcutaneous Tissue and Fascia, Abdomen** **9 Subcutaneous Tissue and Fascia, Buttock** **D Subcutaneous Tissue and Fascia, Right Upper Arm** Axillary fascia Deltoid fascia Infraspinatus fascia Subscapular aponeurosis Supraspinatus fascia **F Subcutaneous Tissue and Fascia, Left Upper Arm** *See D Subcutaneous Tissue and Fascia, Right Upper Arm* **G Subcutaneous Tissue and Fascia, Right Lower Arm** Antebrachial fascia Bicipital aponeurosis **H Subcutaneous Tissue and Fascia, Left Lower Arm** *See G Subcutaneous Tissue and Fascia, Right Lower Arm* **L Subcutaneous Tissue and Fascia, Right Upper Leg** Crural fascia Fascia lata Iliac fascia Iliotibial tract (band) **M Subcutaneous Tissue and Fascia, Left Upper Leg** *See L Subcutaneous Tissue and Fascia, Right Upper Leg* **N Subcutaneous Tissue and Fascia, Right Lower Leg** **P Subcutaneous Tissue and Fascia, Left Lower Leg**	**Ø Open** **3 Percutaneous**	**Z No Device**	**Z No Qualifier**

Ø Medical and Surgical
J Subcutaneous Tissue and Fascia
2 Change Definition: Taking out or off a device from a body part and putting back an identical or similar device in or on the same body part without cutting or puncturing the skin or a mucous membrane
Explanation: All CHANGE procedures are coded using the approach EXTERNAL

Body Part Character 4	Approach Character 5	Device Character 6	Qualifier Character 7
S Subcutaneous Tissue and Fascia, Head and Neck **T Subcutaneous Tissue and Fascia, Trunk** External oblique aponeurosis Transversalis fascia **V Subcutaneous Tissue and Fascia, Upper Extremity** **W Subcutaneous Tissue and Fascia, Lower Extremity**	**X External**	**Ø Drainage Device** **Y Other Device**	**Z No Qualifier**

Non-OR All body part, approach, device, and qualifier values

Ø Medical and Surgical
J Subcutaneous Tissue and Fascia
5 Destruction Definition: Physical eradication of all or a portion of a body part by the direct use of energy, force, or a destructive agent

Explanation: None of the body part is physically taken out

Body Part Character 4		Approach Character 5	Device Character 6	Qualifier Character 7
Ø Subcutaneous Tissue and Fascia, Scalp Galea aponeurotica **1 Subcutaneous Tissue and Fascia, Face** Masseteric fascia Orbital fascia Submandibular space **4 Subcutaneous Tissue and Fascia, Right Neck** Deep cervical fascia Pretracheal fascia Prevertebral fascia **5 Subcutaneous Tissue and Fascia, Left Neck** *See 4 Subcutaneous Tissue and Fascia, Right Neck* **6 Subcutaneous Tissue and Fascia, Chest** Pectoral fascia **7 Subcutaneous Tissue and Fascia, Back** **8 Subcutaneous Tissue and Fascia, Abdomen** **9 Subcutaneous Tissue and Fascia, Buttock** **B Subcutaneous Tissue and Fascia, Perineum** **C Subcutaneous Tissue and Fascia, Pelvic Region** **D Subcutaneous Tissue and Fascia, Right Upper Arm** Axillary fascia Deltoid fascia Infraspinatus fascia Subscapular aponeurosis Supraspinatus fascia **F Subcutaneous Tissue and Fascia, Left Upper Arm** *See D Subcutaneous Tissue and Fascia, Right Upper Arm*	**G Subcutaneous Tissue and Fascia, Right Lower Arm** Antebrachial fascia Bicipital aponeurosis **H Subcutaneous Tissue and Fascia, Left Lower Arm** *See G Subcutaneous Tissue and Fascia, Right Lower Arm* **J Subcutaneous Tissue and Fascia, Right Hand** Palmar fascia (aponeurosis) **K Subcutaneous Tissue and Fascia, Left Hand** *See J Subcutaneous Tissue and Fascia, Right Hand* **L Subcutaneous Tissue and Fascia, Right Upper Leg** Crural fascia Fascia lata Iliac fascia Iliotibial tract (band) **M Subcutaneous Tissue and Fascia, Left Upper Leg** *See L Subcutaneous Tissue and Fascia, Right Upper Leg* **N Subcutaneous Tissue and Fascia, Right Lower Leg** **P Subcutaneous Tissue and Fascia, Left Lower Leg** **Q Subcutaneous Tissue and Fascia, Right Foot** Plantar fascia (aponeurosis) **R Subcutaneous Tissue and Fascia, Left Foot** *See Q Subcutaneous Tissue and Fascia, Right Foot*	**Ø Open** **3 Percutaneous**	**Z No Device**	**Z No Qualifier**

DRG Non-OR All body part, approach, device, and qualifier values

Ø Medical and Surgical
J Subcutaneous Tissue and Fascia
8 Division Definition: Cutting into a body part, without draining fluids and/or gases from the body part, in order to separate or transect a body part
Explanation: All or a portion of the body part is separated into two or more portions

Body Part Character 4	Approach Character 5	Device Character 6	Qualifier Character 7
Ø Subcutaneous Tissue and Fascia, Scalp Galea aponeurotica **1 Subcutaneous Tissue and Fascia, Face** Masseteric fascia Orbital fascia Submandibular space **4 Subcutaneous Tissue and Fascia, Right Neck** Deep cervical fascia Pretracheal fascia Prevertebral fascia **5 Subcutaneous Tissue and Fascia, Left Neck** *See 4 Subcutaneous Tissue and Fascia, Right Neck* **6 Subcutaneous Tissue and Fascia, Chest** Pectoral fascia **7 Subcutaneous Tissue and Fascia, Back** **8 Subcutaneous Tissue and Fascia, Abdomen** **9 Subcutaneous Tissue and Fascia, Buttock** **B Subcutaneous Tissue and Fascia, Perineum** **C Subcutaneous Tissue and Fascia, Pelvic Region** **D Subcutaneous Tissue and Fascia, Right Upper Arm** Axillary fascia Deltoid fascia Infraspinatus fascia Subscapular aponeurosis Supraspinatus fascia **F Subcutaneous Tissue and Fascia, Left Upper Arm** *See D Subcutaneous Tissue and Fascia, Right Upper Arm* **G Subcutaneous Tissue and Fascia, Right Lower Arm** Antebrachial fascia Bicipital aponeurosis **H Subcutaneous Tissue and Fascia, Left Lower Arm** *See G Subcutaneous Tissue and Fascia, Right Lower Arm* **J Subcutaneous Tissue and Fascia, Right Hand** Palmar fascia (aponeurosis) **K Subcutaneous Tissue and Fascia, Left Hand** *See J Subcutaneous Tissue and Fascia, Right Hand* **L Subcutaneous Tissue and Fascia, Right Upper Leg** Crural fascia Fascia lata Iliac fascia Iliotibial tract (band) **M Subcutaneous Tissue and Fascia, Left Upper Leg** *See L Subcutaneous Tissue and Fascia, Right Upper Leg* **N Subcutaneous Tissue and Fascia, Right Lower Leg** **P Subcutaneous Tissue and Fascia, Left Lower Leg** **Q Subcutaneous Tissue and Fascia, Right Foot** Plantar fascia (aponeurosis) **R Subcutaneous Tissue and Fascia, Left Foot** *See Q Subcutaneous Tissue and Fascia, Right Foot* **S Subcutaneous Tissue and Fascia, Head and Neck** **T Subcutaneous Tissue and Fascia, Trunk** External oblique aponeurosis Transversalis fascia **V Subcutaneous Tissue and Fascia, Upper Extremity** **W Subcutaneous Tissue and Fascia, Lower Extremity**	**Ø Open** **3 Percutaneous**	**Z No Device**	**Z No Qualifier**

Ø Medical and Surgical
J Subcutaneous Tissue and Fascia
9 Drainage Definition: Taking or letting out fluids and/or gases from a body part
Explanation: The qualifier DIAGNOSTIC is used to identify drainage procedures that are biopsies

Body Part Character 4	Approach Character 5	Device Character 6	Qualifier Character 7
Ø Subcutaneous Tissue and Fascia, Scalp Galea aponeurotica **1 Subcutaneous Tissue and Fascia, Face** Masseteric fascia Orbital fascia Submandibular space **4 Subcutaneous Tissue and Fascia, Right Neck** Deep cervical fascia Pretracheal fascia Prevertebral fascia **5 Subcutaneous Tissue and Fascia, Left Neck** *See 4 Subcutaneous Tissue and Fascia, Right Neck* **6 Subcutaneous Tissue and Fascia, Chest** Pectoral fascia **7 Subcutaneous Tissue and Fascia, Back** **8 Subcutaneous Tissue and Fascia, Abdomen** **9 Subcutaneous Tissue and Fascia, Buttock** **B Subcutaneous Tissue and Fascia, Perineum** **C Subcutaneous Tissue and Fascia, Pelvic Region** **D Subcutaneous Tissue and Fascia, Right Upper Arm** Axillary fascia Deltoid fascia Infraspinatus fascia Subscapular aponeurosis Supraspinatus fascia **F Subcutaneous Tissue and Fascia, Left Upper Arm** *See D Subcutaneous Tissue and Fascia, Right Upper Arm* **G Subcutaneous Tissue and Fascia, Right Lower Arm** Antebrachial fascia Bicipital aponeurosis **H Subcutaneous Tissue and Fascia, Left Lower Arm** *See G Subcutaneous Tissue and Fascia, Right Lower Arm* **J Subcutaneous Tissue and Fascia, Right Hand** Palmar fascia (aponeurosis) **K Subcutaneous Tissue and Fascia, Left Hand** *See J Subcutaneous Tissue and Fascia, Right Hand* **L Subcutaneous Tissue and Fascia, Right Upper Leg** Crural fascia Fascia lata Iliac fascia Iliotibial tract (band) **M Subcutaneous Tissue and Fascia, Left Upper Leg** *See L Subcutaneous Tissue and Fascia, Right Upper Leg* **N Subcutaneous Tissue and Fascia, Right Lower Leg** **P Subcutaneous Tissue and Fascia, Left Lower Leg** **Q Subcutaneous Tissue and Fascia, Right Foot** Plantar fascia (aponeurosis) **R Subcutaneous Tissue and Fascia, Left Foot** *See Q Subcutaneous Tissue and Fascia, Right Foot*	**Ø** Open **3** Percutaneous	**Ø** Drainage Device	**Z** No Qualifier

Non-OR ØJ9[Ø,1,4,5,6,7,8,9,B,C,D,F,G,H,J,K,L,M,N,P,Q,R][Ø,3]ØZ

ØJ9 Continued on next page

ØJ9 Continued

Ø Medical and Surgical
J Subcutaneous Tissue and Fascia
9 Drainage Definition: Taking or letting out fluids and/or gases from a body part
Explanation: The qualifier DIAGNOSTIC is used to identify drainage procedures that are biopsies

Body Part Character 4		Approach Character 5	Device Character 6	Qualifier Character 7
Ø Subcutaneous Tissue and Fascia, Scalp Galea aponeurotica **1 Subcutaneous Tissue and Fascia, Face** Masseteric fascia Orbital fascia Submandibular space **4 Subcutaneous Tissue and Fascia, Right Neck** Deep cervical fascia Pretracheal fascia Prevertebral fascia **5 Subcutaneous Tissue and Fascia, Left Neck** *See 4 Subcutaneous Tissue and Fascia, Right Neck* **6 Subcutaneous Tissue and Fascia, Chest** Pectoral fascia **7 Subcutaneous Tissue and Fascia, Back** **8 Subcutaneous Tissue and Fascia, Abdomen** **9 Subcutaneous Tissue and Fascia, Buttock** **B Subcutaneous Tissue and Fascia, Perineum** **C Subcutaneous Tissue and Fascia, Pelvic Region** **D Subcutaneous Tissue and Fascia, Right Upper Arm** Axillary fascia Deltoid fascia Infraspinatus fascia Subscapular aponeurosis Supraspinatus fascia **F Subcutaneous Tissue and Fascia, Left Upper Arm** *See D Subcutaneous Tissue and Fascia, Right Upper Arm*	**G Subcutaneous Tissue and Fascia, Right Lower Arm** Antebrachial fascia Bicipital aponeurosis **H Subcutaneous Tissue and Fascia, Left Lower Arm** *See G Subcutaneous Tissue and Fascia, Right Lower Arm* **J Subcutaneous Tissue and Fascia, Right Hand** Palmar fascia (aponeurosis) **K Subcutaenous Tissue and Fascia, Left Hand** *See J Subcutaneous Tissue and Fascia, Right Hand* **L Subcutaneous Tissue and Fascia, Right Upper Leg** Crural fascia Fascia lata Iliac fascia Iliotibial tract (band) **M Subcutaneous Tissue and Fascia, Left Upper Leg** *See L Subcutaneous Tissue and Fascia, Right Upper Leg* **N Subcutaneous Tissue and Fascia, Right Lower Leg** **P Subcutaneous Tissue and Fascia, Left Lower Leg** **Q Subcutaneous Tissue and Fascia, Right Foot** Plantar fascia (aponeurosis) **R Subcutaneous Tissue and Fascia, Left Foot** *See Q Subcutaneous Tissue and Fascia, Right Foot*	**Ø Open** **3 Percutaneous**	**Z No Device**	**X Diagnostic** **Z No Qualifier**

Non-OR ØJ9[Ø,1,4,5,6,7,8,9,B,C,D,F,G,H,J,K,L,M,N,P,Q,R][Ø,3]ZX
Non-OR ØJ9[Ø,1,4,5,6,7,8,9,B,C,D,F,G,H,J,K,L,M,N,P,Q,R]3ZZ

Ø Medical and Surgical
J Subcutaneous Tissue and Fascia
B Excision Definition: Cutting out or off, without replacement, a portion of a body part

Explanation: The qualifier DIAGNOSTIC is used to identify excision procedures that are biopsies

Body Part Character 4	Approach Character 5	Device Character 6	Qualifier Character 7
Ø Subcutaneous Tissue and Fascia, Scalp Galea aponeurotica	**Ø Open** **3 Percutaneous**	**Z No Device**	**X Diagnostic** **Z No Qualifier**
1 Subcutaneous Tissue and Fascia, Face Masseteric fascia Orbital fascia Submandibular space			
4 Subcutaneous Tissue and Fascia, Right Neck Deep cervical fascia Pretracheal fascia Prevertebral fascia			
5 Subcutaneous Tissue and Fascia, Left Neck *See 4 Subcutaneous Tissue and Fascia, Right Neck*			
6 Subcutaneous Tissue and Fascia, Chest Pectoral fascia			
7 Subcutaneous Tissue and Fascia, Back			
8 Subcutaneous Tissue and Fascia, Abdomen			
9 Subcutaneous Tissue and Fascia, Buttock			
B Subcutaneous Tissue and Fascia, Perineum			
C Subcutaneous Tissue and Fascia, Pelvic Region			
D Subcutaneous Tissue and Fascia, Right Upper Arm Axillary fascia Deltoid fascia Infraspinatus fascia Subscapular aponeurosis Supraspinatus fascia			
F Subcutaneous Tissue and Fascia, Left Upper Arm *See D Subcutaneous Tissue and Fascia, Right Upper Arm*			
G Subcutaneous Tissue and Fascia, Right Lower Arm Antebrachial fascia Bicipital aponeurosis			
H Subcutaneous Tissue and Fascia, Left Lower Arm *See G Subcutaneous Tissue and Fascia, Right Lower Arm*			
J Subcutaneous Tissue and Fascia, Right Hand Palmar fascia (aponeurosis)			
K Subcutaneous Tissue and Fascia, Left Hand *See J Subcutaneous Tissue and Fascia, Right Hand*			
L Subcutaneous Tissue and Fascia, Right Upper Leg Crural fascia Fascia lata Iliac fascia Iliotibial tract (band)			
M Subcutaneous Tissue and Fascia, Left Upper Leg *See L Subcutaneous Tissue and Fascia, Right Upper Leg*			
N Subcutaneous Tissue and Fascia, Right Lower Leg			
P Subcutaneous Tissue and Fascia, Left Lower Leg			
Q Subcutaneous Tissue and Fascia, Right Foot Plantar fascia (aponeurosis)			
R Subcutaneous Tissue and Fascia, Left Foot *See Q Subcutaneous Tissue and Fascia, Right Foot*			

DRG Non-OR ØJB[Ø,4,5,6,7,8,9,B,C,D,F,G,H,L,M,N,P,Q,R]3ZZ
Non-OR ØJB[Ø,1,4,5,6,7,8,9,B,C,D,F,G,H,J,K,L,M,N,P,Q,R][Ø,3]ZX

Ø Medical and Surgical
J Subcutaneous Tissue and Fascia
C Extirpation Definition: Taking or cutting out solid matter from a body part

Explanation: The solid matter may be an abnormal byproduct of a biological function or a foreign body; it may be imbedded in a body part or in the lumen of a tubular body part. The solid matter may or may not have been previously broken into pieces.

Body Part Character 4	Approach Character 5	Device Character 6	Qualifier Character 7
Ø Subcutaneous Tissue and Fascia, Scalp Galea aponeurotica 1 Subcutaneous Tissue and Fascia, Face Masseteric fascia Orbital fascia Submandibular space 4 Subcutaneous Tissue and Fascia, Right Neck Deep cervical fascia Pretracheal fascia Prevertebral fascia 5 Subcutaneous Tissue and Fascia, Left Neck *See 4 Subcutaneous Tissue and Fascia, Right Neck* 6 Subcutaneous Tissue and Fascia, Chest Pectoral fascia 7 Subcutaneous Tissue and Fascia, Back 8 Subcutaneous Tissue and Fascia, Abdomen 9 Subcutaneous Tissue and Fascia, Buttock B Subcutaneous Tissue and Fascia, Perineum C Subcutaneous Tissue and Fascia, Pelvic Region D Subcutaneous Tissue and Fascia, Right Upper Arm Axillary fascia Deltoid fascia Infraspinatus fascia Subscapular aponeurosis Supraspinatus fascia F Subcutaneous Tissue and Fascia, Left Upper Arm *See D Subcutaneous Tissue and Fascia, Right Upper Arm* G Subcutaneous Tissue and Fascia, Right Lower Arm Antebrachial fascia Bicipital aponeurosis H Subcutaneous Tissue and Fascia, Left Lower Arm *See G Subcutaneous Tissue and Fascia, Right Lower Arm* J Subcutaneous Tissue and Fascia, Right Hand Palmar fascia (aponeurosis) K Subcutaneous Tissue and Fascia, Left Hand *See J Subcutaneous Tissue and Fascia, Right Hand* L Subcutaneous Tissue and Fascia, Right Upper Leg Crural fascia Fascia lata Iliac fascia Iliotibial tract (band) M Subcutaneous Tissue and Fascia, Left Upper Leg *See L Subcutaneous Tissue and Fascia, Right Upper Leg* N Subcutaneous Tissue and Fascia, Right Lower Leg P Subcutaneous Tissue and Fascia, Left Lower Leg Q Subcutaneous Tissue and Fascia, Right Foot Plantar fascia (aponeurosis) R Subcutaneous Tissue and Fascia, Left Foot *See Q Subcutaneous Tissue and Fascia, Right Foot*	Ø Open 3 Percutaneous	Z No Device	Z No Qualifier

Non-OR All body part, approach, device, and qualifier values

Ø Medical and Surgical
J Subcutaneous Tissue and Fascia
D Extraction Definition: Pulling or stripping out or off all or a portion of a body part by the use of force
Explanation: The qualifier DIAGNOSTIC is used to identify extraction procedures that are biopsies

Body Part Character 4		Approach Character 5	Device Character 6	Qualifier Character 7
Ø Subcutaneous Tissue and Fascia, Scalp Galea aponeurotica **1 Subcutaneous Tissue and Fascia, Face** Masseteric fascia Orbital fascia Submandibular space **4 Subcutaneous Tissue and Fascia, Right Neck** Deep cervical fascia Pretracheal fascia Prevertebral fascia **5 Subcutaneous Tissue and Fascia, Left Neck** *See 4 Subcutaneous Tissue and Fascia, Right Neck* **6 Subcutaneous Tissue and Fascia, Chest** Pectoral fascia **7 Subcutaneous Tissue and Fascia, Back** **8 Subcutaneous Tissue and Fascia, Abdomen** **9 Subcutaneous Tissue and Fascia, Buttock** **B Subcutaneous Tissue and Fascia, Perineum** **C Subcutaneous Tissue and Fascia, Pelvic Region** **D Subcutaneous Tissue and Fascia, Right Upper Arm** Axillary fascia Deltoid fascia Infraspinatus fascia Subscapular aponeurosis Supraspinatus fascia **F Subcutaneous Tissue and Fascia, Left Upper Arm** *See D Subcutaneous Tissue and Fascia, Right Upper Arm*	**G Subcutaneous Tissue and Fascia, Right Lower Arm** Antebrachial fascia Bicipital aponeurosis **H Subcutaneous Tissue and Fascia, Left Lower Arm** *See G Subcutaneous Tissue and Fascia, Right Lower Arm* **J Subcutaneous Tissue and Fascia, Right Hand** Palmar fascia (aponeurosis) **K Subcutaneous Tissue and Fascia, Left Hand** *See J Subcutaneous Tissue and Fascia, Right Hand* **L Subcutaneous Tissue and Fascia, Right Upper Leg** Crural fascia Fascia lata Iliac fascia Iliotibial tract (band) **M Subcutaneous Tissue and Fascia, Left Upper Leg** *See L Subcutaneous Tissue and Fascia, Right Upper Leg* **N Subcutaneous Tissue and Fascia, Right Lower Leg** **P Subcutaneous Tissue and Fascia, Left Lower Leg** **Q Subcutaneous Tissue and Fascia, Right Foot** Plantar fascia (aponeurosis) **R Subcutaneous Tissue and Fascia, Left Foot** *See Q Subcutaneous Tissue and Fascia, Right Foot*	**Ø Open** **3 Percutaneous**	**Z No Device**	**Z No Qualifier**

Non-OR ØJD[Ø,1,4,5,B,C,D,F,G,H,J,K,N,P,Q,R]3ZZ

See Appendix L for Procedure Combinations
Combo-only ØJD[6,7,8,9,L,M]3ZZ

Ø Medical and Surgical
J Subcutaneous Tissue and Fascia
H Insertion Definition: Putting in a nonbiological appliance that monitors, assists, performs, or prevents a physiological function but does not physically take the place of a body part

Explanation: None

Body Part Character 4	Approach Character 5	Device Character 6	Qualifier Character 7
Ø Subcutaneous Tissue and Fascia, Scalp Galea aponeurotica **1 Subcutaneous Tissue and Fascia, Face** Masseteric fascia Orbital fascia Submandibular space **4 Subcutaneous Tissue and Fascia, Right Neck** Deep cervical fascia Pretracheal fascia Prevertebral fascia **5 Subcutaneous Tissue and Fascia, Left Neck** *See 4 Subcutaneous Tissue and Fascia, Right Neck* **9 Subcutaneous Tissue and Fascia, Buttock** **B Subcutaneous Tissue and Fascia, Perineum** **C Subcutaneous Tissue and Fascia, Pelvic Region** **J Subcutaneous Tissue and Fascia, Right Hand** Palmar fascia (aponeurosis) **K Subcutaneous Tissue and Fascia, Left Hand** *See J Subcutaneous Tissue and Fascia, Right Hand* **Q Subcutaneous Tissue and Fascia, Right Foot** Plantar fascia (aponeurosis) **R Subcutaneous Tissue and Fascia, Left Foot** *See Q Subcutaneous Tissue and Fascia, Right Foot*	**Ø Open** **3 Percutaneous**	**N Tissue Expander**	**Z No Qualifier**
6 Subcutaneous Tissue and Fascia, Chest ⊞ Pectoral fascia	**Ø Open** **3 Percutaneous**	**Ø Monitoring Device, Hemodynamic** **2 Monitoring Device** **4 Pacemaker, Single Chamber** **5 Pacemaker, Single Chamber Rate Responsive** **6 Pacemaker, Dual Chamber** **7 Cardiac Resynchronization Pacemaker Pulse Generator** **8 Defibrillator Generator** **9 Cardiac Resynchronization Defibrillator Pulse Generator** **A Contractility Modulation Device** NT **B Stimulator Generator, Single Array** **C Stimulator Generator, Single Array Rechargeable** **D Stimulator Generator, Multiple Array** **E Stimulator Generator, Multiple Array Rechargeable** **F Subcutaneous Defibrillator Lead** **H Contraceptive Device** **M Stimulator Generator** NT **N Tissue Expander** **P Cardiac Rhythm Related Device** **V Infusion Device, Pump** **W Vascular Access Device, Totally Implantable** **X Vascular Access Device, Tunneled** **Y Other Device**	**Z No Qualifier**
7 Subcutaneous Tissue and Fascia, Back NC ⊞	**Ø Open** **3 Percutaneous**	**B Stimulator Generator, Single Array** **C Stimulator Generator, Single Array Rechargeable** **D Stimulator Generator, Multiple Array** **E Stimulator Generator, Multiple Array Rechargeable** **M Stimulator Generator** **N Tissue Expander** **V Infusion Device, Pump** **Y Other Device**	**Z No Qualifier**

DRG Non-OR ØJH6[Ø,3][4,5,6,7,H,P,X]Z
DRG Non-OR ØJH63WX
Non-OR ØJH63YZ
Non-OR ØJH73YZ
HAC ØJH6[Ø,3][4,5,6,7,8,9,P]Z when reported with SDx K68.11 or T81.4Ø-T81.49, T82.6-T82.7 with 7th character A
HAC ØJH63XZ when reported with SDx J95.811

NC ØJH7[Ø,3]MZ
NT ØJH6[Ø,3]AZ
See Appendix H for applicable device trade name
NT ØJH6ØMZ in combination with Ø3HK3MZ or Ø3HL3MZ
See Appendix H for applicable device trade name

See Appendix L for Procedure Combinations
⊞ ØJH6[Ø,3][4,5,6,7,8,9,A,B,C,D,E,F,P]Z
⊞ ØJH7[Ø,3][B,C,D,E]Z

ØJH Continued on next page

Ø Medical and Surgical
J Subcutaneous Tissue and Fascia
H Insertion Definition: Putting in a nonbiological appliance that monitors, assists, performs, or prevents a physiological function but does not physically take the place of a body part

Explanation: None

ØJH Continued

Body Part Character 4	Approach Character 5	Device Character 6	Qualifier Character 7
8 Subcutaneous Tissue and Fascia, Abdomen NC ⊞	**Ø Open** **3 Percutaneous**	**Ø Monitoring Device, Hemodynamic** **2 Monitoring Device** **4 Pacemaker, Single Chamber** **5 Pacemaker, Single Chamber Rate Responsive** **6 Pacemaker, Dual Chamber** **7 Cardiac Resynchronization Pacemaker Pulse Generator** **8 Defibrillator Generator** **9 Cardiac Resynchronization Defibrillator Pulse Generator** **A Contractility Modulation Device** NT **B Stimulator Generator, Single Array** **C Stimulator Generator, Single Array Rechargeable** **D Stimulator Generator, Multiple Array** **E Stimulator Generator, Multiple Array Rechargeable** **H Contraceptive Device** **M Stimulator Generator** **N Tissue Expander** **P Cardiac Rhythm Related Device** **V Infusion Device, Pump** **W Vascular Access Device, Totally Implantable** **X Vascular Access Device, Tunneled** **Y Other Device**	**Z No Qualifier**
D Subcutaneous Tissue and Fascia, Right Upper Arm Axillary fascia Deltoid fascia Infraspinatus fascia Subscapular aponeurosis Supraspinatus fascia **F Subcutaneous Tissue and Fascia, Left Upper Arm** *See D Subcutaneous Tissue and Fascia, Right Upper Arm* **G Subcutaneous Tissue and Fascia, Right Lower Arm** Antebrachial fascia Bicipital aponeurosis **H Subcutaneous Tissue and Fascia, Left Lower Arm** *See G Subcutaneous Tissue and Fascia, Right Lower Arm* **L Subcutaneous Tissue and Fascia, Right Upper Leg** Crural fascia Fascia lata Iliac fascia Iliotibial tract (band) **M Subcutaneous Tissue and Fascia, Left Upper Leg** *See L Subcutaneous Tissue and Fascia, Right Upper Leg* **N Subcutaneous Tissue and Fascia, Right Lower Leg** **P Subcutaneous Tissue and Fascia, Left Lower Leg**	**Ø Open** **3 Percutaneous**	**H Contraceptive Device** **N Tissue Expander** **V Infusion Device, Pump** **W Vascular Access Device, Totally Implantable** **X Vascular Access Device, Tunneled**	**Z No Qualifier**
S Subcutaneous Tissue and Fascia, Head and Neck **V Subcutaneous Tissue and Fascia, Upper Extremity** **W Subcutaneous Tissue and Fascia, Lower Extremity**	**Ø Open** **3 Percutaneous**	**1 Radioactive Element** **3 Infusion Device** **Y Other Device**	**Z No Qualifier**
T Subcutaneous Tissue and Fascia, Trunk External oblique aponeurosis Transversalis fascia	**Ø Open** **3 Percutaneous**	**1 Radioactive Element** **3 Infusion Device** **V Infusion Device, Pump** **Y Other Device**	**Z No Qualifier**

DRG Non-OR ØJH8[Ø,3][2,4,5,6,7,H,P,X]Z
DRG Non-OR ØJH83WX
DRG Non-OR ØJH[D,F,G,H,L,M,N,P]ØXZ
DRG Non-OR ØJH[D,F,G,H,L,M,N,P]3[W,X]Z
DRG Non-OR ØJHN3HZ
DRG Non-OR ØJHP[Ø,3]HZ

Non-OR ØJH83YZ
Non-OR ØJH[D,F,G,H,L,M][Ø,3]HZ
Non-OR ØJHNØHZ
Non-OR ØJH[S,V,W]Ø3Z
Non-OR ØJH[S,V,W]3[3,Y]Z
Non-OR ØJHTØ3Z
Non-OR ØJHT3[3,Y]Z

HAC ØJH8[Ø,3][4,5,6,7,8,9,P]Z when reported with SDx K68.11 or T81.4Ø-T81.49, T82.6-T82.7 with 7th character A
NC ØJH8[Ø,3]MZ
NT ØJHB[Ø,3]AZ *See* Appendix H for applicable device trade name

See Appendix L for Procedure Combinations
⊞ ØJH8[Ø,3][4,5,6,7,8,9,A,B,C,D,E,P]Z

Ø Medical and Surgical
J Subcutaneous Tissue and Fascia
J Inspection Definition: Visually and/or manually exploring a body part

Explanation: Visual exploration may be performed with or without optical instrumentation. Manual exploration may be performed directly or through intervening body layers.

Body Part Character 4	Approach Character 5	Device Character 6	Qualifier Character 7
S Subcutaneous Tissue and Fascia, Head and Neck **T** Subcutaneous Tissue and Fascia, Trunk External oblique aponeurosis Transversalis fascia **V** Subcutaneous Tissue and Fascia, Upper Extremity **W** Subcutaneous Tissue and Fascia, Lower Extremity	**Ø** Open **3** Percutaneous **X** External	**Z** No Device	**Z** No Qualifier

Non-OR All body part, approach, device, and qualifier values

Ø Medical and Surgical
J Subcutaneous Tissue and Fascia
N Release Definition: Freeing a body part from an abnormal physical constraint by cutting or by the use of force

Explanation: Some of the restraining tissue may be taken out but none of the body part is taken out

Body Part Character 4	Approach Character 5	Device Character 6	Qualifier Character 7
Ø Subcutaneous Tissue and Fascia, Scalp Galea aponeurotica **1** Subcutaneous Tissue and Fascia, Face Masseteric fascia Orbital fascia Submandibular space **4** Subcutaneous Tissue and Fascia, Right Neck Deep cervical fascia Pretracheal fascia Prevertebral fascia **5** Subcutaneous Tissue and Fascia, Left Neck *See 4 Subcutaneous Tissue and Fascia, Right Neck* **6** Subcutaneous Tissue and Fascia, Chest Pectoral fascia **7** Subcutaneous Tissue and Fascia, Back **8** Subcutaneous Tissue and Fascia, Abdomen **9** Subcutaneous Tissue and Fascia, Buttock **B** Subcutaneous Tissue and Fascia, Perineum **C** Subcutaneous Tissue and Fascia, Pelvic Region **D** Subcutaneous Tissue and Fascia, Right Upper Arm Axillary fascia Deltoid fascia Infraspinatus fascia Subscapular aponeurosis Supraspinatus fascia **F** Subcutaneous Tissue and Fascia, Left Upper Arm *See D Subcutaneous Tissue and Fascia, Right Upper Arm* **G** Subcutaneous Tissue and Fascia, Right Lower Arm Antebrachial fascia Bicipital aponeurosis **H** Subcutaneous Tissue and Fascia, Left Lower Arm *See G Subcutaneous Tissue and Fascia, Right Lower Arm* **J** Subcutaneous Tissue and Fascia, Right Hand Palmar fascia (aponeurosis) **K** Subcutaneous Tissue and Fascia, Left Hand *See J Subcutaneous Tissue and Fascia, Right Hand* **L** Subcutaneous Tissue and Fascia, Right Upper Leg Crural fascia Fascia lata Iliac fascia Iliotibial tract (band) **M** Subcutaneous Tissue and Fascia, Left Upper Leg *See L Subcutaneous Tissue and Fascia, Right Upper Leg* **N** Subcutaneous Tissue and Fascia, Right Lower Leg **P** Subcutaneous Tissue and Fascia, Left Lower Leg **Q** Subcutaneous Tissue and Fascia, Right Foot Plantar fascia (aponeurosis) **R** Subcutaneous Tissue and Fascia, Left Foot *See Q Subcutaneous Tissue and Fascia, Right Foot*	**Ø** Open **3** Percutaneous **X** External	**Z** No Device	**Z** No Qualifier

Non-OR ØJN[Ø,1,4,5,6,7,8,9,B,C,D,F,G,H,J,K,L,M,N,P,Q,R]XZZ

Ø Medical and Surgical
J Subcutaneous Tissue and Fascia
P Removal Definition: Taking out or off a device from a body part

Explanation: If a device is taken out and a similar device put in without cutting or puncturing the skin or mucous membrane, the procedure is coded to the root operation CHANGE. Otherwise, the procedure for taking out a device is coded to the root operation REMOVAL.

Body Part Character 4	Approach Character 5	Device Character 6	Qualifier Character 7
S Subcutaneous Tissue and Fascia, Head and Neck	**Ø** Open **3** Percutaneous	**Ø** Drainage Device **1** Radioactive Element **3** Infusion Device **7** Autologous Tissue Substitute **J** Synthetic Substitute **K** Nonautologous Tissue Substitute **N** Tissue Expander **Y** Other Device	**Z** No Qualifier
S Subcutaneous Tissue and Fascia, Head and Neck	**X** External	**Ø** Drainage Device **1** Radioactive Element **3** Infusion Device	**Z** No Qualifier
T Subcutaneous Tissue and Fascia, Trunk External oblique aponeurosis Transversalis fascia	**Ø** Open **3** Percutaneous	**Ø** Drainage Device **1** Radioactive Element **2** Monitoring Device **3** Infusion Device **7** Autologous Tissue Substitute **F** Subcutaneous Defibrillator Lead **H** Contraceptive Device **J** Synthetic Substitute **K** Nonautologous Tissue Substitute **M** Stimulator Generator **N** Tissue Expander **P** Cardiac Rhythm Related Device **V** Infusion Device, Pump **W** Vascular Access Device, Totally Implantable **X** Vascular Access Device, Tunneled **Y** Other Device	**Z** No Qualifier
T Subcutaneous Tissue and Fascia, Trunk External oblique aponeurosis Transversalis fascia	**X** External	**Ø** Drainage Device **1** Radioactive Element **2** Monitoring Device **3** Infusion Device **H** Contraceptive Device **V** Infusion Device, Pump **X** Vascular Access Device, Tunneled	**Z** No Qualifier
V Subcutaneous Tissue and Fascia, Upper Extremity **W** Subcutaneous Tissue and Fascia, Lower Extremity	**Ø** Open **3** Percutaneous	**Ø** Drainage Device **1** Radioactive Element **3** Infusion Device **7** Autologous Tissue Substitute **H** Contraceptive Device **J** Synthetic Substitute **K** Nonautologous Tissue Substitute **N** Tissue Expander **V** Infusion Device, Pump **W** Vascular Access Device, Totally Implantable **X** Vascular Access Device, Tunneled **Y** Other Device	**Z** No Qualifier
V Subcutaneous Tissue and Fascia, Upper Extremity **W** Subcutaneous Tissue and Fascia, Lower Extremity	**X** External	**Ø** Drainage Device **1** Radioactive Element **3** Infusion Device **H** Contraceptive Device **V** Infusion Device, Pump **X** Vascular Access Device, Tunneled	**Z** No Qualifier

Non-OR ØJPS[Ø,3][Ø,1,3,7,J,K,N,Y]Z
Non-OR ØJPSX[Ø,1,3]Z
Non-OR ØJPT[Ø,3][Ø,1,2,3,7,H,J,K,M,N,V,W,X,Y]Z
Non-OR ØJPTX[Ø,1,2,3,H,V,X]Z
Non-OR ØJP[V,W][Ø,3][Ø,1,3,7,H,J,K,N,V,W,X,Y]Z
Non-OR ØJP[V,W]X[Ø,1,3,H,V,X]Z
HAC ØJPT[Ø,3][F,P]Z when reported with SDx K68.11 or T81.4Ø-T81.49, T82.6-T82.7 with 7th character A

Ø Medical and Surgical
J Subcutaneous Tissue and Fascia
Q Repair Definition: Restoring, to the extent possible, a body part to its normal anatomic structure and function
Explanation: Used only when the method to accomplish the repair is not one of the other root operations

Body Part Character 4	Approach Character 5	Device Character 6	Qualifier Character 7
Ø Subcutaneous Tissue and Fascia, Scalp Galea aponeurotica **1** Subcutaneous Tissue and Fascia, Face Masseteric fascia Orbital fascia Submandibular space **4** Subcutaneous Tissue and Fascia, Right Neck Deep cervical fascia Pretracheal fascia Prevertebral fascia **5** Subcutaneous Tissue and Fascia, Left Neck ***See*** *4 Subcutaneous Tissue and Fascia, Right Neck* **6** Subcutaneous Tissue and Fascia, Chest Pectoral fascia **7** Subcutaneous Tissue and Fascia, Back **8** Subcutaneous Tissue and Fascia, Abdomen **9** Subcutaneous Tissue and Fascia, Buttock **B** Subcutaneous Tissue and Fascia, Perineum **C** Subcutaneous Tissue and Fascia, Pelvic Region **D** Subcutaneous Tissue and Fascia, Right Upper Arm Axillary fascia Deltoid fascia Infraspinatus fascia Subscapular aponeurosis Supraspinatus fascia **F** Subcutaneous Tissue and Fascia, Left Upper Arm ***See*** *D Subcutaneous Tissue and Fascia, Right Upper Arm* **G** Subcutaneous Tissue and Fascia, Right Lower Arm Antebrachial fascia Bicipital aponeurosis **H** Subcutaneous Tissue and Fascia, Left Lower Arm ***See*** *G Subcutaneous Tissue and Fascia, Right Lower Arm* **J** Subcutaneous Tissue and Fascia, Right Hand Palmar fascia (aponeurosis) **K** Subcutaneous Tissue and Fascia, Left Hand ***See*** *J Subcutaneous Tissue and Fascia, Right Hand* **L** Subcutaneous Tissue and Fascia, Right Upper Leg Crural fascia Fascia lata Iliac fascia Iliotibial tract (band) **M** Subcutaneous Tissue and Fascia, Left Upper Leg ***See*** *L Subcutaneous Tissue and Fascia, Right Upper Leg* **N** Subcutaneous Tissue and Fascia, Right Lower Leg **P** Subcutaneous Tissue and Fascia, Left Lower Leg **Q** Subcutaneous Tissue and Fascia, Right Foot Plantar fascia (aponeurosis) **R** Subcutaneous Tissue and Fascia, Left Foot ***See*** *Q Subcutaneous Tissue and Fascia, Right Foot*	**Ø** Open **3** Percutaneous	**Z** No Device	**Z** No Qualifier

Non-OR ØJQ[Ø,1,4,5,6,7,8,9,B,C,D,F,G,H,J,K,L,M,N,P,Q,R]3ZZ

Subcutaneous Tissue and Fascia

ØJQ–ØJQ

Ø Medical and Surgical
J Subcutaneous Tissue and Fascia
R Replacement Definition: Putting in or on biological or synthetic material that physically takes the place and/or function of all or a portion of a body part

Explanation: The body part may have been taken out or replaced, or may be taken out, physically eradicated, or rendered nonfunctional during the REPLACEMENT procedure. A REMOVAL procedure is coded for taking out the device used in a previous replacement procedure.

Body Part Character 4	Approach Character 5	Device Character 6	Qualifier Character 7
Ø Subcutaneous Tissue and Fascia, Scalp Galea aponeurotica **1 Subcutaneous Tissue and Fascia, Face** Masseteric fascia Orbital fascia Submandibular space **4 Subcutaneous Tissue and Fascia, Right Neck** Deep cervical fascia Pretracheal fascia Prevertebral fascia **5 Subcutaneous Tissue and Fascia, Left Neck** *See 4 Subcutaneous Tissue and Fascia, Right Neck* **6 Subcutaneous Tissue and Fascia, Chest** Pectoral fascia **7 Subcutaneous Tissue and Fascia, Back** **8 Subcutaneous Tissue and Fascia, Abdomen** **9 Subcutaneous Tissue and Fascia, Buttock** **B Subcutaneous Tissue and Fascia, Perineum** **C Subcutaneous Tissue and Fascia, Pelvic Region** **D Subcutaneous Tissue and Fascia, Right Upper Arm** Axillary fascia Deltoid fascia Infraspinatus fascia Subscapular aponeurosis Supraspinatus fascia **F Subcutaneous Tissue and Fascia, Left Upper Arm** *See D Subcutaneous Tissue and Fascia, Right Upper Arm* **G Subcutaneous Tissue and Fascia, Right Lower Arm** Antebrachial fascia Bicipital aponeurosis **H Subcutaneous Tissue and Fascia, Left Lower Arm** *See G Subcutaneous Tissue and Fascia, Right Lower Arm* **J Subcutaneous Tissue and Fascia, Right Hand** Palmar fascia (aponeurosis) **K Subcutaneous Tissue and Fascia, Left Hand** *See J Subcutaneous Tissue and Fascia, Right Hand* **L Subcutaneous Tissue and Fascia, Right Upper Leg** Crural fascia Fascia lata Iliac fascia Iliotibial tract (band) **M Subcutaneous Tissue and Fascia, Left Upper Leg** *See L Subcutaneous Tissue and Fascia, Right Upper Leg* **N Subcutaneous Tissue and Fascia, Right Lower Leg** **P Subcutaneous Tissue and Fascia, Left Lower Leg** **Q Subcutaneous Tissue and Fascia, Right Foot** Plantar fascia (aponeurosis) **R Subcutaneous Tissue and Fascia, Left Foot** *See Q Subcutaneous Tissue and Fascia, Right Foot*	**Ø Open** **3 Percutaneous**	**7 Autologous Tissue Substitute** **J Synthetic Substitute** **K Nonautologous Tissue Substitute**	**Z No Qualifier**

Ø Medical and Surgical
J Subcutaneous Tissue and Fascia
U Supplement: Definition: Putting in or on biological or synthetic material that physically reinforces and/or augments the function of a portion of a body part

Explanation: The biological material is non-living, or is living and from the same individual. The body part may have been previously replaced, and the SUPPLEMENT procedure is performed to physically reinforce and/or augment the function of the replaced body part.

Body Part Character 4		Approach Character 5	Device Character 6	Qualifier Character 7
Ø Subcutaneous Tissue and Fascia, Scalp Galea aponeurotica **1 Subcutaneous Tissue and Fascia, Face** Masseteric fascia Orbital fascia Submandibular space **4 Subcutaneous Tissue and Fascia, Right Neck** Deep cervical fascia Pretracheal fascia Prevertebral fascia **5 Subcutaneous Tissue and Fascia, Left Neck** *See 4 Subcutaneous Tissue and Fascia, Right Neck* **6 Subcutaneous Tissue and Fascia, Chest** Pectoral fascia **7 Subcutaneous Tissue and Fascia, Back** **8 Subcutaneous Tissue and Fascia, Abdomen** **9 Subcutaneous Tissue and Fascia, Buttock** **B Subcutaneous Tissue and Fascia, Perineum** **C Subcutaneous Tissue and Fascia, Pelvic Region** **D Subcutaneous Tissue and Fascia, Right Upper Arm** Axillary fascia Deltoid fascia Infraspinatus fascia Subscapular aponeurosis Supraspinatus fascia **F Subcutaneous Tissue and Fascia, Left Upper Arm** *See D Subcutaneous Tissue and Fascia, Right Upper Arm*	**G Subcutaneous Tissue and Fascia, Right Lower Arm** Antebrachial fascia Bicipital aponeurosis **H Subcutaneous Tissue and Fascia, Left Lower Arm** *See G Subcutaneous Tissue and Fascia, Right Lower Arm* **J Subcutaneous Tissue and Fascia, Right Hand** Palmar fascia (aponeurosis) **K Subcutaneous Tissue and Fascia, Left Hand** *See J Subcutaneous Tissue and Fascia, Right Hand* **L Subcutaneous Tissue and Fascia, Right Upper Leg** Crural fascia Fascia lata Iliac fascia Iliotibial tract (band) **M Subcutaneous Tissue and Fascia, Left Upper Leg** *See L Subcutaneous Tissue and Fascia, Right Upper Leg* **N Subcutaneous Tissue and Fascia, Right Lower Leg** **P Subcutaneous Tissue and Fascia, Left Lower Leg** **Q Subcutaneous Tissue and Fascia, Right Foot** Plantar fascia (aponeurosis) **R Subcutaneous Tissue and Fascia, Left Foot** *See Q Subcutaneous Tissue and Fascia, Right Foot*	**Ø Open** **3 Percutaneous**	**7 Autologous Tissue Substitute** **J Synthetic Substitute** **K Nonautologous Tissue Substitute**	**Z No Qualifier**

Ø Medical and Surgical
J Subcutaneous Tissue and Fascia
W Revision Definition: Correcting, to the extent possible, a portion of a malfunctioning device or the position of a displaced device

Explanation: Revision can include correcting a malfunctioning or displaced device by taking out or putting in components of the device such as a screw or pin

Body Part Character 4	Approach Character 5	Device Character 6	Qualifier Character 7
S Subcutaneous Tissue and Fascia, Head and Neck	Ø Open 3 Percutaneous	Ø Drainage Device 3 Infusion Device 7 Autologous Tissue Substitute J Synthetic Substitute K Nonautologous Tissue Substitute N Tissue Expander Y Other Device	Z No Qualifier
S Subcutaneous Tissue and Fascia, Head and Neck	X External	Ø Drainage Device 3 Infusion Device 7 Autologous Tissue Substitute J Synthetic Substitute K Nonautologous Tissue Substitute N Tissue Expander	Z No Qualifier
T Subcutaneous Tissue and Fascia, Trunk External oblique aponeurosis Transversalis fascia	Ø Open 3 Percutaneous	Ø Drainage Device 2 Monitoring Device 3 Infusion Device 7 Autologous Tissue Substitute F Subcutaneous Defibrillator Lead H Contraceptive Device J Synthetic Substitute K Nonautologous Tissue Substitute M Stimulator Generator N Tissue Expander P Cardiac Rhythm Related Device V Infusion Device, Pump W Vascular Access Device, Totally Implantable X Vascular Access Device, Tunneled Y Other Device	Z No Qualifier
T Subcutaneous Tissue and Fascia, Trunk External oblique aponeurosis Transversalis fascia	X External	Ø Drainage Device 2 Monitoring Device 3 Infusion Device 7 Autologous Tissue Substitute F Subcutaneous Defibrillator Lead H Contraceptive Device J Synthetic Substitute K Nonautologous Tissue Substitute M Stimulator Generator N Tissue Expander P Cardiac Rhythm Related Device V Infusion Device, Pump W Vascular Access Device, Totally Implantable X Vascular Access Device, Tunneled	Z No Qualifier
V Subcutaneous Tissue and Fascia, Upper Extremity W Subcutaneous Tissue and Fascia, Lower Extremity	Ø Open 3 Percutaneous	Ø Drainage Device 3 Infusion Device 7 Autologous Tissue Substitute H Contraceptive Device J Synthetic Substitute K Nonautologous Tissue Substitute N Tissue Expander V Infusion Device, Pump W Vascular Access Device, Totally Implantable X Vascular Access Device, Tunneled Y Other Device	Z No Qualifier
V Subcutaneous Tissue and Fascia, Upper Extremity W Subcutaneous Tissue and Fascia, Lower Extremity	X External	Ø Drainage Device 3 Infusion Device 7 Autologous Tissue Substitute H Contraceptive Device J Synthetic Substitute K Nonautologous Tissue Substitute N Tissue Expander V Infusion Device, Pump W Vascular Access Device, Totally Implantable X Vascular Access Device, Tunneled	Z No Qualifier

DRG Non-OR ØJWS[Ø,3][Ø,3,7,J,K,N,Y]Z
DRG Non-OR ØJWT[Ø,3][Ø,3,7,H,J,K,M,N,V,W,X]Z
DRG Non-OR ØJWTXMZ
DRG Non-OR ØJW[V,W][Ø,3][Ø,3,7,H,J,K,N,V,W,X,Y]Z
Non-OR ØJWSX[Ø,3,7,J,K,N]Z
Non-OR ØJWT3YZ
Non-OR ØJWTX[Ø,2,3,7,F,H,J,K,N,P,V,W,X]Z
Non-OR ØJW[V,W]X[Ø,3,7,H,J,K,N,V,W,X]Z

HAC ØJWT[Ø,3][F,P]Z when reported with SDx K68.11 or T81.4Ø-T81.49, T82.6-T82.7 with 7th character A

Ø Medical and Surgical
J Subcutaneous Tissue and Fascia
X Transfer Definition: Moving, without taking out, all or a portion of a body part to another location to take over the function of all or a portion of a body part
Explanation: The body part transferred remains connected to its vascular and nervous supply

Body Part Character 4	Approach Character 5	Device Character 6	Qualifier Character 7
Ø Subcutaneous Tissue and Fascia, Scalp Galea aponeurotica **1 Subcutaneous Tissue and Fascia, Face** Masseteric fascia; Orbital fascia; Submandibular space **4 Subcutaneous Tissue and Fascia, Right Neck** Deep cervical fascia; Pretracheal fascia; Prevertebral fascia **5 Subcutaneous Tissue and Fascia, Left Neck** *See 4 Subcutaneous Tissue and Fascia, Right Neck* **6 Subcutaneous Tissue and Fascia, Chest** Pectoral fascia **7 Subcutaneous Tissue and Fascia, Back** **8 Subcutaneous Tissue and Fascia, Abdomen** **9 Subcutaneous Tissue and Fascia, Buttock** **B Subcutaneous Tissue and Fascia, Perineum** **C Subcutaneous Tissue and Fascia, Pelvic Region** **D Subcutaneous Tissue and Fascia, Right Upper Arm** Axillary fascia; Deltoid fascia; Infraspinatus fascia; Subscapular aponeurosis; Supraspinatus fascia **F Subcutaneous Tissue and Fascia, Left Upper Arm** *See D Subcutaneous Tissue and Fascia, Right Upper Arm* **G Subcutaneous Tissue and Fascia, Right Lower Arm** Antebrachial fascia; Bicipital aponeurosis **H Subcutaneous Tissue and Fascia, Left Lower Arm** *See G Subcutaneous Tissue and Fascia, Right Lower Arm* **J Subcutaneous Tissue and Fascia, Right Hand** Palmar fascia (aponeurosis) **K Subcutaneous Tissue and Fascia, Left Hand** *See J Subcutaneous Tissue and Fascia, Right Hand* **L Subcutaneous Tissue and Fascia, Right Upper Leg** Crural fascia; Fascia lata; Iliac fascia; Iliotibial tract (band) **M Subcutaneous Tissue and Fascia, Left Upper Leg** *See L Subcutaneous Tissue and Fascia, Right Upper Leg* **N Subcutaneous Tissue and Fascia, Right Lower Leg** **P Subcutaneous Tissue and Fascia, Left Lower Leg** **Q Subcutaneous Tissue and Fascia, Right Foot** Plantar fascia (aponeurosis) **R Subcutaneous Tissue and Fascia, Left Foot** *See Q Subcutaneous Tissue and Fascia, Right Foot*	**Ø Open** **3 Percutaneous**	**Z No Device**	**B Skin and Subcutaneous Tissue** **C Skin, Subcutaneous Tissue and Fascia** **Z No Qualifier**

Muscles ØK2–ØKX

Character Meanings

This Character Meaning table is provided as a guide to assist the user in the identification of character members that may be found in this section of code tables. It **SHOULD NOT** be used to build a PCS code.

Operation–Character 3	Body Part–Character 4	Approach–Character 5	Device–Character 6	Qualifier–Character 7
2 Change	Ø Head Muscle	Ø Open	Ø Drainage Device	Ø Skin
5 Destruction	1 Facial Muscle	3 Percutaneous	7 Autologous Tissue Substitute	1 Subcutaneous Tissue
8 Division	2 Neck Muscle, Right	4 Percutaneous Endoscopic	J Synthetic Substitute	2 Skin and Subcutaneous Tissue
9 Drainage	3 Neck Muscle, Left	7 Via Natural or Artificial Opening	K Nonautologous Tissue Substitute	5 Latissimus Dorsi Myocutaneous Flap
B Excision	4 Tongue, Palate, Pharynx Muscle	8 Via Natural or Artificial Opening Endoscopic	M Stimulator Lead	6 Transverse Rectus Abdominis Myocutaneous Flap
C Extirpation	5 Shoulder Muscle, Right	X External	Y Other Device	7 Deep Inferior Epigastric Artery Perforator Flap
D Extraction	6 Shoulder Muscle, Left		Z No Device	8 Superficial Inferior Epigastric Artery Flap
H Insertion	7 Upper Arm Muscle, Right			9 Gluteal Artery Perforator Flap
J Inspection	8 Upper Arm Muscle, Left			X Diagnostic
M Reattachment	9 Lower Arm and Wrist Muscle, Right			Z No Qualifier
N Release	B Lower Arm and Wrist Muscle, Left			
P Removal	C Hand Muscle, Right			
Q Repair	D Hand Muscle, Left			
R Replacement	F Trunk Muscle, Right			
S Reposition	G Trunk Muscle, Left			
T Resection	H Thorax Muscle, Right			
U Supplement	J Thorax Muscle, Left			
W Revision	K Abdomen Muscle, Right			
X Transfer	L Abdomen Muscle, Left			
	M Perineum Muscle			
	N Hip Muscle, Right			
	P Hip Muscle, Left			
	Q Upper Leg Muscle, Right			
	R Upper Leg Muscle, Left			
	S Lower Leg Muscle, Right			
	T Lower Leg Muscle, Left			
	V Foot Muscle, Right			
	W Foot Muscle, Left			
	X Upper Muscle			
	Y Lower Muscle			

AHA Coding Clinic for table ØK8
2020, 2Q, 25 Endoscopic Stapling of Zenker's Diverticulum

AHA Coding Clinic for table ØKB
2020, 1Q, 27 Delayed reconstruction following mastectomy using gracilis musculocutaneous free flap
2016, 3Q, 20 Excisional debridement of sacrum
2015, 3Q, 3-8 Excisional and nonexcisional debridement

AHA Coding Clinic for table ØKD
2017, 4Q, 41-42 Extraction procedures

AHA Coding Clinic for table ØKH
2020, 4Q, 63 Intercompartmental pressure measurement

AHA Coding Clinic for table ØKN
2017, 2Q, 12 Compartment syndrome and fasciotomy of foot
2017, 2Q, 13 Compartment syndrome and fasciotomy of leg
2015, 2Q, 22 Arthroscopic subacromial decompression
2014, 4Q, 39 Abdominal component release with placement of mesh for hernia repair

AHA Coding Clinic for table ØKQ
2018, 2Q, 25 Third and fourth degree obstetric lacerations
2016, 2Q, 34 Assisted vaginal delivery
2016, 1Q, 7 Obstetrical perineal laceration repair
2014, 4Q, 43 Second degree obstetric perineal laceration
2013, 4Q, 120 Repair of second degree perineum obstetric laceration

AHA Coding Clinic for table ØKS
2017, 1Q, 41 Manual reduction of hernia

AHA Coding Clinic for table ØKT
2016, 2Q, 12 Resection of malignant neoplasm of infratemporal fossa
2015, 1Q, 38 Abdominoperineal resection with flap closure of the perineum and colostomy

AHA Coding Clinic for table ØKX
2018, 2Q, 18 Transverse rectus abdominis myocutaneous (TRAM) delay
2017, 4Q, 67 New qualifier values - Pedicle flap procedures
2016, 3Q, 30 Resection of femur with interposition arthroplasty
2015, 3Q, 33 Cleft lip repair using Millard rotation advancement
2015, 2Q, 26 Pharyngeal flap to soft palate
2014, 4Q, 41 Abdominoperineal resection (APR) with flap closure of perineum and colostomy
2014, 2Q, 10 Transverse abdominomyocutaneous (TRAM) breast reconstruction
2014, 2Q, 12 Pedicle latissimus myocutaneous flap with placement of breast tissue expanders

Muscles

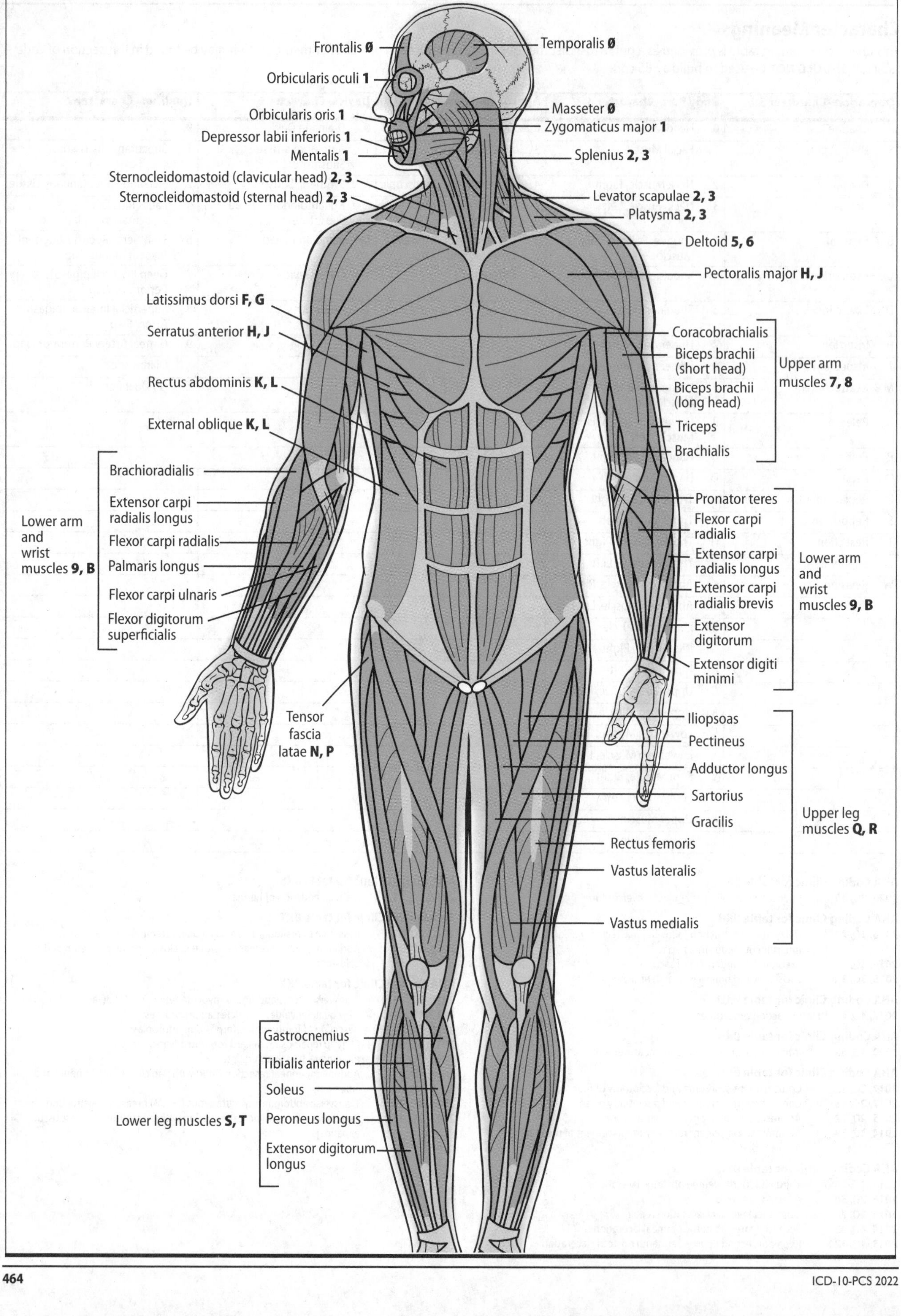
Frontalis Ø
Temporalis Ø
Orbicularis oculi 1
Orbicularis oris 1
Masseter Ø
Zygomaticus major 1
Depressor labii inferioris 1
Mentalis 1
Splenius 2, 3
Sternocleidomastoid (clavicular head) 2, 3
Sternocleidomastoid (sternal head) 2, 3
Levator scapulae 2, 3
Platysma 2, 3
Deltoid 5, 6
Pectoralis major H, J
Latissimus dorsi F, G
Serratus anterior H, J
Coracobrachialis
Biceps brachii (short head)
Biceps brachii (long head)
Triceps
Brachialis
Upper arm muscles 7, 8
Rectus abdominis K, L
External oblique K, L
Brachioradialis
Extensor carpi radialis longus
Flexor carpi radialis
Palmaris longus
Flexor carpi ulnaris
Flexor digitorum superficialis
Lower arm and wrist muscles 9, B
Pronator teres
Flexor carpi radialis
Extensor carpi radialis longus
Extensor carpi radialis brevis
Extensor digitorum
Extensor digiti minimi
Lower arm and wrist muscles 9, B
Tensor fascia latae N, P
Iliopsoas
Pectineus
Adductor longus
Sartorius
Gracilis
Rectus femoris
Vastus lateralis
Vastus medialis
Upper leg muscles Q, R
Gastrocnemius
Tibialis anterior
Soleus
Peroneus longus
Extensor digitorum longus
Lower leg muscles S, T

Ø Medical and Surgical
K Muscles
2 Change Definition: Taking out or off a device from a body part and putting back an identical or similar device in or on the same body part without cutting or puncturing the skin or a mucous membrane

Explanation: All CHANGE procedures are coded using the approach EXTERNAL

Body Part Character 4	Approach Character 5	Device Character 6	Qualifier Character 7
X Upper Muscle **Y** Lower Muscle	**X** External	**Ø** Drainage Device **Y** Other Device	**Z** No Qualifier

Non-OR All body part, approach, device, and qualifier values

Ø Medical and Surgical
K Muscles
5 Destruction Definition: Physical eradication of all or a portion of a body part by the direct use of energy, force, or a destructive agent

Explanation: None of the body part is physically taken out

Body Part Character 4	Approach Character 5	Device Character 6	Qualifier Character 7
Ø Head Muscle Auricularis muscle Masseter muscle Pterygoid muscle Splenius capitis muscle Temporalis muscle Temporoparietalis muscle **1 Facial Muscle** Buccinator muscle Corrugator supercilii muscle Depressor anguli oris muscle Depressor labii inferioris muscle Depressor septi nasi muscle Depressor supercilii muscle Levator anguli oris muscle Levator labii superioris alaeque nasi muscle Levator labii superioris muscle Mentalis muscle Nasalis muscle Occipitofrontalis muscle Orbicularis oris muscle Procerus muscle Risorius muscle Zygomaticus muscle **2 Neck Muscle, Right** Anterior vertebral muscle Arytenoid muscle Cricothyroid muscle Infrahyoid muscle Levator scapulae muscle Platysma muscle Scalene muscle Splenius cervicis muscle Sternocleidomastoid muscle Suprahyoid muscle Thyroarytenoid muscle **3 Neck Muscle, Left** *See 2 Neck Muscle, Right* **4 Tongue, Palate, Pharynx Muscle** Chondroglossus muscle Genioglossus muscle Hyoglossus muscle Inferior longitudinal muscle Levator veli palatini muscle Palatoglossal muscle Palatopharyngeal muscle Pharyngeal constrictor muscle Salpingopharyngeus muscle Styloglossus muscle Stylopharyngeus muscle Superior longitudinal muscle Tensor veli palatini muscle **5 Shoulder Muscle, Right** Deltoid muscle Infraspinatus muscle Subscapularis muscle Supraspinatus muscle Teres major muscle Teres minor muscle **6 Shoulder Muscle, Left** *See 5 Shoulder Muscle, Right* **7 Upper Arm Muscle, Right** Biceps brachii muscle Brachialis muscle Coracobrachialis muscle Triceps brachii muscle **8 Upper Arm Muscle, Left** *See 7 Upper Arm Muscle, Right* **9 Lower Arm and Wrist Muscle, Right** Anatomical snuffbox Brachioradialis muscle Extensor carpi radialis muscle Extensor carpi ulnaris muscle Flexor carpi radialis muscle Flexor carpi ulnaris muscle Flexor pollicis longus muscle Palmaris longus muscle Pronator quadratus muscle Pronator teres muscle **B Lower Arm and Wrist Muscle, Left** *See 9 Lower Arm and Wrist Muscle, Right* **C Hand Muscle, Right** Hypothenar muscle Palmar interosseous muscle Thenar muscle **D Hand Muscle, Left** *See C Hand Muscle, Right* **F Trunk Muscle, Right** Coccygeus muscle Erector spinae muscle Interspinalis muscle Intertransversarius muscle Latissimus dorsi muscle Quadratus lumborum muscle Rhomboid major muscle Rhomboid minor muscle Serratus posterior muscle Transversospinalis muscle Trapezius muscle **G Trunk Muscle, Left** *See F Trunk Muscle, Right* **H Thorax Muscle, Right** Intercostal muscle Levatores costarum muscle Pectoralis major muscle Pectoralis minor muscle Serratus anterior muscle Subclavius muscle Subcostal muscle Transverse thoracis muscle **J Thorax Muscle, Left** *See H Thorax Muscle, Right* **K Abdomen Muscle, Right** External oblique muscle Internal oblique muscle Pyramidalis muscle Rectus abdominis muscle Transversus abdominis muscle **L Abdomen Muscle, Left** *See K Abdomen Muscle, Right* **M Perineum Muscle** Bulbospongiosus muscle Cremaster muscle Deep transverse perineal muscle Ischiocavernosus muscle Levator ani muscle Superficial transverse perineal muscle **N Hip Muscle, Right** Gemellus muscle Gluteus maximus muscle Gluteus medius muscle Gluteus minimus muscle Iliacus muscle Obturator muscle Piriformis muscle Psoas muscle Quadratus femoris muscle Tensor fasciae latae muscle **P Hip Muscle, Left** *See N Hip Muscle, Right* **Q Upper Leg Muscle, Right** Adductor brevis muscle Adductor longus muscle Adductor magnus muscle Biceps femoris muscle Gracilis muscle Pectineus muscle Quadriceps (femoris) Rectus femoris muscle Sartorius muscle Semimembranosus muscle Semitendinosus muscle Vastus intermedius muscle Vastus lateralis muscle Vastus medialis muscle **R Upper Leg Muscle, Left** *See Q Upper Leg Muscle, Right* **S Lower Leg Muscle, Right** Extensor digitorum longus muscle Extensor hallucis longus muscle Fibularis brevis muscle Fibularis longus muscle Flexor digitorum longus muscle Flexor hallucis longus muscle Gastrocnemius muscle Peroneus brevis muscle Peroneus longus muscle Popliteus muscle Soleus muscle Tibialis anterior muscle Tibialis posterior muscle **T Lower Leg Muscle, Left** *See S Lower Leg Muscle, Right* **V Foot Muscle, Right** Abductor hallucis muscle Adductor hallucis muscle Extensor digitorum brevis muscle Extensor hallucis brevis muscle Flexor digitorum brevis muscle Flexor hallucis brevis muscle Quadratus plantae muscle **W Foot Muscle, Left** *See V Foot Muscle, Right*	**Ø** Open **3** Percutaneous **4** Percutaneous Endoscopic	**Z** No Device	**Z** No Qualifier

Ø Medical and Surgical
K Muscles
8 Division

Definition: Cutting into a body part, without draining fluids and/or gases from the body part, in order to separate or transect a body part

Explanation: All or a portion of the body part is separated into two or more portions

Body Part Character 4	Approach Character 5	Device Character 6	Qualifier Character 7
Ø Head Muscle Auricularis muscle Masseter muscle Pterygoid muscle Splenius capitis muscle Temporalis muscle Temporoparietalis muscle **1 Facial Muscle** Buccinator muscle Corrugator supercilii muscle Depressor anguli oris muscle Depressor labii inferioris muscle Depressor septi nasi muscle Depressor supercilii muscle Levator anguli oris muscle Levator labii superioris alaeque nasi muscle Levator labii superioris muscle Mentalis muscle Nasalis muscle Occipitofrontalis muscle Orbicularis oris muscle Procerus muscle Risorius muscle Zygomaticus muscle **2 Neck Muscle, Right** Anterior vertebral muscle Arytenoid muscle Cricothyroid muscle Infrahyoid muscle Levator scapulae muscle Platysma muscle Scalene muscle Splenius cervicis muscle Sternocleidomastoid muscle Suprahyoid muscle Thyroarytenoid muscle **3 Neck Muscle, Left** *See 2 Neck Muscle, Right* Tensor veli palatini muscle **5 Shoulder Muscle, Right** Deltoid muscle Infraspinatus muscle Subscapularis muscle Supraspinatus muscle Teres major muscle Teres minor muscle **6 Shoulder Muscle, Left** *See 5 Shoulder Muscle, Right* **7 Upper Arm Muscle, Right** Biceps brachii muscle Brachialis muscle Coracobrachialis muscle Triceps brachii muscle **8 Upper Arm Muscle, Left** *See 7 Upper Arm Muscle, Right* **9 Lower Arm and Wrist Muscle, Right** Anatomical snuffbox Brachioradialis muscle Extensor carpi radialis muscle Extensor carpi ulnaris muscle Flexor carpi radialis muscle Flexor carpi ulnaris muscle Flexor pollicis longus muscle Palmaris longus muscle Pronator quadratus muscle Pronator teres muscle **B Lower Arm and Wrist Muscle, Left** *See 9 Lower Arm and Wrist Muscle, Right* **C Hand Muscle, Right** Hypothenar muscle Palmar interosseous muscle Thenar muscle **D Hand Muscle, Left** *See C Hand Muscle, Right* **F Trunk Muscle, Right** Coccygeus muscle Erector spinae muscle Interspinalis muscle Intertransversarius muscle Latissimus dorsi muscle Quadratus lumborum muscle Rhomboid major muscle Rhomboid minor muscle Serratus posterior muscle Transversospinalis muscle Trapezius muscle **G Trunk Muscle, Left** *See F Trunk Muscle, Right* **H Thorax Muscle, Right** Intercostal muscle Levatores costarum muscle Pectoralis major muscle Pectoralis minor muscle Serratus anterior muscle Subclavius muscle Subcostal muscle Transverse thoracis muscle **J Thorax Muscle, Left** *See H Thorax Muscle, Right* **K Abdomen Muscle, Right** External oblique muscle Internal oblique muscle Pyramidalis muscle Rectus abdominis muscle Transversus abdominis muscle **L Abdomen Muscle, Left** *See K Abdomen Muscle, Right* **M Perineum Muscle** Bulbospongiosus muscle Cremaster muscle Deep transverse perineal muscle Ischiocavernosus muscle Levator ani muscle Superficial transverse perineal muscle **N Hip Muscle, Right** Gemellus muscle Gluteus maximus muscle Gluteus medius muscle Gluteus minimus muscle Iliacus muscle Obturator muscle Piriformis muscle Psoas muscle Quadratus femoris muscle Tensor fasciae latae muscle **P Hip Muscle, Left** *See N Hip Muscle, Right* **Q Upper Leg Muscle, Right** Adductor brevis muscle Adductor longus muscle Adductor magnus muscle Biceps femoris muscle Gracilis muscle Pectineus muscle Quadriceps (femoris) Rectus femoris muscle Sartorius muscle Semimembranosus muscle Semitendinosus muscle Vastus intermedius muscle Vastus lateralis muscle Vastus medialis muscle **R Upper Leg Muscle, Left** *See Q Upper Leg Muscle, Right* **S Lower Leg Muscle, Right** Extensor digitorum longus muscle Extensor hallucis longus muscle Fibularis brevis muscle Fibularis longus muscle Flexor digitorum longus muscle Flexor hallucis longus muscle Gastrocnemius muscle Peroneus brevis muscle Peroneus longus muscle Popliteus muscle Soleus muscle Tibialis anterior muscle Tibialis posterior muscle **T Lower Leg Muscle, Left** *See S Lower Leg Muscle, Right* **V Foot Muscle, Right** Abductor hallucis muscle Adductor hallucis muscle Extensor digitorum brevis muscle Extensor hallucis brevis muscle Flexor digitorum brevis muscle Flexor hallucis brevis muscle Quadratus plantae muscle **W Foot Muscle, Left** *See V Foot Muscle, Right*	**Ø Open** **3 Percutaneous** **4 Percutaneous Endoscopic**	**Z No Device**	**Z No Qualifier**
4 Tongue, Palate, Pharynx Muscle Chondroglossus muscle Genioglossus muscle Hyoglossus muscle Inferior longitudinal muscle Levator veli palatini muscle Palatoglossal muscle Palatopharyngeal muscle Pharyngeal constrictor muscle Salpingopharyngeus muscle Styloglossus muscle Stylopharyngeus muscle Superior longitudinal muscle Tensor veli palatini muscle	**Ø Open** **3 Percutaneous** **4 Percutaneous Endoscopic** **7 Via Natural or Artificial Opening** **8 Via Natural or Artificial Opening Endoscopic**	**Z No Device**	**Z No Qualifier**

Ø Medical and Surgical
K Muscles
9 Drainage Definition: Taking or letting out fluids and/or gases from a body part
Explanation: The qualifier DIAGNOSTIC is used to identify drainage procedures that are biopsies

Body Part Character 4	Approach Character 5	Device Character 6	Qualifier Character 7
Ø Head Muscle Auricularis muscle Masseter muscle Pterygoid muscle Splenius capitis muscle Temporalis muscle Temporoparietalis muscle **1 Facial Muscle** Buccinator muscle Corrugator supercilii muscle Depressor anguli oris muscle Depressor labii inferioris muscle Depressor septi nasi muscle Depressor supercilii muscle Levator anguli oris muscle Levator labii superioris alaeque nasi muscle Levator labii superioris muscle Mentalis muscle Nasalis muscle Occipitofrontalis muscle Orbicularis oris muscle Procerus muscle Risorius muscle Zygomaticus muscle **2 Neck Muscle, Right** Anterior vertebral muscle Arytenoid muscle Cricothyroid muscle Infrahyoid muscle Levator scapulae muscle Platysma muscle Scalene muscle Splenius cervicis muscle Sternocleidomastoid muscle Suprahyoid muscle Thyroarytenoid muscle **3 Neck Muscle, Left** *See 2 Neck Muscle, Right* **4 Tongue, Palate, Pharynx Muscle** Chondroglossus muscle Genioglossus muscle Hyoglossus muscle Inferior longitudinal muscle Levator veli palatini muscle Palatoglossal muscle Palatopharyngeal muscle Pharyngeal constrictor muscle Salpingopharyngeus muscle Styloglossus muscle Stylopharyngeus muscle Superior longitudinal muscle Tensor veli palatini muscle **5 Shoulder Muscle, Right** Deltoid muscle Infraspinatus muscle Subscapularis muscle Supraspinatus muscle Teres major muscle Teres minor muscle **6 Shoulder Muscle, Left** *See 5 Shoulder Muscle, Right* **7 Upper Arm Muscle, Right** Biceps brachii muscle Brachialis muscle Coracobrachialis muscle Triceps brachii muscle **8 Upper Arm Muscle, Left** *See 7 Upper Arm Muscle, Right* **9 Lower Arm and Wrist Muscle, Right** Anatomical snuffbox Brachioradialis muscle Extensor carpi radialis muscle Extensor carpi ulnaris muscle Flexor carpi radialis muscle Flexor carpi ulnaris muscle Flexor pollicis longus muscle Palmaris longus muscle Pronator quadratus muscle Pronator teres muscle **B Lower Arm and Wrist Muscle, Left** *See 9 Lower Arm and Wrist Muscle, Right* **C Hand Muscle, Right** Hypothenar muscle Palmar interosseous muscle Thenar muscle **D Hand Muscle, Left** *See C Hand Muscle, Right* **F Trunk Muscle, Right** Coccygeus muscle Erector spinae muscle Interspinalis muscle Intertransversarius muscle Latissimus dorsi muscle Quadratus lumborum muscle Rhomboid major muscle Rhomboid minor muscle Serratus posterior muscle Transversospinalis muscle Trapezius muscle **G Trunk Muscle, Left** *See F Trunk Muscle, Right* **H Thorax Muscle, Right** Intercostal muscle Levatores costarum muscle Pectoralis major muscle Pectoralis minor muscle Serratus anterior muscle Subclavius muscle Subcostal muscle Transverse thoracis muscle **J Thorax Muscle, Left** *See H Thorax Muscle, Right* **K Abdomen Muscle, Right** External oblique muscle Internal oblique muscle Pyramidalis muscle Rectus abdominis muscle Transversus abdominis muscle **L Abdomen Muscle, Left** *See K Abdomen Muscle, Right* **M Perineum Muscle** Bulbospongiosus muscle Cremaster muscle Deep transverse perineal muscle Ischiocavernosus muscle Levator ani muscle Superficial transverse perineal muscle **N Hip Muscle, Right** Gemellus muscle Gluteus maximus muscle Gluteus medius muscle Gluteus minimus muscle Iliacus muscle Obturator muscle Piriformis muscle Psoas muscle Quadratus femoris muscle Tensor fasciae latae muscle **P Hip Muscle, Left** *See N Hip Muscle, Right* **Q Upper Leg Muscle, Right** Adductor brevis muscle Adductor longus muscle Adductor magnus muscle Biceps femoris muscle Gracilis muscle Pectineus muscle Quadriceps (femoris) Rectus femoris muscle Sartorius muscle Semimembranosus muscle Semitendinosus muscle Vastus intermedius muscle Vastus lateralis muscle Vastus medialis muscle **R Upper Leg Muscle, Left** *See Q Upper Leg Muscle, Right* **S Lower Leg Muscle, Right** Extensor digitorum longus muscle Extensor hallucis longus muscle Fibularis brevis muscle Fibularis longus muscle Flexor digitorum longus muscle Flexor hallucis longus muscle Gastrocnemius muscle Peroneus brevis muscle Peroneus longus muscle Popliteus muscle Soleus muscle Tibialis anterior muscle Tibialis posterior muscle **T Lower Leg Muscle, Left** *See S Lower Leg Muscle, Right* **V Foot Muscle, Right** Abductor hallucis muscle Adductor hallucis muscle Extensor digitorum brevis muscle Extensor hallucis brevis muscle Flexor digitorum brevis muscle Flexor hallucis brevis muscle Quadratus plantae muscle **W Foot Muscle, Left** *See V Foot Muscle, Right*	**Ø Open** **3 Percutaneous** **4 Percutaneous Endoscopic**	**Ø Drainage Device**	**Z No Qualifier**

ØK9 Continued on next page

Non-OR ØK9[Ø,1,2,3,4,5,6,7,8,9,B,C,D,F,G,H,J,K,L,M,N,P,Q,R,S,T,V,W]3ØZ

Ø Medical and Surgical
K Muscles
9 Drainage

ØK9 Continued

Definition: Taking or letting out fluids and/or gases from a body part

Explanation: The qualifier DIAGNOSTIC is used to identify drainage procedures that are biopsies

Body Part Character 4	Approach Character 5	Device Character 6	Qualifier Character 7
Ø Head Muscle Auricularis muscle Masseter muscle Pterygoid muscle Splenius capitis muscle Temporalis muscle Temporoparietalis muscle	**Ø** Open	**Z** No Device	**X** Diagnostic
1 Facial Muscle Buccinator muscle Corrugator supercilii muscle Depressor anguli oris muscle Depressor labii inferioris muscle Depressor septi nasi muscle Depressor supercilii muscle Levator anguli oris muscle Levator labii superioris alaeque nasi muscle Levator labii superioris muscle Mentalis muscle Nasalis muscle Occipitofrontalis muscle Orbicularis oris muscle Procerus muscle Risorius muscle Zygomaticus muscle	**3** Percutaneous		**Z** No Qualifier
2 Neck Muscle, Right Anterior vertebral muscle Arytenoid muscle Cricothyroid muscle Infrahyoid muscle Levator scapulae muscle Platysma muscle Scalene muscle Splenius cervicis muscle Sternocleidomastoid muscle Suprahyoid muscle Thyroarytenoid muscle	**4** Percutaneous Endoscopic		
3 Neck Muscle, Left *See 2 Neck Muscle, Right*			
4 Tongue, Palate, Pharynx Muscle Chondroglossus muscle Genioglossus muscle Hyoglossus muscle Inferior longitudinal muscle Levator veli palatini muscle Palatoglossal muscle Palatopharyngeal muscle Pharyngeal constrictor muscle Salpingopharyngeus muscle Styloglossus muscle Stylopharyngeus muscle Superior longitudinal muscle Tensor veli palatini muscle			
5 Shoulder Muscle, Right Deltoid muscle Infraspinatus muscle Subscapularis muscle Supraspinatus muscle Teres major muscle Teres minor muscle			
6 Shoulder Muscle, Left *See 5 Shoulder Muscle, Right*			
7 Upper Arm Muscle, Right Biceps brachii muscle Brachialis muscle Coracobrachialis muscle Triceps brachii muscle			
8 Upper Arm Muscle, Left *See 7 Upper Arm Muscle, Right*			
9 Lower Arm and Wrist Muscle, Right Anatomical snuffbox Brachioradialis muscle Extensor carpi radialis muscle Extensor carpi ulnaris muscle Flexor carpi radialis muscle Flexor carpi ulnaris muscle Flexor pollicis longus muscle Palmaris longus muscle Pronator quadratus muscle Pronator teres muscle			
B Lower Arm and Wrist Muscle, Left *See 9 Lower Arm and Wrist Muscle, Right*			
C Hand Muscle, Right Hypothenar muscle Palmar interosseous muscle Thenar muscle			
D Hand Muscle, Left *See C Hand Muscle, Right*			
F Trunk Muscle, Right Coccygeus muscle Erector spinae muscle Interspinalis muscle Intertransversarius muscle Latissimus dorsi muscle Quadratus lumborum muscle Rhomboid major muscle Rhomboid minor muscle Serratus posterior muscle Transversospinalis muscle Trapezius muscle			
G Trunk Muscle, Left *See F Trunk Muscle, Right*			
H Thorax Muscle, Right Intercostal muscle Levatores costarum muscle Pectoralis major muscle Pectoralis minor muscle Serratus anterior muscle Subclavius muscle Subcostal muscle Transverse thoracis muscle			
J Thorax Muscle, Left *See H Thorax Muscle, Right*			
K Abdomen Muscle, Right External oblique muscle Internal oblique muscle Pyramidalis muscle Rectus abdominis muscle Transversus abdominis muscle			
L Abdomen Muscle, Left *See K Abdomen Muscle, Right*			
M Perineum Muscle Bulbospongiosus muscle Cremaster muscle Deep transverse perineal muscle Ischiocavernosus muscle Levator ani muscle Superficial transverse perineal muscle			
N Hip Muscle, Right Gemellus muscle Gluteus maximus muscle Gluteus medius muscle Gluteus minimus muscle Iliacus muscle Obturator muscle Piriformis muscle Psoas muscle Quadratus femoris muscle Tensor fasciae latae muscle			
P Hip Muscle, Left *See N Hip Muscle, Right*			
Q Upper Leg Muscle, Right Adductor brevis muscle Adductor longus muscle Adductor magnus muscle Biceps femoris muscle Gracilis muscle Pectineus muscle Quadriceps (femoris) Rectus femoris muscle Sartorius muscle Semimembranosus muscle Semitendinosus muscle Vastus intermedius muscle Vastus lateralis muscle Vastus medialis muscle			
R Upper Leg Muscle, Left *See Q Upper Leg Muscle, Right*			
S Lower Leg Muscle, Right Extensor digitorum longus muscle Extensor hallucis longus muscle Fibularis brevis muscle Fibularis longus muscle Flexor digitorum longus muscle Flexor hallucis longus muscle Gastrocnemius muscle Peroneus brevis muscle Peroneus longus muscle Popliteus muscle Soleus muscle Tibialis anterior muscle Tibialis posterior muscle			
T Lower Leg Muscle, Left *See S Lower Leg Muscle, Right*			
V Foot Muscle, Right Abductor hallucis muscle Adductor hallucis muscle Extensor digitorum brevis muscle Extensor hallucis brevis muscle Flexor digitorum brevis muscle Flexor hallucis brevis muscle Quadratus plantae muscle			
W Foot Muscle, Left *See V Foot Muscle, Right*			

Non-OR ØK9[Ø,1,2,3,4,5,6,7,8,9,B,F,G,H,J,K,L,M,N,P,Q,R,S,T,V,W]3ZZ
Non-OR ØK9[C,D][3,4]ZZ

Ø Medical and Surgical
K Muscles
B Excision Definition: Cutting out or off, without replacement, a portion of a body part
Explanation: The qualifier DIAGNOSTIC is used to identify excision procedures that are biopsies

Body Part Character 4	Approach Character 5	Device Character 6	Qualifier Character 7
Ø Head Muscle Auricularis muscle Masseter muscle Pterygoid muscle Splenius capitis muscle Temporalis muscle Temporoparietalis muscle **1 Facial Muscle** Buccinator muscle Corrugator supercilii muscle Depressor anguli oris muscle Depressor labii inferioris muscle Depressor septi nasi muscle Depressor supercilii muscle Levator anguli oris muscle Levator labii superioris alaeque nasi muscle Levator labii superioris muscle Mentalis muscle Nasalis muscle Occipitofrontalis muscle Orbicularis oris muscle Procerus muscle Risorius muscle Zygomaticus muscle **2 Neck Muscle, Right** Anterior vertebral muscle Arytenoid muscle Cricothyroid muscle Infrahyoid muscle Levator scapulae muscle Platysma muscle Scalene muscle Splenius cervicis muscle Sternocleidomastoid muscle Suprahyoid muscle Thyroarytenoid muscle **3 Neck Muscle, Left** *See 2 Neck Muscle, Right* **4 Tongue, Palate, Pharynx Muscle** Chondroglossus muscle Genioglossus muscle Hyoglossus muscle Inferior longitudinal muscle Levator veli palatini muscle Palatoglossal muscle Palatopharyngeal muscle Pharyngeal constrictor muscle Salpingopharyngeus muscle Styloglossus muscle Stylopharyngeus muscle Superior longitudinal muscle Tensor veli palatini muscle **5 Shoulder Muscle, Right** Deltoid muscle Infraspinatus muscle Subscapularis muscle Supraspinatus muscle Teres major muscle Teres minor muscle **6 Shoulder Muscle, Left** *See 5 Shoulder Muscle, Right* **7 Upper Arm Muscle, Right** Biceps brachii muscle Brachialis muscle Coracobrachialis muscle Triceps brachii muscle **8 Upper Arm Muscle, Left** *See 7 Upper Arm Muscle, Right* **9 Lower Arm and Wrist Muscle, Right** Anatomical snuffbox Brachioradialis muscle Extensor carpi radialis muscle Extensor carpi ulnaris muscle Flexor carpi radialis muscle Flexor carpi ulnaris muscle Flexor pollicis longus muscle Palmaris longus muscle Pronator quadratus muscle Pronator teres muscle **B Lower Arm and Wrist Muscle, Left** *See 9 Lower Arm and Wrist Muscle, Right* **C Hand Muscle, Right** Hypothenar muscle Palmar interosseous muscle Thenar muscle **D Hand Muscle, Left** *See C Hand Muscle, Right* **F Trunk Muscle, Right** Coccygeus muscle Erector spinae muscle Interspinalis muscle Intertransversarius muscle Latissimus dorsi muscle Quadratus lumborum muscle Rhomboid major muscle Rhomboid minor muscle Serratus posterior muscle Transversospinalis muscle Trapezius muscle **G Trunk Muscle, Left** *See F Trunk Muscle, Right* **H Thorax Muscle, Right** Intercostal muscle Levatores costarum muscle Pectoralis major muscle Pectoralis minor muscle Serratus anterior muscle Subclavius muscle Subcostal muscle Transverse thoracis muscle **J Thorax Muscle, Left** *See H Thorax Muscle, Right* **K Abdomen Muscle, Right** External oblique muscle Internal oblique muscle Pyramidalis muscle Rectus abdominis muscle Transversus abdominis muscle **L Abdomen Muscle, Left** *See K Abdomen Muscle, Right* **M Perineum Muscle** Bulbospongiosus muscle Cremaster muscle Deep transverse perineal muscle Ischiocavernosus muscle Levator ani muscle Superficial transverse perineal muscle **N Hip Muscle, Right** Gemellus muscle Gluteus maximus muscle Gluteus medius muscle Gluteus minimus muscle Iliacus muscle Obturator muscle Piriformis muscle Psoas muscle Quadratus femoris muscle Tensor fasciae latae muscle **P Hip Muscle, Left** *See N Hip Muscle, Right* **Q Upper Leg Muscle, Right** Adductor brevis muscle Adductor longus muscle Adductor magnus muscle Biceps femoris muscle Gracilis muscle Pectineus muscle Quadriceps (femoris) Rectus femoris muscle Sartorius muscle Semimembranosus muscle Semitendinosus muscle Vastus intermedius muscle Vastus lateralis muscle Vastus medialis muscle **R Upper Leg Muscle, Left** *See Q Upper Leg Muscle, Right* **S Lower Leg Muscle, Right** Extensor digitorum longus muscle Extensor hallucis longus muscle Fibularis brevis muscle Fibularis longus muscle Flexor digitorum longus muscle Flexor hallucis longus muscle Gastrocnemius muscle Peroneus brevis muscle Peroneus longus muscle Popliteus muscle Soleus muscle Tibialis anterior muscle Tibialis posterior muscle **T Lower Leg Muscle, Left** *See S Lower Leg Muscle, Right* **V Foot Muscle, Right** Abductor hallucis muscle Adductor hallucis muscle Extensor digitorum brevis muscle Extensor hallucis brevis muscle Flexor digitorum brevis muscle Flexor hallucis brevis muscle Quadratus plantae muscle **W Foot Muscle, Left** *See V Foot Muscle, Right*	**Ø Open** **3 Percutaneous** **4 Percutaneous Endoscopic**	**Z No Device**	**X Diagnostic** **Z No Qualifier**

Ø Medical and Surgical
K Muscles
C Extirpation Definition: Taking or cutting out solid matter from a body part

Explanation: The solid matter may be an abnormal byproduct of a biological function or a foreign body; it may be imbedded in a body part or in the lumen of a tubular body part. The solid matter may or may not have been previously broken into pieces.

Body Part Character 4	Approach Character 5	Device Character 6	Qualifier Character 7
Ø Head Muscle Auricularis muscle Masseter muscle Pterygoid muscle Splenius capitis muscle Temporalis muscle Temporoparietalis muscle **1 Facial Muscle** Buccinator muscle Corrugator supercilii muscle Depressor anguli oris muscle Depressor labii inferioris muscle Depressor septi nasi muscle Depressor supercilii muscle Levator anguli oris muscle Levator labii superioris alaeque nasi muscle Levator labii superioris muscle Mentalis muscle Nasalis muscle Occipitofrontalis muscle Orbicularis oris muscle Procerus muscle Risorius muscle Zygomaticus muscle **2 Neck Muscle, Right** Anterior vertebral muscle Arytenoid muscle Cricothyroid muscle Infrahyoid muscle Levator scapulae muscle Platysma muscle Scalene muscle Splenius cervicis muscle Sternocleidomastoid muscle Suprahyoid muscle Thyroarytenoid muscle **3 Neck Muscle, Left** *See 2 Neck Muscle, Right* **4 Tongue, Palate, Pharynx Muscle** Chondroglossus muscle Genioglossus muscle Hyoglossus muscle Inferior longitudinal muscle Levator veli palatini muscle Palatoglossal muscle Palatopharyngeal muscle Pharyngeal constrictor muscle Salpingopharyngeus muscle Styloglossus muscle Stylopharyngeus muscle Superior longitudinal muscle Tensor veli palatini muscle **5 Shoulder Muscle, Right** Deltoid muscle Infraspinatus muscle Subscapularis muscle Supraspinatus muscle Teres major muscle Teres minor muscle **6 Shoulder Muscle, Left** *See 5 Shoulder Muscle, Right* **7 Upper Arm Muscle, Right** Biceps brachii muscle Brachialis muscle Coracobrachialis muscle Triceps brachii muscle **8 Upper Arm Muscle, Left** *See 7 Upper Arm Muscle, Right* **9 Lower Arm and Wrist Muscle, Right** Anatomical snuffbox Brachioradialis muscle Extensor carpi radialis muscle Extensor carpi ulnaris muscle Flexor carpi radialis muscle Flexor carpi ulnaris muscle Flexor pollicis longus muscle Palmaris longus muscle Pronator quadratus muscle Pronator teres muscle **B Lower Arm and Wrist Muscle, Left** *See 9 Lower Arm and Wrist Muscle, Right* **C Hand Muscle, Right** Hypothenar muscle Palmar interosseous muscle Thenar muscle **D Hand Muscle, Left** *See C Hand Muscle, Right* **F Trunk Muscle, Right** Coccygeus muscle Erector spinae muscle Interspinalis muscle Intertransversarius muscle Latissimus dorsi muscle Quadratus lumborum muscle Rhomboid major muscle Rhomboid minor muscle Serratus posterior muscle Transversospinalis muscle Trapezius muscle **G Trunk Muscle, Left** *See F Trunk Muscle, Right* **H Thorax Muscle, Right** Intercostal muscle Levatores costarum muscle Pectoralis major muscle Pectoralis minor muscle Serratus anterior muscle Subclavius muscle Subcostal muscle Transverse thoracis muscle **J Thorax Muscle, Left** *See H Thorax Muscle, Right* **K Abdomen Muscle, Right** External oblique muscle Internal oblique muscle Pyramidalis muscle Rectus abdominis muscle Transversus abdominis muscle **L Abdomen Muscle, Left** *See K Abdomen Muscle, Right* **M Perineum Muscle** Bulbospongiosus muscle Cremaster muscle Deep transverse perineal muscle Ischiocavernosus muscle Levator ani muscle Superficial transverse perineal muscle **N Hip Muscle, Right** Gemellus muscle Gluteus maximus muscle Gluteus medius muscle Gluteus minimus muscle Iliacus muscle Obturator muscle Piriformis muscle Psoas muscle Quadratus femoris muscle Tensor fasciae latae muscle **P Hip Muscle, Left** *See N Hip Muscle, Right* **Q Upper Leg Muscle, Right** Adductor brevis muscle Adductor longus muscle Adductor magnus muscle Biceps femoris muscle Gracilis muscle Pectineus muscle Quadriceps (femoris) Rectus femoris muscle Sartorius muscle Semimembranosus muscle Semitendinosus muscle Vastus intermedius muscle Vastus lateralis muscle Vastus medialis muscle **R Upper Leg Muscle, Left** *See Q Upper Leg Muscle, Right* **S Lower Leg Muscle, Right** Extensor digitorum longus muscle Extensor hallucis longus muscle Fibularis brevis muscle Fibularis longus muscle Flexor digitorum longus muscle Flexor hallucis longus muscle Gastrocnemius muscle Peroneus brevis muscle Peroneus longus muscle Popliteus muscle Soleus muscle Tibialis anterior muscle Tibialis posterior muscle **T Lower Leg Muscle, Left** *See S Lower Leg Muscle, Right* **V Foot Muscle, Right** Abductor hallucis muscle Adductor hallucis muscle Extensor digitorum brevis muscle Extensor hallucis brevis muscle Flexor digitorum brevis muscle Flexor hallucis brevis muscle Quadratus plantae muscle **W Foot Muscle, Left** *See V Foot Muscle, Right*	**Ø Open** **3 Percutaneous** **4 Percutaneous Endoscopic**	**Z No Device**	**Z No Qualifier**

Ø Medical and Surgical
K Muscles
D Extraction Definition: Pulling or stripping out or off all or a portion of a body part by the use of force
Explanation: The qualifier DIAGNOSTIC is used to identify extraction procedures that are biopsies

Body Part Character 4	Approach Character 5	Device Character 6	Qualifier Character 7
Ø Head Muscle Auricularis muscle Masseter muscle Pterygoid muscle Splenius capitis muscle Temporalis muscle Temporoparietalis muscle **1 Facial Muscle** Buccinator muscle Corrugator supercilii muscle Depressor anguli oris muscle Depressor labii inferioris muscle Depressor septi nasi muscle Depressor supercilii muscle Levator anguli oris muscle Levator labii superioris alaeque nasi muscle Levator labii superioris muscle Mentalis muscle Nasalis muscle Occipitofrontalis muscle Orbicularis oris muscle Procerus muscle Risorius muscle Zygomaticus muscle **2 Neck Muscle, Right** Anterior vertebral muscle Arytenoid muscle Cricothyroid muscle Infrahyoid muscle Levator scapulae muscle Platysma muscle Scalene muscle Splenius cervicis muscle Sternocleidomastoid muscle Suprahyoid muscle Thyroarytenoid muscle **3 Neck Muscle, Left** ***See*** *2 Neck Muscle, Right* **4 Tongue, Palate, Pharynx Muscle** Chondroglossus muscle Genioglossus muscle Hyoglossus muscle Inferior longitudinal muscle Levator veli palatini muscle Palatoglossal muscle Palatopharyngeal muscle Pharyngeal constrictor muscle Salpingopharyngeus muscle Styloglossus muscle Stylopharyngeus muscle Superior longitudinal muscle Tensor veli palatini muscle **5 Shoulder Muscle, Right** Deltoid muscle Infraspinatus muscle Subscapularis muscle Supraspinatus muscle Teres major muscle Teres minor muscle **6 Shoulder Muscle, Left** ***See*** *5 Shoulder Muscle, Right* **7 Upper Arm Muscle, Right** Biceps brachii muscle Brachialis muscle Coracobrachialis muscle Triceps brachii muscle **8 Upper Arm Muscle, Left** ***See*** *7 Upper Arm Muscle, Right* **9 Lower Arm and Wrist Muscle, Right** Anatomical snuffbox Brachioradialis muscle Extensor carpi radialis muscle Extensor carpi ulnaris muscle Flexor carpi radialis muscle Flexor carpi ulnaris muscle Flexor pollicis longus muscle Palmaris longus muscle Pronator quadratus muscle Pronator teres muscle **B Lower Arm and Wrist Muscle, Left** ***See*** *9 Lower Arm and Wrist Muscle, Right* **C Hand Muscle, Right** Hypothenar muscle Palmar interosseous muscle Thenar muscle **D Hand Muscle, Left** ***See*** *C Hand Muscle, Right* **F Trunk Muscle, Right** Coccygeus muscle Erector spinae muscle Interspinalis muscle Intertransversarius muscle Latissimus dorsi muscle Quadratus lumborum muscle Rhomboid major muscle Rhomboid minor muscle Serratus posterior muscle Transversospinalis muscle Trapezius muscle **G Trunk Muscle, Left** ***See*** *F Trunk Muscle, Right* **H Thorax Muscle, Right** Intercostal muscle Levatores costarum muscle Pectoralis major muscle Pectoralis minor muscle Serratus anterior muscle Subclavius muscle Subcostal muscle Transverse thoracis muscle **J Thorax Muscle, Left** ***See*** *H Thorax Muscle, Right* **K Abdomen Muscle, Right** External oblique muscle Internal oblique muscle Pyramidalis muscle Rectus abdominis muscle Transversus abdominis muscle **L Abdomen Muscle, Left** ***See*** *K Abdomen Muscle, Right* **M Perineum Muscle** Bulbospongiosus muscle Cremaster muscle Deep transverse perineal muscle Ischiocavernosus muscle Levator ani muscle Superficial transverse perineal muscle **N Hip Muscle, Right** Gemellus muscle Gluteus maximus muscle Gluteus medius muscle Gluteus minimus muscle Iliacus muscle Obturator muscle Piriformis muscle Psoas muscle Quadratus femoris muscle Tensor fasciae latae muscle **P Hip Muscle, Left** ***See*** *N Hip Muscle, Right* **Q Upper Leg Muscle, Right** Adductor brevis muscle Adductor longus muscle Adductor magnus muscle Biceps femoris muscle Gracilis muscle Pectineus muscle Quadriceps (femoris) Rectus femoris muscle Sartorius muscle Semimembranosus muscle Semitendinosus muscle Vastus intermedius muscle Vastus lateralis muscle Vastus medialis muscle **R Upper Leg Muscle, Left** ***See*** *Q Upper Leg Muscle, Right* **S Lower Leg Muscle, Right** Extensor digitorum longus muscle Extensor hallucis longus muscle Fibularis brevis muscle Fibularis longus muscle Flexor digitorum longus muscle Flexor hallucis longus muscle Gastrocnemius muscle Peroneus brevis muscle Peroneus longus muscle Popliteus muscle Soleus muscle Tibialis anterior muscle Tibialis posterior muscle **T Lower Leg Muscle, Left** ***See*** *S Lower Leg Muscle, Right* **V Foot Muscle, Right** Abductor hallucis muscle Adductor hallucis muscle Extensor digitorum brevis muscle Extensor hallucis brevis muscle Flexor digitorum brevis muscle Flexor hallucis brevis muscle Quadratus plantae muscle **W Foot Muscle, Left** ***See*** *V Foot Muscle, Right*	**Ø** Open	**Z** No Device	**Z** No Qualifier

Ø Medical and Surgical
K Muscles
H Insertion

Definition: Putting in a nonbiological appliance that monitors, assists, performs, or prevents a physiological function but does not physically take the place of a body part

Explanation: None

Body Part Character 4	Approach Character 5	Device Character 6	Qualifier Character 7
X Upper Muscle Y Lower Muscle	Ø Open 3 Percutaneous 4 Percutaneous Endoscopic	M Stimulator Lead Y Other Device	Z No Qualifier

Non-OR ØKH[X,Y][3,4]YZ

Ø Medical and Surgical
K Muscles
J Inspection

Definition: Visually and/or manually exploring a body part

Explanation: Visual exploration may be performed with or without optical instrumentation. Manual exploration may be performed directly or through intervening body layers.

Body Part Character 4	Approach Character 5	Device Character 6	Qualifier Character 7
X Upper Muscle Y Lower Muscle	Ø Open 3 Percutaneous 4 Percutaneous Endoscopic X External	Z No Device	Z No Qualifier

Non-OR ØKJ[X,Y][3,X]ZZ

Ø Medical and Surgical
K Muscles
M Reattachment Definition: Putting back in or on all or a portion of a separated body part to its normal location or other suitable location
Explanation: Vascular circulation and nervous pathways may or may not be reestablished

Body Part Character 4	Approach Character 5	Device Character 6	Qualifier Character 7
Ø Head Muscle Auricularis muscle Masseter muscle Pterygoid muscle Splenius capitis muscle Temporalis muscle Temporoparietalis muscle **1 Facial Muscle** Buccinator muscle Corrugator supercilii muscle Depressor anguli oris muscle Depressor labii inferioris muscle Depressor septi nasi muscle Depressor supercilii muscle Levator anguli oris muscle Levator labii superioris alaeque nasi muscle Levator labii superioris muscle Mentalis muscle Nasalis muscle Occipitofrontalis muscle Orbicularis oris muscle Procerus muscle Risorius muscle Zygomaticus muscle **2 Neck Muscle, Right** Anterior vertebral muscle Arytenoid muscle Cricothyroid muscle Infrahyoid muscle Levator scapulae muscle Platysma muscle Scalene muscle Splenius cervicis muscle Sternocleidomastoid muscle Suprahyoid muscle Thyroarytenoid muscle **3 Neck Muscle, Left** *See 2 Neck Muscle, Right* **4 Tongue, Palate, Pharynx Muscle** Chondroglossus muscle Genioglossus muscle Hyoglossus muscle Inferior longitudinal muscle Levator veli palatini muscle Palatoglossal muscle Palatopharyngeal muscle Pharyngeal constrictor muscle Salpingopharyngeus muscle Styloglossus muscle Stylopharyngeus muscle Superior longitudinal muscle Tensor veli palatini muscle **5 Shoulder Muscle, Right** Deltoid muscle Infraspinatus muscle Subscapularis muscle Supraspinatus muscle Teres major muscle Teres minor muscle **6 Shoulder Muscle, Left** *See 5 Shoulder Muscle, Right* **7 Upper Arm Muscle, Right** Biceps brachii muscle Brachialis muscle Coracobrachialis muscle Triceps brachii muscle **8 Upper Arm Muscle, Left** *See 7 Upper Arm Muscle, Right* **9 Lower Arm and Wrist Muscle, Right** Anatomical snuffbox Brachioradialis muscle Extensor carpi radialis muscle Extensor carpi ulnaris muscle Flexor carpi radialis muscle Flexor carpi ulnaris muscle Flexor pollicis longus muscle Palmaris longus muscle Pronator quadratus muscle Pronator teres muscle **B Lower Arm and Wrist Muscle, Left** *See 9 Lower Arm and Wrist Muscle, Right* **C Hand Muscle, Right** Hypothenar muscle Palmar interosseous muscle Thenar muscle **D Hand Muscle, Left** *See C Hand Muscle, Right* **F Trunk Muscle, Right** Coccygeus muscle Erector spinae muscle Interspinalis muscle Intertransversarius muscle Latissimus dorsi muscle Quadratus lumborum muscle Rhomboid major muscle Rhomboid minor muscle Serratus posterior muscle Transversospinalis muscle Trapezius muscle **G Trunk Muscle, Left** *See F Trunk Muscle, Right* **H Thorax Muscle, Right** Intercostal muscle Levatores costarum muscle Pectoralis major muscle Pectoralis minor muscle Serratus anterior muscle Subclavius muscle Subcostal muscle Transverse thoracis muscle **J Thorax Muscle, Left** *See H Thorax Muscle, Right* **K Abdomen Muscle, Right** External oblique muscle Internal oblique muscle Pyramidalis muscle Rectus abdominis muscle Transversus abdominis muscle **L Abdomen Muscle, Left** *See K Abdomen Muscle, Right* **M Perineum Muscle** Bulbospongiosus muscle Cremaster muscle Deep transverse perineal muscle Ischiocavernosus muscle Levator ani muscle Superficial transverse perineal muscle **N Hip Muscle, Right** Gemellus muscle Gluteus maximus muscle Gluteus medius muscle Gluteus minimus muscle Iliacus muscle Obturator muscle Piriformis muscle Psoas muscle Quadratus femoris muscle Tensor fasciae latae muscle **P Hip Muscle, Left** *See N Hip Muscle, Right* **Q Upper Leg Muscle, Right** Adductor brevis muscle Adductor longus muscle Adductor magnus muscle Biceps femoris muscle Gracilis muscle Pectineus muscle Quadriceps (femoris) Rectus femoris muscle Sartorius muscle Semimembranosus muscle Semitendinosus muscle Vastus intermedius muscle Vastus lateralis muscle Vastus medialis muscle **R Upper Leg Muscle, Left** *See Q Upper Leg Muscle, Right* **S Lower Leg Muscle, Right** Extensor digitorum longus muscle Extensor hallucis longus muscle Fibularis brevis muscle Fibularis longus muscle Flexor digitorum longus muscle Flexor hallucis longus muscle Gastrocnemius muscle Peroneus brevis muscle Peroneus longus muscle Popliteus muscle Soleus muscle Tibialis anterior muscle Tibialis posterior muscle **T Lower Leg Muscle, Left** *See S Lower Leg Muscle, Right* **V Foot Muscle, Right** Abductor hallucis muscle Adductor hallucis muscle Extensor digitorum brevis muscle Extensor hallucis brevis muscle Flexor digitorum brevis muscle Flexor hallucis brevis muscle Quadratus plantae muscle **W Foot Muscle, Left** *See V Foot Muscle, Right*	**Ø Open** **4 Percutaneous Endoscopic**	**Z No Device**	**Z No Qualifier**

Ø Medical and Surgical
K Muscles
N Release

Definition: Freeing a body part from an abnormal physical constraint by cutting or by the use of force

Explanation: Some of the restraining tissue may be taken out but none of the body part is taken out

Body Part Character 4	Approach Character 5	Device Character 6	Qualifier Character 7
Ø Head Muscle Auricularis muscle Masseter muscle Pterygoid muscle Splenius capitis muscle Temporalis muscle Temporoparietalis muscle **1 Facial Muscle** Buccinator muscle Corrugator supercilii muscle Depressor anguli oris muscle Depressor labii inferioris muscle Depressor septi nasi muscle Depressor supercilii muscle Levator anguli oris muscle Levator labii superioris alaeque nasi muscle Levator labii superioris muscle Mentalis muscle Nasalis muscle Occipitofrontalis muscle Orbicularis oris muscle Procerus muscle Risorius muscle Zygomaticus muscle **2 Neck Muscle, Right** Anterior vertebral muscle Arytenoid muscle Cricothyroid muscle Infrahyoid muscle Levator scapulae muscle Platysma muscle Scalene muscle Splenius cervicis muscle Sternocleidomastoid muscle Suprahyoid muscle Thyroarytenoid muscle **3 Neck Muscle, Left** ***See*** *2 Neck Muscle, Right* **4 Tongue, Palate, Pharynx Muscle** Chondroglossus muscle Genioglossus muscle Hyoglossus muscle Inferior longitudinal muscle Levator veli palatini muscle Palatoglossal muscle Palatopharyngeal muscle Pharyngeal constrictor muscle Salpingopharyngeus muscle Styloglossus muscle Stylopharyngeus muscle Superior longitudinal muscle Tensor veli palatini muscle **5 Shoulder Muscle, Right** Deltoid muscle Infraspinatus muscle Subscapularis muscle Supraspinatus muscle Teres major muscle Teres minor muscle **6 Shoulder Muscle, Left** ***See*** *5 Shoulder Muscle, Right* **7 Upper Arm Muscle, Right** Biceps brachii muscle Brachialis muscle Coracobrachialis muscle Triceps brachii muscle **8 Upper Arm Muscle, Left** ***See*** *7 Upper Arm Muscle, Right* **9 Lower Arm and Wrist Muscle, Right** Anatomical snuffbox Brachioradialis muscle Extensor carpi radialis muscle Extensor carpi ulnaris muscle Flexor carpi radialis muscle Flexor carpi ulnaris muscle Flexor pollicis longus muscle Palmaris longus muscle Pronator quadratus muscle Pronator teres muscle **B Lower Arm and Wrist Muscle, Left** ***See*** *9 Lower Arm and Wrist Muscle, Right* **C Hand Muscle, Right** Hypothenar muscle Palmar interosseous muscle Thenar muscle **D Hand Muscle, Left** ***See*** *C Hand Muscle, Right* **F Trunk Muscle, Right** Coccygeus muscle Erector spinae muscle Interspinalis muscle Intertransversarius muscle Latissimus dorsi muscle Quadratus lumborum muscle Rhomboid major muscle Rhomboid minor muscle Serratus posterior muscle Transversospinalis muscle Trapezius muscle **G Trunk Muscle, Left** ***See*** *F Trunk Muscle, Right* **H Thorax Muscle, Right** Intercostal muscle Levatores costarum muscle Pectoralis major muscle Pectoralis minor muscle Serratus anterior muscle Subclavius muscle Subcostal muscle Transverse thoracis muscle **J Thorax Muscle, Left** ***See*** *H Thorax Muscle, Right* **K Abdomen Muscle, Right** External oblique muscle Internal oblique muscle Pyramidalis muscle Rectus abdominis muscle Transversus abdominis muscle **L Abdomen Muscle, Left** ***See*** *K Abdomen Muscle, Right* **M Perineum Muscle** Bulbospongiosus muscle Cremaster muscle Deep transverse perineal muscle Ischiocavernosus muscle Levator ani muscle Superficial transverse perineal muscle **N Hip Muscle, Right** Gemellus muscle Gluteus maximus muscle Gluteus medius muscle Gluteus minimus muscle Iliacus muscle Obturator muscle Piriformis muscle Psoas muscle Quadratus femoris muscle Tensor fasciae latae muscle **P Hip Muscle, Left** ***See*** *N Hip Muscle, Right* **Q Upper Leg Muscle, Right** Adductor brevis muscle Adductor longus muscle Adductor magnus muscle Biceps femoris muscle Gracilis muscle Pectineus muscle Quadriceps (femoris) Rectus femoris muscle Sartorius muscle Semimembranosus muscle Semitendinosus muscle Vastus intermedius muscle Vastus lateralis muscle Vastus medialis muscle **R Upper Leg Muscle, Left** ***See*** *Q Upper Leg Muscle, Right* **S Lower Leg Muscle, Right** Extensor digitorum longus muscle Extensor hallucis longus muscle Fibularis brevis muscle Fibularis longus muscle Flexor digitorum longus muscle Flexor hallucis longus muscle Gastrocnemius muscle Peroneus brevis muscle Peroneus longus muscle Popliteus muscle Soleus muscle Tibialis anterior muscle Tibialis posterior muscle **T Lower Leg Muscle, Left** ***See*** *S Lower Leg Muscle, Right* **V Foot Muscle, Right** Abductor hallucis muscle Adductor hallucis muscle Extensor digitorum brevis muscle Extensor hallucis brevis muscle Flexor digitorum brevis muscle Flexor hallucis brevis muscle Quadratus plantae muscle **W Foot Muscle, Left** ***See*** *V Foot Muscle, Right*	**Ø Open** **3 Percutaneous** **4 Percutaneous Endoscopic** **X External**	**Z No Device**	**Z No Qualifier**

Non-OR ØKN[Ø,1,2,3,4,5,6,7,8,9,B,C,D,F,G,H,J,K,L,M,N,P,Q,R,S,T,V,W]XZZ

Ø Medical and Surgical
K Muscles
P Removal Definition: Taking out or off a device from a body part

Explanation: If a device is taken out and a similar device put in without cutting or puncturing the skin or mucous membrane, the procedure is coded to the root operation CHANGE. Otherwise, the procedure for taking out a device is coded to the root operation REMOVAL.

Body Part Character 4	Approach Character 5	Device Character 6	Qualifier Character 7
X Upper Muscle Y Lower Muscle	Ø Open 3 Percutaneous 4 Percutaneous Endoscopic	Ø Drainage Device 7 Autologous Tissue Substitute J Synthetic Substitute K Nonautologous Tissue Substitute M Stimulator Lead Y Other Device	Z No Qualifier
X Upper Muscle Y Lower Muscle	X External	Ø Drainage Device M Stimulator Lead	Z No Qualifier

Non-OR ØKP[X,Y][3,4]YZ
Non-OR ØKP[X,Y]X[Ø,M]Z

Ø Medical and Surgical
K Muscles
Q Repair Definition: Restoring, to the extent possible, a body part to its normal anatomic structure and function

Explanation: Used only when the method to accomplish the repair is not one of the other root operations

Body Part Character 4	Approach Character 5	Device Character 6	Qualifier Character 7
Ø Head Muscle Auricularis muscle Masseter muscle Pterygoid muscle Splenius capitis muscle Temporalis muscle Temporoparietalis muscle **1 Facial Muscle** Buccinator muscle Corrugator supercilii muscle Depressor anguli oris muscle Depressor labii inferioris muscle Depressor septi nasi muscle Depressor supercilii muscle Levator anguli oris muscle Levator labii superioris alaeque nasi muscle Levator labii superioris muscle Mentalis muscle Nasalis muscle Occipitofrontalis muscle Orbicularis oris muscle Procerus muscle Risorius muscle Zygomaticus muscle **2 Neck Muscle, Right** Anterior vertebral muscle Arytenoid muscle Cricothyroid muscle Infrahyoid muscle Levator scapulae muscle Platysma muscle Scalene muscle Splenius cervicis muscle Sternocleidomastoid muscle Suprahyoid muscle Thyroarytenoid muscle **3 Neck Muscle, Left** ***See*** *2 Neck Muscle, Right* **4 Tongue, Palate, Pharynx Muscle** Chondroglossus muscle Genioglossus muscle Hyoglossus muscle Inferior longitudinal muscle Levator veli palatini muscle Palatoglossal muscle Palatopharyngeal muscle Pharyngeal constrictor muscle Salpingopharyngeus muscle Styloglossus muscle Stylopharyngeus muscle Superior longitudinal muscle Tensor veli palatini muscle **5 Shoulder Muscle, Right** Deltoid muscle Infraspinatus muscle Subscapularis muscle Supraspinatus muscle Teres major muscle Teres minor muscle **6 Shoulder Muscle, Left** ***See*** *5 Shoulder Muscle, Right* **7 Upper Arm Muscle, Right** Biceps brachii muscle Brachialis muscle Coracobrachialis muscle Triceps brachii muscle **8 Upper Arm Muscle, Left** ***See*** *7 Upper Arm Muscle, Right* **9 Lower Arm and Wrist Muscle, Right** Anatomical snuffbox Brachioradialis muscle Extensor carpi radialis muscle Extensor carpi ulnaris muscle Flexor carpi radialis muscle Flexor carpi ulnaris muscle Flexor pollicis longus muscle Palmaris longus muscle Pronator quadratus muscle Pronator teres muscle **B Lower Arm and Wrist Muscle, Left** ***See*** *9 Lower Arm and Wrist Muscle, Right* **C Hand Muscle, Right** Hypothenar muscle Palmar interosseous muscle Thenar muscle **D Hand Muscle, Left** ***See*** *C Hand Muscle, Right* **F Trunk Muscle, Right** Coccygeus muscle Erector spinae muscle Interspinalis muscle Intertransversarius muscle Latissimus dorsi muscle Quadratus lumborum muscle Rhomboid major muscle Rhomboid minor muscle Serratus posterior muscle Transversospinalis muscle Trapezius muscle **G Trunk Muscle, Left** ***See*** *F Trunk Muscle, Right* **H Thorax Muscle, Right** Intercostal muscle Levatores costarum muscle Pectoralis major muscle Pectoralis minor muscle Serratus anterior muscle Subclavius muscle Subcostal muscle Transverse thoracis muscle **J Thorax Muscle, Left** ***See*** *H Thorax Muscle, Right* **K Abdomen Muscle, Right** External oblique muscle Internal oblique muscle Pyramidalis muscle Rectus abdominis muscle Transversus abdominis muscle **L Abdomen Muscle, Left** ***See*** *K Abdomen Muscle, Right* **M Perineum Muscle** Bulbospongiosus muscle Cremaster muscle Deep transverse perineal muscle Ischiocavernosus muscle Levator ani muscle Superficial transverse perineal muscle **N Hip Muscle, Right** Gemellus muscle Gluteus maximus muscle Gluteus medius muscle Gluteus minimus muscle Iliacus muscle Obturator muscle Piriformis muscle Psoas muscle Quadratus femoris muscle Tensor fasciae latae muscle **P Hip Muscle, Left** ***See*** *N Hip Muscle, Right* **Q Upper Leg Muscle, Right** Adductor brevis muscle Adductor longus muscle Adductor magnus muscle Biceps femoris muscle Gracilis muscle Pectineus muscle Quadriceps (femoris) Rectus femoris muscle Sartorius muscle Semimembranosus muscle Semitendinosus muscle Vastus intermedius muscle Vastus lateralis muscle Vastus medialis muscle **R Upper Leg Muscle, Left** ***See*** *Q Upper Leg Muscle, Right* **S Lower Leg Muscle, Right** Extensor digitorum longus muscle Extensor hallucis longus muscle Fibularis brevis muscle Fibularis longus muscle Flexor digitorum longus muscle Flexor hallucis longus muscle Gastrocnemius muscle Peroneus brevis muscle Peroneus longus muscle Popliteus muscle Soleus muscle Tibialis anterior muscle Tibialis posterior muscle **T Lower Leg Muscle, Left** ***See*** *S Lower Leg Muscle, Right* **V Foot Muscle, Right** Abductor hallucis muscle Adductor hallucis muscle Extensor digitorum brevis muscle Extensor hallucis brevis muscle Flexor digitorum brevis muscle Flexor hallucis brevis muscle Quadratus plantae muscle **W Foot Muscle, Left** ***See*** *V Foot Muscle, Right*	**Ø Open** **3 Percutaneous** **4 Percutaneous Endoscopic**	**Z No Device**	**Z No Qualifier**

Ø Medical and Surgical
K Muscles
R Replacement Definition: Putting in or on biological or synthetic material that physically takes the place and/or function of all or a portion of a body part

Explanation: The body part may have been taken out or replaced, or may be taken out, physically eradicated, or rendered nonfunctional during the REPLACEMENT procedure. A REMOVAL procedure is coded for taking out the device used in a previous replacement procedure.

Body Part Character 4	Approach Character 5	Device Character 6	Qualifier Character 7
Ø Head Muscle Auricularis muscle Masseter muscle Pterygoid muscle Splenius capitis muscle Temporalis muscle Temporoparietalis muscle **1 Facial Muscle** Buccinator muscle Corrugator supercilii muscle Depressor anguli oris muscle Depressor labii inferioris muscle Depressor septi nasi muscle Depressor supercilii muscle Levator anguli oris muscle Levator labii superioris alaeque nasi muscle Levator labii superioris muscle Mentalis muscle Nasalis muscle Occipitofrontalis muscle Orbicularis oris muscle Procerus muscle Risorius muscle Zygomaticus muscle **2 Neck Muscle, Right** Anterior vertebral muscle Arytenoid muscle Cricothyroid muscle Infrahyoid muscle Levator scapulae muscle Platysma muscle Scalene muscle Splenius cervicis muscle Sternocleidomastoid muscle Suprahyoid muscle Thyroarytenoid muscle **3 Neck Muscle, Left** ***See*** *2 Neck Muscle, Right* **4 Tongue, Palate, Pharynx Muscle** Chondroglossus muscle Genioglossus muscle Hyoglossus muscle Inferior longitudinal muscle Levator veli palatini muscle Palatoglossal muscle Palatopharyngeal muscle Pharyngeal constrictor muscle Salpingopharyngeus muscle Styloglossus muscle Stylopharyngeus muscle Superior longitudinal muscle Tensor veli palatini muscle **5 Shoulder Muscle, Right** Deltoid muscle Infraspinatus muscle Subscapularis muscle Supraspinatus muscle Teres major muscle Teres minor muscle **6 Shoulder Muscle, Left** ***See*** *5 Shoulder Muscle, Right* **7 Upper Arm Muscle, Right** Biceps brachii muscle Brachialis muscle Coracobrachialis muscle Triceps brachii muscle **8 Upper Arm Muscle, Left** ***See*** *7 Upper Arm Muscle, Right* **9 Lower Arm and Wrist Muscle, Right** Anatomical snuffbox Brachioradialis muscle Extensor carpi radialis muscle Extensor carpi ulnaris muscle Flexor carpi radialis muscle Flexor carpi ulnaris muscle Flexor pollicis longus muscle Palmaris longus muscle Pronator quadratus muscle Pronator teres muscle **B Lower Arm and Wrist Muscle, Left** ***See*** *9 Lower Arm and Wrist Muscle, Right* **C Hand Muscle, Right** Hypothenar muscle Palmar interosseous muscle Thenar muscle **D Hand Muscle, Left** ***See*** *C Hand Muscle, Right* **F Trunk Muscle, Right** Coccygeus muscle Erector spinae muscle Interspinalis muscle Intertransversarius muscle Latissimus dorsi muscle Quadratus lumborum muscle Rhomboid major muscle Rhomboid minor muscle Serratus posterior muscle Transversospinalis muscle Trapezius muscle **G Trunk Muscle, Left** ***See*** *F Trunk Muscle, Right* **H Thorax Muscle, Right** Intercostal muscle Levatores costarum muscle Pectoralis major muscle Pectoralis minor muscle Serratus anterior muscle Subclavius muscle Subcostal muscle Transverse thoracis muscle **J Thorax Muscle, Left** ***See*** *H Thorax Muscle, Right* **K Abdomen Muscle, Right** External oblique muscle Internal oblique muscle Pyramidalis muscle Rectus abdominis muscle Transversus abdominis muscle **L Abdomen Muscle, Left** ***See*** *K Abdomen Muscle, Right* **M Perineum Muscle** Bulbospongiosus muscle Cremaster muscle Deep transverse perineal muscle Ischiocavernosus muscle Levator ani muscle Superficial transverse perineal muscle **N Hip Muscle, Right** Gemellus muscle Gluteus maximus muscle Gluteus medius muscle Gluteus minimus muscle Iliacus muscle Obturator muscle Piriformis muscle Psoas muscle Quadratus femoris muscle Tensor fasciae latae muscle **P Hip Muscle, Left** ***See*** *N Hip Muscle, Right* **Q Upper Leg Muscle, Right** Adductor brevis muscle Adductor longus muscle Adductor magnus muscle Biceps femoris muscle Gracilis muscle Pectineus muscle Quadriceps (femoris) Rectus femoris muscle Sartorius muscle Semimembranosus muscle Semitendinosus muscle Vastus intermedius muscle Vastus lateralis muscle Vastus medialis muscle **R Upper Leg Muscle, Left** ***See*** *Q Upper Leg Muscle, Right* **S Lower Leg Muscle, Right** Extensor digitorum longus muscle Extensor hallucis longus muscle Fibularis brevis muscle Fibularis longus muscle Flexor digitorum longus muscle Flexor hallucis longus muscle Gastrocnemius muscle Peroneus brevis muscle Peroneus longus muscle Popliteus muscle Soleus muscle Tibialis anterior muscle Tibialis posterior muscle **T Lower Leg Muscle, Left** ***See*** *S Lower Leg Muscle, Right* **V Foot Muscle, Right** Abductor hallucis muscle Adductor hallucis muscle Extensor digitorum brevis muscle Extensor hallucis brevis muscle Flexor digitorum brevis muscle Flexor hallucis brevis muscle Quadratus plantae muscle **W Foot Muscle, Left** ***See*** *V Foot Muscle, Right*	**Ø Open** **4 Percutaneous Endoscopic**	**7 Autologous Tissue Substitute** **J Synthetic Substitute** **K Nonautologous Tissue Substitute**	**Z No Qualifier**

Ø Medical and Surgical
K Muscles
S Reposition Definition: Moving to its normal location, or other suitable location, all or a portion of a body part

Explanation: The body part is moved to a new location from an abnormal location, or from a normal location where it is not functioning correctly. The body part may or may not be cut out or off to be moved to the new location.

Body Part Character 4	Approach Character 5	Device Character 6	Qualifier Character 7
Ø Head Muscle Auricularis muscle Masseter muscle Pterygoid muscle Splenius capitis muscle Temporalis muscle Temporoparietalis muscle **1 Facial Muscle** Buccinator muscle Corrugator supercilii muscle Depressor anguli oris muscle Depressor labii inferioris muscle Depressor septi nasi muscle Depressor supercilii muscle Levator anguli oris muscle Levator labii superioris alaeque nasi muscle Levator labii superioris muscle Mentalis muscle Nasalis muscle Occipitofrontalis muscle Orbicularis oris muscle Procerus muscle Risorius muscle Zygomaticus muscle **2 Neck Muscle, Right** Anterior vertebral muscle Arytenoid muscle Cricothyroid muscle Infrahyoid muscle Levator scapulae muscle Platysma muscle Scalene muscle Splenius cervicis muscle Sternocleidomastoid muscle Suprahyoid muscle Thyroarytenoid muscle **3 Neck Muscle, Left** **See** *2 Neck Muscle, Right* **4 Tongue, Palate, Pharynx Muscle** Chondroglossus muscle Genioglossus muscle Hyoglossus muscle Inferior longitudinal muscle Levator veli palatini muscle Palatoglossal muscle Palatopharyngeal muscle Pharyngeal constrictor muscle Salpingopharyngeus muscle Styloglossus muscle Stylopharyngeus muscle Superior longitudinal muscle Tensor veli palatini muscle **5 Shoulder Muscle, Right** Deltoid muscle Infraspinatus muscle Subscapularis muscle Supraspinatus muscle Teres major muscle Teres minor muscle **6 Shoulder Muscle, Left** **See** *5 Shoulder Muscle, Right* **7 Upper Arm Muscle, Right** Biceps brachii muscle Brachialis muscle Coracobrachialis muscle Triceps brachii muscle **8 Upper Arm Muscle, Left** **See** *7 Upper Arm Muscle, Right* **9 Lower Arm and Wrist Muscle, Right** Anatomical snuffbox Brachioradialis muscle Extensor carpi radialis muscle Extensor carpi ulnaris muscle Flexor carpi radialis muscle Flexor carpi ulnaris muscle Flexor pollicis longus muscle Palmaris longus muscle Pronator quadratus muscle Pronator teres muscle **B Lower Arm and Wrist Muscle, Left** **See** *9 Lower Arm and Wrist Muscle, Right* **C Hand Muscle, Right** Hypothenar muscle Palmar interosseous muscle Thenar muscle **D Hand Muscle, Left** **See** *C Hand Muscle, Right* **F Trunk Muscle, Right** Coccygeus muscle Erector spinae muscle Interspinalis muscle Intertransversarius muscle Latissimus dorsi muscle Quadratus lumborum muscle Rhomboid major muscle Rhomboid minor muscle Serratus posterior muscle Transversospinalis muscle Trapezius muscle **G Trunk Muscle, Left** **See** *F Trunk Muscle, Right* **H Thorax Muscle, Right** Intercostal muscle Levatores costarum muscle Pectoralis major muscle Pectoralis minor muscle Serratus anterior muscle Subclavius muscle Subcostal muscle Transverse thoracis muscle **J Thorax Muscle, Left** **See** *H Thorax Muscle, Right* **K Abdomen Muscle, Right** External oblique muscle Internal oblique muscle Pyramidalis muscle Rectus abdominis muscle Transversus abdominis muscle **L Abdomen Muscle, Left** **See** *K Abdomen Muscle, Right* **M Perineum Muscle** Bulbospongiosus muscle Cremaster muscle Deep transverse perineal muscle Ischiocavernosus muscle Levator ani muscle Superficial transverse perineal muscle **N Hip Muscle, Right** Gemellus muscle Gluteus maximus muscle Gluteus medius muscle Gluteus minimus muscle Iliacus muscle Obturator muscle Piriformis muscle Psoas muscle Quadratus femoris muscle Tensor fasciae latae muscle **P Hip Muscle, Left** **See** *N Hip Muscle, Right* **Q Upper Leg Muscle, Right** Adductor brevis muscle Adductor longus muscle Adductor magnus muscle Biceps femoris muscle Gracilis muscle Pectineus muscle Quadriceps (femoris) Rectus femoris muscle Sartorius muscle Semimembranosus muscle Semitendinosus muscle Vastus intermedius muscle Vastus lateralis muscle Vastus medialis muscle **R Upper Leg Muscle, Left** **See** *Q Upper Leg Muscle, Right* **S Lower Leg Muscle, Right** Extensor digitorum longus muscle Extensor hallucis longus muscle Fibularis brevis muscle Fibularis longus muscle Flexor digitorum longus muscle Flexor hallucis longus muscle Gastrocnemius muscle Peroneus brevis muscle Peroneus longus muscle Popliteus muscle Soleus muscle Tibialis anterior muscle Tibialis posterior muscle **T Lower Leg Muscle, Left** **See** *S Lower Leg Muscle, Right* **V Foot Muscle, Right** Abductor hallucis muscle Adductor hallucis muscle Extensor digitorum brevis muscle Extensor hallucis brevis muscle Flexor digitorum brevis muscle Flexor hallucis brevis muscle Quadratus plantae muscle **W Foot Muscle, Left** **See** *V Foot Muscle, Right*	**Ø Open** **4 Percutaneous Endoscopic**	**Z No Device**	**Z No Qualifier**

Ø Medical and Surgical
K Muscles
T Resection Definition: Cutting out or off, without replacement, all of a body part
Explanation: None

Body Part Character 4	Approach Character 5	Device Character 6	Qualifier Character 7
Ø Head Muscle Auricularis muscle Masseter muscle Pterygoid muscle Splenius capitis muscle Temporalis muscle Temporoparietalis muscle	**Ø Open**	**Z No Device**	**Z No Qualifier**
1 Facial Muscle Buccinator muscle Corrugator supercilii muscle Depressor anguli oris muscle Depressor labii inferioris muscle Depressor septi nasi muscle Depressor supercilii muscle Levator anguli oris muscle Levator labii superioris alaeque nasi muscle Levator labii superioris muscle Mentalis muscle Nasalis muscle Occipitofrontalis muscle Orbicularis oris muscle Procerus muscle Risorius muscle Zygomaticus muscle	**4 Percutaneous Endoscopic**		
2 Neck Muscle, Right Anterior vertebral muscle Arytenoid muscle Cricothyroid muscle Infrahyoid muscle Levator scapulae muscle Platysma muscle Scalene muscle Splenius cervicis muscle Sternocleidomastoid muscle Suprahyoid muscle Thyroarytenoid muscle			
3 Neck Muscle, Left *See 2 Neck Muscle, Right*			
4 Tongue, Palate, Pharynx Muscle Chondroglossus muscle Genioglossus muscle Hyoglossus muscle Inferior longitudinal muscle Levator veli palatini muscle Palatoglossal muscle Palatopharyngeal muscle Pharyngeal constrictor muscle Salpingopharyngeus muscle Styloglossus muscle Stylopharyngeus muscle Superior longitudinal muscle Tensor veli palatini muscle			
5 Shoulder Muscle, Right Deltoid muscle Infraspinatus muscle Subscapularis muscle Supraspinatus muscle Teres major muscle Teres minor muscle			
6 Shoulder Muscle, Left *See 5 Shoulder Muscle, Right*			
7 Upper Arm Muscle, Right Biceps brachii muscle Brachialis muscle Coracobrachialis muscle Triceps brachii muscle			
8 Upper Arm Muscle, Left *See 7 Upper Arm Muscle, Right*			
9 Lower Arm and Wrist Muscle, Right Anatomical snuffbox Brachioradialis muscle Extensor carpi radialis muscle Extensor carpi ulnaris muscle Flexor carpi radialis muscle Flexor carpi ulnaris muscle Flexor pollicis longus muscle Palmaris longus muscle Pronator quadratus muscle Pronator teres muscle			
B Lower Arm and Wrist Muscle, Left *See 9 Lower Arm and Wrist Muscle, Right*			
C Hand Muscle, Right Hypothenar muscle Palmar interosseous muscle Thenar muscle			
D Hand Muscle, Left *See C Hand Muscle, Right*			
F Trunk Muscle, Right Coccygeus muscle Erector spinae muscle Interspinalis muscle Intertransversarius muscle Latissimus dorsi muscle Quadratus lumborum muscle Rhomboid major muscle Rhomboid minor muscle Serratus posterior muscle Transversospinalis muscle Trapezius muscle			
G Trunk Muscle, Left *See F Trunk Muscle, Right*			
H Thorax Muscle, Right ⊞ Intercostal muscle Levatores costarum muscle Pectoralis major muscle Pectoralis minor muscle Serratus anterior muscle Subclavius muscle Subcostal muscle Transverse thoracis muscle			
J Thorax Muscle, Left ⊞ *See H Thorax Muscle, Right*			
K Abdomen Muscle, Right External oblique muscle Internal oblique muscle Pyramidalis muscle Rectus abdominis muscle Transversus abdominis muscle			
L Abdomen Muscle, Left *See K Abdomen Muscle, Right*			
M Perineum Muscle Bulbospongiosus muscle Cremaster muscle Deep transverse perineal muscle Ischiocavernosus muscle Levator ani muscle Superficial transverse perineal muscle			
N Hip Muscle, Right Gemellus muscle Gluteus maximus muscle Gluteus medius muscle Gluteus minimus muscle Iliacus muscle Obturator muscle Piriformis muscle Psoas muscle Quadratus femoris muscle Tensor fasciae latae muscle			
P Hip Muscle, Left *See N Hip Muscle, Right*			
Q Upper Leg Muscle, Right Adductor brevis muscle Adductor longus muscle Adductor magnus muscle Biceps femoris muscle Gracilis muscle Pectineus muscle Quadriceps (femoris) Rectus femoris muscle Sartorius muscle Semimembranosus muscle Semitendinosus muscle Vastus intermedius muscle Vastus lateralis muscle Vastus medialis muscle			
R Upper Leg Muscle, Left *See Q Upper Leg Muscle, Right*			
S Lower Leg Muscle, Right Extensor digitorum longus muscle Extensor hallucis longus muscle Fibularis brevis muscle Fibularis longus muscle Flexor digitorum longus muscle Flexor hallucis longus muscle Gastrocnemius muscle Peroneus brevis muscle Peroneus longus muscle Popliteus muscle Soleus muscle Tibialis anterior muscle Tibialis posterior muscle			
T Lower Leg Muscle, Left *See S Lower Leg Muscle, Right*			
V Foot Muscle, Right Abductor hallucis muscle Adductor hallucis muscle Extensor digitorum brevis muscle Extensor hallucis brevis muscle Flexor digitorum brevis muscle Flexor hallucis brevis muscle Quadratus plantae muscle			
W Foot Muscle, Left *See V Foot Muscle, Right*			

See Appendix L for Procedure Combinations
⊞ ØKT[H,J]ØZZ

Ø Medical and Surgical
K Muscles
U Supplement Definition: Putting in or on biological or synthetic material that physically reinforces and/or augments the function of a portion of a body part

Explanation: The biological material is non-living, or is living and from the same individual. The body part may have been previously replaced, and the SUPPLEMENT procedure is performed to physically reinforce and/or augment the function of the replaced body part.

Body Part Character 4	Approach Character 5	Device Character 6	Qualifier Character 7
Ø Head Muscle Auricularis muscle Masseter muscle Pterygoid muscle Splenius capitis muscle Temporalis muscle Temporoparietalis muscle **1 Facial Muscle** Buccinator muscle Corrugator supercilii muscle Depressor anguli oris muscle Depressor labii inferioris muscle Depressor septi nasi muscle Depressor supercilii muscle Levator anguli oris muscle Levator labii superioris alaeque nasi muscle Levator labii superioris muscle Mentalis muscle Nasalis muscle Occipitofrontalis muscle Orbicularis oris muscle Procerus muscle Risorius muscle Zygomaticus muscle **2 Neck Muscle, Right** Anterior vertebral muscle Arytenoid muscle Cricothyroid muscle Infrahyoid muscle Levator scapulae muscle Platysma muscle Scalene muscle Splenius cervicis muscle Sternocleidomastoid muscle Suprahyoid muscle Thyroarytenoid muscle **3 Neck Muscle, Left** *See 2 Neck Muscle, Right* **4 Tongue, Palate, Pharynx Muscle** Chondroglossus muscle Genioglossus muscle Hyoglossus muscle Inferior longitudinal muscle Levator veli palatini muscle Palatoglossal muscle Palatopharyngeal muscle Pharyngeal constrictor muscle Salpingopharyngeus muscle Styloglossus muscle Stylopharyngeus muscle Superior longitudinal muscle Tensor veli palatini muscle **5 Shoulder Muscle, Right** Deltoid muscle Infraspinatus muscle Subscapularis muscle Supraspinatus muscle Teres major muscle Teres minor muscle **6 Shoulder Muscle, Left** *See 5 Shoulder Muscle, Right* **7 Upper Arm Muscle, Right** Biceps brachii muscle Brachialis muscle Coracobrachialis muscle Triceps brachii muscle **8 Upper Arm Muscle, Left** *See 7 Upper Arm Muscle, Right* **9 Lower Arm and Wrist Muscle, Right** Anatomical snuffbox Brachioradialis muscle Extensor carpi radialis muscle Extensor carpi ulnaris muscle Flexor carpi radialis muscle Flexor carpi ulnaris muscle Flexor pollicis longus muscle Palmaris longus muscle Pronator quadratus muscle Pronator teres muscle **B Lower Arm and Wrist Muscle, Left** *See 9 Lower Arm and Wrist Muscle, Right* **C Hand Muscle, Right** Hypothenar muscle Palmar interosseous muscle Thenar muscle **D Hand Muscle, Left** *See C Hand Muscle, Right* **F Trunk Muscle, Right** Coccygeus muscle Erector spinae muscle Interspinalis muscle Intertransversarius muscle Latissimus dorsi muscle Quadratus lumborum muscle Rhomboid major muscle Rhomboid minor muscle Serratus posterior muscle Transversospinalis muscle Trapezius muscle **G Trunk Muscle, Left** *See F Trunk Muscle, Right* **H Thorax Muscle, Right** Intercostal muscle Levatores costarum muscle Pectoralis major muscle Pectoralis minor muscle Serratus anterior muscle Subclavius muscle Subcostal muscle Transverse thoracis muscle **J Thorax Muscle, Left** *See H Thorax Muscle, Right* **K Abdomen Muscle, Right** External oblique muscle Internal oblique muscle Pyramidalis muscle Rectus abdominis muscle Transversus abdominis muscle **L Abdomen Muscle, Left** *See K Abdomen Muscle, Right* **M Perineum Muscle** Bulbospongiosus muscle Cremaster muscle Deep transverse perineal muscle Ischiocavernosus muscle Levator ani muscle Superficial transverse perineal muscle **N Hip Muscle, Right** Gemellus muscle Gluteus maximus muscle Gluteus medius muscle Gluteus minimus muscle Iliacus muscle Obturator muscle Piriformis muscle Psoas muscle Quadratus femoris muscle Tensor fasciae latae muscle **P Hip Muscle, Left** *See N Hip Muscle, Right* **Q Upper Leg Muscle, Right** Adductor brevis muscle Adductor longus muscle Adductor magnus muscle Biceps femoris muscle Gracilis muscle Pectineus muscle Quadriceps (femoris) Rectus femoris muscle Sartorius muscle Semimembranosus muscle Semitendinosus muscle Vastus intermedius muscle Vastus lateralis muscle Vastus medialis muscle **R Upper Leg Muscle, Left** *See Q Upper Leg Muscle, Right* **S Lower Leg Muscle, Right** Extensor digitorum longus muscle Extensor hallucis longus muscle Fibularis brevis muscle Fibularis longus muscle Flexor digitorum longus muscle Flexor hallucis longus muscle Gastrocnemius muscle Peroneus brevis muscle Peroneus longus muscle Popliteus muscle Soleus muscle Tibialis anterior muscle Tibialis posterior muscle **T Lower Leg Muscle, Left** *See S Lower Leg Muscle, Right* **V Foot Muscle, Right** Abductor hallucis muscle Adductor hallucis muscle Extensor digitorum brevis muscle Extensor hallucis brevis muscle Flexor digitorum brevis muscle Flexor hallucis brevis muscle Quadratus plantae muscle **W Foot Muscle, Left** *See V Foot Muscle, Right*	**Ø Open** **4 Percutaneous Endoscopic**	**7 Autologous Tissue Substitute** **J Synthetic Substitute** **K Nonautologous Tissue Substitute**	**Z No Qualifier**

Ø Medical and Surgical
K Muscles
W Revision

Definition: Correcting, to the extent possible, a portion of a malfunctioning device or the position of a displaced device

Explanation: Revision can include correcting a malfunctioning or displaced device by taking out or putting in components of the device such as a screw or pin

Body Part Character 4	Approach Character 5	Device Character 6	Qualifier Character 7
X Upper Muscle **Y** Lower Muscle	**Ø** Open **3** Percutaneous **4** Percutaneous Endoscopic	**Ø** Drainage Device **7** Autologous Tissue Substitute **J** Synthetic Substitute **K** Nonautologous Tissue Substitute **M** Stimulator Lead **Y** Other Device	**Z** No Qualifier
X Upper Muscle **Y** Lower Muscle	**X** External	**Ø** Drainage Device **7** Autologous Tissue Substitute **J** Synthetic Substitute **K** Nonautologous Tissue Substitute **M** Stimulator Lead	**Z** No Qualifier

Non-OR ØKW[X,Y][3,4]YZ
Non-OR ØKW[X,Y]X[Ø,7,J,K,M]Z

Ø Medical and Surgical
K Muscles
X Transfer

Definition: Moving, without taking out, all or a portion of a body part to another location to take over the function of all or a portion of a body part

Explanation: The body part transferred remains connected to its vascular and nervous supply

Body Part Character 4	Approach Character 5	Device Character 6	Qualifier Character 7
Ø Head Muscle Auricularis muscle Masseter muscle Pterygoid muscle Splenius capitis muscle Temporalis muscle Temporoparietalis muscle **1 Facial Muscle** Buccinator muscle Corrugator supercilii muscle Depressor anguli oris muscle Depressor labii inferioris muscle Depressor septi nasi muscle Depressor supercilii muscle Levator anguli oris muscle Levator labii superioris alaeque nasi muscle Levator labii superioris muscle Mentalis muscle Nasalis muscle Occipitofrontalis muscle Orbicularis oris muscle Procerus muscle Risorius muscle Zygomaticus muscle **2 Neck Muscle, Right** Anterior vertebral muscle Arytenoid muscle Cricothyroid muscle Infrahyoid muscle Levator scapulae muscle Platysma muscle Scalene muscle Splenius cervicis muscle Sternocleidomastoid muscle Suprahyoid muscle Thyroarytenoid muscle **3 Neck Muscle, Left** ***See*** *2 Neck Muscle, Right* **4 Tongue, Palate, Pharynx Muscle** Chondroglossus muscle Genioglossus muscle Hyoglossus muscle Inferior longitudinal muscle Levator veli palatini muscle Palatoglossal muscle Palatopharyngeal muscle Pharyngeal constrictor muscle Salpingopharyngeus muscle Styloglossus muscle Stylopharyngeus muscle Superior longitudinal muscle Tensor veli palatini muscle **5 Shoulder Muscle, Right** Deltoid muscle Infraspinatus muscle Subscapularis muscle Supraspinatus muscle Teres major muscle Teres minor muscle **6 Shoulder Muscle, Left** ***See*** *5 Shoulder Muscle, Right* **7 Upper Arm Muscle, Right** Biceps brachii muscle Brachialis muscle Coracobrachialis muscle Triceps brachii muscle **8 Upper Arm Muscle, Left** ***See*** *7 Upper Arm Muscle, Right* **9 Lower Arm and Wrist Muscle, Right** Anatomical snuffbox Brachioradialis muscle Extensor carpi radialis muscle Extensor carpi ulnaris muscle Flexor carpi radialis muscle Flexor carpi ulnaris muscle Flexor pollicis longus muscle Palmaris longus muscle Pronator quadratus muscle Pronator teres muscle **B Lower Arm and Wrist Muscle, Left** ***See*** *9 Lower Arm and Wrist Muscle, Right* **C Hand Muscle, Right** Hypothenar muscle Palmar interosseous muscle Thenar muscle **D Hand Muscle, Left** ***See*** *C Hand Muscle, Right* **H Thorax Muscle, Right** Intercostal muscle Levatores costarum muscle Pectoralis major muscle Pectoralis minor muscle Serratus anterior muscle Subclavius muscle Subcostal muscle Transverse thoracis muscle **J Thorax Muscle, Left** ***See*** *H Thorax Muscle, Right* **M Perineum Muscle** Bulbospongiosus muscle Cremaster muscle Deep transverse perineal muscle Ischiocavernosus muscle Levator ani muscle Superficial transverse perineal muscle **N Hip Muscle, Right** Gemellus muscle Gluteus maximus muscle Gluteus medius muscle Gluteus minimus muscle Iliacus muscle Obturator muscle Piriformis muscle Psoas muscle Quadratus femoris muscle Tensor fasciae latae muscle **P Hip Muscle, Left** ***See*** *N Hip Muscle, Right* **Q Upper Leg Muscle, Right** Adductor brevis muscle Adductor longus muscle Adductor magnus muscle Biceps femoris muscle Gracilis muscle Pectineus muscle Quadriceps (femoris) Rectus femoris muscle Sartorius muscle Semimembranosus muscle Semitendinosus muscle Vastus intermedius muscle Vastus lateralis muscle Vastus medialis muscle **R Upper Leg Muscle, Left** ***See*** *Q Upper Leg Muscle, Right* **S Lower Leg Muscle, Right** Extensor digitorum longus muscle Extensor hallucis longus muscle Fibularis brevis muscle Fibularis longus muscle Flexor digitorum longus muscle Flexor hallucis longus muscle Gastrocnemius muscle Peroneus brevis muscle Peroneus longus muscle Popliteus muscle Soleus muscle Tibialis anterior muscle Tibialis posterior muscle **T Lower Leg Muscle, Left** ***See*** *S Lower Leg Muscle, Right* **V Foot Muscle, Right** Abductor hallucis muscle Adductor hallucis muscle Extensor digitorum brevis muscle Extensor hallucis brevis muscle Flexor digitorum brevis muscle Flexor hallucis brevis muscle Quadratus plantae muscle **W Foot Muscle, Left** ***See*** *V Foot Muscle, Right*	**Ø Open** **4 Percutaneous Endoscopic**	**Z No Device**	**Ø Skin** **1 Subcutaneous Tissue** **2 Skin and Subcutaneous Tissue** **Z No Qualifier**

ØKX Continued on next page

ØKX Continued

Ø Medical and Surgical
K Muscles
X Transfer

Definition: Moving, without taking out, all or a portion of a body part to another location to take over the function of all or a portion of a body part

Explanation: The body part transferred remains connected to its vascular and nervous supply

Body Part Character 4	Approach Character 5	Device Character 6	Qualifier Character 7
F Trunk Muscle, Right Coccygeus muscle Erector spinae muscle Interspinalis muscle Intertransversarius muscle Latissimus dorsi muscle Quadratus lumborum muscle Rhomboid major muscle Rhomboid minor muscle Serratus posterior muscle Transversospinalis muscle Trapezius muscle **G Trunk Muscle, Left** *See F Trunk Muscle, Right*	**Ø Open** **4 Percutaneous Endoscopic**	**Z No Device**	**Ø Skin** **1 Subcutaneous Tissue** **2 Skin and Subcutaneous Tissue** **5 Latissimus Dorsi Myocutaneous Flap** **7 Deep Inferior Epigastric Artery Perforator Flap** **8 Superficial Inferior Epigastric Artery Flap** **9 Gluteal Artery Perforator Flap** **Z No Qualifier**
K Abdomen Muscle, Right External oblique muscle Internal oblique muscle Pyramidalis muscle Rectus abdominis muscle Transversus abdominis muscle **L Abdomen Muscle, Left** *See K Abdomen Muscle, Right*	**Ø Open** **4 Percutaneous Endoscopic**	**Z No Device**	**Ø Skin** **1 Subcutaneous Tissue** **2 Skin and Subcutaneous Tissue** **6 Transverse Rectus Abdominis Myocutaneous Flap** **Z No Qualifier**

Tendons ØL2–ØLX

Character Meanings*

This Character Meaning table is provided as a guide to assist the user in the identification of character members that may be found in this section of code tables. It **SHOULD NOT** be used to build a PCS code.

Operation–Character 3		Body Part–Character 4		Approach–Character 5		Device–Character 6		Qualifier–Character 7	
2	Change	Ø	Head and Neck Tendon	Ø	Open	Ø	Drainage Device	X	Diagnostic
5	Destruction	1	Shoulder Tendon, Right	3	Percutaneous	7	Autologous Tissue Substitute	Z	No Qualifier
8	Division	2	Shoulder Tendon, Left	4	Percutaneous Endoscopic	J	Synthetic Substitute		
9	Drainage	3	Upper Arm Tendon, Right	X	External	K	Nonautologous Tissue Substitute		
B	Excision	4	Upper Arm Tendon, Left			Y	Other Device		
C	Extirpation	5	Lower Arm and Wrist Tendon, Right			Z	No Device		
D	Extraction	6	Lower Arm and Wrist Tendon, Left						
H	Insertion	7	Hand Tendon, Right						
J	Inspection	8	Hand Tendon, Left						
M	Reattachment	9	Trunk Tendon, Right						
N	Release	B	Trunk Tendon, Left						
P	Removal	C	Thorax Tendon, Right						
Q	Repair	D	Thorax Tendon, Left						
R	Replacement	F	Abdomen Tendon, Right						
S	Reposition	G	Abdomen Tendon, Left						
T	Resection	H	Perineum Tendon						
U	Supplement	J	Hip Tendon, Right						
W	Revision	K	Hip Tendon, Left						
X	Transfer	L	Upper Leg Tendon, Right						
		M	Upper Leg Tendon, Left						
		N	Lower Leg Tendon, Right						
		P	Lower Leg Tendon, Left						
		Q	Knee Tendon, Right						
		R	Knee Tendon, Left						
		S	Ankle Tendon, Right						
		T	Ankle Tendon, Left						
		V	Foot Tendon, Right						
		W	Foot Tendon, Left						
		X	Upper Tendon						
		Y	Lower Tendon						

* Includes synovial membrane.

AHA Coding Clinic for table ØL8
2016, 3Q, 30 Resection of femur with interposition arthroplasty

AHA Coding Clinic for table ØLB
2017, 2Q, 21 Arthroscopic anterior cruciate ligament revision using autograft with anterolateral ligament reconstruction
2015, 3Q, 26 Thumb arthroplasty with resection of trapezium
2014, 3Q, 14 Application of TheraSkin® and excisional debridement
2014, 3Q, 18 Placement of reverse sural fasciocutaneous pedicle flap

AHA Coding Clinic for table ØLD
2017, 4Q, 41 Extraction procedures

AHA Coding Clinic for table ØLQ
2016, 3Q, 32 Rotator cuff repair, tenodesis, decompression, acromioplasty and coracoplasty
2015, 2Q, 11 Repair of patellar and quadriceps tendons with allograft
2013, 3Q, 20 Superior labrum anterior posterior (SLAP) repair and subacromial decompression

AHA Coding Clinic for table ØLS
2016, 3Q, 32 Rotator cuff repair, tenodesis, decompression, acromioplasty and coracoplasty
2015, 3Q, 14 Endoprosthetic replacement of humerus and tendon reattachment

AHA Coding Clinic for table ØLU
2015, 2Q, 11 Repair of patellar and quadriceps tendons with allograft

Foot Tendons

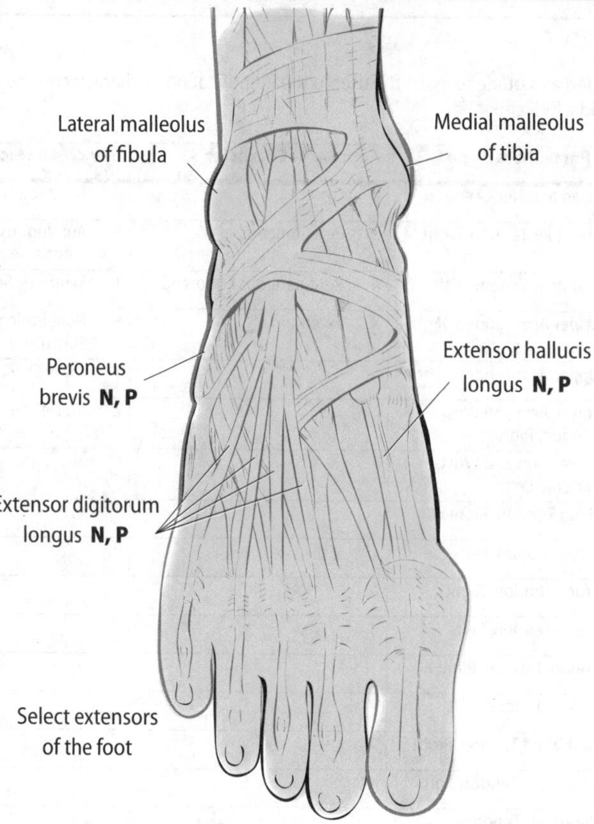

Shoulder Tendons

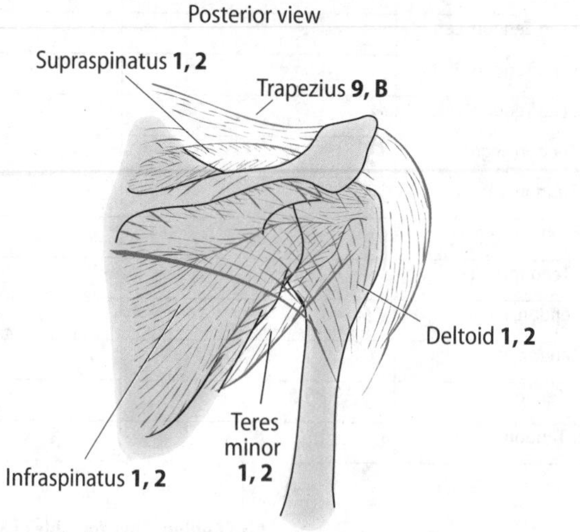

Tendons of Wrist and Hand

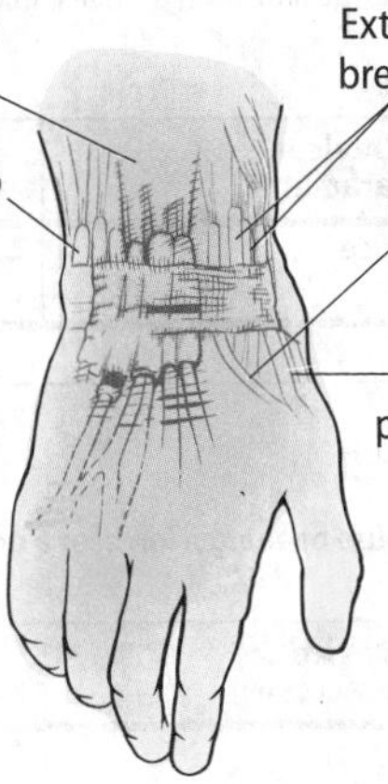

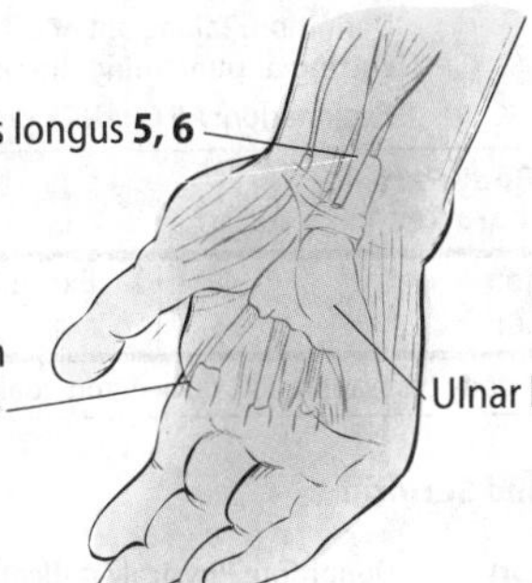

The extensor tendons act to open the hand and extend the fingers. The flexors provide grasping action to the hands.

Leg Muscles and Tendons

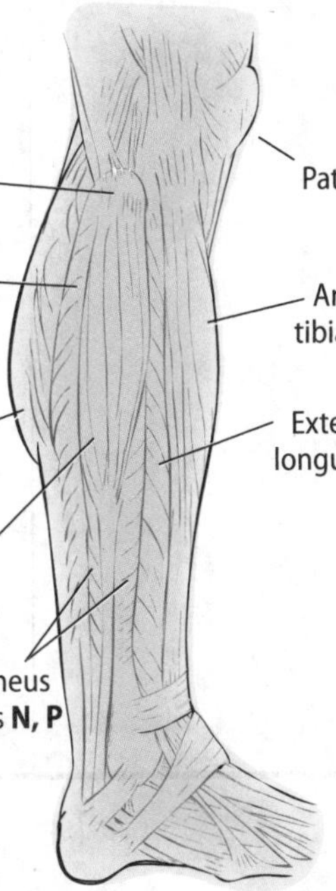

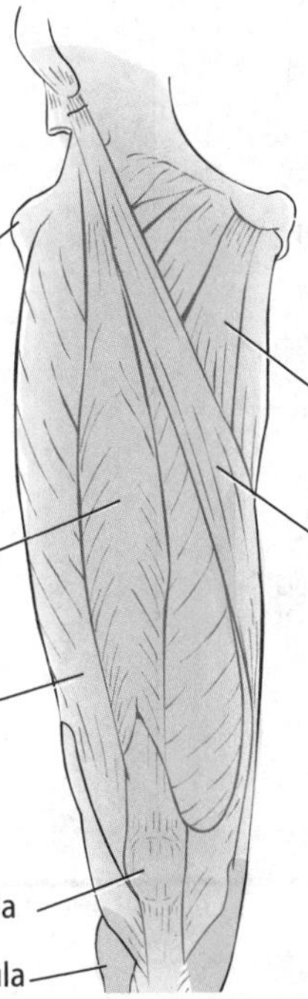

Ø Medical and Surgical
L Tendons
2 Change

Definition: Taking out or off a device from a body part and putting back an identical or similar device in or on the same body part without cutting or puncturing the skin or a mucous membrane

Explanation: All CHANGE procedures are coded using the approach EXTERNAL

Body Part Character 4	Approach Character 5	Device Character 6	Qualifier Character 7
X Upper Tendon **Y** Lower Tendon	**X** External	**Ø** Drainage Device **Y** Other Device	**Z** No Qualifier

Non-OR All body part, approach, device, and qualifier values

Ø Medical and Surgical
L Tendons
5 Destruction

Definition: Physical eradication of all or a portion of a body part by the direct use of energy, force, or a destructive agent

Explanation: None of the body part is physically taken out

Body Part Character 4	Approach Character 5	Device Character 6	Qualifier Character 7
Ø Head and Neck Tendon **1** Shoulder Tendon, Right **2** Shoulder Tendon, Left **3** Upper Arm Tendon, Right **4** Upper Arm Tendon, Left **5** Lower Arm and Wrist Tendon, Right **6** Lower Arm and Wrist Tendon, Left **7** Hand Tendon, Right **8** Hand Tendon, Left **9** Trunk Tendon, Right **B** Trunk Tendon, Left **C** Thorax Tendon, Right **D** Thorax Tendon, Left **F** Abdomen Tendon, Right **G** Abdomen Tendon, Left **H** Perineum Tendon **J** Hip Tendon, Right **K** Hip Tendon, Left **L** Upper Leg Tendon, Right **M** Upper Leg Tendon, Left **N** Lower Leg Tendon, Right Achilles tendon **P** Lower Leg Tendon, Left *See N Lower Leg Tendon, Right* **Q** Knee Tendon, Right Patellar tendon **R** Knee Tendon, Left *See Q Knee Tendon, Right* **S** Ankle Tendon, Right **T** Ankle Tendon, Left **V** Foot Tendon, Right **W** Foot Tendon, Left	**Ø** Open **3** Percutaneous **4** Percutaneous Endoscopic	**Z** No Device	**Z** No Qualifier

Ø Medical and Surgical
L Tendons
8 Division

Definition: Cutting into a body part, without draining fluids and/or gases from the body part, in order to separate or transect a body part
Explanation: All or a portion of the body part is separated into two or more portions

Body Part Character 4	Approach Character 5	Device Character 6	Qualifier Character 7
Ø Head and Neck Tendon **1 Shoulder Tendon, Right** **2 Shoulder Tendon, Left** **3 Upper Arm Tendon, Right** **4 Upper Arm Tendon, Left** **5 Lower Arm and Wrist Tendon, Right** **6 Lower Arm and Wrist Tendon, Left** **7 Hand Tendon, Right** **8 Hand Tendon, Left** **9 Trunk Tendon, Right** **B Trunk Tendon, Left** **C Thorax Tendon, Right** **D Thorax Tendon, Left** **F Abdomen Tendon, Right** **G Abdomen Tendon, Left** **H Perineum Tendon** **J Hip Tendon, Right** **K Hip Tendon, Left** **L Upper Leg Tendon, Right** **M Upper Leg Tendon, Left** **N Lower Leg Tendon, Right** Achilles tendon **P Lower Leg Tendon, Left** *See N Lower Leg Tendon, Right* **Q Knee Tendon, Right** Patellar tendon **R Knee Tendon, Left** *See Q Knee Tendon, Right* **S Ankle Tendon, Right** **T Ankle Tendon, Left** **V Foot Tendon, Right** **W Foot Tendon, Left**	**Ø Open** **3 Percutaneous** **4 Percutaneous Endoscopic**	**Z No Device**	**Z No Qualifier**

Ø Medical and Surgical
L Tendons
9 Drainage Definition: Taking or letting out fluids and/or gases from a body part
Explanation: The qualifier DIAGNOSTIC is used to identify drainage procedures that are biopsies

Body Part Character 4	Approach Character 5	Device Character 6	Qualifier Character 7
Ø Head and Neck Tendon 1 Shoulder Tendon, Right 2 Shoulder Tendon, Left 3 Upper Arm Tendon, Right 4 Upper Arm Tendon, Left 5 Lower Arm and Wrist Tendon, Right 6 Lower Arm and Wrist Tendon, Left 7 Hand Tendon, Right 8 Hand Tendon, Left 9 Trunk Tendon, Right B Trunk Tendon, Left C Thorax Tendon, Right D Thorax Tendon, Left F Abdomen Tendon, Right G Abdomen Tendon, Left H Perineum Tendon J Hip Tendon, Right K Hip Tendon, Left L Upper Leg Tendon, Right M Upper Leg Tendon, Left N Lower Leg Tendon, Right Achilles tendon P Lower Leg Tendon, Left *See N Lower Leg Tendon, Right* Q Knee Tendon, Right Patellar tendon R Knee Tendon, Left *See Q Knee Tendon, Right* S Ankle Tendon, Right T Ankle Tendon, Left V Foot Tendon, Right W Foot Tendon, Left	Ø Open 3 Percutaneous 4 Percutaneous Endoscopic	Ø Drainage Device	Z No Qualifier
Ø Head and Neck Tendon 1 Shoulder Tendon, Right 2 Shoulder Tendon, Left 3 Upper Arm Tendon, Right 4 Upper Arm Tendon, Left 5 Lower Arm and Wrist Tendon, Right 6 Lower Arm and Wrist Tendon, Left 7 Hand Tendon, Right 8 Hand Tendon, Left 9 Trunk Tendon, Right B Trunk Tendon, Left C Thorax Tendon, Right D Thorax Tendon, Left F Abdomen Tendon, Right G Abdomen Tendon, Left H Perineum Tendon J Hip Tendon, Right K Hip Tendon, Left L Upper Leg Tendon, Right M Upper Leg Tendon, Left N Lower Leg Tendon, Right Achilles tendon P Lower Leg Tendon, Left *See N Lower Leg Tendon, Right* Q Knee Tendon, Right Patellar tendon R Knee Tendon, Left *See Q Knee Tendon, Right* S Ankle Tendon, Right T Ankle Tendon, Left V Foot Tendon, Right W Foot Tendon, Left	Ø Open 3 Percutaneous 4 Percutaneous Endoscopic	Z No Device	X Diagnostic Z No Qualifier

Non-OR ØL9[Ø,1,2,3,4,5,6,7,8,9,B,C,D,F,G,H,J,K,L,M,N,P,Q,R,S,T,V,W]3ØZ
Non-OR ØL9[Ø,1,2,3,4,5,6,7,8,9,B,C,D,F,G,H,J,K,L,M,N,P,Q,R,S,T,V,W]3ZZ
Non-OR ØL9[7,8]4ZZ

Ø Medical and Surgical
L Tendons
B Excision Definition: Cutting out or off, without replacement, a portion of a body part
Explanation: The qualifier DIAGNOSTIC is used to identify excision procedures that are biopsies

Body Part Character 4	Approach Character 5	Device Character 6	Qualifier Character 7
Ø Head and Neck Tendon **1 Shoulder Tendon, Right** **2 Shoulder Tendon, Left** **3 Upper Arm Tendon, Right** **4 Upper Arm Tendon, Left** **5 Lower Arm and Wrist Tendon, Right** **6 Lower Arm and Wrist Tendon, Left** **7 Hand Tendon, Right** **8 Hand Tendon, Left** **9 Trunk Tendon, Right** **B Trunk Tendon, Left** **C Thorax Tendon, Right** **D Thorax Tendon, Left** **F Abdomen Tendon, Right** **G Abdomen Tendon, Left** **H Perineum Tendon** **J Hip Tendon, Right** **K Hip Tendon, Left** **L Upper Leg Tendon, Right** **M Upper Leg Tendon, Left** **N Lower Leg Tendon, Right** Achilles tendon **P Lower Leg Tendon, Left** *See N Lower Leg Tendon, Right* **Q Knee Tendon, Right** Patellar tendon **R Knee Tendon, Left** *See Q Knee Tendon, Right* **S Ankle Tendon, Right** **T Ankle Tendon, Left** **V Foot Tendon, Right** **W Foot Tendon, Left**	**Ø Open** **3 Percutaneous** **4 Percutaneous Endoscopic**	**Z No Device**	**X Diagnostic** **Z No Qualifier**

Ø Medical and Surgical
L Tendons
C Extirpation Definition: Taking or cutting out solid matter from a body part

Explanation: The solid matter may be an abnormal byproduct of a biological function or a foreign body; it may be imbedded in a body part or in the lumen of a tubular body part. The solid matter may or may not have been previously broken into pieces.

Body Part Character 4	Approach Character 5	Device Character 6	Qualifier Character 7
Ø Head and Neck Tendon 1 Shoulder Tendon, Right 2 Shoulder Tendon, Left 3 Upper Arm Tendon, Right 4 Upper Arm Tendon, Left 5 Lower Arm and Wrist Tendon, Right 6 Lower Arm and Wrist Tendon, Left 7 Hand Tendon, Right 8 Hand Tendon, Left 9 Trunk Tendon, Right B Trunk Tendon, Left C Thorax Tendon, Right D Thorax Tendon, Left F Abdomen Tendon, Right G Abdomen Tendon, Left H Perineum Tendon J Hip Tendon, Right K Hip Tendon, Left L Upper Leg Tendon, Right M Upper Leg Tendon, Left N Lower Leg Tendon, Right Achilles tendon P Lower Leg Tendon, Left *See N Lower Leg Tendon, Right* Q Knee Tendon, Right Patellar tendon R Knee Tendon, Left *See Q Knee Tendon, Right* S Ankle Tendon, Right T Ankle Tendon, Left V Foot Tendon, Right W Foot Tendon, Left	Ø Open 3 Percutaneous 4 Percutaneous Endoscopic	Z No Device	Z No Qualifier

Ø Medical and Surgical
L Tendons
D Extraction Definition: Pulling or stripping out or off all or a portion of a body part by the use of force
Explanation: The qualifier DIAGNOSTIC is used to identify extraction procedures that are biopsies

Body Part Character 4	Approach Character 5	Device Character 6	Qualifier Character 7
Ø Head and Neck Tendon 1 Shoulder Tendon, Right 2 Shoulder Tendon, Left 3 Upper Arm Tendon, Right 4 Upper Arm Tendon, Left 5 Lower Arm and Wrist Tendon, Right 6 Lower Arm and Wrist Tendon, Left 7 Hand Tendon, Right 8 Hand Tendon, Left 9 Trunk Tendon, Right B Trunk Tendon, Left C Thorax Tendon, Right D Thorax Tendon, Left F Abdomen Tendon, Right G Abdomen Tendon, Left H Perineum Tendon J Hip Tendon, Right K Hip Tendon, Left L Upper Leg Tendon, Right M Upper Leg Tendon, Left N Lower Leg Tendon, Right Achilles tendon P Lower Leg Tendon, Left *See N Lower Leg Tendon, Right* Q Knee Tendon, Right Patellar tendon R Knee Tendon, Left *See Q Knee Tendon, Right* S Ankle Tendon, Right T Ankle Tendon, Left V Foot Tendon, Right W Foot Tendon, Left	Ø Open	Z No Device	Z No Qualifier

Ø Medical and Surgical
L Tendons
H Insertion Definition: Putting in a nonbiological appliance that monitors, assists, performs, or prevents a physiological function but does not physically take the place of a body part
Explanation: None

Body Part Character 4	Approach Character 5	Device Character 6	Qualifier Character 7
X Upper Tendon Y Lower Tendon	Ø Open 3 Percutaneous 4 Percutaneous Endoscopic	Y Other Device	Z No Qualifier

Non-OR ØLH[X,Y][3,4]YZ

Ø Medical and Surgical
L Tendons
J Inspection Definition: Visually and/or manually exploring a body part
Explanation: Visual exploration may be performed with or without optical instrumentation. Manual exploration may be performed directly or through intervening body layers.

Body Part Character 4	Approach Character 5	Device Character 6	Qualifier Character 7
X Upper Tendon Y Lower Tendon	Ø Open 3 Percutaneous 4 Percutaneous Endoscopic X External	Z No Device	Z No Qualifier

Non-OR ØLJ[X,Y][3,X]ZZ

Ø Medical and Surgical
L Tendons
M Reattachment Definition: Putting back in or on all or a portion of a separated body part to its normal location or other suitable location
Explanation: Vascular circulation and nervous pathways may or may not be reestablished

Body Part Character 4	Approach Character 5	Device Character 6	Qualifier Character 7
Ø Head and Neck Tendon 1 Shoulder Tendon, Right 2 Shoulder Tendon, Left 3 Upper Arm Tendon, Right 4 Upper Arm Tendon, Left 5 Lower Arm and Wrist Tendon, Right 6 Lower Arm and Wrist Tendon, Left 7 Hand Tendon, Right 8 Hand Tendon, Left 9 Trunk Tendon, Right B Trunk Tendon, Left C Thorax Tendon, Right D Thorax Tendon, Left F Abdomen Tendon, Right G Abdomen Tendon, Left H Perineum Tendon J Hip Tendon, Right K Hip Tendon, Left L Upper Leg Tendon, Right M Upper Leg Tendon, Left N Lower Leg Tendon, Right Achilles tendon P Lower Leg Tendon, Left *See N Lower Leg Tendon, Right* Q Knee Tendon, Right Patellar tendon R Knee Tendon, Left *See Q Knee Tendon, Right* S Ankle Tendon, Right T Ankle Tendon, Left V Foot Tendon, Right W Foot Tendon, Left	Ø Open 4 Percutaneous Endoscopic	Z No Device	Z No Qualifier

Ø Medical and Surgical
L Tendons
N Release Definition: Freeing a body part from an abnormal physical constraint by cutting or by the use of force
Explanation: Some of the restraining tissue may be taken out but none of the body part is taken out

Body Part Character 4	Approach Character 5	Device Character 6	Qualifier Character 7
Ø Head and Neck Tendon 1 Shoulder Tendon, Right 2 Shoulder Tendon, Left 3 Upper Arm Tendon, Right 4 Upper Arm Tendon, Left 5 Lower Arm and Wrist Tendon, Right 6 Lower Arm and Wrist Tendon, Left 7 Hand Tendon, Right 8 Hand Tendon, Left 9 Trunk Tendon, Right B Trunk Tendon, Left C Thorax Tendon, Right D Thorax Tendon, Left F Abdomen Tendon, Right G Abdomen Tendon, Left H Perineum Tendon J Hip Tendon, Right K Hip Tendon, Left L Upper Leg Tendon, Right M Upper Leg Tendon, Left N Lower Leg Tendon, Right Achilles tendon P Lower Leg Tendon, Left *See N Lower Leg Tendon, Right* Q Knee Tendon, Right Patellar tendon R Knee Tendon, Left *See Q Knee Tendon, Right* S Ankle Tendon, Right T Ankle Tendon, Left V Foot Tendon, Right W Foot Tendon, Left	Ø Open 3 Percutaneous 4 Percutaneous Endoscopic X External	Z No Device	Z No Qualifier

Non-OR ØLN[Ø,1,2,3,4,5,6,7,8,9,B,C,D,F,G,H,J,K,L,M,N,P,Q,R,S,T,V,W]XZZ

Ø Medical and Surgical
L Tendons
P Removal Definition: Taking out or off a device from a body part

Explanation: If a device is taken out and a similar device put in without cutting or puncturing the skin or mucous membrane, the procedure is coded to the root operation CHANGE. Otherwise, the procedure for taking out a device is coded to the root operation REMOVAL.

Body Part Character 4	Approach Character 5	Device Character 6	Qualifier Character 7
X Upper Tendon Y Lower Tendon	Ø Open 3 Percutaneous 4 Percutaneous Endoscopic	Ø Drainage Device 7 Autologous Tissue Substitute J Synthetic Substitute K Nonautologous Tissue Substitute Y Other Device	Z No Qualifier
X Upper Tendon Y Lower Tendon	X External	Ø Drainage Device	Z No Qualifier

Non-OR ØLP[X,Y]3ØZ
Non-OR ØLP[X,Y][3,4]YZ
Non-OR ØLP[X,Y]XØZ

Ø Medical and Surgical
L Tendons
Q Repair Definition: Restoring, to the extent possible, a body part to its normal anatomic structure and function

Explanation: Used only when the method to accomplish the repair is not one of the other root operations

Body Part Character 4	Approach Character 5	Device Character 6	Qualifier Character 7
Ø Head and Neck Tendon 1 Shoulder Tendon, Right 2 Shoulder Tendon, Left 3 Upper Arm Tendon, Right 4 Upper Arm Tendon, Left 5 Lower Arm and Wrist Tendon, Right 6 Lower Arm and Wrist Tendon, Left 7 Hand Tendon, Right 8 Hand Tendon, Left 9 Trunk Tendon, Right B Trunk Tendon, Left C Thorax Tendon, Right D Thorax Tendon, Left F Abdomen Tendon, Right G Abdomen Tendon, Left H Perineum Tendon J Hip Tendon, Right K Hip Tendon, Left L Upper Leg Tendon, Right M Upper Leg Tendon, Left N Lower Leg Tendon, Right Achilles tendon P Lower Leg Tendon, Left *See N Lower Leg Tendon, Right* Q Knee Tendon, Right Patellar tendon R Knee Tendon, Left *See Q Knee Tendon, Right* S Ankle Tendon, Right T Ankle Tendon, Left V Foot Tendon, Right W Foot Tendon, Left	Ø Open 3 Percutaneous 4 Percutaneous Endoscopic	Z No Device	Z No Qualifier

Ø Medical and Surgical
L Tendons
R Replacement Definition: Putting in or on biological or synthetic material that physically takes the place and/or function of all or a portion of a body part

Explanation: The body part may have been taken out or replaced, or may be taken out, physically eradicated, or rendered nonfunctional during the REPLACEMENT procedure. A REMOVAL procedure is coded for taking out the device used in a previous replacement procedure.

Body Part Character 4	Approach Character 5	Device Character 6	Qualifier Character 7
Ø Head and Neck Tendon **1** Shoulder Tendon, Right **2** Shoulder Tendon, Left **3** Upper Arm Tendon, Right **4** Upper Arm Tendon, Left **5** Lower Arm and Wrist Tendon, Right **6** Lower Arm and Wrist Tendon, Left **7** Hand Tendon, Right **8** Hand Tendon, Left **9** Trunk Tendon, Right **B** Trunk Tendon, Left **C** Thorax Tendon, Right **D** Thorax Tendon, Left **F** Abdomen Tendon, Right **G** Abdomen Tendon, Left **H** Perineum Tendon **J** Hip Tendon, Right **K** Hip Tendon, Left **L** Upper Leg Tendon, Right **M** Upper Leg Tendon, Left **N** Lower Leg Tendon, Right Achilles tendon **P** Lower Leg Tendon, Left *See N Lower Leg Tendon, Right* **Q** Knee Tendon, Right Patellar tendon **R** Knee Tendon, Left *See Q Knee Tendon, Right* **S** Ankle Tendon, Right **T** Ankle Tendon, Left **V** Foot Tendon, Right **W** Foot Tendon, Left	**Ø** Open **4** Percutaneous Endoscopic	**7** Autologous Tissue Substitute **J** Synthetic Substitute **K** Nonautologous Tissue Substitute	**Z** No Qualifier

Ø Medical and Surgical
L Tendons
S Reposition Definition: Moving to its normal location, or other suitable location, all or a portion of a body part

Explanation: The body part is moved to a new location from an abnormal location, or from a normal location where it is not functioning correctly. The body part may or may not be cut out or off to be moved to the new location.

Body Part Character 4	Approach Character 5	Device Character 6	Qualifier Character 7
Ø Head and Neck Tendon **1** Shoulder Tendon, Right **2** Shoulder Tendon, Left **3** Upper Arm Tendon, Right **4** Upper Arm Tendon, Left **5** Lower Arm and Wrist Tendon, Right **6** Lower Arm and Wrist Tendon, Left **7** Hand Tendon, Right **8** Hand Tendon, Left **9** Trunk Tendon, Right **B** Trunk Tendon, Left **C** Thorax Tendon, Right **D** Thorax Tendon, Left **F** Abdomen Tendon, Right **G** Abdomen Tendon, Left **H** Perineum Tendon **J** Hip Tendon, Right **K** Hip Tendon, Left **L** Upper Leg Tendon, Right **M** Upper Leg Tendon, Left **N** Lower Leg Tendon, Right Achilles tendon **P** Lower Leg Tendon, Left *See N Lower Leg Tendon, Right* **Q** Knee Tendon, Right Patellar tendon **R** Knee Tendon, Left *See Q Knee Tendon, Right* **S** Ankle Tendon, Right **T** Ankle Tendon, Left **V** Foot Tendon, Right **W** Foot Tendon, Left	**Ø** Open **4** Percutaneous Endoscopic	**Z** No Device	**Z** No Qualifier

Ø Medical and Surgical
L Tendons
T Resection Definition: Cutting out or off, without replacement, all of a body part

Explanation: None

Body Part Character 4	Approach Character 5	Device Character 6	Qualifier Character 7
Ø Head and Neck Tendon 1 Shoulder Tendon, Right 2 Shoulder Tendon, Left 3 Upper Arm Tendon, Right 4 Upper Arm Tendon, Left 5 Lower Arm and Wrist Tendon, Right 6 Lower Arm and Wrist Tendon, Left 7 Hand Tendon, Right 8 Hand Tendon, Left 9 Trunk Tendon, Right B Trunk Tendon, Left C Thorax Tendon, Right D Thorax Tendon, Left F Abdomen Tendon, Right G Abdomen Tendon, Left H Perineum Tendon J Hip Tendon, Right K Hip Tendon, Left L Upper Leg Tendon, Right M Upper Leg Tendon, Left N Lower Leg Tendon, Right Achilles tendon P Lower Leg Tendon, Left *See N Lower Leg Tendon, Right* Q Knee Tendon, Right Patellar tendon R Knee Tendon, Left *See Q Knee Tendon, Right* S Ankle Tendon, Right T Ankle Tendon, Left V Foot Tendon, Right W Foot Tendon, Left	Ø Open 4 Percutaneous Endoscopic	Z No Device	Z No Qualifier

Ø Medical and Surgical
L Tendons
U Supplement Definition: Putting in or on biological or synthetic material that physically reinforces and/or augments the function of a portion of a body part

Explanation: The biological material is non-living, or is living and from the same individual. The body part may have been previously replaced, and the SUPPLEMENT procedure is performed to physically reinforce and/or augment the function of the replaced body part.

Body Part Character 4	Approach Character 5	Device Character 6	Qualifier Character 7
Ø Head and Neck Tendon 1 Shoulder Tendon, Right 2 Shoulder Tendon, Left 3 Upper Arm Tendon, Right 4 Upper Arm Tendon, Left 5 Lower Arm and Wrist Tendon, Right 6 Lower Arm and Wrist Tendon, Left 7 Hand Tendon, Right 8 Hand Tendon, Left 9 Trunk Tendon, Right B Trunk Tendon, Left C Thorax Tendon, Right D Thorax Tendon, Left F Abdomen Tendon, Right G Abdomen Tendon, Left H Perineum Tendon J Hip Tendon, Right K Hip Tendon, Left L Upper Leg Tendon, Right M Upper Leg Tendon, Left N Lower Leg Tendon, Right Achilles tendon P Lower Leg Tendon, Left *See N Lower Leg Tendon, Right* Q Knee Tendon, Right Patellar tendon R Knee Tendon, Left *See Q Knee Tendon, Right* S Ankle Tendon, Right T Ankle Tendon, Left V Foot Tendon, Right W Foot Tendon, Left	Ø Open 4 Percutaneous Endoscopic	7 Autologous Tissue Substitute J Synthetic Substitute K Nonautologous Tissue Substitute	Z No Qualifier

Ø Medical and Surgical
L Tendons
W Revision

Definition: Correcting, to the extent possible, a portion of a malfunctioning device or the position of a displaced device

Explanation: Revision can include correcting a malfunctioning or displaced device by taking out or putting in components of the device such as a screw or pin

Body Part Character 4	Approach Character 5	Device Character 6	Qualifier Character 7
X Upper Tendon Y Lower Tendon	Ø Open 3 Percutaneous 4 Percutaneous Endoscopic	Ø Drainage Device 7 Autologous Tissue Substitute J Synthetic Substitute K Nonautologous Tissue Substitute Y Other Device	Z No Qualifier
X Upper Tendon Y Lower Tendon	X External	Ø Drainage Device 7 Autologous Tissue Substitute J Synthetic Substitute K Nonautologous Tissue Substitute	Z No Qualifier

Non-OR ØLW[X,Y][3,4]YZ
Non-OR ØLW[X,Y]X[Ø,7,J,K]Z

Ø Medical and Surgical
L Tendons
X Transfer

Definition: Moving, without taking out, all or a portion of a body part to another location to take over the function of all or a portion of a body part

Explanation: The body part transferred remains connected to its vascular and nervous supply

Body Part Character 4	Approach Character 5	Device Character 6	Qualifier Character 7
Ø Head and Neck Tendon 1 Shoulder Tendon, Right 2 Shoulder Tendon, Left 3 Upper Arm Tendon, Right 4 Upper Arm Tendon, Left 5 Lower Arm and Wrist Tendon, Right 6 Lower Arm and Wrist Tendon, Left 7 Hand Tendon, Right 8 Hand Tendon, Left 9 Trunk Tendon, Right B Trunk Tendon, Left C Thorax Tendon, Right D Thorax Tendon, Left F Abdomen Tendon, Right G Abdomen Tendon, Left H Perineum Tendon J Hip Tendon, Right K Hip Tendon, Left L Upper Leg Tendon, Right M Upper Leg Tendon, Left N Lower Leg Tendon, Right Achilles tendon P Lower Leg Tendon, Left *See N Lower Leg Tendon, Right* Q Knee Tendon, Right Patellar tendon R Knee Tendon, Left *See Q Knee Tendon, Right* S Ankle Tendon, Right T Ankle Tendon, Left V Foot Tendon, Right W Foot Tendon, Left	Ø Open 4 Percutaneous Endoscopic	Z No Device	Z No Qualifier

Bursae and Ligaments ØM2–ØMX

Character Meanings*

This Character Meaning table is provided as a guide to assist the user in the identification of character members that may be found in this section of code tables. It **SHOULD NOT** be used to build a PCS code.

Operation–Character 3	Body Part–Character 4	Approach–Character 5	Device–Character 6	Qualifier–Character 7
2 Change	Ø Head and Neck Bursa and Ligament	Ø Open	Ø Drainage Device	X Diagnostic
5 Destruction	1 Shoulder Bursa and Ligament, Right	3 Percutaneous	7 Autologous Tissue Substitute	Z No Qualifier
8 Division	2 Shoulder Bursa and Ligament, Left	4 Percutaneous Endoscopic	J Synthetic Substitute	
9 Drainage	3 Elbow Bursa and Ligament, Right	X External	K Nonautologous Tissue Substitute	
B Excision	4 Elbow Bursa and Ligament, Left		Y Other Device	
C Extirpation	5 Wrist Bursa and Ligament, Right		Z No Device	
D Extraction	6 Wrist Bursa and Ligament, Left			
H Insertion	7 Hand Bursa and Ligament, Right			
J Inspection	8 Hand Bursa and Ligament, Left			
M Reattachment	9 Upper Extremity Bursa and Ligament, Right			
N Release	B Upper Extremity Bursa and Ligament, Left			
P Removal	C Upper Spine Bursa and Ligament			
Q Repair	D Lower Spine Bursa and Ligament			
R Replacement	F Sternum Bursa and Ligament			
S Reposition	G Rib(s) Bursa and Ligament			
T Resection	H Abdomen Bursa and Ligament, Right			
U Supplement	J Abdomen Bursa and Ligament, Left			
W Revision	K Perineum Bursa and Ligament			
X Transfer	L Hip Bursa and Ligament, Right			
	M Hip Bursa and Ligament, Left			
	N Knee Bursa and Ligament, Right			
	P Knee Bursa and Ligament, Left			
	Q Ankle Bursa and Ligament, Right			
	R Ankle Bursa and Ligament, Left			
	S Foot Bursa and Ligament, Right			
	T Foot Bursa and Ligament, Left			
	V Lower Extremity Bursa and Ligament, Right			
	W Lower Extremity Bursa and Ligament, Left			
	X Upper Bursa and Ligament			
	Y Lower Bursa and Ligament			

* Includes synovial membrane.

AHA Coding Clinic for table ØMB
2018, 3Q, 17 Excisional debridement of periosteum

AHA Coding Clinic for table ØMM
2013, 3Q, 20 Superior labrum anterior posterior (SLAP) repair and subacromial decompression

AHA Coding Clinic for table ØMQ
2014, 3Q, 9 Interspinous ligamentoplasty

AHA Coding Clinic for table ØMT
2017, 2Q, 21 Arthroscopic anterior cruciate ligament revision using autograft with anterolateral ligament reconstruction

AHA Coding Clinic for table ØMU
2017, 2Q, 21 Arthroscopic anterior cruciate ligament revision using autograft with anterolateral ligament reconstruction

Shoulder Ligaments

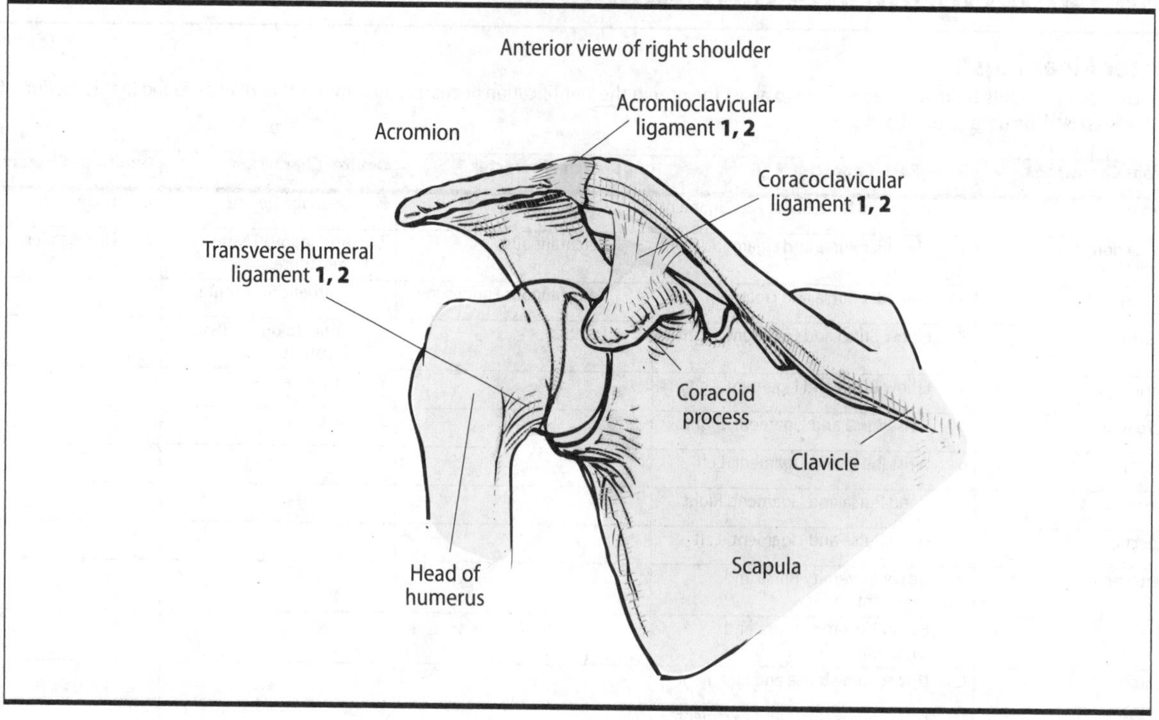

Knee Bursae

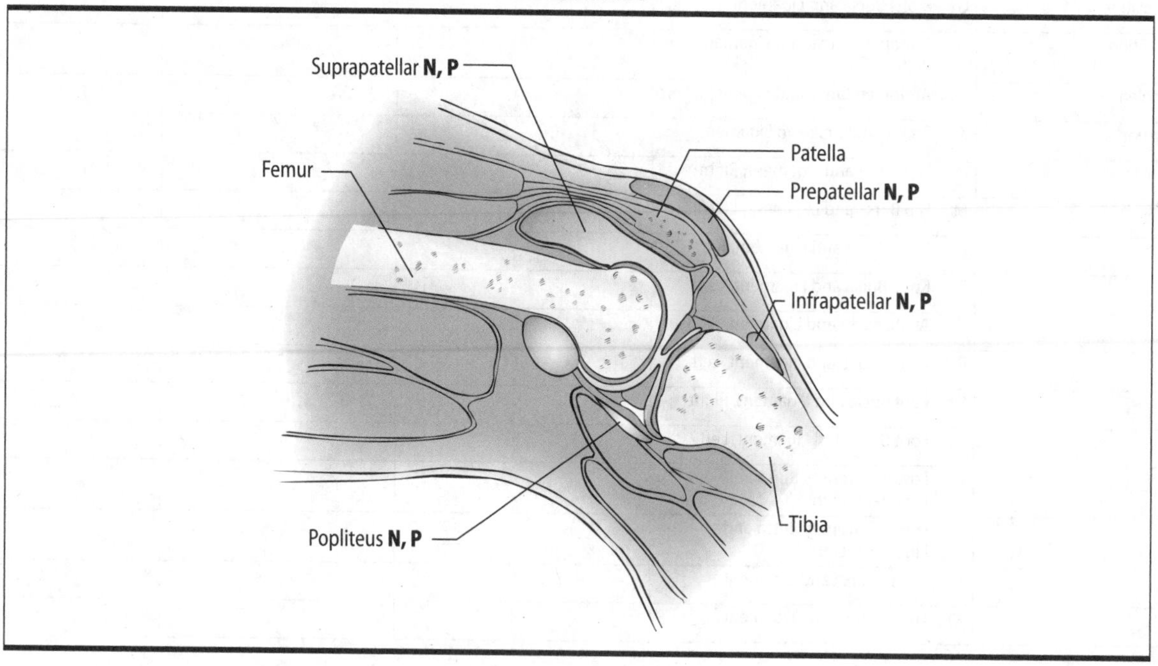

Knee Ligaments

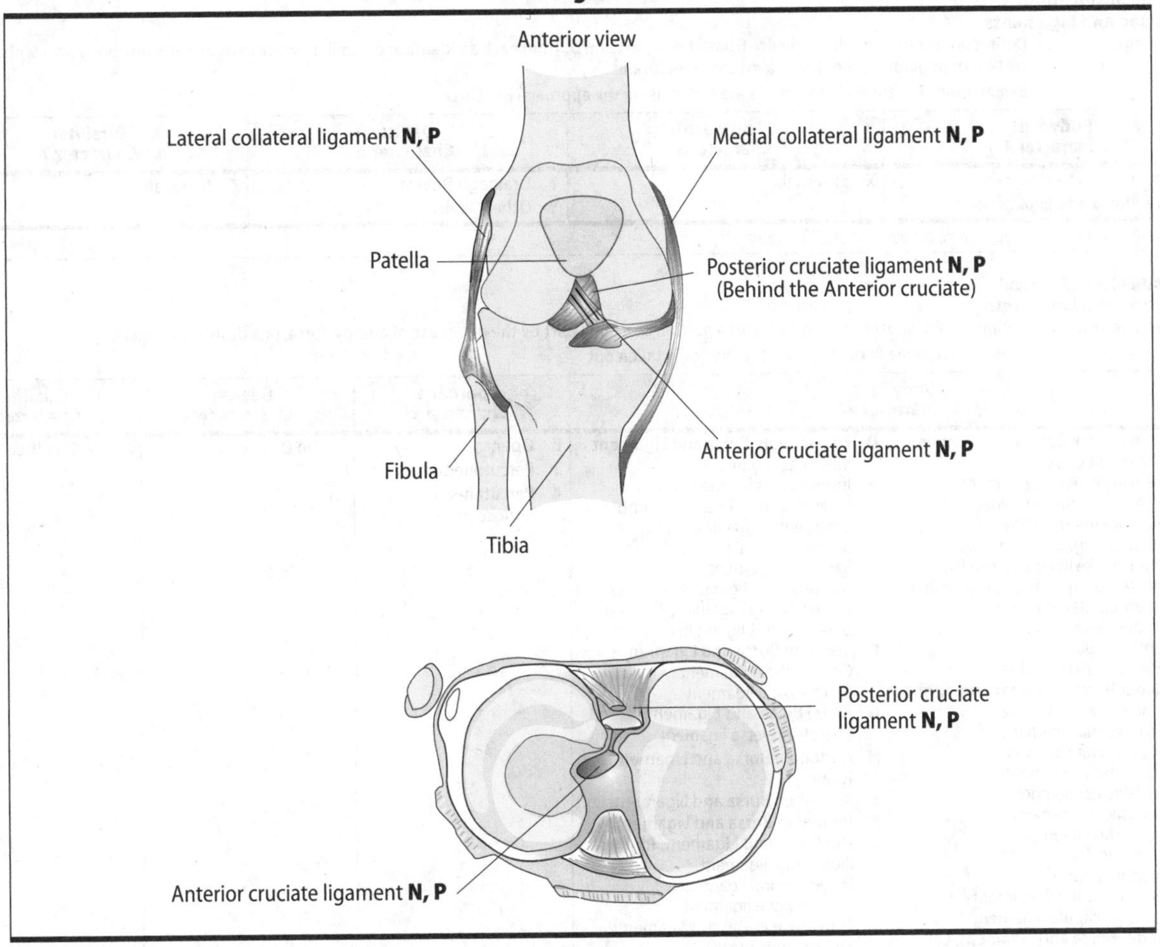

Wrist Ligaments

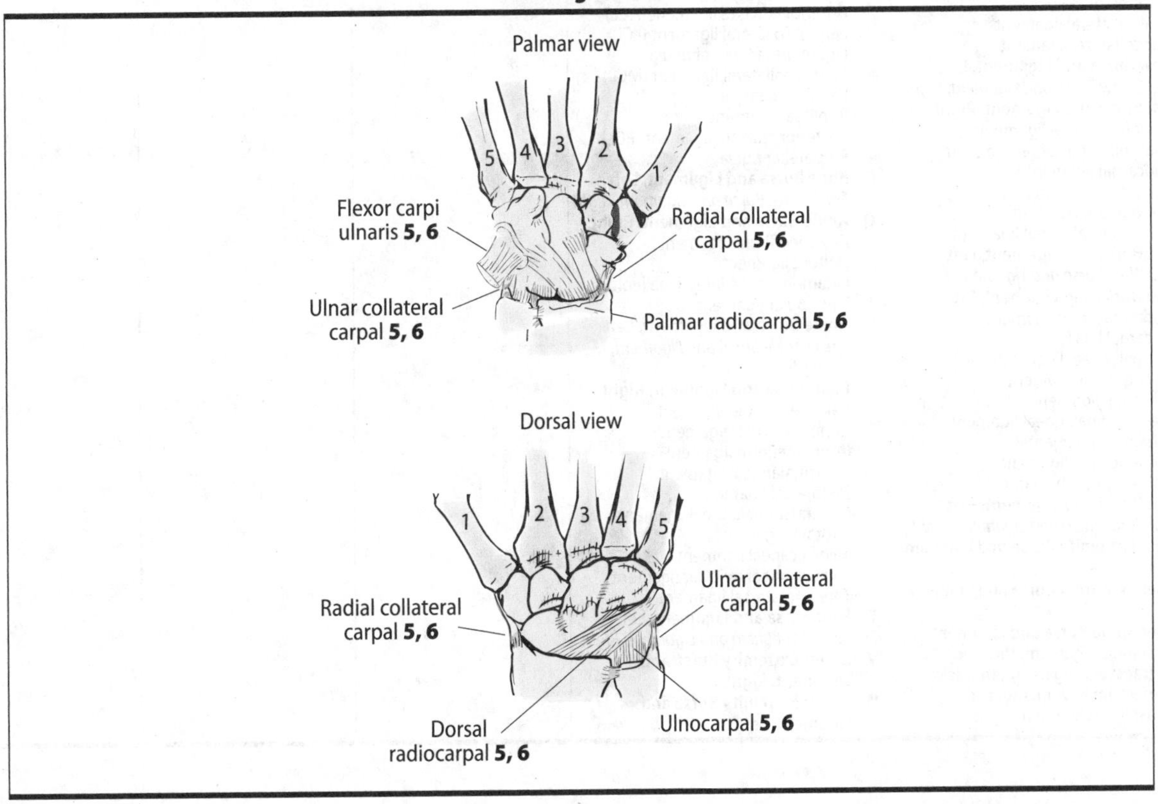

Ø Medical and Surgical
M Bursae and Ligaments
2 Change Definition: Taking out or off a device from a body part and putting back an identical or similar device in or on the same body part without cutting or puncturing the skin or a mucous membrane

Explanation: All CHANGE procedures are coded using the approach EXTERNAL

Body Part Character 4	Approach Character 5	Device Character 6	Qualifier Character 7
X Upper Bursa and Ligament **Y** Lower Bursa and Ligament	**X** External	**Ø** Drainage Device **Y** Other Device	**Z** No Qualifier

Non-OR All body part, approach, device, and qualifier values

Ø Medical and Surgical
M Bursae and Ligaments
5 Destruction Definition: Physical eradication of all or a portion of a body part by the direct use of energy, force, or a destructive agent

Explanation: None of the body part is physically taken out

Body Part Character 4	Approach Character 5	Device Character 6	Qualifier Character 7
Ø Head and Neck Bursa and Ligament Alar ligament of axis Cervical interspinous ligament Cervical intertransverse ligament Cervical ligamentum flavum Interspinous ligament, cervical Intertransverse ligament, cervical Lateral temporomandibular ligament Ligamentum flavum, cervical Sphenomandibular ligament Stylomandibular ligament Transverse ligament of atlas **1 Shoulder Bursa and Ligament, Right** Acromioclavicular ligament Coracoacromial ligament Coracoclavicular ligament Coracohumeral ligament Costoclavicular ligament Glenohumeral ligament Interclavicular ligament Sternoclavicular ligament Subacromial bursa Transverse humeral ligament Transverse scapular ligament **2 Shoulder Bursa and Ligament, Left** **See** *1 Shoulder Bursa and Ligament, Right* **3 Elbow Bursa and Ligfament, Right** Annular ligament Olecranon bursa Radial collateral ligament Ulnar collateral ligament **4 Elbow Bursa and Ligament, Left** **See** *3 Elbow Bursa and Ligament, Right* **5 Wrist Bursa and Ligament, Right** Palmar ulnocarpal ligament Radial collateral carpal ligament Radiocarpal ligament Radioulnar ligament Scapholunate ligament Ulnar collateral carpal ligament **6 Wrist Bursa and Ligament, Left** **See** *5 Wrist Bursa and Ligament, Right* **7 Hand Bursa and Ligament, Right** Carpometacarpal ligament Intercarpal ligament Interphalangeal ligament Lunotriquetral ligament Metacarpal ligament Metacarpophalangeal ligament Pisohamate ligament Pisometacarpal ligament Scaphotrapezium ligament **8 Hand Bursa and Ligament, Left** **See** *7 Hand Bursa and Ligament, Right* **9 Upper Extremity Bursa and Ligament, Right** **B Upper Extremity Bursa and Ligament, Left** **C Upper Spine Bursa and Ligament** Interspinous ligament, thoracic Intertransverse ligament, thoracic Ligamentum flavum, thoracic Supraspinous ligament **D Lower Spine Bursa and Ligament** Iliolumbar ligament Interspinous ligament, lumbar Intertransverse ligament, lumbar Ligamentum flavum, lumbar Sacrococcygeal ligament Sacroiliac ligament Sacrospinous ligament Sacrotuberous ligament Supraspinous ligament **F Sternum Bursa and Ligament** Costoxiphoid ligament Sternocostal ligament **G Rib(s) Bursa and Ligament** Costotransverse ligament **H Abdomen Bursa and Ligament, Right** **J Abdomen Bursa and Ligament, Left** **K Perineum Bursa and Ligament** **L Hip Bursa and Ligament, Right** Iliofemoral ligament Ischiofemoral ligament Pubofemoral ligament Transverse acetabular ligament Trochanteric bursa **M Hip Bursa and Ligament, Left** **See** *L Hip Bursa and Ligament, Right* **N Knee Bursa and Ligament, Right** Anterior cruciate ligament (ACL) Lateral collateral ligament (LCL) Ligament of head of fibula Medial collateral ligament (MCL) Patellar ligament Popliteal ligament Posterior cruciate ligament (PCL) Prepatellar bursa **P Knee Bursa and Ligament, Left** **See** *N Knee Bursa and Ligament, Right* **Q Ankle Bursa and Ligament, Right** Calcaneofibular ligament Deltoid ligament Ligament of the lateral malleolus Talofibular ligament **R Ankle Bursa and Ligament, Left** **See** *Q Ankle Bursa and Ligament, Right* **S Foot Bursa and Ligament, Right** Calcaneocuboid ligament Cuneonavicular ligament Intercuneiform ligament Interphalangeal ligament Metatarsal ligament Metatarsophalangeal ligament Subtalar ligament Talocalcaneal ligament Talocalcaneonavicular ligament Tarsometatarsal ligament **T Foot Bursa and Ligament, Left** **See** *S Foot Bursa and Ligament, Right* **V Lower Extremity Bursa and Ligament, Right** **W Lower Extremity Bursa and Ligament, Left**	**Ø** Open **3** Percutaneous **4** Percutaneous Endoscopic	**Z** No Device	**Z** No Qualifier

Ø Medical and Surgical
M Bursae and Ligaments
8 Division Definition: Cutting into a body part, without draining fluids and/or gases from the body part, in order to separate or transect a body part
Explanation: All or a portion of the body part is separated into two or more portions

Body Part Character 4		Approach Character 5	Device Character 6	Qualifier Character 7
Ø Head and Neck Bursa and Ligament Alar ligament of axis Cervical interspinous ligament Cervical intertransverse ligament Cervical ligamentum flavum Interspinous ligament, cervical Intertransverse ligament, cervical Lateral temporomandibular ligament Ligamentum flavum, cervical Sphenomandibular ligament Stylomandibular ligament Transverse ligament of atlas **1 Shoulder Bursa and Ligament, Right** Acromioclavicular ligament Coracoacromial ligament Coracoclavicular ligament Coracohumeral ligament Costoclavicular ligament Glenohumeral ligament Interclavicular ligament Sternoclavicular ligament Subacromial bursa Transverse humeral ligament Transverse scapular ligament **2 Shoulder Bursa and Ligament, Left** **See** *1 Shoulder Bursa and Ligament, Right* **3 Elbow Bursa and Ligament, Right** Annular ligament Olecranon bursa Radial collateral ligament Ulnar collateral ligament **4 Elbow Bursa and Ligament, Left** **See** *3 Elbow Bursa and Ligament, Right* **5 Wrist Bursa and Ligament, Right** Palmar ulnocarpal ligament Radial collateral carpal ligament Radiocarpal ligament Radioulnar ligament Scapholunate ligament Ulnar collateral carpal ligament **6 Wrist Bursa and Ligament, Left** **See** *5 Wrist Bursa and Ligament, Right* **7 Hand Bursa and Ligament, Right** Carpometacarpal ligament Intercarpal ligament Interphalangeal ligament Lunotriquetral ligament Metacarpal ligament Metacarpophalangeal ligament Pisohamate ligament Pisometacarpal ligament Scaphotrapezium ligament **8 Hand Bursa and Ligament, Left** **See** *7 Hand Bursa and Ligament, Right* **9 Upper Extremity Bursa and Ligament, Right** **B Upper Extremity Bursa and Ligament, Left** **C Upper Spine Bursa and Ligament** Interspinous ligament, thoracic Intertransverse ligament, thoracic Ligamentum flavum, thoracic Supraspinous ligament	**D Lower Spine Bursa and Ligament** Iliolumbar ligament Interspinous ligament, lumbar Intertransverse ligament, lumbar Ligamentum flavum, lumbar Sacrococcygeal ligament Sacroiliac ligament Sacrospinous ligament Sacrotuberous ligament Supraspinous ligament **F Sternum Bursa and Ligament** Costoxiphoid ligament Sternocostal ligament **G Rib(s) Bursa and Ligament** Costotransverse ligament **H Abdomen Bursa and Ligament, Right** **J Abdomen Bursa and Ligament, Left** **K Perineum Bursa and Ligament** **L Hip Bursa and Ligament, Right** Iliofemoral ligament Ischiofemoral ligament Pubofemoral ligament Transverse acetabular ligament Trochanteric bursa **M Hip Bursa and Ligament, Left** **See** *L Hip Bursa and Ligament, Right* **N Knee Bursa and Ligament, Right** Anterior cruciate ligament (ACL) Lateral collateral ligament (LCL) Ligament of head of fibula Medial collateral ligament (MCL) Patellar ligament Popliteal ligament Posterior cruciate ligament (PCL) Prepatellar bursa **P Knee Bursa and Ligament, Left** **See** *N Knee Bursa and Ligament, Right* **Q Ankle Bursa and Ligament, Right** Calcaneofibular ligament Deltoid ligament Ligament of the lateral malleolus Talofibular ligament **R Ankle Bursa and Ligament, Left** **See** *Q Ankle Bursa and Ligament, Right* **S Foot Bursa and Ligament, Right** Calcaneocuboid ligament Cuneonavicular ligament Intercuneiform ligament Interphalangeal ligament Metatarsal ligament Metatarsophalangeal ligament Subtalar ligament Talocalcaneal ligament Talocalcaneonavicular ligament Tarsometatarsal ligament **T Foot Bursa and Ligament, Left** **See** *S Foot Bursa and Ligament, Right* **V Lower Extremity Bursa and Ligament, Right** **W Lower Extremity Bursa and Ligament, Left**	**Ø Open** **3 Percutaneous** **4 Percutaneous Endoscopic**	**Z No Device**	**Z No Qualifier**

Ø Medical and Surgical
M Bursae and Ligaments
9 Drainage Definition: Taking or letting out fluids and/or gases from a body part
Explanation: The qualifier DIAGNOSTIC is used to identify drainage procedures that are biopsies

Body Part Character 4	Approach Character 5	Device Character 6	Qualifier Character 7
Ø Head and Neck Bursa and Ligament Alar ligament of axis Cervical interspinous ligament Cervical intertransverse ligament Cervical ligamentum flavum Interspinous ligament, cervical Intertransverse ligament, cervical Lateral temporomandibular ligament Ligamentum flavum, cervical Sphenomandibular ligament Stylomandibular ligament Transverse ligament of atlas	**Ø Open** **3 Percutaneous** **4 Percutaneous Endoscopic**	**Ø Drainage Device**	**Z No Qualifier**
1 Shoulder Bursa and Ligament, Right Acromioclavicular ligament Coracoacromial ligament Coracoclavicular ligament Coracohumeral ligament Costoclavicular ligament Glenohumeral ligament Interclavicular ligament Sternoclavicular ligament Subacromial bursa Transverse humeral ligament Transverse scapular ligament			
2 Shoulder Bursa and Ligament, Left *See 1 Shoulder Bursa and Ligament, Right*			
3 Elbow Bursa and Ligament, Right Annular ligament Olecranon bursa Radial collateral ligament Ulnar collateral ligament			
4 Elbow Bursa and Ligament, Left *See 3 Elbow Bursa and Ligament, Right*			
5 Wrist Bursa and Ligament, Right Palmar ulnocarpal ligament Radial collateral carpal ligament Radiocarpal ligament Radioulnar ligament Scapholunate ligament Ulnar collateral carpal ligament			
6 Wrist Bursa and Ligament, Left *See 5 Wrist Bursa and Ligament, Right*			
7 Hand Bursa and Ligament, Right Carpometacarpal ligament Intercarpal ligament Interphalangeal ligament Lunotriquetral ligament Metacarpal ligament Metacarpophalangeal ligament Pisohamate ligament Pisometacarpal ligament Scaphotrapezium ligament			
8 Hand Bursa and Ligament, Left *See 7 Hand Bursa and Ligament, Right*			
9 Upper Extremity Bursa and Ligament, Right			
B Upper Extremity Bursa and Ligament, Left			
C Upper Spine Bursa and Ligament Interspinous ligament, thoracic Intertransverse ligament, thoracic Ligamentum flavum, thoracic Supraspinous ligament			
D Lower Spine Bursa and Ligament Iliolumbar ligament Interspinous ligament, lumbar Intertransverse ligament, lumbar Ligamentum flavum, lumbar Sacrococcygeal ligament Sacroiliac ligament Sacrospinous ligament Sacrotuberous ligament Supraspinous ligament			
F Sternum Bursa and Ligament Costoxiphoid ligament Sternocostal ligament			
G Rib(s) Bursa and Ligament Costotransverse ligament			
H Abdomen Bursa and Ligament, Right			
J Abdomen Bursa and Ligament, Left			
K Perineum Bursa and Ligament			
L Hip Bursa and Ligament, Right Iliofemoral ligament Ischiofemoral ligament Pubofemoral ligament Transverse acetabular ligament Trochanteric bursa			
M Hip Bursa and Ligament, Left *See L Hip Bursa and Ligament, Right*			
N Knee Bursa and Ligament, Right Anterior cruciate ligament (ACL) Lateral collateral ligament (LCL) Ligament of head of fibula Medial collateral ligament (MCL) Patellar ligament Popliteal ligament Posterior cruciate ligament (PCL) Prepatellar bursa			
P Knee Bursa and Ligament, Left *See N Knee Bursa and Ligament, Right*			
Q Ankle Bursa and Ligament, Right Calcaneofibular ligament Deltoid ligament Ligament of the lateral malleolus Talofibular ligament			
R Ankle Bursa and Ligament, Left *See Q Ankle Bursa and Ligament, Right*			
S Foot Bursa and Ligament, Right Calcaneocuboid ligament Cuneonavicular ligament Intercuneiform ligament Interphalangeal ligament Metatarsal ligament Metatarsophalangeal ligament Subtalar ligament Talocalcaneal ligament Talocalcaneonavicular ligament Tarsometatarsal ligament			
T Foot Bursa and Ligament, Left *See S Foot Bursa and Ligament, Right*			
V Lower Extremity Bursa and Ligament, Right			
W Lower Extremity Bursa and Ligament, Left			

Non-OR ØM9[Ø,1,2,3,4,5,6,7,8,9,B,C,D,F,G,H,J,K,L,M,N,P,Q,R,S,T,V,W]3ØZ
Non-OR ØM9[1,2,3,4,7,8,9,B,C,D,F,G,H,J,K,L,M,V,W]4ØZ

ØM9 Continued on next page

ØM9 Continued

Ø Medical and Surgical
M Bursae and Ligaments
9 Drainage Definition: Taking or letting out fluids and/or gases from a body part
Explanation: The qualifier DIAGNOSTIC is used to identify drainage procedures that are biopsies

Body Part Character 4	Approach Character 5	Device Character 6	Qualifier Character 7
Ø Head and Neck Bursa and Ligament Alar ligament of axis Cervical interspinous ligament Cervical intertransverse ligament Cervical ligamentum flavum Interspinous ligament, cervical Intertransverse ligament, cervical Lateral temporomandibular ligament Ligamentum flavum, cervical Sphenomandibular ligament Stylomandibular ligament Transverse ligament of atlas	**Ø** Open **3** Percutaneous **4** Percutaneous Endoscopic	**Z** No Device	**X** Diagnostic **Z** No Qualifier
1 Shoulder Bursa and Ligament, Right Acromioclavicular ligament Coracoacromial ligament Coracoclavicular ligament Coracohumeral ligament Costoclavicular ligament Glenohumeral ligament Interclavicular ligament Sternoclavicular ligament Subacromial bursa Transverse humeral ligament Transverse scapular ligament			
2 Shoulder Bursa and Ligament, Left *See 1 Shoulder Bursa and Ligament, Right*			
3 Elbow Bursa and Ligament, Right Annular ligament Olecranon bursa Radial collateral ligament Ulnar collateral ligament			
4 Elbow Bursa and Ligament, Left *See 3 Elbow Bursa and Ligament, Right*			
5 Wrist Bursa and Ligament, Right Palmar ulnocarpal ligament Radial collateral carpal ligament Radiocarpal ligament Radioulnar ligament Scapholunate ligament Ulnar collateral carpal ligament			
6 Wrist Bursa and Ligament, Left *See 5 Wrist Bursa and Ligament, Right*			
7 Hand Bursa and Ligament, Right Carpometacarpal ligament Intercarpal ligament Interphalangeal ligament Lunotriquetral ligament Metacarpal ligament Metacarpophalangeal ligament Pisohamate ligament Pisometacarpal ligament Scaphotrapezium ligament			
8 Hand Bursa and Ligament, Left *See 7 Hand Bursa and Ligament, Right*			
9 Upper Extremity Bursa and Ligament, Right			
B Upper Extremity Bursa and Ligament, Left			
C Upper Spine Bursa and Ligament Interspinous ligament, thoracic Intertransverse ligament, thoracic Ligamentum flavum, thoracic Supraspinous ligament			
D Lower Spine Bursa and Ligament Iliolumbar ligament Interspinous ligament, lumbar Intertransverse ligament, lumbar Ligamentum flavum, lumbar Sacrococcygeal ligament Sacroiliac ligament Sacrospinous ligament Sacrotuberous ligament Supraspinous ligament			
F Sternum Bursa and Ligament Costoxiphoid ligament Sternocostal ligament			
G Rib(s) Bursa and Ligament Costotransverse ligament			
H Abdomen Bursa and Ligament, Right			
J Abdomen Bursa and Ligament, Left			
K Perineum Bursa and Ligament			
L Hip Bursa and Ligament, Right Iliofemoral ligament Ischiofemoral ligament Pubofemoral ligament Transverse acetabular ligament Trochanteric bursa			
M Hip Bursa and Ligament, Left *See L Hip Bursa and Ligament, Right*			
N Knee Bursa and Ligament, Right Anterior cruciate ligament (ACL) Lateral collateral ligament (LCL) Ligament of head of fibula Medial collateral ligament (MCL) Patellar ligament Popliteal ligament Posterior cruciate ligament (PCL) Prepatellar bursa			
P Knee Bursa and Ligament, Left *See N Knee Bursa and Ligament, Right*			
Q Ankle Bursa and Ligament, Right Calcaneofibular ligament Deltoid ligament Ligament of the lateral malleolus Talofibular ligament			
R Ankle Bursa and Ligament, Left *See Q Ankle Bursa and Ligament, Right*			
S Foot Bursa and Ligament, Right Calcaneocuboid ligament Cuneonavicular ligament Intercuneiform ligament Interphalangeal ligament Metatarsal ligament Metatarsophalangeal ligament Subtalar ligament Talocalcaneal ligament Talocalcaneonavicular ligament Tarsometatarsal ligament			
T Foot Bursa and Ligament, Left *See S Foot Bursa and Ligament, Right*			
V Lower Extremity Bursa and Ligament, Right			
W Lower Extremity Bursa and Ligament, Left			

Non-OR ØM9[Ø,1,2,3,4,5,6,7,8,C,D,F,G,L,M,N,P,Q,R,S,T][Ø,3,4]ZX
Non-OR ØM9[Ø,1,2,3,4,5,6,7,8,9,B,C,D,F,G,H,J,K,L,M,N,P,Q,R,S,T,V,W]3ZZ
Non-OR ØM9[Ø,5,6,7,8,9,B,C,D,F,G,H,J,K,N,P,Q,R,S,T,V,W]4ZZ

Ø Medical and Surgical
M Bursae and Ligaments
B Excision Definition: Cutting out or off, without replacement, a portion of a body part

Explanation: The qualifier DIAGNOSTIC is used to identify excision procedures that are biopsies

Body Part Character 4		Approach Character 5	Device Character 6	Qualifier Character 7
Ø Head and Neck Bursa and Ligament Alar ligament of axis Cervical interspinous ligament Cervical intertransverse ligament Cervical ligamentum flavum Interspinous ligament, cervical Intertransverse ligament, cervical Lateral temporomandibular ligament Ligamentum flavum, cervical Sphenomandibular ligament Stylomandibular ligament Transverse ligament of atlas **1 Shoulder Bursa and Ligament, Right** Acromioclavicular ligament Coracoacromial ligament Coracoclavicular ligament Coracohumeral ligament Costoclavicular ligament Glenohumeral ligament Interclavicular ligament Sternoclavicular ligament Subacromial bursa Transverse humeral ligament Transverse scapular ligament **2 Shoulder Bursa and Ligament, Left** **See** *1 Shoulder Bursa and Ligament, Right* **3 Elbow Bursa and Ligament, Right** Annular ligament Olecranon bursa Radial collateral ligament Ulnar collateral ligament **4 Elbow Bursa and Ligament, Left** **See** *3 Elbow Bursa and Ligament, Right* **5 Wrist Bursa and Ligament, Right** Palmar ulnocarpal ligament Radial collateral carpal ligament Radiocarpal ligament Radioulnar ligament Scapholunate ligament Ulnar collateral carpal ligament **6 Wrist Bursa and Ligament, Left** **See** *5 Wrist Bursa and Ligament, Right* **7 Hand Bursa and Ligament, Right** Carpometacarpal ligament Intercarpal ligament Interphalangeal ligament Lunotriquetral ligament Metacarpal ligament Metacarpophalangeal ligament Pisohamate ligament Pisometacarpal ligament Scaphotrapezium ligament **8 Hand Bursa and Ligament, Left** **See** *7 Hand Bursa and Ligament, Right* **9 Upper Extremity Bursa and Ligament, Right** **B Upper Extremity Bursa and Ligament, Left** **C Upper Spine Bursa and Ligament** Interspinous ligament, thoracic Intertransverse ligament, thoracic Ligamentum flavum, thoracic Supraspinous ligament	**D Lower Spine Bursa and Ligament** Iliolumbar ligament Interspinous ligament, lumbar Intertransverse ligament, lumbar Ligamentum flavum, lumbar Sacrococcygeal ligament Sacroiliac ligament Sacrospinous ligament Sacrotuberous ligament Supraspinous ligament **F Sternum Bursa and Ligament** Costoxiphoid ligament Sternocostal ligament **G Rib(s) Bursa and Ligament** Costotransverse ligament **H Abdomen Bursa and Ligament, Right** **J Abdomen Bursa and Ligament, Left** **K Perineum Bursa and Ligament** **L Hip Bursa and Ligament, Right** Iliofemoral ligament Ischiofemoral ligament Pubofemoral ligament Transverse acetabular ligament Trochanteric bursa **M Hip Bursa and Ligament, Left** **See** *L Hip Bursa and Ligament, Right* **N Knee Bursa and Ligament, Right** Anterior cruciate ligament (ACL) Lateral collateral ligament (LCL) Ligament of head of fibula Medial collateral ligament (MCL) Patellar ligament Popliteal ligament Posterior cruciate ligament (PCL) Prepatellar bursa **P Knee Bursa and Ligament, Left** **See** *N Knee Bursa and Ligament, Right* **Q Ankle Bursa and Ligament, Right** Calcaneofibular ligament Deltoid ligament Ligament of the lateral malleolus Talofibular ligament **R Ankle Bursa and Ligament, Left** **See** *Q Ankle Bursa and Ligament, Right* **S Foot Bursa and Ligament, Right** Calcaneocuboid ligament Cuneonavicular ligament Intercuneiform ligament Interphalangeal ligament Metatarsal ligament Metatarsophalangeal ligament Subtalar ligament Talocalcaneal ligament Talocalcaneonavicular ligament Tarsometatarsal ligament **T Foot Bursa and Ligament, Left** **See** *S Foot Bursa and Ligament, Right* **V Lower Extremity Bursa and Ligament, Right** **W Lower Extremity Bursa and Ligament, Left**	**Ø Open** **3 Percutaneous** **4 Percutaneous Endoscopic**	**Z No Device**	**X Diagnostic** **Z No Qualifier**

Non-OR ØMB[Ø,1,2,3,4,5,6,7,8,B,C,D,F,G,L,M,N,P,Q,R,S,T][Ø,3,4]ZX
Non-OR ØMB94ZX

Ø Medical and Surgical
M Bursae and Ligaments
C Extirpation Definition: Taking or cutting out solid matter from a body part

Explanation: The solid matter may be an abnormal byproduct of a biological function or a foreign body; it may be imbedded in a body part or in the lumen of a tubular body part. The solid matter may or may not have been previously broken into pieces.

Body Part Character 4	Approach Character 5	Device Character 6	Qualifier Character 7
Ø Head and Neck Bursa and Ligament Alar ligament of axis Cervical interspinous ligament Cervical intertransverse ligament Cervical ligamentum flavum Interspinous ligament, cervical Intertransverse ligament, cervical Lateral temporomandibular ligament Ligamentum flavum, cervical Sphenomandibular ligament Stylomandibular ligament Transverse ligament of atlas **1 Shoulder Bursa and Ligament, Right** Acromioclavicular ligament Coracoacromial ligament Coracoclavicular ligament Coracohumeral ligament Costoclavicular ligament Glenohumeral ligament Interclavicular ligament Sternoclavicular ligament Subacromial bursa Transverse humeral ligament Transverse scapular ligament **2 Shoulder Bursa and Ligament, Left** *See 1 Shoulder Bursa and Ligament, Right* **3 Elbow Bursa and Ligament, Right** Annular ligament Olecranon bursa Radial collateral ligament Ulnar collateral ligament **4 Elbow Bursa and Ligament, Left** *See 3 Elbow Bursa and Ligament, Right* **5 Wrist Bursa and Ligament, Right** Palmar ulnocarpal ligament Radial collateral carpal ligament Radiocarpal ligament Radioulnar ligament Scapholunate ligament Ulnar collateral carpal ligament **6 Wrist Bursa and Ligament, Left** *See 5 Wrist Bursa and Ligament, Right* **7 Hand Bursa and Ligament, Right** Carpometacarpal ligament Intercarpal ligament Interphalangeal ligament Lunotriquetral ligament Metacarpal ligament Metacarpophalangeal ligament Pisohamate ligament Pisometacarpal ligament Scaphotrapezium ligament **8 Hand Bursa and Ligament, Left** *See 7 Hand Bursa and Ligament, Right* **9 Upper Extremity Bursa and Ligament, Right** **B Upper Extremity Bursa and Ligament, Left** **C Upper Spine Bursa and Ligament** Interspinous ligament, thoracic Intertransverse ligament, thoracic Ligamentum flavum, thoracic Supraspinous ligament **D Lower Spine Bursa and Ligament** Iliolumbar ligament Interspinous ligament, lumbar Intertransverse ligament, lumbar Ligamentum flavum, lumbar Sacrococcygeal ligament Sacroiliac ligament Sacrospinous ligament Sacrotuberous ligament Supraspinous ligament **F Sternum Bursa and Ligament** Costoxiphoid ligament Sternocostal ligament **G Rib(s) Bursa and Ligament** Costotransverse ligament **H Abdomen Bursa and Ligament, Right** **J Abdomen Bursa and Ligament, Left** **K Perineum Bursa and Ligament** **L Hip Bursa and Ligament, Right** Iliofemoral ligament Ischiofemoral ligament Pubofemoral ligament Transverse acetabular ligament Trochanteric bursa **M Hip Bursa and Ligament, Left** *See L Hip Bursa and Ligament, Right* **N Knee Bursa and Ligament, Right** Anterior cruciate ligament (ACL) Lateral collateral ligament (LCL) Ligament of head of fibula Medial collateral ligament (MCL) Patellar ligament Popliteal ligament Posterior cruciate ligament (PCL) Prepatellar bursa **P Knee Bursa and Ligament, Left** *See N Knee Bursa and Ligament, Right* **Q Ankle Bursa and Ligament, Right** Calcaneofibular ligament Deltoid ligament Ligament of the lateral malleolus Talofibular ligament **R Ankle Bursa and Ligament, Left** *See Q Ankle Bursa and Ligament, Right* **S Foot Bursa and Ligament, Right** Calcaneocuboid ligament Cuneonavicular ligament Intercuneiform ligament Interphalangeal ligament Metatarsal ligament Metatarsophalangeal ligament Subtalar ligament Talocalcaneal ligament Talocalcaneonavicular ligament Tarsometatarsal ligament **T Foot Bursa and Ligament, Left** *See S Foot Bursa and Ligament, Right* **V Lower Extremity Bursa and Ligament, Right** **W Lower Extremity Bursa and Ligament, Left**	**Ø Open** **3 Percutaneous** **4 Percutaneous Endoscopic**	**Z No Device**	**Z No Qualifier**

Ø Medical and Surgical
M Bursae and Ligaments
D Extraction Definition: Pulling or stripping out or off all or a portion of a body part by the use of force

Explanation: The qualifier DIAGNOSTIC is used to identify extraction procedures that are biopsies

Body Part Character 4		Approach Character 5	Device Character 6	Qualifier Character 7
Ø Head and Neck Bursa and Ligament Alar ligament of axis Cervical interspinous ligament Cervical intertransverse ligament Cervical ligamentum flavum Interspinous ligament, cervical Intertransverse ligament, cervical Lateral temporomandibular ligament Ligamentum flavum, cervical Sphenomandibular ligament Stylomandibular ligament Transverse ligament of atlas **1 Shoulder Bursa and Ligament, Right** Acromioclavicular ligament Coracoacromial ligament Coracoclavicular ligament Coracohumeral ligament Costoclavicular ligament Glenohumeral ligament Interclavicular ligament Sternoclavicular ligament Subacromial bursa Transverse humeral ligament Transverse scapular ligament **2 Shoulder Bursa and Ligament, Left** *See 1 Shoulder Bursa and Ligament, Right* **3 Elbow Bursa and Ligament, Right** Annular ligament Olecranon bursa Radial collateral ligament Ulnar collateral ligament **4 Elbow Bursa and Ligament, Left** *See 3 Elbow Bursa and Ligament, Right* **5 Wrist Bursa and Ligament, Right** Palmar ulnocarpal ligament Radial collateral carpal ligament Radiocarpal ligament Radioulnar ligament Scapholunate ligament Ulnar collateral carpal ligament **6 Wrist Bursa and Ligament, Left** *See 5 Wrist Bursa and Ligament, Right* **7 Hand Bursa and Ligament, Right** Carpometacarpal ligament Intercarpal ligament Interphalangeal ligament Lunotriquetral ligament Metacarpal ligament Metacarpophalangeal ligament Pisohamate ligament Pisometacarpal ligament Scaphotrapezium ligament **8 Hand Bursa and Ligament, Left** *See 7 Hand Bursa and Ligament, Right* **9 Upper Extremity Bursa and Ligament, Right** **B Upper Extremity Bursa and Ligament, Left** **C Upper Spine Bursa and Ligament** Interspinous ligament, thoracic Intertransverse ligament, thoracic Ligamentum flavum, thoracic Supraspinous ligament	**D Lower Spine Bursa and Ligament** Iliolumbar ligament Interspinous ligament, lumbar Intertransverse ligament, lumbar Ligamentum flavum, lumbar Sacrococcygeal ligament Sacroiliac ligament Sacrospinous ligament Sacrotuberous ligament Supraspinous ligament **F Sternum Bursa and Ligament** Costoxiphoid ligament Sternocostal ligament **G Rib(s) Bursa and Ligament** Costotransverse ligament **H Abdomen Bursa and Ligament, Right** **J Abdomen Bursa and Ligament, Left** **K Perineum Bursa and Ligament** **L Hip Bursa and Ligament, Right** Iliofemoral ligament Ischiofemoral ligament Pubofemoral ligament Transverse acetabular ligament Trochanteric bursa **M Hip Bursa and Ligament, Left** *See L Hip Bursa and Ligament, Right* **N Knee Bursa and Ligament, Right** Anterior cruciate ligament (ACL) Lateral collateral ligament (LCL) Ligament of head of fibula Medial collateral ligament (MCL) Patellar ligament Popliteal ligament Posterior cruciate ligament (PCL) Prepatellar bursa **P Knee Bursa and Ligament, Left** *See N Knee Bursa and Ligament, Right* **Q Ankle Bursa and Ligament, Right** Calcaneofibular ligament Deltoid ligament Ligament of the lateral malleolus Talofibular ligament **R Ankle Bursa and Ligament, Left** *See Q Ankle Bursa and Ligament, Right* **S Foot Bursa and Ligament, Right** Calcaneocuboid ligament Cuneonavicular ligament Intercuneiform ligament Interphalangeal ligament Metatarsal ligament Metatarsophalangeal ligament Subtalar ligament Talocalcaneal ligament Talocalcaneonavicular ligament Tarsometatarsal ligament **T Foot Bursa and Ligament, Left** *See S Foot Bursa and Ligament, Right* **V Lower Extremity Bursa and Ligament, Right** **W Lower Extremity Bursa and Ligament, Left**	**Ø Open** **3 Percutaneous** **4 Percutaneous Endoscopic**	**Z No Device**	**Z No Qualifier**

Ø Medical and Surgical
M Bursae and Ligaments
H Insertion Definition: Putting in a nonbiological appliance that monitors, assists, performs, or prevents a physiological function but does not physically take the place of a body part

Explanation: None

Body Part Character 4	Approach Character 5	Device Character 6	Qualifier Character 7
X Upper Bursa and Ligament Y Lower Bursa and Ligament	Ø Open 3 Percutaneous 4 Percutaneous Endoscopic	Y Other Device	Z No Qualifier

Non-OR ØMH[X,Y][3,4]YZ

Ø Medical and Surgical
M Bursae and Ligaments
J Inspection Definition: Visually and/or manually exploring a body part

Explanation: Visual exploration may be performed with or without optical instrumentation. Manual exploration may be performed directly or through intervening body layers.

Body Part Character 4	Approach Character 5	Device Character 6	Qualifier Character 7
X Upper Bursa and Ligament Y Lower Bursa and Ligament	Ø Open 3 Percutaneous 4 Percutaneous Endoscopic X External	Z No Device	Z No Qualifier

Non-OR ØMJ[X,Y][3,X]ZZ

Ø Medical and Surgical
M Bursae and Ligaments
M Reattachment Definition: Putting back in or on all or a portion of a separated body part to its normal location or other suitable location
Explanation: Vascular circulation and nervous pathways may or may not be reestablished

Body Part Character 4		Approach Character 5	Device Character 6	Qualifier Character 7
Ø Head and Neck Bursa and Ligament Alar ligament of axis Cervical interspinous ligament Cervical intertransverse ligament Cervical ligamentum flavum Interspinous ligament, cervical Intertransverse ligament, cervical Lateral temporomandibular ligament Ligamentum flavum, cervical Sphenomandibular ligament Stylomandibular ligament Transverse ligament of atlas **1 Shoulder Bursa and Ligament, Right** Acromioclavicular ligament Coracoacromial ligament Coracoclavicular ligament Coracohumeral ligament Costoclavicular ligament Glenohumeral ligament Interclavicular ligament Sternoclavicular ligament Subacromial bursa Transverse humeral ligament Transverse scapular ligament **2 Shoulder Bursa and Ligament, Left** ***See*** *1 Shoulder Bursa and Ligament, Right* **3 Elbow Bursa and Ligament, Right** Annular ligament Olecranon bursa Radial collateral ligament Ulnar collateral ligament **4 Elbow Bursa and Ligament, Left** ***See*** *3 Elbow Bursa and Ligament, Right* **5 Wrist Bursa and Ligament, Right** Palmar ulnocarpal ligament Radial collateral carpal ligament Radiocarpal ligament Radioulnar ligament Scapholunate ligament Ulnar collateral carpal ligament **6 Wrist Bursa and Ligament, Left** ***See*** *5 Wrist Bursa and Ligament, Right* **7 Hand Bursa and Ligament, Right** Carpometacarpal ligament Intercarpal ligament Interphalangeal ligament Lunotriquetral ligament Metacarpal ligament Metacarpophalangeal ligament Pisohamate ligament Pisometacarpal ligament Scaphotrapezium ligament **8 Hand Bursa and Ligament, Left** ***See*** *7 Hand Bursa and Ligament, Right* **9 Upper Extremity Bursa and Ligament, Right** **B Upper Extremity Bursa and Ligament, Left** **C Upper Spine Bursa and Ligament** Interspinous ligament, thoracic Intertransverse ligament, thoracic Ligamentum flavum, thoracic Supraspinous ligament	**D Lower Spine Bursa and Ligament** Iliolumbar ligament Interspinous ligament, lumbar Intertransverse ligament, lumbar Ligamentum flavum, lumbar Sacrococcygeal ligament Sacroiliac ligament Sacrospinous ligament Sacrotuberous ligament Supraspinous ligament **F Sternum Bursa and Ligament** Costoxiphoid ligament Sternocostal ligament **G Rib(s) Bursa and Ligament** Costotransverse ligament **H Abdomen Bursa and Ligament, Right** **J Abdomen Bursa and Ligament, Left** **K Perineum Bursa and Ligament** **L Hip Bursa and Ligament, Right** Iliofemoral ligament Ischiofemoral ligament Pubofemoral ligament Transverse acetabular ligament Trochanteric bursa **M Hip Bursa and Ligament, Left** ***See*** *L Hip Bursa and Ligament, Right* **N Knee Bursa and Ligament, Right** Anterior cruciate ligament (ACL) Lateral collateral ligament (LCL) Ligament of head of fibula Medial collateral ligament (MCL) Patellar ligament Popliteal ligament Posterior cruciate ligament (PCL) Prepatellar bursa **P Knee Bursa and Ligament, Left** ***See*** *N Knee Bursa and Ligament, Right* **Q Ankle Bursa and Ligament, Right** Calcaneofibular ligament Deltoid ligament Ligament of the lateral malleolus Talofibular ligament **R Ankle Bursa and Ligament, Left** ***See*** *Q Ankle Bursa and Ligament, Right* **S Foot Bursa and Ligament, Right** Calcaneocuboid ligament Cuneonavicular ligament Intercuneiform ligament Interphalangeal ligament Metatarsal ligament Metatarsophalangeal ligament Subtalar ligament Talocalcaneal ligament Talocalcaneonavicular ligament Tarsometatarsal ligament **T Foot Bursa and Ligament, Left** ***See*** *S Foot Bursa and Ligament, Right* **V Lower Extremity Bursa and Ligament, Right** **W Lower Extremity Bursa and Ligament, Left**	**Ø Open** **4 Percutaneous Endoscopic**	**Z No Device**	**Z No Qualifier**

Ø Medical and Surgical
M Bursae and Ligaments
N Release Definition: Freeing a body part from an abnormal physical constraint by cutting or by the use of force
Explanation: Some of the restraining tissue may be taken out but none of the body part is taken out

Body Part Character 4	Approach Character 5	Device Character 6	Qualifier Character 7
Ø Head and Neck Bursa and Ligament Alar ligament of axis Cervical interspinous ligament Cervical intertransverse ligament Cervical ligamentum flavum Interspinous ligament, cervical Intertransverse ligament, cervical Lateral temporomandibular ligament Ligamentum flavum, cervical Sphenomandibular ligament Stylomandibular ligament Transverse ligament of atlas **1 Shoulder Bursa and Ligament, Right** Acromioclavicular ligament Coracoacromial ligament Coracoclavicular ligament Coracohumeral ligament Costoclavicular ligament Glenohumeral ligament Interclavicular ligament Sternoclavicular ligament Subacromial bursa Transverse humeral ligament Transverse scapular ligament **2 Shoulder Bursa and Ligament, Left** *See 1 Shoulder Bursa and Ligament, Right* **3 Elbow Bursa and Ligament, Right** Annular ligament Olecranon bursa Radial collateral ligament Ulnar collateral ligament **4 Elbow Bursa and Ligament, Left** *See 3 Elbow Bursa and Ligament, Right* **5 Wrist Bursa and Ligament, Right** Palmar ulnocarpal ligament Radial collateral carpal ligament Radiocarpal ligament Radioulnar ligament Scapholunate ligament Ulnar collateral carpal ligament **6 Wrist Bursa and Ligament, Left** *See 5 Wrist Bursa and Ligament, Right* **7 Hand Bursa and Ligament, Right** Carpometacarpal ligament Intercarpal ligament Interphalangeal ligament Lunotriquetral ligament Metacarpal ligament Metacarpophalangeal ligament Pisohamate ligament Pisometacarpal ligament Scaphotrapezium ligament **8 Hand Bursa and Ligament, Left** *See 7 Hand Bursa and Ligament, Right* **9 Upper Extremity Bursa and Ligament, Right** **B Upper Extremity Bursa and Ligament, Left** **C Upper Spine Bursa and Ligament** Interspinous ligament, thoracic Intertransverse ligament, thoracic Ligamentum flavum, thoracic Supraspinous ligament **D Lower Spine Bursa and Ligament** Iliolumbar ligament Interspinous ligament, lumbar Intertransverse ligament, lumbar Ligamentum flavum, lumbar Sacrococcygeal ligament Sacroiliac ligament Sacrospinous ligament Sacrotuberous ligament Supraspinous ligament **F Sternum Bursa and Ligament** Costoxiphoid ligament Sternocostal ligament **G Rib(s) Bursa and Ligament** Costotransverse ligament **H Abdomen Bursa and Ligament, Right** **J Abdomen Bursa and Ligament, Left** **K Perineum Bursa and Ligament** **L Hip Bursa and Ligament, Right** Iliofemoral ligament Ischiofemoral ligament Pubofemoral ligament Transverse acetabular ligament Trochanteric bursa **M Hip Bursa and Ligament, Left** *See L Hip Bursa and Ligament, Right* **N Knee Bursa and Ligament, Right** Anterior cruciate ligament (ACL) Lateral collateral ligament (LCL) Ligament of head of fibula Medial collateral ligament (MCL) Patellar ligament Popliteal ligament Posterior cruciate ligament (PCL) Prepatellar bursa **P Knee Bursa and Ligament, Left** *See N Knee Bursa and Ligament, Right* **Q Ankle Bursa and Ligament, Right** Calcaneofibular ligament Deltoid ligament Ligament of the lateral malleolus Talofibular ligament **R Ankle Bursa and Ligament, Left** *See Q Ankle Bursa and Ligament, Right* **S Foot Bursa and Ligament, Right** Calcaneocuboid ligament Cuneonavicular ligament Intercuneiform ligament Interphalangeal ligament Metatarsal ligament Metatarsophalangeal ligament Subtalar ligament Talocalcaneal ligament Talocalcaneonavicular ligament Tarsometatarsal ligament **T Foot Bursa and Ligament, Left** *See S Foot Bursa and Ligament, Right* **V Lower Extremity Bursa and Ligament, Right** **W Lower Extremity Bursa and Ligament, Left**	**Ø Open** **3 Percutaneous** **4 Percutaneous Endoscopic** **X External**	**Z No Device**	**Z No Qualifier**

Non-OR ØMN[Ø,1,2,3,4,5,6,7,8,9,B,C,D,F,G,H,J,K,L,M,N,P,Q,R,S,T,V,W]XZZ

Ø Medical and Surgical
M Bursae and Ligaments
P Removal Definition: Taking out or off a device from a body part

Explanation: If a device is taken out and a similar device put in without cutting or puncturing the skin or mucous membrane, the procedure is coded to the root operation CHANGE. Otherwise, the procedure for taking out a device is coded to the root operation REMOVAL.

Body Part Character 4	Approach Character 5	Device Character 6	Qualifier Character 7
X Upper Bursa and Ligament Y Lower Bursa and Ligament	Ø Open 3 Percutaneous 4 Percutaneous Endoscopic	Ø Drainage Device 7 Autologous Tissue Substitute J Synthetic Substitute K Nonautologous Tissue Substitute Y Other Device	Z No Qualifier
X Upper Bursa and Ligament Y Lower Bursa and Ligament	X External	Ø Drainage Device	Z No Qualifier

Non-OR ØMP[X,Y]3ØZ
Non-OR ØMP[X,Y][3,4]YZ
Non-OR ØMP[X,Y]XØZ

Ø Medical and Surgical
M Bursae and Ligaments
Q Repair Definition: Restoring, to the extent possible, a body part to its normal anatomic structure and function
Explanation: Used only when the method to accomplish the repair is not one of the other root operations

Body Part Character 4		Approach Character 5	Device Character 6	Qualifier Character 7
Ø Head and Neck Bursa and Ligament Alar ligament of axis Cervical interspinous ligament Cervical intertransverse ligament Cervical ligamentum flavum Interspinous ligament, cervical Intertransverse ligament, cervical Lateral temporomandibular ligament Ligamentum flavum, cervical Sphenomandibular ligament Stylomandibular ligament Transverse ligament of atlas **1 Shoulder Bursa and Ligament, Right** Acromioclavicular ligament Coracoacromial ligament Coracoclavicular ligament Coracohumeral ligament Costoclavicular ligament Glenohumeral ligament Interclavicular ligament Sternoclavicular ligament Subacromial bursa Transverse humeral ligament Transverse scapular ligament **2 Shoulder Bursa and Ligament, Left** ***See*** *1 Shoulder Bursa and Ligament, Right* **3 Elbow Bursa and Ligament, Right** Annular ligament Olecranon bursa Radial collateral ligament Ulnar collateral ligament **4 Elbow Bursa and Ligament, Left** ***See*** *3 Elbow Bursa and Ligament, Right* **5 Wrist Bursa and Ligament, Right** Palmar ulnocarpal ligament Radial collateral carpal ligament Radiocarpal ligament Radioulnar ligament Scapholunate ligament Ulnar collateral carpal ligament **6 Wrist Bursa and Ligament, Left** ***See*** *5 Wrist Bursa and Ligament, Right* **7 Hand Bursa and Ligament, Right** Carpometacarpal ligament Intercarpal ligament Interphalangeal ligament Lunotriquetral ligament Metacarpal ligament Metacarpophalangeal ligament Pisohamate ligament Pisometacarpal ligament Scaphotrapezium ligament **8 Hand Bursa and Ligament, Left** ***See*** *7 Hand Bursa and Ligament, Right* **9 Upper Extremity Bursa and Ligament, Right** **B Upper Extremity Bursa and Ligament, Left** **C Upper Spine Bursa and Ligament** Interspinous ligament, thoracic Intertransverse ligament, thoracic Ligamentum flavum, thoracic Supraspinous ligament	**D Lower Spine Bursa and Ligament** Iliolumbar ligament Interspinous ligament, lumbar Intertransverse ligament, lumbar Ligamentum flavum, lumbar Sacrococcygeal ligament Sacroiliac ligament Sacrospinous ligament Sacrotuberous ligament Supraspinous ligament **F Sternum Bursa and Ligament** Costoxiphoid ligament Sternocostal ligament **G Rib(s) Bursa and Ligament** Costotransverse ligament **H Abdomen Bursa and Ligament, Right** **J Abdomen Bursa and Ligament, Left** **K Perineum Bursa and Ligament** **L Hip Bursa and Ligament, Right** Iliofemoral ligament Ischiofemoral ligament Pubofemoral ligament Transverse acetabular ligament Trochanteric bursa **M Hip Bursa and Ligament, Left** ***See*** *L Hip Bursa and Ligament, Right* **N Knee Bursa and Ligament, Right** Anterior cruciate ligament (ACL) Lateral collateral ligament (LCL) Ligament of head of fibula Medial collateral ligament (MCL) Patellar ligament Popliteal ligament Posterior cruciate ligament (PCL) Prepatellar bursa **P Knee Bursa and Ligament, Left** ***See*** *N Knee Bursa and Ligament, Right* **Q Ankle Bursa and Ligament, Right** Calcaneofibular ligament Deltoid ligament Ligament of the lateral malleolus Talofibular ligament **R Ankle Bursa and Ligament, Left** ***See*** *Q Ankle Bursa and Ligament, Right* **S Foot Bursa and Ligament, Right** Calcaneocuboid ligament Cuneonavicular ligament Intercuneiform ligament Interphalangeal ligament Metatarsal ligament Metatarsophalangeal ligament Subtalar ligament Talocalcaneal ligament Talocalcaneonavicular ligament Tarsometatarsal ligament **T Foot Bursa and Ligament, Left** ***See*** *S Foot Bursa and Ligament, Right* **V Lower Extremity Bursa and Ligament, Right** **W Lower Extremity Bursa and Ligament, Left**	**Ø Open** **3 Percutaneous** **4 Percutaneous Endoscopic**	**Z No Device**	**Z No Qualifier**

Ø Medical and Surgical
M Bursae and Ligaments
R Replacement Definition: Putting in or on biological or synthetic material that physically takes the place and/or function of all or a portion of a body part

Explanation: The body part may have been taken out or replaced, or may be taken out, physically eradicated, or rendered nonfunctional during the REPLACEMENT procedure. A REMOVAL procedure is coded for taking out the device used in a previous replacement procedure.

Body Part Character 4	Approach Character 5	Device Character 6	Qualifier Character 7
Ø Head and Neck Bursa and Ligament Alar ligament of axis Cervical interspinous ligament Cervical intertransverse ligament Cervical ligamentum flavum Interspinous ligament, cervical Intertransverse ligament, cervical Lateral temporomandibular ligament Ligamentum flavum, cervical Sphenomandibular ligament Stylomandibular ligament Transverse ligament of atlas **1 Shoulder Bursa and Ligament, Right** Acromioclavicular ligament Coracoacromial ligament Coracoclavicular ligament Coracohumeral ligament Costoclavicular ligament Glenohumeral ligament Interclavicular ligament Sternoclavicular ligament Subacromial bursa Transverse humeral ligament Transverse scapular ligament **2 Shoulder Bursa and Ligament, Left** *See 1 Shoulder Bursa and Ligament, Right* **3 Elbow Bursa and Ligament, Right** Annular ligament Olecranon bursa Radial collateral ligament Ulnar collateral ligament **4 Elbow Bursa and Ligament, Left** *See 3 Elbow Bursa and Ligament, Right* **5 Wrist Bursa and Ligament, Right** Palmar ulnocarpal ligament Radial collateral carpal ligament Radiocarpal ligament Radioulnar ligament Scapholunate ligament Ulnar collateral carpal ligament **6 Wrist Bursa and Ligament, Left** *See 5 Wrist Bursa and Ligament, Right* **7 Hand Bursa and Ligament, Right** Carpometacarpal ligament Intercarpal ligament Interphalangeal ligament Lunotriquetral ligament Metacarpal ligament Metacarpophalangeal ligament Pisohamate ligament Pisometacarpal ligament Scaphotrapezium ligament **8 Hand Bursa and Ligament, Left** *See 7 Hand Bursa and Ligament, Right* **9 Upper Extremity Bursa and Ligament, Right** **B Upper Extremity Bursa and Ligament, Left** **C Upper Spine Bursa and Ligament** Interspinous ligament, thoracic Intertransverse ligament, thoracic Ligamentum flavum, thoracic Supraspinous ligament **D Lower Spine Bursa and Ligament** Iliolumbar ligament Interspinous ligament, lumbar Intertransverse ligament, lumbar Ligamentum flavum, lumbar Sacrococcygeal ligament Sacroiliac ligament Sacrospinous ligament Sacrotuberous ligament Supraspinous ligament **F Sternum Bursa and Ligament** Costoxiphoid ligament Sternocostal ligament **G Rib(s) Bursa and Ligament** Costotransverse ligament **H Abdomen Bursa and Ligament, Right** **J Abdomen Bursa and Ligament, Left** **K Perineum Bursa and Ligament** **L Hip Bursa and Ligament, Right** Iliofemoral ligament Ischiofemoral ligament Pubofemoral ligament Transverse acetabular ligament Trochanteric bursa **M Hip Bursa and Ligament, Left** *See L Hip Bursa and Ligament, Right* **N Knee Bursa and Ligament, Right** Anterior cruciate ligament (ACL) Lateral collateral ligament (LCL) Ligament of head of fibula Medial collateral ligament (MCL) Patellar ligament Popliteal ligament Posterior cruciate ligament (PCL) Prepatellar bursa **P Knee Bursa and Ligament, Left** *See N Knee Bursa and Ligament, Right* **Q Ankle Bursa and Ligament, Right** Calcaneofibular ligament Deltoid ligament Ligament of the lateral malleolus Talofibular ligament **R Ankle Bursa and Ligament, Left** *See Q Ankle Bursa and Ligament, Right* **S Foot Bursa and Ligament, Right** Calcaneocuboid ligament Cuneonavicular ligament Intercuneiform ligament Interphalangeal ligament Metatarsal ligament Metatarsophalangeal ligament Subtalar ligament Talocalcaneal ligament Talocalcaneonavicular ligament Tarsometatarsal ligament **T Foot Bursa and Ligament, Left** *See S Foot Bursa and Ligament, Right* **V Lower Extremity Bursa and Ligament, Right** **W Lower Extremity Bursa and Ligament, Left**	**Ø Open** **4 Percutaneous Endoscopic**	**7 Autologous Tissue Substitute** **J Synthetic Substitute** **K Nonautologous Tissue Substitute**	**Z No Qualifier**

Ø Medical and Surgical
M Bursae and Ligaments
S Reposition Definition: Moving to its normal location, or other suitable location, all or a portion of a body part

Explanation: The body part is moved to a new location from an abnormal location, or from a normal location where it is not functioning correctly. The body part may or may not be cut out or off to be moved to the new location.

Body Part Character 4		Approach Character 5	Device Character 6	Qualifier Character 7
Ø Head and Neck Bursa and Ligament Alar ligament of axis Cervical interspinous ligament Cervical intertransverse ligament Cervical ligamentum flavum Interspinous ligament, cervical Intertransverse ligament, cervical Lateral temporomandibular ligament Ligamentum flavum, cervical Sphenomandibular ligament Stylomandibular ligament Transverse ligament of atlas **1 Shoulder Bursa and Ligament, Right** Acromioclavicular ligament Coracoacromial ligament Coracoclavicular ligament Coracohumeral ligament Costoclavicular ligament Glenohumeral ligament Interclavicular ligament Sternoclavicular ligament Subacromial bursa Transverse humeral ligament Transverse scapular ligament **2 Shoulder Bursa and Ligament, Left** **See** *1 Shoulder Bursa and Ligament, Right* **3 Elbow Bursa and Ligament, Right** Annular ligament Olecranon bursa Radial collateral ligament Ulnar collateral ligament **4 Elbow Bursa and Ligament, Left** **See** *3 Elbow Bursa and Ligament, Right* **5 Wrist Bursa and Ligament, Right** Palmar ulnocarpal ligament Radial collateral carpal ligament Radiocarpal ligament Radioulnar ligament Scapholunate ligament Ulnar collateral carpal ligament **6 Wrist Bursa and Ligament, Left** **See** *5 Wrist Bursa and Ligament, Right* **7 Hand Bursa and Ligament, Right** Carpometacarpal ligament Intercarpal ligament Interphalangeal ligament Lunotriquetral ligament Metacarpal ligament Metacarpophalangeal ligament Pisohamate ligament Pisometacarpal ligament Scaphotrapezium ligament **8 Hand Bursa and Ligament, Left** **See** *7 Hand Bursa and Ligament, Right* **9 Upper Extremity Bursa and Ligament, Right** **B Upper Extremity Bursa and Ligament, Left** **C Upper Spine Bursa and Ligament** Interspinous ligament, thoracic Intertransverse ligament, thoracic Ligamentum flavum, thoracic Supraspinous ligament	**D Lower Spine Bursa and Ligament** Iliolumbar ligament Interspinous ligament, lumbar Intertransverse ligament, lumbar Ligamentum flavum, lumbar Sacrococcygeal ligament Sacroiliac ligament Sacrospinous ligament Sacrotuberous ligament Supraspinous ligament **F Sternum Bursa and Ligament** Costoxiphoid ligament Sternocostal ligament **G Rib(s) Bursa and Ligament** Costotransverse ligament **H Abdomen Bursa and Ligament, Right** **J Abdomen Bursa and Ligament, Left** **K Perineum Bursa and Ligament** **L Hip Bursa and Ligament, Right** Iliofemoral ligament Ischiofemoral ligament Pubofemoral ligament Transverse acetabular ligament Trochanteric bursa **M Hip Bursa and Ligament, Left** **See** *L Hip Bursa and Ligament, Right* **N Knee Bursa and Ligament, Right** Anterior cruciate ligament (ACL) Lateral collateral ligament (LCL) Ligament of head of fibula Medial collateral ligament (MCL) Patellar ligament Popliteal ligament Posterior cruciate ligament (PCL) Prepatellar bursa **P Knee Bursa and Ligament, Left** **See** *N Knee Bursa and Ligament, Right* **Q Ankle Bursa and Ligament, Right** Calcaneofibular ligament Deltoid ligament Ligament of the lateral malleolus Talofibular ligament **R Ankle Bursa and Ligament, Left** **See** *Q Ankle Bursa and Ligament, Right* **S Foot Bursa and Ligament, Right** Calcaneocuboid ligament Cuneonavicular ligament Intercuneiform ligament Interphalangeal ligament Metatarsal ligament Metatarsophalangeal ligament Subtalar ligament Talocalcaneal ligament Talocalcaneonavicular ligament Tarsometatarsal ligament **T Foot Bursa and Ligament, Left** **See** *S Foot Bursa and Ligament, Right* **V Lower Extremity Bursa and Ligament, Right** **W Lower Extremity Bursa and Ligament, Left**	**Ø Open** **4 Percutaneous Endoscopic**	**Z No Device**	**Z No Qualifier**

Ø Medical and Surgical
M Bursae and Ligaments
T Resection Definition: Cutting out or off, without replacement, all of a body part

Explanation: None

Body Part Character 4	Approach Character 5	Device Character 6	Qualifier Character 7
Ø Head and Neck Bursa and Ligament Alar ligament of axis Cervical interspinous ligament Cervical intertransverse ligament Cervical ligamentum flavum Interspinous ligament, cervical Intertransverse ligament, cervical Lateral temporomandibular ligament Ligamentum flavum, cervical Sphenomandibular ligament Stylomandibular ligament Transverse ligament of atlas **1 Shoulder Bursa and Ligament, Right** Acromioclavicular ligament Coracoacromial ligament Coracoclavicular ligament Coracohumeral ligament Costoclavicular ligament Glenohumeral ligament Interclavicular ligament Sternoclavicular ligament Subacromial bursa Transverse humeral ligament Transverse scapular ligament **2 Shoulder Bursa and Ligament, Left** **See** *1 Shoulder Bursa and Ligament, Right* **3 Elbow Bursa and Ligament, Right** Annular ligament Olecranon bursa Radial collateral ligament Ulnar collateral ligament **4 Elbow Bursa and Ligament, Left** **See** *3 Elbow Bursa and Ligament, Right* **5 Wrist Bursa and Ligament, Right** Palmar ulnocarpal ligament Radial collateral carpal ligament Radiocarpal ligament Radioulnar ligament Scapholunate ligament Ulnar collateral carpal ligament **6 Wrist Bursa and Ligament, Left** **See** *5 Wrist Bursa and Ligament, Right* **7 Hand Bursa and Ligament, Right** Carpometacarpal ligament Intercarpal ligament Interphalangeal ligament Lunotriquetral ligament Metacarpal ligament Metacarpophalangeal ligament Pisohamate ligament Pisometacarpal ligament Scaphotrapezium ligament **8 Hand Bursa and Ligament, Left** **See** *7 Hand Bursa and Ligament, Right* **9 Upper Extremity Bursa and Ligament, Right** **B Upper Extremity Bursa and Ligament, Left** **C Upper Spine Bursa and Ligament** Interspinous ligament, thoracic Intertransverse ligament, thoracic Ligamentum flavum, thoracic Supraspinous ligament **D Lower Spine Bursa and Ligament** Iliolumbar ligament Interspinous ligament, lumbar Intertransverse ligament, lumbar Ligamentum flavum, lumbar Sacrococcygeal ligament Sacroiliac ligament Sacrospinous ligament Sacrotuberous ligament Supraspinous ligament **F Sternum Bursa and Ligament** Costoxiphoid ligament Sternocostal ligament **G Rib(s) Bursa and Ligament** Costotransverse ligament **H Abdomen Bursa and Ligament, Right** **J Abdomen Bursa and Ligament, Left** **K Perineum Bursa and Ligament** **L Hip Bursa and Ligament, Right** Iliofemoral ligament Ischiofemoral ligament Pubofemoral ligament Transverse acetabular ligament Trochanteric bursa **M Hip Bursa and Ligament, Left** **See** *L Hip Bursa and Ligament, Right* **N Knee Bursa and Ligament, Right** Anterior cruciate ligament (ACL) Lateral collateral ligament (LCL) Ligament of head of fibula Medial collateral ligament (MCL) Patellar ligament Popliteal ligament Posterior cruciate ligament (PCL) Prepatellar bursa **P Knee Bursa and Ligament, Left** **See** *N Knee Bursa and Ligament, Right* **Q Ankle Bursa and Ligament, Right** Calcaneofibular ligament Deltoid ligament Ligament of the lateral malleolus Talofibular ligament **R Ankle Bursa and Ligament, Left** **See** *Q Ankle Bursa and Ligament, Right* **S Foot Bursa and Ligament, Right** Calcaneocuboid ligament Cuneonavicular ligament Intercuneiform ligament Interphalangeal ligament Metatarsal ligament Metatarsophalangeal ligament Subtalar ligament Talocalcaneal ligament Talocalcaneonavicular ligament Tarsometatarsal ligament **T Foot Bursa and Ligament, Left** **See** *S Foot Bursa and Ligament, Right* **V Lower Extremity Bursa and Ligament, Right** **W Lower Extremity Bursa and Ligament, Left**	**Ø Open** **4 Percutaneous Endoscopic**	**Z No Device**	**Z No Qualifier**

Ø Medical and Surgical
M Bursae and Ligaments
U Supplement Definition: Putting in or on biological or synthetic material that physically reinforces and/or augments the function of a portion of a body part

Explanation: The biological material is non-living, or is living and from the same individual. The body part may have been previously replaced, and the SUPPLEMENT procedure is performed to physically reinforce and/or augment the function of the replaced body part.

Body Part Character 4	Approach Character 5	Device Character 6	Qualifier Character 7
Ø Head and Neck Bursa and Ligament Alar ligament of axis Cervical interspinous ligament Cervical intertransverse ligament Cervical ligamentum flavum Interspinous ligament, cervical Intertransverse ligament, cervical Lateral temporomandibular ligament Ligamentum flavum, cervical Sphenomandibular ligament Stylomandibular ligament Transverse ligament of atlas **1 Shoulder Bursa and Ligament, Right** Acromioclavicular ligament Coracoacromial ligament Coracoclavicular ligament Coracohumeral ligament Costoclavicular ligament Glenohumeral ligament Interclavicular ligament Sternoclavicular ligament Subacromial bursa Transverse humeral ligament Transverse scapular ligament **2 Shoulder Bursa and Ligament, Left** ***See*** *1 Shoulder Bursa and Ligament, Right* **3 Elbow Bursa and Ligament, Right** Annular ligament Olecranon bursa Radial collateral ligament Ulnar collateral ligament **4 Elbow Bursa and Ligament, Left** ***See*** *3 Elbow Bursa and Ligament, Right* **5 Wrist Bursa and Ligament, Right** Palmar ulnocarpal ligament Radial collateral carpal ligament Radiocarpal ligament Radioulnar ligament Scapholunate ligament Ulnar collateral carpal ligament **6 Wrist Bursa and Ligament, Left** ***See*** *5 Wrist Bursa and Ligament, Right* **7 Hand Bursa and Ligament, Right** Carpometacarpal ligament Intercarpal ligament Interphalangeal ligament Lunotriquetral ligament Metacarpal ligament Metacarpophalangeal ligament Pisohamate ligament Pisometacarpal ligament Scaphotrapezium ligament **8 Hand Bursa and Ligament, Left** ***See*** *7 Hand Bursa and Ligament, Right* **9 Upper Extremity Bursa and Ligament, Right** **B Upper Extremity Bursa and Ligament, Left** **C Upper Spine Bursa and Ligament** Interspinous ligament, thoracic Intertransverse ligament, thoracic Ligamentum flavum, thoracic Supraspinous ligament **D Lower Spine Bursa and Ligament** Iliolumbar ligament Interspinous ligament, lumbar Intertransverse ligament, lumbar Ligamentum flavum, lumbar Sacrococcygeal ligament Sacroiliac ligament Sacrospinous ligament Sacrotuberous ligament Supraspinous ligament **F Sternum Bursa and Ligament** Costoxiphoid ligament Sternocostal ligament **G Rib(s) Bursa and Ligament** Costotransverse ligament **H Abdomen Bursa and Ligament, Right** **J Abdomen Bursa and Ligament, Left** **K Perineum Bursa and Ligament** **L Hip Bursa and Ligament, Right** Iliofemoral ligament Ischiofemoral ligament Pubofemoral ligament Transverse acetabular ligament Trochanteric bursa **M Hip Bursa and Ligament, Left** ***See*** *L Hip Bursa and Ligament, Right* **N Knee Bursa and Ligament, Right** Anterior cruciate ligament (ACL) Lateral collateral ligament (LCL) Ligament of head of fibula Medial collateral ligament (MCL) Patellar ligament Popliteal ligament Posterior cruciate ligament (PCL) Prepatellar bursa **P Knee Bursa and Ligament, Left** ***See*** *N Knee Bursa and Ligament, Right* **Q Ankle Bursa and Ligament, Right** Calcaneofibular ligament Deltoid ligament Ligament of the lateral malleolus Talofibular ligament **R Ankle Bursa and Ligament, Left** ***See*** *Q Ankle Bursa and Ligament, Right* **S Foot Bursa and Ligament, Right** Calcaneocuboid ligament Cuneonavicular ligament Intercuneiform ligament Interphalangeal ligament Metatarsal ligament Metatarsophalangeal ligament Subtalar ligament Talocalcaneal ligament Talocalcaneonavicular ligament Tarsometatarsal ligament **T Foot Bursa and Ligament, Left** ***See*** *S Foot Bursa and Ligament, Right* **V Lower Extremity Bursa and Ligament, Right** **W Lower Extremity Bursa and Ligament, Left**	**Ø Open** **4 Percutaneous Endoscopic**	**7 Autologous Tissue Substitute** **J Synthetic Substitute** **K Nonautologous Tissue Substitute**	**Z No Qualifier**

Ø Medical and Surgical
M Bursae and Ligaments
W Revision Definition: Correcting, to the extent possible, a portion of a malfunctioning device or the position of a displaced device

Explanation: Revision can include correcting a malfunctioning or displaced device by taking out or putting in components of the device such as a screw or pin

Body Part Character 4	Approach Character 5	Device Character 6	Qualifier Character 7
X Upper Bursa and Ligament Y Lower Bursa and Ligament	Ø Open 3 Percutaneous 4 Percutaneous Endoscopic	Ø Drainage Device 7 Autologous Tissue Substitute J Synthetic Substitute K Nonautologous Tissue Substitute Y Other Device	Z No Qualifier
X Upper Bursa and Ligament Y Lower Bursa and Ligament	X External	Ø Drainage Device 7 Autologous Tissue Substitute J Synthetic Substitute K Nonautologous Tissue Substitute	Z No Qualifier

Non-OR ØMW[X,Y][3,4]YZ
Non-OR ØMW[X,Y]X[Ø,7,J,K]Z

Ø Medical and Surgical
M Bursae and Ligaments
X Transfer Definition: Moving, without taking out, all or a portion of a body part to another location to take over the function of all or a portion of a body part
Explanation: The body part transferred remains connected to its vascular and nervous supply

Body Part Character 4	Approach Character 5	Device Character 6	Qualifier Character 7
Ø Head and Neck Bursa and Ligament Alar ligament of axis Cervical interspinous ligament Cervical intertransverse ligament Cervical ligamentum flavum Interspinous ligament, cervical Intertransverse ligament, cervical Lateral temporomandibular ligament Ligamentum flavum, cervical Sphenomandibular ligament Stylomandibular ligament Transverse ligament of atlas **1 Shoulder Bursa and Ligament, Right** Acromioclavicular ligament Coracoacromial ligament Coracoclavicular ligament Coracohumeral ligament Costoclavicular ligament Glenohumeral ligament Interclavicular ligament Sternoclavicular ligament Subacromial bursa Transverse humeral ligament Transverse scapular ligament **2 Shoulder Bursa and Ligament, Left** *See 1 Shoulder Bursa and Ligament, Right* **3 Elbow Bursa and Ligament, Right** Annular ligament Olecranon bursa Radial collateral ligament Ulnar collateral ligament **4 Elbow Bursa and Ligament, Left** *See 3 Elbow Bursa and Ligament, Right* **5 Wrist Bursa and Ligament, Right** Palmar ulnocarpal ligament Radial collateral carpal ligament Radiocarpal ligament Radioulnar ligament Scapholunate ligament Ulnar collateral carpal ligament **6 Wrist Bursa and Ligament, Left** *See 5 Wrist Bursa and Ligament, Right* **7 Hand Bursa and Ligament, Right** Carpometacarpal ligament Intercarpal ligament Interphalangeal ligament Lunotriquetral ligament Metacarpal ligament Metacarpophalangeal ligament Pisohamate ligament Pisometacarpal ligament Scaphotrapezium ligament **8 Hand Bursa and Ligament, Left** *See 7 Hand Bursa and Ligament, Right* **9 Upper Extremity Bursa and Ligament, Right** **B Upper Extremity Bursa and Ligament, Left** **C Upper Spine Bursa and Ligament** Interspinous ligament, thoracic Intertransverse ligament, thoracic Ligamentum flavum, thoracic Supraspinous ligament **D Lower Spine Bursa and Ligament** Iliolumbar ligament Interspinous ligament, lumbar Intertransverse ligament, lumbar Ligamentum flavum, lumbar Sacrococcygeal ligament Sacroiliac ligament Sacrospinous ligament Sacrotuberous ligament Supraspinous ligament **F Sternum Bursa and Ligament** Costoxiphoid ligament Sternocostal ligament **G Rib(s) Bursa and Ligament** Costotransverse ligament **H Abdomen Bursa and Ligament, Right** **J Abdomen Bursa and Ligament, Left** **K Perineum Bursa and Ligament** **L Hip Bursa and Ligament, Right** Iliofemoral ligament Ischiofemoral ligament Pubofemoral ligament Transverse acetabular ligament Trochanteric bursa **M Hip Bursa and Ligament, Left** *See L Hip Bursa and Ligament, Right* **N Knee Bursa and Ligament, Right** Anterior cruciate ligament (ACL) Lateral collateral ligament (LCL) Ligament of head of fibula Medial collateral ligament (MCL) Patellar ligament Popliteal ligament Posterior cruciate ligament (PCL) Prepatellar bursa **P Knee Bursa and Ligament, Left** *See N Knee Bursa and Ligament, Right* **Q Ankle Bursa and Ligament, Right** Calcaneofibular ligament Deltoid ligament Ligament of the lateral malleolus Talofibular ligament **R Ankle Bursa and Ligament, Left** *See Q Ankle Bursa and Ligament, Right* **S Foot Bursa and Ligament, Right** Calcaneocuboid ligament Cuneonavicular ligament Intercuneiform ligament Interphalangeal ligament Metatarsal ligament Metatarsophalangeal ligament Subtalar ligament Talocalcaneal ligament Talocalcaneonavicular ligament Tarsometatarsal ligament **T Foot Bursa and Ligament, Left** *See S Foot Bursa and Ligament, Right* **V Lower Extremity Bursa and Ligament, Right** **W Lower Extremity Bursa and Ligament, Left**	**Ø Open** **4 Percutaneous Endoscopic**	**Z No Device**	**Z No Qualifier**

Head and Facial Bones ØN2–ØNW

Character Meanings

This Character Meaning table is provided as a guide to assist the user in the identification of character members that may be found in this section of code tables. It **SHOULD NOT** be used to build a PCS code.

Operation–Character 3	Body Part–Character 4	Approach–Character 5	Device–Character 6	Qualifier–Character 7
2 Change	Ø Skull	Ø Open	Ø Drainage Device	X Diagnostic
5 Destruction	1 Frontal Bone	3 Percutaneous	3 Infusion Device	Z No Qualifier
8 Division	3 Parietal Bone, Right	4 Percutaneous Endoscopic	4 Internal Fixation Device	
9 Drainage	4 Parietal Bone, Left	X External	5 External Fixation Device	
B Excision	5 Temporal Bone, Right		7 Autologous Tissue Substitute	
C Extirpation	6 Temporal Bone, Left		J Synthetic Substitute	
D Extraction	7 Occipital Bone		K Nonautologous Tissue Substitute	
H Insertion	B Nasal Bone		M Bone Growth Stimulator	
J Inspection	C Sphenoid Bone		N Neurostimulator Generator	
N Release	F Ethmoid Bone, Right		S Hearing Device	
P Removal	G Ethmoid Bone, Left		Y Other Device	
Q Repair	H Lacrimal Bone, Right		Z No Device	
R Replacement	J Lacrimal Bone, Left			
S Reposition	K Palatine Bone, Right			
T Resection	L Palatine Bone, Left			
U Supplement	M Zygomatic Bone, Right			
W Revision	N Zygomatic Bone, Left			
	P Orbit, Right			
	Q Orbit, Left			
	R Maxilla			
	T Mandible, Right			
	V Mandible, Left			
	W Facial Bone			
	X Hyoid Bone			

AHA Coding Clinic for table ØNB
2021, 1Q, 21 Maxillectomy with reconstruction of maxilla
2017, 1Q, 20 Preparatory nasal adhesion repair before definitive cleft palate repair
2015, 3Q, 3-8 Excisional and nonexcisional debridement
2015, 2Q, 12 Orbital exenteration

AHA Coding Clinic for table ØND
2017, 4Q, 41 Extraction procedures

AHA Coding Clinic for table ØNH
2015, 3Q, 13 Nonexcisional debridement of cranial wound with removal and replacement of hardware

AHA Coding Clinic for table ØNP
2015, 3Q, 13 Nonexcisional debridement of cranial wound with removal and replacement of hardware

AHA Coding Clinic for table ØNQ
2016, 3Q, 29 Closure of bilateral alveolar clefts

AHA Coding Clinic for table ØNR
2021, 1Q, 21 Maxillectomy with reconstruction of maxilla
2017, 3Q, 17 Resection of schwannoma and placement of DuraGen and Lorenz cranial plating system
2017, 3Q, 22 Replacement of native skull bone flap
2017, 1Q, 23 Reconstruction of mandible using titanium and bone
2014, 3Q, 7 Hemi-cranioplasty for repair of cranial defect

AHA Coding Clinic for table ØNS
2017, 3Q, 22 Replacement of native skull bone flap
2017, 1Q, 20 Preparatory nasal adhesion repair before definitive cleft palate repair
2016, 2Q, 30 Clipping (occlusion) of cerebral artery, decompressive craniectomy and storage of bone flap in abdominal wall
2015, 3Q, 17 Craniosynostosis with cranial vault reconstruction
2015, 3Q, 27 Moyamoya disease and hemispheric pial synagiosis with craniotomy
2014, 3Q, 23 Le Fort I osteotomy
2013, 3Q, 24 Distraction osteogenesis
2013, 3Q, 25 Fracture of frontal bone with repair and coagulation for hemostasis

AHA Coding Clinic for table ØNU
2016, 3Q, 29 Closure of bilateral alveolar clefts
2013, 3Q, 24 Distraction osteogenesis

Head and Facial Bones

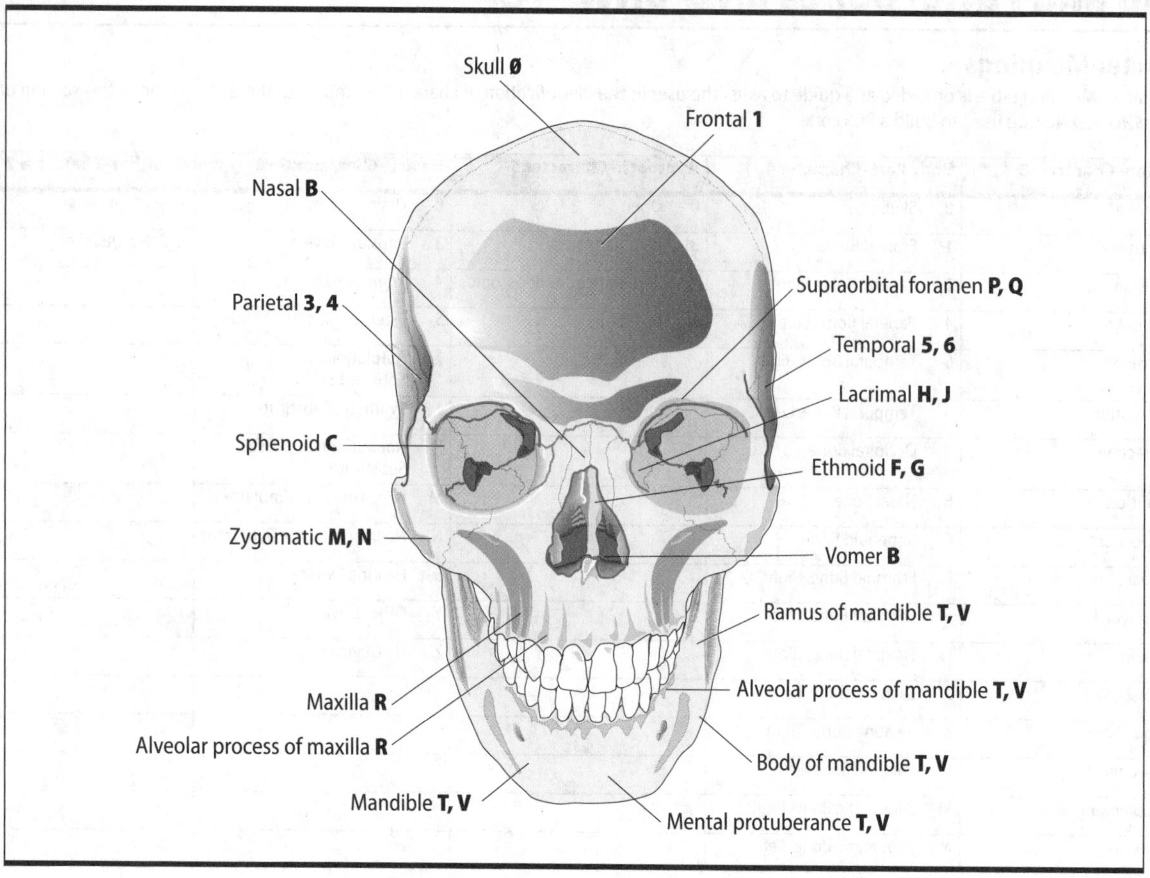

Skull Bones

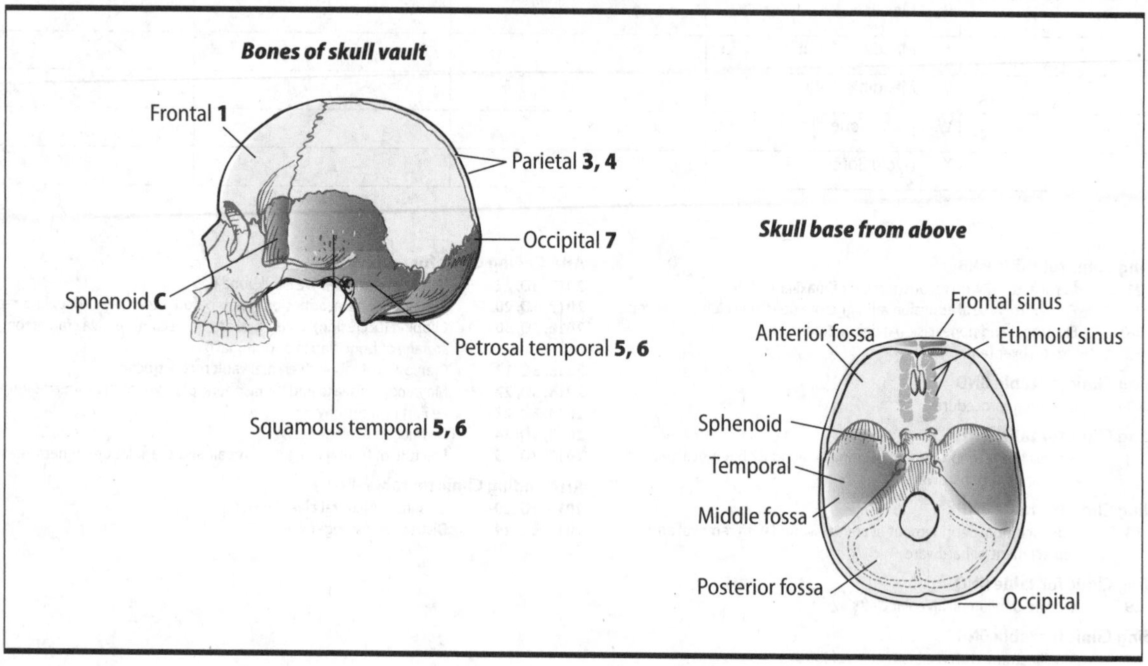

Ø Medical and Surgical
N Head and Facial Bones
2 Change Definition: Taking out or off a device from a body part and putting back an identical or similar device in or on the same body part without cutting or puncturing the skin or a mucous membrane

Explanation: All CHANGE procedures are coded using the approach EXTERNAL

Body Part Character 4	Approach Character 5	Device Character 6	Qualifier Character 7
Ø Skull **B** Nasal Bone Vomer of nasal septum **W** Facial Bone	**X** External	**Ø** Drainage Device **Y** Other Device	**Z** No Qualifier

Non-OR All body part, approach, device, and qualifier values

Ø Medical and Surgical
N Head and Facial Bones
5 Destruction Definition: Physical eradication of all or a portion of a body part by the direct use of energy, force, or a destructive agent

Explanation: None of the body part is physically taken out

Body Part Character 4	Approach Character 5	Device Character 6	Qualifier Character 7
Ø Skull **1 Frontal Bone** Zygomatic process of frontal bone **3 Parietal Bone, Right** **4 Parietal Bone, Left** **5 Temporal Bone, Right** Mastoid process Petrous part of temporal bone Tympanic part of temporal bone Zygomatic process of temporal bone **6 Temporal Bone, Left** *See 5 Temporal Bone, Right* **7 Occipital Bone** Foramen magnum **B Nasal Bone** Vomer of nasal septum **C Sphenoid Bone** Greater wing Lesser wing Optic foramen Pterygoid process Sella turcica **F Ethmoid Bone, Right** Cribriform plate **G Ethmoid Bone, Left** *See F Ethmoid Bone, Right* **H Lacrimal Bone, Right** **J Lacrimal Bone, Left** **K Palatine Bone, Right** **L Palatine Bone, Left** **M Zygomatic Bone, Right** **N Zygomatic Bone, Left** **P Orbit, Right** Bony orbit Orbital portion of ethmoid bone Orbital portion of frontal bone Orbital portion of lacrimal bone Orbital portion of maxilla Orbital portion of palatine bone Orbital portion of sphenoid bone Orbital portion of zygomatic bone **Q Orbit, Left** *See P Orbit, Right* **R Maxilla** Alveolar process of maxilla **T Mandible, Right** Alveolar process of mandible Condyloid process Mandibular notch Mental foramen **V Mandible, Left** *See T Mandible, Right* **X Hyoid Bone**	**Ø Open** **3 Percutaneous** **4 Percutaneous Endoscopic**	**Z** No Device	**Z** No Qualifier

Ø Medical and Surgical
N Head and Facial Bones
8 Division Definition: Cutting into a body part, without draining fluids and/or gases from the body part, in order to separate or transect a body part
Explanation: All or a portion of the body part is separated into two or more portions

Body Part Character 4	Approach Character 5	Device Character 6	Qualifier Character 7
Ø Skull **1 Frontal Bone** Zygomatic process of frontal bone **3 Parietal Bone, Right** **4 Parietal Bone, Left** **5 Temporal Bone, Right** Mastoid process Petrous part of temporal bone Tympanic part of temporal bone Zygomatic process of temporal bone **6 Temporal Bone, Left** *See 5 Temporal Bone, Right* **7 Occipital Bone** Foramen magnum **B Nasal Bone** Vomer of nasal septum **C Sphenoid Bone** Greater wing Lesser wing Optic foramen Pterygoid process Sella turcica **F Ethmoid Bone, Right** Cribriform plate **G Ethmoid Bone, Left** *See F Ethmoid Bone, Right* **H Lacrimal Bone, Right** **J Lacrimal Bone, Left** **K Palatine Bone, Right** **L Palatine Bone, Left** **M Zygomatic Bone, Right** **N Zygomatic Bone, Left** **P Orbit, Right** Bony orbit Orbital portion of ethmoid bone Orbital portion of frontal bone Orbital portion of lacrimal bone Orbital portion of maxilla Orbital portion of palatine bone Orbital portion of sphenoid bone Orbital portion of zygomatic bone **Q Orbit, Left** *See P Orbit, Right* **R Maxilla** Alveolar process of maxilla **T Mandible, Right** Alveolar process of mandible Condyloid process Mandibular notch Mental foramen **V Mandible, Left** *See T Mandible, Right* **X Hyoid Bone**	**Ø Open** **3 Percutaneous** **4 Percutaneous Endoscopic**	**Z No Device**	**Z No Qualifier**

Non-OR ØN8B[Ø,3,4]ZZ

Ø Medical and Surgical
N Head and Facial Bones
9 Drainage Definition: Taking or letting out fluids and/or gases from a body part
Explanation: The qualifier DIAGNOSTIC is used to identify drainage procedures that are biopsies

Body Part Character 4	Approach Character 5	Device Character 6	Qualifier Character 7
Ø Skull **1 Frontal Bone** Zygomatic process of frontal bone **3 Parietal Bone, Right** **4 Parietal Bone, Left** **5 Temporal Bone, Right** Mastoid process Petrous part of temporal bone Tympanic part of temporal bone Zygomatic process of temporal bone **6 Temporal Bone, Left** *See 5 Temporal Bone, Right* **7 Occipital Bone** Foramen magnum **B Nasal Bone** Vomer of nasal septum **C Sphenoid Bone** Greater wing Lesser wing Optic foramen Pterygoid process Sella turcica **F Ethmoid Bone, Right** Cribriform plate **G Ethmoid Bone, Left** *See F Ethmoid Bone, Right* **H Lacrimal Bone, Right** **J Lacrimal Bone, Left** **K Palatine Bone, Right** **L Palatine Bone, Left** **M Zygomatic Bone, Right** **N Zygomatic Bone, Left** **P Orbit, Right** Bony orbit Orbital portion of ethmoid bone Orbital portion of frontal bone Orbital portion of lacrimal bone Orbital portion of maxilla Orbital portion of palatine bone Orbital portion of sphenoid bone Orbital portion of zygomatic bone **Q Orbit, Left** *See P Orbit, Right* **R Maxilla** Alveolar process of maxilla **T Mandible, Right** Alveolar process of mandible Condyloid process Mandibular notch Mental foramen **V Mandible, Left** *See T Mandible, Right* **X Hyoid Bone**	**Ø Open** **3 Percutaneous** **4 Percutaneous Endoscopic**	**Ø Drainage Device**	**Z No Qualifier**

Non-OR ØN9[Ø,1,3,4,5,6,7,C,F,G,H,J,K,L,M,N,P,Q,X]3ØZ
Non-OR ØN9[B,R,T,V][Ø,3,4]ØZ

ØN9 Continued on next page

ØN9 Continued

Ø Medical and Surgical
N Head and Facial Bones
9 Drainage Definition: Taking or letting out fluids and/or gases from a body part
Explanation: The qualifier DIAGNOSTIC is used to identify drainage procedures that are biopsies

Body Part Character 4	Approach Character 5	Device Character 6	Qualifier Character 7
Ø Skull **1** Frontal Bone Zygomatic process of frontal bone **3** Parietal Bone, Right **4** Parietal Bone, Left **5** Temporal Bone, Right Mastoid process Petrous part of temporal bone Tympanic part of temporal bone Zygomatic process of temporal bone **6** Temporal Bone, Left *See 5 Temporal Bone, Right* **7** Occipital Bone Foramen magnum **B** Nasal Bone Vomer of nasal septum **C** Sphenoid Bone Greater wing Lesser wing Optic foramen Pterygoid process Sella turcica **F** Ethmoid Bone, Right Cribriform plate **G** Ethmoid Bone, Left *See F Ethmoid Bone, Right* **H** Lacrimal Bone, Right **J** Lacrimal Bone, Left **K** Palatine Bone, Right **L** Palatine Bone, Left **M** Zygomatic Bone, Right **N** Zygomatic Bone, Left **P** Orbit, Right Bony orbit Orbital portion of ethmoid bone Orbital portion of frontal bone Orbital portion of lacrimal bone Orbital portion of maxilla Orbital portion of palatine bone Orbital portion of sphenoid bone Orbital portion of zygomatic bone **Q** Orbit, Left *See P Orbit, Right* **R** Maxilla Alveolar process of maxilla **T** Mandible, Right Alveolar process of mandible Condyloid process Mandibular notch Mental foramen **V** Mandible, Left *See T Mandible, Right* **X** Hyoid Bone	**Ø** Open **3** Percutaneous **4** Percutaneous Endoscopic	**Z** No Device	**X** Diagnostic **Z** No Qualifier

Non-OR ØN9[Ø,1,3,4,5,6,7,C,F,G,H,J,K,L,M,N,P,Q,X]3ZZ
Non-OR ØN9B[Ø,3,4]Z[X,Z]
Non-OR ØN9[R,T,V][Ø,3,4]ZZ

Ø Medical and Surgical
N Head and Facial Bones
B Excision Definition: Cutting out or off, without replacement, a portion of a body part
Explanation: The qualifier DIAGNOSTIC is used to identify excision procedures that are biopsies

Body Part Character 4	Approach Character 5	Device Character 6	Qualifier Character 7
Ø Skull **1 Frontal Bone** Zygomatic process of frontal bone **3 Parietal Bone, Right** **4 Parietal Bone, Left** **5 Temporal Bone, Right** Mastoid process Petrous part of temporal bone Tympanic part of temporal bone Zygomatic process of temporal bone **6 Temporal Bone, Left** *See 5 Temporal Bone, Right* **7 Occipital Bone** Foramen magnum **B Nasal Bone** Vomer of nasal septum **C Sphenoid Bone** Greater wing Lesser wing Optic foramen Pterygoid process Sella turcica **F Ethmoid Bone, Right** Cribriform plate **G Ethmoid Bone, Left** *See F Ethmoid Bone, Right* **H Lacrimal Bone, Right** **J Lacrimal Bone, Left** **K Palatine Bone, Right** **L Palatine Bone, Left** **M Zygomatic Bone, Right** **N Zygomatic Bone, Left** **P Orbit, Right** Bony orbit Orbital portion of ethmoid bone Orbital portion of frontal bone Orbital portion of lacrimal bone Orbital portion of maxilla Orbital portion of palatine bone Orbital portion of sphenoid bone Orbital portion of zygomatic bone **Q Orbit, Left** *See P Orbit, Right* **R Maxilla** Alveolar process of maxilla **T Mandible, Right** Alveolar process of mandible Condyloid process Mandibular notch Mental foramen **V Mandible, Left** *See T Mandible, Right* **X Hyoid Bone**	**Ø Open** **3 Percutaneous** **4 Percutaneous Endoscopic**	**Z** No Device	**X** Diagnostic **Z** No Qualifier

Non-OR ØNB[B,R,T,V][Ø,3,4]ZX

Ø Medical and Surgical
N Head and Facial Bones
C Extirpation Definition: Taking or cutting out solid matter from a body part

Explanation: The solid matter may be an abnormal byproduct of a biological function or a foreign body; it may be imbedded in a body part or in the lumen of a tubular body part. The solid matter may or may not have been previously broken into pieces.

Body Part Character 4	Approach Character 5	Device Character 6	Qualifier Character 7
1 Frontal Bone Zygomatic process of frontal bone **3 Parietal Bone, Right** **4 Parietal Bone, Left** **5 Temporal Bone, Right** Mastoid process Petrous part of temporal bone Tympanic part of temporal bone Zygomatic process of temporal bone **6 Temporal Bone, Left** ***See*** *5 Temporal Bone, Right* **7 Occipital Bone** Foramen magnum **B Nasal Bone** Vomer of nasal septum **C Sphenoid Bone** Greater wing Lesser wing Optic foramen Pterygoid process Sella turcica **F Ethmoid Bone, Right** Cribriform plate **G Ethmoid Bone, Left** ***See*** *F Ethmoid Bone, Right* **H Lacrimal Bone, Right** **J Lacrimal Bone, Left** **K Palatine Bone, Right** **L Palatine Bone, Left** **M Zygomatic Bone, Right** **N Zygomatic Bone, Left** **P Orbit, Right** Bony orbit Orbital portion of ethmoid bone Orbital portion of frontal bone Orbital portion of lacrimal bone Orbital portion of maxilla Orbital portion of palatine bone Orbital portion of sphenoid bone Orbital portion of zygomatic bone **Q Orbit, Left** ***See*** *P Orbit, Right* **R Maxilla** Alveolar process of maxilla **T Mandible, Right** Alveolar process of mandible Condyloid process Mandibular notch Mental foramen **V Mandible, Left** ***See*** *T Mandible, Right* **X Hyoid Bone**	**Ø Open** **3 Percutaneous** **4 Percutaneous Endoscopic**	**Z No Device**	**Z No Qualifier**

Non-OR ØNC[B,R,T,V][Ø,3,4]ZZ

Ø Medical and Surgical
N Head and Facial Bones
D Extraction Definition: Pulling or stripping out or off all or a portion of a body part by the use of force
Explanation: The qualifier DIAGNOSTIC is used to identify extraction procedures that are biopsies

Body Part Character 4	Approach Character 5	Device Character 6	Qualifier Character 7
Ø Skull **1 Frontal Bone** Zygomatic process of frontal bone **3 Parietal Bone, Right** **4 Parietal Bone, Left** **5 Temporal Bone, Right** Mastoid process Petrous part of temporal bone Tympanic part of temporal bone Zygomatic process of temporal bone **6 Temporal Bone, Left** *See 5 Temporal Bone, Right* **7 Occipital Bone** Foramen magnum **B Nasal Bone** Vomer of nasal septum **C Sphenoid Bone** Greater wing Lesser wing Optic foramen Pterygoid process Sella turcica **F Ethmoid Bone, Right** Cribriform plate **G Ethmoid Bone, Left** *See F Ethmoid Bone, Right* **H Lacrimal Bone, Right** **J Lacrimal Bone, Left** **K Palatine Bone, Right** **L Palatine Bone, Left** **M Zygomatic Bone, Right** **N Zygomatic Bone, Left** **P Orbit, Right** Bony orbit Orbital portion of ethmoid bone Orbital portion of frontal bone Orbital portion of lacrimal bone Orbital portion of maxilla Orbital portion of palatine bone Orbital portion of sphenoid bone Orbital portion of zygomatic bone **Q Orbit, Left** *See P Orbit, Right* **R Maxilla** Alveolar process of maxilla **T Mandible, Right** Alveolar process of mandible Condyloid process Mandibular notch Mental foramen **V Mandible, Left** *See T Mandible, Right* **X Hyoid Bone**	**Ø Open**	**Z No Device**	**Z No Qualifier**

Ø Medical and Surgical
N Head and Facial Bones
H Insertion Definition: Putting in a nonbiological appliance that monitors, assists, performs, or prevents a physiological function but does not physically take the place of a body part

Explanation: None

Body Part Character 4	Approach Character 5	Device Character 6	Qualifier Character 7
Ø Skull ⊞	**Ø Open**	3 Infusion Device **4 Internal Fixation Device** **5 External Fixation Device** **M Bone Growth Stimulator** **N Neurostimulator Generator**	**Z No Qualifier**
Ø Skull	**3 Percutaneous** **4 Percutaneous Endoscopic**	3 Infusion Device **4 Internal Fixation Device** **5 External Fixation Device** **M Bone Growth Stimulator**	**Z No Qualifier**
1 Frontal Bone Zygomatic process of frontal bone **3 Parietal Bone, Right** **4 Parietal Bone, Left** **7 Occipital Bone** Foramen magnum **C Sphenoid Bone** Greater wing Lesser wing Optic foramen Pterygoid process Sella turcica **F Ethmoid Bone, Right** Cribriform plate **G Ethmoid Bone, Left** *See F Ethmoid Bone, Right* **H Lacrimal Bone, Right** **J Lacrimal Bone, Left** **K Palatine Bone, Right** **L Palatine Bone, Left** **M Zygomatic Bone, Right** **N Zygomatic Bone, Left** **P Orbit, Right** Bony orbit Orbital portion of ethmoid bone Orbital portion of frontal bone Orbital portion of lacrimal bone Orbital portion of maxilla Orbital portion of palatine bone Orbital portion of sphenoid bone Orbital portion of zygomatic bone **Q Orbit, Left** *See P Orbit, Right* **X Hyoid Bone**	**Ø Open** **3 Percutaneous** **4 Percutaneous Endoscopic**	**4 Internal Fixation Device**	**Z No Qualifier**
5 Temporal Bone, Right Mastoid process Petrous part of temporal bone Tympanic part of temporal bone Zygomatic process of temporal bone **6 Temporal Bone, Left** *See 5 Temporal Bone, Right*	**Ø Open** **3 Percutaneous** **4 Percutaneous Endoscopic**	**4 Internal Fixation Device** **S Hearing Device**	**Z No Qualifier**
B Nasal Bone Vomer of nasal septum	**Ø Open** **3 Percutaneous** **4 Percutaneous Endoscopic**	**4 Internal Fixation Device** **M Bone Growth Stimulator**	**Z No Qualifier**
R Maxilla Alveolar process of maxilla **T Mandible, Right** Alveolar process of mandible Condyloid process Mandibular notch Mental foramen **V Mandible, Left** *See T Mandible, Right*	**Ø Open** **3 Percutaneous** **4 Percutaneous Endoscopic**	**4 Internal Fixation Device** **5 External Fixation Device**	**Z No Qualifier**
W Facial Bone	**Ø Open** **3 Percutaneous** **4 Percutaneous Endoscopic**	**M Bone Growth Stimulator**	**Z No Qualifier**

Non-OR ØNHØØ5Z
Non-OR ØNHØ[3,4]5Z
Non-OR ØNHB[Ø,3,4][4,M]Z

See Appendix L for Procedure Combinations
⊞ ØNHØØNZ

Ø Medical and Surgical
N Head and Facial Bones
J Inspection Definition: Visually and/or manually exploring a body part

Explanation: Visual exploration may be performed with or without optical instrumentation. Manual exploration may be performed directly or through intervening body layers.

Body Part Character 4	Approach Character 5	Device Character 6	Qualifier Character 7
Ø Skull B Nasal Bone Vomer of nasal septum W Facial Bone	Ø Open 3 Percutaneous 4 Percutaneous Endoscopic X External	Z No Device	Z No Qualifier

Non-OR ØNJ[Ø,B,W][3,X]ZZ

Ø Medical and Surgical
N Head and Facial Bones
N Release Definition: Freeing a body part from an abnormal physical constraint by cutting or by the use of force

Explanation: Some of the restraining tissue may be taken out but none of the body part is taken out

Body Part Character 4	Approach Character 5	Device Character 6	Qualifier Character 7
1 Frontal Bone Zygomatic process of frontal bone 3 Parietal Bone, Right 4 Parietal Bone, Left 5 Temporal Bone, Right Mastoid process Petrous part of temporal bone Tympanic part of temporal bone Zygomatic process of temporal bone 6 Temporal Bone, Left *See 5 Temporal Bone, Right* 7 Occipital Bone Foramen magnum B Nasal Bone Vomer of nasal septum C Sphenoid Bone Greater wing Lesser wing Optic foramen Pterygoid process Sella turcica F Ethmoid Bone, Right Cribriform plate G Ethmoid Bone, Left *See F Ethmoid Bone, Right* H Lacrimal Bone, Right J Lacrimal Bone, Left K Palatine Bone, Right L Palatine Bone, Left M Zygomatic Bone, Right N Zygomatic Bone, Left P Orbit, Right Bony orbit Orbital portion of ethmoid bone Orbital portion of frontal bone Orbital portion of lacrimal bone Orbital portion of maxilla Orbital portion of palatine bone Orbital portion of sphenoid bone Orbital portion of zygomatic bone Q Orbit, Left *See P Orbit, Right* R Maxilla Alveolar process of maxilla T Mandible, Right Alveolar process of mandible Condyloid process Mandibular notch Mental foramen V Mandible, Left *See T Mandible, Right* X Hyoid Bone	Ø Open 3 Percutaneous 4 Percutaneous Endoscopic	Z No Device	Z No Qualifier

Non-OR ØNNB[Ø,3,4]ZZ

Ø Medical and Surgical
N Head and Facial Bones
P Removal Definition: Taking out or off a device from a body part

Explanation: If a device is taken out and a similar device put in without cutting or puncturing the skin or mucous membrane, the procedure is coded to the root operation CHANGE. Otherwise, the procedure for taking out a device is coded to the root operation REMOVAL.

Body Part Character 4	Approach Character 5	Device Character 6	Qualifier Character 7
Ø Skull	Ø Open	Ø Drainage Device 4 Internal Fixation Device 5 External Fixation Device 7 Autologous Tissue Substitute J Synthetic Substitute K Nonautologous Tissue Substitute M Bone Growth Stimulator N Neurostimulator Generator S Hearing Device	Z No Qualifier
Ø Skull	3 Percutaneous 4 Percutaneous Endoscopic	Ø Drainage Device 4 Internal Fixation Device 5 External Fixation Device 7 Autologous Tissue Substitute J Synthetic Substitute K Nonautologous Tissue Substitute M Bone Growth Stimulator S Hearing Device	Z No Qualifier
Ø Skull	X External	Ø Drainage Device 4 Internal Fixation Device 5 External Fixation Device M Bone Growth Stimulator S Hearing Device	Z No Qualifier
B Nasal Bone Vomer of nasal septum W Facial Bone	Ø Open 3 Percutaneous 4 Percutaneous Endoscopic	Ø Drainage Device 4 Internal Fixation Device 7 Autologous Tissue Substitute J Synthetic Substitute K Nonautologous Tissue Substitute M Bone Growth Stimulator	Z No Qualifier
B Nasal Bone Vomer of nasal septum W Facial Bone	X External	Ø Drainage Device 4 Internal Fixation Device M Bone Growth Stimulator	Z No Qualifier

Non-OR ØNPØ[3,4]5Z
Non-OR ØNPØX[Ø,5]Z
Non-OR ØNPB[Ø,3,4][Ø,4,7,J,K,M]Z
Non-OR ØNPBX[Ø,4,M]Z
Non-OR ØNPWX[Ø,M]Z

Ø Medical and Surgical
N Head and Facial Bones
Q Repair Definition: Restoring, to the extent possible, a body part to its normal anatomic structure and function
Explanation: Used only when the method to accomplish the repair is not one of the other root operations

Body Part Character 4	Approach Character 5	Device Character 6	Qualifier Character 7
Ø Skull 1 Frontal Bone Zygomatic process of frontal bone 3 Parietal Bone, Right 4 Parietal Bone, Left 5 Temporal Bone, Right Mastoid process Petrous part of temporal bone Tympanic part of temporal bone Zygomatic process of temporal bone 6 Temporal Bone, Left *See 5 Temporal Bone, Right* 7 Occipital Bone Foramen magnum B Nasal Bone Vomer of nasal septum C Sphenoid Bone Greater wing Lesser wing Optic foramen Pterygoid process Sella turcica F Ethmoid Bone, Right Cribriform plate G Ethmoid Bone, Left *See F Ethmoid Bone, Right* H Lacrimal Bone, Right J Lacrimal Bone, Left K Palatine Bone, Right L Palatine Bone, Left M Zygomatic Bone, Right N Zygomatic Bone, Left P Orbit, Right Bony orbit Orbital portion of ethmoid bone Orbital portion of frontal bone Orbital portion of lacrimal bone Orbital portion of maxilla Orbital portion of palatine bone Orbital portion of sphenoid bone Orbital portion of zygomatic bone Q Orbit, Left *See P Orbit, Right* R Maxilla Alveolar process of maxilla T Mandible, Right Alveolar process of mandible Condyloid process Mandibular notch Mental foramen V Mandible, Left *See T Mandible, Right* X Hyoid Bone	Ø Open 3 Percutaneous 4 Percutaneous Endoscopic X External	Z No Device	Z No Qualifier

Non-OR ØNQ[Ø,1,3,4,5,6,7,B,C,F,G,H,J,K,L,M,N,P,Q,R,T,V,X]XZZ

Ø Medical and Surgical
N Head and Facial Bones
R Replacement Definition: Putting in or on biological or synthetic material that physically takes the place and/or function of all or a portion of a body part

Explanation: The body part may have been taken out or replaced, or may be taken out, physically eradicated, or rendered nonfunctional during the REPLACEMENT procedure. A REMOVAL procedure is coded for taking out the device used in a previous replacement procedure.

Body Part Character 4	Approach Character 5	Device Character 6	Qualifier Character 7
Ø Skull **1 Frontal Bone** Zygomatic process of frontal bone **3 Parietal Bone, Right** **4 Parietal Bone, Left** **5 Temporal Bone, Right** Mastoid process Petrous part of temporal bone Tympanic part of temporal bone Zygomatic process of temporal bone **6 Temporal Bone, Left** *See 5 Temporal Bone, Right* **7 Occipital Bone** Foramen magnum **B Nasal Bone** Vomer of nasal septum **C Sphenoid Bone** Greater wing Lesser wing Optic foramen Pterygoid process Sella turcica **F Ethmoid Bone, Right** Cribriform plate **G Ethmoid Bone, Left** *See F Ethmoid Bone, Right* **H Lacrimal Bone, Right** **J Lacrimal Bone, Left** **K Palatine Bone, Right** **L Palatine Bone, Left** **M Zygomatic Bone, Right** **N Zygomatic Bone, Left** **P Orbit, Right** Bony orbit Orbital portion of ethmoid bone Orbital portion of frontal bone Orbital portion of lacrimal bone Orbital portion of maxilla Orbital portion of palatine bone Orbital portion of sphenoid bone Orbital portion of zygomatic bone **Q Orbit, Left** *See P Orbit, Right* **R Maxilla** Alveolar process of maxilla **T Mandible, Right** Alveolar process of mandible Condyloid process Mandibular notch Mental foramen **V Mandible, Left** *See T Mandible, Right* **X Hyoid Bone**	**Ø Open** **3 Percutaneous** **4 Percutaneous Endoscopic**	**7 Autologous Tissue Substitute** **J Synthetic Substitute** **K Nonautologous Tissue Substitute**	**Z No Qualifier**

Ø Medical and Surgical
N Head and Facial Bones
S Reposition Definition: Moving to its normal location, or other suitable location, all or a portion of a body part

Explanation: The body part is moved to a new location from an abnormal location, or from a normal location where it is not functioning correctly. The body part may or may not be cut out or off to be moved to the new location.

Body Part Character 4	Approach Character 5	Device Character 6	Qualifier Character 7
Ø Skull R Maxilla Alveolar process of maxilla T Mandible, Right Alveolar process of mandible Condyloid process Mandibular notch Mental foramen V Mandible, Left *See T Mandible, Right*	Ø Open 3 Percutaneous 4 Percutaneous Endoscopic	4 Internal Fixation Device 5 External Fixation Device Z No Device	Z No Qualifier
Ø Skull R Maxilla Alveolar process of maxilla T Mandible, Right Alveolar process of mandible Condyloid process Mandibular notch Mental foramen V Mandible, Left *See T Mandible, Right*	X External	Z No Device	Z No Qualifier
1 Frontal Bone Zygomatic process of frontal bone 3 Parietal Bone, Right 4 Parietal Bone, Left 5 Temporal Bone, Right Mastoid process Petrous part of temporal bone Tympanic part of temporal bone Zygomatic process of temporal bone 6 Temporal Bone, Left *See 5 Temporal Bone, Right* 7 Occipital Bone Foramen magnum B Nasal Bone Vomer of nasal septum C Sphenoid Bone Greater wing Lesser wing Optic foramen Pterygoid process Sella turcica F Ethmoid Bone, Right Cribriform plate G Ethmoid Bone, Left *See F Ethmoid Bone, Right* H Lacrimal Bone, Right J Lacrimal Bone, Left K Palatine Bone, Right L Palatine Bone, Left M Zygomatic Bone, Right N Zygomatic Bone, Left P Orbit, Right Bony orbit Orbital portion of ethmoid bone Orbital portion of frontal bone Orbital portion of lacrimal bone Orbital portion of maxilla Orbital portion of palatine bone Orbital portion of sphenoid bone Orbital portion of zygomatic bone Q Orbit, Left *See P Orbit, Right* X Hyoid Bone	Ø Open 3 Percutaneous 4 Percutaneous Endoscopic	4 Internal Fixation Device Z No Device	Z No Qualifier

Non-OR ØNS[R,T,V][3,4][4,5,Z]Z
Non-OR ØNS[Ø,R,T,V]XZZ
Non-OR ØNS[B,C,F,G,H,J,K,L,M,N,P,Q,X][3,4][4,Z]Z

ØNS Continued on next page

Ø Medical and Surgical
N Head and Facial Bones
S Reposition Definition: Moving to its normal location, or other suitable location, all or a portion of a body part

Explanation: The body part is moved to a new location from an abnormal location, or from a normal location where it is not functioning correctly. The body part may or may not be cut out or off to be moved to the new location.

ØNS Continued

Body Part Character 4	Approach Character 5	Device Character 6	Qualifier Character 7
1 Frontal Bone Zygomatic process of frontal bone 3 Parietal Bone, Right 4 Parietal Bone, Left 5 Temporal Bone, Right Mastoid process Petrous part of temporal bone Tympanic part of temporal bone Zygomatic process of temporal bone 6 Temporal Bone, Left *See 5 Temporal Bone, Right* 7 Occipital Bone Foramen magnum B Nasal Bone Vomer of nasal septum C Sphenoid Bone Greater wing Lesser wing Optic foramen Pterygoid process Sella turcica F Ethmoid Bone, Right Cribriform plate G Ethmoid Bone, Left *See F Ethmoid Bone, Right* H Lacrimal Bone, Right J Lacrimal Bone, Left K Palatine Bone, Right L Palatine Bone, Left M Zygomatic Bone, Right N Zygomatic Bone, Left P Orbit, Right Bony orbit Orbital portion of ethmoid bone Orbital portion of frontal bone Orbital portion of lacrimal bone Orbital portion of maxilla Orbital portion of palatine bone Orbital portion of sphenoid bone Orbital portion of zygomatic bone Q Orbit, Left *See P Orbit, Right* X Hyoid Bone	X External	Z No Device	Z No Qualifier

Non-OR ØNS[1,3,4,5,6,7,B,C,F,G,H,J,K,L,M,N,P,Q,X]XZZ

Ø Medical and Surgical
N Head and Facial Bones
T Resection Definition: Cutting out or off, without replacement, all of a body part

Explanation: None

Body Part Character 4	Approach Character 5	Device Character 6	Qualifier Character 7
1 Frontal Bone Zygomatic process of frontal bone **3 Parietal Bone, Right** **4 Parietal Bone, Left** **5 Temporal Bone, Right** Mastoid process Petrous part of temporal bone Tympanic part of temporal bone Zygomatic process of temporal bone **6 Temporal Bone, Left** *See 5 Temporal Bone, Right* **7 Occipital Bone** Foramen magnum **B Nasal Bone** Vomer of nasal septum **C Sphenoid Bone** Greater wing Lesser wing Optic foramen Pterygoid process Sella turcica **F Ethmoid Bone, Right** Cribriform plate **G Ethmoid Bone, Left** *See F Ethmoid Bone, Right* **H Lacrimal Bone, Right** **J Lacrimal Bone, Left** **K Palatine Bone, Right** **L Palatine Bone, Left** **M Zygomatic Bone, Right** **N Zygomatic Bone, Left** **P Orbit, Right** Bony orbit Orbital portion of ethmoid bone Orbital portion of frontal bone Orbital portion of lacrimal bone Orbital portion of maxilla Orbital portion of palatine bone Orbital portion of sphenoid bone Orbital portion of zygomatic bone **Q Orbit, Left** *See P Orbit, Right* **R Maxilla** Alveolar process of maxilla **T Mandible, Right** Alveolar process of mandible Condyloid process Mandibular notch Mental foramen **V Mandible, Left** *See T Mandible, Right* **X Hyoid Bone**	**Ø Open**	**Z No Device**	**Z No Qualifier**

Ø Medical and Surgical
N Head and Facial Bones
U Supplement Definition: Putting in or on biological or synthetic material that physically reinforces and/or augments the function of a portion of a body part

Explanation: The biological material is non-living, or is living and from the same individual. The body part may have been previously replaced, and the SUPPLEMENT procedure is performed to physically reinforce and/or augment the function of the replaced body part.

Body Part Character 4	Approach Character 5	Device Character 6	Qualifier Character 7
Ø Skull **1 Frontal Bone** Zygomatic process of frontal bone **3 Parietal Bone, Right** **4 Parietal Bone, Left** **5 Temporal Bone, Right** Mastoid process Petrous part of temporal bone Tympanic part of temporal bone Zygomatic process of temporal bone **6 Temporal Bone, Left** *See 5 Temporal Bone, Right* **7 Occipital Bone** Foramen magnum **B Nasal Bone** Vomer of nasal septum **C Sphenoid Bone** Greater wing Lesser wing Optic foramen Pterygoid process Sella turcica **F Ethmoid Bone, Right** Cribriform plate **G Ethmoid Bone, Left** *See F Ethmoid Bone, Right* **H Lacrimal Bone, Right** **J Lacrimal Bone, Left** **K Palatine Bone, Right** **L Palatine Bone, Left** **M Zygomatic Bone, Right** **N Zygomatic Bone, Left** **P Orbit, Right** Bony orbit Orbital portion of ethmoid bone Orbital portion of frontal bone Orbital portion of lacrimal bone Orbital portion of maxilla Orbital portion of palatine bone Orbital portion of sphenoid bone Orbital portion of zygomatic bone **Q Orbit, Left** *See P Orbit, Right* **R Maxilla** Alveolar process of maxilla **T Mandible, Right** Alveolar process of mandible Condyloid process Mandibular notch Mental foramen **V Mandible, Left** *See T Mandible, Right* **X Hyoid Bone**	**Ø Open** **3 Percutaneous** **4 Percutaneous Endoscopic**	**7 Autologous Tissue Substitute** **J Synthetic Substitute** **K Nonautologous Tissue Substitute**	**Z No Qualifier**

Ø Medical and Surgical
N Head and Facial Bones
W Revision Definition: Correcting, to the extent possible, a portion of a malfunctioning device or the position of a displaced device

Explanation: Revision can include correcting a malfunctioning or displaced device by taking out or putting in components of the device such as a screw or pin

Body Part Character 4	Approach Character 5	Device Character 6	Qualifier Character 7
Ø Skull	**Ø** Open	**Ø** Drainage Device **4** Internal Fixation Device **5** External Fixation Device **7** Autologous Tissue Substitute **J** Synthetic Substitute **K** Nonautologous Tissue Substitute **M** Bone Growth Stimulator **N** Neurostimulator Generator **S** Hearing Device	**Z** No Qualifier
Ø Skull	**3** Percutaneous **4** Percutaneous Endoscopic **X** External	**Ø** Drainage Device **4** Internal Fixation Device **5** External Fixation Device **7** Autologous Tissue Substitute **J** Synthetic Substitute **K** Nonautologous Tissue Substitute **M** Bone Growth Stimulator **S** Hearing Device	**Z** No Qualifier
B Nasal Bone Vomer of nasal septum **W** Facial Bone	**Ø** Open **3** Percutaneous **4** Percutaneous Endoscopic **X** External	**Ø** Drainage Device **4** Internal Fixation Device **7** Autologous Tissue Substitute **J** Synthetic Substitute **K** Nonautologous Tissue Substitute **M** Bone Growth Stimulator	**Z** No Qualifier

Non-OR ØNWØX[Ø,4,5,7,J,K,M,S]Z
Non-OR ØNWB[Ø,3,4,X][Ø,4,7,J,K,M]Z
Non-OR ØNWWX[Ø,4,7,J,K,M]Z

Upper Bones ØP2–ØPW

Character Meanings

This Character Meaning table is provided as a guide to assist the user in the identification of character members that may be found in this section of code tables. It **SHOULD NOT** be used to build a PCS code.

Operation–Character 3	Body Part–Character 4	Approach–Character 5	Device–Character 6	Qualifier–Character 7
2 Change	Ø Sternum	Ø Open	Ø Drainage Device OR Internal Fixation Device, Rigid Plate	X Diagnostic
5 Destruction	1 Ribs, 1 to 2	3 Percutaneous	3 Spinal Stabilization Device, Vertebral Body Tether	Z No Qualifier
8 Division	2 Ribs, 3 or more	4 Percutaneous Endoscopic	4 Internal Fixation Device	
9 Drainage	3 Cervical Vertebra	X External	5 External Fixation Device	
B Excision	4 Thoracic Vertebra		6 Internal Fixation Device, Intramedullary	
C Extirpation	5 Scapula, Right		7 Autologous Tissue Substitute OR Internal Fixation Device, Intramedullary Limb Lengthening	
D Extraction	6 Scapula, Left		8 External Fixation Device, Limb Lengthening	
H Insertion	7 Glenoid Cavity, Right		B External Fixation Device, Monoplanar	
J Inspection	8 Glenoid Cavity, Left		C External Fixation Device, Ring	
N Release	9 Clavicle, Right		D External Fixation Device, Hybrid	
P Removal	B Clavicle, Left		J Synthetic Substitute	
Q Repair	C Humeral Head, Right		K Nonautologous Tissue Substitute	
R Replacement	D Humeral Head, Left		M Bone Growth Stimulator	
S Reposition	F Humeral Shaft, Right		Y Other Device	
T Resection	G Humeral Shaft, Left		Z No Device	
U Supplement	H Radius, Right			
W Revision	J Radius, Left			
	K Ulna, Right			
	L Ulna, Left			
	M Carpal, Right			
	N Carpal, Left			
	P Metacarpal, Right			
	Q Metacarpal, Left			
	R Thumb Phalanx, Right			
	S Thumb Phalanx, Left			
	T Finger Phalanx, Right			
	V Finger Phalanx, Left			
	Y Upper Bone			

AHA Coding Clinic for table ØPB
2015, 3Q, 3-8 Excisional and nonexcisional debridement
2015, 2Q, 34 Decompressive laminectomy
2013, 4Q, 109 Separating conjoined twins
2013, 4Q, 116 Spinal decompression
2013, 3Q, 20 Superior labrum anterior posterior (SLAP) repair and subacromialdecompression
2012, 4Q, 101 Rib resection with reconstruction of anterior chest wall
2012, 2Q, 19 Multiple decompressive cervical laminectomies

AHA Coding Clinic for table ØPC
2019, 3Q, 19 Removal of sternal wire

AHA Coding Clinic for table ØPD
2017, 4Q, 41 Extraction procedures

AHA Coding Clinic for table ØPH
2020, 1Q, 29 Repair of sternal dehiscence using Sternal Talon® device
2019, 4Q, 34 Intramedullary limb lengthening internal fixation device
2019, 2Q, 40 Decompression of spinal cord and placement of instrumentation
2018, 3Q, 26 Anterior vertebral tethering using Dynesys Tethering System
2017, 2Q, 20 Exchange of intramedullary antibiotic impregnated spacer
2016, 4Q, 117 Placement of magnetic growth rods
2014, 4Q, 28 Removal and replacement of displaced growing rods

AHA Coding Clinic for table ØPP
2019, 3Q, 19 Removal of sternal wire
2017, 2Q, 20 Exchange of intramedullary antibiotic impregnated spacer
2016, 4Q, 117 Placement of magnetic growth rods
2014, 4Q, 28 Removal and replacement of displaced growing rods

AHA Coding Clinic for table ØPR
2018, 4Q, 92 Radial head arthroplasty

AHA Coding Clinic for table ØPS
2020, 1Q, 33 Spinal fusion without use of bone graft
2018, 3Q, 26 Anterior vertebral tethering using Dynesys Tethering System
2017, 4Q, 53 New and revised body part values - Ribs
2016, 1Q, 21 Elongation derotation flexion casting
2015, 4Q, 33 Ravitch operation
2015, 2Q, 35 Application of tongs to reduce and stabilize cervical fracture
2014, 4Q, 26 Placement of vertical expandable prosthetic titanium rib (VEPTR)
2014, 4Q, 32 Open reduction internal fixation of fracture with debridement
2014, 3Q, 33 Radial fracture treatment with open reduction internal fixation, and release of carpal ligament

AHA Coding Clinic for table ØPT
2015, 3Q, 26 Thumb arthroplasty with resection of trapezium

AHA Coding Clinic for table ØPU
2015, 2Q, 20 Cervical laminoplasty
2013, 4Q, 109 Separating conjoined twins

AHA Coding Clinic for table ØPW
2014, 4Q, 26 Adjustment of VEPTR lengthening mechanism
2014, 4Q, 27 Bilateral lengthening of growing rods

Upper Bones

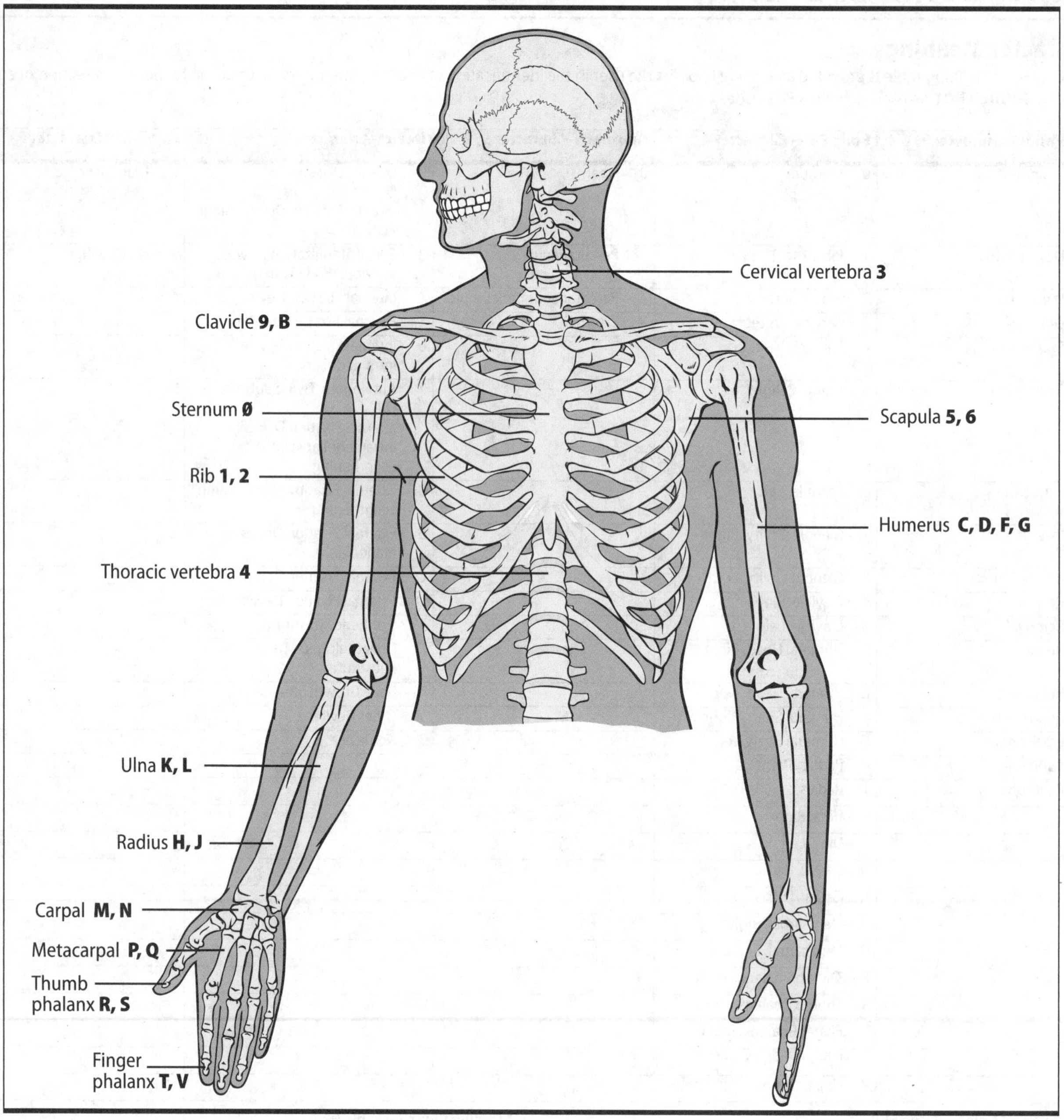
Cervical vertebra **3**
Clavicle **9, B**
Sternum **Ø**
Scapula **5, 6**
Rib **1, 2**
Humerus **C, D, F, G**
Thoracic vertebra **4**
Ulna **K, L**
Radius **H, J**
Carpal **M, N**
Metacarpal **P, Q**
Thumb phalanx **R, S**
Finger phalanx **T, V**

Humerus and Scapula

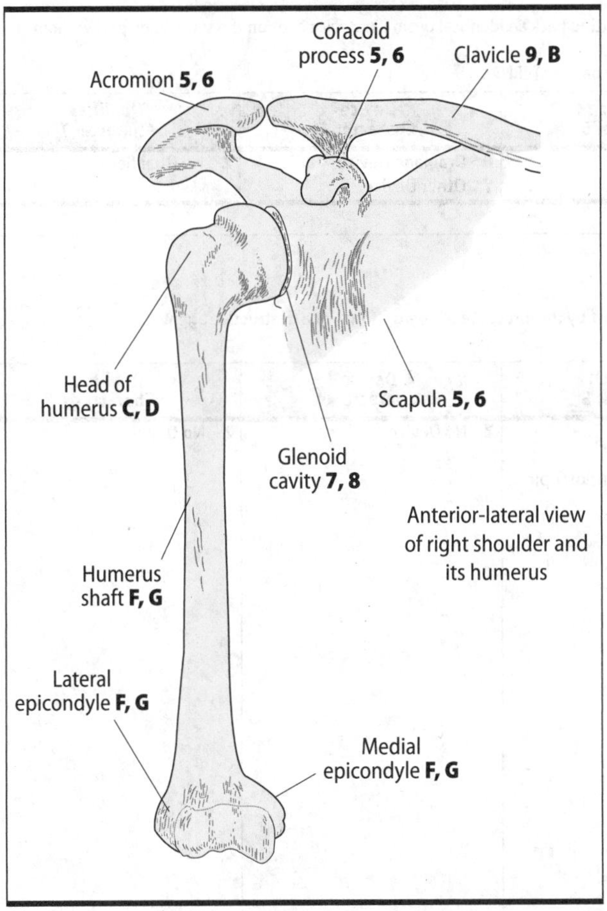

Radius and Ulna

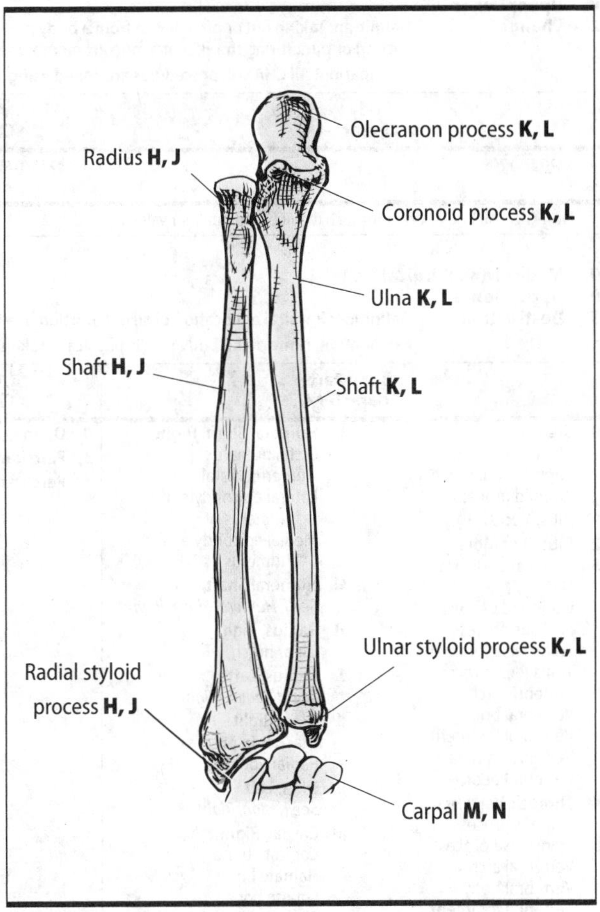

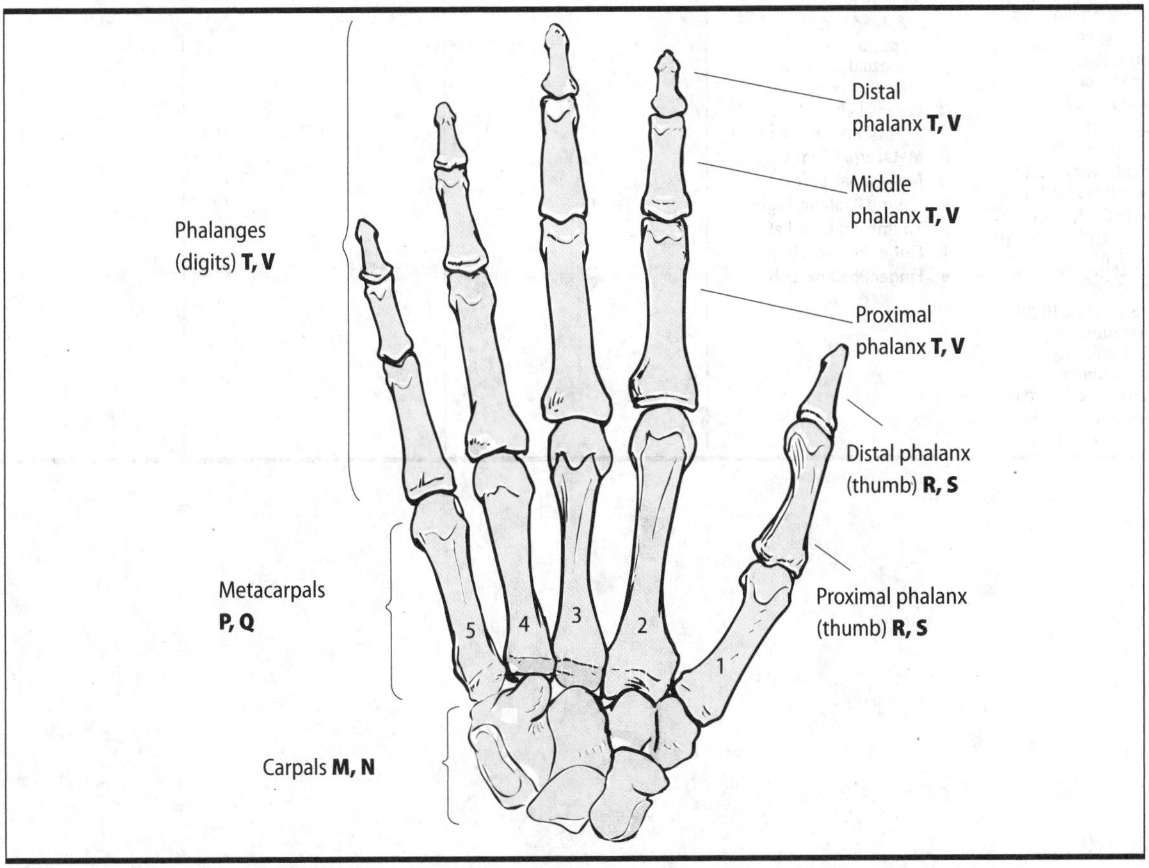

Ø Medical and Surgical
P Upper Bones
2 Change Definition: Taking out or off a device from a body part and putting back an identical or similar device in or on the same body part without cutting or puncturing the skin or a mucous membrane

Explanation: All CHANGE procedures are coded using the approach EXTERNAL

Body Part Character 4	Approach Character 5	Device Character 6	Qualifier Character 7
Y Upper Bone	X External	Ø Drainage Device Y Other Device	Z No Qualifier

Non-OR All body part, approach, device, and qualifier values

Ø Medical and Surgical
P Upper Bones
5 Destruction Definition: Physical eradication of all or a portion of a body part by the direct use of energy, force, or a destructive agent

Explanation: None of the body part is physically taken out

Body Part Character 4	Body Part Character 4 (cont.)	Approach Character 5	Device Character 6	Qualifier Character 7
Ø Sternum Manubrium Suprasternal notch Xiphoid process **1 Ribs, 1 to 2** **2 Ribs, 3 or More** **3 Cervical Vertebra** Dens Odontoid process Spinous process Transverse foramen Transverse process Vertebral arch Vertebral body Vertebral foramen Vertebral lamina Vertebral pedicle **4 Thoracic Vertebra** Spinous process Transverse process Vertebral arch Vertebral body Vertebral foramen Vertebral lamina Vertebral pedicle **5 Scapula, Right** Acromion (process) Coracoid process **6 Scapula, Left** *See 5 Scapula, Right* **7 Glenoid Cavity, Right** Glenoid fossa (of scapula) **8 Glenoid Cavity, Left** *See 7 Glenoid Cavity, Right* **9 Clavicle, Right** **B Clavicle, Left** **C Humeral Head, Right** Greater tuberosity Lesser tuberosity Neck of humerus (anatomical)(surgical) **D Humeral Head, Left** *See C Humeral Head, Right*	**F Humeral Shaft, Right** Distal humerus Humerus, distal Lateral epicondyle of humerus Medial epicondyle of humerus **G Humeral Shaft, Left** *See F Humeral Shaft, Right* **H Radius, Right** Ulnar notch **J Radius, Left** *See H Radius, Right* **K Ulna, Right** Olecranon process Radial notch **L Ulna, Left** *See K Ulna, Right* **M Carpal, Right** Capitate bone Hamate bone Lunate bone Pisiform bone Scaphoid bone Trapezium bone Trapezoid bone Triquetral bone **N Carpal, Left** *See M Carpal, Right* **P Metacarpal, Right** **Q Metacarpal, Left** **R Thumb Phalanx, Right** **S Thumb Phalanx, Left** **T Finger Phalanx, Right** **V Finger Phalanx, Left**	Ø Open 3 Percutaneous 4 Percutaneous Endoscopic	Z No Device	Z No Qualifier

Ø Medical and Surgical
P Upper Bones
8 Division Definition: Cutting into a body part, without draining fluids and/or gases from the body part, in order to separate or transect a body part
Explanation: All or a portion of the body part is separated into two or more portions

Body Part Character 4	Approach Character 5	Device Character 6	Qualifier Character 7
Ø Sternum Manubrium Suprasternal notch Xiphoid process **1 Ribs, 1 to 2** **2 Ribs, 3 or More** **3 Cervical Vertebra** Dens Odontoid process Spinous process Transverse foramen Transverse process Vertebral arch Vertebral body Vertebral foramen Vertebral lamina Vertebral pedicle **4 Thoracic Vertebra** Spinous process Transverse process Vertebral arch Vertebral body Vertebral foramen Vertebral lamina Vertebral pedicle **5 Scapula, Right** Acromion (process) Coracoid process **6 Scapula, Left** *See 5 Scapula, Right* **7 Glenoid Cavity, Right** Glenoid fossa (of scapula) **8 Glenoid Cavity, Left** *See 7 Glenoid Cavity, Right* **9 Clavicle, Right** **B Clavicle, Left** **C Humeral Head, Right** Greater tuberosity Lesser tuberosity Neck of humerus (anatomical)(surgical) **D Humeral Head, Left** *See C Humeral Head, Right* **F Humeral Shaft, Right** Distal humerus Humerus, distal Lateral epicondyle of humerus Medial epicondyle of humerus **G Humeral Shaft, Left** *See F Humeral Shaft, Right* **H Radius, Right** Ulnar notch **J Radius, Left** *See H Radius, Right* **K Ulna, Right** Olecranon process Radial notch **L Ulna, Left** *See K Ulna, Right* **M Carpal, Right** Capitate bone Hamate bone Lunate bone Pisiform bone Scaphoid bone Trapezium bone Trapezoid bone Triquetral bone **N Carpal, Left** *See M Carpal, Right* **P Metacarpal, Right** **Q Metacarpal, Left** **R Thumb Phalanx, Right** **S Thumb Phalanx, Left** **T Finger Phalanx, Right** **V Finger Phalanx, Left**	**Ø Open** **3 Percutaneous** **4 Percutaneous Endoscopic**	**Z No Device**	**Z No Qualifier**

Ø Medical and Surgical
P Upper Bones
9 Drainage Definition: Taking or letting out fluids and/or gases from a body part
Explanation: The qualifier DIAGNOSTIC is used to identify drainage procedures that are biopsies

Body Part Character 4	Approach Character 5	Device Character 6	Qualifier Character 7
Ø Sternum Manubrium Suprasternal notch Xiphoid process **1 Ribs, 1 to 2** **2 Ribs, 3 or More** **3 Cervical Vertebra** Dens Odontoid process Spinous process Transverse foramen Transverse process Vertebral arch Vertebral body Vertebral foramen Vertebral lamina Vertebral pedicle **4 Thoracic Vertebra** Spinous process Transverse process Vertebral arch Vertebral body Vertebral foramen Vertebral lamina Vertebral pedicle **5 Scapula, Right** Acromion (process) Coracoid process **6 Scapula, Left** *See 5 Scapula, Right* **7 Glenoid Cavity, Right** Glenoid fossa (of scapula) **8 Glenoid Cavity, Left** *See 7 Glenoid Cavity, Right* **9 Clavicle, Right** **B Clavicle, Left** **C Humeral Head, Right** Greater tuberosity Lesser tuberosity Neck of humerus (anatomical)(surgical) **D Humeral Head, Left** *See C Humeral Head, Right* **F Humeral Shaft, Right** Distal humerus Humerus, distal Lateral epicondyle of humerus Medial epicondyle of humerus **G Humeral Shaft, Left** *See F Humeral Shaft, Right* **H Radius, Right** Ulnar notch **J Radius, Left** *See H Radius, Right* **K Ulna, Right** Olecranon process Radial notch **L Ulna, Left** *See K Ulna, Right* **M Carpal, Right** Capitate bone Hamate bone Lunate bone Pisiform bone Scaphoid bone Trapezium bone Trapezoid bone Triquetral bone **N Carpal, Left** *See M Carpal, Right* **P Metacarpal, Right** **Q Metacarpal, Left** **R Thumb Phalanx, Right** **S Thumb Phalanx, Left** **T Finger Phalanx, Right** **V Finger Phalanx, Left**	**Ø Open** **3 Percutaneous** **4 Percutaneous Endoscopic**	**Ø Drainage Device**	**Z No Qualifier**

Non-OR ØP9[Ø,1,2,3,4,5,6,7,8,9,B,C,D,F,G,H,J,K,L,M,N,P,Q,R,S,T,V]3ØZ

ØP9 Continued on next page

ØP9 Continued

Ø Medical and Surgical
P Upper Bones
9 Drainage Definition: Taking or letting out fluids and/or gases from a body part
Explanation: The qualifier DIAGNOSTIC is used to identify drainage procedures that are biopsies

Body Part Character 4		Approach Character 5	Device Character 6	Qualifier Character 7
Ø Sternum Manubrium Suprasternal notch Xiphoid process **1 Ribs, 1 to 2** **2 Ribs, 3 or More** **3 Cervical Vertebra** Dens Odontoid process Spinous process Transverse foramen Transverse process Vertebral arch Vertebral body Vertebral foramen Vertebral lamina Vertebral pedicle **4 Thoracic Vertebra** Spinous process Transverse process Vertebral arch Vertebral body Vertebral foramen Vertebral lamina Vertebral pedicle **5 Scapula, Right** Acromion (process) Coracoid process **6 Scapula, Left** ***See*** *5 Scapula, Right* **7 Glenoid Cavity, Right** Glenoid fossa (of scapula) **8 Glenoid Cavity, Left** ***See*** *7 Glenoid Cavity, Right* **9 Clavicle, Right** **B Clavicle, Left** **C Humeral Head, Right** Greater tuberosity Lesser tuberosity Neck of humerus (anatomical)(surgical)	**D Humeral Head, Left** ***See*** *C Humeral Head, Right* **F Humeral Shaft, Right** Distal humerus Humerus, distal Lateral epicondyle of humerus Medial epicondyle of humerus **G Humeral Shaft, Left** ***See*** *F Humeral Shaft, Right* **H Radius, Right** Ulnar notch **J Radius, Left** ***See*** *H Radius, Right* **K Ulna, Right** Olecranon process Radial notch **L Ulna, Left** ***See*** *K Ulna, Right* **M Carpal, Right** Capitate bone Hamate bone Lunate bone Pisiform bone Scaphoid bone Trapezium bone Trapezoid bone Triquetral bone **N Carpal, Left** ***See*** *M Carpal, Right* **P Metacarpal, Right** **Q Metacarpal, Left** **R Thumb Phalanx, Right** **S Thumb Phalanx, Left** **T Finger Phalanx, Right** **V Finger Phalanx, Left**	**Ø Open** **3 Percutaneous** **4 Percutaneous Endoscopic**	**Z No Device**	**X Diagnostic** **Z No Qualifier**

Non-OR ØP9[Ø,1,2,3,4,5,6,7,8,9,B,C,D,F,G,H,J,K,L,M,N,P,Q,R,S,T,V]3ZZ

Ø Medical and Surgical
P Upper Bones
B Excision Definition: Cutting out or off, without replacement, a portion of a body part
Explanation: The qualifier DIAGNOSTIC is used to identify excision procedures that are biopsies

Body Part Character 4	Approach Character 5	Device Character 6	Qualifier Character 7
Ø Sternum Manubrium Suprasternal notch Xiphoid process **1 Ribs, 1 to 2** **2 Ribs, 3 or More** **3 Cervical Vertebra** Dens Odontoid process Spinous process Transverse foramen Transverse process Vertebral arch Vertebral body Vertebral foramen Vertebral lamina Vertebral pedicle **4 Thoracic Vertebra** Spinous process Transverse process Vertebral arch Vertebral body Vertebral foramen Vertebral lamina Vertebral pedicle **5 Scapula, Right** Acromion (process) Coracoid process **6 Scapula, Left** ***See* *5 Scapula, Right*** **7 Glenoid Cavity, Right** Glenoid fossa (of scapula) **8 Glenoid Cavity, Left** ***See* *7 Glenoid Cavity, Right*** **9 Clavicle, Right** **B Clavicle, Left** **C Humeral Head, Right** Greater tuberosity Lesser tuberosity Neck of humerus (anatomical)(surgical) **D Humeral Head, Left** ***See* *C Humeral Head, Right*** **F Humeral Shaft, Right** Distal humerus Humerus, distal Lateral epicondyle of humerus Medial epicondyle of humerus **G Humeral Shaft, Left** ***See* *F Humeral Shaft, Right*** **H Radius, Right** Ulnar notch **J Radius, Left** ***See* *H Radius, Right*** **K Ulna, Right** Olecranon process Radial notch **L Ulna, Left** ***See* *K Ulna, Right*** **M Carpal, Right** Capitate bone Hamate bone Lunate bone Pisiform bone Scaphoid bone Trapezium bone Trapezoid bone Triquetral bone **N Carpal, Left** ***See* *M Carpal, Right*** **P Metacarpal, Right** **Q Metacarpal, Left** **R Thumb Phalanx, Right** **S Thumb Phalanx, Left** **T Finger Phalanx, Right** **V Finger Phalanx, Left**	**Ø Open** **3 Percutaneous** **4 Percutaneous Endoscopic**	**Z No Device**	**X Diagnostic** **Z No Qualifier**

Ø Medical and Surgical
P Upper Bones
C Extirpation Definition: Taking or cutting out solid matter from a body part

Explanation: The solid matter may be an abnormal byproduct of a biological function or a foreign body; it may be imbedded in a body part or in the lumen of a tubular body part. The solid matter may or may not have been previously broken into pieces.

Body Part Character 4	Approach Character 5	Device Character 6	Qualifier Character 7
Ø Sternum Manubrium Suprasternal notch Xiphoid process **1 Ribs, 1 to 2** **2 Ribs, 3 or More** **3 Cervical Vertebra** Dens Odontoid process Spinous process Transverse foramen Transverse process Vertebral arch Vertebral body Vertebral foramen Vertebral lamina Vertebral pedicle **4 Thoracic Vertebra** Spinous process Transverse process Vertebral arch Vertebral body Vertebral foramen Vertebral lamina Vertebral pedicle **5 Scapula, Right** Acromion (process) Coracoid process **6 Scapula, Left** *See 5 Scapula, Right* **7 Glenoid Cavity, Right** Glenoid fossa (of scapula) **8 Glenoid Cavity, Left** *See 7 Glenoid Cavity, Right* **9 Clavicle, Right** **B Clavicle, Left** **C Humeral Head, Right** Greater tuberosity Lesser tuberosity Neck of humerus (anatomical)(surgical) **D Humeral Head, Left** *See C Humeral Head, Right* **F Humeral Shaft, Right** Distal humerus Humerus, distal Lateral epicondyle of humerus Medial epicondyle of humerus **G Humeral Shaft, Left** *See F Humeral Shaft, Right* **H Radius, Right** Ulnar notch **J Radius, Left** *See H Radius, Right* **K Ulna, Right** Olecranon process Radial notch **L Ulna, Left** *See K Ulna, Right* **M Carpal, Right** Capitate bone Hamate bone Lunate bone Pisiform bone Scaphoid bone Trapezium bone Trapezoid bone Triquetral bone **N Carpal, Left** *See M Carpal, Right* **P Metacarpal, Right** **Q Metacarpal, Left** **R Thumb Phalanx, Right** **S Thumb Phalanx, Left** **T Finger Phalanx, Right** **V Finger Phalanx, Left**	**Ø Open** **3 Percutaneous** **4 Percutaneous Endoscopic**	**Z No Device**	**Z No Qualifier**

Ø Medical and Surgical
P Upper Bones
D Extraction

Definition: Pulling or stripping out or off all or a portion of a body part by the use of force
Explanation: The qualifier DIAGNOSTIC is used to identify extraction procedures that are biopsies

Body Part Character 4	Approach Character 5	Device Character 6	Qualifier Character 7
Ø Sternum Manubrium Suprasternal notch Xiphoid process **1 Ribs, 1 to 2** **2 Ribs, 3 or More** **3 Cervical Vertebra** Dens Odontoid process Spinous process Transverse foramen Transverse process Vertebral arch Vertebral body Vertebral foramen Vertebral lamina Vertebral pedicle **4 Thoracic Vertebra** Spinous process Transverse process Vertebral arch Vertebral body Vertebral foramen Vertebral lamina Vertebral pedicle **5 Scapula, Right** Acromion (process) Coracoid process **6 Scapula, Left** *See 5 Scapula, Right* **7 Glenoid Cavity, Right** Glenoid fossa (of scapula) **8 Glenoid Cavity, Left** *See 7 Glenoid Cavity, Right* **9 Clavicle, Right** **B Clavicle, Left** **C Humeral Head, Right** Greater tuberosity Lesser tuberosity Neck of humerus (anatomical)(surgical) **D Humeral Head, Left** *See C Humeral Head, Right* **F Humeral Shaft, Right** Distal humerus Humerus, distal Lateral epicondyle of humerus Medial epicondyle of humerus **G Humeral Shaft, Left** *See F Humeral Shaft, Right* **H Radius, Right** Ulnar notch **J Radius, Left** *See H Radius, Right* **K Ulna, Right** Olecranon process Radial notch **L Ulna, Left** *See K Ulna, Right* **M Carpal, Right** Capitate bone Hamate bone Lunate bone Pisiform bone Scaphoid bone Trapezium bone Trapezoid bone Triquetral bone **N Carpal, Left** *See M Carpal, Right* **P Metacarpal, Right** **Q Metacarpal, Left** **R Thumb Phalanx, Right** **S Thumb Phalanx, Left** **T Finger Phalanx, Right** **V Finger Phalanx, Left**	**Ø Open**	**Z No Device**	**Z No Qualifier**

Ø Medical and Surgical
P Upper Bones
H Insertion

Definition: Putting in a nonbiological appliance that monitors, assists, performs, or prevents a physiological function but does not physically take the place of a body part

Explanation: None

Body Part Character 4		Approach Character 5	Device Character 6	Qualifier Character 7
Ø Sternum Manubrium Suprasternal notch Xiphoid process		**Ø Open** **3 Percutaneous** **4 Percutaneous Endoscopic**	**Ø Internal Fixation Device, Rigid Plate** **4 Internal Fixation Device**	**Z No Qualifier**
1 Ribs, 1 to 2 **2 Ribs, 3 or More** **3 Cervical Vertebra** Dens Odontoid process Spinous process Transverse foramen Transverse process Vertebral arch Vertebral body Vertebral foramen Vertebral lamina Vertebral pedicle **4 Thoracic Vertebra** Spinous process Transverse process Vertebral arch Vertebral body Vertebral foramen Vertebral lamina Vertebral pedicle	**5 Scapula, Right** Acromion (process) Coracoid process **6 Scapula, Left** *See 5 Scapula, Right* **7 Glenoid Cavity, Right** Glenoid fossa (of scapula) **8 Glenoid Cavity, Left** *See 7 Glenoid Cavity, Right* **9 Clavicle, Right** **B Clavicle, Left**	**Ø Open** **3 Percutaneous** **4 Percutaneous Endoscopic**	**4 Internal Fixation Device**	**Z No Qualifier**
C Humeral Head, Right Greater tuberosity Lesser tuberosity Neck of humerus (anatomical)(surgical) **D Humeral Head, Left** *See C Humeral Head, Right*	**H Radius, Right** Ulnar notch **J Radius, Left** *See H Radius, Right* **K Ulna, Right** Olecranon process Radial notch **L Ulna, Left** *See K Ulna, Right*	**Ø Open** **3 Percutaneous** **4 Percutaneous Endoscopic**	**4 Internal Fixation Device** **5 External Fixation Device** **6 Internal Fixation Device, Intramedullary** **8 External Fixation Device, Limb Lengthening** **B External Fixation Device, Monoplanar** **C External Fixation Device, Ring** **D External Fixation Device, Hybrid**	**Z No Qualifier**
F Humeral Shaft, Right Distal humerus Humerus, distal Lateral epicondyle of humerus Medial epicondyle of humerus	**G Humeral Shaft, Left** *See F Humeral Shaft, Right*	**Ø Open** **3 Percutaneous** **4 Percutaneous Endoscopic**	**4 Internal Fixation Device** **5 External Fixation Device** **6 Internal Fixation Device, Intramedullary** **7 Internal Fixation Device, Intramedullary Limb Lengthening** **8 External Fixation Device, Limb Lengthening** **B External Fixation Device, Monoplanar** **C External Fixation Device, Ring** **D External Fixation Device, Hybrid**	**Z No Qualifier**
M Carpal, Right Capitate bone Hamate bone Lunate bone Pisiform bone Scaphoid bone Trapezium bone Trapezoid bone Triquetral bone **N Carpal, Left** *See M Carpal, Right*	**P Metacarpal, Right** **Q Metacarpal, Left** **R Thumb Phalanx, Right** **S Thumb Phalanx, Left** **T Finger Phalanx, Right** **V Finger Phalanx, Left**	**Ø Open** **3 Percutaneous** **4 Percutaneous Endoscopic**	**4 Internal Fixation Device** **5 External Fixation Device**	**Z No Qualifier**
Y Upper Bone		**Ø Open** **3 Percutaneous** **4 Percutaneous Endoscopic**	**M Bone Growth Stimulator**	**Z No Qualifier**

Non-OR ØPH[C,D,H,J,K,L][Ø,3,4]8Z
Non-OR ØPH[F,G][Ø,3,4]8Z

Ø Medical and Surgical
P Upper Bones
J Inspection Definition: Visually and/or manually exploring a body part

Explanation: Visual exploration may be performed with or without optical instrumentation. Manual exploration may be performed directly or through intervening body layers.

Body Part Character 4	Approach Character 5	Device Character 6	Qualifier Character 7
Y Upper Bone	Ø Open 3 Percutaneous 4 Percutaneous Endoscopic X External	Z No Device	Z No Qualifier

Non-OR ØPJY[3,X]ZZ

Ø Medical and Surgical
P Upper Bones
N Release Definition: Freeing a body part from an abnormal physical constraint by cutting or by the use of force

Explanation: Some of the restraining tissue may be taken out but none of the body part is taken out

Body Part Character 4		Approach Character 5	Device Character 6	Qualifier Character 7
Ø Sternum Manubrium Suprasternal notch Xiphoid process **1 Ribs, 1 to 2** **2 Ribs, 3 or More** **3 Cervical Vertebra** Dens Odontoid process Spinous process Transverse foramen Transverse process Vertebral arch Vertebral body Vertebral foramen Vertebral lamina Vertebral pedicle **4 Thoracic Vertebra** Spinous process Transverse process Vertebral arch Vertebral body Vertebral foramen Vertebral lamina Vertebral pedicle **5 Scapula, Right** Acromion (process) Coracoid process **6 Scapula, Left** *See 5 Scapula, Right* **7 Glenoid Cavity, Right** Glenoid fossa (of scapula) **8 Glenoid Cavity, Left** *See 7 Glenoid Cavity, Right* **9 Clavicle, Right** **B Clavicle, Left** **C Humeral Head, Right** Greater tuberosity Lesser tuberosity Neck of humerus (anatomical) (surgical) **D Humeral Head, Left** *See C Humeral Head, Right*	**F Humeral Shaft, Right** Distal humerus Humerus, distal Lateral epicondyle of humerus Medial epicondyle of humerus **G Humeral Shaft, Left** *See F Humeral Shaft, Right* **H Radius, Right** Ulnar notch **J Radius, Left** *See H Radius, Right* **K Ulna, Right** Olecranon process Radial notch **L Ulna, Left** *See K Ulna, Right* **M Carpal, Right** Capitate bone Hamate bone Lunate bone Pisiform bone Scaphoid bone Trapezium bone Trapezoid bone Triquetral bone **N Carpal, Left** *See M Carpal, Right* **P Metacarpal, Right** **Q Metacarpal, Left** **R Thumb Phalanx, Right** **S Thumb Phalanx, Left** **T Finger Phalanx, Right** **V Finger Phalanx, Left**	Ø Open 3 Percutaneous 4 Percutaneous Endoscopic	Z No Device	Z No Qualifier

Ø Medical and Surgical
P Upper Bones
P Removal Definition: Taking out or off a device from a body part

Explanation: If a device is taken out and a similar device put in without cutting or puncturing the skin or mucous membrane, the procedure is coded to the root operation CHANGE. Otherwise, the procedure for taking out a device is coded to the root operation REMOVAL.

Body Part Character 4	Approach Character 5	Device Character 6	Qualifier Character 7
Ø Sternum Manubrium, Suprasternal notch, Xiphoid process **1 Ribs, 1 to 2** **2 Ribs, 3 or More** **3 Cervical Vertebra** Dens, Odontoid process, Spinous process, Transverse foramen, Transverse process, Vertebral arch, Vertebral body, Vertebral foramen, Vertebral lamina, Vertebral pedicle **4 Thoracic Vertebra** Spinous process, Transverse process, Vertebral arch, Vertebral body, Vertebral foramen, Vertebral lamina, Vertebral pedicle **5 Scapula, Right** Acromion (process), Coracoid process **6 Scapula, Left** *See 5 Scapula, Right* **7 Glenoid Cavity, Right** Glenoid fossa (of scapula) **8 Glenoid Cavity, Left** *See 7 Glenoid Cavity, Right* **9 Clavicle, Right** **B Clavicle, Left**	**Ø Open** **3 Percutaneous** **4 Percutaneous Endoscopic**	**4 Internal Fixation Device** **7 Autologous Tissue Substitute** **J Synthetic Substitute** **K Nonautologous Tissue Substitute**	**Z No Qualifier**
Ø Sternum Manubrium, Suprasternal notch, Xiphoid process **1 Ribs, 1 to 2** **2 Ribs, 3 or More** **3 Cervical Vertebra** Dens, Odontoid process, Spinous process, Transverse foramen, Transverse process, Vertebral arch, Vertebral body, Vertebral foramen, Vertebral lamina, Vertebral pedicle **4 Thoracic Vertebra** Spinous process, Transverse process, Vertebral arch, Vertebral body, Vertebral foramen, Vertebral lamina, Vertebral pedicle **5 Scapula, Right** Acromion (process), Coracoid process **6 Scapula, Left** *See 5 Scapula, Right* **7 Glenoid Cavity, Right** Glenoid fossa (of scapula) **8 Glenoid Cavity, Left** *See 7 Glenoid Cavity, Right* **9 Clavicle, Right** **B Clavicle, Left**	**X External**	**4 Internal Fixation Device**	**Z No Qualifier**
C Humeral Head, Right Greater tuberosity, Lesser tuberosity, Neck of humerus (anatomical) (surgical) **D Humeral Head, Left** *See C Humeral Head, Right* **F Humeral Shaft, Right** Distal humerus, Humerus, distal, Lateral epicondyle of humerus, Medial epicondyle of humerus **G Humeral Shaft, Left** *See F Humeral Shaft, Right* **H Radius, Right** Ulnar notch **J Radius, Left** *See H Radius, Right* **K Ulna, Right** Olecranon process, Radial notch **L Ulna, Left** *See K Ulna, Right* **M Carpal, Right** Capitate bone, Hamate bone, Lunate bone, Pisiform bone, Scaphoid bone, Trapezium bone, Trapezoid bone, Triquetral bone **N Carpal, Left** *See M Carpal, Right* **P Metacarpal, Right** **Q Metacarpal, Left** **R Thumb Phalanx, Right** **S Thumb Phalanx, Left** **T Finger Phalanx, Right** **V Finger Phalanx, Left**	**Ø Open** **3 Percutaneous** **4 Percutaneous Endoscopic**	**4 Internal Fixation Device** **5 External Fixation Device** **7 Autologous Tissue Substitute** **J Synthetic Substitute** **K Nonautologous Tissue Substitute**	**Z No Qualifier**

Non-OR ØPP[Ø,1,2,3,4,5,6,7,8,9,B]X4Z

ØPP Continued on next page

Ø Medical and Surgical
P Upper Bones
P Removal

ØPP Continued

Definition: Taking out or off a device from a body part

Explanation: If a device is taken out and a similar device put in without cutting or puncturing the skin or mucous membrane, the procedure is coded to the root operation CHANGE. Otherwise, the procedure for taking out a device is coded to the root operation REMOVAL.

Body Part Character 4	Approach Character 5	Device Character 6	Qualifier Character 7
C Humeral Head, Right Greater tuberosity Lesser tuberosity Neck of humerus (anatomical) (surgical) **D Humeral Head, Left** *See C Humeral Head, Right* **F Humeral Shaft, Right** Distal humerus Humerus, distal Lateral epicondyle of humerus Medial epicondyle of humerus **G Humeral Shaft, Left** *See F Humeral Shaft, Right* **H Radius, Right** Ulnar notch **J Radius, Left** *See H Radius, Right* **K Ulna, Right** Olecranon process **Radial notch** **L Ulna, Left** *See K Ulna, Right* **M Carpal, Right** Capitate bone Hamate bone Lunate bone Pisiform bone Scaphoid bone Trapezium bone Trapezoid bone Triquetral bone **N Carpal, Left** *See M Carpal, Right* **P Metacarpal, Right** **Q Metacarpal, Left** **R Thumb Phalanx, Right** **S Thumb Phalanx, Left** **T Finger Phalanx, Right** **V Finger Phalanx, Left**	**X External**	**4 Internal Fixation Device** **5 External Fixation Device**	**Z No Qualifier**
Y Upper Bone	**Ø Open** **3 Percutaneous** **4 Percutaneous Endoscopic** **X External**	**Ø Drainage Device** **M Bone Growth Stimulator**	**Z No Qualifier**

Non-OR ØPP[C,D,F,G,H,J,K,L,M,N,P,Q,R,S,T,V]X[4,5]Z
Non-OR ØPPY3ØZ
Non-OR ØPPYX[Ø,M]Z

Ø Medical and Surgical
P Upper Bones
Q Repair Definition: Restoring, to the extent possible, a body part to its normal anatomic structure and function
Explanation: Used only when the method to accomplish the repair is not one of the other root operations

Body Part Character 4	Approach Character 5	Device Character 6	Qualifier Character 7
Ø Sternum Manubrium Suprasternal notch Xiphoid process **1 Ribs, 1 to 2** **2 Ribs, 3 or More** **3 Cervical Vertebra** Dens Odontoid process Spinous process Transverse foramen Transverse process Vertebral arch Vertebral body Vertebral foramen Vertebral lamina Vertebral pedicle **4 Thoracic Vertebra** Spinous process Transverse process Vertebral arch Vertebral body Vertebral foramen Vertebral lamina Vertebral pedicle **5 Scapula, Right** Acromion (process) Coracoid process **6 Scapula, Left** ***See*** *5 Scapula, Right* **7 Glenoid Cavity, Right** Glenoid fossa (of scapula) **8 Glenoid Cavity, Left** ***See*** *7 Glenoid Cavity, Right* **9 Clavicle, Right** **B Clavicle, Left** **C Humeral Head, Right** Greater tuberosity Lesser tuberosity Neck of humerus (anatomical)(surgical) **D Humeral Head, Left** ***See*** *C Humeral Head, Right* **F Humeral Shaft, Right** Distal humerus Humerus, distal Lateral epicondyle of humerus Medial epicondyle of humerus **G Humeral Shaft, Left** ***See*** *F Humeral Shaft, Right* **H Radius, Right** Ulnar notch **J Radius, Left** ***See*** *H Radius, Right* **K Ulna, Right** Olecranon process Radial notch **L Ulna, Left** ***See*** *K Ulna, Right* **M Carpal, Right** Capitate bone Hamate bone Lunate bone Pisiform bone Scaphoid bone Trapezium bone Trapezoid bone Triquetral bone **N Carpal, Left** ***See*** *M Carpal, Right* **P Metacarpal, Right** **Q Metacarpal, Left** **R Thumb Phalanx, Right** **S Thumb Phalanx, Left** **T Finger Phalanx, Right** **V Finger Phalanx, Left**	**Ø Open** **3 Percutaneous** **4 Percutaneous Endoscopic** **X External**	**Z No Device**	**Z No Qualifier**

Non-OR ØPQ[Ø,1,2,3,4,5,6,7,8,9,B,C,D,F,G,H,J,K,L,M,N,P,Q,R,S,T,V]XZZ

Ø Medical and Surgical
P Upper Bones
R Replacement

Definition: Putting in or on biological or synthetic material that physically takes the place and/or function of all or a portion of a body part

Explanation: The body part may have been taken out or replaced, or may be taken out, physically eradicated, or rendered nonfunctional during the REPLACEMENT procedure. A REMOVAL procedure is coded for taking out the device used in a previous replacement procedure.

Body Part Character 4	Approach Character 5	Device Character 6	Qualifier Character 7
Ø Sternum Manubrium Suprasternal notch Xiphoid process **1 Ribs, 1 to 2** **2 Ribs, 3 or More** **3 Cervical Vertebra** Dens Odontoid process Spinous process Transverse foramen Transverse process Vertebral arch Vertebral body Vertebral foramen Vertebral lamina Vertebral pedicle **4 Thoracic Vertebra** Spinous process Transverse process Vertebral arch Vertebral body Vertebral foramen Vertebral lamina Vertebral pedicle **5 Scapula, Right** Acromion (process) Coracoid process **6 Scapula, Left** *See 5 Scapula, Right* **7 Glenoid Cavity, Right** Glenoid fossa (of scapula) **8 Glenoid Cavity, Left** *See 7 Glenoid Cavity, Right* **9 Clavicle, Right** **B Clavicle, Left** **C Humeral Head, Right** Greater tuberosity Lesser tuberosity Neck of humerus (anatomical)(surgical) **D Humeral Head, Left** *See C Humeral Head, Right* **F Humeral Shaft, Right** Distal humerus Humerus, distal Lateral epicondyle of humerus Medial epicondyle of humerus **G Humeral Shaft, Left** *See F Humeral Shaft, Right* **H Radius, Right** Ulnar notch **J Radius, Left** *See H Radius, Right* **K Ulna, Right** Olecranon process Radial notch **L Ulna, Left** *See K Ulna, Right* **M Carpal, Right** Capitate bone Hamate bone Lunate bone Pisiform bone Scaphoid bone Trapezium bone Trapezoid bone Triquetral bone **N Carpal, Left** *See M Carpal, Right* **P Metacarpal, Right** **Q Metacarpal, Left** **R Thumb Phalanx, Right** **S Thumb Phalanx, Left** **T Finger Phalanx, Right** **V Finger Phalanx, Left**	**Ø Open** **3 Percutaneous** **4 Percutaneous Endoscopic**	**7 Autologous Tissue Substitute** **J Synthetic Substitute** **K Nonautologous Tissue Substitute**	**Z No Qualifier**

Ø Medical and Surgical
P Upper Bones
S Reposition

Definition: Moving to its normal location, or other suitable location, all or a portion of a body part

Explanation: The body part is moved to a new location from an abnormal location, or from a normal location where it is not functioning correctly. The body part may or may not be cut out or off to be moved to the new location.

Body Part Character 4		Approach Character 5	Device Character 6	Qualifier Character 7
Ø Sternum Manubrium Suprasternal notch Xiphoid process		**Ø Open** **3 Percutaneous** **4 Percutaneous Endoscopic**	**Ø Internal Fixation Device, Rigid Plate** **4 Internal Fixation Device** **Z No Device**	**Z No Qualifier**
Ø Sternum Manubrium Suprasternal notch Xiphoid process		**X External**	**Z No Device**	**Z No Qualifier**
1 Ribs, 1 to 2 **2 Ribs, 3 or More** **3 Cervical Vertebra** ⊞ Dens Odontoid process Spinous process Transverse foramen Transverse process Vertebral arch Vertebral body Vertebral foramen Vertebral lamina Vertebral pedicle	**5 Scapula, Right** Acromion (process) Coracoid process **6 Scapula, Left** *See 5 Scapula, Right* **7 Glenoid Cavity, Right** Glenoid fossa (of scapula) **8 Glenoid Cavity, Left** *See 7 Glenoid Cavity, Right* **9 Clavicle, Right** **B Clavicle, Left**	**Ø Open** **3 Percutaneous** **4 Percutaneous Endoscopic**	**4 Internal Fixation Device** **Z No Device**	**Z No Qualifier**
1 Ribs, 1 to 2 **2 Ribs, 3 or More** **3 Cervical Vertebra** Dens Odontoid process Spinous process Transverse foramen Transverse process Vertebral arch Vertebral body Vertebral foramen Vertebral lamina Vertebral pedicle	**5 Scapula, Right** Acromion (process) Coracoid process **6 Scapula, Left** *See 5 Scapula, Right* **7 Glenoid Cavity, Right** Glenoid fossa (of scapula) **8 Glenoid Cavity, Left** *See 7 Glenoid Cavity, Right* **9 Clavicle, Right** **B Clavicle, Left**	**X External**	**Z No Device**	**Z No Qualifier**
4 Thoracic Vertebra ⊞ Spinous process Transverse process Vertebral arch Vertebral body Vertebral foramen Vertebral lamina Vertebral pedicle		**Ø Open** **4 Percutaneous Endoscopic**	**3 Spinal Stabilization Device, Vertebral Body Tether** **4 Internal Fixation Device** **Z No Device**	**Z No Qualifier**
4 Thoracic Vertebra Spinous process Transverse process Vertebral arch Vertebral body Vertebral foramen Vertebral lamina Vertebral pedicle		**3 Percutaneous**	**4 Internal Fixation Device** **Z No Device**	**Z No Qualifier**
4 Thoracic Vertebra Spinous process Transverse process Vertebral arch Vertebral body Vertebral foramen Vertebral lamina Vertebral pedicle		**X External**	**Z No Device**	**Z No Qualifier**
C Humeral Head, Right Greater tuberosity Lesser tuberosity Neck of humerus (anatomical)(surgical) **D Humeral Head, Left** *See C Humeral Head, Right* **F Humeral Shaft, Right** Distal humerus Humerus, distal Lateral epicondyle of humerus Medial epicondyle of humerus	**G Humeral Shaft, Left** *See F Humeral Shaft, Right* **H Radius, Right** Ulnar notch **J Radius, Left** *See H Radius, Right* **K Ulna, Right** Olecranon process Radial notch **L Ulna, Left** *See K Ulna, Right*	**Ø Open** **3 Percutaneous** **4 Percutaneous Endoscopic**	**4 Internal Fixation Device** **5 External Fixation Device** **6 Internal Fixation Device, Intramedullary** **B External Fixation Device, Monoplanar** **C External Fixation Device, Ring** **D External Fixation Device, Hybrid** **Z No Device**	**Z No Qualifier**

Non-OR ØPSØ[3,4]ZZ
Non-OR ØPSØXZZ
Non-OR ØPS[1,2,5,6,7,8,9,B][3,4]ZZ
Non-OR ØPS[1,2,3,5,6,7,8,9,B]XZZ
Non-OR ØPS4XZZ
Non-OR ØPS[C,D,F,G,H,J,K,L][3,4]ZZ

See Appendix L for Procedure Combinations
⊞ ØPS[3,4]3ZZ

ØPS Continued on next page

ØPS Continued

Ø Medical and Surgical
P Upper Bones
S Reposition

Definition: Moving to its normal location, or other suitable location, all or a portion of a body part

Explanation: The body part is moved to a new location from an abnormal location, or from a normal location where it is not functioning correctly. The body part may or may not be cut out or off to be moved to the new location.

Body Part Character 4		Approach Character 5	Device Character 6	Qualifier Character 7
C Humeral Head, Right Greater tuberosity Lesser tuberosity Neck of humerus (anatomical)(surgical) **D Humeral Head, Left** *See C Humeral Head, Right* **F Humeral Shaft, Right** Distal humerus Humerus, distal Lateral epicondyle of humerus Medial epicondyle of humerus	**G Humeral Shaft, Left** *See F Humeral Shaft, Right* **H Radius, Right** Ulnar notch **J Radius, Left** *See H Radius, Right* **K Ulna, Right** Olecranon process Radial notch **L Ulna, Left** *See K Ulna, Right*	**X External**	**Z No Device**	**Z No Qualifier**
M Carpal, Right Capitate bone Hamate bone Lunate bone Pisiform bone Scaphoid bone Trapezium bone Trapezoid bone Triquetral bone	**N Carpal, Left** *See M Carpal, Right* **P Metacarpal, Right** **Q Metacarpal, Left** **R Thumb Phalanx, Right** **S Thumb Phalanx, Left** **T Finger Phalanx, Right** **V Finger Phalanx, Left**	**Ø Open** **3 Percutaneous** **4 Percutaneous Endoscopic**	**4 Internal Fixation Device** **5 External Fixation Device** **Z No Device**	**Z No Qualifier**
M Carpal, Right Capitate bone Hamate bone Lunate bone Pisiform bone Scaphoid bone Trapezium bone Trapezoid bone Triquetral bone	**N Carpal, Left** *See M Carpal, Right* **P Metacarpal, Right** **Q Metacarpal, Left** **R Thumb Phalanx, Right** **S Thumb Phalanx, Left** **T Finger Phalanx, Right** **V Finger Phalanx, Left**	**X External**	**Z No Device**	**Z No Qualifier**

Non-OR ØPS[C,D,F,G,H,J,K,L]XZZ
Non-OR ØPS[M,N,P,Q,R,S,T,V][3,4]ZZ
Non-OR ØPS[M,N,P,Q,R,S,T,V]XZZ

Ø Medical and Surgical
P Upper Bones
T Resection

Definition: Cutting out or off, without replacement, all of a body part

Explanation: None

Body Part Character 4		Approach Character 5	Device Character 6	Qualifier Character 7
Ø Sternum Manubrium Suprasternal notch Xiphoid process **1 Ribs, 1 to 2** **2 Ribs, 3 or More** **5 Scapula, Right** Acromion (process) Coracoid process **6 Scapula, Left** *See 5 Scapula, Right* **7 Glenoid Cavity, Right** Glenoid fossa (of scapula) **8 Glenoid Cavity, Left** *See 7 Glenoid Cavity, Right* **9 Clavicle, Right** **B Clavicle, Left** **C Humeral Head, Right** Greater tuberosity Lesser tuberosity Neck of humerus (anatomical) (surgical) **D Humeral Head, Left** *See C Humeral Head, Right* **F Humeral Shaft, Right** Distal humerus Humerus, distal Lateral epicondyle of humerus Medial epicondyle of humerus	**G Humeral Shaft, Left** *See F Humeral Shaft, Right* **H Radius, Right** Ulnar notch **J Radius, Left** *See H Radius, Right* **K Ulna, Right** Olecranon process Radial notch **L Ulna, Left** *See K Ulna, Right* **M Carpal, Right** Capitate bone Hamate bone Lunate bone Pisiform bone Scaphoid bone Trapezium bone Trapezoid bone Triquetral bone **N Carpal, Left** *See M Carpal, Right* **P Metacarpal, Right** **Q Metacarpal, Left** **R Thumb Phalanx, Right** **S Thumb Phalanx, Left** **T Finger Phalanx, Right** **V Finger Phalanx, Left**	**Ø Open**	**Z No Device**	**Z No Qualifier**

Ø Medical and Surgical
P Upper Bones
U Supplement

Definition: Putting in or on biological or synthetic material that physically reinforces and/or augments the function of a portion of a body part

Explanation: The biological material is non-living, or is living and from the same individual. The body part may have been previously replaced, and the SUPPLEMENT procedure is performed to physically reinforce and/or augment the function of the replaced body part.

Body Part Character 4		Approach Character 5	Device Character 6	Qualifier Character 7
Ø Sternum Manubrium Suprasternal notch Xiphoid process **1 Ribs, 1 to 2** **2 Ribs, 3 or More** **3 Cervical Vertebra** ⊞ Dens Odontoid process Spinous process Transverse foramen Transverse process Vertebral arch Vertebral body Vertebral foramen Vertebral lamina Vertebral pedicle **4 Thoracic Vertebra** ⊞ Spinous process Transverse process Vertebral arch Vertebral body Vertebral foramen Vertebral lamina Vertebral pedicle **5 Scapula, Right** Acromion (process) Coracoid process **6 Scapula, Left** ***See*** *5 Scapula, Right* **7 Glenoid Cavity, Right** Glenoid fossa (of scapula) **8 Glenoid Cavity, Left** ***See*** *7 Glenoid Cavity, Right* **9 Clavicle, Right** **B Clavicle, Left** **C Humeral Head, Right** Greater tuberosity Lesser tuberosity Neck of humerus (anatomical) (surgical)	**D Humeral Head, Left** ***See*** *C Humeral Head, Right* **F Humeral Shaft, Right** Distal humerus Humerus, distal Lateral epicondyle of humerus Medial epicondyle of humerus **G Humeral Shaft, Left** ***See*** *F Humeral Shaft, Right* **H Radius, Right** Ulnar notch **J Radius, Left** ***See*** *H Radius, Right* **K Ulna, Right** Olecranon process Radial notch **L Ulna, Left** ***See*** *K Ulna, Right* **M Carpal, Right** Capitate bone Hamate bone Lunate bone Pisiform bone Scaphoid bone Trapezium bone Trapezoid bone Triquetral bone **N Carpal, Left** ***See*** *M Carpal, Right* **P Metacarpal, Right** **Q Metacarpal, Left** **R Thumb Phalanx, Right** **S Thumb Phalanx, Left** **T Finger Phalanx, Right** **V Finger Phalanx, Left**	**Ø Open** **3 Percutaneous** **4 Percutaneous Endoscopic**	**7 Autologous Tissue Substitute** **J Synthetic Substitute** **K Nonautologous Tissue Substitute**	**Z No Qualifier**

See Appendix L for Procedure Combinations
⊞ ØPU[3,4]3JZ

Ø Medical and Surgical
P Upper Bones
W Revision

Definition: Correcting, to the extent possible, a portion of a malfunctioning device or the position of a displaced device

Explanation: Revision can include correcting a malfunctioning or displaced device by taking out or putting in components of the device such as a screw or pin

Body Part Character 4		Approach Character 5	Device Character 6	Qualifier Character 7
Ø Sternum Manubrium Suprasternal notch Xiphoid process **1 Ribs, 1 to 2** **2 Ribs, 3 or More** **3 Cervical Vertebra** Dens Odontoid process Spinous process Transverse foramen Transverse process Vertebral arch Vertebral body Vertebral foramen Vertebral lamina Vertebral pedicle **4 Thoracic Vertebra** Spinous process Transverse process Vertebral arch Vertebral body Vertebral foramen Vertebral lamina Vertebral pedicle	**5 Scapula, Right** Acromion (process) Coracoid process **6 Scapula, Left** *See 5 Scapula, Right* **7 Glenoid Cavity, Right** Glenoid fossa (of scapula) **8 Glenoid Cavity, Left** *See 7 Glenoid Cavity, Right* **9 Clavicle, Right** **B Clavicle, Left**	**Ø Open** **3 Percutaneous** **4 Percutaneous Endoscopic** **X External**	**4 Internal Fixation Device** **7 Autologous Tissue Substitute** **J Synthetic Substitute** **K Nonautologous Tissue Substitute**	**Z No Qualifier**
C Humeral Head, Right Greater tuberosity Lesser tuberosity Neck of humerus (anatomical)(surgical) **D Humeral Head, Left** *See C Humeral Head, Right* **F Humeral Shaft, Right** Distal humerus Humerus, distal Lateral epicondyle of humerus Medial epicondyle of humerus **G Humeral Shaft, Left** *See F Humeral Shaft, Right* **H Radius, Right** Ulnar notch **J Radius, Left** *See H Radius, Right* **K Ulna, Right** Olecranon process Radial notch	**L Ulna, Left** *See K Ulna, Right* **M Carpal, Right** Capitate bone Hamate bone Lunate bone Pisiform bone Scaphoid bone Trapezium bone Trapezoid bone Triquetral bone **N Carpal, Left** *See M Carpal, Right* **P Metacarpal, Right** **Q Metacarpal, Left** **R Thumb Phalanx, Right** **S Thumb Phalanx, Left** **T Finger Phalanx, Right** **V Finger Phalanx, Left**	**Ø Open** **3 Percutaneous** **4 Percutaneous Endoscopic** **X External**	**4 Internal Fixation Device** **5 External Fixation Device** **7 Autologous Tissue Substitute** **J Synthetic Substitute** **K Nonautologous Tissue Substitute**	**Z No Qualifier**
Y Upper Bone		**Ø Open** **3 Percutaneous** **4 Percutaneous Endoscopic** **X External**	**Ø Drainage Device** **M Bone Growth Stimulator**	**Z No Qualifier**

Non-OR ØPW[Ø,1,2,3,4,5,6,7,8,9,B]X[4,7,J,K]Z
Non-OR ØPW[C,D,F,G,H,J,K,L,M,N,P,Q,R,S,T,V]X[4,5,7,J,K]Z
Non-OR ØPWYX[Ø,M]Z

Lower Bones ØQ2–ØQW

Character Meanings

This Character Meaning table is provided as a guide to assist the user in the identification of character members that may be found in this section of code tables. It **SHOULD NOT** be used to build a PCS code.

Operation–Character 3	Body Part–Character 4	Approach–Character 5	Device–Character 6	Qualifier–Character 7
2 Change	Ø Lumbar Vertebra	Ø Open	Ø Drainage Device	2 Sesamoid Bone(s) 1st Toe
5 Destruction	1 Sacrum	3 Percutaneous	3 Spinal Stabilization Device, Vertebral Body Tether	X Diagnostic
8 Division	2 Pelvic Bone, Right	4 Percutaneous Endoscopic	4 Internal Fixation Device	Z No Qualifier
9 Drainage	3 Pelvic Bone, Left	X External	5 External Fixation Device	
B Excision	4 Acetabulum, Right		6 Internal Fixation Device, Intramedullary	
C Extirpation	5 Acetabulum, Left		7 Autologous Tissue Substitute OR Internal Fixation Device, Intramedullary Limb Lengthening	
D Extraction	6 Upper Femur, Right		8 External Fixation Device, Limb Lengthening	
H Insertion	7 Upper Femur, Left		B External Fixation Device, Monoplanar	
J Inspection	8 Femoral Shaft, Right		C External Fixation Device, Ring	
N Release	9 Femoral Shaft, Left		D External Fixation Device, Hybrid	
P Removal	B Lower Femur, Right		J Synthetic Substitute	
Q Repair	C Lower Femur, Left		K Nonautologous Tissue Substitute	
R Replacement	D Patella, Right		M Bone Growth Stimulator	
S Reposition	F Patella, Left		Y Other Device	
T Resection	G Tibia, Right		Z No Device	
U Supplement	H Tibia, Left			
W Revision	J Fibula, Right			
	K Fibula, Left			
	L Tarsal, Right			
	M Tarsal, Left			
	N Metatarsal, Right			
	P Metatarsal, Left			
	Q Toe Phalanx, Right			
	R Toe Phalanx, Left			
	S Coccyx			
	Y Lower Bone			

AHA Coding Clinic for table ØQ8

2018, 1Q, 25 Periacetabular osteotomy for repair of congenital hip dysplasia
2016, 2Q, 31 Periacetabular ostectomy for repair of congenital hip dysplasia

AHA Coding Clinic for table ØQB

2021, 2Q, 18 Excision of tibial sesamoid
2020, 2Q, 26 Sacral Pressure Ulcer with Excisional and Nonexcisional Debridement of Same Site
2019, 2Q, 19 Cervical spinal fusion, decompression and placement of interfacet stabilization device
2018, 3Q, 17 Excisional debridement of periosteum
2017, 1Q, 23 Reconstruction of mandible using titanium and bone
2016, 3Q, 30 Resection of femur with interposition arthroplasty
2015, 3Q, 3-8 Excisional and nonexcisional debridement
2015, 3Q, 26 Femoral head resection
2015, 2Q, 34 Decompressive laminectomy
2014, 4Q, 25 Femoroacetabular impingement and labral tear with repair
2014, 2Q, 6 Posterior lumbar fusion with discectomy
2013, 4Q, 116 Spinal decompression
2013, 2Q, 39 Ankle fusion, osteotomy, and removal of hardware
2012, 2Q, 19 Multiple decompressive cervical laminectomies

AHA Coding Clinic for table ØQD

2017, 4Q, 41 Extraction procedures

AHA Coding Clinic for table ØQH

2019, 4Q, 34 Intramedullary limb lengthening internal fixation device
2017, 1Q, 21 Staged scoliosis surgery with iliac fixation and spinal fusion
2016, 3Q, 34 Tibial/fibula epiphysiodesis

AHA Coding Clinic for table ØQP

2020, 4Q, 56 Removal of external fixation device
2017, 4Q, 74-75 Magnetic growth rods
2015, 2Q, 6 Planned implant break

AHA Coding Clinic for table ØQQ

2018, 1Q, 15 Pubic symphysis fusion
2014, 3Q, 24 Repair of lipomyelomeningocele and tethered cord

AHA Coding Clinic for table ØQR

2017, 1Q, 22 Total knee replacement and patellar component
2016, 3Q, 30 Resection of femur with interposition arthroplasty

AHA Coding Clinic for table ØQS

2020, 1Q, 33 Spinal fusion without use of bone graft
2019, 3Q, 26 Open reduction with internal fixation and placement of strut allograft
2018, 1Q, 13 Bilateral cuboid osteotomy for repair of congenital talipes equinovarus
2018, 1Q, 25 Periacetabular osteotomy for repair of congenital hip dysplasia
2016, 3Q, 34 Tibial/fibula epiphysiodesis
2014, 4Q, 29 Rotational osteosynthesis
2014, 4Q, 31 Reposition of femur for correction of valgus and recurvatum deformities

AHA Coding Clinic for table ØQT

2017, 1Q, 22 Chopart amputation of foot
2016, 3Q, 30 Resection of femur with interposition arthroplasty
2015, 3Q, 26 Femoral head resection
2014, 4Q, 29 Rotational osteosynthesis

AHA Coding Clinic for table ØQU

2019, 3Q, 26 Open reduction with internal fixation and placement of strut allograft
2019, 2Q, 35 Kiva® kyphoplasty
2015, 3Q, 18 Total hip replacement with acetabular reconstruction
2014, 4Q, 31 Reposition of femur for correction of valgus and recurvatum deformities
2014, 2Q, 12 Percutaneous vertebroplasty using cement
2013, 2Q, 35 Use of bone void filler in grafting

AHA Coding Clinic for table ØQW

2017, 4Q, 74-75 Magnetic growth rods

Lower Bones

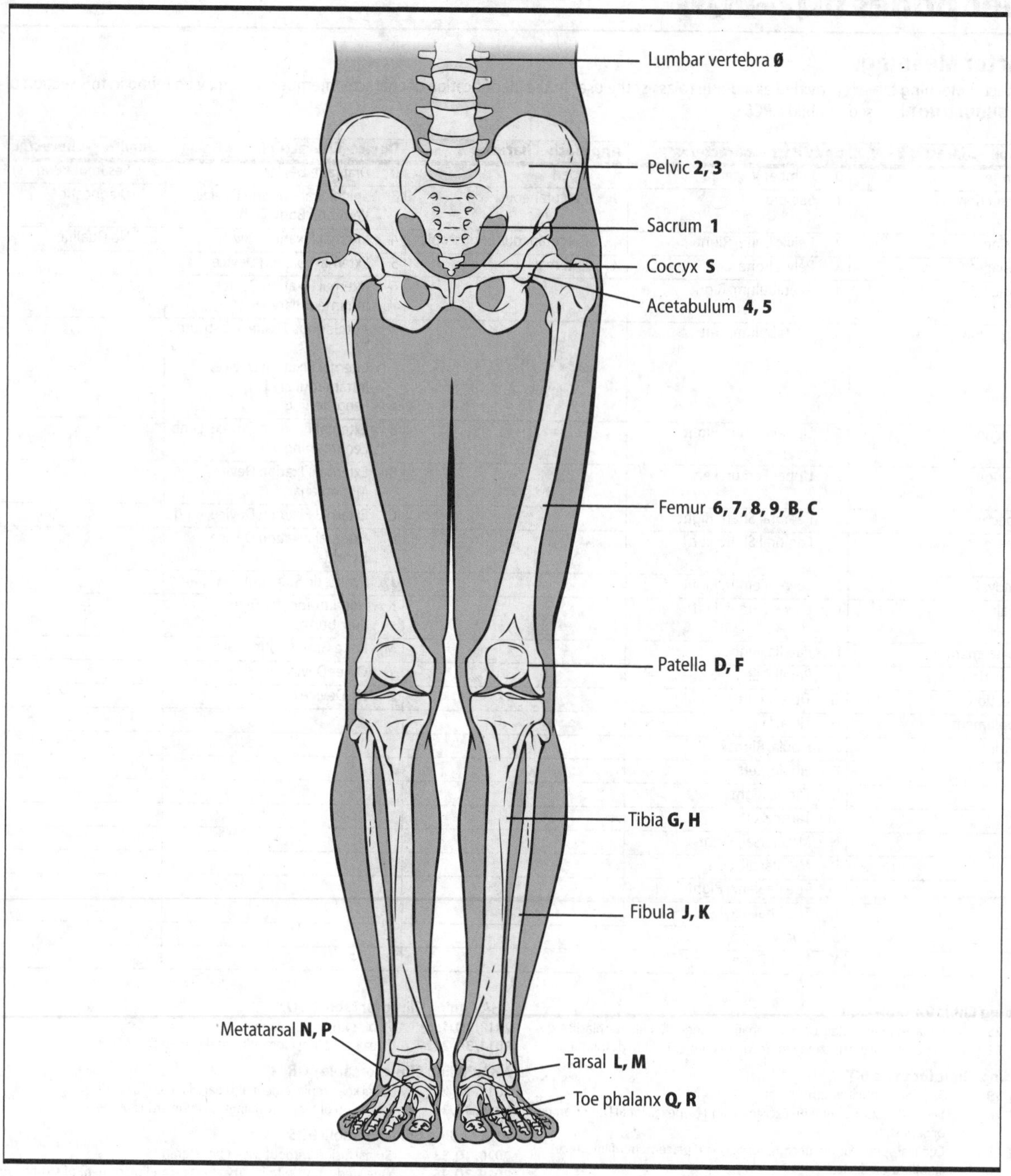
Lumbar vertebra Ø
Pelvic 2, 3
Sacrum 1
Coccyx S
Acetabulum 4, 5
Femur 6, 7, 8, 9, B, C
Patella D, F
Tibia G, H
Fibula J, K
Metatarsal N, P
Tarsal L, M
Toe phalanx Q, R

Hip Bone Anatomy

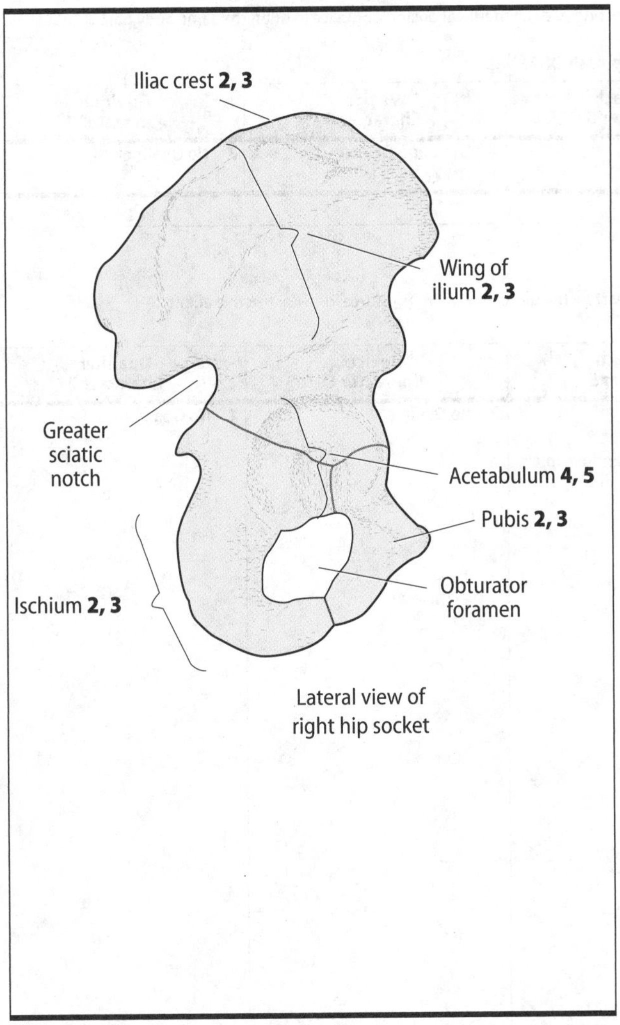

Pelvic and Lower Extremity Bones

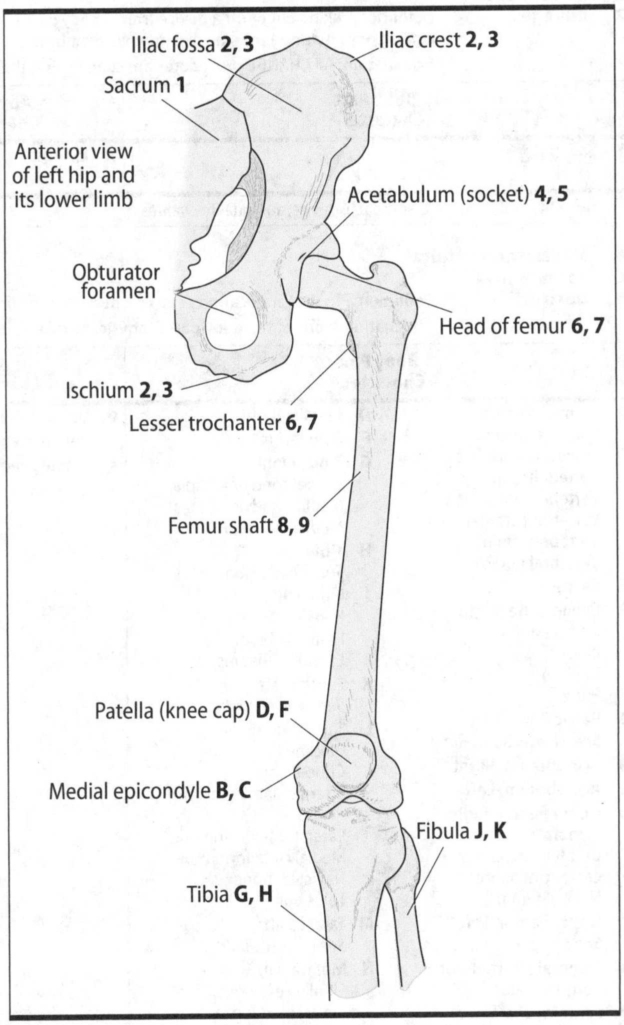

Foot Bones

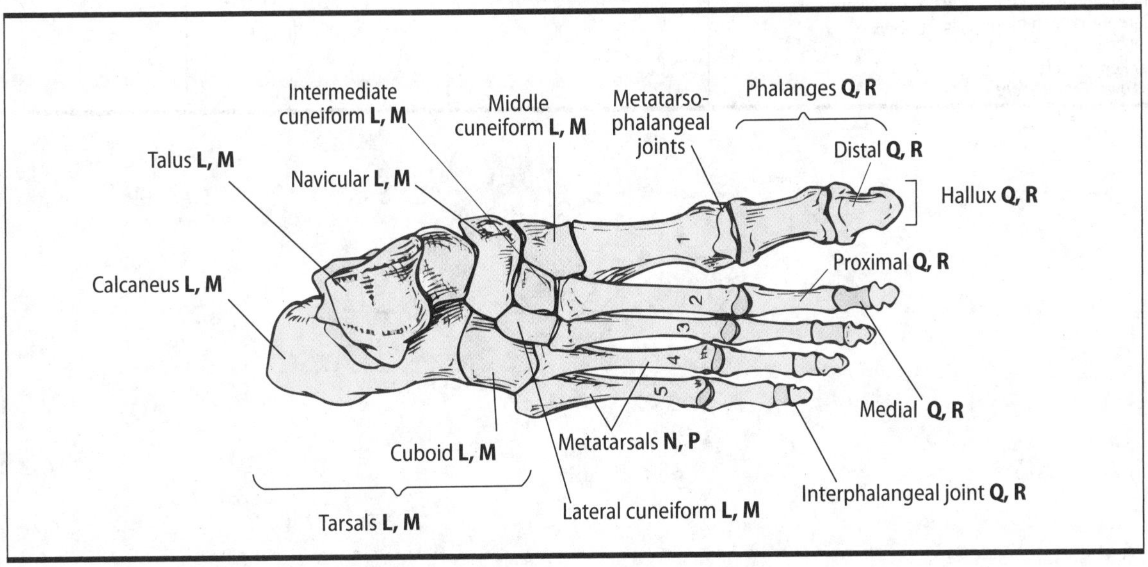

Ø Medical and Surgical
Q Lower Bones
2 Change

Definition: Taking out or off a device from a body part and putting back an identical or similar device in or on the same body part without cutting or puncturing the skin or a mucous membrane

Explanation: All CHANGE procedures are coded using the approach EXTERNAL

Body Part Character 4	Approach Character 5	Device Character 6	Qualifier Character 7
Y Lower Bone	X External	Ø Drainage Device Y Other Device	Z No Qualifier

Non-OR All body part, approach, device, and qualifier values

Ø Medical and Surgical
Q Lower Bones
5 Destruction

Definition: Physical eradication of all or a portion of a body part by the direct use of energy, force, or a destructive agent

Explanation: None of the body part is physically taken out

Body Part Character 4		Approach Character 5	Device Character 6	Qualifier Character 7
Ø Lumbar Vertebra Spinous process Transverse process Vertebral arch Vertebral body Vertebral foramen Vertebral lamina Vertebral pedicle **1 Sacrum** **2 Pelvic Bone, Right** Iliac crest Ilium Ischium Pubis **3 Pelvic Bone, Left** *See 2 Pelvic Bone, Right* **4 Acetabulum, Right** **5 Acetabulum, Left** **6 Upper Femur, Right** Femoral head Greater trochanter Lesser trochanter Neck of femur **7 Upper Femur, Left** *See 6 Upper Femur, Right* **8 Femoral Shaft, Right** Body of femur **9 Femoral Shaft, Left** *See 8 Femoral Shaft, Right* **B Lower Femur, Right** Lateral condyle of femur Lateral epicondyle of femur Medial condyle of femur Medial epicondyle of femur **C Lower Femur, Left** *See B Lower Femur, Right*	**D Patella, Right** **F Patella, Left** **G Tibia, Right** Lateral condyle of tibia Medial condyle of tibia Medial malleolus **H Tibia, Left** *See G Tibia, Right* **J Fibula, Right** Body of fibula Head of fibula Lateral malleolus **K Fibula, Left** *See J Fibula, Right* **L Tarsal, Right** Calcaneus Cuboid bone Intermediate cuneiform bone Lateral cuneiform bone Medial cuneiform bone Navicular bone Talus bone **M Tarsal, Left** *See L Tarsal, Right* **N Metatarsal, Right** Fibular sesamoid Tibial sesamoid **P Metatarsal, Left** *See N Metatarsal, Right* **Q Toe Phalanx, Right** **R Toe Phalanx, Left** **S Coccyx**	Ø Open 3 Percutaneous 4 Percutaneous Endoscopic	Z No Device	Z No Qualifier

Ø Medical and Surgical
Q Lower Bones
8 Division Definition: Cutting into a body part, without draining fluids and/or gases from the body part, in order to separate or transect a body part
Explanation: All or a portion of the body part is separated into two or more portions

Body Part Character 4	Approach Character 5	Device Character 6	Qualifier Character 7
Ø Lumbar Vertebra Spinous process Transverse process Vertebral arch Vertebral body Vertebral foramen Vertebral lamina Vertebral pedicle **1 Sacrum** **2 Pelvic Bone, Right** Iliac crest Ilium Ischium Pubis **3 Pelvic Bone, Left** *See 2 Pelvic Bone, Right* **4 Acetabulum, Right** **5 Acetabulum, Left** **6 Upper Femur, Right** Femoral head Greater trochanter Lesser trochanter Neck of femur **7 Upper Femur, Left** *See 6 Upper Femur, Right* **8 Femoral Shaft, Right** Body of femur **9 Femoral Shaft, Left** *See 8 Femoral Shaft, Right* **B Lower Femur, Right** Lateral condyle of femur Lateral epicondyle of femur Medial condyle of femur Medial epicondyle of femur **C Lower Femur, Left** *See B Lower Femur, Right* **D Patella, Right** **F Patella, Left** **G Tibia, Right** Lateral condyle of tibia Medial condyle of tibia Medial malleolus **H Tibia, Left** *See G Tibia, Right* **J Fibula, Right** Body of fibula Head of fibula Lateral malleolus **K Fibula, Left** *See J Fibula, Right* **L Tarsal, Right** Calcaneus Cuboid bone Intermediate cuneiform bone Lateral cuneiform bone Medial cuneiform bone Navicular bone Talus bone **M Tarsal, Left** *See L Tarsal, Right* **N Metatarsal, Right** Fibular sesamoid Tibial sesamoid **P Metatarsal, Left** *See N Metatarsal, Right* **Q Toe Phalanx, Right** **R Toe Phalanx, Left** **S Coccyx**	**Ø Open** **3 Percutaneous** **4 Percutaneous Endoscopic**	**Z No Device**	**Z No Qualifier**

Ø Medical and Surgical
Q Lower Bones
9 Drainage Definition: Taking or letting out fluids and/or gases from a body part
Explanation: The qualifier DIAGNOSTIC is used to identify drainage procedures that are biopsies

Body Part Character 4	Approach Character 5	Device Character 6	Qualifier Character 7
Ø Lumbar Vertebra Spinous process Transverse process Vertebral arch Vertebral body Vertebral foramen Vertebral lamina Vertebral pedicle **1 Sacrum** **2 Pelvic Bone, Right** Iliac crest Ilium Ischium Pubis **3 Pelvic Bone, Left** *See 2 Pelvic Bone, Right* **4 Acetabulum, Right** **5 Acetabulum, Left** **6 Upper Femur, Right** Femoral head Greater trochanter Lesser trochanter Neck of femur **7 Upper Femur, Left** *See 6 Upper Femur, Right* **8 Femoral Shaft, Right** Body of femur **9 Femoral Shaft, Left** *See 8 Femoral Shaft, Right* **B Lower Femur, Right** Lateral condyle of femur Lateral epicondyle of femur Medial condyle of femur Medial epicondyle of femur **C Lower Femur, Left** *See B Lower Femur, Right* **D Patella, Right** **F Patella, Left** **G Tibia, Right** Lateral condyle of tibia Medial condyle of tibia Medial malleolus **H Tibia, Left** *See G Tibia, Right* **J Fibula, Right** Body of fibula Head of fibula Lateral malleolus **K Fibula, Left** *See J Fibula, Right* **L Tarsal, Right** Calcaneus Cuboid bone Intermediate cuneiform bone Lateral cuneiform bone Medial cuneiform bone Navicular bone Talus bone **M Tarsal, Left** *See L Tarsal, Right* **N Metatarsal, Right** Fibular sesamoid Tibial sesamoid **P Metatarsal, Left** *See N Metatarsal, Right* **Q Toe Phalanx, Right** **R Toe Phalanx, Left** **SCoccyx**	**Ø Open** **3 Percutaneous** **4 Percutaneous Endoscopic**	**Ø Drainage Device**	**Z No Qualifier**
Ø Lumbar Vertebra Spinous process Transverse process Vertebral arch Vertebral body Vertebral foramen Vertebral lamina Vertebral pedicle **1 Sacrum** **2 Pelvic Bone, Right** Iliac crest Ilium Ischium Pubis **3 Pelvic Bone, Left** *See 2 Pelvic Bone, Right* **4 Acetabulum, Right** **5 Acetabulum, Left** **6 Upper Femur, Right** Femoral head Greater trochanter Lesser trochanter Neck of femur **7 Upper Femur, Left** *See 6 Upper Femur, Right* **8 Femoral Shaft, Right** Body of femur **9 Femoral Shaft, Left** *See 8 Femoral Shaft, Right* **B Lower Femur, Right** Lateral condyle of femur Lateral epicondyle of femur Medial condyle of femur Medial epicondyle of femur **C Lower Femur, Left** *See B Lower Femur, Right* **D Patella, Right** **F Patella, Left** **G Tibia, Right** Lateral condyle of tibia Medial condyle of tibia Medial malleolus **H Tibia, Left** *See G Tibia, Right* **J Fibula, Right** Body of fibula Head of fibula Lateral malleolus **K Fibula, Left** *See J Fibula, Right* **L Tarsal, Right** Calcaneus Cuboid bone Intermediate cuneiform bone Lateral cuneiform bone Medial cuneiform bone Navicular bone Talus bone **M Tarsal, Left** *See L Tarsal, Right* **N Metatarsal, Right** Fibular sesamoid Tibial sesamoid **P Metatarsal, Left** *See N Metatarsal, Right* **Q Toe Phalanx, Right** **R Toe Phalanx, Left** **S Coccyx**	**Ø Open** **3 Percutaneous** **4 Percutaneous Endoscopic**	**Z No Device**	**X Diagnostic** **Z No Qualifier**

Non-OR ØQ9[Ø,1,2,3,4,5,6,7,8,9,B,C,D,F,G,H,J,K,L,M,P,Q,R,S]3ØZ
Non-OR ØQ9[Ø,1,2,3,4,5,6,7,8,9,B,C,D,F,G,H,J,K,L,M,P,Q,R,S]3ZZ

Ø Medical and Surgical
Q Lower Bones
B Excision Definition: Cutting out or off, without replacement, a portion of a body part
Explanation: The qualifier DIAGNOSTIC is used to identify excision procedures that are biopsies

Body Part Character 4	Approach Character 5	Device Character 6	Qualifier Character 7
Ø Lumbar Vertebra Spinous process Transverse process Vertebral arch Vertebral body Vertebral foramen Vertebral lamina Vertebral pedicle **1 Sacrum** **2 Pelvic Bone, Right** Iliac crest Ilium Ischium Pubis **3 Pelvic Bone, Left** *See 2 Pelvic Bone, Right* **4 Acetabulum, Right** **5 Acetabulum, Left** **6 Upper Femur, Right** Femoral head Greater trochanter Lesser trochanter Neck of femur **7 Upper Femur, Left** *See 6 Upper Femur, Right* **8 Femoral Shaft, Right** Body of femur **9 Femoral Shaft, Left** *See 8 Femoral Shaft, Right* **B Lower Femur, Right** Lateral condyle of femur Lateral epicondyle of femur Medial condyle of femur Medial epicondyle of femur **C Lower Femur, Left** *See B Lower Femur, Right* **D Patella, Right** **F Patella, Left** **G Tibia, Right** Lateral condyle of tibia Medial condyle of tibia Medial malleolus **H Tibia, Left** *See G Tibia, Right* **J Fibula, Right** Body of fibula Head of fibula Lateral malleolus **K Fibula, Left** *See J Fibula, Right* **L Tarsal, Right** Calcaneus Cuboid bone Intermediate cuneiform bone Lateral cuneiform bone Medial cuneiform bone Navicular bone Talus bone **M Tarsal, Left** *See L Tarsal, Right* **Q Toe Phalanx, Right** **R Toe Phalanx, Left** **S Coccyx**	**Ø Open** **3 Percutaneous** **4 Percutaneous Endoscopic**	**Z No Device**	**X Diagnostic** **Z No Qualifier**
N Metatarsal, Right Fibular sesamoid Tibial sesamoid **P Metatarsal, Left** *See N Metatarsal, Right*	**Ø Open** **3 Percutaneous** **4 Percutaneous Endoscopic**	**Z No Device**	**2 Sesamoid Bone(s) 1st Toe** **X Diagnostic** **Z No Qualifier**

Ø Medical and Surgical
Q Lower Bones
C Extirpation Definition: Taking or cutting out solid matter from a body part

Explanation: The solid matter may be an abnormal byproduct of a biological function or a foreign body; it may be imbedded in a body part or in the lumen of a tubular body part. The solid matter may or may not have been previously broken into pieces.

Body Part Character 4	Approach Character 5	Device Character 6	Qualifier Character 7
Ø Lumbar Vertebra Spinous process Transverse process Vertebral arch Vertebral body Vertebral foramen Vertebral lamina Vertebral pedicle **1 Sacrum** **2 Pelvic Bone, Right** Iliac crest Ilium Ischium Pubis **3 Pelvic Bone, Left** *See 2 Pelvic Bone, Right* **4 Acetabulum, Right** **5 Acetabulum, Left** **6 Upper Femur, Right** Femoral head Greater trochanter Lesser trochanter Neck of femur **7 Upper Femur, Left** *See 6 Upper Femur, Right* **8 Femoral Shaft, Right** Body of femur **9 Femoral Shaft, Left** *See 8 Femoral Shaft, Right* **B Lower Femur, Right** Lateral condyle of femur Lateral epicondyle of femur Medial condyle of femur Medial epicondyle of femur **C Lower Femur, Left** *See B Lower Femur, Right* **D Patella, Right** **F Patella, Left** **G Tibia, Right** Lateral condyle of tibia Medial condyle of tibia Medial malleolus **H Tibia, Left** *See G Tibia, Right* **J Fibula, Right** Body of fibula Head of fibula Lateral malleolus **K Fibula, Left** *See J Fibula, Right* **L Tarsal, Right** Calcaneus Cuboid bone Intermediate cuneiform bone Lateral cuneiform bone Medial cuneiform bone Navicular bone Talus bone **M Tarsal, Left** *See L Tarsal, Right* **N Metatarsal, Right** Fibular sesamoid Tibial sesamoid **P Metatarsal, Left** *See N Metatarsal, Right* **Q Toe Phalanx, Right** **R Toe Phalanx, Left** **S Coccyx**	**Ø Open** **3 Percutaneous** **4 Percutaneous Endoscopic**	**Z No Device**	**Z No Qualifier**

Ø Medical and Surgical
Q Lower Bones
D Extraction Definition: Pulling or stripping out or off all or a portion of a body part by the use of force
Explanation: The qualifier DIAGNOSTIC is used to identify extraction procedures that are biopsies

Body Part Character 4	Approach Character 5	Device Character 6	Qualifier Character 7
Ø Lumbar Vertebra Spinous process Transverse process Vertebral arch Vertebral body Vertebral foramen Vertebral lamina Vertebral pedicle **1 Sacrum** **2 Pelvic Bone, Right** Iliac crest Ilium Ischium Pubis **3 Pelvic Bone, Left** *See 2 Pelvic Bone, Right* **4 Acetabulum, Right** **5 Acetabulum, Left** **6 Upper Femur, Right** Femoral head Greater trochanter Lesser trochanter Neck of femur **7 Upper Femur, Left** *See 6 Upper Femur, Right* **8 Femoral Shaft, Right** Body of femur **9 Femoral Shaft, Left** *See 8 Femoral Shaft, Right* **B Lower Femur, Right** Lateral condyle of femur Lateral epicondyle of femur Medial condyle of femur Medial epicondyle of femur **C Lower Femur, Left** *See B Lower Femur, Right* **D Patella, Right** **F Patella, Left** **G Tibia, Right** Lateral condyle of tibia Medial condyle of tibia Medial malleolus **H Tibia, Left** *See G Tibia, Right* **J Fibula, Right** Body of fibula Head of fibula Lateral malleolus **K Fibula, Left** *See J Fibula, Right* **L Tarsal, Right** Calcaneus Cuboid bone Intermediate cuneiform bone Lateral cuneiform bone Medial cuneiform bone Navicular bone Talus bone **M Tarsal, Left** *See L Tarsal, Right* **N Metatarsal, Right** Fibular sesamoid Tibial sesamoid **P Metatarsal, Left** *See N Metatarsal, Right* **Q Toe Phalanx, Right** **R Toe Phalanx, Left** **S Coccyx**	**Ø Open**	**Z No Device**	**Z No Qualifier**

Ø Medical and Surgical
Q Lower Bones
H Insertion

Definition: Putting in a nonbiological appliance that monitors, assists, performs, or prevents a physiological function but does not physically take the place of a body part

Explanation: None

Body Part Character 4		Approach Character 5	Device Character 6	Qualifier Character 7
Ø Lumbar Vertebra Spinous process Transverse process Vertebral arch Vertebral body Vertebral foramen Vertebral lamina Vertebral pedicle **1 Sacrum** **2 Pelvic Bone, Right** Iliac crest Ilium Ischium Pubis **3 Pelvic Bone, Left** *See 2 Pelvic Bone, Right* **4 Acetabulum, Right** **5 Acetabulum, Left**	**D Patella, Right** **F Patella, Left** **L Tarsal, Right** Calcaneus Cuboid bone Intermediate cuneiform bone Lateral cuneiform bone Medial cuneiform bone Navicular bone Talus bone **M Tarsal, Left** *See L Tarsal, Right* **N Metatarsal, Right** Fibular sesamoid Tibial sesamoid **P Metatarsal, Left** *See N Metatarsal, Right* **Q Toe Phalanx, Right** **R Toe Phalanx, Left** **S Coccyx**	**Ø Open** **3 Percutaneous** **4 Percutaneous Endoscopic**	**4 Internal Fixation Device** **5 External Fixation Device**	**Z No Qualifier**
6 Upper Femur, Right Femoral head Greater trochanter Lesser trochanter Neck of femur **7 Upper Femur, Left** *See 6 Upper Femur, Right* **B Lower Femur, Right** Lateral condyle of femur Lateral epicondyle of femur Medial condyle of femur Medial epicondyle of femur	**C Lower Femur, Left** *See B Lower Femur, Right* **J Fibula, Right** Body of fibula Head of fibula Lateral malleolus **K Fibula, Left** *See J Fibula, Right*	**Ø Open** **3 Percutaneous** **4 Percutaneous Endoscopic**	**4 Internal Fixation Device** **5 External Fixation Device** **6 Internal Fixation Device, Intramedullary** **8 External Fixation Device, Limb Lengthening** **B External Fixation Device, Monoplanar** **C External Fixation Device, Ring** **D External Fixation Device, Hybrid**	**Z No Qualifier**
8 Femoral Shaft, Right Body of femur **9 Femoral Shaft, Left** *See 8 Femoral Shaft, Right*	**G Tibia, Right** Lateral condyle of tibia Medial condyle of tibia Medial malleolus **H Tibia, Left** *See G Tibia, Right*	**Ø Open** **3 Percutaneous** **4 Percutaneous Endoscopic**	**4 Internal Fixation Device** **5 External Fixation Device** **6 Internal Fixation Device, Intramedullary** **7 Internal Fixation Device, Intramedullary Limb Lengthening** **8 External Fixation Device, Limb Lengthening** **B External Fixation Device, Monoplanar** **C External Fixation Device, Ring** **D External Fixation Device, Hybrid**	**Z No Qualifier**
Y Lower Bone		**Ø Open** **3 Percutaneous** **4 Percutaneous Endoscopic**	**M Bone Growth Stimulator**	**Z No Qualifier**

Non-OR ØQH[6,7,B,C,J,K][Ø,3,4]8Z
Non-OR ØQH[8,9,G,H][Ø,3,4]8Z

Ø Medical and Surgical
Q Lower Bones
J Inspection

Definition: Visually and/or manually exploring a body part

Explanation: Visual exploration may be performed with or without optical instrumentation. Manual exploration may be performed directly or through intervening body layers.

Body Part Character 4	Approach Character 5	Device Character 6	Qualifier Character 7
Y Lower Bone	**Ø Open** **3 Percutaneous** **4 Percutaneous Endoscopic** **X External**	**Z No Device**	**Z No Qualifier**

Non-OR ØQJY[3,X]ZZ

Ø Medical and Surgical
Q Lower Bones
N Release Definition: Freeing a body part from an abnormal physical constraint by cutting or by the use of force
Explanation: Some of the restraining tissue may be taken out but none of the body part is taken out

Body Part Character 4	Approach Character 5	Device Character 6	Qualifier Character 7
Ø Lumbar Vertebra Spinous process Transverse process Vertebral arch Vertebral body Vertebral foramen Vertebral lamina Vertebral pedicle **1 Sacrum** **2 Pelvic Bone, Right** Iliac crest Ilium Ischium Pubis **3 Pelvic Bone, Left** *See 2 Pelvic Bone, Right* **4 Acetabulum, Right** **5 Acetabulum, Left** **6 Upper Femur, Right** Femoral head Greater trochanter Lesser trochanter Neck of femur **7 Upper Femur, Left** *See 6 Upper Femur, Right* **8 Femoral Shaft, Right** Body of femur **9 Femoral Shaft, Left** *See 8 Femoral Shaft, Right* **B Lower Femur, Right** Lateral condyle of femur Lateral epicondyle of femur Medial condyle of femur Medial epicondyle of femur **C Lower Femur, Left** *See B Lower Femur, Right* **D Patella, Right** **F Patella, Left** **G Tibia, Right** Lateral condyle of tibia Medial condyle of tibia Medial malleolus **H Tibia, Left** *See G Tibia, Right* **J Fibula, Right** Body of fibula Head of fibula Lateral malleolus **K Fibula, Left** *See J Fibula, Right* **L Tarsal, Right** Calcaneus Cuboid bone Intermediate cuneiform bone Lateral cuneiform bone Medial cuneiform bone Navicular bone Talus bone **M Tarsal, Left** *See L Tarsal, Right* **N Metatarsal, Right** Fibular sesamoid Tibial sesamoid **P Metatarsal, Left** *See N Metatarsal, Right* **Q Toe Phalanx, Right** **R Toe Phalanx, Left** **SCoccyx**	**Ø Open** **3 Percutaneous** **4 Percutaneous Endoscopic**	**Z No Device**	**Z No Qualifier**

Ø Medical and Surgical
Q Lower Bones
P Removal Definition: Taking out or off a device from a body part

Explanation: If a device is taken out and a similar device put in without cutting or puncturing the skin or mucous membrane, the procedure is coded to the root operation CHANGE. Otherwise, the procedure for taking out a device is coded to the root operation REMOVAL.

Body Part Character 4		Approach Character 5	Device Character 6	Qualifier Character 7
Ø Lumbar Vertebra Spinous process Transverse process Vertebral arch Vertebral body Vertebral foramen Vertebral lamina Vertebral pedicle **1 Sacrum** **2 Pelvic Bone, Right** Iliac crest Ilium Ischium Pubis **3 Pelvic Bone, Left** *See 2 Pelvic Bone, Right* **4 Acetabulum, Right** **5 Acetabulum, Left** **6 Upper Femur, Right** Femoral head Greater trochanter Lesser trochanter Neck of femur **7 Upper Femur, Left** *See 6 Upper Femur, Right* **8 Femoral Shaft, Right** Body of femur **9 Femoral Shaft, Left** *See 8 Femoral Shaft, Right* **B Lower Femur, Right** Lateral condyle of femur Lateral epicondyle of femur Medial condyle of femur Medial epicondyle of femur	**C Lower Femur, Left** *See B Lower Femur, Right* **D Patella, Right** **F Patella, Left** **G Tibia, Right** Lateral condyle of tibia Medial condyle of tibia Medial malleolus **H Tibia, Left** *See G Tibia, Right* **J Fibula, Right** Body of fibula Head of fibula Lateral malleolus **K Fibula, Left** *See J Fibula, Right* **L Tarsal, Right** Calcaneus Cuboid bone Intermediate cuneiform bone Lateral cuneiform bone Medial cuneiform bone Navicular bone Talus bone **M Tarsal, Left** *See L Tarsal, Right* **N Metatarsal, Right** Fibular sesamoid Tibial sesamoid **P Metatarsal, Left** *See N Metatarsal, Right* **Q Toe Phalanx, Right** **R Toe Phalanx, Left** **S Coccyx**	**Ø Open** **3 Percutaneous** **4 Percutaneous Endoscopic**	**4 Internal Fixation Device** **5 External Fixation Device** **7 Autologous Tissue Substitute** **J Synthetic Substitute** **K Nonautologous Tissue Substitute**	**Z No Qualifier**
Ø Lumbar Vertebra Spinous process Transverse process Vertebral arch Vertebral body Vertebral foramen Vertebral lamina Vertebral pedicle **1 Sacrum** **2 Pelvic Bone, Right** Iliac crest Ilium Ischium Pubis **3 Pelvic Bone, Left** *See 2 Pelvic Bone, Right* **4 Acetabulum, Right** **5 Acetabulum, Left** **6 Upper Femur, Right** Femoral head Greater trochanter Lesser trochanter Neck of femur **7 Upper Femur, Left** *See 6 Upper Femur, Right* **8 Femoral Shaft, Right** Body of femur **9 Femoral Shaft, Left** *See 8 Femoral Shaft, Right* **B Lower Femur, Right** Lateral condyle of femur Lateral epicondyle of femur Medial condyle of femur Medial epicondyle of femur	**C Lower Femur, Left** *See B Lower Femur, Right* **D Patella, Right** **F Patella, Left** **G Tibia, Right** Lateral condyle of tibia Medial condyle of tibia Medial malleolus **H Tibia, Left** *See G Tibia, Right* **J Fibula, Right** Body of fibula Head of fibula Lateral malleolus **K Fibula, Left** *See J Fibula, Right* **L Tarsal, Right** Calcaneus Cuboid bone Intermediate cuneiform bone Lateral cuneiform bone Medial cuneiform bone Navicular bone Talus bone **M Tarsal, Left** *See L Tarsal, Right* **N Metatarsal, Right** Fibular sesamoid Tibial sesamoid **P Metatarsal, Left** *See N Metatarsal, Right* **Q Toe Phalanx, Right** **R Toe Phalanx, Left** **S Coccyx**	**X External**	**4 Internal Fixation Device** **5 External Fixation Device**	**Z No Qualifier**
Y Lower Bone		**Ø Open** **3 Percutaneous** **4 Percutaneous Endoscopic** **X External**	**Ø Drainage Device** **M Bone Growth Stimulator**	**Z No Qualifier**

Non-OR ØQPYX[Ø,M]Z **Non-OR** ØQPY3ØZ **Non-OR** ØQP[Ø,1,2,3,4,5,6,7,8,9,B,C,D,F,G,H,J,K,L,M,N,P,Q,R,S]X[4,5]Z

Ø Medical and Surgical
Q Lower Bones
Q Repair Definition: Restoring, to the extent possible, a body part to its normal anatomic structure and function
Explanation: Used only when the method to accomplish the repair is not one of the other root operations

Body Part Character 4	Approach Character 5	Device Character 6	Qualifier Character 7
Ø Lumbar Vertebra Spinous process Transverse process Vertebral arch Vertebral body Vertebral foramen Vertebral lamina Vertebral pedicle **1 Sacrum** **2 Pelvic Bone, Right** Iliac crest Ilium Ischium Pubis **3 Pelvic Bone, Left** *See 2 Pelvic Bone, Right* **4 Acetabulum, Right** **5 Acetabulum, Left** **6 Upper Femur, Right** Femoral head Greater trochanter Lesser trochanter Neck of femur **7 Upper Femur, Left** *See 6 Upper Femur, Right* **8 Femoral Shaft, Right** Body of femur **9 Femoral Shaft, Left** *See 8 Femoral Shaft, Right* **B Lower Femur, Right** Lateral condyle of femur Lateral epicondyle of femur Medial condyle of femur Medial epicondyle of femur **C Lower Femur, Left** *See B Lower Femur, Right* **D Patella, Right** **F Patella, Left** **G Tibia, Right** Lateral condyle of tibia Medial condyle of tibia Medial malleolus **H Tibia, Left** *See G Tibia, Right* **J Fibula, Right** Body of fibula Head of fibula Lateral malleolus **K Fibula, Left** *See J Fibula, Right* **L Tarsal, Right** Calcaneus Cuboid bone Intermediate cuneiform bone Lateral cuneiform bone Medial cuneiform bone Navicular bone Talus bone **M Tarsal, Left** *See L Tarsal, Right* **N Metatarsal, Right** Fibular sesamoid Tibial sesamoid **P Metatarsal, Left** *See N Metatarsal, Right* **Q Toe Phalanx, Right** **R Toe Phalanx, Left** **S Coccyx**	**Ø Open** **3 Percutaneous** **4 Percutaneous Endoscopic** **X External**	**Z No Device**	**Z No Qualifier**

Non-OR ØQQ[Ø,1,2,3,4,5,6,7,8,9,B,C,D,F,G,H,J,K,L,M,N,P,Q,R,S]XZZ

Ø Medical and Surgical
Q Lower Bones
R Replacement Definition: Putting in or on biological or synthetic material that physically takes the place and/or function of all or a portion of a body part

Explanation: The body part may have been taken out or replaced, or may be taken out, physically eradicated, or rendered nonfunctional during the REPLACEMENT procedure. A REMOVAL procedure is coded for taking out the device used in a previous replacement procedure.

Body Part Character 4	Approach Character 5	Device Character 6	Qualifier Character 7
Ø Lumbar Vertebra Spinous process Transverse process Vertebral arch Vertebral body Vertebral foramen Vertebral lamina Vertebral pedicle **1 Sacrum** **2 Pelvic Bone, Right** Iliac crest Ilium Ischium Pubis **3 Pelvic Bone, Left** *See 2 Pelvic Bone, Right* **4 Acetabulum, Right** **5 Acetabulum, Left** **6 Upper Femur, Right** Femoral head Greater trochanter Lesser trochanter Neck of femur **7 Upper Femur, Left** *See 6 Upper Femur, Right* **8 Femoral Shaft, Right** Body of femur **9 Femoral Shaft, Left** *See 8 Femoral Shaft, Right* **B Lower Femur, Right** Lateral condyle of femur Lateral epicondyle of femur Medial condyle of femur Medial epicondyle of femur **C Lower Femur, Left** *See B Lower Femur, Right* **D Patella, Right** **F Patella, Left** **G Tibia, Right** Lateral condyle of tibia Medial condyle of tibia Medial malleolus **H Tibia, Left** *See G Tibia, Right* **J Fibula, Right** Body of fibula Head of fibula Lateral malleolus **K Fibula, Left** *See J Fibula, Right* **L Tarsal, Right** Calcaneus Cuboid bone Intermediate cuneiform bone Lateral cuneiform bone Medial cuneiform bone Navicular bone Talus bone **M Tarsal, Left** *See L Tarsal, Right* **N Metatarsal, Right** Fibular sesamoid Tibial sesamoid **P Metatarsal, Left** *See N Metatarsal, Right* **Q Toe Phalanx, Right** **R Toe Phalanx, Left** **S Coccyx**	**Ø Open** **3 Percutaneous** **4 Percutaneous Endoscopic**	**7 Autologous Tissue Substitute** **J Synthetic Substitute** **K Nonautologous Tissue Substitute**	**Z No Qualifier**

Ø Medical and Surgical
Q Lower Bones
S Reposition Definition: Moving to its normal location, or other suitable location, all or a portion of a body part

Explanation: The body part is moved to a new location from an abnormal location, or from a normal location where it is not functioning correctly. The body part may or may not be cut out or off to be moved to the new location.

Body Part Character 4	Approach Character 5	Device Character 6	Qualifier Character 7
Ø Lumbar Vertebra Spinous process Transverse process Vertebral arch Vertebral body Vertebral foramen Vertebral lamina Vertebral pedicle	**Ø Open** **4 Percutaneous Endoscopic**	**3 Spinal Stabilization Device, Vertebral Body Tether** **4 Internal Fixation Device** **Z No Device**	**Z No Qualifier**
Ø Lumbar Vertebra ⊞ Spinous process Transverse process Vertebral arch Vertebral body Vertebral foramen Vertebral lamina Vertebral pedicle	**3 Percutaneous**	**4 Internal Fixation Device** **Z No Device**	**Z No Qualifier**
Ø Lumbar Vertebra Spinous process Transverse process Vertebral arch Vertebral body Vertebral foramen Vertebral lamina Vertebral pedicle	**X External**	**Z No Device**	**Z No Qualifier**
1 Sacrum ⊞ **4 Acetabulum, Right** **5 Acetabulum, Left** **S Coccyx** ⊞	**Ø Open** **3 Percutaneous** **4 Percutaneous Endoscopic**	**4 Internal Fixation Device** **Z No Device**	**Z No Qualifier**
1 Sacrum **4 Acetabulum, Right** **5 Acetabulum, Left** **S Coccyx**	**X External**	**Z No Device**	**Z No Qualifier**
2 Pelvic Bone, Right Iliac crest Ilium Ischium Pubis **3 Pelvic Bone, Left** *See 2 Pelvic Bone, Right* **D Patella, Right** **F Patella, Left** **L Tarsal, Right** Calcaneus Cuboid bone Intermediate cuneiform bone Lateral cuneiform bone Medial cuneiform bone Navicular bone Talus bone **M Tarsal, Left** *See L Tarsal, Right* **Q Toe Phalanx, Right** **R Toe Phalanx, Left**	**Ø Open** **3 Percutaneous** **4 Percutaneous Endoscopic**	**4 Internal Fixation Device** **5 External Fixation Device** **Z No Device**	**Z No Qualifier**
2 Pelvic Bone, Right Iliac crest Ilium Ischium Pubis **3 Pelvic Bone, Left** *See 2 Pelvic Bone, Right* **D Patella, Right** **F Patella, Left** **L Tarsal, Right** Calcaneus Cuboid bone Intermediate cuneiform bone Lateral cuneiform bone Medial cuneiform bone Navicular bone Talus bone **M Tarsal, Left** *See L Tarsal, Right* **Q Toe Phalanx, Right** **R Toe Phalanx, Left**	**X External**	**Z No Device**	**Z No Qualifier**

Non-OR ØQSØXZZ
Non-OR ØQS[4,5][3,4]ZZ
Non-OR ØQS[1,4,5,S]XZZ
Non-OR ØQS[2,3,D,F,L,M,Q,R][3,4]ZZ
Non-OR ØQS[2,3,D,F,L,M,Q,R]XZZ

See Appendix L for Procedure Combinations
⊞ ØQSØ3ZZ
⊞ ØQS[1,S]3ZZ

ØQS Continued on next page

Ø Medical and Surgical
Q Lower Bones
S Reposition Definition: Moving to its normal location, or other suitable location, all or a portion of a body part

ØQS Continued

Explanation: The body part is moved to a new location from an abnormal location, or from a normal location where it is not functioning correctly. The body part may or may not be cut out or off to be moved to the new location.

Body Part Character 4	Approach Character 5	Device Character 6	Qualifier Character 7
6 Upper Femur, Right Femoral head Greater trochanter Lesser trochanter Neck of femur **7 Upper Femur, Left** *See 6 Upper Femur, Right* **8 Femoral Shaft, Right** Body of femur **9 Femoral Shaft, Left** *See 8 Femoral Shaft, Right* **B Lower Femur, Right** Lateral condyle of femur Lateral epicondyle of femur Medial condyle of femur Medial epicondyle of femur **C Lower Femur, Left** *See B Lower Femur, Right* **G Tibia, Right** Lateral condyle of tibia Medial condyle of tibia Medial malleolus **H Tibia, Left** *See G Tibia, Right* **J Fibula, Right** Body of fibula Head of fibula Lateral malleolus **K Fibula, Left** *See J Fibula, Right*	**Ø Open** **3 Percutaneous** **4 Percutaneous Endoscopic**	**4 Internal Fixation Device** **5 External Fixation Device** **6 Internal Fixation Device, Intramedullary** **B External Fixation Device, Monoplanar** **C External Fixation Device, Ring** **D External Fixation Device, Hybrid** **Z No Device**	**Z No Qualifier**
6 Upper Femur, Right Femoral head Greater trochanter Lesser trochanter Neck of femur **7 Upper Femur, Left** *See 6 Upper Femur, Right* **8 Femoral Shaft, Right** Body of femur **9 Femoral Shaft, Left** *See 8 Femoral Shaft, Right* **B Lower Femur, Right** Lateral condyle of femur Lateral epicondyle of femur Medial condyle of femur Medial epicondyle of femur **C Lower Femur, Left** *See B Lower Femur, Right* **G Tibia, Right** Lateral condyle of tibia Medial condyle of tibia Medial malleolus **H Tibia, Left** *See G Tibia, Right* **J Fibula, Right** Body of fibula Head of fibula Lateral malleolus **K Fibula, Left** *See J Fibula, Right*	**X External**	**Z No Device**	**Z No Qualifier**
N Metatarsal, Right Fibular sesamoid Tibial sesamoid **P Metatarsal, Left** *See N Metatarsal, Right*	**Ø Open** **3 Percutaneous** **4 Percutaneous Endoscopic**	**4 Internal Fixation Device** **5 External Fixation Device** **Z No Device**	**2 Sesamoid Bone(s) 1st Toe** **Z No Qualifier**
N Metatarsal, Right Fibular sesamoid Tibial sesamoid **P Metatarsal, Left** *See N Metatarsal, Right*	**X External**	**Z No Device**	**2 Sesamoid Bone(s) 1st Toe** **Z No Qualifier**

Non-OR ØQS[6,7,8,9,B,C,G,H,J,K][3,4]ZZ
Non-OR ØQS[6,7,8,9,B,C,G,H,J,K]XZZ
Non-OR ØQS[N,P][3,4]Z[2,Z]
Non-OR ØQS[N,P]XZ[2,Z]

Ø Medical and Surgical
Q Lower Bones
T Resection Definition: Cutting out or off, without replacement, all of a body part
Explanation: None

Body Part Character 4		Approach Character 5	Device Character 6	Qualifier Character 7
2 Pelvic Bone, Right Iliac crest Ilium Ischium Pubis **3 Pelvic Bone, Left** *See 2 Pelvic Bone, Right* **4 Acetabulum, Right** **5 Acetabulum, Left** **6 Upper Femur, Right** Femoral head Greater trochanter Lesser trochanter Neck of femur **7 Upper Femur, Left** *See 6 Upper Femur, Right* **8 Femoral Shaft, Right** Body of femur **9 Femoral Shaft, Left** *See 8 Femoral Shaft, Right* **B Lower Femur, Right** Lateral condyle of femur Lateral epicondyle of femur Medial condyle of femur Medial epicondyle of femur **C Lower Femur, Left** *See B Lower Femur, Right* **D Patella, Right**	**F Patella, Left** **G Tibia, Right** Lateral condyle of tibia Medial condyle of tibia Medial malleolus **H Tibia, Left** *See G Tibia, Right* **J Fibula, Right** Body of fibula Head of fibula Lateral malleolus **K Fibula, Left** *See J Fibula, Right* **L Tarsal, Right** Calcaneus Cuboid bone Intermediate cuneiform bone Lateral cuneiform bone Medial cuneiform bone Navicular bone Talus bone **M Tarsal, Left** *See L Tarsal, Right* **N Metatarsal, Right** Fibular sesamoid Tibial sesamoid **P Metatarsal, Left** *See N Metatarsal, Right* **Q Toe Phalanx, Right** **R Toe Phalanx, Left** **S Coccyx**	**Ø Open**	**Z No Device**	**Z No Qualifier**

Ø Medical and Surgical
Q Lower Bones
U Supplement Definition: Putting in or on biological or synthetic material that physically reinforces and/or augments the function of a portion of a body part
Explanation: The biological material is non-living, or is living and from the same individual. The body part may have been previously replaced, and the SUPPLEMENT procedure is performed to physically reinforce and/or augment the function of the replaced body part.

Body Part Character 4		Approach Character 5	Device Character 6	Qualifier Character 7
Ø Lumbar Vertebra ⊞ Spinous process Transverse process Vertebral arch Vertebral body Vertebral foramen Vertebral lamina Vertebral pedicle **1 Sacrum** ⊞ **2 Pelvic Bone, Right** Iliac crest Ilium Ischium Pubis **3 Pelvic Bone, Left** *See 2 Pelvic Bone, Right* **4 Acetabulum, Right** **5 Acetabulum, Left** **6 Upper Femur, Right** Femoral head Greater trochanter Lesser trochanter Neck of femur **7 Upper Femur, Left** *See 6 Upper Femur, Right* **8 Femoral Shaft, Right** Body of femur **9 Femoral Shaft, Left** *See 8 Femoral Shaft, Right* **B Lower Femur, Right** Lateral condyle of femur Lateral epicondyle of femur Medial condyle of femur Medial epicondyle of femur	**C Lower Femur, Left** *See B Lower Femur, Right* **D Patella, Right** **F Patella, Left** **G Tibia, Right** Lateral condyle of tibia Medial condyle of tibia Medial malleolus **H Tibia, Left** *See G Tibia, Right* **J Fibula, Right** Body of fibula Head of fibula Lateral malleolus **K Fibula, Left** *See J Fibula, Right* **L Tarsal, Right** Calcaneus Cuboid bone Intermediate cuneiform bone Lateral cuneiform bone Medial cuneiform bone Navicular bone Talus bone **M Tarsal, Left** *See L Tarsal, Right* **N Metatarsal, Right** Fibular sesamoid Tibial sesamoid **P Metatarsal, Left** *See N Metatarsal, Right* **Q Toe Phalanx, Right** **R Toe Phalanx, Left** **S Coccyx** ⊞	**Ø Open** **3 Percutaneous** **4 Percutaneous Endoscopic**	**7 Autologous Tissue Substitute** **J Synthetic Substitute** **K Nonautologous Tissue Substitute**	**Z No Qualifier**

See Appendix L for Procedure Combinations
⊞ ØQU[Ø,1,S]3JZ

Ø Medical and Surgical
Q Lower Bones
W Revision Definition: Correcting, to the extent possible, a portion of a malfunctioning device or the position of a displaced device

Explanation: Revision can include correcting a malfunctioning or displaced device by taking out or putting in components of the device such as a screw or pin

Body Part Character 4	Approach Character 5	Device Character 6	Qualifier Character 7
Ø Lumbar Vertebra Spinous process Transverse process Vertebral arch Vertebral body Vertebral foramen Vertebral lamina Vertebral pedicle **1 Sacrum** **4 Acetabulum, Right** **5 Acetabulum, Left** **S Coccyx**	**Ø Open** **3 Percutaneous** **4 Percutaneous Endoscopic** **X External**	**4 Internal Fixation Device** **7 Autologous Tissue Substitute** **J Synthetic Substitute** **K Nonautologous Tissue Substitute**	**Z No Qualifier**
2 Pelvic Bone, Right Iliac crest Ilium Ischium Pubis **3 Pelvic Bone, Left** *See 2 Pelvic Bone, Right* **6 Upper Femur, Right** Femoral head Greater trochanter Lesser trochanter Neck of femur **7 Upper Femur, Left** *See 6 Upper Femur, Right* **8 Femoral Shaft, Right** Body of femur **9 Femoral Shaft, Left** *See 8 Femoral Shaft, Right* **B Lower Femur, Right** Lateral condyle of femur Lateral epicondyle of femur Medial condyle of femur Medial epicondyle of femur **C Lower Femur, Left** *See B Lower Femur, Right* **D Patella, Right** **F Patella, Left** **G Tibia, Right** Lateral condyle of tibia Medial condyle of tibia Medial malleolus **H Tibia, Left** *See G Tibia, Right* **J Fibula, Right** Body of fibula Head of fibula Lateral malleolus **K Fibula, Left** *See J Fibula, Right* **L Tarsal, Right** Calcaneus Cuboid bone Intermediate cuneiform bone Lateral cuneiform bone Medial cuneiform bone Navicular bone Talus bone **M Tarsal, Left** *See L Tarsal, Right* **N Metatarsal, Right** Fibular sesamoid Tibial sesamoid **P Metatarsal, Left** *See N Metatarsal, Right* **Q Toe Phalanx, Right** **R Toe Phalanx, Left**	**Ø Open** **3 Percutaneous** **4 Percutaneous Endoscopic** **X External**	**4 Internal Fixation Device** **5 External Fixation Device** **7 Autologous Tissue Substitute** **J Synthetic Substitute** **K Nonautologous Tissue Substitute**	**Z No Qualifier**
Y Lower Bone	**Ø Open** **3 Percutaneous** **4 Percutaneous Endoscopic** **X External**	**Ø Drainage Device** **M Bone Growth Stimulator**	**Z No Qualifier**

Non-OR ØQW[Ø,1,4,5,S]X[4,7,J,K]Z
Non-OR ØQW[2,3,6,7,8,9,B,C,D,F,G,H,J,K,L,M,N,P,Q,R]X[4,5,7,J,K]Z
Non-OR ØQWYX[Ø,M]Z

Upper Joints ØR2–ØRW

Character Meanings*

This Character Meaning table is provided as a guide to assist the user in the identification of character members that may be found in this section of code tables. It **SHOULD NOT** be used to build a PCS code.

Operation–Character 3	Body Part–Character 4	Approach–Character 5	Device–Character 6	Qualifier–Character 7
2 Change	Ø Occipital-cervical Joint	Ø Open	Ø Drainage Device OR Synthetic Substitute, Reverse Ball and Socket	Ø Anterior Approach, Anterior Column
5 Destruction	1 Cervical Vertebral Joint	3 Percutaneous	3 Infusion Device OR Internal Fixation Device, Sustained Compression	1 Posterior Approach, Posterior Column
9 Drainage	2 Cervical Vertebral Joint, 2 or more	4 Percutaneous Endoscopic	4 Internal Fixation Device	6 Humeral Surface
B Excision	3 Cervical Vertebral Disc	X External	5 External Fixation Device	7 Glenoid Surface
C Extirpation	4 Cervicothoracic Vertebral Joint		7 Autologous Tissue Substitute	J Posterior Approach, Anterior Column
G Fusion	5 Cervicothoracic Vertebral Disc		8 Spacer	X Diagnostic
H Insertion	6 Thoracic Vertebral Joint		A Interbody Fusion Device	Z No Qualifier
J Inspection	7 Thoracic Vertebral Joint, 2 to 7		B Spinal Stabilization Device, Interspinous Process	
N Release	8 Thoracic Vertebral Joint, 8 or more		C Spinal Stabilization Device, Pedicle-Based	
P Removal	9 Thoracic Vertebral Disc		D Spinal Stabilization Device, Facet Replacement	
Q Repair	A Thoracolumbar Vertebral Joint		J Synthetic Substitute	
R Replacement	B Thoracolumbar Vertebral Disc		K Nonautologous Tissue Substitute	
S Reposition	C Temporomandibular Joint, Right		Y Other Device	
T Resection	D Temporomandibular Joint, Left		Z No Device	
U Supplement	E Sternoclavicular Joint, Right			
W Revision	F Sternoclavicular Joint, Left			
	G Acromioclavicular Joint, Right			
	H Acromioclavicular Joint, Left			
	J Shoulder Joint, Right			
	K Shoulder Joint, Left			
	L Elbow Joint, Right			
	M Elbow Joint, Left			
	N Wrist Joint, Right			
	P Wrist Joint, Left			
	Q Carpal Joint, Right			
	R Carpal Joint, Left			
	S Carpometacarpal Joint, Right			
	T Carpometacarpal Joint, Left			
	U Metacarpophalangeal Joint, Right			
	V Metacarpophalangeal Joint, Left			
	W Finger Phalangeal Joint, Right			
	X Finger Phalangeal Joint, Left			
	Y Upper Joint			

* Includes synovial membrane.

AHA Coding Clinic for table ØRB

2019, 3Q, 26	Acromioclavicular joint reconstruction using allograft

AHA Coding Clinic for table ØRG

2021, 1Q, 18	Placement of interspinous distraction device (spacer) for decompression
2021, 1Q, 53	Official guidelines for coding and reporting for interbody fusion device B3.10c
2020, 4Q, 56-58	Intramedullary sustained compression joint fusion
2020, 2Q, 27	Spinal Fusion with NuVasive® VersaTie®
2020, 1Q, 33	Spinal fusion without use of bone graft
2019, 3Q, 28	Use of VERTE-STACK™ implant with fusion
2019, 3Q, 35	Fusion procedures of the spine (guideline B3.1Øc)
2019, 2Q, 19	Cervical spinal fusion, decompression and placement of interfacet stabilization device
2019, 1Q, 30	Spinal fusion performed at same level as decompressive laminectomy
2018, 4Q, 43	Joint fusion device value
2018, 1Q, 22	Spinal fusion procedures without bone graft
2017, 4Q, 62	Added and revised device values - Nerve substitutes
2017, 4Q, 76	Radiolucent porous interbody fusion device
2017, 2Q, 23	Decompression of spinal cord and placement of instrumentation
2014, 3Q, 30	Spinal fusion and fixation instrumentation
2014, 2Q, 7	Anterior cervical thoracic fusion with total discectomy
2013, 1Q, 21-23	Spinal fusion of thoracic and lumbar vertebrae
2013, 1Q, 29	Cervical and thoracic spinal fusion

AHA Coding Clinic for table ØRH

2021, 1Q, 18	Placement of interspinous distraction device (spacer) for decompression
2019, 2Q, 40	Decompression of spinal cord and placement of instrumentation
2018, 3Q, 26	Anterior vertebral tethering using Dynesys Tethering System
2017, 2Q, 23	Decompression of spinal cord and placement of instrumentation
2016, 3Q, 32	Rotator cuff repair, tenodesis, decompression, acromioplasty and coracoplasty

AHA Coding Clinic for table ØRN

2019, 1Q, 30	Spinal fusion performed at same level as decompressive laminectomy
2016, 3Q, 32	Rotator cuff repair, tenodesis, decompression, acromioplasty and coracoplasty
2015, 2Q, 22	Arthroscopic subacromial decompression
2015, 2Q, 23	Arthroscopic release of shoulder joint

AHA Coding Clinic for table ØRP

2017, 4Q, 107	Total ankle replacement versus revision

AHA Coding Clinic for table ØRQ

2016, 1Q, 30	Thermal capsulorrhapy of shoulder

AHA Coding Clinic for table ØRR

2018, 4Q, 92	Radial head arthroplasty
2017, 4Q, 107	Total ankle replacement versus revision
2015, 3Q, 14	Endoprosthetic replacement of humerus and tendon reattachment
2015, 1Q, 27	Reverse total shoulder arthroplasty

AHA Coding Clinic for table ØRS

2019, 3Q, 26	Acromioclavicular joint reconstruction using allograft
2018, 3Q, 26	Anterior vertebral tethering using Dynesys Tethering System
2015, 2Q, 35	Application of tongs to reduce and stabilize cervical fracture
2014, 4Q, 32	Open reduction internal fixation of fracture with debridement
2014, 3Q, 33	Radial fracture treatment with open reduction internal fixation, and release of carpal ligament
2013, 2Q, 39	Application of cervical tongs for reduction of cervical fracture

AHA Coding Clinic for table ØRT

2019, 3Q, 26	Acromioclavicular joint reconstruction using allograft
2014, 2Q, 7	Anterior cervical thoracic fusion with total discectomy

AHA Coding Clinic for table ØRU

2019, 3Q, 26	Acromioclavicular joint reconstruction using allograft
2015, 3Q, 26	Thumb arthroplasty with resection of trapezium

AHA Coding Clinic for table ØRW

2017, 4Q, 107	Total ankle replacement versus revision

Upper Joints

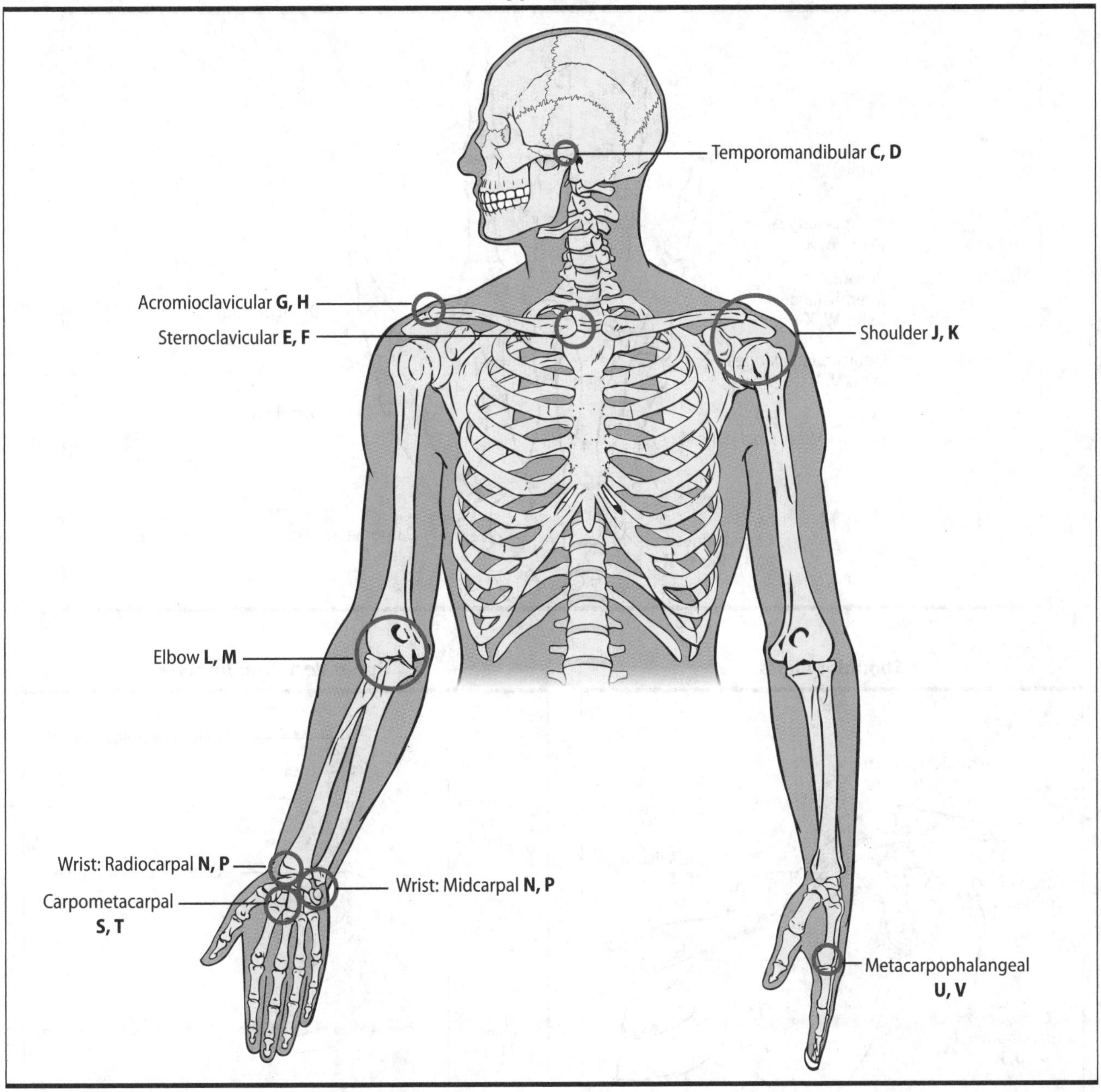

Hand Joints

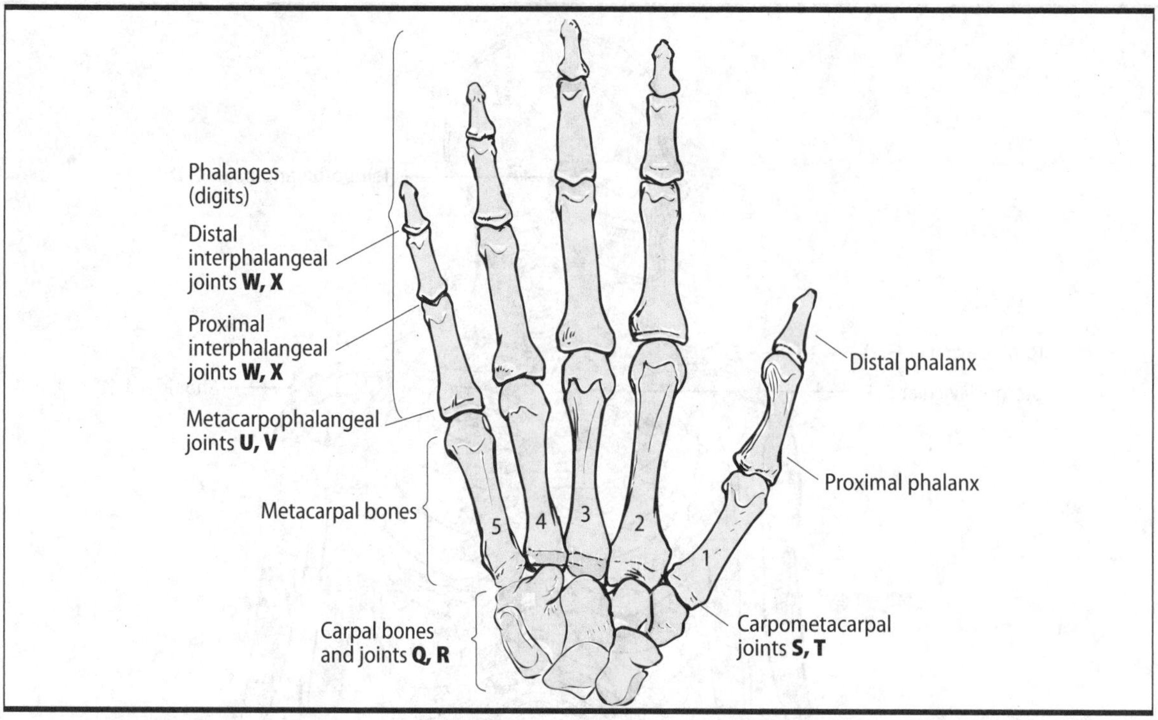

Shoulder Joints

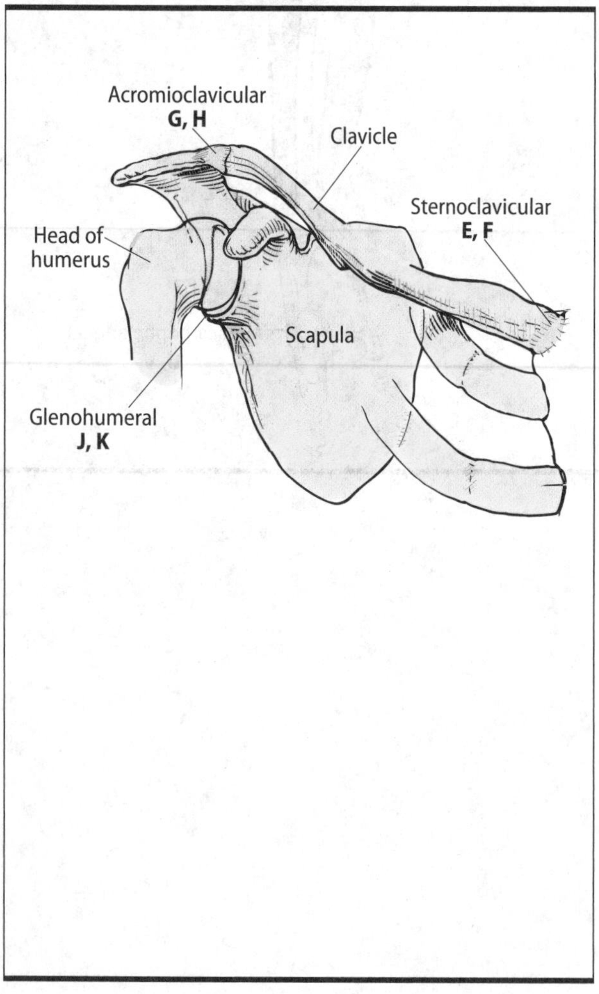

Upper Vertebral Joints

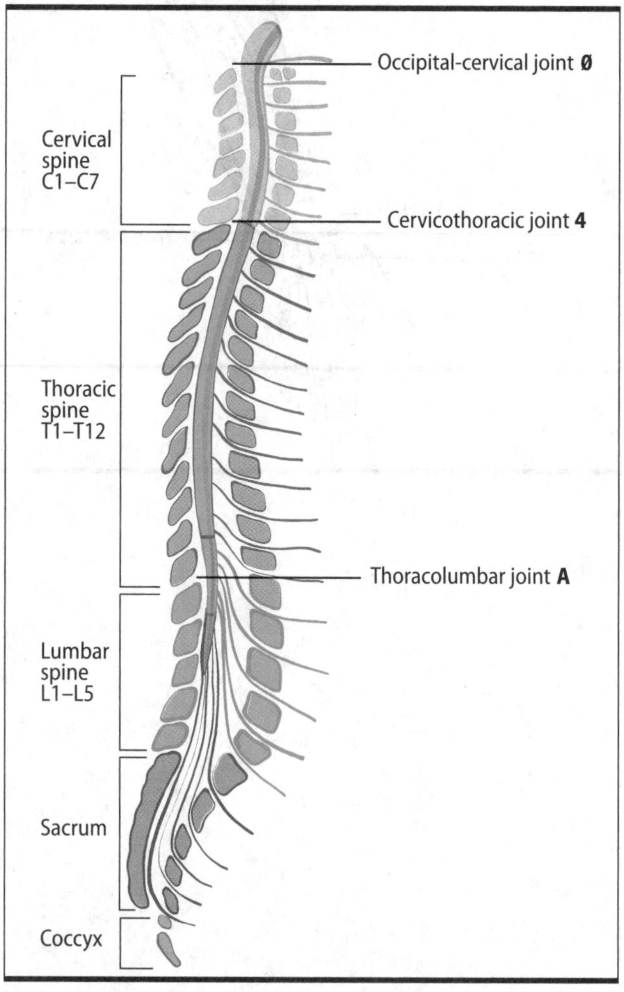

Ø Medical and Surgical
R Upper Joints
2 Change Definition: Taking out or off a device from a body part and putting back an identical or similar device in or on the same body part without cutting or puncturing the skin or a mucous membrane

Explanation: All CHANGE procedures are coded using the approach EXTERNAL

Body Part Character 4	Approach Character 5	Device Character 6	Qualifier Character 7
Y Upper Joint	X External	Ø Drainage Device Y Other Device	Z No Qualifier

Non-OR All body part, approach, device, and qualifier values

Ø Medical and Surgical
R Upper Joints
5 Destruction Definition: Physical eradication of all or a portion of a body part by the direct use of energy, force, or a destructive agent

Explanation: None of the body part is physically taken out

Body Part Character 4	Approach Character 5	Device Character 6	Qualifier Character 7
Ø Occipital-cervical Joint **1 Cervical Vertebral Joint** Atlantoaxial joint Cervical facet joint **3 Cervical Vertebral Disc** **4 Cervicothoracic Vertebral Joint** Cervicothoracic facet joint **5 Cervicothoracic Vertebral Disc** **6 Thoracic Vertebral Joint** Costotransverse joint Costovertebral joint Thoracic facet joint **9 Thoracic Vertebral Disc** **A Thoracolumbar Vertebral Joint** Thoracolumbar facet joint **B Thoracolumbar Vertebral Disc** **C Temporomandibular Joint, Right** **D Temporomandibular Joint, Left** **E Sternoclavicular Joint, Right** **F Sternoclavicular Joint, Left** **G Acromioclavicular Joint, Right** **H Acromioclavicular Joint, Left** **J Shoulder Joint, Right** Glenohumeral joint Glenoid ligament (labrum) **K Shoulder Joint, Left** *See J Shoulder Joint, Right* **L Elbow Joint, Right** Distal humerus, involving joint Humeroradial joint Humeroulnar joint Proximal radioulnar joint **M Elbow Joint, Left** *See L Elbow Joint, Right* **N Wrist Joint, Right** Distal radioulnar joint Radiocarpal joint **P Wrist Joint, Left** *See N Wrist Joint, Right* **Q Carpal Joint, Right** Intercarpal joint Midcarpal joint **R Carpal Joint, Left** *See Q Carpal Joint, Right* **S Carpometacarpal Joint, Right** **T Carpometacarpal Joint, Left** **U Metacarpophalangeal Joint, Right** **V Metacarpophalangeal Joint, Left** **W Finger Phalangeal Joint, Right** Interphalangeal (IP) joint **X Finger Phalangeal Joint, Left** *See W Finger Phalangeal Joint, Right*	Ø Open 3 Percutaneous 4 Percutaneous Endoscopic	Z No Device	Z No Qualifier

Non-OR ØR5[3,5,9,B][3,4]ZZ

Ø Medical and Surgical
R Upper Joints
9 Drainage Definition: Taking or letting out fluids and/or gases from a body part
Explanation: The qualifier DIAGNOSTIC is used to identify drainage procedures that are biopsies

Body Part Character 4	Approach Character 5	Device Character 6	Qualifier Character 7
Ø Occipital-cervical Joint **1 Cervical Vertebral Joint** Atlantoaxial joint Cervical facet joint **3 Cervical Vertebral Disc** **4 Cervicothoracic Vertebral Joint** Cervicothoracic facet joint **5 Cervicothoracic Vertebral Disc** **6 Thoracic Vertebral Joint** Costotransverse joint Costovertebral joint Thoracic facet joint **9 Thoracic Vertebral Disc** **A Thoracolumbar Vertebral Joint** Thoracolumbar facet joint **B Thoracolumbar Vertebral Disc** **C Temporomandibular Joint, Right** **D Temporomandibular Joint, Left** **E Sternoclavicular Joint, Right** **F Sternoclavicular Joint, Left** **G Acromioclavicular Joint, Right** **H Acromioclavicular Joint, Left** **J Shoulder Joint, Right** Glenohumeral joint Glenoid ligament (labrum) **K Shoulder Joint, Left** *See J Shoulder Joint, Right* **L Elbow Joint, Right** Distal humerus, involving joint Humeroradial joint Humeroulnar joint Proximal radioulnar joint **M Elbow Joint, Left** *See L Elbow Joint, Right* **N Wrist Joint, Right** Distal radioulnar joint Radiocarpal joint **P Wrist Joint, Left** *See N Wrist Joint, Right* **Q Carpal Joint, Right** Intercarpal joint Midcarpal joint **R Carpal Joint, Left** *See Q Carpal Joint, Right* **S Carpometacarpal Joint, Right** **T Carpometacarpal Joint, Left** **U Metacarpophalangeal Joint, Right** **V Metacarpophalangeal Joint, Left** **W Finger Phalangeal Joint, Right** Interphalangeal (IP) joint **X Finger Phalangeal Joint, Left** *See W Finger Phalangeal Joint, Right*	**Ø** Open **3** Percutaneous **4** Percutaneous Endoscopic	**Ø** Drainage Device	**Z** No Qualifier
Ø Occipital-cervical Joint **1 Cervical Vertebral Joint** Atlantoaxial joint Cervical facet joint **3 Cervical Vertebral Disc** **4 Cervicothoracic Vertebral Joint** Cervicothoracic facet joint **5 Cervicothoracic Vertebral Disc** **6 Thoracic Vertebral Joint** Costotransverse joint Costovertebral joint Thoracic facet joint **9 Thoracic Vertebral Disc** **A Thoracolumbar Vertebral Joint** Thoracolumbar facet joint **B Thoracolumbar Vertebral Disc** **C Temporomandibular Joint, Right** **D Temporomandibular Joint, Left** **E Sternoclavicular Joint, Right** **F Sternoclavicular Joint, Left** **G Acromioclavicular Joint, Right** **H Acromioclavicular Joint, Left** **J Shoulder Joint, Right** Glenohumeral joint Glenoid ligament (labrum) **K Shoulder Joint, Left** *See J Shoulder Joint, Right* **L Elbow Joint, Right** Distal humerus, involving joint Humeroradial joint Humeroulnar joint Proximal radioulnar joint **M Elbow Joint, Left** *See L Elbow Joint, Right* **N Wrist Joint, Right** Distal radioulnar joint Radiocarpal joint **P Wrist Joint, Left** *See N Wrist Joint, Right* **Q Carpal Joint, Right** Intercarpal joint Midcarpal joint **R Carpal Joint, Left** *See Q Carpal Joint, Right* **S Carpometacarpal Joint, Right** **T Carpometacarpal Joint, Left** **U Metacarpophalangeal Joint, Right** **V Metacarpophalangeal Joint, Left** **W Finger Phalangeal Joint, Right** Interphalangeal (IP) joint **X Finger Phalangeal Joint, Left** *See W Finger Phalangeal Joint, Right*	**Ø** Open **3** Percutaneous **4** Percutaneous Endoscopic	**Z** No Device	**X** Diagnostic **Z** No Qualifier

Non-OR ØR9[Ø,1,3,4,5,6,9,A,B,E,F,G,H,J,K,L,M,N,P,Q,R,S,T,U,V,W,X][3,4]ØZ
Non-OR ØR9[C,D]3ØZ
Non-OR ØR9[Ø,1,3,4,5,6,9,A,B,E,F,G,H,J,K,L,M,N,P,Q,R,S,T,U,V,W,X][Ø,3,4]ZX
Non-OR ØR9[Ø,1,3,4,5,6,9,A,B,E,F,G,H,J,K,L,M,N,P,Q,R,S,T,U,V,W,X][3,4]ZZ
Non-OR ØR9[C,D]3ZZ

Ø Medical and Surgical
R Upper Joints
B Excision Definition: Cutting out or off, without replacement, a portion of a body part
Explanation: The qualifier DIAGNOSTIC is used to identify excision procedures that are biopsies

Body Part Character 4	Approach Character 5	Device Character 6	Qualifier Character 7
Ø Occipital-cervical Joint **1 Cervical Vertebral Joint** Atlantoaxial joint Cervical facet joint **3 Cervical Vertebral Disc** **4 Cervicothoracic Vertebral Joint** Cervicothoracic facet joint **5 Cervicothoracic Vertebral Disc** **6 Thoracic Vertebral Joint** Costotransverse joint Costovertebral joint Thoracic facet joint **9 Thoracic Vertebral Disc** **A Thoracolumbar Vertebral Joint** Thoracolumbar facet joint **B Thoracolumbar Vertebral Disc** **C Temporomandibular Joint, Right** **D Temporomandibular Joint, Left** **E Sternoclavicular Joint, Right** **F Sternoclavicular Joint, Left** **G Acromioclavicular Joint, Right** **H Acromioclavicular Joint, Left** **J Shoulder Joint, Right** Glenohumeral joint Glenoid ligament (labrum) **K Shoulder Joint, Left** *See J Shoulder Joint, Right* **L Elbow Joint, Right** Distal humerus, involving joint Humeroradial joint Humeroulnar joint Proximal radioulnar joint **M Elbow Joint, Left** *See L Elbow Joint, Right* **N Wrist Joint, Right** Distal radioulnar joint Radiocarpal joint **P Wrist Joint, Left** *See N Wrist Joint, Right* **Q Carpal Joint, Right** Intercarpal joint Midcarpal joint **R Carpal Joint, Left** *See Q Carpal Joint, Right* **S Carpometacarpal Joint, Right** **T Carpometacarpal Joint, Left** **U Metacarpophalangeal Joint, Right** **V Metacarpophalangeal Joint, Left** **W Finger Phalangeal Joint, Right** Interphalangeal (IP) joint **X Finger Phalangeal Joint, Left** *See W Finger Phalangeal Joint, Right*	**Ø Open** **3 Percutaneous** **4 Percutaneous Endoscopic**	**Z No Device**	**X Diagnostic** **Z No Qualifier**

Non-OR ØRB[Ø,1,3,4,5,6,9,A,B,E,F,G,H,J,K,L,M,N,P,Q,R,S,T,U,V,W,X][Ø,3,4]ZX

Ø Medical and Surgical
R Upper Joints
C Extirpation Definition: Taking or cutting out solid matter from a body part

Explanation: The solid matter may be an abnormal byproduct of a biological function or a foreign body; it may be imbedded in a body part or in the lumen of a tubular body part. The solid matter may or may not have been previously broken into pieces.

Body Part Character 4	Approach Character 5	Device Character 6	Qualifier Character 7
Ø Occipital-cervical Joint **1 Cervical Vertebral Joint** Atlantoaxial joint Cervical facet joint **3 Cervical Vertebral Disc** **4 Cervicothoracic Vertebral Joint** Cervicothoracic facet joint **5 Cervicothoracic Vertebral Disc** **6 Thoracic Vertebral Joint** Costotransverse joint Costovertebral joint Thoracic facet joint **9 Thoracic Vertebral Disc** **A Thoracolumbar Vertebral Joint** Thoracolumbar facet joint **B Thoracolumbar Vertebral Disc** **C Temporomandibular Joint, Right** **D Temporomandibular Joint, Left** **E Sternoclavicular Joint, Right** **F Sternoclavicular Joint, Left** **G Acromioclavicular Joint, Right** **H Acromioclavicular Joint, Left** **J Shoulder Joint, Right** Glenohumeral joint Glenoid ligament (labrum) **K Shoulder Joint, Left** *See J Shoulder Joint, Right* **L Elbow Joint, Right** Distal humerus, involving joint Humeroradial joint Humeroulnar joint Proximal radioulnar joint **M Elbow Joint, Left** *See L Elbow Joint, Right* **N Wrist Joint, Right** Distal radioulnar joint Radiocarpal joint **P Wrist Joint, Left** *See N Wrist Joint, Right* **Q Carpal Joint, Right** Intercarpal joint Midcarpal joint **R Carpal Joint, Left** *See Q Carpal Joint, Right* **S Carpometacarpal Joint, Right** **T Carpometacarpal Joint, Left** **U Metacarpophalangeal Joint, Right** **V Metacarpophalangeal Joint, Left** **W Finger Phalangeal Joint, Right** Interphalangeal (IP) joint **X Finger Phalangeal Joint, Left** *See W Finger Phalangeal Joint, Right*	**Ø Open** **3 Percutaneous** **4 Percutaneous Endoscopic**	**Z No Device**	**Z No Qualifier**

Ø Medical and Surgical
R Upper Joints
G Fusion Definition: Joining together portions of an articular body part rendering the articular body part immobile
Explanation: The body part is joined together by fixation device, bone graft, or other means

Body Part Character 4	Approach Character 5	Device Character 6	Qualifier Character 7
Ø Occipital-cervical Joint **1 Cervical Vertebral Joint** Atlantoaxial joint Cervical facet joint **2 Cervical Vertebral Joints, 2 or more** Cervical facet joint **4 Cervicothoracic Vertebral Joint** Cervicothoracic facet joint **6 Thoracic Vertebral Joint** Costotransverse joint Costovertebral joint Thoracic facet joint **7 Thoracic Vertebral Joints, 2 to 7** ⊞ **8 Thoracic Vertebral Joints, 8 or more** **A Thoracolumbar Vertebral Joint** Thoracolumbar facet joint	**Ø Open** **3 Percutaneous** **4 Percutaneous Endoscopic**	**7 Autologous Tissue Substitute** **J Synthetic Substitute** **K Nonautologous Tissue Substitute**	**Ø Anterior Approach, Anterior Column** **1 Posterior Approach, Posterior Column** **J Posterior Approach, Anterior Column**
Ø Occipital-cervical Joint **1 Cervical Vertebral Joint** Atlantoaxial joint Cervical facet joint **2 Cervical Vertebral Joints, 2 or more** Cervical facet joint **4 Cervicothoracic Vertebral Joint** Cervicothoracic facet joint **6 Thoracic Vertebral Joint** Costotransverse joint Costovertebral joint Thoracic facet joint **7 Thoracic Vertebral Joints, 2 to 7** ⊞ **8 Thoracic Vertebral Joints, 8 or more** **A Thoracolumbar Vertebral Joint** Thoracolumbar facet joint	**Ø Open** **3 Percutaneous** **4 Percutaneous Endoscopic**	**A Interbody Fusion Device**	**Ø Anterior Approach, Anterior Column** **J Posterior Approach, Anterior Column**
C Temporomandibular Joint, Right **D Temporomandibular Joint, Left** **E Sternoclavicular Joint, Right** **F Sternoclavicular Joint, Left** **G Acromioclavicular Joint, Right** **H Acromioclavicular Joint, Left** **J Shoulder Joint, Right** Glenohumeral joint Glenoid ligament (labrum) **K Shoulder Joint, Left** *See J Shoulder Joint, Right*	**Ø Open** **3 Percutaneous** **4 Percutaneous Endoscopic**	**4 Internal Fixation Device** **7 Autologous Tissue Substitute** **J Synthetic Substitute** **K Nonautologous Tissue Substitute**	**Z No Qualifier**
L Elbow Joint, Right Distal humerus, involving joint Humeroradial joint Humeroulnar joint Proximal radioulnar joint **M Elbow Joint, Left** *See L Elbow Joint, Right* **N Wrist Joint, Right** Distal radioulnar joint Radiocarpal joint **P Wrist Joint, Left** *See N Wrist Joint, Right* **Q Carpal Joint, Right** Intercarpal joint Midcarpal joint **R Carpal Joint, Left** *See Q Carpal Joint, Right* **S Carpometacarpal Joint, Right** **T Carpometacarpal Joint, Left** **U Metacarpophalangeal Joint, Right** **V Metacarpophalangeal Joint, Left** **W Finger Phalangeal Joint, Right** Interphalangeal (IP) joint **X Finger Phalangeal Joint, Left** *See W Finger Phalangeal Joint, Right*	**Ø Open** **3 Percutaneous** **4 Percutaneous Endoscopic**	**3 Internal Fixation Device, Sustained Compression** **4 Internal Fixation Device** **5 External Fixation Device** **7 Autologous Tissue Substitute** **J Synthetic Substitute** **K Nonautologous Tissue Substitute**	**Z No Qualifier**

HAC ØRG[Ø,1,2,4,6,7,8,A][Ø,3,4][7,J,K][Ø,1,J] when reported with SDx K68.11 or T81.4Ø–T81.49, T84.6Ø-T84.619, T84.63-T84.7 with 7th character A

HAC ØRG[Ø,1,2,4,6,7,8,A][Ø,3,4]A[Ø,J] when reported with SDx K68.11 or T81.4Ø–T81.49, T84.6Ø-T84.619, T84.63-T84.7 with 7th character A

HAC ØRG[E,F,G,H,J,K][Ø,3,4][4,7,J,K]Z when reported with SDx K68.11 or T81.4Ø–T81.49, T84.6Ø-T84.619, T84.63-T84.7 with 7th character A

HAC ØRG[L,M][Ø,3,4][3,4,5,7,J,K]Z when reported with SDx K68.11 or T81.4Ø–T81.49, T84.6Ø-T84.619, T84.63-T84.7 with 7th character A

See Appendix L for Procedure Combinations
⊞ ØRG7[Ø,3,4][7,J,K][Ø,1,J]
⊞ ØRG7[Ø,3,4]A[Ø,J]

Ø Medical and Surgical
R Upper Joints
H Insertion

Definition: Putting in a nonbiological appliance that monitors, assists, performs, or prevents a physiological function but does not physically take the place of a body part

Explanation: None

Body Part Character 4	Approach Character 5	Device Character 6	Qualifier Character 7
Ø Occipital-cervical Joint **1 Cervical Vertebral Joint** Atlantoaxial joint Cervical facet joint **4 Cervicothoracic Vertebral Joint** Cervicothoracic facet joint **6 Thoracic Vertebral Joint** Costotransverse joint Costovertebral joint Thoracic facet joint **A Thoracolumbar Vertebral Joint** Thoracolumbar facet joint	**Ø** Open **3** Percutaneous **4** Percutaneous Endoscopic	**3** Infusion Device **4** Internal Fixation Device **8** Spacer **B** Spinal Stabilization Device, Interspinous Process **C** Spinal Stabilization Device, Pedicle-Based **D** Spinal Stabilization Device, Facet Replacement	**Z** No Qualifier
3 Cervical Vertebral Disc **5 Cervicothoracic Vertebral Disc** **9 Thoracic Vertebral Disc** **B Thoracolumbar Vertebral Disc**	**Ø** Open **3** Percutaneous **4** Percutaneous Endoscopic	**3** Infusion Device	**Z** No Qualifier
C Temporomandibular Joint, Right **D Temporomandibular Joint, Left** **E Sternoclavicular Joint, Right** **F Sternoclavicular Joint, Left** **G Acromioclavicular Joint, Right** **H Acromioclavicular Joint, Left** **J Shoulder Joint, Right** Glenohumeral joint Glenoid ligament (labrum) **K Shoulder Joint, Left** *See J Shoulder Joint, Right*	**Ø** Open **3** Percutaneous **4** Percutaneous Endoscopic	**3** Infusion Device **4** Internal Fixation Device **8** Spacer	**Z** No Qualifier
L Elbow Joint, Right Distal humerus, involving joint Humeroradial joint Humeroulnar joint Proximal radioulnar joint **M Elbow Joint, Left** *See L Elbow Joint, Right* **N Wrist Joint, Right** Distal radioulnar joint Radiocarpal joint **P Wrist Joint, Left** *See N Wrist Joint, Right* **Q Carpal Joint, Right** Intercarpal joint Midcarpal joint **R Carpal Joint, Left** *See Q Carpal Joint, Right* **S Carpometacarpal Joint, Right** **T Carpometacarpal Joint, Left** **U Metacarpophalangeal Joint, Right** **V Metacarpophalangeal Joint, Left** **W Finger Phalangeal Joint, Right** Interphalangeal (IP) joint **X Finger Phalangeal Joint, Left** *See W Finger Phalangeal Joint, Right*	**Ø** Open **3** Percutaneous **4** Percutaneous Endoscopic	**3** Infusion Device **4** Internal Fixation Device **5** External Fixation Device **8** Spacer	**Z** No Qualifier

Non-OR ØRH[Ø,1,4,6,A][Ø,3,4][3,8]Z
Non-OR ØRH[3,5,9,B][Ø,3,4]3Z
Non-OR ØRH[C,D][Ø,4]8Z
Non-OR ØRH[C,D]3[3,8]Z
Non-OR ØRH[E,F,G,H,J,K][Ø,3,4][3,8]Z
Non-OR ØRH[L,M,N,P,Q,R,S,T,U,V,W,X][Ø,3,4][3,8]Z

Ø Medical and Surgical
R Upper Joints
J Inspection Definition: Visually and/or manually exploring a body part

Explanation: Visual exploration may be performed with or without optical instrumentation. Manual exploration may be performed directly or through intervening body layers.

Body Part Character 4	Approach Character 5	Device Character 6	Qualifier Character 7
Ø Occipital-cervical Joint **1 Cervical Vertebral Joint** Atlantoaxial joint Cervical facet joint **3 Cervical Vertebral Disc** **4 Cervicothoracic Vertebral Joint** Cervicothoracic facet joint **5 Cervicothoracic Vertebral Disc** **6 Thoracic Vertebral Joint** Costotransverse joint Costovertebral joint Thoracic facet joint **9 Thoracic Vertebral Disc** **A Thoracolumbar Vertebral Joint** Thoracolumbar facet joint **B Thoracolumbar Vertebral Disc** **C Temporomandibular Joint, Right** **D Temporomandibular Joint, Left** **E Sternoclavicular Joint, Right** **F Sternoclavicular Joint, Left** **G Acromioclavicular Joint, Right** **H Acromioclavicular Joint, Left** **J Shoulder Joint, Right** Glenohumeral joint Glenoid ligament (labrum) **K Shoulder Joint, Left** ***See** J Shoulder Joint, Right* **L Elbow Joint, Right** Distal humerus, involving joint Humeroradial joint Humeroulnar joint Proximal radioulnar joint **M Elbow Joint, Left** ***See** L Elbow Joint, Right* **N Wrist Joint, Right** Distal radioulnar joint Radiocarpal joint **P Wrist Joint, Left** ***See** N Wrist Joint, Right* **Q Carpal Joint, Right** Intercarpal joint Midcarpal joint **R Carpal Joint, Left** ***See** Q Carpal Joint, Right* **S Carpometacarpal Joint, Right** **T Carpometacarpal Joint, Left** **U Metacarpophalangeal Joint, Right** **V Metacarpophalangeal Joint, Left** **W Finger Phalangeal Joint, Right** Interphalangeal (IP) joint **X Finger Phalangeal Joint, Left** ***See** W Finger Phalangeal Joint, Right*	**Ø Open** **3 Percutaneous** **4 Percutaneous Endoscopic** **X External**	**Z No Device**	**Z No Qualifier**

Non-OR ØRJ[Ø,1,3,4,5,6,9,A,B,C,D,E,F,G,H,J,K,L,M,N,P,Q,R,S,T,U,V,W,X][3,X]ZZ

Ø Medical and Surgical
R Upper Joints
N Release Definition: Freeing a body part from an abnormal physical constraint by cutting or by the use of force

Explanation: Some of the restraining tissue may be taken out but none of the body part is taken out

Body Part Character 4	Approach Character 5	Device Character 6	Qualifier Character 7
Ø Occipital-cervical Joint 1 Cervical Vertebral Joint Atlantoaxial joint Cervical facet joint 3 Cervical Vertebral Disc 4 Cervicothoracic Vertebral Joint Cervicothoracic facet joint 5 Cervicothoracic Vertebral Disc 6 Thoracic Vertebral Joint Costotransverse joint Costovertebral joint Thoracic facet joint 9 Thoracic Vertebral Disc A Thoracolumbar Vertebral Joint Thoracolumbar facet joint B Thoracolumbar Vertebral Disc C Temporomandibular Joint, Right D Temporomandibular Joint, Left E Sternoclavicular Joint, Right F Sternoclavicular Joint, Left G Acromioclavicular Joint, Right H Acromioclavicular Joint, Left J Shoulder Joint, Right Glenohumeral joint Glenoid ligament (labrum) K Shoulder Joint, Left *See J Shoulder Joint, Right* L Elbow Joint, Right Distal humerus, involving joint Humeroradial joint Humeroulnar joint Proximal radioulnar joint M Elbow Joint, Left *See L Elbow Joint, Right* N Wrist Joint, Right Distal radioulnar joint Radiocarpal joint P Wrist Joint, Left *See N Wrist Joint, Right* Q Carpal Joint, Right Intercarpal joint Midcarpal joint R Carpal Joint, Left *See Q Carpal Joint, Right* S Carpometacarpal Joint, Right T Carpometacarpal Joint, Left U Metacarpophalangeal Joint, Right V Metacarpophalangeal Joint, Left W Finger Phalangeal Joint, Right Interphalangeal (IP) joint X Finger Phalangeal Joint, Left *See W Finger Phalangeal Joint, Right*	Ø Open 3 Percutaneous 4 Percutaneous Endoscopic X External	Z No Device	Z No Qualifier

Non-OR ØRN[Ø,1,3,4,5,6,9,A,B,C,D,E,F,G,H,J,K,L,M,N,P,Q,R,S,T,U,V,W,X]XZZ

Ø Medical and Surgical
R Upper Joints
P Removal Definition: Taking out or off a device from a body part

Explanation: If a device is taken out and a similar device put in without cutting or puncturing the skin or mucous membrane, the procedure is coded to the root operation CHANGE. Otherwise, the procedure for taking out the device is coded to the root operation REMOVAL.

Body Part Character 4	Approach Character 5	Device Character 6	Qualifier Character 7
Ø Occipital-cervical Joint 1 Cervical Vertebral Joint Atlantoaxial joint Cervical facet joint 4 Cervicothoracic Vertebral Joint Cervicothoracic facet joint 6 Thoracic Vertebral Joint Costotransverse joint Costovertebral joint Thoracic facet joint A Thoracolumbar Vertebral Joint Thoracolumbar facet joint	Ø Open 3 Percutaneous 4 Percutaneous Endoscopic	Ø Drainage Device 3 Infusion Device 4 Internal Fixation Device 7 Autologous Tissue Substitute 8 Spacer A Interbody Fusion Device J Synthetic Substitute K Nonautologous Tissue Substitute	Z No Qualifier
Ø Occipital-cervical Joint 1 Cervical Vertebral Joint Atlantoaxial joint Cervical facet joint 4 Cervicothoracic Vertebral Joint Cervicothoracic facet joint 6 Thoracic Vertebral Joint Costotransverse joint Costovertebral joint Thoracic facet joint A Thoracolumbar Vertebral Joint Thoracolumbar facet joint	X External	Ø Drainage Device 3 Infusion Device 4 Internal Fixation Device	Z No Qualifier
3 Cervical Vertebral Disc 5 Cervicothoracic Vertebral Disc 9 Thoracic Vertebral Disc B Thoracolumbar Vertebral Disc	Ø Open 3 Percutaneous 4 Percutaneous Endoscopic	Ø Drainage Device 3 Infusion Device 7 Autologous Tissue Substitute J Synthetic Substitute K Nonautologous Tissue Substitute	Z No Qualifier
3 Cervical Vertebral Disc 5 Cervicothoracic Vertebral Disc 9 Thoracic Vertebral Disc B Thoracolumbar Vertebral Disc	X External	Ø Drainage Device 3 Infusion Device	Z No Qualifier
C Temporomandibular Joint, Right D Temporomandibular Joint, Left E Sternoclavicular Joint, Right F Sternoclavicular Joint, Left G Acromioclavicular Joint, Right H Acromioclavicular Joint, Left	Ø Open 3 Percutaneous 4 Percutaneous Endoscopic	Ø Drainage Device 3 Infusion Device 4 Internal Fixation Device 7 Autologous Tissue Substitute 8 Spacer J Synthetic Substitute K Nonautologous Tissue Substitute	Z No Qualifier
C Temporomandibular Joint, Right D Temporomandibular Joint, Left E Sternoclavicular Joint, Right F Sternoclavicular Joint, Left G Acromioclavicular Joint, Right H Acromioclavicular Joint, Left	X External	Ø Drainage Device 3 Infusion Device 4 Internal Fixation Device	Z No Qualifier
J Shoulder Joint, Right Glenohumeral joint Glenoid ligament (labrum) K Shoulder Joint, Left *See J Shoulder Joint, Right*	Ø Open 3 Percutaneous 4 Percutaneous Endoscopic	Ø Drainage Device 3 Infusion Device 4 Internal Fixation Device 7 Autologous Tissue Substitute 8 Spacer K Nonautologous Tissue Substitute	Z No Qualifier
J Shoulder Joint, Right Glenohumeral joint Glenoid ligament (labrum) K Shoulder Joint, Left *See J Shoulder Joint, Right*	Ø Open 3 Percutaneous 4 Percutaneous Endoscopic	J Synthetic Substitute	6 Humeral Surface 7 Glenoid Surface Z No Qualifier
J Shoulder Joint, Right Glenohumeral joint Glenoid ligament (labrum) K Shoulder Joint, Left *See J Shoulder Joint, Right*	X External	Ø Drainage Device 3 Infusion Device 4 Internal Fixation Device	Z No Qualifier

Non-OR ØRP[Ø,1,4,6,A]3[Ø,3,8]Z
Non-OR ØRP[Ø,1,4,6,A][Ø,4]8Z
Non-OR ØRP[Ø,1,4,6,A]X[Ø,3,4]Z
Non-OR ØRP[3,5,9,B]3[Ø,3]Z
Non-OR ØRP[3,5,9,B]X[Ø,3]Z
Non-OR ØRP[C,D,E,F,G,H]3[Ø,3,8]Z
Non-OR ØRP[C,D,E,F,G,H][Ø,4]8Z
Non-OR ØRP[C,D]X[Ø,3]Z
Non-OR ØRP[E,F,G,H,J,K]X[Ø,3,4]Z
Non-OR ØRP[J,K]3[Ø,3,8]Z
Non-OR ØRP[J,K][Ø,4]8Z
Non-OR ØRP[J,K]X[Ø,3,4]Z

ØRP Continued on next page

Ø Medical and Surgical
R Upper Joints
P Removal Definition: Taking out or off a device from a body part

Explanation: If a device is taken out and a similar device put in without cutting or puncturing the skin or mucous membrane, the procedure is coded to the root operation CHANGE. Otherwise, the procedure for taking out the device is coded to the root operation REMOVAL.

ØRP Continued

Body Part Character 4	Approach Character 5	Device Character 6	Qualifier Character 7
L Elbow Joint, Right Distal humerus, involving joint Humeroradial joint Humeroulnar joint Proximal radioulnar joint **M Elbow Joint, Left** *See L Elbow Joint, Right* **N Wrist Joint, Right** Distal radioulnar joint Radiocarpal joint **P Wrist Joint, Left** *See N Wrist Joint, Right* **Q Carpal Joint, Right** Intercarpal joint Midcarpal joint **R Carpal Joint, Left** *See Q Carpal Joint, Right* **S Carpometacarpal Joint, Right** **T Carpometacarpal Joint, Left** **U Metacarpophalangeal Joint, Right** **V Metacarpophalangeal Joint, Left** **W Finger Phalangeal Joint, Right** Interphalangeal (IP) joint **X Finger Phalangeal Joint, Left** *See W Finger Phalangeal Joint, Right*	**Ø Open** **3 Percutaneous** **4 Percutaneous Endoscopic**	**Ø Drainage Device** **3 Infusion Device** **4 Internal Fixation Device** **5 External Fixation Device** **7 Autologous Tissue Substitute** **8 Spacer** **J Synthetic Substitute** **K Nonautologous Tissue Substitute**	**Z No Qualifier**
L Elbow Joint, Right Distal humerus, involving joint Humeroradial joint Humeroulnar joint Proximal radioulnar joint **M Elbow Joint, Left** *See L Elbow Joint, Right* **N Wrist Joint, Right** Distal radioulnar joint Radiocarpal joint **P Wrist Joint, Left** *See N Wrist Joint, Right* **Q Carpal Joint, Right** Intercarpal joint Midcarpal joint **R Carpal Joint, Left** *See Q Carpal Joint, Right* **S Carpometacarpal Joint, Right** **T Carpometacarpal Joint, Left** **U Metacarpophalangeal Joint, Right** **V Metacarpophalangeal Joint, Left** **W Finger Phalangeal Joint, Right** Interphalangeal (IP) joint **X Finger Phalangeal Joint, Left** *See W Finger Phalangeal Joint, Right*	**X External**	**Ø Drainage Device** **3 Infusion Device** **4 Internal Fixation Device** **5 External Fixation Device**	**Z No Qualifier**

Non-OR ØRP[L,M,N,P,Q,R,S,T,U,V,W,X]3[Ø,3,8]Z
Non-OR ØRP[L,M,N,P,Q,R,S,T,U,V,W,X][Ø,4]8Z
Non-OR ØRP[L,M,N,P,Q,R,S,T,U,V,W,X]X[Ø,3,4,5]Z

Ø Medical and Surgical
R Upper Joints
Q Repair Definition: Restoring, to the extent possible, a body part to its normal anatomic structure and function
Explanation: Used only when the method to accomplish the repair is not one of the other root operations

Body Part Character 4	Approach Character 5	Device Character 6	Qualifier Character 7
Ø Occipital-cervical Joint **1 Cervical Vertebral Joint** Atlantoaxial joint Cervical facet joint **3 Cervical Vertebral Disc** **4 Cervicothoracic Vertebral Joint** Cervicothoracic facet joint **5 Cervicothoracic Vertebral Disc** **6 Thoracic Vertebral Joint** Costotransverse joint Costovertebral joint Thoracic facet joint **9 Thoracic Vertebral Disc** **A Thoracolumbar Vertebral Joint** Thoracolumbar facet joint **B Thoracolumbar Vertebral Disc** **C Temporomandibular Joint, Right** **D Temporomandibular Joint, Left** **E Sternoclavicular Joint, Right** **F Sternoclavicular Joint, Left** **G Acromioclavicular Joint, Right** **H Acromioclavicular Joint, Left** **J Shoulder Joint, Right** Glenohumeral joint Glenoid ligament (labrum) **K Shoulder Joint, Left** *See J Shoulder Joint, Right* **L Elbow Joint, Right** Distal humerus, involving joint Humeroradial joint Humeroulnar joint Proximal radioulnar joint **M Elbow Joint, Left** *See L Elbow Joint, Right* **N Wrist Joint, Right** Distal radioulnar joint Radiocarpal joint **P Wrist Joint, Left** *See N Wrist Joint, Right* **Q Carpal Joint, Right** Intercarpal joint Midcarpal joint **R Carpal Joint, Left** *See Q Carpal Joint, Right* **S Carpometacarpal Joint, Right** **T Carpometacarpal Joint, Left** **U Metacarpophalangeal Joint, Right** **V Metacarpophalangeal Joint, Left** **W Finger Phalangeal Joint, Right** Interphalangeal (IP) joint **X Finger Phalangeal Joint, Left** *See W Finger Phalangeal Joint, Right*	**Ø Open** **3 Percutaneous** **4 Percutaneous Endoscopic** **X External**	**Z No Device**	**Z No Qualifier**

Non-OR ØRQ[Ø,1,3,4,5,6,9,A,B,C,D,E,F,G,H,J,K,L,M,N,P,Q,R,S,T,U,V,W,X]XZZ
HAC ØRQ[E,F,G,H,J,K,L,M][Ø,3,4]ZZ when reported with SDx K68.11 or T81.4Ø–T81.49, T84.6Ø-T84.619, T84.63-T84.7 with 7th character A

Ø Medical and Surgical
R Upper Joints
R Replacement Definition: Putting in or on biological or synthetic material that physically takes the place and/or function of all or a portion of a body part

Explanation: The body part may have been taken out or replaced, or may be taken out, physically eradicated, or rendered nonfunctional during the REPLACEMENT procedure. A REMOVAL procedure is coded for taking out the device used in a previous replacement procedure.

Body Part Character 4	Approach Character 5	Device Character 6	Qualifier Character 7
Ø Occipital-cervical Joint **1 Cervical Vertebral Joint** Atlantoaxial joint Cervical facet joint **3 Cervical Vertebral Disc** **4 Cervicothoracic Vertebral Joint** Cervicothoracic facet joint **5 Cervicothoracic Vertebral Disc** **6 Thoracic Vertebral Joint** Costotransverse joint Costovertebral joint Thoracic facet joint **9 Thoracic Vertebral Disc** **A Thoracolumbar Vertebral Joint** Thoracolumbar facet joint **B Thoracolumbar Vertebral Disc** **C Temporomandibular Joint, Right** **D Temporomandibular Joint, Left** **E Sternoclavicular Joint, Right** **F Sternoclavicular Joint, Left** **G Acromioclavicular Joint, Right** **H Acromioclavicular Joint, Left** **L Elbow Joint, Right** Distal humerus, involving joint Humeroradial joint Humeroulnar joint Proximal radioulnar joint **M Elbow Joint, Left** *See L Elbow Joint, Right* **N Wrist Joint, Right** Distal radioulnar joint Radiocarpal joint **P Wrist Joint, Left** *See N Wrist Joint, Right* **Q Carpal Joint, Right** Intercarpal joint Midcarpal joint **R Carpal Joint, Left** *See Q Carpal Joint, Right* **S Carpometacarpal Joint, Right** **T Carpometacarpal Joint, Left** **U Metacarpophalangeal Joint, Right** **V Metacarpophalangeal Joint, Left** **W Finger Phalangeal Joint, Right** Interphalangeal (IP) joint **X Finger Phalangeal Joint, Left** *See W Finger Phalangeal Joint, Right*	**Ø Open**	**7 Autologous Tissue Substitute** **J Synthetic Substitute** **K Nonautologous Tissue Substitute**	**Z No Qualifier**
J Shoulder Joint, Right Glenohumeral joint Glenoid ligament (labrum) **K Shoulder Joint, Left** *See J Shoulder Joint, Right*	**Ø Open**	**Ø Synthetic Substitute, Reverse Ball and Socket** **7 Autologous Tissue Substitute** **K Nonautologous Tissue Substitute**	**Z No Qualifier**
J Shoulder Joint, Right Glenohumeral joint Glenoid ligament (labrum) **K Shoulder Joint, Left** *See J Shoulder Joint, Right*	**Ø Open**	**J Synthetic Substitute**	**6 Humeral Surface** **7 Glenoid Surface** **Z No Qualifier**

Ø Medical and Surgical
R Upper Joints
S Reposition

Definition: Moving to its normal location, or other suitable location, all or a portion of a body part

Explanation: The body part is moved to a new location from an abnormal location, or from a normal location where it is not functioning correctly. The body part may or may not be cut out or off to be moved to the new location.

Body Part Character 4	Approach Character 5	Device Character 6	Qualifier Character 7
Ø Occipital-cervical Joint **1 Cervical Vertebral Joint** Atlantoaxial joint Cervical facet joint **4 Cervicothoracic Vertebral Joint** Cervicothoracic facet joint **6 Thoracic Vertebral Joint** Costotransverse joint Costovertebral joint Thoracic facet joint **A Thoracolumbar Vertebral Joint** Thoracolumbar facet joint **C Temporomandibular Joint, Right** **D Temporomandibular Joint, Left** **E Sternoclavicular Joint, Right** **F Sternoclavicular Joint, Left** **G Acromioclavicular Joint, Right** **H Acromioclavicular Joint, Left** **J Shoulder Joint, Right** Glenohumeral joint Glenoid ligament (labrum) **K Shoulder Joint, Left** *See J Shoulder Joint, Right*	**Ø Open** **3 Percutaneous** **4 Percutaneous Endoscopic** **X External**	**4 Internal Fixation Device** **Z No Device**	**Z No Qualifier**
L Elbow Joint, Right Distal humerus, involving joint Humeroradial joint Humeroulnar joint Proximal radioulnar joint **M Elbow Joint, Left** *See L Elbow Joint, Right* **N Wrist Joint, Right** Distal radioulnar joint Radiocarpal joint **P Wrist Joint, Left** *See N Wrist Joint, Right* **Q Carpal Joint, Right** Intercarpal joint Midcarpal joint **R Carpal Joint, Left** *See Q Carpal Joint, Right* **S Carpometacarpal Joint, Right** **T Carpometacarpal Joint, Left** **U Metacarpophalangeal Joint, Right** **V Metacarpophalangeal Joint, Left** **W Finger Phalangeal Joint, Right** Interphalangeal (IP) joint **X Finger Phalangeal Joint, Left** *See W Finger Phalangeal Joint, Right*	**Ø Open** **3 Percutaneous** **4 Percutaneous Endoscopic** **X External**	**4 Internal Fixation Device** **5 External Fixation Device** **Z No Device**	**Z No Qualifier**

Non-OR ØRS[Ø,1,4,6,A,C,D,E,F,G,H,J,K][3,4,X][4,Z]Z
Non-OR ØRS[L,M,N,P,Q,R,S,T,U,V,W,X][3,4,X][4,5,Z]Z

Ø Medical and Surgical
R Upper Joints
T Resection Definition: Cutting out or off, without replacement, all of a body part
Explanation: None

Body Part Character 4	Approach Character 5	Device Character 6	Qualifier Character 7
3 Cervical Vertebral Disc **4 Cervicothoracic Vertebral Joint** Cervicothoracic facet joint **5 Cervicothoracic Vertebral Disc** **9 Thoracic Vertebral Disc** **B Thoracolumbar Vertebral Disc** **C Temporomandibular Joint, Right** **D Temporomandibular Joint, Left** **E Sternoclavicular Joint, Right** **F Sternoclavicular Joint, Left** **G Acromioclavicular Joint, Right** **H Acromioclavicular Joint, Left** **J Shoulder Joint, Right** Glenohumeral joint Glenoid ligament (labrum) **K Shoulder Joint, Left** *See J Shoulder Joint, Right* **L Elbow Joint, Right** Distal humerus, involving joint Humeroradial joint Humeroulnar joint Proximal radioulnar joint **M Elbow Joint, Left** *See L Elbow Joint, Right* **N Wrist Joint, Right** Distal radioulnar joint Radiocarpal joint **P Wrist Joint, Left** *See N Wrist Joint, Right* **Q Carpal Joint, Right** Intercarpal joint Midcarpal joint **R Carpal Joint, Left** *See Q Carpal Joint, Right* **S Carpometacarpal Joint, Right** **T Carpometacarpal Joint, Left** **U Metacarpophalangeal Joint, Right** **V Metacarpophalangeal Joint, Left** **W Finger Phalangeal Joint, Right** Interphalangeal (IP) joint **X Finger Phalangeal Joint, Left** *See W Finger Phalangeal Joint, Right*	**Ø Open**	**Z No Device**	**Z No Qualifier**

Ø Medical and Surgical
R Upper Joints
U Supplement Definition: Putting in or on biological or synthetic material that physically reinforces and/or augments the function of a portion of a body part

Explanation: The biological material is non-living, or is living and from the same individual. The body part may have been previously replaced, and the SUPPLEMENT procedure is performed to physically reinforce and/or augment the function of the replaced body part.

Body Part Character 4	Approach Character 5	Device Character 6	Qualifier Character 7
Ø Occipital-cervical Joint **1 Cervical Vertebral Joint** Atlantoaxial joint Cervical facet joint **3 Cervical Vertebral Disc** **4 Cervicothoracic Vertebral Joint** Cervicothoracic facet joint **5 Cervicothoracic Vertebral Disc** **6 Thoracic Vertebral Joint** Costotransverse joint Costovertebral joint Thoracic facet joint **9 Thoracic Vertebral Disc** **A Thoracolumbar Vertebral Joint** Thoracolumbar facet joint **B Thoracolumbar Vertebral Disc** **C Temporomandibular Joint, Right** **D Temporomandibular Joint, Left** **E Sternoclavicular Joint, Right** **F Sternoclavicular Joint, Left** **G Acromioclavicular Joint, Right** **H Acromioclavicular Joint, Left** **J Shoulder Joint, Right** Glenohumeral joint Glenoid ligament (labrum) **K Shoulder Joint, Left** *See J Shoulder Joint, Right* **L Elbow Joint, Right** Distal humerus, involving joint Humeroradial joint Humeroulnar joint Proximal radioulnar joint **M Elbow Joint, Left** *See L Elbow Joint, Right* **N Wrist Joint, Right** Distal radioulnar joint Radiocarpal joint **P Wrist Joint, Left** *See N Wrist Joint, Right* **Q Carpal Joint, Right** Intercarpal joint Midcarpal joint **R Carpal Joint, Left** *See Q Carpal Joint, Right* **S Carpometacarpal Joint, Right** **T Carpometacarpal Joint, Left** **U Metacarpophalangeal Joint, Right** **V Metacarpophalangeal Joint, Left** **W Finger Phalangeal Joint, Right** Interphalangeal (IP) joint **X Finger Phalangeal Joint, Left** *See W Finger Phalangeal Joint, Right*	**Ø Open** **3 Percutaneous** **4 Percutaneous Endoscopic**	**7 Autologous Tissue Substitute** **J Synthetic Substitute** **K Nonautologous Tissue Substitute**	**Z No Qualifier**

HAC ØRU[E,F,G,H,J,K,L,M][Ø,3,4][7,J,K]Z when reported with SDx K68.11 or T81.4Ø–T81.49, T84.6Ø-T84.619, T84.63-T84.7 with 7th character A

Ø Medical and Surgical
R Upper Joints
W Revision Definition: Correcting, to the extent possible, a portion of a malfunctioning device or the position of a displaced device
Explanation: Revision can include correcting a malfunctioning or displaced device by taking out or putting in components of the device such as a screw or pin

Body Part Character 4	Approach Character 5	Device Character 6	Qualifier Character 7
Ø Occipital-cervical Joint 1 Cervical Vertebral Joint Atlantoaxial joint Cervical facet joint 4 Cervicothoracic Vertebral Joint Cervicothoracic facet joint 6 Thoracic Vertebral Joint Costotransverse joint Costovertebral joint Thoracic facet joint A Thoracolumbar Vertebral Joint Thoracolumbar facet joint	Ø Open 3 Percutaneous 4 Percutaneous Endoscopic X External	Ø Drainage Device 3 Infusion Device 4 Internal Fixation Device 7 Autologous Tissue Substitute 8 Spacer A Interbody Fusion Device J Synthetic Substitute K Nonautologous Tissue Substitute	Z No Qualifier
3 Cervical Vertebral Disc 5 Cervicothoracic Vertebral Disc 9 Thoracic Vertebral Disc B Thoracolumbar Vertebral Disc	Ø Open 3 Percutaneous 4 Percutaneous Endoscopic X External	Ø Drainage Device 3 Infusion Device 7 Autologous Tissue Substitute J Synthetic Substitute K Nonautologous Tissue Substitute	Z No Qualifier
C Temporomandibular Joint, Right D Temporomandibular Joint, Left E Sternoclavicular Joint, Right F Sternoclavicular Joint, Left G Acromioclavicular Joint, Right H Acromioclavicular Joint, Left	Ø Open 3 Percutaneous 4 Percutaneous Endoscopic X External	Ø Drainage Device 3 Infusion Device 4 Internal Fixation Device 7 Autologous Tissue Substitute 8 Spacer J Synthetic Substitute K Nonautologous Tissue Substitute	Z No Qualifier
J Shoulder Joint, Right Glenohumeral joint Glenoid ligament (labrum) K Shoulder Joint, Left *See J Shoulder Joint, Right*	Ø Open 3 Percutaneous 4 Percutaneous Endoscopic X External	Ø Drainage Device 3 Infusion Device 4 Internal Fixation Device 7 Autologous Tissue Substitute 8 Spacer J Synthetic Substitute K Nonautologous Tissue Substitute	Z No Qualifier
J Shoulder Joint, Right Glenohumeral joint Glenoid ligament (labrum) K Shoulder Joint, Left *See J Shoulder Joint, Right*	Ø Open 3 Percutaneous 4 Percutaneous Endoscopic X External	J Synthetic Substitute	6 Humeral Surgace 7 Glenoid Surface Z No Qualifier
L Elbow Joint, Right Distal humerus, involving joint Humeroradial joint Humeroulnar joint Proximal radioulnar joint M Elbow Joint, Left *See L Elbow Joint, Right* N Wrist Joint, Right Distal radioulnar joint Radiocarpal joint P Wrist Joint, Left *See N Wrist Joint, Right* Q Carpal Joint, Right Intercarpal joint Midcarpal joint R Carpal Joint, Left *See Q Carpal Joint, Right* S Carpometacarpal Joint, Right T Carpometacarpal Joint, Left U Metacarpophalangeal Joint, Right V Metacarpophalangeal Joint, Left W Finger Phalangeal Joint, Right Interphalangeal (IP) joint X Finger Phalangeal Joint, Left *See W Finger Phalangeal Joint, Right*	Ø Open 3 Percutaneous 4 Percutaneous Endoscopic X External	Ø Drainage Device 3 Infusion Device 4 Internal Fixation Device 5 External Fixation Device 7 Autologous Tissue Substitute 8 Spacer J Synthetic Substitute K Nonautologous Tissue Substitute	Z No Qualifier

Non-OR ØRW[Ø,1,4,6,A]X[Ø,3,4,7,8,A,J,K]Z
Non-OR ØRW[3,5,9,B]X[Ø,3,7,J,K]Z
Non-OR ØRW[C,D,E,F,G,H]X[Ø,3,4,7,8,J,K]Z
Non-OR ØRW[J,K]X[Ø,3,4,7,8,J,K]Z
Non-OR ØRW[J,K]XJ[6,7]
Non-OR ØRW[L,M,N,P,Q,R,S,T,U,V,W,X]X[Ø,3,4,5,7,8,J,K]Z

Lower Joints ØS2–ØSW

Character Meanings*

This Character Meaning table is provided as a guide to assist the user in the identification of character members that may be found in this section of code tables. It **SHOULD NOT** be used to build a PCS code.

Operation–Character 3	Body Part–Character 4	Approach–Character 5	Device–Character 6	Qualifier–Character 7
2 Change	Ø Lumbar Vertebral Joint	Ø Open	Ø Drainage Device OR Synthetic Substitute, Polyethylene	Ø Anterior Approach, Anterior Column
5 Destruction	1 Lumbar Vertebral Joint, 2 or more	3 Percutaneous	1 Synthetic Substitute, Metal	1 Posterior Approach, Posterior Column
9 Drainage	2 Lumbar Vertebral Disc	4 Percutaneous Endoscopic	2 Synthetic Substitute, Metal on Polyethylene	9 Cemented
B Excision	3 Lumbosacral Joint	X External	3 Infusion Device OR Internal Fixation Device, Sustained Compression OR Synthetic Substitute, Ceramic	A Uncemented
C Extirpation	4 Lumbosacral Disc		4 Internal Fixation Device OR Synthetic Substitute, Ceramic on Polyethylene	C Patellar Surface
G Fusion	5 Sacrococcygeal Joint		5 External Fixation Device	J Posterior Approach, Anterior Column
H Insertion	6 Coccygeal Joint		6 Synthetic Substitute, Oxidized Zirconium on Polyethylene	X Diagnostic
J Inspection	7 Sacroiliac Joint, Right		7 Autologous Tissue Substitute	Z No Qualifier
N Release	8 Sacroiliac Joint, Left		8 Spacer	
P Removal	9 Hip Joint, Right		9 Liner	
Q Repair	A Hip Joint, Acetabular Surface, Right		A Interbody Fusion Device	
R Replacement	B Hip Joint, Left		B Resurfacing Device OR Spinal Stabilization Device, Interspinous Process	
S Reposition	C Knee Joint, Right		C Spinal Stabilization Device, Pedicle-Based	
T Resection	D Knee Joint, Left		D Spinal Stabilization Device, Facet Replacement	
U Supplement	E Hip Joint, Acetabular Surface, Left		E Articulating Spacer	
W Revision	F Ankle Joint, Right		J Synthetic Substitute	
	G Ankle Joint, Left		K Nonautologous Tissue Substitute	
	H Tarsal Joint, Right		L Synthetic Substitute, Unicondylar Medial	
	J Tarsal Joint, Left		M Synthetic Substitute, Unicondylar Lateral	
	K Tarsometatarsal Joint, Right		N Synthetic Substitute, Patellofemoral	
	L Tarsometatarsal Joint, Left		Y Other Device	
	M Metatarsal-Phalangeal Joint, Right		Z No Device	
	N Metatarsal-Phalangeal Joint, Left			
	P Toe Phalangeal Joint, Right			
	Q Toe Phalangeal Joint, Left			
	R Hip Joint, Femoral Surface, Right			
	S Hip Joint, Femoral Surface, Left			
	T Knee Joint, Femoral Surface, Right			
	U Knee Joint, Femoral Surface, Left			
	V Knee Joint, Tibial Surface, Right			
	W Knee Joint, Tibial Surface, Left			
	Y Lower Joint			

* Includes synovial membrane.

AHA Coding Clinic for table ØS9

2018, 2Q, 17	Arthroscopic drainage of knee and nonexcisional debridement
2017, 1Q, 50	Dry aspiration of ankle joint

AHA Coding Clinic for table ØSB

2017, 4Q, 76	Radiolucent porous interbody fusion device
2016, 2Q, 16	Decompressive laminectomy/foraminotomy and lumbar discectomy
2016, 1Q, 20	Metatarsophalangeal joint resection arthroplasty
2015, 1Q, 34	Arthroscopic meniscectomy with debridement and abrasion chondroplasty
2014, 2Q, 6	Posterior lumbar fusion with discectomy

AHA Coding Clinic for table ØSG

2021, 1Q, 18	Placement of interspinous distraction device (spacer) for decompression
2021, 1Q, 53	Official guidelines for coding and reporting for interbody fusion device B3.10c
2020, 4Q, 56-58	Intramedullary sustained compression joint fusion
2020, 2Q, 27	Spinal Fusion with NuVasive® VersaTie®
2020, 1Q, 33	Spinal fusion without use of bone graft
2019, 3Q, 35	Fusion procedures of the spine (guideline B3.1Øc)
2019, 1Q, 30	Spinal fusion performed at same level as decompressive laminectomy
2018, 4Q, 43	Joint fusion device value
2018, 1Q, 22	Spinal fusion procedures without bone graft
2017, 4Q, 76	Radiolucent porous interbody fusion device
2017, 2Q, 23	Decompression of spinal cord and placement of instrumentation
2014, 3Q, 30	Spinal fusion and fixation instrumentation
2014, 3Q, 36	Lumbar interbody fusion of two vertebral levels
2014, 2Q, 6	Posterior lumbar fusion with discectomy
2013, 3Q, 25	36Ø-degree spinal fusion
2013, 2Q, 39	Ankle fusion, osteotomy, and removal of hardware
2013, 1Q, 21-23	Spinal fusion of thoracic and lumbar vertebrae

AHA Coding Clinic for table ØSH

2021, 1Q, 18	Placement of interspinous distraction device (spacer) for decompression
2017, 2Q, 23	Decompression of spinal cord and placement of instrumentation

AHA Coding Clinic for table ØSJ

2017, 1Q, 50	Dry aspiration of ankle joint

AHA Coding Clinic for table ØSN

2020, 2Q, 26	Arthroscopic Manipulation and Nonexcisional Debridement of Knee Joint
2019, 1Q, 30	Spinal fusion performed at same level as decompressive laminectomy

AHA Coding Clinic for table ØSP

2021, 1Q, 17	Revision of ankle arthroplasty with placement of tibial insert
2018, 4Q, 43	Articulating spacer for hip and knee joint
2018, 2Q, 16	Exchange of tibial polyethylene component with stabilizing insert (tibial tray)
2017, 4Q, 107	Total ankle replacement versus revision
2016, 4Q, 110-112	Removal and revision of hip and knee devices
2015, 2Q, 18	Total knee revision
2015, 2Q, 19	Revision of femoral head and acetabular liner
2013, 2Q, 39	Ankle fusion, osteotomy, and removal of hardware

AHA Coding Clinic for table ØSQ

2014, 4Q, 25	Femoroacetabular impingement and labral tear with repair

AHA Coding Clinic for table ØSR

2021, 1Q, 17	Revision of ankle arthroplasty with placement of tibial insert
2020, 3Q, 33	Total hip arthroplasty using dual mobility components
2018, 4Q, 43	Articulating spacer for hip and knee joint
2018, 2Q, 16	Exchange of tibial polyethylene component with stabilizing insert (tibial tray)
2017, 4Q, 38-39	Oxidized zirconium on polyethylene bearing surface
2017, 4Q, 107	Total ankle replacement versus revision
2017, 1Q, 22	Total knee replacement and patellar component
2016, 4Q, 110-111	Partial (unicondylar) knee replacement
2016, 4Q, 111-112	Removal and revision of hip and knee devices
2016, 3Q, 35	Use of cemented versus uncemented qualifier for joint replacement
2015, 3Q, 18	Total hip replacement with acetabular reconstruction
2015, 2Q, 18	Total knee revision
2015, 2Q, 19	Revision of femoral head and acetabular liner

AHA Coding Clinic for table ØSS

2016, 2Q, 31	Periacetabular ostectomy for repair of congenital hip dysplasia

AHA Coding Clinic for table ØST

2016, 1Q, 20	Metatarsophalangeal joint resection arthroplasty
2014, 4Q, 29	Rotational osteosynthesis

AHA Coding Clinic for table ØSU

2021, 1Q, 17	Revision of ankle arthroplasty with placement of tibial insert
2018, 2Q, 16	Exchange of tibial polyethylene component with stabilizing insert (tibial tray)
2016, 4Q, 111	Removal and revision of hip and knee devices
2015, 2Q, 19	Revision of femoral head and acetabular liner

AHA Coding Clinic for table ØSW

2017, 4Q, 107	Total ankle replacement versus revision
2016, 4Q, 110-112	Removal and revision of hip and knee devices
2015, 2Q, 18	Total knee revision
2015, 2Q, 19	Revision of femoral head and acetabular liner

Lower Joints

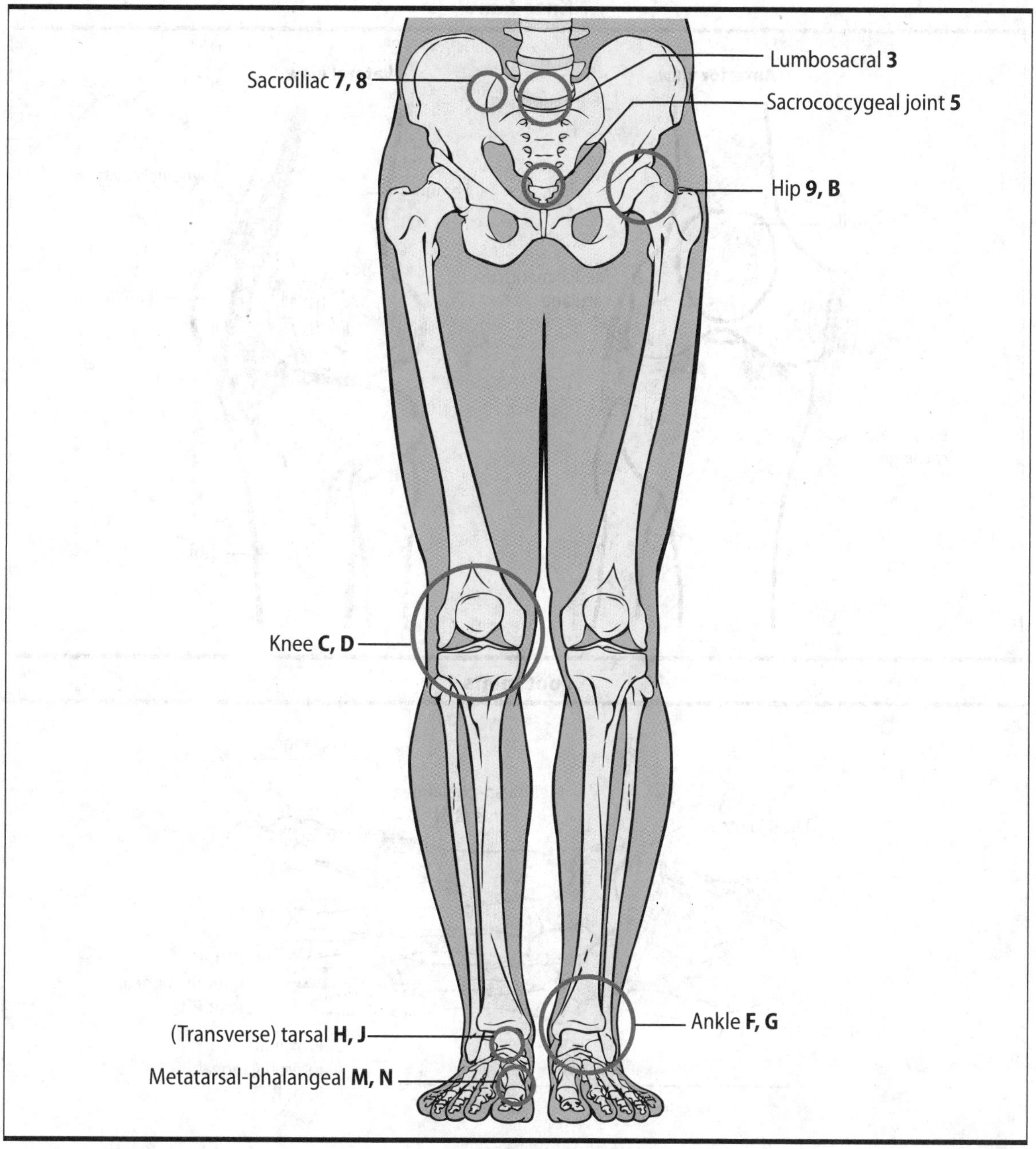

Hip Joint

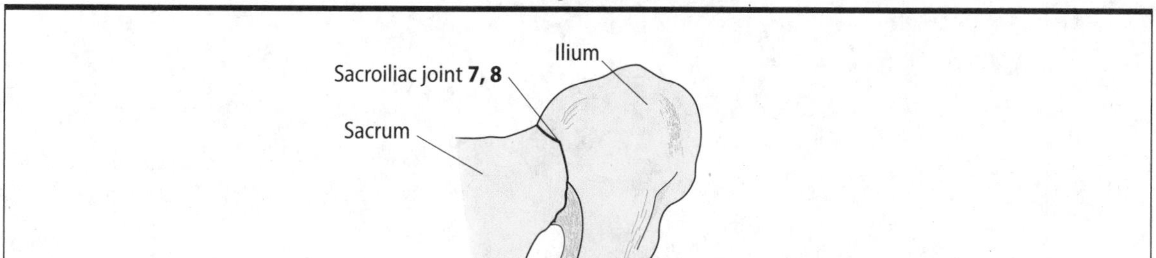

Knee Joint

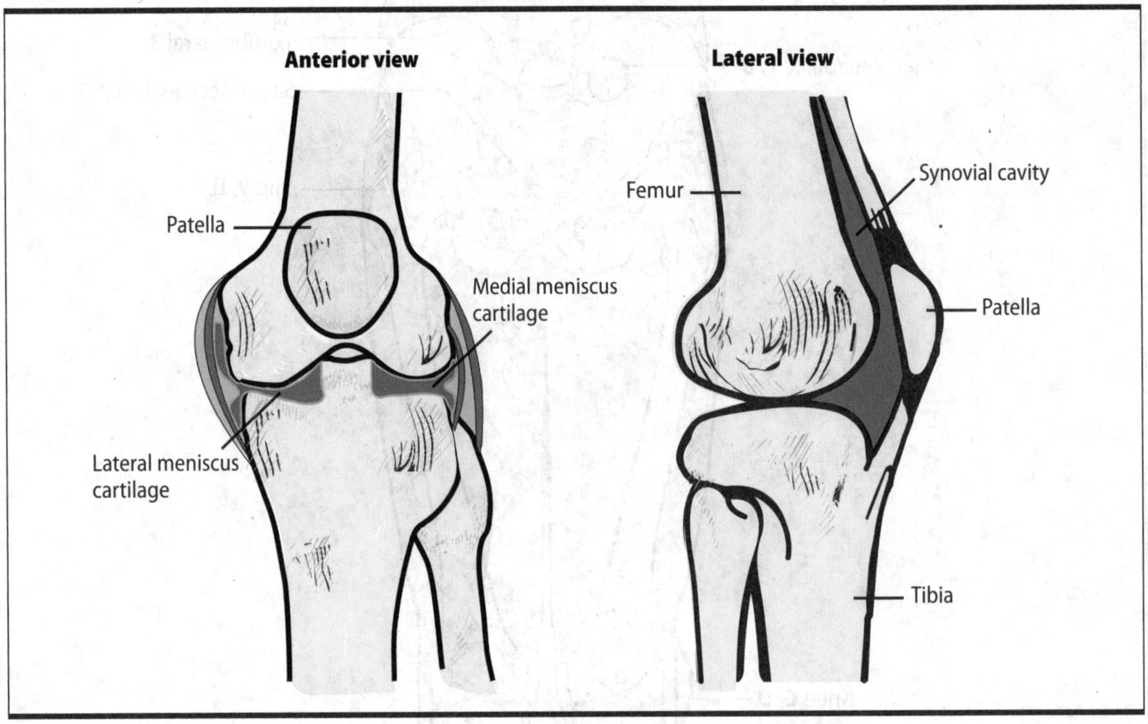

Foot Joints

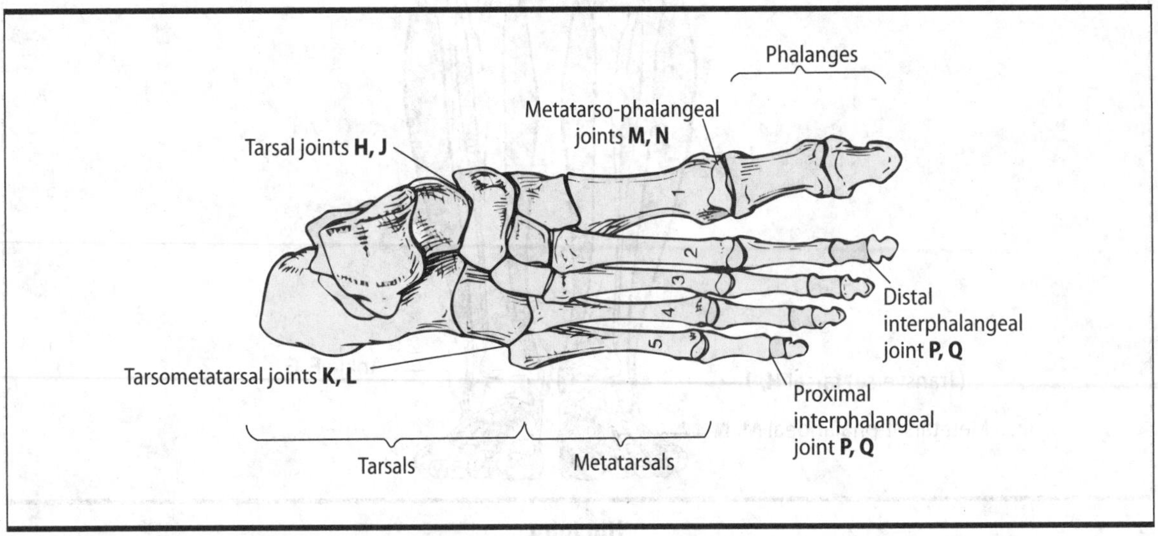

Ø Medical and Surgical
S Lower Joints
2 Change Definition: Taking out or off a device from a body part and putting back an identical or similar device in or on the same body part without cutting or puncturing the skin or a mucous membrane

Explanation: All CHANGE procedures are coded using the approach EXTERNAL

Body Part Character 4	Approach Character 5	Device Character 6	Qualifier Character 7
Y Lower Joint	X External	Ø Drainage Device Y Other Device	Z No Qualifier

Non-OR All body part, approach, device, and qualifier values

Ø Medical and Surgical
S Lower Joints
5 Destruction Definition: Physical eradication of all or a portion of a body part by the direct use of energy, force, or a destructive agent

Explanation: None of the body part is physically taken out

Body Part Character 4	Approach Character 5	Device Character 6	Qualifier Character 7
Ø Lumbar Vertebral Joint Lumbar facet joint **2 Lumbar Vertebral Disc** **3 Lumbosacral Joint** Lumbosacral facet joint **4 Lumbosacral Disc** **5 Sacrococcygeal Joint** Sacrococcygeal symphysis **6 Coccygeal Joint** **7 Sacroiliac Joint, Right** **8 Sacroiliac Joint, Left** **9 Hip Joint, Right** Acetabulofemoral joint **B Hip Joint, Left** *See 9 Hip Joint, Right* **C Knee Joint, Right** Femoropatellar joint Femorotibial joint Lateral meniscus Medial meniscus Patellofemoral joint Tibiofemoral joint **D Knee Joint, Left** *See C Knee Joint, Right* **F Ankle Joint, Right** Inferior tibiofibular joint Talocrural joint **G Ankle Joint, Left** *See F Ankle Joint, Right* **H Tarsal Joint, Right** Calcaneocuboid joint Cuboideonavicular joint Cuneonavicular joint Intercuneiform joint Subtalar (talocalcaneal) joint Talocalcaneal (subtalar) joint Talocalcaneonavicular joint **J Tarsal Joint, Left** *See H Tarsal Joint, Right* **K Tarsometatarsal Joint, Right** **L Tarsometatarsal Joint, Left** **M Metatarsal-Phalangeal Joint, Right** Metatarsophalangeal (MTP) joint **N Metatarsal-Phalangeal Joint, Left** *See M Metatarsal-Phalangeal Joint, Right* **P Toe Phalangeal Joint, Right** Interphalangeal (IP) joint **Q Toe Phalangeal Joint, Left** *See P Toe Phalangeal Joint, Right*	Ø Open 3 Percutaneous 4 Percutaneous Endoscopic	Z No Device	Z No Qualifier

Ø Medical and Surgical
S Lower Joints
9 Drainage Definition: Taking or letting out fluids and/or gases from a body part
Explanation: The qualifier DIAGNOSTIC is used to identify drainage procedures that are biopsies

Body Part Character 4	Approach Character 5	Device Character 6	Qualifier Character 7
Ø Lumbar Vertebral Joint Lumbar facet joint **2 Lumbar Vertebral Disc** **3 Lumbosacral Joint** Lumbosacral facet joint **4 Lumbosacral Disc** **5 Sacrococcygeal Joint** Sacrococcygeal symphysis **6 Coccygeal Joint** **7 Sacroiliac Joint, Right** **8 Sacroiliac Joint, Left** **9 Hip Joint, Right** Acetabulofemoral joint **B Hip Joint, Left** *See 9 Hip Joint, Right* **C Knee Joint, Right** Femoropatellar joint Femorotibial joint Lateral meniscus Medial meniscus Patellofemoral joint Tibiofemoral joint **D Knee Joint, Left** *See C Knee Joint, Right* **F Ankle Joint, Right** Inferior tibiofibular joint Talocrural joint **G Ankle Joint, Left** *See F Ankle Joint, Right* **H Tarsal Joint, Right** Calcaneocuboid joint Cuboideonavicular joint Cuneonavicular joint Intercuneiform joint Subtalar (talocalcaneal) joint Talocalcaneal (subtalar) joint Talocalcaneonavicular joint **J Tarsal Joint, Left** *See H Tarsal Joint, Right* **K Tarsometatarsal Joint, Right** **L Tarsometatarsal Joint, Left** **M Metatarsal-Phalangeal Joint, Right** Metatarsophalangeal (MTP) joint **N Metatarsal-Phalangeal Joint, Left** *See M Metatarsal-Phalangeal Joint, Right* **P Toe Phalangeal Joint, Right** Interphalangeal (IP) joint **Q Toe Phalangeal Joint, Left** *See P Toe Phalangeal Joint, Right*	**Ø Open** **3 Percutaneous** **4 Percutaneous Endoscopic**	**Ø Drainage Device**	**Z No Qualifier**
Ø Lumbar Vertebral Joint Lumbar facet joint **2 Lumbar Vertebral Disc** **3 Lumbosacral Joint** Lumbosacral facet joint **4 Lumbosacral Disc** **5 Sacrococcygeal Joint** Sacrococcygeal symphysis **6 Coccygeal Joint** **7 Sacroiliac Joint, Right** **8 Sacroiliac Joint, Left** **9 Hip Joint, Right** Acetabulofemoral joint **B Hip Joint, Left** *See 9 Hip Joint, Right* **C Knee Joint, Right** Femoropatellar joint Femorotibial joint Lateral meniscus Medial meniscus Patellofemoral joint Tibiofemoral joint **D Knee Joint, Left** *See C Knee Joint, Right* **F Ankle Joint, Right** Inferior tibiofibular joint Talocrural joint **G Ankle Joint, Left** *See F Ankle Joint, Right* **H Tarsal Joint, Right** Calcaneocuboid joint Cuboideonavicular joint Cuneonavicular joint Intercuneiform joint Subtalar (talocalcaneal) joint Talocalcaneal (subtalar) joint Talocalcaneonavicular joint **J Tarsal Joint, Left** *See H Tarsal Joint, Right* **K Tarsometatarsal Joint, Right** **L Tarsometatarsal Joint, Left** **M Metatarsal-Phalangeal Joint, Right** Metatarsophalangeal (MTP) joint **N Metatarsal-Phalangeal Joint, Left** *See M Metatarsal-Phalangeal Joint, Right* **P Toe Phalangeal Joint, Right** Interphalangeal (IP) joint **Q Toe Phalangeal Joint, Left** *See P Toe Phalangeal Joint, Right*	**Ø Open** **3 Percutaneous** **4 Percutaneous Endoscopic**	**Z No Device**	**X Diagnostic** **Z No Qualifier**

Non-OR ØS9[Ø,2,3,4,5,6,7,8,9,B,C,D,F,G,H,J,K,L,M,N,P,Q][3,4]ØZ
Non-OR ØS9[Ø,2,3,4,5,6,7,8,9,B,C,D,F,G,H,J,K,L,M,N,P,Q][Ø,3,4]ZX
Non-OR ØS9[Ø,2,3,4,5,6,7,8,9,B,C,D,F,G,H,J,K,L,M,N,P,Q][3,4]ZZ

Ø Medical and Surgical
S Lower Joints
B Excision Definition: Cutting out or off, without replacement, a portion of a body part
Explanation: The qualifier DIAGNOSTIC is used to identify excision procedures that are biopsies

Body Part Character 4	Approach Character 5	Device Character 6	Qualifier Character 7
Ø Lumbar Vertebral Joint Lumbar facet joint **2 Lumbar Vertebral Disc** **3 Lumbosacral Joint** Lumbosacral facet joint **4 Lumbosacral Disc** **5 Sacrococcygeal Joint** Sacrococcygeal symphysis **6 Coccygeal Joint** **7 Sacroiliac Joint, Right** **8 Sacroiliac Joint, Left** **9 Hip Joint, Right** Acetabulofemoral joint **B Hip Joint, Left** *See 9 Hip Joint, Right* **C Knee Joint, Right** Femoropatellar joint Femorotibial joint Lateral meniscus Medial meniscus Patellofemoral joint Tibiofemoral joint **D Knee Joint, Left** *See C Knee Joint, Right* **F Ankle Joint, Right** Inferior tibiofibular joint Talocrural joint **G Ankle Joint, Left** *See F Ankle Joint, Right* **H Tarsal Joint, Right** Calcaneocuboid joint Cuboideonavicular joint Cuneonavicular joint Intercuneiform joint Subtalar (talocalcaneal) joint Talocalcaneal (subtalar) joint Talocalcaneonavicular joint **J Tarsal Joint, Left** *See H Tarsal Joint, Right* **K Tarsometatarsal Joint, Right** **L Tarsometatarsal Joint, Left** **M Metatarsal-Phalangeal Joint, Right** Metatarsophalangeal (MTP) joint **N Metatarsal-Phalangeal Joint, Left** *See M Metatarsal-Phalangeal Joint, Right* **P Toe Phalangeal Joint, Right** Interphalangeal (IP) joint **Q Toe Phalangeal Joint, Left** *See P Toe Phalangeal Joint, Right*	**Ø Open** **3 Percutaneous** **4 Percutaneous Endoscopic**	**Z No Device**	**X Diagnostic** **Z No Qualifier**

Non-OR ØSB[Ø,2,3,4,5,6,7,8,9,B,C,D,F,G,H,J,K,L,M,N,P,Q][Ø,3,4]ZX

Ø Medical and Surgical
S Lower Joints
C Extirpation Definition: Taking or cutting out solid matter from a body part

Explanation: The solid matter may be an abnormal byproduct of a biological function or a foreign body; it may be imbedded in a body part or in the lumen of a tubular body part. The solid matter may or may not have been previously broken into pieces.

Body Part Character 4	Approach Character 5	Device Character 6	Qualifier Character 7
Ø Lumbar Vertebral Joint Lumbar facet joint **2 Lumbar Vertebral Disc** **3 Lumbosacral Joint** Lumbosacral facet joint **4 Lumbosacral Disc** **5 Sacrococcygeal Joint** Sacrococcygeal symphysis **6 Coccygeal Joint** **7 Sacroiliac Joint, Right** **8 Sacroiliac Joint, Left** **9 Hip Joint, Right** Acetabulofemoral joint **B Hip Joint, Left** *See 9 Hip Joint, Right* **C Knee Joint, Right** Femoropatellar joint Femorotibial joint Lateral meniscus Medial meniscus Patellofemoral joint Tibiofemoral joint **D Knee Joint, Left** *See C Knee Joint, Right* **F Ankle Joint, Right** Inferior tibiofibular joint Talocrural joint **G Ankle Joint, Left** *See F Ankle Joint, Right* **H Tarsal Joint, Right** Calcaneocuboid joint Cuboideonavicular joint Cuneonavicular joint Intercuneiform joint Subtalar (talocalcaneal) joint Talocalcaneal (subtalar) joint Talocalcaneonavicular joint **J Tarsal Joint, Left** *See H Tarsal Joint, Right* **K Tarsometatarsal Joint, Right** **L Tarsometatarsal Joint, Left** **M Metatarsal-Phalangeal Joint, Right** Metatarsophalangeal (MTP) joint **N Metatarsal-Phalangeal Joint, Left** *See M Metatarsal-Phalangeal Joint, Right* **P Toe Phalangeal Joint, Right** Interphalangeal (IP) joint **Q Toe Phalangeal Joint, Left** *See P Toe Phalangeal Joint, Right*	**Ø Open** **3 Percutaneous** **4 Percutaneous Endoscopic**	**Z No Device**	**Z No Qualifier**

Ø Medical and Surgical
S Lower Joints
G Fusion Definition: Joining together portions of an articular body part rendering the articular body part immobile
Explanation: The body part is joined together by fixation device, bone graft, or other means

Body Part Character 4	Approach Character 5	Device Character 6	Qualifier Character 7
Ø Lumbar Vertebral Joint Lumbar facet joint **1 Lumbar Vertebral Joints, 2 or more** ⊞ **3 Lumbosacral Joint** Lumbosacral facet joint	**Ø Open** **3 Percutaneous** **4 Percutaneous Endoscopic**	**7 Autologous Tissue Substitute** **J Synthetic Substitute** **K Nonautologous Tissue Substitute**	**Ø Anterior Approach, Anterior Column** **1 Posterior Approach, Posterior Column** **J Posterior Approach, Anterior Column**
Ø Lumbar Vertebral Joint Lumbar facet joint **1 Lumbar Vertebral Joints, 2 or more** ⊞ **3 Lumbosacral Joint** Lumbosacral facet joint	**Ø Open** **3 Percutaneous** **4 Percutaneous Endoscopic**	**A Interbody Fusion Device**	**Ø Anterior Approach, Anterior Column** **J Posterior Approach, Anterior Column**
5 Sacrococcygeal Joint Sacrococcygeal symphysis **6 Coccygeal Joint** **7 Sacroiliac Joint, Right** **8 Sacroiliac Joint, Left**	**Ø Open** **3 Percutaneous** **4 Percutaneous Endoscopic**	**4 Internal Fixation Device** **7 Autologous Tissue Substitute** **J Synthetic Substitute** **K Nonautologous Tissue Substitute**	**Z No Qualifier**
9 Hip Joint, Right Acetabulofemoral joint **B Hip Joint, Left** *See 9 Hip Joint, Right* **C Knee Joint, Right** Femoropatellar joint Femorotibial joint Lateral meniscus Medial meniscus Patellofemoral joint Tibiofemoral joint **D Knee Joint, Left** *See C Knee Joint, Right* **F Ankle Joint, Right** Inferior tibiofibular joint Talocrural joint **G Ankle Joint, Left** *See F Ankle Joint, Right* **H Tarsal Joint, Right** Calcaneocuboid joint Cuboideonavicular joint Cuneonavicular joint Intercuneiform joint Subtalar (talocalcaneal) joint Talocalcaneal (subtalar) joint Talocalcaneonavicular joint **J Tarsal Joint, Left** *See H Tarsal Joint, Right* **K Tarsometatarsal Joint, Right** **L Tarsometatarsal Joint, Left** **M Metatarsal-Phalangeal Joint, Right** Metatarsophalangeal (MTP) joint **N Metatarsal-Phalangeal Joint, Left** *See M Metatarsal-Phalangeal Joint, Right* **P Toe Phalangeal Joint, Right** Interphalangeal (IP) joint **Q Toe Phalangeal Joint, Left** *See P Toe Phalangeal Joint, Right*	**Ø Open** **3 Percutaneous** **4 Percutaneous Endoscopic**	**3 Internal Fixation Device, Sustained Compression** **4 Internal Fixation Device** **5 External Fixation Device** **7 Autologous Tissue Substitute** **J Synthetic Substitute** **K Nonautologous Tissue Substitute**	**Z No Qualifier**

HAC ØSG[Ø,1,3][Ø,3,4][7,J,K][Ø,1,J] when reported with SDx K68.11 or T81.4Ø–T81.49, T84.6Ø-T84.619, T84.63-T84.7 with 7th character A
HAC ØSG[Ø,1,3][Ø,3,4]A[Ø,J] when reported with SDx K68.11 or T81.4Ø–T81.49, T84.6Ø-T84.619, T84.63-T84.7 with 7th character A
HAC ØSG[7,8][Ø,3,4][4,7,J,K]Z when reported with SDx K68.11 or T81.4Ø–T81.49, T84.6Ø-T84.619, T84.63-T84.7 with 7th character A

See Appendix L for Procedure Combinations
⊞ ØSG1[Ø,3,4][7,J,K][Ø,1,J]
⊞ ØSG1[Ø,3,4]A[Ø,J]

Lower Joints
ØSG–ØSG

Ø Medical and Surgical
S Lower Joints
H Insertion Definition: Putting in a nonbiological appliance that monitors, assists, performs, or prevents a physiological function but does not physically take the place of a body part

Explanation: None

Body Part Character 4	Approach Character 5	Device Character 6	Qualifier Character 7
Ø Lumbar Vertebral Joint Lumbar facet joint **3 Lumbosacral Joint** Lumbosacral facet joint	**Ø Open** **3 Percutaneous** **4 Percutaneous Endoscopic**	**3 Infusion Device** **4 Internal Fixation Device** **8 Spacer** **B Spinal Stabilization Device, Interspinous Process** **C Spinal Stabilization Device, Pedicle-Based** **D Spinal Stabilization Device, Facet Replacement**	**Z No Qualifier**
2 Lumbar Vertebral Disc **4 Lumbosacral Disc**	**Ø Open** **3 Percutaneous** **4 Percutaneous Endoscopic**	**3 Infusion Device** **8 Spacer**	**Z No Qualifier**
5 Sacrococcygeal Joint Sacrococcygeal symphysis **6 Coccygeal Joint** **7 Sacroiliac Joint, Right** **8 Sacroiliac Joint, Left**	**Ø Open** **3 Percutaneous** **4 Percutaneous Endoscopic**	**3 Infusion Device** **4 Internal Fixation Device** **8 Spacer**	**Z No Qualifier**
9 Hip Joint, Right Acetabulofemoral joint **B Hip Joint, Left** *See 9 Hip Joint, Right* **C Knee Joint, Right** Femoropatellar joint Femorotibial joint Lateral meniscus Medial meniscus Patellofemoral joint Tibiofemoral joint **D Knee Joint, Left** *See C Knee Joint, Right* **F Ankle Joint, Right** Inferior tibiofibular joint Talocrural joint **G Ankle Joint, Left** *See F Ankle Joint, Right* **H Tarsal Joint, Right** Calcaneocuboid joint Cuboideonavicular joint Cuneonavicular joint Intercuneiform joint Subtalar (talocalcaneal) joint Talocalcaneal (subtalar) joint Talocalcaneonavicular joint **J Tarsal Joint, Left** *See H Tarsal Joint, Right* **K Tarsometatarsal Joint, Right** **L Tarsometatarsal Joint, Left** **M Metatarsal-Phalangeal Joint, Right** Metatarsophalangeal (MTP) joint **N Metatarsal-Phalangeal Joint, Left** *See M Metatarsal-Phalangeal Joint, Right* **P Toe Phalangeal Joint, Right** Interphalangeal (IP) joint **Q Toe Phalangeal Joint, Left** *See P Toe Phalangeal Joint, Right*	**Ø Open** **3 Percutaneous** **4 Percutaneous Endoscopic**	**3 Infusion Device** **4 Internal Fixation Device** **5 External Fixation Device** **8 Spacer**	**Z No Qualifier**

Non-OR ØSH[Ø,3][Ø,3,4][3,8]Z
Non-OR ØSH[2,4][Ø,3,4][3,8]Z
Non-OR ØSH[5,6,7,8][Ø,3,4][3,8]Z
Non-OR ØSH[9,B,C,D][Ø,3,4]3Z
Non-OR ØSH[9,B,C,D][3,4]8Z
Non-OR ØSH[F,G,H,J,K,L,M,N,P,Q][Ø,3,4][3,8]Z

Ø Medical and Surgical
S Lower Joints
J Inspection Definition: Visually and/or manually exploring a body part

Explanation: Visual exploration may be performed with or without optical instrumentation. Manual exploration may be performed directly or through intervening body layers.

Body Part Character 4		Approach Character 5	Device Character 6	Qualifier Character 7
Ø Lumbar Vertebral Joint Lumbar facet joint **2 Lumbar Vertebral Disc** **3 Lumbosacral Joint** Lumbosacral facet joint **4 Lumbosacral Disc** **5 Sacrococcygeal Joint** Sacrococcygeal symphysis **6 Coccygeal Joint** **7 Sacroiliac Joint, Right** **8 Sacroiliac Joint, Left** **9 Hip Joint, Right** Acetabulofemoral joint **B Hip Joint, Left** *See 9 Hip Joint, Right* **C Knee Joint, Right** Femoropatellar joint Femorotibial joint Lateral meniscus Medial meniscus Patellofemoral joint Tibiofemoral joint **D Knee Joint, Left** *See C Knee Joint, Right* **F Ankle Joint, Right** Inferior tibiofibular joint Talocrural joint **G Ankle Joint, Left** *See F Ankle Joint, Right*	**H Tarsal Joint, Right** Calcaneocuboid joint Cuboideonavicular joint Cuneonavicular joint Intercuneiform joint Subtalar (talocalcaneal) joint Talocalcaneal (subtalar) joint Talocalcaneonavicular joint **J Tarsal Joint, Left** *See H Tarsal Joint, Right* **K Tarsometatarsal Joint, Right** **L Tarsometatarsal Joint, Left** **M Metatarsal-Phalangeal Joint, Right** Metatarsophalangeal (MTP) joint **N Metatarsal-Phalangeal Joint, Left** *See M Metatarsal-Phalangeal Joint, Right* **P Toe Phalangeal Joint, Right** Interphalangeal (IP) joint **Q Toe Phalangeal Joint, Left** *See P Toe Phalangeal Joint, Right*	**Ø** Open **3** Percutaneous **4** Percutaneous Endoscopic **X** External	**Z** No Device	**Z** No Qualifier

Non-OR ØSJ[Ø,2,3,4,5,6,7,8,9,B,C,D,F,G,H,J,K,L,M,N,P,Q][3,X]ZZ

Ø Medical and Surgical
S Lower Joints
N Release Definition: Freeing a body part from an abnormal physical constraint by cutting or by the use of force

Explanation: Some of the restraining tissue may be taken out but none of the body part is taken out

Body Part Character 4		Approach Character 5	Device Character 6	Qualifier Character 7
Ø Lumbar Vertebral Joint Lumbar facet joint **2 Lumbar Vertebral Disc** **3 Lumbosacral Joint** Lumbosacral facet joint **4 Lumbosacral Disc** **5 Sacrococcygeal Joint** Sacrococcygeal symphysis **6 Coccygeal Joint** **7 Sacroiliac Joint, Right** **8 Sacroiliac Joint, Left** **9 Hip Joint, Right** Acetabulofemoral joint **B Hip Joint, Left** *See 9 Hip Joint, Right* **C Knee Joint, Right** Femoropatellar joint Femorotibial joint Lateral meniscus Medial meniscus Patellofemoral joint Tibiofemoral joint **D Knee Joint, Left** *See C Knee Joint, Right* **F Ankle Joint, Right** Inferior tibiofibular joint Talocrural joint **G Ankle Joint, Left** *See F Ankle Joint, Right*	**H Tarsal Joint, Right** Calcaneocuboid joint Cuboideonavicular joint Cuneonavicular joint Intercuneiform joint Subtalar (talocalcaneal) joint Talocalcaneal (subtalar) joint Talocalcaneonavicular joint **J Tarsal Joint, Left** *See H Tarsal Joint, Right* **K Tarsometatarsal Joint, Right** **L Tarsometatarsal Joint, Left** **M Metatarsal-Phalangeal Joint, Right** Metatarsophalangeal (MTP) joint **N Metatarsal-Phalangeal Joint, Left** *See M Metatarsal-Phalangeal Joint, Right* **P Toe Phalangeal Joint, Right** Interphalangeal (IP) joint **Q Toe Phalangeal Joint, Left** *See P Toe Phalangeal Joint, Right*	**Ø** Open **3** Percutaneous **4** Percutaneous Endoscopic **X** External	**Z** No Device	**Z** No Qualifier

Non-OR ØSN[Ø,2,3,4,5,6,7,8,9,B,C,D,F,G,H,J,K,L,M,N,P,Q]XZZ

Lower Joints

Ø Medical and Surgical
S Lower Joints
P Removal Definition: Taking out or off a device from a body part

Explanation: If a device is taken out and a similar device put in without cutting or puncturing the skin or mucous membrane, the procedure is coded to the root operation CHANGE. Otherwise, the procedure for taking out the device is coded to the root operation REMOVAL.

Body Part Character 4	Approach Character 5	Device Character 6	Qualifier Character 7
Ø Lumbar Vertebral Joint Lumbar facet joint 3 Lumbosacral Joint Lumbosacral facet joint	Ø Open 3 Percutaneous 4 Percutaneous Endoscopic	Ø Drainage Device 3 Infusion Device 4 Internal Fixation Device 7 Autologous Tissue Substitute 8 Spacer A Interbody Fusion Device J Synthetic Substitute K Nonautologous Tissue Substitute	Z No Qualifier
Ø Lumbar Vertebral Joint Lumbar facet joint 3 Lumbosacral Joint Lumbosacral facet joint	X External	Ø Drainage Device 3 Infusion Device 4 Internal Fixation Device	Z No Qualifier
2 Lumbar Vertebral Disc 4 Lumbosacral Disc	Ø Open 3 Percutaneous 4 Percutaneous Endoscopic	Ø Drainage Device 3 Infusion Device 7 Autologous Tissue Substitute J Synthetic Substitute K Nonautologous Tissue Substitute	Z No Qualifier
2 Lumbar Vertebral Disc 4 Lumbosacral Disc	X External	Ø Drainage Device 3 Infusion Device	Z No Qualifier
5 Sacrococcygeal Joint Sacrococcygeal symphysis 6 Coccygeal Joint 7 Sacroiliac Joint, Right 8 Sacroiliac Joint, Left	Ø Open 3 Percutaneous 4 Percutaneous Endoscopic	Ø Drainage Device 3 Infusion Device 4 Internal Fixation Device 7 Autologous Tissue Substitute 8 Spacer J Synthetic Substitute K Nonautologous Tissue Substitute	Z No Qualifier
5 Sacrococcygeal Joint Sacrococcygeal symphysis 6 Coccygeal Joint 7 Sacroiliac Joint, Right 8 Sacroiliac Joint, Left	X External	Ø Drainage Device 3 Infusion Device 4 Internal Fixation Device	Z No Qualifier
9 Hip Joint, Right ⊞ Acetabulofemoral joint B Hip Joint, Left ⊞ *See 9 Hip Joint, Right*	Ø Open	Ø Drainage Device 3 Infusion Device 4 Internal Fixation Device 5 External Fixation Device 7 Autologous Tissue Substitute 8 Spacer 9 Liner B Resurfacing Device E Articulating Spacer J Synthetic Substitute K Nonautologous Tissue Substitute	Z No Qualifier
9 Hip Joint, Right ⊞ Acetabulofemoral joint B Hip Joint, Left ⊞ *See 9 Hip Joint, Right*	3 Percutaneous 4 Percutaneous Endoscopic	Ø Drainage Device 3 Infusion Device 4 Internal Fixation Device 5 External Fixation Device 7 Autologous Tissue Substitute 8 Spacer J Synthetic Substitute K Nonautologous Tissue Substitute	Z No Qualifier
9 Hip Joint, Right Acetabulofemoral joint B Hip Joint, Left *See 9 Hip Joint, Right*	X External	Ø Drainage Device 3 Infusion Device 4 Internal Fixation Device 5 External Fixation Device	Z No Qualifier

Non-OR ØSP[Ø,3][Ø,3,4]8Z
Non-OR ØSP[Ø,3]3[Ø,3]Z
Non-OR ØSP[Ø,3]X[Ø,3,4]Z
Non-OR ØSP[2,4]3[Ø,3]Z
Non-OR ØSP[2,4]X[Ø,3]Z
Non-OR ØSP[5,6,7,8][Ø,3,4]8Z
Non-OR ØSP[5,6,7,8]3[Ø,3]Z
Non-OR ØSP[5,6,7,8]X[Ø,3,4]Z
Non-OR ØSP[9,B]3[Ø,3,8]Z
Non-OR ØSP[9,B]X[Ø,3,4,5]Z

See Appendix L for Procedure Combinations
Combo-only ØSP[9,B]48Z
⊞ ØSP[9,B]Ø[8,9,B,E,J]Z
⊞ ØSP[9,B]4JZ

ØSP Continued on next page

ØSP Continued

Ø Medical and Surgical
S Lower Joints
P Removal Definition: Taking out or off a device from a body part

Explanation: If a device is taken out and a similar device put in without cutting or puncturing the skin or mucous membrane, the procedure is coded to the root operation CHANGE. Otherwise, the procedure for taking out the device is coded to the root operation REMOVAL.

Body Part Character 4	Approach Character 5	Device Character 6	Qualifier Character 7
A Hip Joint, Acetabular Surface, Right ⊞ **E Hip Joint, Acetabular Surface, Left** ⊞ **R Hip Joint, Femoral Surface, Right** ⊞ **S Hip Joint, Femoral Surface, Left** ⊞ **T Knee Joint, Femoral Surface, Right** ⊞ Femoropatellar joint Patellofemoral joint **U Knee Joint, Femoral Surface, Left** ⊞ *See T Knee Joint, Femoral Surface, Right* **V Knee Joint, Tibial Surface, Right** ⊞ Femorotibial joint Tibiofemoral joint **W Knee Joint, Tibial Surface, Left** ⊞ *See V Knee Joint, Tibial Surface, Right*	**Ø Open** **3 Percutaneous** **4 Percutaneous Endoscopic**	**J Synthetic Substitute**	**Z No Qualifier**
C Knee Joint, Right ⊞ Femoropatellar joint Femorotibial joint Lateral meniscus Medial meniscus Patellofemoral joint Tibiofemoral joint **D Knee Joint, Left** ⊞ *See C Knee Joint, Right*	**Ø Open**	**Ø Drainage Device** **3 Infusion Device** **4 Internal Fixation Device** **5 External Fixation Device** **7 Autologous Tissue Substitute** **8 Spacer** **9 Liner** **E Articulating Spacer** **K Nonautologous Tissue Substitute** **L Synthetic Substitute, Unicondylar Medial** **M Synthetic Substitute, Unicondylar Lateral** **N Synthetic Substitute, Patellofemoral**	**Z No Qualifier**
C Knee Joint, Right ⊞ Femoropatellar joint Femorotibial joint Lateral meniscus Medial meniscus Patellofemoral joint Tibiofemoral joint **D Knee Joint, Left** ⊞ *See C Knee Joint, Right*	**Ø Open**	**J Synthetic Substitute**	**C Patellar Surface** **Z No Qualifier**
C Knee Joint, Right ⊞ Femoropatellar joint Femorotibial joint Lateral meniscus Medial meniscus Patellofemoral joint Tibiofemoral joint **D Knee Joint, Left** ⊞ *See C Knee Joint, Right*	**3 Percutaneous** **4 Percutaneous Endoscopic**	**Ø Drainage Device** **3 Infusion Device** **4 Internal Fixation Device** **5 External Fixation Device** **7 Autologous Tissue Substitute** **8 Spacer** **K Nonautologous Tissue Substitute** **L Synthetic Substitute, Unicondylar Medial** **M Synthetic Substitute, Unicondylar Lateral** **N Synthetic Substitute, Patellofemoral**	**Z No Qualifier**
C Knee Joint, Right ⊞ Femoropatellar joint Femorotibial joint Lateral meniscus Medial meniscus Patellofemoral joint Tibiofemoral joint **D Knee Joint, Left** ⊞ *See C Knee Joint, Right*	**3 Percutaneous** **4 Percutaneous Endoscopic**	**J Synthetic Substitute**	**C Patellar Surface** **Z No Qualifier**

Non-OR ØSP[C,D]3[Ø,3]Z

See Appendix L for Procedure Combinations

Combo-only ØSP[C,D][3,4]8Z
⊞ ØSP[A,E,R,S,T,U,V,W][Ø,4]JZ
⊞ ØSP[C,D]Ø[8,9,E,L,M,N]Z
⊞ ØSP[C,D]ØJ[C,Z]
⊞ ØSP[C,D]4[L,M,N]Z
⊞ ØSP[C,D]4J[C,Z]

ØSP Continued on next page

Ø Medical and Surgical
S Lower Joints
P Removal Definition: Taking out or off a device from a body part

Explanation: If a device is taken out and a similar device put in without cutting or puncturing the skin or mucous membrane, the procedure is coded to the root operation CHANGE. Otherwise, the procedure for taking out the device is coded to the root operation REMOVAL.

ØSP Continued

Body Part Character 4	Approach Character 5	Device Character 6	Qualifier Character 7
C Knee Joint, Right Femoropatellar joint Femorotibial joint Lateral meniscus Medial meniscus Patellofemoral joint Tibiofemoral joint **D Knee Joint, Left** *See C Knee Joint, Right*	**X External**	**Ø Drainage Device** **3 Infusion Device** **4 Internal Fixation Device** **5 External Fixation Device**	**Z No Qualifier**
F Ankle Joint, Right Inferior tibiofibular joint Talocrural joint **G Ankle Joint, Left** *See F Ankle Joint, Right* **H Tarsal Joint, Right** Calcaneocuboid joint Cuboideonavicular joint Cuneonavicular joint Intercuneiform joint Subtalar (talocalcaneal) joint Talocalcaneal (subtalar) joint Talocalcaneonavicular joint **J Tarsal Joint, Left** *See H Tarsal Joint, Right* **K Tarsometatarsal Joint, Right** **L Tarsometatarsal Joint, Left** **M Metatarsal-Phalangeal Joint, Right** Metatarsophalangeal (MTP) joint **N Metatarsal-Phalangeal Joint, Left** *See M Metatarsal-Phalangeal Joint, Right* **P Toe Phalangeal Joint, Right** Interphalangeal (IP) joint **Q Toe Phalangeal Joint, Left** *See P Toe Phalangeal Joint, Right*	**Ø Open** **3 Percutaneous** **4 Percutaneous Endoscopic**	**Ø Drainage Device** **3 Infusion Device** **4 Internal Fixation Device** **5 External Fixation Device** **7 Autologous Tissue Substitute** **8 Spacer** **J Synthetic Substitute** **K Nonautologous Tissue Substitute**	**Z No Qualifier**
F Ankle Joint, Right Inferior tibiofibular joint Talocrural joint **G Ankle Joint, Left** *See F Ankle Joint, Right* **H Tarsal Joint, Right** Calcaneocuboid joint Cuboideonavicular joint Cuneonavicular joint Intercuneiform joint Subtalar (talocalcaneal) joint Talocalcaneal (subtalar) joint Talocalcaneonavicular joint **J Tarsal Joint, Left** *See H Tarsal Joint, Right* **K Tarsometatarsal Joint, Right** **L Tarsometatarsal Joint, Left** **M Metatarsal-Phalangeal Joint, Right** Metatarsophalangeal (MTP) joint **N Metatarsal-Phalangeal Joint, Left** *See M Metatarsal-Phalangeal Joint, Right* **P Toe Phalangeal Joint, Right** Interphalangeal (IP) joint **Q Toe Phalangeal Joint, Left** *See P Toe Phalangeal Joint, Right*	**X External**	**Ø Drainage Device** **3 Infusion Device** **4 Internal Fixation Device** **5 External Fixation Device**	**Z No Qualifier**

Non-OR ØSP[C,D]X[Ø,3,4,5]Z
Non-OR ØSP[F,G,H,J,K,L,M,N,P,Q]3[Ø,3,8]Z
Non-OR ØSP[F,G,H,J,K,L,M,N,P,Q][Ø,4]8Z
Non-OR ØSP[F,G,H,J,K,L,M,N,P,Q]X[Ø,3,4,5]Z

Ø Medical and Surgical
S Lower Joints
Q Repair Definition: Restoring, to the extent possible, a body part to its normal anatomic structure and function
Explanation: Used only when the method to accomplish the repair is not one of the other root operations

Body Part Character 4	Approach Character 5	Device Character 6	Qualifier Character 7
Ø Lumbar Vertebral Joint Lumbar facet joint **2 Lumbar Vertebral Disc** **3 Lumbosacral Joint** Lumbosacral facet joint **4 Lumbosacral Disc** **5 Sacrococcygeal Joint** Sacrococcygeal symphysis **6 Coccygeal Joint** **7 Sacroiliac Joint, Right** **8 Sacroiliac Joint, Left** **9 Hip Joint, Right** Acetabulofemoral joint **B Hip Joint, Left** *See 9 Hip Joint, Right* **C Knee Joint, Right** Femoropatellar joint Femorotibial joint Lateral meniscus Medial meniscus Patellofemoral joint Tibiofemoral joint **D Knee Joint, Left** *See C Knee Joint, Right* **F Ankle Joint, Right** Inferior tibiofibular joint Talocrural joint **G Ankle Joint, Left** *See F Ankle Joint, Right* **H Tarsal Joint, Right** Calcaneocuboid joint Cuboideonavicular joint Cuneonavicular joint Intercuneiform joint Subtalar (talocalcaneal) joint Talocalcaneal (subtalar) joint Talocalcaneonavicular joint **J Tarsal Joint, Left** *See H Tarsal Joint, Right* **K Tarsometatarsal Joint, Right** **L Tarsometatarsal Joint, Left** **M Metatarsal-Phalangeal Joint, Right** Metatarsophalangeal (MTP) joint **N Metatarsal-Phalangeal Joint, Left** *See M Metatarsal-Phalangeal Joint, Right* **P Toe Phalangeal Joint, Right** Interphalangeal (IP) joint **Q Toe Phalangeal Joint, Left** *See P Toe Phalangeal Joint, Right*	**Ø Open** **3 Percutaneous** **4 Percutaneous Endoscopic** **X External**	**Z No Device**	**Z No Qualifier**

Non-OR ØSQ[Ø,2,3,4,5,6,7,8,9,B,C,D,F,G,H,J,K,L,M,N,P,Q]XZZ

Ø Medical and Surgical
S Lower Joints
R Replacement

Definition: Putting in or on biological or synthetic material that physically takes the place and/or function of all or a portion of a body part

Explanation: The body part may have been taken out or replaced, or may be taken out, physically eradicated, or rendered nonfunctional during the REPLACEMENT procedure. A REMOVAL procedure is coded for taking out the device used in a previous replacement procedure.

Body Part Character 4	Approach Character 5	Device Character 6	Qualifier Character 7
Ø Lumbar Vertebral Joint Lumbar facet joint **2 Lumbar Vertebral Disc** NC **3 Lumbosacral Joint** Lumbosacral facet joint **4 Lumbosacral Disc** NC **5 Sacrococcygeal Joint** Sacrococcygeal symphysis **6 Coccygeal Joint** **7 Sacroiliac Joint, Right** **8 Sacroiliac Joint, Left** **H Tarsal Joint, Right** Calcaneocuboid joint, Cuboideonavicular joint, Cuneonavicular joint, Intercuneiform joint, Subtalar (talocalcaneal) joint, Talocalcaneal (subtalar) joint, Talocalcaneonavicular joint **J Tarsal Joint, Left** *See H Tarsal Joint, Right* **K Tarsometatarsal Joint, Right** **L Tarsometatarsal Joint, Left** **M Metatarsal-Phalangeal Joint, Right** Metatarsophalangeal (MTP) joint **N Metatarsal-Phalangeal Joint, Left** *See M Metatarsal-Phalangeal Joint, Right* **P Toe Phalangeal Joint, Right** Interphalangeal (IP) joint **Q Toe Phalangeal Joint, Left** *See P Toe Phalangeal Joint, Right*	Ø Open	7 Autologous Tissue Substitute J Synthetic Substitute K Nonautologous Tissue Substitute	Z No Qualifier
9 Hip Joint, Right ⊞ Acetabulofemoral joint **B Hip Joint, Left** ⊞ *See 9 Hip Joint, Right*	Ø Open	1 Synthetic Substitute, Metal 2 Synthetic Substitute, Metal on Polyethylene 3 Synthetic Substitute, Ceramic 4 Synthetic Substitute, Ceramic on Polyethylene 6 Synthetic Substitute, Oxidized Zirconium on Polyethylene J Synthetic Substitute	9 Cemented A Uncemented Z No Qualifier
9 Hip Joint, Right ⊞ Acetabulofemoral joint **B Hip Joint, Left** ⊞ *See 9 Hip Joint, Right*	Ø Open	7 Autologous Tissue Substitute E Articulating Spacer K Nonautologous Tissue Substitute	Z No Qualifier
A Hip Joint, Acetabular Surface, Right ⊞ **E Hip Joint, Acetabular Surface, Left** ⊞	Ø Open	Ø Synthetic Substitute, Polyethylene 1 Synthetic Substitute, Metal 3 Synthetic Substitute, Ceramic J Synthetic Substitute	9 Cemented A Uncemented Z No Qualifier
A Hip Joint, Acetabular Surface, Right **E Hip Joint, Acetabular Surface, Left**	Ø Open	7 Autologous Tissue Substitute K Nonautologous Tissue Substitute	Z No Qualifier

HAC ØSR[9,B]Ø[1,2,3,4,6,J][9,A,Z] when reported with SDx of I26.Ø2-I26.Ø9, I26.92-I26.99, or I82.4Ø1-I82.4Z9

HAC ØSR[9,B]Ø[7,E,K]Z when reported with SDx of I26.Ø2-I26.Ø9, I26.92-I26.99, or I82.4Ø1-I82.4Z9

HAC ØSR[A,E]Ø[Ø,1,3,J][9,A,Z] when reported with SDx of I26.Ø2-I26.Ø9, I26.92-I26.99, or I82.4Ø1-I82.4Z9

HAC ØSR[A,E]Ø[7,K]Z when reported with SDx of I26.Ø2-I26.Ø9, I26.92-I26.99, or I82.4Ø1-I82.4Z9

NC ØSR[2,4]ØJZ when beneficiary age is over 6Ø

See Appendix L for Procedure Combinations
⊞ ØSR[9,B]Ø[1,2,3,4,6,J][9,A,Z]
⊞ ØSR[9,B]ØEZ
⊞ ØSR[A,E]Ø[Ø,1,3,J][9,A,Z]

ØSR Continued on next page

ØSR Continued

Ø Medical and Surgical
S Lower Joints
R Replacement Definition: Putting in or on biological or synthetic material that physically takes the place and/or function of all or a portion of a body part

Explanation: The body part may have been taken out or replaced, or may be taken out, physically eradicated, or rendered nonfunctional during the REPLACEMENT procedure. A REMOVAL procedure is coded for taking out the device used in a previous replacement procedure.

Body Part Character 4	Approach Character 5	Device Character 6	Qualifier Character 7
C Knee Joint, Right ⊞ Femoropatellar joint Femorotibial joint Lateral meniscus Medial meniscus Patellofemoral joint Tibiofemoral joint **D Knee Joint, Left** ⊞ *See C Knee Joint, Right*	**Ø Open**	**6 Synthetic Substitute, Oxidized Zirconium on Polyethylene** **J Synthetic Substitute** **L Synthetic Substitute, Unicondylar Medial** **M Synthetic Substitute, Unicondylar Lateral** **N Synthetic Substitute, Patellofemoral**	**9 Cemented** **A Uncemented** **Z No Qualifier**
C Knee Joint, Right ⊞ Femoropatellar joint Femorotibial joint Lateral meniscus Medial meniscus Patellofemoral joint Tibiofemoral joint **D Knee Joint, Left** ⊞ *See C Knee Joint, Right*	**Ø Open**	**7 Autologous Tissue Substitute** **E Articulating Spacer** **K Nonautologous Tissue Substitute**	**Z No Qualifier**
F Ankle Joint, Right Inferior tibiofibular joint Talocrural joint **G Ankle Joint, Left** *See F Ankle Joint, Right* **T Knee Joint, Femoral Surface, Right** Femoropatellar joint Patellofemoral joint **U Knee Joint, Femoral Surface, Left** *See T Knee Joint, Femoral Surface, Right* **V Knee Joint, Tibial Surface, Right** Femorotibial joint Tibiofemoral joint **W Knee Joint, Tibial Surface, Left** *See V Knee Joint, Tibial Surface, Right*	**Ø Open**	**7 Autologous Tissue Substitute** **K Nonautologous Tissue Substitute**	**Z No Qualifier**
F Ankle Joint, Right Inferior tibiofibular joint Talocrural joint **G Ankle Joint, Left** *See F Ankle Joint, Right* **T Knee Joint, Femoral Surface, Right** ⊞ Femoropatellar joint Patellofemoral joint **U Knee Joint, Femoral Surface, Left** ⊞ *See T Knee Joint, Femoral Surface, Right* **V Knee Joint, Tibial Surface, Right** ⊞ Femorotibial joint Tibiofemoral joint **W Knee Joint, Tibial Surface, Left** ⊞ *See V Knee Joint, Tibial Surface, Right*	**Ø Open**	**J Synthetic Substitute**	**9 Cemented** **A Uncemented** **Z No Qualifier**
R Hip Joint, Femoral Surface, Right ⊞ **S Hip Joint, Femoral Surface, Left** ⊞	**Ø Open**	**1 Synthetic Substitute, Metal** **3 Synthetic Substitute, Ceramic** **J Synthetic Substitute**	**9 Cemented** **A Uncemented** **Z No Qualifier**
R Hip Joint, Femoral Surface, Right **S Hip Joint, Femoral Surface, Left**	**Ø Open**	**7 Autologous Tissue Substitute** **K Nonautologous Tissue Substitute**	**Z No Qualifier**

HAC ØSR[C,D]Ø[6,J,L,M,N][9,A,Z] when reported with SDx of I26.Ø2-I26.Ø9, I26.92-I26.99 or I82.4Ø1-I82.4Z9

HAC ØSR[C,D]Ø[7,E,K]Z when reported with SDx of I26.Ø2-I26.Ø9, I26.92-I26.99 or I82.4Ø1-I82.4Z9

HAC ØSR[T,U,V,W]Ø[7,K]Z when reported with SDx of I26.Ø2-I26.Ø9, I26.92-I26.99 or I82.4Ø1-I82.4Z9

HAC ØSR[T,U,V,W]ØJ[9,A,Z] when reported with SDx of I26.Ø2-I26.Ø9, I26.92-I26.99 or I82.4Ø1-I82.4Z9

HAC ØSR[R,S]Ø[1,3,J][9,A,Z] when reported with SDx of I26.Ø2-I26.Ø9, I26.92-I26.99, or I82.4Ø1-I82.4Z9

HAC ØSR[R,S]Ø[7,K]Z when reported with SDx of I26.Ø2-I26.Ø9, I26.92-I26.99, or I82.4Ø1-I82.4Z9

See Appendix L for Procedure Combinations

⊞ ØSR[C,D]Ø[6,J,L,M,N][9,A,Z]
⊞ ØSR[C,D]ØEZ
⊞ ØSR[T,U,V,W]ØJ[9,A,Z]
⊞ ØSR[R,S]Ø[1,3,J][9,A,Z]

Ø Medical and Surgical
S Lower Joints
S Reposition

Definition: Moving to its normal location, or other suitable location, all or a portion of a body part

Explanation: The body part is moved to a new location from an abnormal location, or from a normal location where it is not functioning correctly. The body part may or may not be cut out or off to be moved to the new location.

Body Part Character 4	Approach Character 5	Device Character 6	Qualifier Character 7
Ø Lumbar Vertebral Joint Lumbar facet joint **3 Lumbosacral Joint** Lumbosacral facet joint **5 Sacrococcygeal Joint** Sacrococcygeal symphysis **6 Coccygeal Joint** **7 Sacroiliac Joint, Right** **8 Sacroiliac Joint, Left**	**Ø** Open **3** Percutaneous **4** Percutaneous Endoscopic **X** External	**4** Internal Fixation Device **Z** No Device	**Z** No Qualifier
9 Hip Joint, Right Acetabulofemoral joint **B Hip Joint, Left** *See 9 Hip Joint, Right* **C Knee Joint, Right** Femoropatellar joint Femorotibial joint Lateral meniscus Medial meniscus Patellofemoral joint Tibiofemoral joint **D Knee Joint, Left** *See C Knee Joint, Right* **F Ankle Joint, Right** Inferior tibiofibular joint Talocrural joint **G Ankle Joint, Left** *See F Ankle Joint, Right* **H Tarsal Joint, Right** Calcaneocuboid joint Cuboideonavicular joint Cuneonavicular joint Intercuneiform joint Subtalar (talocalcaneal) joint Talocalcaneal (subtalar) joint Talocalcaneonavicular joint **J Tarsal Joint, Left** *See H Tarsal Joint, Right* **K Tarsometatarsal Joint, Right** **L Tarsometatarsal Joint, Left** **M Metatarsal-Phalangeal Joint, Right** Metatarsophalangeal (MTP) joint **N Metatarsal-Phalangeal Joint, Left** *See M Metatarsal-Phalangeal Joint, Right* **P Toe Phalangeal Joint, Right** Interphalangeal (IP) joint **Q Toe Phalangeal Joint, Left** *See P Toe Phalangeal Joint, Right*	**Ø** Open **3** Percutaneous **4** Percutaneous Endoscopic **X** External	**4** Internal Fixation Device **5** External Fixation Device **Z** No Device	**Z** No Qualifier

Non-OR ØSS[Ø,3,5,6,7,8][3,4,X][4,Z]Z
Non-OR ØSS[9,B,C,D,F,G,H,J,K,L,M,N,P,Q][3,4,X][4,5,Z]Z

Ø Medical and Surgical
S Lower Joints
T Resection

Definition: Cutting out or off, without replacement, all of a body part

Explanation: None

Body Part Character 4	Approach Character 5	Device Character 6	Qualifier Character 7
2 Lumbar Vertebral Disc **4 Lumbosacral Disc** **5 Sacrococcygeal Joint** Sacrococcygeal symphysis **6 Coccygeal Joint** **7 Sacroiliac Joint, Right** **8 Sacroiliac Joint, Left** **9 Hip Joint, Right** Acetabulofemoral joint **B Hip Joint, Left** *See 9 Hip Joint, Right* **C Knee Joint, Right** Femoropatellar joint Femorotibial joint Lateral meniscus Medial meniscus Patellofemoral joint Tibiofemoral joint **D Knee Joint, Left** *See C Knee Joint, Right* **F Ankle Joint, Right** Inferior tibiofibular joint Talocrural joint **G Ankle Joint, Left** *See F Ankle Joint, Right* **H Tarsal Joint, Right** Calcaneocuboid joint Cuboideonavicular joint Cuneonavicular joint Intercuneiform joint Subtalar (talocalcaneal) joint Talocalcaneal (subtalar) joint Talocalcaneonavicular joint **J Tarsal Joint, Left** *See H Tarsal Joint, Right* **K Tarsometatarsal Joint, Right** **L Tarsometatarsal Joint, Left** **M Metatarsal-Phalangeal Joint, Right** Metatarsophalangeal (MTP) joint **N Metatarsal-Phalangeal Joint, Left** *See M Metatarsal-Phalangeal Joint, Right* **P Toe Phalangeal Joint, Right** Interphalangeal (IP) joint **Q Toe Phalangeal Joint, Left** *See P Toe Phalangeal Joint, Right*	**Ø** Open	**Z** No Device	**Z** No Qualifier

Ø Medical and Surgical
S Lower Joints
U Supplement Definition: Putting in or on biological or synthetic material that physically reinforces and/or augments the function of a portion of a body part

Explanation: The biological material is non-living, or is living and from the same individual. The body part may have been previously replaced, and the SUPPLEMENT procedure is performed to physically reinforce and/or augment the function of the replaced body part.

Body Part Character 4	Approach Character 5	Device Character 6	Qualifier Character 7
Ø Lumbar Vertebral Joint Lumbar facet joint **2 Lumbar Vertebral Disc** **3 Lumbosacral Joint** Lumbosacral facet joint **4 Lumbosacral Disc** **5 Sacrococcygeal Joint** Sacrococcygeal symphysis **6 Coccygeal Joint** **7 Sacroiliac Joint, Right** **8 Sacroiliac Joint, Left** **F Ankle Joint, Right** Inferior tibiofibular joint Talocrural joint **G Ankle Joint, Left** *See F Ankle Joint, Right* **H Tarsal Joint, Right** Calcaneocuboid joint Cuboideonavicular joint Cuneonavicular joint Intercuneiform joint Subtalar (talocalcaneal) joint Talocalcaneal (subtalar) joint Talocalcaneonavicular joint **J Tarsal Joint, Left** *See H Tarsal Joint, Right* **K Tarsometatarsal Joint, Right** **L Tarsometatarsal Joint, Left** **M Metatarsal-Phalangeal Joint, Right** Metatarsophalangeal (MTP) joint **N Metatarsal-Phalangeal Joint, Left** *See M Metatarsal-Phalangeal Joint, Right* **P Toe Phalangeal Joint, Right** Interphalangeal (IP) joint **Q Toe Phalangeal Joint, Left** *See P Toe Phalangeal Joint, Right*	**Ø Open** **3 Percutaneous** **4 Percutaneous Endoscopic**	**7 Autologous Tissue Substitute** **J Synthetic Substitute** **K Nonautologous Tissue Substitute**	**Z No Qualifier**
9 Hip Joint, Right ⊞ Acetabulofemoral joint **B Hip Joint, Left** ⊞ *See 9 Hip Joint, Right*	**Ø Open**	**7 Autologous Tissue Substitute** **9 Liner** **B Resurfacing Device** **J Synthetic Substitute** **K Nonautologous Tissue Substitute**	**Z No Qualifier**
9 Hip Joint, Right Acetabulofemoral joint **B Hip Joint, Left** *See 9 Hip Joint, Right*	**3 Percutaneous** **4 Percutaneous Endoscopic**	**7 Autologous Tissue Substitute** **J Synthetic Substitute** **K Nonautologous Tissue Substitute**	**Z No Qualifier**
A Hip Joint, Acetabular Surface, Right ⊞ **E Hip Joint, Acetabular Surface, Left** ⊞ **R Hip Joint, Femoral Surface, Right** ⊞ **S Hip Joint, Femoral Surface, Left** ⊞	**Ø Open**	**9 Liner** **B Resurfacing Device**	**Z No Qualifier**
C Knee Joint, Right Femoropatellar joint Femorotibial joint Lateral meniscus Medial meniscus Patellofemoral joint Tibiofemoral joint **D Knee Joint, Left** *See C Knee Joint, Right*	**Ø Open**	**7 Autologous Tissue Substitute** **J Synthetic Substitute** **K Nonautologous Tissue Substitute**	**Z No Qualifier**
C Knee Joint, Right Femoropatellar joint Femorotibial joint Lateral meniscus Medial meniscus Patellofemoral joint Tibiofemoral joint **D Knee Joint, Left** *See C Knee Joint, Right*	**Ø Open**	**9 Liner**	**C Patellar Surface** **Z No Qualifier**

HAC ØSU[9,B]ØBZ when reported with SDx of I26.Ø2-I26.Ø9, I26.92-I26.99, or I82.4Ø1-I82.4Z9

HAC ØSU[A,E,R,S]ØBZ when reported with SDx of I26.Ø2-I26.Ø9, I26.92-I26.99, or I82.4Ø1-I82.4Z9

See Appendix L for Procedure Combinations
⊞ ØSU[9,B]Ø9Z
⊞ ØSU[A,E,R,S]Ø9Z

ØSU Continued on next page

Ø Medical and Surgical
S Lower Joints
U Supplement

Definition: Putting in or on biological or synthetic material that physically reinforces and/or augments the function of a portion of a body part

Explanation: The biological material is non-living, or is living and from the same individual. The body part may have been previously replaced, and the SUPPLEMENT procedure is performed to physically reinforce and/or augment the function of the replaced body part.

ØSU Continued

Body Part Character 4	Approach Character 5	Device Character 6	Qualifier Character 7
C Knee Joint, Right Femoropatellar joint Femorotibial joint Lateral meniscus Medial meniscus Patellofemoral joint Tibiofemoral joint **D Knee Joint, Left** *See C Knee Joint, Right*	**3 Percutaneous** **4 Percutaneous Endoscopic**	**7 Autologous Tissue Substitute** **J Synthetic Substitute** **K Nonautologous Tissue Substitute**	**Z No Qualifier**
T Knee Joint, Femoral Surface, Right Femoropatellar joint Patellofemoral joint **U Knee Joint, Femoral Surface, Left** *See T Knee Joint, Femoral Surface, Right* **V Knee Joint, Tibial Surface, Right** ⊞ Femorotibial joint Tibiofemoral joint **W Knee Joint, Tibial Surface, Left** ⊞ *See V Knee Joint, Tibial Surface, Right*	**Ø Open**	**9 Liner**	**Z No Qualifier**

See Appendix L for Procedure Combinations

⊞ ØSU[V,W]Ø9Z

Ø Medical and Surgical
S Lower Joints
W Revision

Definition: Correcting, to the extent possible, a portion of a malfunctioning device or the position of a displaced device

Explanation: Revision can include correcting a malfunctioning or displaced device by taking out or putting in components of the device such as a screw or pin

Body Part Character 4	Approach Character 5	Device Character 6	Qualifier Character 7
Ø Lumbar Vertebral Joint Lumbar facet joint **3 Lumbosacral Joint** Lumbosacral facet joint	**Ø Open** **3 Percutaneous** **4 Percutaneous Endoscopic** **X External**	**Ø Drainage Device** **3 Infusion Device** **4 Internal Fixation Device** **7 Autologous Tissue Substitute** **8 Spacer** **A Interbody Fusion Device** **J Synthetic Substitute** **K Nonautologous Tissue Substitute**	**Z No Qualifier**
2 Lumbar Vertebral Disc **4 Lumbosacral Disc**	**Ø Open** **3 Percutaneous** **4 Percutaneous Endoscopic** **X External**	**Ø Drainage Device** **3 Infusion Device** **7 Autologous Tissue Substitute** **J Synthetic Substitute** **K Nonautologous Tissue Substitute**	**Z No Qualifier**
5 Sacrococcygeal Joint Sacrococcygeal symphysis **6 Coccygeal Joint** **7 Sacroiliac Joint, Right** **8 Sacroiliac Joint, Left**	**Ø Open** **3 Percutaneous** **4 Percutaneous Endoscopic** **X External**	**Ø Drainage Device** **3 Infusion Device** **4 Internal Fixation Device** **7 Autologous Tissue Substitute** **8 Spacer** **J Synthetic Substitute** **K Nonautologous Tissue Substitute**	**Z No Qualifier**
9 Hip Joint, Right Acetabulofemoral joint **B Hip Joint, Left** *See 9 Hip Joint, Right*	**Ø Open**	**Ø Drainage Device** **3 Infusion Device** **4 Internal Fixation Device** **5 External Fixation Device** **7 Autologous Tissue Substitute** **8 Spacer** **9 Liner** **B Resurfacing Device** **J Synthetic Substitute** **K Nonautologous Tissue Substitute**	**Z No Qualifier**
9 Hip Joint, Right Acetabulofemoral joint **B Hip Joint, Left** *See 9 Hip Joint, Right*	**3 Percutaneous** **4 Percutaneous Endoscopic** **X External**	**Ø Drainage Device** **3 Infusion Device** **4 Internal Fixation Device** **5 External Fixation Device** **7 Autologous Tissue Substitute** **8 Spacer** **J Synthetic Substitute** **K Nonautologous Tissue Substitute**	**Z No Qualifier**
A Hip Joint, Acetabular Surface, Right **E Hip Joint, Acetabular Surface, Left** **R Hip Joint, Femoral Surface, Right** **S Hip Joint, Femoral Surface, Left** **T Knee Joint, Femoral Surface, Right** Femoropatellar joint Patellofemoral joint **U Knee Joint, Femoral Surface, Left** *See T Knee Joint, Femoral Surface, Right* **V Knee Joint, Tibial Surface, Right** Femorotibial joint Tibiofemoral joint **W Knee Joint, Tibial Surface, Left** *See V Knee Joint, Tibial Surface, Right*	**Ø Open** **3 Percutaneous** **4 Percutaneous Endoscopic** **X External**	**J Synthetic Substitute**	**Z No Qualifier**
C Knee Joint, Right Femoropatellar joint Femorotibial joint Lateral meniscus Medial meniscus Patellofemoral joint Tibiofemoral joint **D Knee Joint, Left** *See C Knee Joint, Right*	**Ø Open**	**Ø Drainage Device** **3 Infusion Device** **4 Internal Fixation Device** **5 External Fixation Device** **7 Autologous Tissue Substitute** **8 Spacer** **9 Liner** **K Nonautologous Tissue Substitute**	**Z No Qualifier**

Non-OR ØSW[Ø,3]X[Ø,3,4,7,8,A,J,K]Z
Non-OR ØSW[2,4]X[Ø,3,7,J,K]Z
Non-OR ØSW[5,6,7,8]X[Ø,3,4,7,8,J,K]Z
Non-OR ØSW[9,B]X[Ø,3,4,5,7,8,J,K]Z
Non-OR ØSW[A,E,R,S,T,U,V,W]XJZ

ØSW Continued on next page

Ø Medical and Surgical
S Lower Joints
W Revision Definition: Correcting, to the extent possible, a portion of a malfunctioning device or the position of a displaced device
Explanation: Revision can include correcting a malfunctioning or displaced device by taking out or putting in components of the device such as a screw or pin

ØSW Continued

Body Part Character 4	Approach Character 5	Device Character 6	Qualifier Character 7
C Knee Joint, Right Femoropatellar joint Femorotibial joint Lateral meniscus Medial meniscus Patellofemoral joint Tibiofemoral joint **D Knee Joint, Left** *See C Knee Joint, Right*	**Ø Open**	**J Synthetic Substitute**	**C Patellar Surface** **Z No Qualifier**
C Knee Joint, Right Femoropatellar joint Femorotibial joint Lateral meniscus Medial meniscus Patellofemoral joint Tibiofemoral joint **D Knee Joint, Left** *See C Knee Joint, Right*	**3 Percutaneous** **4 Percutaneous Endoscopic** **X External**	**Ø Drainage Device** **3 Infusion Device** **4 Internal Fixation Device** **5 External Fixation Device** **7 Autologous Tissue Substitute** **8 Spacer** **K Nonautologous Tissue Substitute**	**Z No Qualifier**
C Knee Joint, Right Femoropatellar joint Femorotibial joint Lateral meniscus Medial meniscus Patellofemoral joint Tibiofemoral joint **D Knee Joint, Left** *See C Knee Joint, Right*	**3 Percutaneous** **4 Percutaneous Endoscopic** **X External**	**J Synthetic Substitute**	**C Patellar Surface** **Z No Qualifier**
F Ankle Joint, Right Inferior tibiofibular joint Talocrural joint **G Ankle Joint, Left** *See F Ankle Joint, Right* **H Tarsal Joint, Right** Calcaneocuboid joint Cuboideonavicular joint Cuneonavicular joint Intercuneiform joint Subtalar (talocalcaneal) joint Talocalcaneal (subtalar) joint Talocalcaneonavicular joint **J Tarsal Joint, Left** *See H Tarsal Joint, Right* **K Tarsometatarsal Joint, Right** **L Tarsometatarsal Joint, Left** **M Metatarsal-Phalangeal Joint, Right** Metatarsophalangeal (MTP) joint **N Metatarsal-Phalangeal Joint, Left** *See M Metatarsal-Phalangeal Joint, Right* **P Toe Phalangeal Joint, Right** Interphalangeal (IP) joint **Q Toe Phalangeal Joint, Left** *See P Toe Phalangeal Joint, Right*	**Ø Open** **3 Percutaneous** **4 Percutaneous Endoscopic** **X External**	**Ø Drainage Device** **3 Infusion Device** **4 Internal Fixation Device** **5 External Fixation Device** **7 Autologous Tissue Substitute** **8 Spacer** **J Synthetic Substitute** **K Nonautologous Tissue Substitute**	**Z No Qualifier**

Non-OR ØSW[C,D]X[Ø,3,4,5,7,8,K]Z
Non-OR ØSW[C,D]XJ[C,Z]
Non-OR ØSW[F,G,H,J,K,L,M,N,P,Q]X[Ø,3,4,5,7,8,J,K]Z

Urinary System ØT1–ØTY

Character Meanings

This Character Meaning table is provided as a guide to assist the user in the identification of character members that may be found in this section of code tables. It **SHOULD NOT** be used to build a PCS code.

Operation–Character 3	Body Part–Character 4	Approach–Character 5	Device–Character 6	Qualifier–Character 7
1 Bypass	Ø Kidney, Right	Ø Open	Ø Drainage Device	Ø Allogeneic
2 Change	1 Kidney, Left	3 Percutaneous	1 Radioactive Element	1 Syngeneic
5 Destruction	2 Kidneys, Bilateral	4 Percutaneous Endoscopic	2 Monitoring Device	2 Zooplastic
7 Dilation	3 Kidney Pelvis, Right	7 Via Natural or Artificial Opening	3 Infusion Device	3 Kidney Pelvis, Right
8 Division	4 Kidney Pelvis, Left	8 Via Natural or Artificial Opening Endoscopic	7 Autologous Tissue Substitute	4 Kidney Pelvis, Left
9 Drainage	5 Kidney	X External	C Extraluminal Device	6 Ureter, Right
B Excision	6 Ureter, Right		D Intraluminal Device	7 Ureter, Left
C Extirpation	7 Ureter, Left		J Synthetic Substitute	8 Colon
D Extraction	8 Ureters, Bilateral		K Nonautologous Tissue Substitute	9 Colocutaneous
F Fragmentation	9 Ureter		L Artificial Sphincter	A Ileum
H Insertion	B Bladder		M Stimulator Lead	B Bladder
J Inspection	C Bladder Neck		Y Other Device	C Ileocutaneous
L Occlusion	D Urethra		Z No Device	D Cutaneous
M Reattachment				X Diagnostic
N Release				Z No Qualifier
P Removal				
Q Repair				
R Replacement				
S Reposition				
T Resection				
U Supplement				
V Restriction				
W Revision				
Y Transplantation				

AHA Coding Clinic for table ØT1
2017, 3Q, 20 Creation of Indiana pouch
2017, 3Q, 21 Augmentation cystoplasty with Indiana pouch and continent urinary diversion
2017, 1Q, 37 Perineal urethrostomy
2015, 3Q, 34 Redo urinary diversion surgery via left ureteral reimplantation

AHA Coding Clinic for table ØT7
2019, 2Q, 16 Reimplantation of ureters with insertion of tubes
2017, 4Q, 111 Exchange of ureteral stent
2016, 2Q, 27 Exchange of ureteral stents
2015, 2Q, 8 Urinary calculi fragmentation and evacuation
2013, 4Q, 123 Urolift® procedure

AHA Coding Clinic for table ØT9
2017, 3Q, 19 Ureteral stent placement for urinary leakage
2017, 3Q, 20 Creation of Indiana pouch
2017, 3Q, 21 Augmentation cystoplasty with Indiana pouch and continent urinary diversion

AHA Coding Clinic for table ØTB
2016, 1Q, 19 Biopsy of neobladder malignancy
2015, 3Q, 34 Excision of Mitrofanoff polyp
2014, 2Q, 8 Ileoscopy with excision of polyp of ileal loop urinary diversion

AHA Coding Clinic for table ØTC
2019, 3Q, 4 Evacuation of clots from bladder dome
2016, 3Q, 23 Ureteral stone migrating into bladder
2015, 2Q, 7 Urinary calculi fragmentation and evacuation
2015, 2Q, 8 Urinary calculi fragmentation and evacuation
2013, 4Q, 122 Laser lithotripsy with removal of fragments

AHA Coding Clinic for table ØTF
2015, 2Q, 7 Urinary calculi fragmentation and evacuation
2013, 4Q, 122 Extracorporeal shock wave lithotripsy
2013, 4Q, 122 Laser lithotripsy with removal of fragments

AHA Coding Clinic for table ØTH
2020, 4Q, 43-44 Insertion of radioactive element
2019, 2Q, 16 Reimplantation of ureters with insertion of tubes

AHA Coding Clinic for table ØTP
2017, 4Q, 111 Exchange of ureteral stent
2016, 2Q, 27 Exchange of ureteral stents

AHA Coding Clinic for table ØTQ
2018, 2Q, 27 Dismembered pyeloplasty
2017, 1Q, 37 Perineal urethrostomy

AHA Coding Clinic for table ØTR
2017, 3Q, 20 Creation of Indiana pouch

AHA Coding Clinic for table ØTS
2019, 1Q, 29 Young-Dees-Leadbetter bladder neck reconstruction
2018, 2Q, 27 Dismembered pyeloplasty
2017, 1Q, 36 Dismembered pyeloplasty
2016, 1Q, 15 Pubovaginal sling placement

AHA Coding Clinic for table ØTT
2014, 3Q, 16 Hand-assisted laparoscopy nephroureterectomy

AHA Coding Clinic for table ØTU
2019, 1Q, 29 Young-Dees-Leadbetter bladder neck reconstruction
2017, 3Q, 21 Augmentation cystoplasty with Indiana pouch and continent urinary diversion

AHA Coding Clinic for table ØTV
2015, 2Q, 11 Cystourethroscopic Deflux® injection

Urinary System

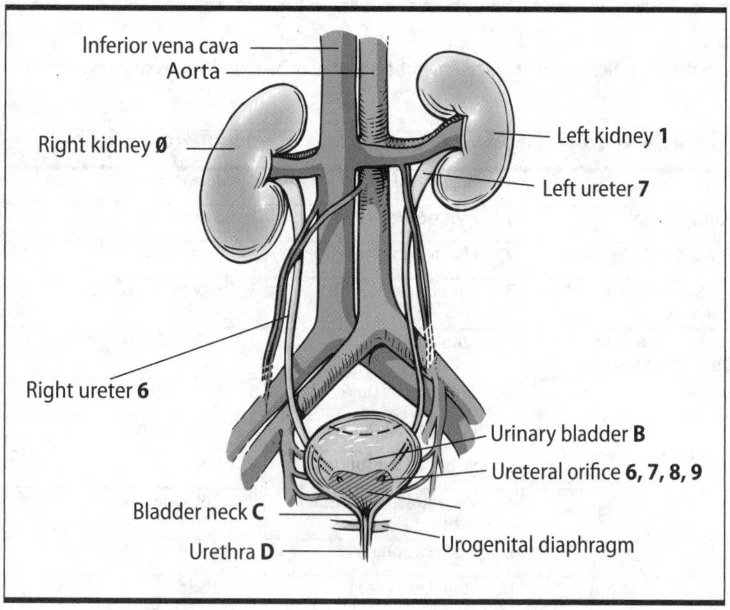

Kidney

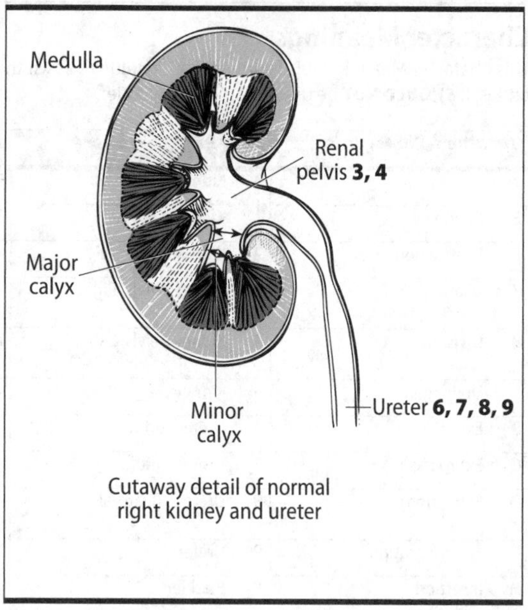

Cutaway detail of normal right kidney and ureter

Bladder

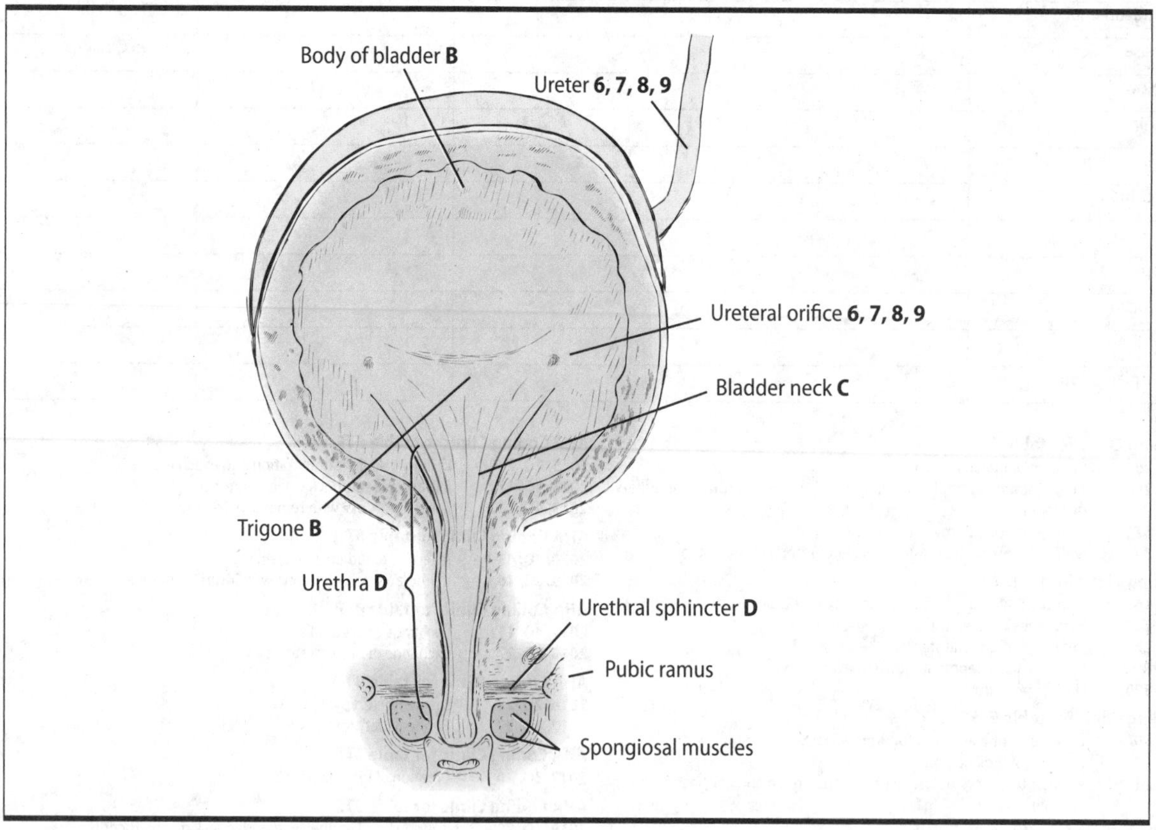

Ø Medical and Surgical
T Urinary System
1 Bypass Definition: Altering the route of passage of the contents of a tubular body part

Explanation: Rerouting contents of a body part to a downstream area of the normal route, to a similar route and body part, or to an abnormal route and dissimilar body part. Includes one or more anastomoses, with or without the use of a device.

Body Part Character 4	Approach Character 5	Device Character 6	Qualifier Character 7
3 Kidney Pelvis, Right Ureteropelvic junction (UPJ) **4 Kidney Pelvis, Left** *See 3 Kidney Pelvis, Right*	**Ø Open** **4 Percutaneous Endoscopic**	**7 Autologous Tissue Substitute** **J Synthetic Substitute** **K Nonautologous Tissue Substitute** **Z No Device**	**3 Kidney Pelvis, Right** **4 Kidney Pelvis, Left** **6 Ureter, Right** **7 Ureter, Left** **8 Colon** **9 Colocutaneous** **A Ileum** **B Bladder** **C Ileocutaneous** **D Cutaneous**
3 Kidney Pelvis, Right Ureteropelvic junction (UPJ) **4 Kidney Pelvis, Left** *See 3 Kidney Pelvis, Right*	**3 Percutaneous**	**J Synthetic Substitute**	**D Cutaneous**
6 Ureter, Right Ureteral orifice Ureterovesical orifice **7 Ureter, Left** *See 6 Ureter, Right* **8 Ureters, Bilateral** *See 6 Ureter, Right*	**Ø Open** **4 Percutaneous Endoscopic**	**7 Autologous Tissue Substitute** **J Synthetic Substitute** **K Nonautologous Tissue Substitute** **Z No Device**	**6 Ureter, Right** **7 Ureter, Left** **8 Colon** **9 Colocutaneous** **A Ileum** **B Bladder** **C Ileocutaneous** **D Cutaneous**
6 Ureter, Right Ureteral orifice Ureterovesical orifice **7 Ureter, Left** *See 6 Ureter, Right* **8 Ureters, Bilateral** *See 6 Ureter, Right*	**3 Percutaneous**	**J Synthetic Substitute**	**D Cutaneous**
B Bladder Trigone of bladder	**Ø Open** **4 Percutaneous Endoscopic**	**7 Autologous Tissue Substitute** **J Synthetic Substitute** **K Nonautologous Tissue Substitute** **Z No Device**	**9 Colocutaneous** **C Ileocutaneous** **D Cutaneous**
B Bladder Trigone of bladder	**3 Percutaneous**	**J Synthetic Substitute**	**D Cutaneous**

Ø Medical and Surgical
T Urinary System
2 Change Definition: Taking out or off a device from a body part and putting back an identical or similar device in or on the same body part without cutting or puncturing the skin or a mucous membrane

Explanation: All CHANGE procedures are coded using the approach EXTERNAL

Body Part Character 4	Approach Character 5	Device Character 6	Qualifier Character 7
5 Kidney Renal calyx Renal capsule Renal cortex Renal segment **9 Ureter** Ureteral orifice Ureterovesical orifice **B Bladder** Trigone of bladder **D Urethra** Bulbourethral (Cowper's) gland Cowper's (bulbourethral) gland External urethral sphincter Internal urethral sphincter Membranous urethra Penile urethra Prostatic urethra	**X External**	**Ø Drainage Device** **Y Other Device**	**Z No Qualifier**

Non-OR All body part, approach, device, and qualifier values

Ø Medical and Surgical
T Urinary System
5 Destruction Definition: Physical eradication of all or a portion of a body part by the direct use of energy, force, or a destructive agent
Explanation: None of the body part is physically taken out

Body Part Character 4	Approach Character 5	Device Character 6	Qualifier Character 7
Ø Kidney, Right Renal calyx Renal capsule Renal cortex Renal segment **1 Kidney, Left** *See Ø Kidney, Right* **3 Kidney Pelvis, Right** Ureteropelvic junction (UPJ) **4 Kidney Pelvis, Left** *See 3 Kidney Pelvis, Right* **6 Ureter, Right** Ureteral orifice Ureterovesical orifice **7 Ureter, Left** *See 6 Ureter, Right* **B Bladder** Trigone of bladder **C Bladder Neck**	**Ø Open** **3 Percutaneous** **4 Percutaneous Endoscopic** **7 Via Natural or Artificial Opening** **8 Via Natural or Artificial Opening Endoscopic**	**Z No Device**	**Z No Qualifier**
D Urethra Bulbourethral (Cowper's) gland Cowper's (bulbourethral) gland External urethral sphincter Internal urethral sphincter Membranous urethra Penile urethra Prostatic urethra	**Ø Open** **3 Percutaneous** **4 Percutaneous Endoscopic** **7 Via Natural or Artificial Opening** **8 Via Natural or Artificial Opening Endoscopic** **X External**	**Z No Device**	**Z No Qualifier**

Non-OR ØT5D[Ø,3,4,7,8,X]ZZ

Ø Medical and Surgical
T Urinary System
7 Dilation Definition: Expanding an orifice or the lumen of a tubular body part
Explanation: The orifice can be a natural orifice or an artificially created orifice. Accomplished by stretching a tubular body part using intraluminal pressure or by cutting part of the orifice or wall of the tubular body part.

Body Part Character 4	Approach Character 5	Device Character 6	Qualifier Character 7
3 Kidney Pelvis, Right Ureteropelvic junction (UPJ) **4 Kidney Pelvis, Left** *See 3 Kidney Pelvis, Right* **6 Ureter, Right** Ureteral orifice Ureterovesical orifice **7 Ureter, Left** *See 6 Ureter, Right* **8 Ureters, Bilateral** *See 6 Ureter, Right* **B Bladder** Trigone of bladder **C Bladder Neck** **D Urethra** Bulbourethral (Cowper's) gland Cowper's (bulbourethral) gland External urethral sphincter Internal urethral sphincter Membranous urethra Penile urethra Prostatic urethra	**Ø Open** **3 Percutaneous** **4 Percutaneous Endoscopic** **7 Via Natural or Artificial Opening** **8 Via Natural or Artificial Opening Endoscopic**	**D Intraluminal Device** **Z No Device**	**Z No Qualifier**

Non-OR ØT7[6,7,8][Ø,3,4,7]DZ
Non-OR ØT7[6,7,8]7ZZ
Non-OR ØT788ZZ
Non-OR ØT7B7[D,Z]Z
Non-OR ØT7C[Ø,3,4]ZZ
Non-OR ØT7[C,D][Ø,3,4]DZ
Non-OR ØT7[C,D][7,8][D,Z]Z

Ø Medical and Surgical
T Urinary System
8 Division Definition: Cutting into a body part, without draining fluids and/or gases from the body part, in order to separate or transect a body part
Explanation: All or a portion of the body part is separated into two or more portions

Body Part Character 4	Approach Character 5	Device Character 6	Qualifier Character 7
2 Kidneys, Bilateral Renal calyx Renal capsule Renal cortex Renal segment **C Bladder Neck**	**Ø Open** **3 Percutaneous** **4 Percutaneous Endoscopic**	**Z No Device**	**Z No Qualifier**

Ø Medical and Surgical
T Urinary System
9 Drainage Definition: Taking or letting out fluids and/or gases from a body part

Explanation: The qualifier DIAGNOSTIC is used to identify drainage procedures that are biopsies

Body Part Character 4	Approach Character 5	Device Character 6	Qualifier Character 7
Ø Kidney, Right Renal calyx Renal capsule Renal cortex Renal segment **1 Kidney, Left** *See Ø Kidney, Right* **3 Kidney Pelvis, Right** Ureteropelvic junction (UPJ) **4 Kidney Pelvis, Left** *See 3 Kidney Pelvis, Right* **6 Ureter, Right** Ureteral orifice Ureterovesical orifice **7 Ureter, Left** *See 6 Ureter, Right* **8 Ureters, Bilateral** *See 6 Ureter, Right* **B Bladder** Trigone of bladder **C Bladder Neck**	**Ø Open** **3 Percutaneous** **4 Percutaneous Endoscopic** **7 Via Natural or Artificial Opening** **8 Via Natural or Artificial Opening Endoscopic**	**Ø Drainage Device**	**Z No Qualifier**
Ø Kidney, Right Renal calyx Renal capsule Renal cortex Renal segment **1 Kidney, Left** *See Ø Kidney, Right* **3 Kidney Pelvis, Right** Ureteropelvic junction (UPJ) **4 Kidney Pelvis, Left** *See 3 Kidney Pelvis, Right* **6 Ureter, Right** Ureteral orifice Ureterovesical orifice **7 Ureter, Left** *See 6 Ureter, Right* **8 Ureters, Bilateral** *See 6 Ureter, Right* **B Bladder** Trigone of bladder **C Bladder Neck**	**Ø Open** **3 Percutaneous** **4 Percutaneous Endoscopic** **7 Via Natural or Artificial Opening** **8 Via Natural or Artificial Opening Endoscopic**	**Z No Device**	**X Diagnostic** **Z No Qualifier**
D Urethra Bulbourethral (Cowper's) gland Cowper's (bulbourethral) gland External urethral sphincter Internal urethral sphincter Membranous urethra Penile urethra Prostatic urethra	**Ø Open** **3 Percutaneous** **4 Percutaneous Endoscopic** **7 Via Natural or Artificial Opening** **8 Via Natural or Artificial Opening Endoscopic** **X External**	**Ø Drainage Device**	**Z No Qualifier**
D Urethra Bulbourethral (Cowper's) gland Cowper's (bulbourethral) gland External urethral sphincter Internal urethral sphincter Membranous urethra Penile urethra Prostatic urethra	**Ø Open** **3 Percutaneous** **4 Percutaneous Endoscopic** **7 Via Natural or Artificial Opening** **8 Via Natural or Artificial Opening Endoscopic** **X External**	**Z No Device**	**X Diagnostic** **Z No Qualifier**

Non-OR ØT9[Ø,1,3,4]3ØZ
Non-OR ØT9[6,7,8][Ø,3,4,7,8]ØZ
Non-OR ØT9[B,C][3,4,7,8]ØZ
Non-OR ØT9[Ø,1,3,4,6,7,8][3,4,7,8]ZX
Non-OR ØT9[Ø,1,3,4][3,4]ZZ
Non-OR ØT9[6,7,8]3ZZ
Non-OR ØT9[B,C][3,4,7,8]ZZ
Non-OR ØT9D3ØZ
Non-OR ØT9D[Ø,3,4,7,8,X]ZX
Non-OR ØT9D3ZZ

Ø Medical and Surgical
T Urinary System
B Excision

Definition: Cutting out or off, without replacement, a portion of a body part
Explanation: The qualifier DIAGNOSTIC is used to identify excision procedures that are biopsies

Body Part Character 4	Approach Character 5	Device Character 6	Qualifier Character 7
Ø Kidney, Right Renal calyx Renal capsule Renal cortex Renal segment **1 Kidney, Left** *See Ø Kidney, Right* **3 Kidney Pelvis, Right** Ureteropelvic junction (UPJ) **4 Kidney Pelvis, Left** *See 3 Kidney Pelvis, Right* **6 Ureter, Right** Ureteral orifice Ureterovesical orifice **7 Ureter, Left** *See 6 Ureter, Right* **B Bladder** Trigone of bladder **C Bladder Neck**	**Ø Open** **3 Percutaneous** **4 Percutaneous Endoscopic** **7 Via Natural or Artificial Opening** **8 Via Natural or Artificial Opening Endoscopic**	**Z No Device**	**X Diagnostic** **Z No Qualifier**
D Urethra Bulbourethral (Cowper's) gland Cowper's (bulbourethral) gland External urethral sphincter Internal urethral sphincter Membranous urethra Penile urethra Prostatic urethra	**Ø Open** **3 Percutaneous** **4 Percutaneous Endoscopic** **7 Via Natural or Artificial Opening** **8 Via Natural or Artificial Opening Endoscopic** **X External**	**Z No Device**	**X Diagnostic** **Z No Qualifier**

Non-OR ØTB[Ø,1,3,4,6,7][3,4,7,8]ZX
Non-OR ØTBD[Ø,3,4,7,8,X]ZX

Ø Medical and Surgical
T Urinary System
C Extirpation

Definition: Taking or cutting out solid matter from a body part
Explanation: The solid matter may be an abnormal byproduct of a biological function or a foreign body; it may be imbedded in a body part or in the lumen of a tubular body part. The solid matter may or may not have been previously broken into pieces.

Body Part Character 4	Approach Character 5	Device Character 6	Qualifier Character 7
Ø Kidney, Right Renal calyx Renal capsule Renal cortex Renal segment **1 Kidney, Left** *See Ø Kidney, Right* **3 Kidney Pelvis, Right** Ureteropelvic junction (UPJ) **4 Kidney Pelvis, Left** *See 3 Kidney Pelvis, Right* **6 Ureter, Right** Ureteral orifice Ureterovesical orifice **7 Ureter, Left** *See 6 Ureter, Right* **B Bladder** Trigone of bladder **C Bladder Neck**	**Ø Open** **3 Percutaneous** **4 Percutaneous Endoscopic** **7 Via Natural or Artificial Opening** **8 Via Natural or Artificial Opening Endoscopic**	**Z No Device**	**Z No Qualifier**
D Urethra Bulbourethral (Cowper's) gland Cowper's (bulbourethral) gland External urethral sphincter Internal urethral sphincter Membranous urethra Penile urethra Prostatic urethra	**Ø Open** **3 Percutaneous** **4 Percutaneous Endoscopic** **7 Via Natural or Artificial Opening** **8 Via Natural or Artificial Opening Endoscopic** **X External**	**Z No Device**	**Z No Qualifier**

Non-OR ØTC[B,C][7,8]ZZ
Non-OR ØTCD[7,8,X]ZZ

Ø Medical and Surgical
T Urinary System
D Extraction Definition: Pulling or stripping out or off all or a portion of a body part by the use of force

Explanation: The qualifier DIAGNOSTIC is used to identify extraction procedures that are biopsies

Body Part Character 4	Approach Character 5	Device Character 6	Qualifier Character 7
Ø Kidney, Right Renal calyx Renal capsule Renal cortex Renal segment **1 Kidney, Left** *See Ø Kidney, Right*	**Ø Open** **3 Percutaneous** **4 Percutaneous Endoscopic**	**Z No Device**	**Z No Qualifier**

Ø Medical and Surgical
T Urinary System
F Fragmentation Definition: Breaking solid matter in a body part into pieces

Explanation: Physical force (e.g., manual, ultrasonic) applied directly or indirectly is used to break the solid matter into pieces. The solid matter may be an abnormal byproduct of a biological function or a foreign body. The pieces of solid matter are not taken out.

Body Part Character 4	Approach Character 5	Device Character 6	Qualifier Character 7
3 Kidney Pelvis, Right Ureteropelvic junction (UPJ) **4 Kidney Pelvis, Left** *See 3 Kidney Pelvis, Right* **6 Ureter, Right** Ureteral orifice Ureterovesical orifice **7 Ureter, Left** *See 6 Ureter, Right* **B Bladder** Trigone of bladder **C Bladder Neck** **D Urethra** NC Bulbourethral (Cowper's) gland Cowper's (bulbourethral) gland External urethral sphincter Internal urethral sphincter Membranous urethra Penile urethra Prostatic urethra	**Ø Open** **3 Percutaneous** **4 Percutaneous Endoscopic** **7 Via Natural or Artificial Opening** **8 Via Natural or Artificial Opening Endoscopic** **X External**	**Z No Device**	**Z No Qualifier**

Non-OR ØTF[3,4][Ø,7,8]ZZ
Non-OR ØTF[6,7,B,C,D][Ø,3,4,7,8]ZZ
Non-OR ØTF[3,4,6,7,B,C,D]XZZ
NC ØTFDXZZ

Ø Medical and Surgical
T Urinary System
H Insertion Definition: Putting in a nonbiological appliance that monitors, assists, performs, or prevents a physiological function but does not physically take the place of a body part

Explanation: None

Body Part Character 4	Approach Character 5	Device Character 6	Qualifier Character 7
5 Kidney Renal calyx Renal capsule Renal cortex Renal segment	Ø Open 3 Percutaneous 4 Percutaneous Endoscopic 7 Via Natural or Artificial Opening 8 Via Natural or Artificial Opening Endoscopic	1 Radioactive Element 2 Monitoring Device 3 Infusion Device Y Other Device	Z No Qualifier
9 Ureter Ureteral orifice Ureterovesical orifice	Ø Open 3 Percutaneous 4 Percutaneous Endoscopic 7 Via Natural or Artificial Opening 8 Via Natural or Artificial Opening Endoscopic	1 Radioactive Element 2 Monitoring Device 3 Infusion Device M Stimulator Lead Y Other Device	Z No Qualifier
B Bladder NC Trigone of bladder	Ø Open 3 Percutaneous 4 Percutaneous Endoscopic 7 Via Natural or Artificial Opening 8 Via Natural or Artificial Opening Endoscopic	1 Radioactive Element 2 Monitoring Device 3 Infusion Device L Artificial Sphincter M Stimulator Lead Y Other Device	Z No Qualifier
C Bladder Neck	Ø Open 3 Percutaneous 4 Percutaneous Endoscopic 7 Via Natural or Artificial Opening 8 Via Natural or Artificial Opening Endoscopic	L Artificial Sphincter	Z No Qualifier
D Urethra Bulbourethral (Cowper's) gland Cowper's (bulbourethral) gland External urethral sphincter Internal urethral sphincter Membranous urethra Penile urethra Prostatic urethra	Ø Open 3 Percutaneous 4 Percutaneous Endoscopic 7 Via Natural or Artificial Opening 8 Via Natural or Artificial Opening Endoscopic	1 Radioactive Element 2 Monitoring Device 3 Infusion Device L Artificial Sphincter Y Other Device	Z No Qualifier
D Urethra Bulbourethral (Cowper's) gland Cowper's (bulbourethral) gland External urethral sphincter Internal urethral sphincter Membranous urethra Penile urethra Prostatic urethra	X External	2 Monitoring Device 3 Infusion Device L Artificial Sphincter	Z No Qualifier

Non-OR ØTH5Ø3Z
Non-OR ØTH53[1,3,Y]Z
Non-OR ØTH54[3,Y]Z
Non-OR ØTH57[1,2,3,Y]Z
Non-OR ØTH58[2,3]Z
Non-OR ØTH9Ø3Z
Non-OR ØTH93[1,3,Y]Z
Non-OR ØTH94[3,Y]Z
Non-OR ØTH97[1,2,3,Y]Z
Non-OR ØTH98[2,3]Z
Non-OR ØTHBØ3Z
Non-OR ØTHB3[1,3,Y]Z
Non-OR ØTHB4[3,Y]Z
Non-OR ØTHB7[1,2,3,Y]Z
Non-OR ØTHB8[2,3]Z
Non-OR ØTHDØ3Z
Non-OR ØTHD3[1,3,Y]Z
Non-OR ØTHD4[3,Y]Z
Non-OR ØTHD7[1,2,3,Y]Z
Non-OR ØTHD8[2,3,Y]Z
Non-OR ØTHDX3Z
NC ØTHB[Ø,3,4,7,8]MZ

Ø Medical and Surgical
T Urinary System
J Inspection Definition: Visually and/or manually exploring a body part

Explanation: Visual exploration may be performed with or without optical instrumentation. Manual exploration may be performed directly or through intervening body layers.

Body Part Character 4	Approach Character 5	Device Character 6	Qualifier Character 7
5 Kidney Renal calyx Renal capsule Renal cortex Renal segment **9 Ureter** Ureteral orifice Ureterovesical orifice **B Bladder** Trigone of bladder **D Urethra** Bulbourethral (Cowper's) gland Cowper's (bulbourethral) gland External urethral sphincter Internal urethral sphincter Membranous urethra Penile urethra Prostatic urethra	**Ø Open** **3 Percutaneous** **4 Percutaneous Endoscopic** **7 Via Natural or Artificial Opening** **8 Via Natural or Artificial Opening Endoscopic** **X External**	**Z No Device**	**Z No Qualifier**

Non-OR ØTJ[5,9,D][3,4,7,8,X]ZZ
Non-OR ØTJB[3,7,8,X]ZZ

Ø Medical and Surgical
T Urinary System
L Occlusion Definition: Completely closing an orifice or the lumen of a tubular body part

Explanation: The orifice can be a natural orifice or an artificially created orifice

Body Part Character 4	Approach Character 5	Device Character 6	Qualifier Character 7
3 Kidney Pelvis, Right Ureteropelvic junction (UPJ) **4 Kidney Pelvis, Left** ***See*** *3 Kidney Pelvis, Right* **6 Ureter, Right** Ureteral orifice Ureterovesical orifice **7 Ureter, Left** ***See*** *6 Ureter, Right* **B Bladder** Trigone of bladder **C Bladder Neck**	**Ø Open** **3 Percutaneous** **4 Percutaneous Endoscopic**	**C Extraluminal Device** **D Intraluminal Device** **Z No Device**	**Z No Qualifier**
3 Kidney Pelvis, Right Ureteropelvic junction (UPJ) **4 Kidney Pelvis, Left** ***See*** *3 Kidney Pelvis, Right* **6 Ureter, Right** Ureteral orifice Ureterovesical orifice **7 Ureter, Left** ***See*** *6 Ureter, Right* **B Bladder** Trigone of bladder **C Bladder Neck**	**7 Via Natural or Artificial Opening** **8 Via Natural or Artificial Opening Endoscopic**	**D Intraluminal Device** **Z No Device**	**Z No Qualifier**
D Urethra Bulbourethral (Cowper's) gland Cowper's (bulbourethral) gland External urethral sphincter Internal urethral sphincter Membranous urethra Penile urethra Prostatic urethra	**Ø Open** **3 Percutaneous** **4 Percutaneous Endoscopic** **X External**	**C Extraluminal Device** **D Intraluminal Device** **Z No Device**	**Z No Qualifier**
D Urethra Bulbourethral (Cowper's) gland Cowper's (bulbourethral) gland External urethral sphincter Internal urethral sphincter Membranous urethra Penile urethra Prostatic urethra	**7 Via Natural or Artificial Opening** **8 Via Natural or Artificial Opening Endoscopic**	**D Intraluminal Device** **Z No Device**	**Z No Qualifier**

Urinary System

Ø Medical and Surgical
T Urinary System
M Reattachment Definition: Putting back in or on all or a portion of a separated body part to its normal location or other suitable location
Explanation: Vascular circulation and nervous pathways may or may not be reestablished

Body Part Character 4	Approach Character 5	Device Character 6	Qualifier Character 7
Ø Kidney, Right Renal calyx Renal capsule Renal cortex Renal segment **1 Kidney, Left** *See Ø Kidney, Right* **2 Kidneys, Bilateral** *See Ø Kidney, Right* **3 Kidney Pelvis, Right** Ureteropelvic junction (UPJ) **4 Kidney Pelvis, Left** *See 3 Kidney Pelvis, Right* **6 Ureter, Right** Ureteral orifice Ureterovesical orifice **7 Ureter, Left** *See 6 Ureter, Right* **8 Ureters, Bilateral** *See 6 Ureter, Right* **B Bladder** Trigone of bladder **C Bladder Neck** **D Urethra** Bulbourethral (Cowper's) gland Cowper's (bulbourethral) gland External urethral sphincter Internal urethral sphincter Membranous urethra Penile urethra Prostatic urethra	**Ø Open** **4 Percutaneous Endoscopic**	**Z No Device**	**Z No Qualifier**

Ø Medical and Surgical
T Urinary System
N Release Definition: Freeing a body part from an abnormal physical constraint by cutting or by the use of force
Explanation: Some of the restraining tissue may be taken out but none of the body part is taken out

Body Part Character 4	Approach Character 5	Device Character 6	Qualifier Character 7
Ø Kidney, Right Renal calyx Renal capsule Renal cortex Renal segment **1 Kidney, Left** *See Ø Kidney, Right* **3 Kidney Pelvis, Right** Ureteropelvic junction (UPJ) **4 Kidney Pelvis, Left** *See 3 Kidney Pelvis, Right* **6 Ureter, Right** Ureteral orifice Ureterovesical orifice **7 Ureter, Left** *See 6 Ureter, Right* **B Bladder** Trigone of bladder **C Bladder Neck**	**Ø Open** **3 Percutaneous** **4 Percutaneous Endoscopic** **7 Via Natural or Artificial Opening** **8 Via Natural or Artificial Opening Endoscopic**	**Z No Device**	**Z No Qualifier**
D Urethra Bulbourethral (Cowper's) gland Cowper's (bulbourethral) gland External urethral sphincter Internal urethral sphincter Membranous urethra Penile urethra Prostatic urethra	**Ø Open** **3 Percutaneous** **4 Percutaneous Endoscopic** **7 Via Natural or Artificial Opening** **8 Via Natural or Artificial Opening Endoscopic** **X External**	**Z No Device**	**Z No Qualifier**

Ø Medical and Surgical
T Urinary System
P Removal Definition: Taking out or off a device from a body part

Explanation: If a device is taken out and a similar device put in without cutting or puncturing the skin or mucous membrane, the procedure is coded to the root operation CHANGE. Otherwise, the procedure for taking out the device is coded to the root operation REMOVAL.

Body Part Character 4	Approach Character 5	Device Character 6	Qualifier Character 7
5 Kidney Renal calyx Renal capsule Renal cortex Renal segment	**Ø Open** **3 Percutaneous** **4 Percutaneous Endoscopic** **7 Via Natural or Artificial Opening** **8 Via Natural or Artificial Opening Endoscopic**	**Ø Drainage Device** **2 Monitoring Device** **3 Infusion Device** **7 Autologous Tissue Substitute** **C Extraluminal Device** **D Intraluminal Device** **J Synthetic Substitute** **K Nonautologous Tissue Substitute** **Y Other Device**	**Z No Qualifier**
5 Kidney Renal calyx Renal capsule Renal cortex Renal segment	**X External**	**Ø Drainage Device** **2 Monitoring Device** **3 Infusion Device** **D Intraluminal Device**	**Z No Qualifier**
9 Ureter Ureteral orifice Ureterovesical orifice	**Ø Open** **3 Percutaneous** **4 Percutaneous Endoscopic** **7 Via Natural or Artificial Opening** **8 Via Natural or Artificial Opening Endoscopic**	**Ø Drainage Device** **2 Monitoring Device** **3 Infusion Device** **7 Autologous Tissue Substitute** **C Extraluminal Device** **D Intraluminal Device** **J Synthetic Substitute** **K Nonautologous Tissue Substitute** **M Stimulator Lead** **Y Other Device**	**Z No Qualifier**
9 Ureter Ureteral orifice Ureterovesical orifice	**X External**	**Ø Drainage Device** **2 Monitoring Device** **3 Infusion Device** **D Intraluminal Device** **M Stimulator Lead**	**Z No Qualifier**
B Bladder NC Trigone of bladder	**Ø Open** **3 Percutaneous** **4 Percutaneous Endoscopic** **7 Via Natural or Artificial Opening** **8 Via Natural or Artificial Opening Endoscopic**	**Ø Drainage Device** **2 Monitoring Device** **3 Infusion Device** **7 Autologous Tissue Substitute** **C Extraluminal Device** **D Intraluminal Device** **J Synthetic Substitute** **K Nonautologous Tissue Substitute** **L Artificial Sphincter** **M Stimulator Lead** **Y Other Device**	**Z No Qualifier**
B Bladder Trigone of bladder	**X External**	**Ø Drainage Device** **2 Monitoring Device** **3 Infusion Device** **D Intraluminal Device** **L Artificial Sphincter** **M Stimulator Lead**	**Z No Qualifier**
D Urethra Bulbourethral (Cowper's) gland Cowper's (bulbourethral) gland External urethral sphincter Internal urethral sphincter Membranous urethra Penile urethra Prostatic urethra	**Ø Open** **3 Percutaneous** **4 Percutaneous Endoscopic** **7 Via Natural or Artificial Opening** **8 Via Natural or Artificial Opening Endoscopic**	**Ø Drainage Device** **2 Monitoring Device** **3 Infusion Device** **7 Autologous Tissue Substitute** **C Extraluminal Device** **D Intraluminal Device** **J Synthetic Substitute** **K Nonautologous Tissue Substitute** **L Artificial Sphincter** **Y Other Device**	**Z No Qualifier**
D Urethra Bulbourethral (Cowper's) gland Cowper's (bulbourethral) gland External urethral sphincter Internal urethral sphincter Membranous urethra Penile urethra Prostatic urethra	**X External**	**Ø Drainage Device** **2 Monitoring Device** **3 Infusion Device** **D Intraluminal Device** **L Artificial Sphincter**	**Z No Qualifier**

Non-OR ØTP5[3,4,7]YZ
Non-OR ØTP5[7,8][Ø,2,3,D]Z
Non-OR ØTP5X[Ø,2,3,D]Z
Non-OR ØTP9[3,4,7]YZ
Non-OR ØTP9[7,8][Ø,2,3,D]Z
Non-OR ØTP9X[Ø,2,3,D]Z
Non-OR ØTPB[3,4,7]YZ
Non-OR ØTPB[7,8][Ø,2,3,D]Z
Non-OR ØTPBX[Ø,2,3,D,L]Z
Non-OR ØTPD[3,4]YZ
Non-OR ØTPD[7,8][Ø,2,3,D,Y]Z
Non-OR ØTPDX[Ø,2,3,D]Z
NC ØTPB[Ø,3,4,7,8]MZ

Ø Medical and Surgical
T Urinary System
Q Repair Definition: Restoring, to the extent possible, a body part to its normal anatomic structure and function

Explanation: Used only when the method to accomplish the repair is not one of the other root operations

Body Part Character 4	Approach Character 5	Device Character 6	Qualifier Character 7
Ø Kidney, Right Renal calyx Renal capsule Renal cortex Renal segment **1 Kidney, Left** *See Ø Kidney, Right* **3 Kidney Pelvis, Right** Ureteropelvic junction (UPJ) **4 Kidney Pelvis, Left** *See 3 Kidney Pelvis, Right* **6 Ureter, Right** Ureteral orifice Ureterovesical orifice **7 Ureter, Left** *See 6 Ureter, Right* **B Bladder** ⊞ Trigone of bladder **C Bladder Neck**	**Ø Open** **3 Percutaneous** **4 Percutaneous Endoscopic** **7 Via Natural or Artificial Opening** **8 Via Natural or Artificial Opening Endoscopic**	**Z No Device**	**Z No Qualifier**
D Urethra Bulbourethral (Cowper's) gland Cowper's (bulbourethral) gland External urethral sphincter Internal urethral sphincter Membranous urethra Penile urethra Prostatic urethra	**Ø Open** **3 Percutaneous** **4 Percutaneous Endoscopic** **7 Via Natural or Artificial Opening** **8 Via Natural or Artificial Opening Endoscopic** **X External**	**Z No Device**	**Z No Qualifier**

See Appendix L for Procedure Combinations

⊞ ØTQB[Ø,3,4]ZZ

Ø Medical and Surgical
T Urinary System
R Replacement Definition: Putting in or on biological or synthetic material that physically takes the place and/or function of all or a portion of a body part

Explanation: The body part may have been taken out or replaced, or may be taken out, physically eradicated, or rendered nonfunctional during the REPLACEMENT procedure. A REMOVAL procedure is coded for taking out the device used in a previous replacement procedure.

Body Part Character 4	Approach Character 5	Device Character 6	Qualifier Character 7
3 Kidney Pelvis, Right Ureteropelvic junction (UPJ) **4 Kidney Pelvis, Left** *See 3 Kidney Pelvis, Right* **6 Ureter, Right** Ureteral orifice Ureterovesical orifice **7 Ureter, Left** *See 6 Ureter, Right* **B Bladder** Trigone of bladder **C Bladder Neck**	**Ø Open** **4 Percutaneous Endoscopic** **7 Via Natural or Artificial Opening** **8 Via Natural or Artificial Opening Endoscopic**	**7 Autologous Tissue Substitute** **J Synthetic Substitute** **K Nonautologous Tissue Substitute**	**Z No Qualifier**
D Urethra Bulbourethral (Cowper's) gland Cowper's (bulbourethral) gland External urethral sphincter Internal urethral sphincter Membranous urethra Penile urethra Prostatic urethra	**Ø Open** **4 Percutaneous Endoscopic** **7 Via Natural or Artificial Opening** **8 Via Natural or Artificial Opening Endoscopic** **X External**	**7 Autologous Tissue Substitute** **J Synthetic Substitute** **K Nonautologous Tissue Substitute**	**Z No Qualifier**

Ø Medical and Surgical
T Urinary System
S Reposition Definition: Moving to its normal location, or other suitable location, all or a portion of a body part

Explanation: The body part is moved to a new location from an abnormal location, or from a normal location where it is not functioning correctly. The body part may or may not be cut out or off to be moved to the new location.

Body Part Character 4	Approach Character 5	Device Character 6	Qualifier Character 7
Ø Kidney, Right Renal calyx Renal capsule Renal cortex Renal segment **1 Kidney, Left** *See Ø Kidney, Right* **2 Kidneys, Bilateral** *See Ø Kidney, Right* **3 Kidney Pelvis, Right** Ureteropelvic junction (UPJ) **4 Kidney Pelvis, Left** *See 3 Kidney Pelvis, Right* **6 Ureter, Right** Ureteral orifice Ureterovesical orifice **7 Ureter, Left** *See 6 Ureter, Right* **8 Ureters, Bilateral** *See 6 Ureter, Right* **B Bladder** Trigone of bladder **C Bladder Neck** **D Urethra** Bulbourethral (Cowper's) gland Cowper's (bulbourethral) gland External urethral sphincter Internal urethral sphincter Membranous urethra Penile urethra Prostatic urethra	**Ø Open** **4 Percutaneous Endoscopic**	**Z No Device**	**Z No Qualifier**

Ø Medical and Surgical
T Urinary System
T Resection Definition: Cutting out or off, without replacement, all of a body part

Explanation: None

Body Part Character 4	Approach Character 5	Device Character 6	Qualifier Character 7
Ø Kidney, Right Renal calyx Renal capsule Renal cortex Renal segment **1 Kidney, Left** *See Ø Kidney, Right* **2 Kidneys, Bilateral** *See Ø Kidney, Right*	**Ø Open** **4 Percutaneous Endoscopic**	**Z No Device**	**Z No Qualifier**
3 Kidney Pelvis, Right Ureteropelvic junction (UPJ) **4 Kidney Pelvis, Left** *See 3 Kidney Pelvis, Right* **6 Ureter, Right** Ureteral orifice Ureterovesical orifice **7 Ureter, Left** *See 6 Ureter, Right* **B Bladder** ⊞ Trigone of bladder **C Bladder Neck** **D Urethra** Bulbourethral (Cowper's) gland Cowper's (bulbourethral) gland External urethral sphincter Internal urethral sphincter Membranous urethra Penile urethra Prostatic urethra	**Ø Open** **4 Percutaneous Endoscopic** **7 Via Natural or Artificial Opening** **8 Via Natural or Artificial Opening Endoscopic**	**Z No Device**	**Z No Qualifier**

Non-OR ØTTD[4,7,8]ZZ

See Appendix L for Procedure Combinations

Combo-only ØTTDØZZ
⊞ ØTTBØZZ

Ø Medical and Surgical
T Urinary System
U Supplement Definition: Putting in or on biological or synthetic material that physically reinforces and/or augments the function of a portion of a body part

Explanation: The biological material is non-living, or is living and from the same individual. The body part may have been previously replaced, and the SUPPLEMENT procedure is performed to physically reinforce and/or augment the function of the replaced body part.

Body Part Character 4	Approach Character 5	Device Character 6	Qualifier Character 7
3 Kidney Pelvis, Right Ureteropelvic junction (UPJ) **4 Kidney Pelvis, Left** *See 3 Kidney Pelvis, Right* **6 Ureter, Right** Ureteral orifice Ureterovesical orifice **7 Ureter, Left** *See 6 Ureter, Right* **B Bladder** Trigone of bladder **C Bladder Neck**	**Ø Open** **4 Percutaneous Endoscopic** **7 Via Natural or Artificial Opening** **8 Via Natural or Artificial Opening Endoscopic**	**7 Autologous Tissue Substitute** **J Synthetic Substitute** **K Nonautologous Tissue Substitute**	**Z No Qualifier**
D Urethra Bulbourethral (Cowper's) gland Cowper's (bulbourethral) gland External urethral sphincter Internal urethral sphincter Membranous urethra Penile urethra Prostatic urethra	**Ø Open** **4 Percutaneous Endoscopic** **7 Via Natural or Artificial Opening** **8 Via Natural or Artificial Opening Endoscopic** **X External**	**7 Autologous Tissue Substitute** **J Synthetic Substitute** **K Nonautologous Tissue Substitute**	**Z No Qualifier**

Ø Medical and Surgical
T Urinary System
V Restriction Definition: Partially closing an orifice or the lumen of a tubular body part

Explanation: The orifice can be a natural orifice or an artificially created orifice

Body Part Character 4	Approach Character 5	Device Character 6	Qualifier Character 7
3 Kidney Pelvis, Right Ureteropelvic junction (UPJ) **4 Kidney Pelvis, Left** *See 3 Kidney Pelvis, Right* **6 Ureter, Right** Ureteral orifice Ureterovesical orifice **7 Ureter, Left** *See 6 Ureter, Right* **B Bladder** Trigone of bladder **C Bladder Neck**	**Ø Open** **3 Percutaneous** **4 Percutaneous Endoscopic**	**C Extraluminal Device** **D Intraluminal Device** **Z No Device**	**Z No Qualifier**
3 Kidney Pelvis, Right Ureteropelvic junction (UPJ) **4 Kidney Pelvis, Left** *See 3 Kidney Pelvis, Right* **6 Ureter, Right** Ureteral orifice Ureterovesical orifice **7 Ureter, Left** *See 6 Ureter, Right* **B Bladder** Trigone of bladder **C Bladder Neck**	**7 Via Natural or Artificial Opening** **8 Via Natural or Artificial Opening Endoscopic**	**D Intraluminal Device** **Z No Device**	**Z No Qualifier**
D Urethra Bulbourethral (Cowper's) gland Cowper's (bulbourethral) gland External urethral sphincter Internal urethral sphincter Membranous urethra Penile urethra Prostatic urethra	**Ø Open** **3 Percutaneous** **4 Percutaneous Endoscopic**	**C Extraluminal Device** **D Intraluminal Device** **Z No Device**	**Z No Qualifier**
D Urethra Bulbourethral (Cowper's) gland Cowper's (bulbourethral) gland External urethral sphincter Internal urethral sphincter Membranous urethra Penile urethra Prostatic urethra	**7 Via Natural or Artificial Opening** **8 Via Natural or Artificial Opening Endoscopic**	**D Intraluminal Device** **Z No Device**	**Z No Qualifier**
D Urethra Bulbourethral (Cowper's) gland Cowper's (bulbourethral) gland External urethral sphincter Internal urethral sphincter Membranous urethra Penile urethra Prostatic urethra	**X External**	**Z No Device**	**Z No Qualifier**

Ø Medical and Surgical
T Urinary System
W Revision

Definition: Correcting, to the extent possible, a portion of a malfunctioning device or the position of a displaced device

Explanation: Revision can include correcting a malfunctioning or displaced device by taking out or putting in components of the device such as a screw or pin

Body Part Character 4	Approach Character 5	Device Character 6	Qualifier Character 7
5 Kidney Renal calyx Renal capsule Renal cortex Renal segment	**Ø Open** **3 Percutaneous** **4 Percutaneous Endoscopic** **7 Via Natural or Artificial Opening** **8 Via Natural or Artificial Opening Endoscopic**	**Ø Drainage Device** **2 Monitoring Device** **3 Infusion Device** **7 Autologous Tissue Substitute** **C Extraluminal Device** **D Intraluminal Device** **J Synthetic Substitute** **K Nonautologous Tissue Substitute** **Y Other Device**	**Z No Qualifier**
5 Kidney Renal calyx Renal capsule Renal cortex Renal segment	**X External**	**Ø Drainage Device** **2 Monitoring Device** **3 Infusion Device** **7 Autologous Tissue Substitute** **C Extraluminal Device** **D Intraluminal Device** **J Synthetic Substitute** **K Nonautologous Tissue Substitute**	**Z No Qualifier**
9 Ureter Ureteral orifice Ureterovesical orifice	**Ø Open** **3 Percutaneous** **4 Percutaneous Endoscopic** **7 Via Natural or Artificial Opening** **8 Via Natural or Artificial Opening Endoscopic**	**Ø Drainage Device** **2 Monitoring Device** **3 Infusion Device** **7 Autologous Tissue Substitute** **C Extraluminal Device** **D Intraluminal Device** **J Synthetic Substitute** **K Nonautologous Tissue Substitute** **M Stimulator Lead** **Y Other Device**	**Z No Qualifier**
9 Ureter Ureteral orifice Ureterovesical orifice	**X External**	**Ø Drainage Device** **2 Monitoring Device** **3 Infusion Device** **7 Autologous Tissue Substitute** **C Extraluminal Device** **D Intraluminal Device** **J Synthetic Substitute** **K Nonautologous Tissue Substitute** **M Stimulator Lead**	**Z No Qualifier**
B Bladder Trigone of bladder	**Ø Open** **3 Percutaneous** **4 Percutaneous Endoscopic** **7 Via Natural or Artificial Opening** **8 Via Natural or Artificial Opening Endoscopic**	**Ø Drainage Device** **2 Monitoring Device** **3 Infusion Device** **7 Autologous Tissue Substitute** **C Extraluminal Device** **D Intraluminal Device** **J Synthetic Substitute** **K Nonautologous Tissue Substitute** **L Artificial Sphincter** **M Stimulator Lead** **Y Other Device**	**Z No Qualifier**
B Bladder Trigone of bladder	**X External**	**Ø Drainage Device** **2 Monitoring Device** **3 Infusion Device** **7 Autologous Tissue Substitute** **C Extraluminal Device** **D Intraluminal Device** **J Synthetic Substitute** **K Nonautologous Tissue Substitute** **L Artificial Sphincter** **M Stimulator Lead**	**Z No Qualifier**

Non-OR ØTW5[3,4,7]YZ
Non-OR ØTW5X[Ø,2,3,7,C,D,J,K]Z
Non-OR ØTW9[3,4,7]YZ
Non-OR ØTW9X[Ø,2,3,7,C,D,J,K,M]Z
Non-OR ØTWB[3,4,7]YZ
Non-OR ØTWBX[Ø,2,3,7,C,D,J,K,L,M]Z

ØTW Continued on next page

ØTW Continued

Ø Medical and Surgical
T Urinary System
W Revision Definition: Correcting, to the extent possible, a portion of a malfunctioning device or the position of a displaced device

Explanation: Revision can include correcting a malfunctioning or displaced device by taking out or putting in components of the device such as a screw or pin

Body Part Character 4	Approach Character 5	Device Character 6	Qualifier Character 7
D Urethra Bulbourethral (Cowper's) gland Cowper's (bulbourethral) gland External urethral sphincter Internal urethral sphincter Membranous urethra Penile urethra Prostatic urethra	**Ø Open** **3 Percutaneous** **4 Percutaneous Endoscopic** **7 Via Natural or Artificial Opening** **8 Via Natural or Artificial Opening Endoscopic**	**Ø Drainage Device** **2 Monitoring Device** **3 Infusion Device** **7 Autologous Tissue Substitute** **C Extraluminal Device** **D Intraluminal Device** **J Synthetic Substitute** **K Nonautologous Tissue Substitute** **L Artificial Sphincter** **Y Other Device**	**Z No Qualifier**
D Urethra Bulbourethral (Cowper's) gland Cowper's (bulbourethral) gland External urethral sphincter Internal urethral sphincter Membranous urethra Penile urethra Prostatic urethra	**X External**	**Ø Drainage Device** **2 Monitoring Device** **3 Infusion Device** **7 Autologous Tissue Substitute** **C Extraluminal Device** **D Intraluminal Device** **J Synthetic Substitute** **K Nonautologous Tissue Substitute** **L Artificial Sphincter**	**Z No Qualifier**

Non-OR ØTWD[3,4,7,8]YZ
Non-OR ØTWDX[Ø,2,3,7,C,D,J,K,L]Z

Ø Medical and Surgical
T Urinary System
Y Transplantation Definition: Putting in or on all or a portion of a living body part taken from another individual or animal to physically take the place and/or function of all or a portion of a similar body part

Explanation: The native body part may or may not be taken out, and the transplanted body part may take over all or a portion of its function

Body Part Character 4	Approach Character 5	Device Character 6	Qualifier Character 7
Ø Kidney, Right LC ⊞ Renal calyx Renal capsule Renal cortex Renal segment **1 Kidney, Left** LC ⊞ *See Ø Kidney, Right*	**Ø Open**	**Z No Device**	**Ø Allogeneic** **1 Syngeneic** **2 Zooplastic**

LC ØTY[Ø,1]ØZ[Ø,1,2]

See Appendix L for Procedure Combinations
⊞ ØTY[Ø,1]ØZ[Ø,1,2]

Female Reproductive System ØU1–ØUY

Character Meanings

This Character Meaning table is provided as a guide to assist the user in the identification of character members that may be found in this section of code tables. It **SHOULD NOT** be used to build a PCS code.

Operation–Character 3	Body Part–Character 4	Approach–Character 5	Device–Character 6	Qualifier–Character 7
1 Bypass	Ø Ovary, Right	Ø Open	Ø Drainage Device	Ø Allogeneic
2 Change	1 Ovary, Left	3 Percutaneous	1 Radioactive Element	1 Syngeneic
5 Destruction	2 Ovaries, Bilateral	4 Percutaneous Endoscopic	3 Infusion Device	2 Zooplastic
7 Dilation	3 Ovary	7 Via Natural or Artificial Opening	7 Autologous Tissue Substitute	5 Fallopian Tube, Right
8 Division	4 Uterine Supporting Structure	8 Via Natural or Artificial Opening Endoscopic	C Extraluminal Device	6 Fallopian Tube, Left
9 Drainage	5 Fallopian Tube, Right	F Via Natural or Artificial Opening With Percutaneous Endoscopic Assistance	D Intraluminal Device	9 Uterus
B Excision	6 Fallopian Tube, Left	X External	G Intraluminal Device, Pessary	L Supracervical
C Extirpation	7 Fallopian Tubes, Bilateral		H Contraceptive Device	X Diagnostic
D Extraction	8 Fallopian Tube		J Synthetic Substitute	Z No Qualifier
F Fragmentation	9 Uterus		K Nonautologous Tissue Substitute	
H Insertion	B Endometrium		Y Other Device	
J Inspection	C Cervix		Z No Device	
L Occlusion	D Uterus and Cervix			
M Reattachment	F Cul-de-sac			
N Release	G Vagina			
P Removal	H Vagina and Cul-de-sac			
Q Repair	J Clitoris			
S Reposition	K Hymen			
T Resection	L Vestibular Gland			
U Supplement	M Vulva			
V Restriction	N Ova			
W Revision				
Y Transplantation				

AHA Coding Clinic for table ØU5
2015, 3Q, 31 Tubal ligation for sterilization

AHA Coding Clinic for table ØU7
2020, 2Q, 30 Duhrssen Cervical Incision

AHA Coding Clinic for table ØU9
2016, 4Q, 58 Longitudinal vaginal septum

AHA Coding Clinic for table ØUB
2018, 1Q, 23 Tubal ligation procedure
2015, 3Q, 31 Laparoscopic partial salpingectomy for ectopic pregnancy
2015, 3Q, 31 Tubal ligation for sterilization
2014, 4Q, 16 Excision of multiple uterine fibroids
2014, 3Q, 12 Excision of skin tag from labia majora

AHA Coding Clinic for table ØUC
2015, 3Q, 30 Removal of cervical cerclage
2013, 2Q, 38 Evacuation of clot post-partum

AHA Coding Clinic for table ØUH
2020, 4Q, 43-44 Insertion of radioactive element
2018, 1Q, 25 Intrauterine brachytherapy & placement of tandems & ovoids
2013, 2Q, 34 Placement of intrauterine device via open approach

AHA Coding Clinic for table ØUJ
2015, 1Q, 33 Robotic-assisted laparoscopic hysterectomy converted to open procedure

AHA Coding Clinic for table ØUL
2018, 1Q, 23 Tubal ligation procedure
2015, 3Q, 31 Tubal ligation for sterilization

AHA Coding Clinic for table ØUQ
2020, 4Q, 59-60 Extraction of ectopic products of conception
2014, 4Q, 18 Obstetrical periurethral laceration
2013, 4Q, 120 Repair of clitoral obstetric laceration

AHA Coding Clinic for table ØUS
2016, 1Q, 9 Anteversion of retroverted pregnant uterus

AHA Coding Clinic for table ØUT
2017, 4Q, 68 New qualifier values - Supracervical hysterectomy
2015, 1Q, 33 Robotic-assisted laparoscopic hysterectomy converted to open procedure
2013, 3Q, 28 Total hysterectomy
2013, 1Q, 24 Excision versus Resection of remaining ovarian remnant following previous excision

AHA Coding Clinic for table ØUV
2015, 3Q, 30 Insertion of cervical cerclage

AHA Coding Clinic for table ØUY
2018, 4Q, 40 Uterus transplant

Female Reproductive System

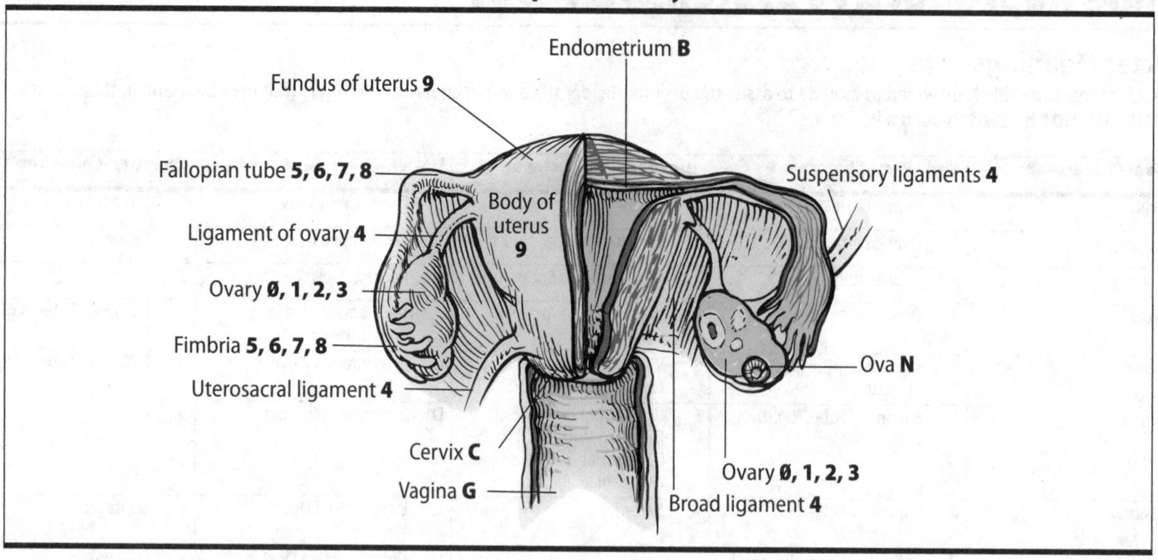

Female Internal/External Structures

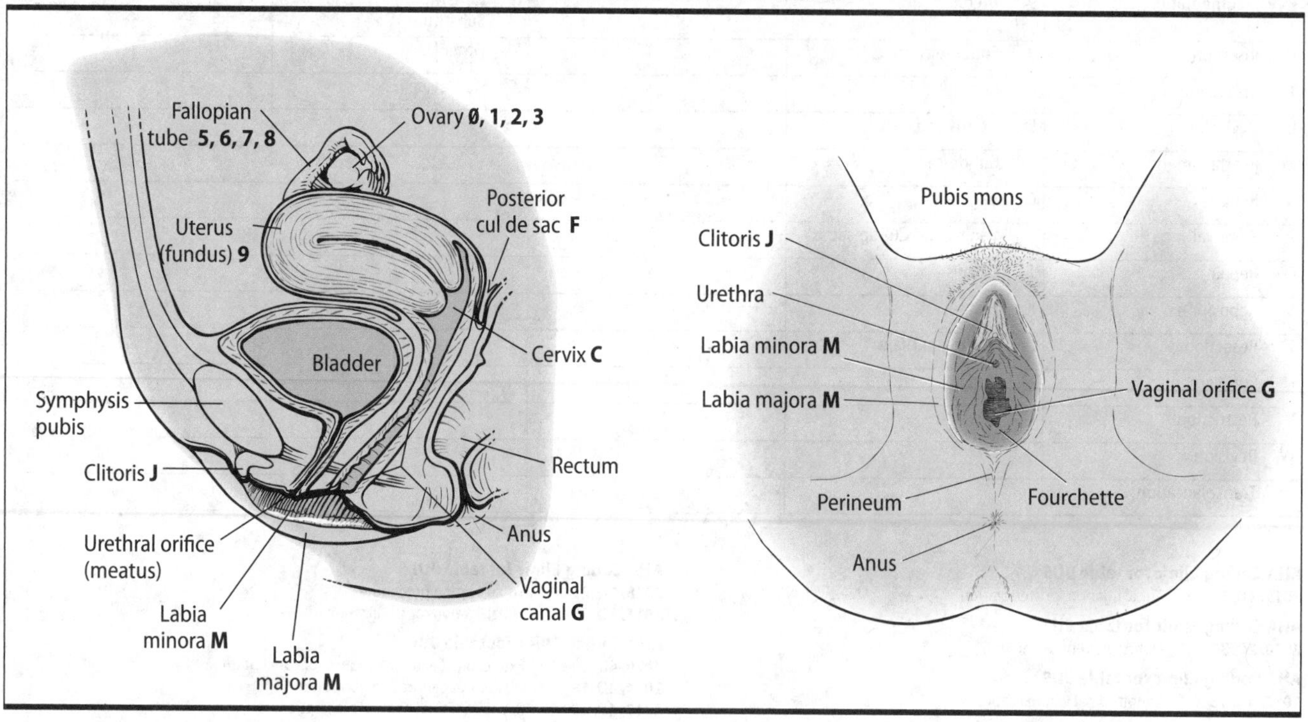

Ø Medical and Surgical
U Female Reproductive System
1 Bypass Definition: Altering the route of passage of the contents of a tubular body part

Explanation: Rerouting contents of a body part to a downstream area of the normal route, to a similar route and body part, or to an abnormal route and dissimilar body part. Includes one or more anastomoses, with or without the use of a device.

Body Part Character 4	Approach Character 5	Device Character 6	Qualifier Character 7
5 Fallopian Tube, Right ♀ Oviduct Salpinx Uterine tube **6 Fallopian Tube, Left** ♀ *See 5 Fallopian Tube, Right*	**Ø Open** **4 Percutaneous Endoscopic**	**7 Autologous Tissue Substitute** **J Synthetic Substitute** **K Nonautologous Tissue Substitute** **Z No Device**	**5 Fallopian Tube, Right** **6 Fallopian Tube, Left** **9 Uterus**

♀ All body part, approach, device, and qualifier values

Ø Medical and Surgical
U Female Reproductive System
2 Change Definition: Taking out or off a device from a body part and putting back an identical or similar device in or on the same body part without cutting or puncturing the skin or a mucous membrane

Explanation: All CHANGE procedures are coded using the approach EXTERNAL

Body Part Character 4	Approach Character 5	Device Character 6	Qualifier Character 7
3 Ovary ♀ **8 Fallopian Tube** ♀ **M Vulva** ♀ Labia majora Labia minora	**X External**	**Ø Drainage Device** **Y Other Device**	**Z No Qualifier**
D Uterus and Cervix ♀	**X External**	**Ø Drainage Device** **H Contraceptive Device** **Y Other Device**	**Z No Qualifier**
H Vagina and Cul-de-sac ♀	**X External**	**Ø Drainage Device** **G Intraluminal Device, Pessary** **Y Other Device**	**Z No Qualifier**

Non-OR All body part, approach, device, and qualifier values
♀ All body part, approach, device, and qualifier values

Ø Medical and Surgical
U Female Reproductive System
5 Destruction Definition: Physical eradication of all or a portion of a body part by the direct use of energy, force, or a destructive agent

Explanation: None of the body part is physically taken out

Body Part Character 4	Approach Character 5	Device Character 6	Qualifier Character 7
Ø Ovary, Right ♀ **1 Ovary, Left** ♀ **2 Ovaries, Bilateral** ♀ **4 Uterine Supporting Structure** ♀ Broad ligament Infundibulopelvic ligament Ovarian ligament Round ligament of uterus	**Ø Open** **3 Percutaneous** **4 Percutaneous Endoscopic** **8 Via Natural or Artificial Opening Endoscopic**	**Z No Device**	**Z No Qualifier**
5 Fallopian Tube, Right ♀ Oviduct Salpinx Uterine tube **6 Fallopian Tube, Left** ♀ *See 5 Fallopian Tube, Right* **7 Fallopian Tubes, Bilateral** NC ♀ **9 Uterus** ♀ Fundus uteri Myometrium Perimetrium Uterine cornu **B Endometrium** ♀ **C Cervix** ♀ **F Cul-de-sac** ♀	**Ø Open** **3 Percutaneous** **4 Percutaneous Endoscopic** **7 Via Natural or Artificial Opening** **8 Via Natural or Artificial Opening Endoscopic**	**Z No Device**	**Z No Qualifier**
G Vagina ♀ **K Hymen** ♀	**Ø Open** **3 Percutaneous** **4 Percutaneous Endoscopic** **7 Via Natural or Artificial Opening** **8 Via Natural or Artificial Opening Endoscopic** **X External**	**Z No Device**	**Z No Qualifier**
J Clitoris ♀ **L Vestibular Gland** ♀ Bartholin's (greater vestibular) gland Greater vestibular (Bartholin's) gland Paraurethral (Skene's) gland Skene's (paraurethral) gland **M Vulva** ♀ Labia majora Labia minora	**Ø Open** **X External**	**Z No Device**	**Z No Qualifier**

NC ØU57[Ø,3,4,7,8]ZZ with principal or secondary diagnosis of Z3Ø.2

♀ All body part, approach, device, and qualifier values

Ø Medical and Surgical
U Female Reproductive System
7 Dilation Definition: Expanding an orifice or the lumen of a tubular body part

Explanation: The orifice can be a natural orifice or an artificially created orifice. Accomplished by stretching a tubular body part using intraluminal pressure or by cutting part of the orifice or wall of the tubular body part.

Body Part Character 4	Approach Character 5	Device Character 6	Qualifier Character 7
5 Fallopian Tube, Right ♀ Oviduct Salpinx Uterine tube **6 Fallopian Tube, Left** ♀ *See 5 Fallopian Tube, Right* **7 Fallopian Tubes, Bilateral** ♀ **9 Uterus** ♀ Fundus uteri Myometrium Perimetrium Uterine cornu **C Cervix** ♀ **G Vagina** ♀	**Ø Open** **3 Percutaneous** **4 Percutaneous Endoscopic** **7 Via Natural or Artificial Opening** **8 Via Natural or Artificial Opening Endoscopic**	**D Intraluminal Device** **Z No Device**	**Z No Qualifier**
K Hymen ♀	**Ø Open** **3 Percutaneous** **4 Percutaneous Endoscopic** **7 Via Natural or Artificial Opening** **8 Via Natural or Artificial Opening Endoscopic** **X External**	**D Intraluminal Device** **Z No Device**	**Z No Qualifier**

Non-OR ØU7C[Ø,3,4,7,8][D,Z]Z
Non-OR ØU7G[7,8][D,Z]Z

♀ All body part, approach, device, and qualifier values

Ø Medical and Surgical
U Female Reproductive System
8 Division Definition: Cutting into a body part, without draining fluids and/or gases from the body part, in order to separate or transect a body part

Explanation: All or a portion of the body part is separated into two or more portions

Body Part Character 4	Approach Character 5	Device Character 6	Qualifier Character 7
Ø Ovary, Right ♀ **1 Ovary, Left** ♀ **2 Ovaries, Bilateral** ♀ **4 Uterine Supporting Structure** ♀ Broad ligament Infundibulopelvic ligament Ovarian ligament Round ligament of uterus	**Ø Open** **3 Percutaneous** **4 Percutaneous Endoscopic**	**Z No Device**	**Z No Qualifier**
K Hymen ♀	**7 Via Natural or Artificial Opening** **8 Via Natural or Artificial Opening Endoscopic** **X External**	**Z No Device**	**Z No Qualifier**

Non-OR ØU8K[7,8,X]ZZ

♀ All body part, approach, device, and qualifier values

Ø Medical and Surgical
U Female Reproductive System
9 Drainage Definition: Taking or letting out fluids and/or gases from a body part
Explanation: The qualifier DIAGNOSTIC is used to identify drainage procedures that are biopsies

Body Part Character 4	Approach Character 5	Device Character 6	Qualifier Character 7
Ø Ovary, Right ♀ **1** Ovary, Left ♀ **2** Ovaries, Bilateral ♀	**Ø** Open **3** Percutaneous **4** Percutaneous Endoscopic **8** Via Natural or Artificial Opening Endoscopic	**Ø** Drainage Device	**Z** No Qualifier
Ø Ovary, Right ♀ **1** Ovary, Left ♀ **2** Ovaries, Bilateral ♀	**Ø** Open **3** Percutaneous **4** Percutaneous Endoscopic **8** Via Natural or Artificial Opening Endoscopic	**Z** No Device	**X** Diagnostic **Z** No Qualifier
Ø Ovary, Right ♀ **1** Ovary, Left ♀ **2** Ovaries, Bilateral ♀	**X** External	**Z** No Device	**Z** No Qualifier
4 Uterine Supporting Structure ♀ Broad ligament Infundibulopelvic ligament Ovarian ligament Round ligament of uterus	**Ø** Open **3** Percutaneous **4** Percutaneous Endoscopic **8** Via Natural or Artificial Opening Endoscopic	**Ø** Drainage Device	**Z** No Qualifier
4 Uterine Supporting Structure ♀ Broad ligament Infundibulopelvic ligament Ovarian ligament Round ligament of uterus	**Ø** Open **3** Percutaneous **4** Percutaneous Endoscopic **8** Via Natural or Artificial Opening Endoscopic	**Z** No Device	**X** Diagnostic **Z** No Qualifier
5 Fallopian Tube, Right ♀ Oviduct Salpinx Uterine tube **6** Fallopian Tube, Left ♀ *See 5 Fallopian Tube, Right* **7** Fallopian Tubes, Bilateral ♀ **9** Uterus ♀ Fundus uteri Myometrium Perimetrium Uterine cornu **C** Cervix ♀ **F** Cul-de-sac ♀	**Ø** Open **3** Percutaneous **4** Percutaneous Endoscopic **7** Via Natural or Artificial Opening **8** Via Natural or Artificial Opening Endoscopic	**Ø** Drainage Device	**Z** No Qualifier
5 Fallopian Tube, Right ♀ Oviduct Salpinx Uterine tube **6** Fallopian Tube, Left ♀ *See 5 Fallopian Tube, Right* **7** Fallopian Tubes, Bilateral ♀ **9** Uterus ♀ Fundus uteri Myometrium Perimetrium Uterine cornu **C** Cervix ♀ **F** Cul-de-sac ♀	**Ø** Open **3** Percutaneous **4** Percutaneous Endoscopic **7** Via Natural or Artificial Opening **8** Via Natural or Artificial Opening Endoscopic	**Z** No Device	**X** Diagnostic **Z** No Qualifier

Non-OR ØU9[Ø,1,2][3,8]ØZ
Non-OR ØU9[Ø,1,2][3,8]ZZ
Non-OR ØU9[Ø,1,2]8ZX
Non-OR ØU94[3,8]ØZ
Non-OR ØU94[3,8]ZZ
Non-OR ØU948ZX
Non-OR ØU9[5,6,7,9,C]3ØZ
Non-OR ØU9F[3,4]ØZ
Non-OR ØU9[5,6,7][3,4,7,8]ZZ
Non-OR ØU9[9,C]3ZZ
Non-OR ØU9F[3,4]ZZ
♀ All body part, approach, device, and qualifier values

ØU9 Continued on next page

ØU9 Continued

Ø Medical and Surgical
U Female Reproductive System
9 Drainage Definition: Taking or letting out fluids and/or gases from a body part
Explanation: The qualifier DIAGNOSTIC is used to identify drainage procedures that are biopsies

Body Part Character 4	Approach Character 5	Device Character 6	Qualifier Character 7
G Vagina ♀ K Hymen ♀	Ø Open 3 Percutaneous 4 Percutaneous Endoscopic 7 Via Natural or Artificial Opening 8 Via Natural or Artificial Opening Endoscopic X External	Ø Drainage Device	Z No Qualifier
G Vagina ♀ K Hymen ♀	Ø Open 3 Percutaneous 4 Percutaneous Endoscopic 7 Via Natural or Artificial Opening 8 Via Natural or Artificial Opening Endoscopic X External	Z No Device	X Diagnostic Z No Qualifier
J Clitoris ♀ L Vestibular Gland ♀ Bartholin's (greater vestibular) gland Greater vestibular (Bartholin's) gland Paraurethral (Skene's) gland Skene's (paraurethral) gland M Vulva ♀ Labia majora Labia minora	Ø Open X External	Ø Drainage Device	Z No Qualifier
J Clitoris ♀ L Vestibular Gland ♀ Bartholin's (greater vestibular) gland Greater vestibular (Bartholin's) gland Paraurethral (Skene's) gland Skene's (paraurethral) gland M Vulva ♀ Labia majora Labia minora	Ø Open X External	Z No Device	X Diagnostic Z No Qualifier

Non-OR ØU9G3ØZ
Non-OR ØU9K[Ø,3,4,7,8,X]ØZ
Non-OR ØU9G3ZZ
Non-OR ØU9K[Ø,3,4,7,8,X]ZZ
Non-OR ØU9L[Ø,X]ØZ
Non-OR ØU9L[Ø,X]ZZ
♀ All body part, approach, device, and qualifier values

Ø Medical and Surgical
U Female Reproductive System
B Excision Definition: Cutting out or off, without replacement, a portion of a body part
Explanation: The qualifier DIAGNOSTIC is used to identify excision procedures that are biopsies

Body Part Character 4	Approach Character 5	Device Character 6	Qualifier Character 7
Ø Ovary, Right ♀ **1 Ovary, Left** ♀ **2 Ovaries, Bilateral** ♀ **4 Uterine Supporting Structure** ♀ Broad ligament Infundibulopelvic ligament Ovarian ligament Round ligament of uterus **5 Fallopian Tube, Right** ♀ Oviduct Salpinx Uterine tube **6 Fallopian Tube, Left** ♀ *See 5 Fallopian Tube, Right* **7 Fallopian Tubes, Bilateral** ♀ **9 Uterus** ♀ Fundus uteri Myometrium Perimetrium Uterine cornu **C Cervix** ♀ **F Cul-de-sac** ♀	**Ø Open** **3 Percutaneous** **4 Percutaneous Endoscopic** **7 Via Natural or Artificial Opening** **8 Via Natural or Artificial Opening Endoscopic**	**Z No Device**	**X Diagnostic** **Z No Qualifier**
G Vagina ♀ **K Hymen** ♀	**Ø Open** **3 Percutaneous** **4 Percutaneous Endoscopic** **7 Via Natural or Artificial Opening** **8 Via Natural or Artificial Opening Endoscopic** **X External**	**Z No Device**	**X Diagnostic** **Z No Qualifier**
J Clitoris ♀ **L Vestibular Gland** ♀ Bartholin's (greater vestibular) gland Greater vestibular (Bartholin's) gland Paraurethral (Skene's) gland Skene's (paraurethral) gland **M Vulva** ♀ Labia majora Labia minora	**Ø Open** **X External**	**Z No Device**	**X Diagnostic** **Z No Qualifier**

♀ All body part, approach, device, and qualifier values

Ø Medical and Surgical
U Female Reproductive System
C Extirpation Definition: Taking or cutting out solid matter from a body part

Explanation: The solid matter may be an abnormal byproduct of a biological function or a foreign body; it may be imbedded in a body part or in the lumen of a tubular body part. The solid matter may or may not have been previously broken into pieces.

Body Part Character 4	Approach Character 5	Device Character 6	Qualifier Character 7
Ø Ovary, Right ♀ **1 Ovary, Left** ♀ **2 Ovaries, Bilateral** ♀ **4 Uterine Supporting Structure** ♀ Broad ligament Infundibulopelvic ligament Ovarian ligament Round ligament of uterus	**Ø Open** **3 Percutaneous** **4 Percutaneous Endoscopic** **8 Via Natural or Artificial Opening Endoscopic**	**Z No Device**	**Z No Qualifier**
5 Fallopian Tube, Right ♀ Oviduct Salpinx Uterine tube **6 Fallopian Tube, Left** ♀ *See 5 Fallopian Tube, Right* **7 Fallopian Tubes, Bilateral** ♀ **9 Uterus** ♀ Fundus uteri Myometrium Perimetrium Uterine cornu **B Endometrium** ♀ **C Cervix** ♀ **F Cul-de-sac** ♀	**Ø Open** **3 Percutaneous** **4 Percutaneous Endoscopic** **7 Via Natural or Artificial Opening** **8 Via Natural or Artificial Opening Endoscopic**	**Z No Device**	**Z No Qualifier**
G Vagina ♀ **K Hymen** ♀	**Ø Open** **3 Percutaneous** **4 Percutaneous Endoscopic** **7 Via Natural or Artificial Opening** **8 Via Natural or Artificial Opening Endoscopic** **X External**	**Z No Device**	**Z No Qualifier**
J Clitoris ♀ **L Vestibular Gland** ♀ Bartholin's (greater vestibular) gland Greater vestibular (Bartholin's) gland Paraurethral (Skene's) gland Skene's (paraurethral) gland **M Vulva** ♀ Labia majora Labia minora	**Ø Open** **X External**	**Z No Device**	**Z No Qualifier**

Non-OR ØUC9[7,8]ZZ
Non-OR ØUCG[7,8,X]ZZ
Non-OR ØUCK[Ø,3,4,7,8,X]ZZ
Non-OR ØUCMXZZ
♀ All body part, approach, device, and qualifier values

Ø Medical and Surgical
U Female Reproductive System
D Extraction Definition: Pulling or stripping out or off all or a portion of a body part by the use of force

Explanation: The qualifier DIAGNOSTIC is used to identify extraction procedures that are biopsies

Body Part Character 4	Approach Character 5	Device Character 6	Qualifier Character 7
B Endometrium ♀	**7 Via Natural or Artificial Opening** **8 Via Natural or Artificial Opening Endoscopic**	**Z No Device**	**X Diagnostic** **Z No Qualifier**
N Ova ♀	**Ø Open** **3 Percutaneous** **4 Percutaneous Endoscopic**	**Z No Device**	**Z No Qualifier**

♀ All body part, approach, device, and qualifier values

Ø Medical and Surgical
U Female Reproductive System
F Fragmentation Definition: Breaking solid matter in a body part into pieces

Explanation: Physical force (e.g., manual, ultrasonic) applied directly or indirectly is used to break the solid matter into pieces. The solid matter may be an abnormal byproduct of a biological function or a foreign body. The pieces of solid matter are not taken out.

Body Part Character 4	Approach Character 5	Device Character 6	Qualifier Character 7
5 Fallopian Tube, Right NC♀ Oviduct Salpinx Uterine tube **6 Fallopian Tube, Left** NC♀ *See 5 Fallopian Tube, Right* **7 Fallopian Tubes, Bilateral** NC♀ **9 Uterus** NC♀ Fundus uteri Myometrium Perimetrium Uterine cornu	**Ø Open** **3 Percutaneous** **4 Percutaneous Endoscopic** **7 Via Natural or Artificial Opening** **8 Via Natural or Artificial Opening Endoscopic** **X External**	**Z No Device**	**Z No Qualifier**

Non-OR ØUF[5,6,7,9]XZZ
NC ØUF[5,6,7,9]XZZ
♀ All body part, approach, device, and qualifier values

Ø Medical and Surgical
U Female Reproductive System
H Insertion Definition: Putting in a nonbiological appliance that monitors, assists, performs, or prevents a physiological function but does not physically take the place of a body part

Explanation: None

Body Part Character 4	Approach Character 5	Device Character 6	Qualifier Character 7
3 Ovary ♀	**Ø Open** **3 Percutaneous** **4 Percutaneous Endoscopic**	**1 Radioactive Element** **3 Infusion Device** **Y Other Device**	**Z No Qualifier**
3 Ovary ♀	**7 Via Natural or Artificial Opening** **8 Via Natural or Artificial Opening Endoscopic**	**1 Radioactive Element** **Y Other Device**	**Z No Qualifier**
8 Fallopian Tube ♀ **D Uterus and Cervix** ♀ **H Vagina and Cul-de-sac** ♀	**Ø Open** **3 Percutaneous** **4 Percutaneous Endoscopic** **7 Via Natural or Artificial Opening** **8 Via Natural or Artificial Opening Endoscopic**	**3 Infusion Device** **Y Other Device**	**Z No Qualifier**
9 Uterus ♀ Fundus uteri Myometrium Perimetrium Uterine cornu	**Ø Open** **7 Via Natural or Artificial Opening** **8 Via Natural or Artificial Opening Endoscopic**	**1 Radioactive Element** **H Contraceptive Device**	**Z No Qualifier**
C Cervix ♀	**Ø Open** **3 Percutaneous** **4 Percutaneous Endoscopic**	**1 Radioactive Element**	**Z No Qualifier**
C Cervix ♀	**7 Via Natural or Artificial Opening** **8 Via Natural or Artificial Opening Endoscopic**	**1 Radioactive Element** **H Contraceptive Device**	**Z No Qualifier**
F Cul-de-sac ♀	**7 Via Natural or Artificial Opening** **8 Via Natural or Artificial Opening Endoscopic**	**G Intraluminal Device, Pessary**	**Z No Qualifier**
G Vagina ♀	**Ø Open** **3 Percutaneous** **4 Percutaneous Endoscopic** **X External**	**1 Radioactive Element**	**Z No Qualifier**
G Vagina ♀	**7 Via Natural or Artificial Opening** **8 Via Natural or Artificial Opening Endoscopic**	**1 Radioactive Element** **G Intraluminal Device, Pessary**	**Z No Qualifier**

Non-OR ØUH3[Ø,4][3,Y]Z
Non-OR ØUH33[1,3,Y]Z
Non-OR ØUH3[7,8][1,Y]Z
Non-OR ØUH[8,D][Ø,3,4,7,8][3,Y]Z
Non-OR ØUHH[3,4]YZ
Non-OR ØUHH[7,8][3,Y]Z
Non-OR ØUH9[Ø,7,8][1,H]Z
Non-OR ØUHC[7,8]HZ
Non-OR ØUHF[7,8]HZ
Non-OR ØUHG[7,8]HZ
♀ All body part, approach, device, and qualifier values

Ø Medical and Surgical
U Female Reproductive System
J Inspection Definition: Visually and/or manually exploring a body part

Explanation: Visual exploration may be performed with or without optical instrumentation. Manual exploration may be performed directly or through intervening body layers.

Body Part Character 4	Approach Character 5	Device Character 6	Qualifier Character 7
3 Ovary ♀	Ø Open 3 Percutaneous 4 Percutaneous Endoscopic 8 Via Natural or Artificial Opening Endoscopic X External	Z No Device	Z No Qualifier
8 Fallopian Tube ♀ D Uterus and Cervix ♀ H Vagina and Cul-de-sac ♀	Ø Open 3 Percutaneous 4 Percutaneous Endoscopic 7 Via Natural or Artificial Opening 8 Via Natural or Artificial Opening Endoscopic X External	Z No Device	Z No Qualifier
M Vulva ♀ Labia majora Labia minora	Ø Open X External	Z No Device	Z No Qualifier

Non-OR ØUJ3[3,8,X]ZZ
Non-OR ØUJ[8,D,H][3,7,8,X]ZZ
Non-OR ØUJMXZZ
♀ All body part, approach, device, and qualifier values

Ø Medical and Surgical
U Female Reproductive System
L Occlusion Definition: Completely closing an orifice or the lumen of a tubular body part

Explanation: The orifice can be a natural orifice or an artificially created orifice

Body Part Character 4	Approach Character 5	Device Character 6	Qualifier Character 7
5 Fallopian Tube, Right ♀ Oviduct Salpinx Uterine tube 6 Fallopian Tube, Left ♀ *See 5 Fallopian Tube, Right* 7 Fallopian Tubes, Bilateral NC ♀	Ø Open 3 Percutaneous 4 Percutaneous Endoscopic	C Extraluminal Device D Intraluminal Device Z No Device	Z No Qualifier
5 Fallopian Tube, Right ♀ Oviduct Salpinx Uterine tube 6 Fallopian Tube, Left ♀ *See 5 Fallopian Tube, Right* 7 Fallopian Tubes, Bilateral NC ♀	7 Via Natural or Artificial Opening 8 Via Natural or Artificial Opening Endoscopic	D Intraluminal Device Z No Device	Z No Qualifier
F Cul-de-sac ♀ G Vagina ♀	7 Via Natural or Artificial Opening 8 Via Natural or Artificial Opening Endoscopic	D Intraluminal Device Z No Device	Z No Qualifier

NC ØUL7[Ø,3,4][C,D,Z]Z with principal or secondary diagnosis of Z30.2
NC ØUL7[7,8][D,Z]Z with principal or secondary diagnosis of Z30.2
♀ All body part, approach, device, and qualifier values

Female Reproductive System

Ø Medical and Surgical
U Female Reproductive System
M Reattachment Definition: Putting back in or on all or a portion of a separated body part to its normal location or other suitable location

Explanation: Vascular circulation and nervous pathways may or may not be reestablished

Body Part Character 4	Approach Character 5	Device Character 6	Qualifier Character 7
Ø Ovary, Right ♀ **1 Ovary, Left** ♀ **2 Ovaries, Bilateral** ♀ **4 Uterine Supporting Structure** ♀ Broad ligament Infundibulopelvic ligament Ovarian ligament Round ligament of uterus **5 Fallopian Tube, Right** ♀ Oviduct Salpinx Uterine tube **6 Fallopian Tube, Left** ♀ *See 5 Fallopian Tube, Right* **7 Fallopian Tubes, Bilateral** ♀ **9 Uterus** ♀ Fundus uteri Myometrium Perimetrium Uterine cornu **C Cervix** ♀ **F Cul-de-sac** ♀ **G Vagina** ♀	**Ø Open** **4 Percutaneous Endoscopic**	**Z No Device**	**Z No Qualifier**
J Clitoris ♀ **M Vulva** ♀ Labia majora Labia minora	**X External**	**Z No Device**	**Z No Qualifier**
K Hymen ♀	**Ø Open** **4 Percutaneous Endoscopic** **X External**	**Z No Device**	**Z No Qualifier**

♀ All body part, approach, device, and qualifier values

ØUM–ØUM

Ø Medical and Surgical
U Female Reproductive System
N Release Definition: Freeing a body part from an abnormal physical constraint by cutting or by the use of force
Explanation: Some of the restraining tissue may be taken out but none of the body part is taken out

Body Part Character 4	Approach Character 5	Device Character 6	Qualifier Character 7
Ø Ovary, Right ♀ **1 Ovary, Left** ♀ **2 Ovaries, Bilateral** ♀ **4 Uterine Supporting Structure** ♀ Broad ligament Infundibulopelvic ligament Ovarian ligament Round ligament of uterus	**Ø Open** **3 Percutaneous** **4 Percutaneous Endoscopic** **8 Via Natural or Artificial Opening Endoscopic**	**Z No Device**	**Z No Qualifier**
5 Fallopian Tube, Right ♀ Oviduct Salpinx Uterine tube **6 Fallopian Tube, Left** ♀ *See 5 Fallopian Tube, Right* **7 Fallopian Tubes, Bilateral** ♀ **9 Uterus** ♀ Fundus uteri Myometrium Perimetrium Uterine cornu **C Cervix** ♀ **F Cul-de-sac** ♀	**Ø Open** **3 Percutaneous** **4 Percutaneous Endoscopic** **7 Via Natural or Artificial Opening** **8 Via Natural or Artificial Opening Endoscopic**	**Z No Device**	**Z No Qualifier**
G Vagina ♀ **K Hymen** ♀	**Ø Open** **3 Percutaneous** **4 Percutaneous Endoscopic** **7 Via Natural or Artificial Opening** **8 Via Natural or Artificial Opening Endoscopic** **X External**	**Z No Device**	**Z No Qualifier**
J Clitoris ♀ **L Vestibular Gland** ♀ Bartholin's (greater vestibular) gland Greater vestibular (Bartholin's) gland Paraurethral (Skene's) gland Skene's (paraurethral) gland **M Vulva** ♀ Labia majora Labia minora	**Ø Open** **X External**	**Z No Device**	**Z No Qualifier**

♀ All body part, approach, device, and qualifier values

Ø Medical and Surgical
U Female Reproductive System
P Removal Definition: Taking out or off a device from a body part

Explanation: If a device is taken out and a similar device put in without cutting or puncturing the skin or mucous membrane, the procedure is coded to the root operation CHANGE. Otherwise, the procedure for taking out the device is coded to the root operation REMOVAL.

Body Part Character 4	Approach Character 5	Device Character 6	Qualifier Character 7
3 Ovary ♀	Ø Open 3 Percutaneous 4 Percutaneous Endoscopic	Ø Drainage Device 3 Infusion Device Y Other Device	Z No Qualifier
3 Ovary ♀	7 Via Natural or Artificial Opening 8 Via Natural or Artificial Opening Endoscopic	Y Other Device	Z No Qualifier
3 Ovary ♀	X External	Ø Drainage Device 3 Infusion Device	Z No Qualifier
8 Fallopian Tube ♀	Ø Open 3 Percutaneous 4 Percutaneous Endoscopic 7 Via Natural or Artificial Opening 8 Via Natural or Artificial Opening Endoscopic	Ø Drainage Device 3 Infusion Device 7 Autologous Tissue Substitute C Extraluminal Device D Intraluminal Device J Synthetic Substitute K Nonautologous Tissue Substitute Y Other Device	Z No Qualifier
8 Fallopian Tube ♀	X External	Ø Drainage Device 3 Infusion Device D Intraluminal Device	Z No Qualifier
D Uterus and Cervix ♀	Ø Open 3 Percutaneous 4 Percutaneous Endoscopic 7 Via Natural or Artificial Opening 8 Via Natural or Artificial Opening Endoscopic	Ø Drainage Device 1 Radioactive Element 3 Infusion Device 7 Autologous Tissue Substitute C Extraluminal Device D Intraluminal Device H Contraceptive Device J Synthetic Substitute K Nonautologous Tissue Substitute Y Other Device	Z No Qualifier
D Uterus and Cervix ♀	X External	Ø Drainage Device 3 Infusion Device D Intraluminal Device H Contraceptive Device	Z No Qualifier
H Vagina and Cul-de-sac ♀	Ø Open 3 Percutaneous 4 Percutaneous Endoscopic 7 Via Natural or Artificial Opening 8 Via Natural or Artificial Opening Endoscopic	Ø Drainage Device 1 Radioactive Element 3 Infusion Device 7 Autologous Tissue Substitute D Intraluminal Device J Synthetic Substitute K Nonautologous Tissue Substitute Y Other Device	Z No Qualifier
H Vagina and Cul-de-sac ♀	X External	Ø Drainage Device 1 Radioactive Element 3 Infusion Device D Intraluminal Device	Z No Qualifier
M Vulva ♀ Labia majora Labia minora	Ø Open	Ø Drainage Device 7 Autologous Tissue Substitute J Synthetic Substitute K Nonautologous Tissue Substitute	Z No Qualifier
M Vulva ♀ Labia majora Labia minora	X External	Ø Drainage Device	Z No Qualifier

Non-OR ØUP3[3,4]YZ
Non-OR ØUP3[7,8]YZ
Non-OR ØUP3X[Ø,3]Z
Non-OR ØUP8[3,4]YZ
Non-OR ØUP8[7,8][Ø,3,D,Y]Z
Non-OR ØUP8X[Ø,3,D]Z
Non-OR ØUPD[3,4][C,Y]Z
Non-OR ØUPD[7,8][Ø,3,C,D,H,Y]Z
Non-OR ØUPDX[Ø,3,D,H]Z
Non-OR ØUPH[3,4]YZ
Non-OR ØUPH[7,8][Ø,3,D,Y]Z
Non-OR ØUPHX[Ø,1,3,D]Z
Non-OR ØUPMXØZ
♀ All body part, approach, device, and qualifier values

Ø Medical and Surgical
U Female Reproductive System
Q Repair Definition: Restoring, to the extent possible, a body part to its normal anatomic structure and function

Explanation: Used only when the method to accomplish the repair is not one of the other root operations

Body Part Character 4	Approach Character 5	Device Character 6	Qualifier Character 7
Ø Ovary, Right ♀ **1 Ovary, Left** ♀ **2 Ovaries, Bilateral** ♀ **4 Uterine Supporting Structure** ♀ Broad ligament Infundibulopelvic ligament Ovarian ligament Round ligament of uterus	**Ø Open** **3 Percutaneous** **4 Percutaneous Endoscopic** **8 Via Natural or Artificial Opening Endoscopic**	**Z No Device**	**Z No Qualifier**
5 Fallopian Tube, Right ♀ Oviduct Salpinx Uterine tube **6 Fallopian Tube, Left** ♀ *See* 5 *Fallopian Tube, Right* **7 Fallopian Tubes, Bilateral** ♀ **9 Uterus** ♀ Fundus uteri Myometrium Perimetrium Uterine cornu **C Cervix** ♀ **F Cul-de-sac** ♀	**Ø Open** **3 Percutaneous** **4 Percutaneous Endoscopic** **7 Via Natural or Artificial Opening** **8 Via Natural or Artificial Opening Endoscopic**	**Z No Device**	**Z No Qualifier**
G Vagina ♀ **K Hymen** ♀	**Ø Open** **3 Percutaneous** **4 Percutaneous Endoscopic** **7 Via Natural or Artificial Opening** **8 Via Natural or Artificial Opening Endoscopic** **X External**	**Z No Device**	**Z No Qualifier**
J Clitoris ♀ **L Vestibular Gland** ♀ Bartholin's (greater vestibular) gland Greater vestibular (Bartholin's) gland Paraurethral (Skene's) gland Skene's (paraurethral) gland **M Vulva** ♀ Labia majora Labia minora	**Ø Open** **X External**	**Z No Device**	**Z No Qualifier**

Non-OR ØUQG[7,X]ZZ
Non-OR ØUQKXZZ
Non-OR ØUQMXZZ
♀ All body part, approach, device, and qualifier values

Ø Medical and Surgical
U Female Reproductive System
S Reposition Definition: Moving to its normal location, or other suitable location, all or a portion of a body part

Explanation: The body part is moved to a new location from an abnormal location, or from a normal location where it is not functioning correctly. The body part may or may not be cut out or off to be moved to the new location.

Body Part Character 4	Approach Character 5	Device Character 6	Qualifier Character 7
Ø Ovary, Right ♀ **1 Ovary, Left** ♀ **2 Ovaries, Bilateral** ♀ **4 Uterine Supporting Structure** ♀ Broad ligament Infundibulopelvic ligament Ovarian ligament Round ligament of uterus **5 Fallopian Tube, Right** ♀ Oviduct Salpinx Uterine tube **6 Fallopian Tube, Left** ♀ *See* 5 *Fallopian Tube, Right* **7 Fallopian Tubes, Bilateral** ♀ **C Cervix** ♀ **F Cul-de-sac** ♀	**Ø Open** **4 Percutaneous Endoscopic** **8 Via Natural or Artificial Opening Endoscopic**	**Z No Device**	**Z No Qualifier**
9 Uterus ♀ Fundus uteri Myometrium Perimetrium Uterine cornu **G Vagina** ♀	**Ø Open** **4 Percutaneous Endoscopic** **7 Via Natural or Artificial Opening** **8 Via Natural or Artificial Opening Endoscopic** **X External**	**Z No Device**	**Z No Qualifier**

Non-OR ØUS9XZZ
♀ All body part, approach, device, and qualifier values

Ø Medical and Surgical
U Female Reproductive System
T Resection Definition: Cutting out or off, without replacement, all of a body part
Explanation: None

Body Part Character 4	Approach Character 5	Device Character 6	Qualifier Character 7
Ø Ovary, Right ♀ **1 Ovary, Left** ♀ **2 Ovaries, Bilateral** ⊞♀ **5 Fallopian Tube, Right** ♀ Oviduct Salpinx Uterine tube **6 Fallopian Tube, Left** ♀ *See 5 Fallopian Tube, Right* **7 Fallopian Tubes, Bilateral** ⊞♀	**Ø Open** **4 Percutaneous Endoscopic** **7 Via Natural or Artificial Opening** **8 Via Natural or Artificial Opening Endoscopic** **F Via Natural or Artificial Opening With Percutaneous Endoscopic Assistance**	**Z No Device**	**Z No Qualifier**
4 Uterine Supporting Structure ⊞♀ Broad ligament Infundibulopelvic ligament Ovarian ligament Round ligament of uterus **C Cervix** ⊞♀ **F Cul-de-sac** ♀ **G Vagina** ⊞♀	**Ø Open** **4 Percutaneous Endoscopic** **7 Via Natural or Artificial Opening** **8 Via Natural or Artificial Opening Endoscopic**	**Z No Device**	**Z No Qualifier**
9 Uterus ⊞♀ Fundus uteri Myometrium Perimetrium Uterine cornu	**Ø Open** **4 Percutaneous Endoscopic** **7 Via Natural or Artificial Opening** **8 Via Natural or Artificial Opening Endoscopic** **F Via Natural or Artificial Opening With Percutaneous Endoscopic Assistance**	**Z No Device**	**L Supracervical** **Z No Qualifier**
J Clitoris ♀ **L Vestibular Gland** ♀ Bartholin's (greater vestibular) gland Greater vestibular (Bartholin's) gland Paraurethral (Skene's) gland Skene's (paraurethral) gland **M Vulva** ⊞♀ Labia majora Labia minora	**Ø Open** **X External**	**Z No Device**	**Z No Qualifier**
K Hymen ♀	**Ø Open** **4 Percutaneous Endoscopic** **7 Via Natural or Artificial Opening** **8 Via Natural or Artificial Opening Endoscopic** **X External**	**Z No Device**	**Z No Device**

♀ All body part, approach, device, and qualifier values

See Appendix L for Procedure Combinations
⊞ ØUT[2,7]ØZZ
⊞ ØUT[4,C][Ø,4,7,8]ZZ
⊞ ØUTGØZZ
⊞ ØUT9[Ø,4,7,8,F]ZZ
⊞ ØUTM[Ø,X]ZZ

Ø Medical and Surgical
U Female Reproductive System
U Supplement Definition: Putting in or on biological or synthetic material that physically reinforces and/or augments the function of a portion of a body part

Explanation: The biological material is non-living, or is living and from the same individual. The body part may have been previously replaced, and the SUPPLEMENT procedure is performed to physically reinforce and/or augment the function of the replaced body part.

Body Part Character 4	Approach Character 5	Device Character 6	Qualifier Character 7
4 Uterine Supporting Structure ♀ Broad ligament Infundibulopelvic ligament Ovarian ligament Round ligament of uterus	**Ø Open** **4 Percutaneous Endoscopic**	**7 Autologous Tissue Substitute** **J Synthetic Substitute** **K Nonautologous Tissue Substitute**	**Z No Qualifier**
5 Fallopian Tube, Right ♀ Oviduct Salpinx Uterine tube **6 Fallopian Tube, Left** ♀ *See 5 Fallopian Tube, Right* **7 Fallopian Tubes, Bilateral** ♀ **F Cul-de-sac** ♀	**Ø Open** **4 Percutaneous Endoscopic** **7 Via Natural or Artificial Opening** **8 Via Natural or Artificial Opening Endoscopic**	**7 Autologous Tissue Substitute** **J Synthetic Substitute** **K Nonautologous Tissue Substitute**	**Z No Qualifier**
G Vagina ♀ **K Hymen** ♀	**Ø Open** **4 Percutaneous Endoscopic** **7 Via Natural or Artificial Opening** **8 Via Natural or Artificial Opening Endoscopic** **X External**	**7 Autologous Tissue Substitute** **J Synthetic Substitute** **K Nonautologous Tissue Substitute**	**Z No Qualifier**
J Clitoris ♀ **M Vulva** ♀ Labia majora Labia minora	**Ø Open** **X External**	**7 Autologous Tissue Substitute** **J Synthetic Substitute** **K Nonautologous Tissue Substitute**	**Z No Qualifier**

♀ All body part, approach, device, and qualifier values

Ø Medical and Surgical
U Female Reproductive System
V Restriction Definition: Partially closing an orifice or the lumen of a tubular body part

Explanation: The orifice can be a natural orifice or an artificially created orifice

Body Part Character 4	Approach Character 5	Device Character 6	Qualifier Character 7
C Cervix ♀	**Ø Open** **3 Percutaneous** **4 Percutaneous Endoscopic**	**C Extraluminal Device** **D Intraluminal Device** **Z No Device**	**Z No Qualifier**
C Cervix ♀	**7 Via Natural or Artificial Opening** **8 Via Natural or Artificial Opening Endoscopic**	**D Intraluminal Device** **Z No Device**	**Z No Qualifier**

♀ All body part, approach, device, and qualifier values

Ø Medical and Surgical
U Female Reproductive System
W Revision Definition: Correcting, to the extent possible, a portion of a malfunctioning device or the position of a displaced device

Explanation: Revision can include correcting a malfunctioning or displaced device by taking out or putting in components of the device such as a screw or pin

Body Part Character 4	Approach Character 5	Device Character 6	Qualifier Character 7
3 Ovary ♀	Ø Open 3 Percutaneous 4 Percutaneous Endoscopic	Ø Drainage Device 3 Infusion Device Y Other Device	Z No Qualifier
3 Ovary ♀	7 Via Natural or Artificial Opening 8 Via Natural or Artificial Opening Endoscopic	Y Other Device	Z No Qualifier
3 Ovary ♀	X External	Ø Drainage Device 3 Infusion Device	Z No Qualifier
8 Fallopian Tube ♀	Ø Open 3 Percutaneous 4 Percutaneous Endoscopic 7 Via Natural or Artificial Opening 8 Via Natural or Artificial Opening Endoscopic	Ø Drainage Device 3 Infusion Device 7 Autologous Tissue Substitute C Extraluminal Device D Intraluminal Device J Synthetic Substitute K Nonautologous Tissue Substitute Y Other Device	Z No Qualifier
8 Fallopian Tube ♀	X External	Ø Drainage Device 3 Infusion Device 7 Autologous Tissue Substitute C Extraluminal Device D Intraluminal Device J Synthetic Substitute K Nonautologous Tissue Substitute	Z No Qualifier
D Uterus and Cervix ♀	Ø Open 3 Percutaneous 4 Percutaneous Endoscopic 7 Via Natural or Artificial Opening 8 Via Natural or Artificial Opening Endoscopic	Ø Drainage Device 1 Radioactive Element 3 Infusion Device 7 Autologous Tissue Substitute C Extraluminal Device D Intraluminal Device H Contraceptive Device J Synthetic Substitute K Nonautologous Tissue Substitute Y Other Device	Z No Qualifier
D Uterus and Cervix ♀	X External	Ø Drainage Device 3 Infusion Device 7 Autologous Tissue Substitute C Extraluminal Device D Intraluminal Device H Contraceptive Device J Synthetic Substitute K Nonautologous Tissue Substitute	Z No Qualifier
H Vagina and Cul-de-sac ♀	Ø Open 3 Percutaneous 4 Percutaneous Endoscopic 7 Via Natural or Artificial Opening 8 Via Natural or Artificial Opening Endoscopic	Ø Drainage Device 1 Radioactive Element 3 Infusion Device 7 Autologous Tissue Substitute D Intraluminal Device J Synthetic Substitute K Nonautologous Tissue Substitute Y Other Device	Z No Qualifier
H Vagina and Cul-de-sac ♀	X External	Ø Drainage Device 3 Infusion Device 7 Autologous Tissue Substitute D Intraluminal Device J Synthetic Substitute K Nonautologous Tissue Substitute	Z No Qualifier
M Vulva ♀ Labia majora Labia minora	Ø Open X External	Ø Drainage Device 7 Autologous Tissue Substitute J Synthetic Substitute K Nonautologous Tissue Substitute	Z No Qualifier

Non-OR ØUW3[3,4]YZ
Non-OR ØUW3[7,8]YZ
Non-OR ØUW3X[Ø,3]Z
Non-OR ØUW8[3,4,7,8]YZ
Non-OR ØUW8X[Ø,3,7,C,D,J,K]Z
Non-OR ØUWD[3,4,7,8]YZ
Non-OR ØUWDX[Ø,3,7,C,D,H,J,K]Z
Non-OR ØUWH[3,4,7,8]YZ
Non-OR ØUWHX[Ø,3,7,D,J,K]Z
Non-OR ØUWMX[Ø,7,J,K]Z
♀ All body part, approach, device, and qualifier values

Ø Medical and Surgical
U Female Reproductive System
Y Transplantation Definition: Putting in or on all or a portion of a living body part taken from another individual or animal to physically take the place and/or function of all or a portion of a similar body part

Explanation: The native body part may or may not be taken out, and the transplanted body part may take over all or a portion of its function

Body Part Character 4	Approach Character 5	Device Character 6	Qualifier Character 7
Ø Ovary, Right ♀ **1** Ovary, Left ♀ **9** Uterus ♀	**Ø** Open	**Z** No Device	**Ø** Allogeneic **1** Syngeneic **2** Zooplastic

♀ All body part, approach, device, and qualifier values

Male Reproductive System ØV1–ØVX

Character Meanings

This Character Meaning table is provided as a guide to assist the user in the identification of character members that may be found in this section of code tables. It **SHOULD NOT** be used to build a PCS code.

Operation–Character 3	Body Part–Character 4	Approach–Character 5	Device–Character 6	Qualifier–Character 7
1 Bypass	Ø Prostate	Ø Open	Ø Drainage Device	Ø Allogeneic
2 Change	1 Seminal Vesicle, Right	3 Percutaneous	1 Radioactive Element	1 Syngeneic
5 Destruction	2 Seminal Vesicle, Left	4 Percutaneous Endoscopic	3 Infusion Device	2 Zooplastic
7 Dilation	3 Seminal Vesicles, Bilateral	7 Via Natural or Artificial Opening	7 Autologous Tissue Substitute	D Urethra
9 Drainage	4 Prostate and Seminal Vesicles	8 Via Natural or Artificial Opening Endoscopic	C Extraluminal Device	J Epididymis, Right
B Excision	5 Scrotum	X External	D Intraluminal Device	K Epididymis, Left
C Extirpation	6 Tunica Vaginalis, Right		J Synthetic Substitute	N Vas Deferens, Right
H Insertion	7 Tunica Vaginalis, Left		K Nonautologous Tissue Substitute	P Vas Deferens, Left
J Inspection	8 Scrotum and Tunica Vaginalis		Y Other Device	S Penis
L Occlusion	9 Testis, Right		Z No Device	X Diagnostic
M Reattachment	B Testis, Left			Z No Qualifier
N Release	C Testes, Bilateral			
P Removal	D Testis			
Q Repair	F Spermatic Cord, Right			
R Replacement	G Spermatic Cord, Left			
S Reposition	H Spermatic Cords, Bilateral			
T Resection	J Epididymis, Right			
U Supplement	K Epididymis, Left			
W Revision	L Epididymis, Bilateral			
X Transfer	M Epididymis and Spermatic Cord			
Y Transplantation	N Vas Deferens, Right			
	P Vas Deferens, Left			
	Q Vas Deferens, Bilateral			
	R Vas Deferens			
	S Penis			
	T Prepuce			

AHA Coding Clinic for table ØV1
2018, 3Q, 12 Al-Ghorab distal penile shunt surgery

AHA Coding Clinic for table ØV9
2018, 3Q, 12 Al-Ghorab distal penile shunt surgery

AHA Coding Clinic for table ØVB
2020, 1Q, 31 Repair of buried penis
2019, 3Q, 18 Radical prostatectomy and lymph node dissection with biopsy of neurovascular bundle
2016, 1Q, 23 Transurethral resection of ejaculatory ducts
2014, 4Q, 33 Radical prostatectomy

AHA Coding Clinic for table ØVH
2020, 4Q, 43-44 Insertion of radioactive element

AHA Coding Clinic for table ØVP
2016, 2Q, 28 Removal of multi-component inflatable penile prosthesis with placement of new malleable device

AHA Coding Clinic for table ØVQ
2018, 3Q, 12 Al-Ghorab distal penile shunt surgery

AHA Coding Clinic for table ØVT
2020, 4Q, 99 Robotic-assisted prostatectomy with extension of incision for specimen removal
2019, 3Q, 18 Radical prostatectomy and lymph node dissection with biopsy of neurovascular bundle
2014, 4Q, 33 Radical prostatectomy

AHA Coding Clinic for table ØVU
2020, 1Q, 31 Repair of buried penis
2016, 2Q, 28 Removal of multi-component inflatable penile prosthesis with placement of new malleable device
2015, 3Q, 25 Placement of inflatable penile prosthesis

AHA Coding Clinic for table ØVX
2018, 4Q, 40 Transfer of prepuce

AHA Coding Clinic for table ØVY
2020, 4Q, 58 Male reproductive organ transplant

Male Reproductive System

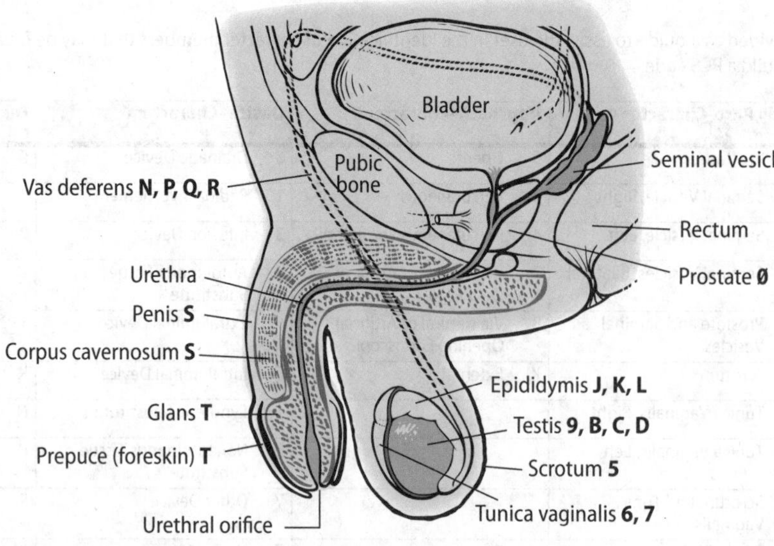

Penis

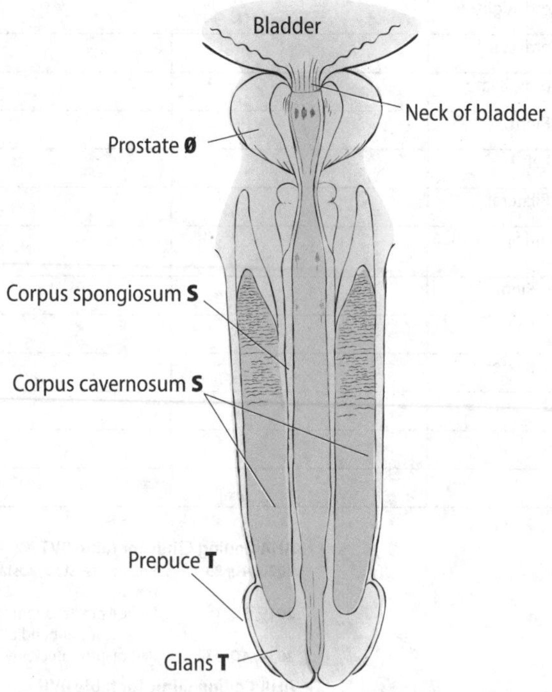

Ø Medical and Surgical
V Male Reproductive System
1 Bypass Definition: Altering the route of passage of the contents of a tubular body part

Explanation: Rerouting contents of a body part to a downstream area of the normal route, to a similar route and body part, or to an abnormal route and dissimilar body part. Includes one or more anastomoses, with or without the use of a device.

Body Part Character 4	Approach Character 5	Device Character 6	Qualifier Character 7
N Vas Deferens, Right ♂ Ductus deferens Ejaculatory duct **P** Vas Deferens, Left ♂ *See N Vas Deferens, Right* **Q** Vas Deferens, Bilateral ♂ *See N Vas Deferens, Right*	**Ø** Open **4** Percutaneous Endoscopic	**7** Autologous Tissue Substitute **J** Synthetic Substitute **K** Nonautologous Tissue Substitute **Z** No Device	**J** Epididymis, Right **K** Epididymis, Left **N** Vas Deferens, Right **P** Vas Deferens, Left

♂ All body part, approach, device, and qualifier values

Ø Medical and Surgical
V Male Reproductive System
2 Change Definition: Taking out or off a device from a body part and putting back an identical or similar device in or on the same body part without cutting or puncturing the skin or a mucous membrane

Explanation: All CHANGE procedures are coded using the approach EXTERNAL

Body Part Character 4	Approach Character 5	Device Character 6	Qualifier Character 7
4 Prostate and Seminal Vesicles ♂ **8** Scrotum and Tunica Vaginalis ♂ **D** Testis ♂ **M** Epididymis and Spermatic Cord ♂ **R** Vas Deferens ♂ Ductus deferens Ejaculatory duct **S** Penis ♂ Corpus cavernosum Corpus spongiosum	**X** External	**Ø** Drainage Device **Y** Other Device	**Z** No Qualifier

Non-OR All body part, approach, device, and qualifier values
♂ All body part, approach, device, and qualifier values

Ø Medical and Surgical
V Male Reproductive System
5 Destruction Definition: Physical eradication of all or a portion of a body part by the direct use of energy, force, or a destructive agent

Explanation: None of the body part is physically taken out

Body Part Character 4	Approach Character 5	Device Character 6	Qualifier Character 7
Ø Prostate ♂	**Ø** Open **3** Percutaneous **4** Percutaneous Endoscopic **7** Via Natural or Artificial Opening **8** Via Natural or Artificial Opening Endoscopic	**Z** No Device	**Z** No Qualifier
1 Seminal Vesicle, Right ♂ **2** Seminal Vesicle, Left ♂ **3** Seminal Vesicles, Bilateral ♂ **6** Tunica Vaginalis, Right ♂ **7** Tunica Vaginalis, Left ♂ **9** Testis, Right ♂ **B** Testis, Left ♂ **C** Testes, Bilateral ♂	**Ø** Open **3** Percutaneous **4** Percutaneous Endoscopic	**Z** No Device	**Z** No Qualifier
5 Scrotum ♂ **S** Penis ♂ Corpus cavernosum Corpus spongiosum **T** Prepuce ♂ Foreskin Glans penis	**Ø** Open **3** Percutaneous **4** Percutaneous Endoscopic **X** External	**Z** No Device	**Z** No Qualifier
F Spermatic Cord, Right ♂ **G** Spermatic Cord, Left ♂ **H** Spermatic Cords, Bilateral ♂ **J** Epididymis, Right ♂ **K** Epididymis, Left ♂ **L** Epididymis, Bilateral ♂ **N** Vas Deferens, Right NC ♂ Ductus deferens Ejaculatory duct **P** Vas Deferens, Left NC ♂ *See N Vas Deferens, Right* **Q** Vas Deferens, Bilateral NC ♂ *See N Vas Deferens, Right*	**Ø** Open **3** Percutaneous **4** Percutaneous Endoscopic **8** Via Natural or Artificial Opening Endoscopic	**Z** No Device	**Z** No Qualifier

Non-OR ØV55[Ø,3,4,X]ZZ
Non-OR ØV5[N,P,Q][Ø,3,4,8]ZZ
NC ØV5[N,P,Q][Ø,3,4]ZZ with principal or secondary diagnosis of Z3Ø.2
♂ All body part, approach, device, and qualifier values

Ø Medical and Surgical
V Male Reproductive System
7 Dilation Definition: Expanding an orifice or the lumen of a tubular body part

Explanation: The orifice can be a natural orifice or an artificially created orifice. Accomplished by stretching a tubular body part using intraluminal pressure or by cutting part of the orifice or wall of the tubular body part.

Body Part Character 4	Approach Character 5	Device Character 6	Qualifier Character 7
N Vas Deferens, Right ♂ Ductus deferens Ejaculatory duct **P Vas Deferens, Left** ♂ *See N Vas Deferens, Right* **Q Vas Deferens, Bilateral** ♂ *See N Vas Deferens, Right*	**Ø Open** **3 Percutaneous** **4 Percutaneous Endoscopic**	**D Intraluminal Device** **Z No Device**	**Z No Qualifier**

♂ All body part, approach, device, and qualifier values

Ø Medical and Surgical
V Male Reproductive System
9 Drainage Definition: Taking or letting out fluids and/or gases from a body part

Explanation: The qualifier DIAGNOSTIC is used to identify drainage procedures that are biopsies

Body Part Character 4	Approach Character 5	Device Character 6	Qualifier Character 7
Ø Prostate ♂	**Ø Open** **3 Percutaneous** **4 Percutaneous Endoscopic** **7 Via Natural or Artificial Opening** **8 Via Natural or Artificial Opening Endoscopic**	**Ø Drainage Device**	**Z No Qualifier**
Ø Prostate ♂	**Ø Open** **3 Percutaneous** **4 Percutaneous Endoscopic** **7 Via Natural or Artificial Opening** **8 Via Natural or Artificial Opening Endoscopic**	**Z No Device**	**X Diagnostic** **Z No Qualifier**
1 Seminal Vesicle, Right ♂ **2 Seminal Vesicle, Left** ♂ **3 Seminal Vesicles, Bilateral** ♂ **6 Tunica Vaginalis, Right** ♂ **7 Tunica Vaginalis, Left** ♂ **9 Testis, Right** ♂ **B Testis, Left** ♂ **C Testes, Bilateral** ♂ **F Spermatic Cord, Right** ♂ **G Spermatic Cord, Left** ♂ **H Spermatic Cords, Bilateral** ♂ **J Epididymis, Right** ♂ **K Epididymis, Left** ♂ **L Epididymis, Bilateral** ♂ **N Vas Deferens, Right** ♂ Ductus deferens Ejaculatory duct **P Vas Deferens, Left** ♂ *See N Vas Deferens, Right* **Q Vas Deferens, Bilateral** ♂ *See N Vas Deferens, Right*	**Ø Open** **3 Percutaneous** **4 Percutaneous Endoscopic**	**Ø Drainage Device**	**Z No Qualifier**

Non-OR ØV9Ø[3,4]ØZ
Non-OR ØV9Ø[3,4]Z[X,Z]
Non-OR ØV9Ø[7,8]ZX
Non-OR ØV9[1,2,3,9,B,C][3,4]ØZ
Non-OR ØV9[6,7,F,G,H,N,P,Q][Ø,3,4]ØZ
Non-OR ØV9[J,K,L]3ØZ
♂ All body part, approach, device, and qualifier values

ØV9 Continued on next page

Ø **Medical and Surgical**
V **Male Reproductive System**
9 **Drainage** Definition: Taking or letting out fluids and/or gases from a body part
Explanation: The qualifier DIAGNOSTIC is used to identify drainage procedures that are biopsies

ØV9 Continued

Body Part Character 4	Approach Character 5	Device Character 6	Qualifier Character 7
1 Seminal Vesicle, Right ♂ 2 Seminal Vesicle, Left ♂ 3 Seminal Vesicles, Bilateral ♂ 6 Tunica Vaginalis, Right ♂ 7 Tunica Vaginalis, Left ♂ 9 Testis, Right ♂ B Testis, Left ♂ C Testes, Bilateral ♂ F Spermatic Cord, Right ♂ G Spermatic Cord, Left ♂ H Spermatic Cords, Bilateral ♂ J Epididymis, Right ♂ K Epididymis, Left ♂ L Epididymis, Bilateral ♂ N Vas Deferens, Right ♂ Ductus deferens Ejaculatory duct P Vas Deferens, Left ♂ *See N Vas Deferens, Right* Q Vas Deferens, Bilateral ♂ *See N Vas Deferens, Right*	Ø Open 3 Percutaneous 4 Percutaneous Endoscopic	Z No Device	X Diagnostic Z No Qualifier
5 Scrotum ♂ S Penis ♂ Corpus cavernosum Corpus spongiosum T Prepuce ♂ Foreskin Glans penis	Ø Open 3 Percutaneous 4 Percutaneous Endoscopic X External	Ø Drainage Device	Z No Qualifier
5 Scrotum ♂ S Penis ♂ Corpus cavernosum Corpus spongiosum T Prepuce ♂ Foreskin Glans penis	Ø Open 3 Percutaneous 4 Percutaneous Endoscopic X External	Z No Device	X Diagnostic Z No Qualifier

Non-OR ØV9[1,2,3,9,B,C][3,4]Z[X,Z]
Non-OR ØV9[6,7,F,G,H,J,K,L,N,P,Q][Ø,3,4]ZX
Non-OR ØV9[6,7,F,G,H,N,P,Q][Ø,3,4]ZZ
Non-OR ØV9[J,K,L]3ZZ
Non-OR ØV95[Ø,3,4,X]ØZ
Non-OR ØV9[S,T]3ØZ
Non-OR ØV95ØZX
Non-OR ØV95[3,4,X]Z[X,Z]
Non-OR ØV9[S,T]3ZZ
♂ All body part, approach, device, and qualifier values

Ø Medical and Surgical
V Male Reproductive System
B Excision Definition: Cutting out or off, without replacement, a portion of a body part

Explanation: The qualifier DIAGNOSTIC is used to identify excision procedures that are biopsies

Body Part Character 4	Approach Character 5	Device Character 6	Qualifier Character 7
Ø Prostate ♂	**Ø Open** **3 Percutaneous** **4 Percutaneous Endoscopic** **7 Via Natural or Artificial Opening** **8 Via Natural or Artificial Opening Endoscopic**	**Z No Device**	**X Diagnostic** **Z No Qualifier**
1 Seminal Vesicle, Right ♂ **2 Seminal Vesicle, Left** ♂ **3 Seminal Vesicles, Bilateral** ♂ **6 Tunica Vaginalis, Right** ♂ **7 Tunica Vaginalis, Left** ♂ **9 Testis, Right** ♂ **B Testis, Left** ♂ **C Testes, Bilateral** ♂	**Ø Open** **3 Percutaneous** **4 Percutaneous Endoscopic**	**Z No Device**	**X Diagnostic** **Z No Qualifier**
5 Scrotum ♂ **S Penis** ♂ Corpus cavernosum Corpus spongiosum **T Prepuce** ♂ Foreskin Glans penis	**Ø Open** **3 Percutaneous** **4 Percutaneous Endoscopic** **X External**	**Z No Device**	**X Diagnostic** **Z No Qualifier**
F Spermatic Cord, Right ♂ **G Spermatic Cord, Left** ♂ **H Spermatic Cords, Bilateral** ♂ **J Epididymis, Right** ♂ **K Epididymis, Left** ♂ **L Epididymis, Bilateral** ♂ **N Vas Deferens, Right** NC ♂ Ductus deferens Ejaculatory duct **P Vas Deferens, Left** NC ♂ *See N Vas Deferens, Right* **Q Vas Deferens, Bilateral** NC ♂ *See N Vas Deferens, Right*	**Ø Open** **3 Percutaneous** **4 Percutaneous Endoscopic** **8 Via Natural or Artificial Opening Endoscopic**	**Z No Device**	**X Diagnostic** **Z No Qualifier**

Non-OR ØVBØ[3,4,7,8]ZX
Non-OR ØVB[1,2,3,9,B,C][3,4]ZX
Non-OR ØVB[6,7][Ø,3,4]ZX
Non-OR ØVB5ØZX
Non-OR ØVB5[3,4,X]Z[X,Z]
Non-OR ØVB[F,G,H,J,K,L][Ø,3,4,8]ZX
Non-OR ØVB[N,P,Q][Ø,3,4,8]Z[X,Z]
NC ØVB[N,P,Q][Ø,3,4]ZZ with principal or secondary diagnosis of Z3Ø.2
♂ All body part, approach, device, and qualifier values

Ø Medical and Surgical
V Male Reproductive System
C Extirpation Definition: Taking or cutting out solid matter from a body part

Explanation: The solid matter may be an abnormal byproduct of a biological function or a foreign body; it may be imbedded in a body part or in the lumen of a tubular body part. The solid matter may or may not have been previously broken into pieces.

Body Part Character 4	Approach Character 5	Device Character 6	Qualifier Character 7
Ø Prostate ♂	**Ø Open** **3 Percutaneous** **4 Percutaneous Endoscopic** **7 Via Natural or Artificial Opening** **8 Via Natural or Artificial Opening Endoscopic**	**Z No Device**	**Z No Qualifier**
1 Seminal Vesicle, Right ♂ **2 Seminal Vesicle, Left** ♂ **3 Seminal Vesicles, Bilateral** ♂ **6 Tunica Vaginalis, Right** ♂ **7 Tunica Vaginalis, Left** ♂ **9 Testis, Right** ♂ **B Testis, Left** ♂ **C Testes, Bilateral** ♂ **F Spermatic Cord, Right** ♂ **G Spermatic Cord, Left** ♂ **H Spermatic Cords, Bilateral** ♂ **J Epididymis, Right** ♂ **K Epididymis, Left** ♂ **L Epididymis, Bilateral** ♂ **N Vas Deferens, Right** ♂ Ductus deferens Ejaculatory duct **P Vas Deferens, Left** ♂ *See N Vas Deferens, Right* **Q Vas Deferens, Bilateral** ♂ *See N Vas Deferens, Right*	**Ø Open** **3 Percutaneous** **4 Percutaneous Endoscopic**	**Z No Device**	**Z No Qualifier**
5 Scrotum ♂ **S Penis** ♂ Corpus cavernosum Corpus spongiosum **T Prepuce** ♂ Foreskin Glans penis	**Ø Open** **3 Percutaneous** **4 Percutaneous Endoscopic** **X External**	**Z No Device**	**Z No Qualifier**

Non-OR ØVC[6,7,N,P,Q][Ø,3,4]ZZ
Non-OR ØVC5[3,4,X]ZZ
Non-OR ØVCSXZZ
♂ All body part, approach, device, and qualifier values

Ø Medical and Surgical
V Male Reproductive System
H Insertion Definition: Putting in a nonbiological appliance that monitors, assists, performs, or prevents a physiological function but does not physically take the place of a body part

Explanation: None

Body Part Character 4	Approach Character 5	Device Character 6	Qualifier Character 7
Ø Prostate ♂	Ø Open 3 Percutaneous 4 Percutaneous Endoscopic 7 Via Natural or Artificial Opening 8 Via Natural or Artificial Opening Endoscopic	1 Radioactive Element	Z No Qualifier
4 Prostate and Seminal Vesicles ♂ 8 Scrotum and Tunica Vaginalis ♂ M Epididymis and Spermatic Cord ♂ R Vas Deferens ♂ Ductus deferens Ejaculatory duct	Ø Open 3 Percutaneous 4 Percutaneous Endoscopic 7 Via Natural or Artificial Opening 8 Via Natural or Artificial Opening Endoscopic	3 Infusion Device Y Other Device	Z No Qualifier
D Testis ♂	Ø Open 3 Percutaneous 4 Percutaneous Endoscopic 7 Via Natural or Artificial Opening 8 Via Natural or Artificial Opening Endoscopic	1 Radioactive Element 3 Infusion Device Y Other Device	Z No Qualifier
S Penis ♂ Corpus cavernosum Corpus spongiosum	Ø Open 3 Percutaneous 4 Percutaneous Endoscopic	3 Infusion Device Y Other Device	Z No Qualifier
S Penis ♂ Corpus cavernosum Corpus spongiosum	7 Via Natural or Artificial Opening 8 Via Natural or Artificial Opening Endoscopic	Y Other Device	Z No Qualifier
S Penis ♂ Corpus cavernosum Corpus spongiosum	X External	3 Infusion Device	Z No Qualifier

Non-OR ØVH[4,8,M,R][Ø,3,4,7,8][3,Y]Z
Non-OR ØVHD[Ø,3,4,7,8][1,3,Y]Z
Non-OR ØVHS[Ø,3,4][3,Y]Z
Non-OR ØVHS[7,8]YZ
Non-OR ØVHSX3Z
♂ All body part, approach, device, and qualifier values

Ø Medical and Surgical
V Male Reproductive System
J Inspection Definition: Visually and/or manually exploring a body part

Explanation: Visual exploration may be performed with or without optical instrumentation. Manual exploration may be performed directly or through intervening body layers.

Body Part Character 4	Approach Character 5	Device Character 6	Qualifier Character 7
4 Prostate and Seminal Vesicles ♂ 8 Scrotum and Tunica Vaginalis ♂ D Testis ♂ M Epididymis and Spermatic Cord ♂ R Vas Deferens ♂ Ductus deferens Ejaculatory duct S Penis ♂ Corpus cavernosum Corpus spongiosum	Ø Open 3 Percutaneous 4 Percutaneous Endoscopic X External	Z No Device	Z No Qualifier

Non-OR ØVJ[4,D,M,R][3,X]ZZ
Non-OR ØVJ8[Ø,3,4,X]ZZ
Non-OR ØVJS[3,4,X]ZZ
♂ All body part, approach, device, and qualifier values

Ø Medical and Surgical
V Male Reproductive System
L Occlusion Definition: Completely closing an orifice or the lumen of a tubular body part

Explanation: The orifice can be a natural orifice or an artificially created orifice

Body Part Character 4	Approach Character 5	Device Character 6	Qualifier Character 7
F Spermatic Cord, Right NC ♂ **G Spermatic Cord, Left** NC ♂ **H Spermatic Cords, Bilateral** NC ♂ **N Vas Deferens, Right** NC ♂ Ductus deferens Ejaculatory duct **P Vas Deferens, Left** NC ♂ *See* N Vas Deferens, Right **Q Vas Deferens, Bilateral** NC ♂ *See* N Vas Deferens, Right	**Ø Open** **3 Percutaneous** **4 Percutaneous Endoscopic** **8 Via Natural or Artificial Opening Endoscopic**	**C Extraluminal Device** **D Intraluminal Device** **Z No Device**	**Z No Qualifier**

Non-OR ØVL[F,G,H][Ø,3,4,8][C,D,Z]Z
Non-OR ØVL[N,P,Q][Ø,3,4,8][C,Z]Z
NC ØVL[F,G,H][Ø,3,4][C,D,Z]Z with principal or secondary diagnosis of Z3Ø.2
NC ØVL[N,P,Q][Ø,3,4][C,Z]Z with principal or secondary diagnosis of Z3Ø.2
♂ All body part, approach, device, and qualifier values

Ø Medical and Surgical
V Male Reproductive System
M Reattachment Definition: Putting back in or on all or a portion of a separated body part to its normal location or other suitable location

Explanation: Vascular circulation and nervous pathways may or may not be reestablished

Body Part Character 4	Approach Character 5	Device Character 6	Qualifier Character 7
5 Scrotum ♂ **S Penis** ♂ Corpus cavernosum Corpus spongiosum	**X External**	**Z No Device**	**Z No Qualifier**
6 Tunica Vaginalis, Right ♂ **7 Tunica Vaginalis, Left** ♂ **9 Testis, Right** ♂ **B Testis, Left** ♂ **C Testes, Bilateral** ♂ **F Spermatic Cord, Right** ♂ **G Spermatic Cord, Left** ♂ **H Spermatic Cords, Bilateral** ♂	**Ø Open** **4 Percutaneous Endoscopic**	**Z No Device**	**Z No Qualifier**

♂ All body part, approach, device, and qualifier values

Ø Medical and Surgical
V Male Reproductive System
N Release Definition: Freeing a body part from an abnormal physical constraint by cutting or by the use of force
Explanation: Some of the restraining tissue may be taken out but none of the body part is taken out

Body Part Character 4	Approach Character 5	Device Character 6	Qualifier Character 7
Ø Prostate ♂	**Ø Open** **3 Percutaneous** **4 Percutaneous Endoscopic** **7 Via Natural or Artificial Opening** **8 Via Natural or Artificial Opening Endoscopic**	**Z No Device**	**Z No Qualifier**
1 Seminal Vesicle, Right ♂ **2 Seminal Vesicle, Left** ♂ **3 Seminal Vesicles, Bilateral** ♂ **6 Tunica Vaginalis, Right** ♂ **7 Tunica Vaginalis, Left** ♂ **9 Testis, Right** ♂ **B Testis, Left** ♂ **C Testes, Bilateral** ♂	**Ø Open** **3 Percutaneous** **4 Percutaneous Endoscopic**	**Z No Device**	**Z No Qualifier**
5 Scrotum ♂ **S Penis** ♂ Corpus cavernosum Corpus spongiosum **T Prepuce** ♂ Foreskin Glans penis	**Ø Open** **3 Percutaneous** **4 Percutaneous Endoscopic** **X External**	**Z No Device**	**Z No Qualifier**
F Spermatic Cord, Right ♂ **G Spermatic Cord, Left** ♂ **H Spermatic Cords, Bilateral** ♂ **J Epididymis, Right** ♂ **K Epididymis, Left** ♂ **L Epididymis, Bilateral** ♂ **N Vas Deferens, Right** ♂ Ductus deferens Ejaculatory duct **P Vas Deferens, Left** ♂ *See N Vas Deferens, Right* **Q Vas Deferens, Bilateral** ♂ *See N Vas Deferens, Right*	**Ø Open** **3 Percutaneous** **4 Percutaneous Endoscopic** **8 Via Natural or Artificial Opening Endoscopic**	**Z No Device**	**Z No Qualifier**

Non-OR ØVN[9,B,C][Ø,3,4]ZZ
Non-OR ØVNT[Ø,3,4,X]ZZ

♂ All body part, approach, device, and qualifier values

Ø Medical and Surgical
V Male Reproductive System
P Removal Definition: Taking out or off a device from a body part

Explanation: If a device is taken out and a similar device put in without cutting or puncturing the skin or mucous membrane, the procedure is coded to the root operation CHANGE. Otherwise, the procedure for taking out the device is coded to the root operation REMOVAL.

Body Part Character 4	Approach Character 5	Device Character 6	Qualifier Character 7
4 Prostate and Seminal Vesicles ♂	Ø Open 3 Percutaneous 4 Percutaneous Endoscopic 7 Via Natural or Artificial Opening 8 Via Natural or Artificial Opening Endoscopic	Ø Drainage Device 1 Radioactive Element 3 Infusion Device 7 Autologous Tissue Substitute J Synthetic Substitute K Nonautologous Tissue Substitute Y Other Device	Z No Qualifier
4 Prostate and Seminal Vesicles ♂	X External	Ø Drainage Device 1 Radioactive Element 3 Infusion Device	Z No Qualifier
8 Scrotum and Tunica Vaginalis ♂ D Testis ♂ S Penis ♂ Corpus cavernosum Corpus spongiosum	Ø Open 3 Percutaneous 4 Percutaneous Endoscopic 7 Via Natural or Artificial Opening 8 Via Natural or Artificial Opening Endoscopic	Ø Drainage Device 3 Infusion Device 7 Autologous Tissue Substitute J Synthetic Substitute K Nonautologous Tissue Substitute Y Other Device	Z No Qualifier
8 Scrotum and Tunica Vaginalis ♂ D Testis ♂ S Penis ♂ Corpus cavernosum Corpus spongiosum	X External	Ø Drainage Device 3 Infusion Device	Z No Qualifier
M Epididymis and Spermatic Cord ♂	Ø Open 3 Percutaneous 4 Percutaneous Endoscopic 7 Via Natural or Artificial Opening 8 Via Natural or Artificial Opening Endoscopic	Ø Drainage Device 3 Infusion Device 7 Autologous Tissue Substitute C Extraluminal Device J Synthetic Substitute K Nonautologous Tissue Substitute Y Other Device	Z No Qualifier
M Epididymis and Spermatic Cord ♂	X External	Ø Drainage Device 3 Infusion Device	Z No Qualifier
R Vas Deferens ♂ Ductus deferens Ejaculatory duct	Ø Open 3 Percutaneous 4 Percutaneous Endoscopic 7 Via Natural or Artificial Opening 8 Via Natural or Artificial Opening Endoscopic	Ø Drainage Device 3 Infusion Device 7 Autologous Tissue Substitute C Extraluminal Device D Intraluminal Device J Synthetic Substitute K Nonautologous Tissue Substitute Y Other Device	Z No Qualifier
R Vas Deferens ♂ Ductus deferens Ejaculatory duct	X External	Ø Drainage Device 3 Infusion Device D Intraluminal Device	Z No Qualifier

Non-OR ØVP4[3,4]YZ
Non-OR ØVP4[7,8][Ø,3,Y]Z
Non-OR ØVP4X[Ø,1,3]Z
Non-OR ØVP8[Ø,3,4,7,8][Ø,3,7,J,K,Y]Z
Non-OR ØVP[D,S][3,4]YZ
Non-OR ØVP[D,S][7,8][Ø,3,Y]Z
Non-OR ØVP[8,D,S]X[Ø,3]Z
Non-OR ØVPM[3,4]YZ
Non-OR ØVPM[7,8][Ø,3,Y]Z
Non-OR ØVPMX[Ø,3]Z
Non-OR ØVPR[Ø,3,4][Ø,3,7,C,J,K,Y]Z
Non-OR ØVPR[7,8][Ø,3,7,C,D,J,K,Y]Z
Non-OR ØVPRX[Ø,3,D]Z
♂ All body part, approach, device, and qualifier values

Ø Medical and Surgical
V Male Reproductive System
Q Repair Definition: Restoring, to the extent possible, a body part to its normal anatomic structure and function

Explanation: Used only when the method to accomplish the repair is not one of the other root operations

Body Part Character 4	Approach Character 5	Device Character 6	Qualifier Character 7
Ø Prostate ♂	Ø Open 3 Percutaneous 4 Percutaneous Endoscopic 7 Via Natural or Artificial Opening 8 Via Natural or Artificial Opening Endoscopic	Z No Device	Z No Qualifier
1 Seminal Vesicle, Right ♂ 2 Seminal Vesicle, Left ♂ 3 Seminal Vesicles, Bilateral ♂ 6 Tunica Vaginalis, Right ♂ 7 Tunica Vaginalis, Left ♂ 9 Testis, Right ♂ B Testis, Left ♂ C Testes, Bilateral ♂	Ø Open 3 Percutaneous 4 Percutaneous Endoscopic	Z No Device	Z No Qualifier
5 Scrotum ♂ S Penis ♂ Corpus cavernosum Corpus spongiosum T Prepuce ♂ Foreskin Glans penis	Ø Open 3 Percutaneous 4 Percutaneous Endoscopic X External	Z No Device	Z No Qualifier
F Spermatic Cord, Right ♂ G Spermatic Cord, Left ♂ H Spermatic Cords, Bilateral ♂ J Epididymis, Right ♂ K Epididymis, Left ♂ L Epididymis, Bilateral ♂ N Vas Deferens, Right ♂ Ductus deferens Ejaculatory duct P Vas Deferens, Left ♂ *See N Vas Deferens, Right* Q Vas Deferens, Bilateral ♂ *See N Vas Deferens, Right*	Ø Open 3 Percutaneous 4 Percutaneous Endoscopic 8 Via Natural or Artificial Opening Endoscopic	Z No Device	Z No Qualifier

Non-OR ØVQ[6,7][Ø,3,4]ZZ
Non-OR ØVQ5[Ø,3,4,X]ZZ

♂ All body part, approach, device, and qualifier values

Ø Medical and Surgical
V Male Reproductive System
R Replacement Definition: Putting in or on biological or synthetic material that physically takes the place and/or function of all or a portion of a body part

Explanation: The body part may have been taken out or replaced, or may be taken out, physically eradicated, or rendered nonfunctional during the REPLACEMENT procedure. A REMOVAL procedure is coded for taking out the device used in a previous replacement procedure.

Body Part Character 4	Approach Character 5	Device Character 6	Qualifier Character 7
9 Testis, Right ♂ B Testis, Left ♂ C Testes, Bilateral ♂	Ø Open	J Synthetic Substitute	Z No Qualifier

♂ All body part, approach, device, and qualifier values

Ø Medical and Surgical
V Male Reproductive System
S Reposition Definition: Moving to its normal location, or other suitable location, all or a portion of a body part

Explanation: The body part is moved to a new location from an abnormal location, or from a normal location where it is not functioning correctly. The body part may or may not be cut out or off to be moved to the new location.

Body Part Character 4	Approach Character 5	Device Character 6	Qualifier Character 7
9 Testis, Right ♂ B Testis, Left ♂ C Testes, Bilateral ♂ F Spermatic Cord, Right ♂ G Spermatic Cord, Left ♂ H Spermatic Cords, Bilateral ♂	Ø Open 3 Percutaneous 4 Percutaneous Endoscopic 8 Via Natural or Artificial Opening Endoscopic	Z No Device	Z No Qualifier

♂ All body part, approach, device, and qualifier values

Ø Medical and Surgical
V Male Reproductive System
T Resection Definition: Cutting out or off, without replacement, all of a body part
Explanation: None

Body Part Character 4	Approach Character 5	Device Character 6	Qualifier Character 7
Ø Prostate ⊞♂	Ø Open 4 Percutaneous Endoscopic 7 Via Natural or Artificial Opening 8 Via Natural or Artificial Opening Endoscopic	Z No Device	Z No Qualifier
1 Seminal Vesicle, Right ♂ 2 Seminal Vesicle, Left ♂ 3 Seminal Vesicles, Bilateral ⊞♂ 6 Tunica Vaginalis, Right ♂ 7 Tunica Vaginalis, Left ♂ 9 Testis, Right ♂ B Testis, Left ♂ C Testes, Bilateral ♂ F Spermatic Cord, Right ♂ G Spermatic Cord, Left ♂ H Spermatic Cords, Bilateral ♂ J Epididymis, Right ♂ K Epididymis, Left ♂ L Epididymis, Bilateral ♂ N Vas Deferens, Right NC♂ Ductus deferens Ejaculatory duct P Vas Deferens, Left NC♂ *See N Vas Deferens, Right* Q Vas Deferens, Bilateral NC♂ *See N Vas Deferens, Right*	Ø Open 4 Percutaneous Endoscopic	Z No Device	Z No Qualifier
5 Scrotum ♂ S Penis ♂ Corpus cavernosum Corpus spongiosum T Prepuce ♂ Foreskin Glans penis	Ø Open 4 Percutaneous Endoscopic X External	Z No Device	Z No Qualifier

Non-OR ØVT[N,P,Q][Ø,4]ZZ
Non-OR ØVT[5,T][Ø,4,X]ZZ
NC ØVT[N,P,Q][Ø,4]ZZ with principal or secondary diagnosis of Z3Ø.2
♂ All body part, approach, device, and qualifier values

See Appendix L for Procedure Combinations
⊞ ØVTØ[Ø,4,7,8]ZZ
⊞ ØVT3[Ø,4]ZZ

Male Reproductive System

Ø Medical and Surgical
V Male Reproductive System
U Supplement Definition: Putting in or on biological or synthetic material that physically reinforces and/or augments the function of a portion of a body part

Explanation: The biological material is non-living, or is living and from the same individual. The body part may have been previously replaced, and the SUPPLEMENT procedure is performed to physically reinforce and/or augment the function of the replaced body part.

Body Part Character 4	Approach Character 5	Device Character 6	Qualifier Character 7
1 Seminal Vesicle, Right ♂ **2 Seminal Vesicle, Left** ♂ **3 Seminal Vesicles, Bilateral** ♂ **6 Tunica Vaginalis, Right** ♂ **7 Tunica Vaginalis, Left** ♂ **F Spermatic Cord, Right** ♂ **G Spermatic Cord, Left** ♂ **H Spermatic Cords, Bilateral** ♂ **J Epididymis, Right** ♂ **K Epididymis, Left** ♂ **L Epididymis, Bilateral** ♂ **N Vas Deferens, Right** ♂ Ductus deferens Ejaculatory duct **P Vas Deferens, Left** ♂ ***See*** *N Vas Deferens, Right* **Q Vas Deferens, Bilateral** ♂ ***See*** *N Vas Deferens, Right*	**Ø Open** **4 Percutaneous Endoscopic** **8 Via Natural or Artificial Opening Endoscopic**	**7 Autologous Tissue Substitute** **J Synthetic Substitute** **K Nonautologous Tissue Substitute**	**Z No Qualifier**
5 Scrotum ♂ **S Penis** ♂ Corpus cavernosum Corpus spongiosum **T Prepuce** ♂ Foreskin Glans penis	**Ø Open** **4 Percutaneous Endoscopic** **X External**	**7 Autologous Tissue Substitute** **J Synthetic Substitute** **K Nonautologous Tissue Substitute**	**Z No Qualifier**
9 Testis, Right ♂ **B Testis, Left** ♂ **C Testes, Bilateral** ♂	**Ø Open**	**7 Autologous Tissue Substitute** **J Synthetic Substitute** **K Nonautologous Tissue Substitute**	**Z No Qualifier**

Non-OR ØVUSX[7,J,K]Z ♂ All body part, approach, device, and qualifier values

ØVU–ØVU

Ø Medical and Surgical
V Male Reproductive System
W Revision Definition: Correcting, to the extent possible, a portion of a malfunctioning device or the position of a displaced device

Explanation: Revision can include correcting a malfunctioning or displaced device by taking out or putting in components of the device such as a screw or pin

Body Part Character 4	Approach Character 5	Device Character 6	Qualifier Character 7
4 Prostate and Seminal Vesicles ♂ 8 Scrotum and Tunica Vaginalis ♂ D Testis ♂ S Penis ♂ Corpus cavernosum Corpus spongiosum	Ø Open 3 Percutaneous 4 Percutaneous Endoscopic 7 Via Natural or Artificial Opening 8 Via Natural or Artificial Opening Endoscopic	Ø Drainage Device 3 Infusion Device 7 Autologous Tissue Substitute J Synthetic Substitute K Nonautologous Tissue Substitute Y Other Device	Z No Qualifier
4 Prostate and Seminal Vesicles ♂ 8 Scrotum and Tunica Vaginalis ♂ D Testis ♂ S Penis ♂ Corpus cavernosum Corpus spongiosum	X External	Ø Drainage Device 3 Infusion Device 7 Autologous Tissue Substitute J Synthetic Substitute K Nonautologous Tissue Substitute	Z No Qualifier
M Epididymis and Spermatic Cord ♂	Ø Open 3 Percutaneous 4 Percutaneous Endoscopic 7 Via Natural or Artificial Opening 8 Via Natural or Artificial Opening Endoscopic	Ø Drainage Device 3 Infusion Device 7 Autologous Tissue Substitute C Extraluminal Device J Synthetic Substitute K Nonautologous Tissue Substitute Y Other Device	Z No Qualifier
M Epididymis and Spermatic Cord ♂	X External	Ø Drainage Device 3 Infusion Device 7 Autologous Tissue Substitute C Extraluminal Device J Synthetic Substitute K Nonautologous Tissue Substitute	Z No Qualifier
R Vas Deferens ♂ Ductus deferens Ejaculatory duct	Ø Open 3 Percutaneous 4 Percutaneous Endoscopic 7 Via Natural or Artificial Opening 8 Via Natural or Artificial Opening Endoscopic	Ø Drainage Device 3 Infusion Device 7 Autologous Tissue Substitute C Extraluminal Device D Intraluminal Device J Synthetic Substitute K Nonautologous Tissue Substitute Y Other Device	Z No Qualifier
R Vas Deferens ♂ Ductus deferens Ejaculatory duct	X External	Ø Drainage Device 3 Infusion Device 7 Autologous Tissue Substitute C Extraluminal Device D Intraluminal Device J Synthetic Substitute K Nonautologous Tissue Substitute	Z No Qualifier

Non-OR ØVW[4,D,S][3,4,7,8]YZ
Non-OR ØVW8[Ø,3,4,7,8][Ø,3,7,J,K,Y]Z
Non-OR ØVW[4,8,D,S]X[Ø,3,7,J,K]Z
Non-OR ØVWM[3,4,7,8]YZ
Non-OR ØVWMX[Ø,3,7,C,J,K]Z
Non-OR ØVWR[Ø,3,4,7,8][Ø,3,7,C,D,J,K,Y]Z
Non-OR ØVWRX[Ø,3,7,C,D,J,K]Z
♂ All body part, approach, device, and qualifier values

Ø Medical and Surgical
V Male Reproductive System
X Transfer Definition: Moving, without taking out, all or a portion of a body part to another location to take over the function of all or a portion of a body part

Explanation: The body part transferred remains connected to its vascular and nervous supply

Body Part Character 4	Approach Character 5	Device Character 6	Qualifier Character 7
T Prepuce Foreskin Glans penis	Ø Open X External	Z No Device	D Urethra S Penis

Ø Medical and Surgical
V Male Reproductive System
Y Transplantation Definition: Putting in or on all or a portion of a living body part taken from another individual or animal to physically take the place and/or function of all or a portion of a similar body part

Explanation: The native body part may or may not be taken out, and the transplanted body part may take over all or a portion of its function

Body Part Character 4	Approach Character 5	Device Character 6	Qualifier Character 7
5 Scrotum ♂ **S Penis** ♂ Corpus cavernosum Corpus spongiosum	**Ø Open**	**Z No Device**	**Ø Allogeneic** **1 Syngeneic** **2 Zooplastic**

♂ All body part, approach, device, and qualifier values

Anatomical Regions, General ØWØ–ØWY

Character Meanings

This Character Meaning table is provided as a guide to assist the user in the identification of character members that may be found in this section of code tables. It **SHOULD NOT** be used to build a PCS code.

Operation–Character 3	Body Region–Character 4	Approach–Character 5	Device–Character 6	Qualifier–Character 7
Ø Alteration	Ø Head	Ø Open	Ø Drainage Device	Ø Vagina OR Allogeneic
1 Bypass	1 Cranial Cavity	3 Percutaneous	1 Radioactive Element	1 Penis OR Syngeneic
2 Change	2 Face	4 Percutaneous Endoscopic	3 Infusion Device	2 Stoma
3 Control	3 Oral Cavity and Throat	7 Via Natural or Artificial Opening	7 Autologous Tissue Substitute	4 Cutaneous
4 Creation	4 Upper Jaw	8 Via Natural or Artificial Opening Endoscopic	J Synthetic Substitute	6 Bladder
8 Division	5 Lower Jaw	X External	K Nonautologous Tissue Substitute	9 Pleural Cavity, Right
9 Drainage	6 Neck		Y Other Device	B Pleural Cavity, Left
B Excision	8 Chest Wall		Z No Device	G Peritoneal Cavity
C Extirpation	9 Pleural Cavity, Right			J Pelvic Cavity
F Fragmentation	B Pleural Cavity, Left			W Upper Vein
H Insertion	C Mediastinum			X Diagnostic
J Inspection	D Pericardial Cavity			Y Lower Vein
M Reattachment	F Abdominal Wall			Z No Qualifier
P Removal	G Peritoneal Cavity			
Q Repair	H Retroperitoneum			
U Supplement	J Pelvic Cavity			
W Revision	K Upper Back			
Y Transplantation	L Lower Back			
	M Perineum, Male			
	N Perineum, Female			
	P Gastrointestinal Tract			
	Q Respiratory Tract			
	R Genitourinary Tract			

AHA Coding Clinic for table ØWØ
2015, 1Q, 31 Bilateral browpexy

AHA Coding Clinic for table ØW1
2020, 4Q, 55 Insertion of subcutaneous pump system for ascites drainage
2018, 4Q, 41-42 Anatomical regions bypass qualifiers
2015, 2Q, 36 Insertion of infusion device into peritoneal cavity
2013, 4Q, 126-127 Creation of percutaneous cutaneoperitoneal fistula

AHA Coding Clinic for table ØW3
2019, 3Q, 4 Evacuation of subdural hematoma and control of bleeding artery
2018, 4Q, 38 Control of epistaxis
2018, 1Q, 19 Argon plasma coagulation of duodenal arteriovenous malformation
2018, 1Q, 19 Control of epistaxis via silver nitrate cauterization
2017, 4Q, 57-58 Added approach values - Transorifice esophageal vein banding
2017, 4Q, 105 Control of gastrointestinal bleeding
2017, 4Q, 106 Control of bleeding of external naris using suture
2017, 4Q, 106 Nasal packing for epistaxis
2016, 4Q, 99-100 Root operation Control
2014, 4Q, 44 Bakri balloon for control of postpartum hemorrhage
2013, 3Q, 23 Control of intraoperative bleeding

AHA Coding Clinic for table ØW4
2019, 4Q, 30 Transfer large intestine to vagina
2016, 4Q, 101 Root operation Creation

AHA Coding Clinic for table ØW9
2020, 4Q, 56 Transvaginal drainage of pelvis
2017, 3Q, 12 Therapeutic and diagnostic paracentesis
2017, 2Q, 16 Incision and drainage of floor of mouth

AHA Coding Clinic for table ØWB
2019, 1Q, 27 Excision of pelvic sidewall mass
2017, 2Q, 16 Excision of floor of mouth
2016, 1Q, 21 Excision of urachal mass
2013, 4Q, 119 Excision of inclusion cyst of perineum

AHA Coding Clinic for table ØWC
2019, 4Q, 35 Extirpation of jaw
2017, 2Q, 16 Excision of floor of mouth

AHA Coding Clinic for table ØWH
2021, 2Q, 14 Peritoneal dialysis catheter placement
2019, 4Q, 43 Unidirectional source brachytherapy
2018, 1Q, 25 Intrauterine brachytherapy & placement of tandems & ovoids
2017, 4Q, 104 Intrauterine brachytherapy & placement of tandems & ovoids
2016, 2Q, 14 Insertion of peritoneal totally implantable venous access device
2015, 2Q, 36 Insertion of infusion device into peritoneal cavity

AHA Coding Clinic for table ØWJ
2021, 2Q, 19 Electromagnetic stealth guided ventriculoperitoneal shunt insertion with endoscopy
2019, 1Q, 3-8 Whipple procedure
2019, 1Q, 25 Laparoscopic appendectomy converted to open procedure
2018, 3Q, 29 Decommissioning of left ventricular assist device with exploration of mediastinum
2016, 4Q, 58 Longitudinal vaginal septum
2013, 2Q, 36 Insertion of ventriculoperitoneal shunt with laparoscopic assistance

AHA Coding Clinic for table ØWP
2021, 2Q, 14 Removal of peritoneal dialysis catheter

AHA Coding Clinic for table ØWQ
2017, 4Q, 106 Control of bleeding of external naris using suture
2017, 3Q, 8 Removal of silo and closure of gastroschisis
2016, 3Q, 3-7 Stoma creation & takedown procedures
2014, 4Q, 38 Abdominoplasty and abdominal wall plication for hernia repair
2014, 3Q, 28 Ileostomy takedown and parastomal hernia repair

AHA Coding Clinic for table ØWU
2017, 3Q, 8 First stage of gastroschisis repair with silo placement
2016, 3Q, 40 Omentoplasty
2015, 2Q, 29 Placement of Ioban™ antimicrobial drape over surgical wound
2014, 4Q, 39 Abdominal component release with placement of mesh for hernia repair
2012, 4Q, 101 Rib resection with reconstruction of anterior chest wall

AHA Coding Clinic for table ØWW
2015, 2Q, 9 Revision of ventriculoperitoneal (VP) shunt

AHA Coding Clinic for table ØWY
2016, 4Q, 112-113 Transplantation

Ø Medical and Surgical
W Anatomical Regions, General
Ø Alteration Definition: Modifying the anatomic structure of a body part without affecting the function of the body part

Explanation: Principal purpose is to improve appearance

Body Part Character 4	Approach Character 5	Device Character 6	Qualifier Character 7
Ø Head **2** Face **4** Upper Jaw **5** Lower Jaw **6** Neck Parapharyngeal space Retropharyngeal space **8** Chest Wall **F** Abdominal Wall **K** Upper Back **L** Lower Back **M** Perineum, Male ♂ **N** Perineum, Female ♀	**Ø** Open **3** Percutaneous **4** Percutaneous Endoscopic	**7** Autologous Tissue Substitute **J** Synthetic Substitute **K** Nonautologous Tissue Substitute **Z** No Device	**Z** No Qualifier

♂ ØWØM[Ø,3,4][7,J,K,Z]Z
♀ ØWØN[Ø,3,4][7,J,K,Z]Z

Ø Medical and Surgical
W Anatomical Regions, General
1 Bypass Definition: Altering the route of passage of the contents of a tubular body part

Explanation: Rerouting contents of a body part to a downstream area of the normal route, to a similar route and body part, or to an abnormal route and dissimilar body part. Includes one or more anastomoses, with or without the use of a device.

Body Part Character 4	Approach Character 5	Device Character 6	Qualifier Character 7
1 Cranial Cavity	**Ø** Open	**J** Synthetic Substitute	**9** Pleural Cavity, Right **B** Pleural Cavity, Left **G** Peritoneal Cavity **J** Pelvic Cavity
9 Pleural Cavity, Right **B** Pleural Cavity, Left **J** Pelvic Cavity Retropubic space	**Ø** Open **3** Percutaneous **4** Percutaneous Endoscopic	**J** Synthetic Substitute	**4** Cutaneous **9** Pleural Cavity, Right **B** Pleural Cavity, Left **G** Peritoneal Cavity **J** Pelvic Cavity **W** Upper Vein **Y** Lower Vein
G Peritoneal Cavity	**Ø** Open **3** Percutaneous **4** Percutaneous Endoscopic	**J** Synthetic Substitute	**4** Cutaneous **6** Bladder **9** Pleural Cavity, Right **B** Pleural Cavity, Left **G** Peritoneal Cavity **J** Pelvic Cavity **W** Upper Vein **Y** Lower Vein

Non-OR ØW1[9,B][Ø,3,4]J[4,G,W,Y]
Non-OR ØW1J[Ø,3,4]J[4,W,Y]
Non-OR ØW1G[Ø,3,4]J[9,B,G,J]

Ø Medical and Surgical
W Anatomical Regions, General
2 Change Definition: Taking out or off a device from a body part and putting back an identical or similar device in or on the same body part without cutting or puncturing the skin or a mucous membrane

Explanation: All CHANGE procedures are coded using the approach EXTERNAL

Body Part Character 4	Approach Character 5	Device Character 6	Qualifier Character 7
Ø Head 1 Cranial Cavity 2 Face 4 Upper Jaw 5 Lower Jaw 6 Neck Parapharyngeal space Retropharyngeal space 8 Chest Wall 9 Pleural Cavity, Right B Pleural Cavity, Left C Mediastinum Mediastinal cavity Mediastinal space D Pericardial Cavity F Abdominal Wall G Peritoneal Cavity H Retroperitoneum Retroperitoneal cavity Retroperitoneal space J Pelvic Cavity Retropubic space K Upper Back L Lower Back M Perineum, Male ♂ N Perineum, Female ♀	X External	Ø Drainage Device Y Other Device	Z No Qualifier

Non-OR All body part, approach, device, and qualifier values
♂ ØW2MX[Ø,Y]Z
♀ ØW2NX[Ø,Y]Z

Ø Medical and Surgical
W Anatomical Regions, General
3 Control Definition: Stopping, or attempting to stop, postprocedural or other acute bleeding

Explanation: None

Body Part Character 4	Approach Character 5	Device Character 6	Qualifier Character 7
Ø Head **1 Cranial Cavity** **2 Face** **4 Upper Jaw** **5 Lower Jaw** **6 Neck** Parapharyngeal space Retropharyngeal space **8 Chest Wall** **9 Pleural Cavity, Right** **B Pleural Cavity, Left** **C Mediastinum** Mediastinal cavity Mediastinal space **D Pericardial Cavity** **F Abdominal Wall** **G Peritoneal Cavity** **H Retroperitoneum** Retroperitoneal cavity Retroperitoneal space **J Pelvic Cavity** Retropubic space **K Upper Back** **L Lower Back** **M Perineum, Male** ♂ **N Perineum, Female** ♀	**Ø Open** **3 Percutaneous** **4 Percutaneous Endoscopic**	**Z No Device**	**Z No Qualifier**
3 Oral Cavity and Throat	**Ø Open** **3 Percutaneous** **4 Percutaneous Endoscopic** **7 Via Natural or Artificial Opening** **8 Via Natural or Artificial Opening Endoscopic** **X External**	**Z No Device**	**Z No Qualifier**
P Gastrointestinal Tract **Q Respiratory Tract** **R Genitourinary Tract**	**Ø Open** **3 Percutaneous** **4 Percutaneous Endoscopic** **7 Via Natural or Artificial Opening** **8 Via Natural or Artificial Opening Endoscopic**	**Z No Device**	**Z No Qualifier**

Non-OR ØW3P8ZZ

♂ ØW3M[Ø,3,4]ZZ
♀ ØW3N[Ø,3,4]ZZ

Ø Medical and Surgical
W Anatomical Regions, General
4 Creation Definition: Putting in or on biological or synthetic material to form a new body part that to the extent possible replicates the anatomic structure or function of an absent body part

Explanation: Used for gender reassignment surgery and corrective procedures in individuals with congenital anomalies

Body Part Character 4	Approach Character 5	Device Character 6	Qualifier Character 7
M Perineum, Male ♂	**Ø Open**	**7 Autologous Tissue Substitute** **J Synthetic Substitute** **K Nonautologous Tissue Substitute**	**Ø Vagina**
N Perineum, Female ♀	**Ø Open**	**7 Autologous Tissue Substitute** **J Synthetic Substitute** **K Nonautologous Tissue Substitute**	**1 Penis**

♂ ØW4MØ[7,J,K]Ø
♀ ØW4NØ[7,J,K]1

Ø Medical and Surgical
W Anatomical Regions, General
8 Division Definition: Cutting into a body part, without draining fluids and/or gases from the body part, in order to separate or transect a body part

Explanation: All or a portion of the body part is separated into two or more portions

Body Part Character 4	Approach Character 5	Device Character 6	Qualifier Character 7
N Perineum, Female ♀	**X External**	**Z No Device**	**Z No Qualifier**

Non-OR ØW8NXZZ

♀ ØW8NXZZ

Ø Medical and Surgical
W Anatomical Regions, General
9 Drainage Definition: Taking or letting out fluids and/or gases from a body part
Explanation: The qualifier DIAGNOSTIC is used to identify drainage procedures that are biopsies

Body Part Character 4	Approach Character 5	Device Character 6	Qualifier Character 7
Ø Head 1 Cranial Cavity 2 Face 3 Oral Cavity and Throat 4 Upper Jaw 5 Lower Jaw 6 Neck Parapharyngeal space Retropharyngeal space 8 Chest Wall 9 Pleural Cavity, Right B Pleural Cavity, Left C Mediastinum Mediastinal cavity Mediastinal space D Pericardial Cavity F Abdominal Wall G Peritoneal Cavity H Retroperitoneum Retroperitoneal cavity Retroperitoneal space K Upper Back L Lower Back M Perineum, Male ♂ N Perineum, Female ♀	Ø Open 3 Percutaneous 4 Percutaneous Endoscopic	Ø Drainage Device	Z No Qualifier
Ø Head 1 Cranial Cavity 2 Face 3 Oral Cavity and Throat 4 Upper Jaw 5 Lower Jaw 6 Neck Parapharyngeal space Retropharyngeal space 8 Chest Wall 9 Pleural Cavity, Right B Pleural Cavity, Left C Mediastinum Mediastinal cavity Mediastinal space D Pericardial Cavity F Abdominal Wall G Peritoneal Cavity H Retroperitoneum Retroperitoneal cavity Retroperitoneal space K Upper Back L Lower Back M Perineum, Male ♂ N Perineum, Female ♀	Ø Open 3 Percutaneous 4 Percutaneous Endoscopic	Z No Device	X Diagnostic Z No Qualifier
J Pelvic Cavity Retropubic space	Ø Open 3 Percutaneous 4 Percutaneous Endoscopic 7 Via Natural or Artificial Opening 8 Via Natural or Artificial Opening Endoscopic	Ø Drainage Device	Z No Qualifier
J Pelvic Cavity Retropubic space	Ø Open 3 Percutaneous 4 Percutaneous Endoscopic 7 Via Natural or Artificial Opening 8 Via Natural or Artificial Opening Endoscopic	Z No Device	X Diagnostic Z No Qualifier

Non-OR ØW9[Ø,8,9,B,K,L,M]ØØZ
Non-OR ØW9[Ø,1,2,3,4,5,6,8,9,B,C,D,F,G,H,K,L,M,N]3ØZ
Non-OR ØW9[Ø,1,8,F,K,L,M]4ØZ
Non-OR ØW9[Ø,2,3,4,5,6,8,9,B,K,L,M,N]ØZX
Non-OR ØW9[Ø,1,2,3,4,5,6,8,9,B,C,D,G,K,L,M,N]3ZX
Non-OR ØW9[Ø,1,2,3,4,5,6,8,C,K,L,M,N]4ZX
Non-OR ØW9[Ø,8,9,B,K,L,M]ØZZ
Non-OR ØW9[Ø,1,2,3,4,5,6,8,9,B,C,D,F,G,H,K,L,M,N]3ZZ
Non-OR ØW9[Ø,1,8,F,K,L,M]4ZZ
Non-OR ØW9J[3,7,8]ØZ
Non-OR ØW9J[3,7,8]Z[X,Z]

♂ ØW9M[Ø,3,4]ØZ
♂ ØW9M[Ø,3,4]Z[X,Z]
♀ ØW9N[Ø,3,4]ØZ
♀ ØW9N[Ø,3]Z[X,Z]
♀ ØW9N4ZZ

Ø Medical and Surgical
W Anatomical Regions, General
B Excision Definition: Cutting out or off, without replacement, a portion of a body part

Explanation: The qualifier DIAGNOSTIC is used to identify excision procedures that are biopsies

Body Part Character 4	Approach Character 5	Device Character 6	Qualifier Character 7
Ø Head 2 Face 3 Oral Cavity and Throat 4 Upper Jaw 5 Lower Jaw 8 Chest Wall K Upper Back L Lower Back M Perineum, Male ♂ N Perineum, Female ♀	Ø Open 3 Percutaneous 4 Percutaneous Endoscopic X External	Z No Device	X Diagnostic Z No Qualifier
6 Neck Parapharyngeal space Retropharyngeal space F Abdominal Wall	Ø Open 3 Percutaneous 4 Percutaneous Endoscopic	Z No Device	X Diagnostic Z No Qualifier
6 Neck Parapharyngeal space Retropharyngeal space F Abdominal Wall	X External	Z No Device	2 Stoma X Diagnostic Z No Qualifier
C Mediastinum Mediastinal cavity Mediastinal space H Retroperitoneum Retroperitoneal cavity Retroperitoneal space	Ø Open 3 Percutaneous 4 Percutaneous Endoscopic	Z No Device	X Diagnostic Z No Qualifier

Non-OR ØWB[Ø,2,4,5,8,K,L,M][Ø,3,4,X]ZX
Non-OR ØWB6[Ø,3,4]ZX
Non-OR ØWB6XZX
Non-OR ØWBH[3,4]ZX
♂ ØWBM[Ø,3,4,X]Z[X,Z]
♀ ØWBN[Ø,3,4,X]Z[X,Z]

Ø Medical and Surgical
W Anatomical Regions, General
C Extirpation Definition: Taking or cutting out solid matter from a body part

Explanation: The solid matter may be an abnormal byproduct of a biological function or a foreign body; it may be imbedded in a body part or in the lumen of a tubular body part. The solid matter may or may not have been previously broken into pieces.

Body Part Character 4	Approach Character 5	Device Character 6	Qualifier Character 7
1 Cranial Cavity 3 Oral Cavity and Throat 9 Pleural Cavity, Right B Pleural Cavity, Left C Mediastinum Mediastinal cavity Mediastinal space D Pericardial Cavity G Peritoneal Cavity H Retroperitoneum Retroperitoneal cavity Retroperitoneal space J Pelvic Cavity Retropubic space	Ø Open 3 Percutaneous 4 Percutaneous Endoscopic X External	Z No Device	Z No Qualifier
4 Upper Jaw 5 Lower Jaw	Ø Open 3 Percutaneous 4 Percutaneous Endoscopic	Z No Device	Z No Qualifier
P Gastrointestinal Tract Q Respiratory Tract R Genitourinary Tract	Ø Open 3 Percutaneous 4 Percutaneous Endoscopic 7 Via Natural or Artificial Opening 8 Via Natural or Artificial Opening Endoscopic X External	Z No Device	Z No Qualifier

Non-OR ØWC[1,3]XZZ
Non-OR ØWC[9,B][Ø,3,4,X]ZZ
Non-OR ØWC[C,D,G,H,J]XZZ
Non-OR ØWC[4,5][Ø,3,4]ZZ
Non-OR ØWC[P,R][7,8,X]ZZ
Non-OR ØWCQ[Ø,3,4,X]ZZ

Ø Medical and Surgical
W Anatomical Regions, General
F Fragmentation Definition: Breaking solid matter in a body part into pieces

Explanation: Physical force (e.g., manual, ultrasonic) applied directly or indirectly is used to break the solid matter into pieces. The solid matter may be an abnormal byproduct of a biological function or a foreign body. The pieces of solid matter are not taken out.

Body Part Character 4	Approach Character 5	Device Character 6	Qualifier Character 7
1 Cranial Cavity NC 3 Oral Cavity and Throat NC 9 Pleural Cavity, Right NC B Pleural Cavity, Left NC C Mediastinum NC Mediastinal cavity Mediastinal space D Pericardial Cavity G Peritoneal Cavity NC J Pelvic Cavity NC Retropubic space	Ø Open 3 Percutaneous 4 Percutaneous Endoscopic X External	Z No Device	Z No Qualifier
P Gastrointestinal Tract NC Q Respiratory Tract NC R Genitourinary Tract	Ø Open 3 Percutaneous 4 Percutaneous Endoscopic 7 Via Natural or Artificial Opening 8 Via Natural or Artificial Opening Endoscopic X External	Z No Device	Z No Qualifier

Non-OR ØWF[1,3,9,B,C,G]XZZ
Non-OR ØWFJ[Ø,3,4,X]ZZ
Non-OR ØWFP[Ø,3,4,7,8,X]ZZ
Non-OR ØWFQXZZ
Non-OR ØWFR[Ø,3,4,7,8,X]ZZ
NC ØWF[1,3,9,B,C,G,J]XZZ
NC ØWF[P,Q]XZZ

Ø Medical and Surgical
W Anatomical Regions, General
H Insertion Definition: Putting in a nonbiological appliance that monitors, assists, performs, or prevents a physiological function but does not physically take the place of a body part

Explanation: None

Body Part Character 4	Approach Character 5	Device Character 6	Qualifier Character 7
Ø Head 1 Cranial Cavity 2 Face 3 Oral Cavity and Throat 4 Upper Jaw 5 Lower Jaw 6 Neck Parapharyngeal space Retropharyngeal space 8 Chest Wall 9 Pleural Cavity, Right B Pleural Cavity, Left C Mediastinum Mediastinal cavity Mediastinal space D Pericardial Cavity F Abdominal Wall G Peritoneal Cavity H Retroperitoneum Retroperitoneal cavity Retroperitoneal space J Pelvic Cavity Retropubic space K Upper Back L Lower Back M Perineum, Male N Perineum, Female ♀	Ø Open 3 Percutaneous 4 Percutaneous Endoscopic	1 Radioactive Element 3 Infusion Device Y Other Device	Z No Qualifier
P Gastrointestinal Tract Q Respiratory Tract R Genitourinary Tract	Ø Open 3 Percutaneous 4 Percutaneous Endoscopic 7 Via Natural or Artificial Opening 8 Via Natural or Artificial Opening Endoscopic	1 Radioactive Element 3 Infusion Device Y Other Device	Z No Qualifier

DRG Non-OR ØWH[Ø,2,4,5,6,K,L,M][Ø,3,4][3,Y]Z
Non-OR ØWH1[Ø,3,4]3Z
Non-OR ØWH[8,9,B][Ø,3,4][3,Y]Z
Non-OR ØWHPØYZ
Non-OR ØWHP[3,4,7,8][3,Y]Z
Non-OR ØWHQ[Ø,7,8][3,Y]Z
Non-OR ØWHR[Ø,3,4,7,8][3,Y]Z
♀ ØWHN[Ø,3,4][3,Y]Z

Ø Medical and Surgical
W Anatomical Regions, General
J Inspection Definition: Visually and/or manually exploring a body part

Explanation: Visual exploration may be performed with or without optical instrumentation. Manual exploration may be performed directly or through intervening body layers.

Body Part Character 4	Approach Character 5	Device Character 6	Qualifier Character 7
Ø Head 2 Face 3 Oral Cavity and Throat 4 Upper Jaw 5 Lower Jaw 6 Neck Parapharyngeal space Retropharyngeal space 8 Chest Wall F Abdominal Wall K Upper Back L Lower Back M Perineum, Male ♂ N Perineum, Female ♀	Ø Open 3 Percutaneous 4 Percutaneous Endoscopic X External	Z No Device	Z No Qualifier
1 Cranial Cavity 9 Pleural Cavity, Right B Pleural Cavity, Left C Mediastinum Mediastinal cavity Mediastinal space D Pericardial Cavity G Peritoneal Cavity H Retroperitoneum Retroperitoneal cavity Retroperitoneal space J Pelvic Cavity Retropubic space	Ø Open 3 Percutaneous 4 Percutaneous Endoscopic	Z No Device	Z No Qualifier
P Gastrointestinal Tract Q Respiratory Tract R Genitourinary Tract	Ø Open 3 Percutaneous 4 Percutaneous Endoscopic 7 Via Natural or Artificial Opening 8 Via Natural or Artificial Opening Endoscopic	Z No Device	Z No Qualifier

DRG Non-OR ØWJ[Ø,2,4,5,K,L]ØZZ
DRG Non-OR ØWJM[Ø,4]ZZ
Non-OR ØWJ3ØZZ
Non-OR ØWJ[Ø,2,3,4,5,6,8,F,K,L,M,N][3,X]ZZ
Non-OR ØWJ[Ø,2,3,4,5,K,L]4ZZ
Non-OR ØWJDØZZ
Non-OR ØWJ[1,9,B,C,D,G,H,J]3ZZ
Non-OR ØWJ[P,Q,R][3,7,8]ZZ

♂ ØWJM[Ø,3,4,X]ZZ
♀ ØWJN[Ø,3,4,X]ZZ

Ø Medical and Surgical
W Anatomical Regions, General
M Reattachment Definition: Putting back in or on all or a portion of a separated body part to its normal location or other suitable location

Explanation: Vascular circulation and nervous pathways may or may not be reestablished

Body Part Character 4	Approach Character 5	Device Character 6	Qualifier Character 7
2 Face 4 Upper Jaw 5 Lower Jaw 6 Neck Parapharyngeal space Retropharyngeal space 8 Chest Wall F Abdominal Wall K Upper Back L Lower Back M Perineum, Male ♂ N Perineum, Female ♀	Ø Open	Z No Device	Z No Qualifier

♂ ØWMMØZZ
♀ ØWMNØZZ

Ø Medical and Surgical
W Anatomical Regions, General
P Removal Definition: Taking out or off a device from a body part

Explanation: If a device is taken out and a similar device put in without cutting or puncturing the skin or mucous membrane, the procedure is coded to the root operation CHANGE. Otherwise, the procedure for taking out the device is coded to the root operation REMOVAL.

Body Part Character 4	Approach Character 5	Device Character 6	Qualifier Character 7
Ø Head 2 Face 4 Upper Jaw 5 Lower Jaw 6 Neck Parapharyngeal space Retropharyngeal space 8 Chest Wall C Mediastinum Mediastinal cavity Mediastinal space F Abdominal Wall K Upper Back L Lower Back M Perineum, Male ♂ N Perineum, Female ♀	Ø Open 3 Percutaneous 4 Percutaneous Endoscopic X External	Ø Drainage Device 1 Radioactive Element 3 Infusion Device 7 Autologous Tissue Substitute J Synthetic Substitute K Nonautologous Tissue Substitute Y Other Device	Z No Qualifier
1 Cranial Cavity 9 Pleural Cavity, Right B Pleural Cavity, Left G Peritoneal Cavity J Pelvic Cavity Retropubic space	Ø Open 3 Percutaneous 4 Percutaneous Endoscopic	Ø Drainage Device 1 Radioactive Element 3 Infusion Device J Synthetic Substitute Y Other Device	Z No Qualifier
1 Cranial Cavity 9 Pleural Cavity, Right B Pleural Cavity, Left G Peritoneal Cavity J Pelvic Cavity Retropubic space	X External	Ø Drainage Device 1 Radioactive Element 3 Infusion Device	Z No Qualifier
D Pericardial Cavity H Retroperitoneum Retroperitoneal cavity Retroperitoneal space	Ø Open 3 Percutaneous 4 Percutaneous Endoscopic	Ø Drainage Device 1 Radioactive Element 3 Infusion Device Y Other Device	Z No Qualifier
D Pericardial Cavity H Retroperitoneum Retroperitoneal cavity Retroperitoneal space	X External	Ø Drainage Device 1 Radioactive Element 3 Infusion Device	Z No Qualifier
P Gastrointestinal Tract Q Respiratory Tract R Genitourinary Tract	Ø Open 3 Percutaneous 4 Percutaneous Endoscopic 7 Via Natural or Artificial Opening 8 Via Natural or Artificial Opening Endoscopic X External	1 Radioactive Element 3 Infusion Device Y Other Device	Z No Qualifier

Non-OR ØWP[Ø,2,4,5,6,8][Ø,3,4,X][Ø,1,3,7,J,K,Y]Z
Non-OR ØWP[C,F]X[Ø,1,3,7,J,K,Y]Z
Non-OR ØWP[K,L][Ø,3,4,X][Ø,1,3,7,J,K,Y]Z
Non-OR ØWPM[Ø,3,4][Ø,1,3,J,Y]Z
Non-OR ØWPMX[Ø,1,3,Y]Z
Non-OR ØWPNX[Ø,1,3,7,J,K,Y]Z
Non-OR ØWP1[Ø,3,4]3Z
Non-OR ØWP[9,B,J][Ø,3,4][Ø,1,3,J,Y]Z
Non-OR ØWP[1,9,B,G,J]X[Ø,1,3]Z
Non-OR ØWP[D,H]X[Ø,1,3]Z
Non-OR ØWPP[3,4,7,8,X][1,3,Y]Z
Non-OR ØWPQ73Z
Non-OR ØWPQ8[3,Y]Z
Non-OR ØWPQ[Ø,X][1,3,Y]Z
Non-OR ØWPR[Ø,3,4,7,8,X][1,3,Y]Z

♂ ØWPM[Ø,3,4,X][Ø,1,3,7,J,K,Y]Z
♀ ØWPN[Ø,3,4,X][Ø,1,3,7,J,K,Y]Z

Ø Medical and Surgical
W Anatomical Regions, General
Q Repair Definition: Restoring, to the extent possible, a body part to its normal anatomic structure and function

Explanation: Used only when the method to accomplish the repair is not one of the other root operations

Body Part Character 4	Approach Character 5	Device Character 6	Qualifier Character 7
Ø Head 2 Face 3 Oral Cavity and Throat 4 Upper Jaw 5 Lower Jaw 8 Chest Wall K Upper Back L Lower Back M Perineum, Male ♂ N Perineum, Female ♀	Ø Open 3 Percutaneous 4 Percutaneous Endoscopic X External	Z No Device	Z No Qualifier
6 Neck Parapharyngeal space Retropharyngeal space F Abdominal Wall	Ø Open 3 Percutaneous 4 Percutaneous Endoscopic	Z No Device	Z No Qualifier
6 Neck Parapharyngeal space Retropharyngeal space F Abdominal Wall ⊞	X External	Z No Device	2 Stoma Z No Qualifier
C Mediastinum Mediastinal cavity Mediastinal space	Ø Open 3 Percutaneous 4 Percutaneous Endoscopic	Z No Device	Z No Qualifier

Non-OR ØWQNXZZ
♂ ØWQM[Ø,3,4,X]ZZ
♀ ØWQN[Ø,3,4,X]ZZ

See Appendix L for Procedure Combinations
⊞ ØWQFXZ[2,Z]

Ø Medical and Surgical
W Anatomical Regions, General
U Supplement Definition: Putting in or on biological or synthetic material that physically reinforces and/or augments the function of a portion of a body part

Explanation: The biological material is non-living, or is living and from the same individual. The body part may have been previously replaced, and the SUPPLEMENT procedure is performed to physically reinforce and/or augment the function of the replaced body part.

Body Part Character 4	Approach Character 5	Device Character 6	Qualifier Character 7
Ø Head 2 Face 4 Upper Jaw 5 Lower Jaw 6 Neck Parapharyngeal space Retropharyngeal space 8 Chest Wall C Mediastinum Mediastinal cavity Mediastinal space F Abdominal Wall K Upper Back L Lower Back M Perineum, Male ♂ N Perineum, Female ♀	Ø Open 4 Percutaneous Endoscopic	7 Autologous Tissue Substitute J Synthetic Substitute K Nonautologous Tissue Substitute	Z No Qualifier

♂ ØWUM[Ø,4][7,J,K]Z
♀ ØWUN[Ø,4][7,J,K]Z

Ø Medical and Surgical
W Anatomical Regions, General
W Revision Definition: Correcting, to the extent possible, a portion of a malfunctioning device or the position of a displaced device

Explanation: Revision can include correcting a malfunctioning or displaced device by taking out or putting in components of the device such as a screw or pin

Body Part Character 4	Approach Character 5	Device Character 6	Qualifier Character 7
Ø Head 2 Face 4 Upper Jaw 5 Lower Jaw 6 Neck Parapharyngeal space Retropharyngeal space 8 Chest Wall C Mediastinum Mediastinal cavity Mediastinal space F Abdominal Wall K Upper Back L Lower Back M Perineum, Male ♂ N Perineum, Female ♀	Ø Open 3 Percutaneous 4 Percutaneous Endoscopic X External	Ø Drainage Device 1 Radioactive Element 3 Infusion Device 7 Autologous Tissue Substitute J Synthetic Substitute K Nonautologous Tissue Substitute Y Other Device	Z No Qualifier
1 Cranial Cavity 9 Pleural Cavity, Right B Pleural Cavity, Left G Peritoneal Cavity J Pelvic Cavity Retropubic space	Ø Open 3 Percutaneous 4 Percutaneous Endoscopic X External	Ø Drainage Device 1 Radioactive Element 3 Infusion Device J Synthetic Substitute Y Other Device	Z No Qualifier
D Pericardial Cavity H Retroperitoneum Retroperitoneal cavity Retroperitoneal space	Ø Open 3 Percutaneous 4 Percutaneous Endoscopic X External	Ø Drainage Device 1 Radioactive Element 3 Infusion Device Y Other Device	Z No Qualifier
P Gastrointestinal Tract Q Respiratory Tract R Genitourinary Tract	Ø Open 3 Percutaneous 4 Percutaneous Endoscopic 7 Via Natural or Artificial Opening 8 Via Natural or Artificial Opening Endoscopic X External	1 Radioactive Element 3 Infusion Device Y Other Device	Z No Qualifier

DRG Non-OR ØWW[Ø,2,4,5,6,K,L][Ø,3,4][Ø,1,3,7,J,K,Y]Z
DRG Non-OR ØWWM[Ø,3,4][Ø,1,3,J,Y]Z
Non-OR ØWW[Ø,2,4,5,6,C,F,K,L,M,N]X[Ø,1,3,7,J,K,Y]Z
Non-OR ØWW8[Ø,3,4,X][Ø,1,3,7,J,K,Y]Z
Non-OR ØWW[1,G,J]X[Ø,1,3,J,Y]Z
Non-OR ØWW[9,B][Ø,3,4,X][Ø,1,3,J,Y]Z
Non-OR ØWW[D,H]X[Ø,1,3,Y]Z
Non-OR ØWWP[3,4,7,8,X][1,3,Y]Z
Non-OR ØWWQ[Ø,X][1,3,Y]Z
Non-OR ØWWR[Ø,3,4,7,8,X][1,3,Y]Z

♂ ØWWM[Ø,3,4,X][Ø,1,3,7,K,Y]Z
♀ ØWWN[Ø,3,4,X][Ø,1,3,7,K,Y]Z

Ø Medical and Surgical
W Anatomical Regions, General
Y Transplantation Definition: Putting in or on all or a portion of a living body part taken from another individual or animal to physically take the place and/or function of all or a portion of a similar body part

Explanation: The native body part may or may not be taken out, and the transplanted body part may take over all or a portion of its function

Body Part Character 4	Approach Character 5	Device Character 6	Qualifier Character 7
2 Face	Ø Open	Z No Device	Ø Allogeneic 1 Syngeneic

Anatomical Regions, Upper Extremities ØXØ–ØXY

Character Meanings

This Character Meaning table is provided as a guide to assist the user in the identification of character members that may be found in this section of code tables. It **SHOULD NOT** be used to build a PCS code.

Operation–Character 3	Body Part–Character 4	Approach–Character 5	Device–Character 6	Qualifier–Character 7
Ø Alteration	Ø Forequarter, Right	Ø Open	Ø Drainage Device	Ø Allogeneic OR Complete
2 Change	1 Forequarter, Left	3 Percutaneous	1 Radioactive Element	1 High OR Syngeneic
3 Control	2 Shoulder Region, Right	4 Percutaneous Endoscopic	3 Infusion Device	2 Mid
6 Detachment	3 Shoulder Region, Left	X External	7 Autologous Tissue Substitute	3 Low
9 Drainage	4 Axilla, Right		J Synthetic Substitute	4 Complete 1st Ray
B Excision	5 Axilla, Left		K Nonautologous Tissue Substitute	5 Complete 2nd Ray
H Insertion	6 Upper Extremity, Right		Y Other Device	6 Complete 3rd Ray
J Inspection	7 Upper Extremity, Left		Z No Device	7 Complete 4th Ray
M Reattachment	8 Upper Arm, Right			8 Complete 5th Ray
P Removal	9 Upper Arm, Left			9 Partial 1st Ray
Q Repair	B Elbow Region, Right			B Partial 2nd Ray
R Replacement	C Elbow Region, Left			C Partial 3rd Ray
U Supplement	D Lower Arm, Right			D Partial 4th Ray
W Revision	F Lower Arm, Left			F Partial 5th Ray
X Transfer	G Wrist Region, Right			L Thumb, Right
Y Transplantation	H Wrist Region, Left			M Thumb, Left
	J Hand, Right			N Toe, Right
	K Hand, Left			P Toe, Left
	L Thumb, Right			X Diagnostic
	M Thumb, Left			Z No Qualifier
	N Index Finger, Right			
	P Index Finger, Left			
	Q Middle Finger, Right			
	R Middle Finger, Left			
	S Ring Finger, Right			
	T Ring Finger, Left			
	V Little Finger, Right			
	W Little Finger, Left			

AHA Coding Clinic for table ØX3
2016, 4Q, 99 Root operation Control
2015, 1Q, 35 Evacuation of hematoma for control of postprocedural bleeding
2013, 3Q, 23 Control of intraoperative bleeding

AHA Coding Clinic for table ØX6
2017, 2Q, 3-4 Qualifiers for the root operation detachment
2017, 2Q, 18 Removal of polydactyl digits
2017, 1Q, 52 Further distal phalangeal amputation
2016, 3Q, 33 Traumatic amputation of fingers with further revision amputation

AHA Coding Clinic for table ØXH
2017, 2Q, 20 Exchange of intramedullary antibiotic impregnated spacer

AHA Coding Clinic for table ØXP
2017, 2Q, 20 Exchange of intramedullary antibiotic impregnated spacer

AHA Coding Clinic for table ØXY
2016, 4Q, 112-113 Transplantation

Detachment Qualifier Descriptions

Qualifier Definition	Upper Arm	Lower Arm
1 **High:** Amputation at the proximal portion of the shaft of the:	Humerus	Radius/Ulna
2 **Mid:** Amputation at the middle portion of the shaft of the:	Humerus	Radius/Ulna
3 **Low:** Amputation at the distal portion of the shaft of the:	Humerus	Radius/Ulna

Qualifier Definition	Hand
Ø Complete 1st through 5th Rays Ray: digit of hand or foot with corresponding metacarpus or metatarsus	Through carpo-metacarpal joint, **Wrist**
4 Complete 1st Ray	Through carpo-metacarpal joint, **Thumb**
5 Complete 2nd Ray	Through carpo-metacarpal joint, **Index Finger**
6 Complete 3rd Ray	Through carpo-metacarpal joint, **Middle Finger**
7 Complete 4th Ray	Through carpo-metacarpal joint, **Ring Finger**
8 Complete 5th Ray	Through carpo-metacarpal joint, **Little Finger**
9 Partial 1st Ray	Anywhere along shaft or head of metacarpal bone, **Thumb**
B Partial 2nd Ray	Anywhere along shaft or head of metacarpal bone, **Index Finger**
C Partial 3rd Ray	Anywhere along shaft or head of metacarpal bone, **Middle Finger**
D Partial 4th Ray	Anywhere along shaft or head of metacarpal bone, **Ring Finger**
F Partial 5th Ray	Anywhere along shaft or head of metacarpal bone, **Little Finger**

Qualifier Definition	Thumb/Finger
Ø Complete	At the metacarpophalangeal joint
1 High	Anywhere along the proximal phalanx
2 Mid	Through the proximal interphalangeal joint or anywhere along the middle phalanx
3 Low	Through the distal interphalangeal joint or anywhere along the distal phalanx

Ø Medical and Surgical
X Anatomical Regions, Upper Extremities
Ø Alteration Definition: Modifying the anatomic structure of a body part without affecting the function of the body part
Explanation: Principal purpose is to improve appearance

Body Part Character 4	Approach Character 5	Device Character 6	Qualifier Character 7
2 Shoulder Region, Right 3 Shoulder Region, Left 4 Axilla, Right 5 Axilla, Left 6 Upper Extremity, Right 7 Upper Extremity, Left 8 Upper Arm, Right 9 Upper Arm, Left B Elbow Region, Right C Elbow Region, Left D Lower Arm, Right F Lower Arm, Left G Wrist Region, Right H Wrist Region, Left	Ø Open 3 Percutaneous 4 Percutaneous Endoscopic	7 Autologous Tissue Substitute J Synthetic Substitute K Nonautologous Tissue Substitute Z No Device	Z No Qualifier

Ø Medical and Surgical
X Anatomical Regions, Upper Extremities
2 Change Definition: Taking out or off a device from a body part and putting back an identical or similar device in or on the same body part without cutting or puncturing the skin or a mucous membrane
Explanation: All CHANGE procedures are coded using the approach EXTERNAL

Body Part Character 4	Approach Character 5	Device Character 6	Qualifier Character 7
6 Upper Extremity, Right 7 Upper Extremity, Left	X External	Ø Drainage Device Y Other Device	Z No Qualifier

Non-OR All body part, approach, device, and qualifier values

Ø Medical and Surgical
X Anatomical Regions, Upper Extremities
3 Control Definition: Stopping, or attempting to stop, postprocedural or other acute bleeding
Explanation: None

Body Part Character 4	Approach Character 5	Device Character 6	Qualifier Character 7
2 Shoulder Region, Right 3 Shoulder Region, Left 4 Axilla, Right 5 Axilla, Left 6 Upper Extremity, Right 7 Upper Extremity, Left 8 Upper Arm, Right 9 Upper Arm, Left B Elbow Region, Right C Elbow Region, Left D Lower Arm, Right F Lower Arm, Left G Wrist Region, Right H Wrist Region, Left J Hand, Right K Hand, Left	Ø Open 3 Percutaneous 4 Percutaneous Endoscopic	Z No Device	Z No Qualifier

Ø Medical and Surgical
X Anatomical Regions, Upper Extremities
6 Detachment Definition: Cutting off all or a portion of the upper or lower extremities

Explanation: The body part value is the site of the detachment, with a qualifier if applicable to further specify the level where the extremity was detached

Body Part Character 4	Approach Character 5	Device Character 6	Qualifier Character 7
Ø Forequarter, Right 1 Forequarter, Left 2 Shoulder Region, Right 3 Shoulder Region, Left B Elbow Region, Right C Elbow Region, Left	Ø Open	Z No Device	Z No Qualifier
8 Upper Arm, Right 9 Upper Arm, Left D Lower Arm, Right F Lower Arm, Left	Ø Open	Z No Device	1 High 2 Mid 3 Low
J Hand, Right K Hand, Left	Ø Open	Z No Device	Ø Complete 4 Complete 1st Ray 5 Complete 2nd Ray 6 Complete 3rd Ray 7 Complete 4th Ray 8 Complete 5th Ray 9 Partial 1st Ray B Partial 2nd Ray C Partial 3rd Ray D Partial 4th Ray F Partial 5th Ray
L Thumb, Right M Thumb, Left N Index Finger, Right P Index Finger, Left Q Middle Finger, Right R Middle Finger, Left S Ring Finger, Right T Ring Finger, Left V Little Finger, Right W Little Finger, Left	Ø Open	Z No Device	Ø Complete 1 High 2 Mid 3 Low

Ø Medical and Surgical
X Anatomical Regions, Upper Extremities
9 Drainage Definition: Taking or letting out fluids and/or gases from a body part
Explanation: The qualifier DIAGNOSTIC is used to identify drainage procedures that are biopsies

Body Part Character 4	Approach Character 5	Device Character 6	Qualifier Character 7
2 Shoulder Region, Right 3 Shoulder Region, Left 4 Axilla, Right 5 Axilla, Left 6 Upper Extremity, Right 7 Upper Extremity, Left 8 Upper Arm, Right 9 Upper Arm, Left B Elbow Region, Right C Elbow Region, Left D Lower Arm, Right F Lower Arm, Left G Wrist Region, Right H Wrist Region, Left J Hand, Right K Hand, Left	Ø Open 3 Percutaneous 4 Percutaneous Endoscopic	Ø Drainage Device	Z No Qualifier
2 Shoulder Region, Right 3 Shoulder Region, Left 4 Axilla, Right 5 Axilla, Left 6 Upper Extremity, Right 7 Upper Extremity, Left 8 Upper Arm, Right 9 Upper Arm, Left B Elbow Region, Right C Elbow Region, Left D Lower Arm, Right F Lower Arm, Left G Wrist Region, Right H Wrist Region, Left J Hand, Right K Hand, Left	Ø Open 3 Percutaneous 4 Percutaneous Endoscopic	Z No Device	X Diagnostic Z No Qualifier

Non-OR All body part, approach, device, and qualifier values

Ø Medical and Surgical
X Anatomical Regions, Upper Extremities
B Excision Definition: Cutting out or off, without replacement, a portion of a body part
Explanation: The qualifier DIAGNOSTIC is used to identify excision procedures that are biopsies

Body Part Character 4	Approach Character 5	Device Character 6	Qualifier Character 7
2 Shoulder Region, Right 3 Shoulder Region, Left 4 Axilla, Right 5 Axilla, Left 6 Upper Extremity, Right 7 Upper Extremity, Left 8 Upper Arm, Right 9 Upper Arm, Left B Elbow Region, Right C Elbow Region, Left D Lower Arm, Right F Lower Arm, Left G Wrist Region, Right H Wrist Region, Left J Hand, Right K Hand, Left	Ø Open 3 Percutaneous 4 Percutaneous Endoscopic	Z No Device	X Diagnostic Z No Qualifier

Non-OR ØXB[2,3,4,5,6,7,8,9,B,C,D,F,G,H,J,K][Ø,3,4]ZX

Ø Medical and Surgical
X Anatomical Regions, Upper Extremities
H Insertion Definition: Putting in a nonbiological appliance that monitors, assists, performs, or prevents a physiological function but does not physically take the place of a body part

Explanation: None

Body Part Character 4	Approach Character 5	Device Character 6	Qualifier Character 7
2 Shoulder Region, Right 3 Shoulder Region, Left 4 Axilla, Right 5 Axilla, Left 6 Upper Extremity, Right 7 Upper Extremity, Left 8 Upper Arm, Right 9 Upper Arm, Left B Elbow Region, Right C Elbow Region, Left D Lower Arm, Right F Lower Arm, Left G Wrist Region, Right H Wrist Region, Left J Hand, Right K Hand, Left	Ø Open 3 Percutaneous 4 Percutaneous Endoscopic	1 Radioactive Element 3 Infusion Device Y Other Device	Z No Qualifier

DRG Non-OR ØXH[2,3,4,5,6,7,8,9,B,C,D,F,G,H,J,K][Ø,3,4][3,Y]Z

Ø Medical and Surgical
X Anatomical Regions, Upper Extremities
J Inspection Definition: Visually and/or manually exploring a body part

Explanation: Visual exploration may be performed with or without optical instrumentation. Manual exploration may be performed directly or through intervening body layers.

Body Part Character 4	Approach Character 5	Device Character 6	Qualifier Character 7
2 Shoulder Region, Right 3 Shoulder Region, Left 4 Axilla, Right 5 Axilla, Left 6 Upper Extremity, Right 7 Upper Extremity, Left 8 Upper Arm, Right 9 Upper Arm, Left B Elbow Region, Right C Elbow Region, Left D Lower Arm, Right F Lower Arm, Left G Wrist Region, Right H Wrist Region, Left J Hand, Right K Hand, Left	Ø Open 3 Percutaneous 4 Percutaneous Endoscopic X External	Z No Device	Z No Qualifier

DRG Non-OR ØXJ[2,3,4,5,6,7,8,9,B,C,D,F,G,H,J,K]ØZZ
Non-OR ØXJ[2,3,4,5,6,7,8,9,B,C,D,F,G,H][3,4,X]ZZ
Non-OR ØXJ[J,K][3,X]ZZ

Ø Medical and Surgical
X Anatomical Regions, Upper Extremities
M Reattachment Definition: Putting back in or on all or a portion of a separated body part to its normal location or other suitable location

Explanation: Vascular circulation and nervous pathways may or may not be reestablished

Body Part Character 4	Approach Character 5	Device Character 6	Qualifier Character 7
Ø Forequarter, Right 1 Forequarter, Left 2 Shoulder Region, Right 3 Shoulder Region, Left 4 Axilla, Right 5 Axilla, Left 6 Upper Extremity, Right 7 Upper Extremity, Left 8 Upper Arm, Right 9 Upper Arm, Left B Elbow Region, Right C Elbow Region, Left D Lower Arm, Right F Lower Arm, Left G Wrist Region, Right H Wrist Region, Left J Hand, Right K Hand, Left L Thumb, Right M Thumb, Left N Index Finger, Right P Index Finger, Left Q Middle Finger, Right R Middle Finger, Left S Ring Finger, Right T Ring Finger, Left V Little Finger, Right W Little Finger, Left	Ø Open	Z No Device	Z No Qualifier

Ø Medical and Surgical
X Anatomical Regions, Upper Extremities
P Removal Definition: Taking out or off a device from a body part

Explanation: If a device is taken out and a similar device put in without cutting or puncturing the skin or mucous membrane, the procedure is coded to the root operation CHANGE. Otherwise, the procedure for taking out the device is coded to the root operation REMOVAL.

Body Part Character 4	Approach Character 5	Device Character 6	Qualifier Character 7
6 Upper Extremity, Right 7 Upper Extremity, Left	Ø Open 3 Percutaneous 4 Percutaneous Endoscopic X External	Ø Drainage Device 1 Radioactive Element 3 Infusion Device 7 Autologous Tissue Substitute J Synthetic Substitute K Nonautologous Tissue Substitute Y Other Device	Z No Qualifier

Non-OR All body part, approach, device, and qualifier values

Ø Medical and Surgical
X Anatomical Regions, Upper Extremities
Q Repair Definition: Restoring, to the extent possible, a body part to its normal anatomic structure and function

Explanation: Used only when the method to accomplish the repair is not one of the other root operations

Body Part Character 4	Approach Character 5	Device Character 6	Qualifier Character 7
2 Shoulder Region, Right **3** Shoulder Region, Left **4** Axilla, Right **5** Axilla, Left **6** Upper Extremity, Right **7** Upper Extremity, Left **8** Upper Arm, Right **9** Upper Arm, Left **B** Elbow Region, Right **C** Elbow Region, Left **D** Lower Arm, Right **F** Lower Arm, Left **G** Wrist Region, Right **H** Wrist Region, Left **J** Hand, Right **K** Hand, Left **L** Thumb, Right **M** Thumb, Left **N** Index Finger, Right **P** Index Finger, Left **Q** Middle Finger, Right **R** Middle Finger, Left **S** Ring Finger, Right **T** Ring Finger, Left **V** Little Finger, Right **W** Little Finger, Left	**Ø** Open **3** Percutaneous **4** Percutaneous Endoscopic **X** External	**Z** No Device	**Z** No Qualifier

Ø Medical and Surgical
X Anatomical Regions, Upper Extremities
R Replacement Definition: Putting in or on biological or synthetic material that physically takes the place and/or function of all or a portion of a body part

Explanation: The body part may have been taken out or replaced, or may be taken out, physically eradicated, or rendered nonfunctional during the REPLACEMENT procedure. A REMOVAL procedure is coded for taking out the device used in a previous replacement procedure.

Body Part Character 4	Approach Character 5	Device Character 6	Qualifier Character 7
L Thumb, Right **M** Thumb, Left	**Ø** Open **4** Percutaneous Endoscopic	**7** Autologous Tissue Substitute	**N** Toe, Right **P** Toe, Left

Ø Medical and Surgical
X Anatomical Regions, Upper Extremities
U Supplement Definition: Putting in or on biological or synthetic material that physically reinforces and/or augments the function of a portion of a body part

Explanation: The biological material is non-living, or is living and from the same individual. The body part may have been previously replaced, and the SUPPLEMENT procedure is performed to physically reinforce and/or augment the function of the replaced body part.

Body Part Character 4	Approach Character 5	Device Character 6	Qualifier Character 7
2 Shoulder Region, Right 3 Shoulder Region, Left 4 Axilla, Right 5 Axilla, Left 6 Upper Extremity, Right 7 Upper Extremity, Left 8 Upper Arm, Right 9 Upper Arm, Left B Elbow Region, Right C Elbow Region, Left D Lower Arm, Right F Lower Arm, Left G Wrist Region, Right H Wrist Region, Left J Hand, Right K Hand, Left L Thumb, Right M Thumb, Left N Index Finger, Right P Index Finger, Left Q Middle Finger, Right R Middle Finger, Left S Ring Finger, Right T Ring Finger, Left V Little Finger, Right W Little Finger, Left	Ø Open 4 Percutaneous Endoscopic	7 Autologous Tissue Substitute J Synthetic Substitute K Nonautologous Tissue Substitute	Z No Qualifier

Ø Medical and Surgical
X Anatomical Regions, Upper Extremities
W Revision Definition: Correcting, to the extent possible, a portion of a malfunctioning device or the position of a displaced device

Explanation: Revision can include correcting a malfunctioning or displaced device by taking out or putting in components of the device such as a screw or pin

Body Part Character 4	Approach Character 5	Device Character 6	Qualifier Character 7
6 Upper Extremity, Right 7 Upper Extremity, Left	Ø Open 3 Percutaneous 4 Percutaneous Endoscopic X External	Ø Drainage Device 3 Infusion Device 7 Autologous Tissue Substitute J Synthetic Substitute K Nonautologous Tissue Substitute Y Other Device	Z No Qualifier

DRG Non-OR ØXW[6,7][Ø,3,4][Ø,3,7,J,K,Y]Z
Non-OR ØXW[6,7]X[Ø,3,7,J,K,Y]Z

Ø Medical and Surgical
X Anatomical Regions, Upper Extremities
X Transfer Definition: Moving, without taking out, all or a portion of a body part to another location to take over the function of all or a portion of a body part

Explanation: The body part transferred remains connected to its vascular and nervous supply

Body Part Character 4	Approach Character 5	Device Character 6	Qualifier Character 7
N Index Finger, Right	Ø Open	Z No Device	L Thumb, Right
P Index Finger, Left	Ø Open	Z No Device	M Thumb, Left

Ø Medical and Surgical
X Anatomical Regions, Upper Extremities
Y Transplantation Definition: Putting in or on all or a portion of a living body part taken from another individual or animal to physically take the place and/or function of all or a portion of a similar body part

Explanation: The native body part may or may not be taken out, and the transplanted body part may take over all or a portion of its function

Body Part Character 4	Approach Character 5	Device Character 6	Qualifier Character 7
J Hand, Right K Hand, Left	Ø Open	Z No Device	Ø Allogeneic 1 Syngeneic

Anatomical Regions, Lower Extremities ØYØ–ØYW

Character Meanings

This Character Meaning table is provided as a guide to assist the user in the identification of character members that may be found in this section of code tables. It **SHOULD NOT** be used to build a PCS code.

Operation–Character 3	Body Part–Character 4	Approach–Character 5	Device–Character 6	Qualifier–Character 7
Ø Alteration	Ø Buttock, Right	Ø Open	Ø Drainage Device	Ø Complete
2 Change	1 Buttock, Left	3 Percutaneous	1 Radioactive Element	1 High
3 Control	2 Hindquarter, Right	4 Percutaneous Endoscopic	3 Infusion Device	2 Mid
6 Detachment	3 Hindquarter, Left	X External	7 Autologous Tissue Substitute	3 Low
9 Drainage	4 Hindquarter, Bilateral		J Synthetic Substitute	4 Complete 1st Ray
B Excision	5 Inguinal Region, Right		K Nonautologous Tissue Substitute	5 Complete 2nd Ray
H Insertion	6 Inguinal Region, Left		Y Other Device	6 Complete 3rd Ray
J Inspection	7 Femoral Region, Right		Z No Device	7 Complete 4th Ray
M Reattachment	8 Femoral Region, Left			8 Complete 5th Ray
P Removal	9 Lower Extremity, Right			9 Partial 1st Ray
Q Repair	A Inguinal Region, Bilateral			B Partial 2nd Ray
U Supplement	B Lower Extremity, Left			C Partial 3rd Ray
W Revision	C Upper Leg, Right			D Partial 4th Ray
	D Upper Leg, Left			F Partial 5th Ray
	E Femoral Region, Bilateral			X Diagnostic
	F Knee Region, Right			Z No Qualifier
	G Knee Region, Left			
	H Lower Leg, Right			
	J Lower Leg, Left			
	K Ankle Region, Right			
	L Ankle Region, Left			
	M Foot, Right			
	N Foot, Left			
	P 1st Toe, Right			
	Q 1st Toe, Left			
	R 2nd Toe, Right			
	S 2nd Toe, Left			
	T 3rd Toe, Right			
	U 3rd Toe, Left			
	V 4th Toe, Right			
	W 4th Toe, Left			
	X 5th Toe, Right			
	Y 5th Toe, Left			

AHA Coding Clinic for table ØY3

2016, 4Q, 99 Root operation Control
2013, 3Q, 23 Control of intraoperative bleeding

AHA Coding Clinic for table ØY6

2019, 2Q, 17 Cryoamputation of lower leg
2017, 2Q, 3-4 Qualifiers for the root operation detachment
2017, 1Q, 22 Chopart amputation of foot
2015, 2Q, 28 Partial amputation of hallux at interphalangeal Joint
2015, 1Q, 28 Mid-foot amputation

AHA Coding Clinic for table ØY9

2015, 1Q, 22 Incision and drainage of abscess of femoropopliteal bypass site
2015, 1Q, 22 Incision and drainage of groin abscess

Detachment Qualifier Descriptions

Qualifier Definition	Upper Leg	Lower Leg
1 **High:** Amputation at the proximal portion of the shaft of the:	Femur	Tibia/Fibula
2 **Mid:** Amputation at the middle portion of the shaft of the:	Femur	Tibia/Fibula
3 **Low:** Amputation at the distal portion of the shaft of the:	Femur	Tibia/Fibula

Qualifier Definition	Foot
Ø Complete 1st through 5th Rays Ray: digit of hand or foot with corresponding metacarpus or metatarsus	Through tarso-metatarsal Joint, **Ankle**
4 Complete 1st Ray	Through tarso-metatarsal joint, **Great Toe**
5 Complete 2nd Ray	Through tarso-metatarsal joint, **2nd Toe**
6 Complete 3rd Ray	Through tarso-metatarsal joint, **3rd Toe**
7 Complete 4th Ray	Through tarso-metatarsal joint, **4th Toe**
8 Complete 5th Ray	Through tarso-metatarsal joint, **Little Toe**
9 Partial 1st Ray	Anywhere along shaft or head of metatarsal bone, **Great Toe**
B Partial 2nd Ray	Anywhere along shaft or head of metatarsal bone, **2nd Toe**
C Partial 3rd Ray	Anywhere along shaft or head of metatarsal bone, **3rd Toe**
D Partial 4th Ray	Anywhere along shaft or head of metatarsal bone, **4th Toe**
F Partial 5th Ray	Anywhere along shaft or head of metatarsal bone, **Little Toe**

Qualifier Definition	Toe
Ø Complete	At the metatarsal-phalangeal joint
1 High	Anywhere along the proximal phalanx
2 Mid	Through the proximal interphalangeal joint or anywhere along the middle phalanx
3 Low	Through the distal interphalangeal joint or anywhere along the distal phalanx

Ø Medical and Surgical
Y Anatomical Regions, Lower Extremities
Ø Alteration Definition: Modifying the anatomic structure of a body part without affecting the function of the body part
Explanation: Principal purpose is to improve appearance

Body Part Character 4	Approach Character 5	Device Character 6	Qualifier Character 7
Ø Buttock, Right 1 Buttock, Left 9 Lower Extremity, Right B Lower Extremity, Left C Upper Leg, Right D Upper Leg, Left F Knee Region, Right G Knee Region, Left H Lower Leg, Right J Lower Leg, Left K Ankle Region, Right L Ankle Region, Left	Ø Open 3 Percutaneous 4 Percutaneous Endoscopic	7 Autologous Tissue Substitute J Synthetic Substitute K Nonautologous Tissue Substitute Z No Device	Z No Qualifier

Ø Medical and Surgical
Y Anatomical Regions, Lower Extremities
2 Change Definition: Taking out or off a device from a body part and putting back an identical or similar device in or on the same body part without cutting or puncturing the skin or a mucous membrane
Explanation: All CHANGE procedures are coded using the approach EXTERNAL

Body Part Character 4	Approach Character 5	Device Character 6	Qualifier Character 7
9 Lower Extremity, Right B Lower Extremity, Left	X External	Ø Drainage Device Y Other Device	Z No Qualifier

Non-OR All body part, approach, device, and qualifier values

Ø Medical and Surgical
Y Anatomical Regions, Lower Extremities
3 Control Definition: Stopping, or attempting to stop, postprocedural or other acute bleeding
Explanation: None

Body Part Character 4	Approach Character 5	Device Character 6	Qualifier Character 7
Ø Buttock, Right 1 Buttock, Left 5 Inguinal Region, Right Inguinal canal Inguinal triangle 6 Inguinal Region, Left *See 5 Inguinal Region, Right* 7 Femoral Region, Right 8 Femoral Region, Left 9 Lower Extremity, Right B Lower Extremity, Left C Upper Leg, Right D Upper Leg, Left F Knee Region, Right G Knee Region, Left H Lower Leg, Right J Lower Leg, Left K Ankle Region, Right L Ankle Region, Left M Foot, Right N Foot, Left	Ø Open 3 Percutaneous 4 Percutaneous Endoscopic	Z No Device	Z No Qualifier

Ø Medical and Surgical
Y Anatomical Regions, Lower Extremities
6 Detachment Definition: Cutting off all or a portion of the upper or lower extremities

Explanation: The body part value is the site of the detachment, with a qualifier if applicable to further specify the level where the extremity was detached

Body Part Character 4	Approach Character 5	Device Character 6	Qualifier Character 7
2 Hindquarter, Right **3** Hindquarter, Left **4** Hindquarter, Bilateral **7** Femoral Region, Right **8** Femoral Region, Left **F** Knee Region, Right **G** Knee Region, Left	**Ø** Open	**Z** No Device	**Z** No Qualifier
C Upper Leg, Right **D** Upper Leg, Left **H** Lower Leg, Right **J** Lower Leg, Left	**Ø** Open	**Z** No Device	**1** High **2** Mid **3** Low
M Foot, Right **N** Foot, Left	**Ø** Open	**Z** No Device	**Ø** Complete **4** Complete 1st Ray **5** Complete 2nd Ray **6** Complete 3rd Ray **7** Complete 4th Ray **8** Complete 5th Ray **9** Partial 1st Ray **B** Partial 2nd Ray **C** Partial 3rd Ray **D** Partial 4th Ray **F** Partial 5th Ray
P 1st Toe, Right Hallux **Q** 1st Toe, Left *See 1st Toe, Right* **R** 2nd Toe, Right **S** 2nd Toe, Left **T** 3rd Toe, Right **U** 3rd Toe, Left **V** 4th Toe, Right **W** 4th Toe, Left **X** 5th Toe, Right **Y** 5th Toe, Left	**Ø** Open	**Z** No Device	**Ø** Complete **1** High **2** Mid **3** Low

Ø Medical and Surgical
Y Anatomical Regions, Lower Extremities
9 Drainage Definition: Taking or letting out fluids and/or gases from a body part
Explanation: The qualifier DIAGNOSTIC is used to identify drainage procedures that are biopsies

Body Part Character 4	Approach Character 5	Device Character 6	Qualifier Character 7
Ø Buttock, Right 1 Buttock, Left 5 Inguinal Region, Right Inguinal canal Inguinal triangle 6 Inguinal Region, Left *See 5 Inguinal Region, Right* 7 Femoral Region, Right 8 Femoral Region, Left 9 Lower Extremity, Right B Lower Extremity, Left C Upper Leg, Right D Upper Leg, Left F Knee Region, Right G Knee Region, Left H Lower Leg, Right J Lower Leg, Left K Ankle Region, Right L Ankle Region, Left M Foot, Right N Foot, Left	Ø Open 3 Percutaneous 4 Percutaneous Endoscopic	Ø Drainage Device	Z No Qualifier
Ø Buttock, Right 1 Buttock, Left 5 Inguinal Region, Right Inguinal canal Inguinal triangle 6 Inguinal Region, Left *See 5 Inguinal Region, Right* 7 Femoral Region, Right 8 Femoral Region, Left 9 Lower Extremity, Right B Lower Extremity, Left C Upper Leg, Right D Upper Leg, Left F Knee Region, Right G Knee Region, Left H Lower Leg, Right J Lower Leg, Left K Ankle Region, Right L Ankle Region, Left M Foot, Right N Foot, Left	Ø Open 3 Percutaneous 4 Percutaneous Endoscopic	Z No Device	X Diagnostic Z No Qualifier

Non-OR ØY9[Ø,1,7,8,9,B,C,D,F,G,H,J,K,L,M,N][Ø,3,4]ØZ
Non-OR ØY9[5,6]3ØZ
Non-OR ØY9[Ø,1,7,8,9,B,C,D,F,G,H,J,K,L,M,N][Ø,3,4]Z[X,Z]
Non-OR ØY9[5,6]3ZZ

Ø Medical and Surgical
Y Anatomical Regions, Lower Extremities
B Excision Definition: Cutting out or off, without replacement, a portion of a body part

Explanation: The qualifier DIAGNOSTIC is used to identify excision procedures that are biopsies

Body Part Character 4	Approach Character 5	Device Character 6	Qualifier Character 7
Ø Buttock, Right 1 Buttock, Left 5 Inguinal Region, Right Inguinal canal Inguinal triangle 6 Inguinal Region, Left *See 5 Inguinal Region, Right* 7 Femoral Region, Right 8 Femoral Region, Left 9 Lower Extremity, Right B Lower Extremity, Left C Upper Leg, Right D Upper Leg, Left F Knee Region, Right G Knee Region, Left H Lower Leg, Right J Lower Leg, Left K Ankle Region, Right L Ankle Region, Left M Foot, Right N Foot, Left	Ø Open 3 Percutaneous 4 Percutaneous Endoscopic	Z No Device	X Diagnostic Z No Qualifier

Non-OR ØYB[Ø,1,9,B,C,D,F,G,H,J,K,L,M,N][Ø,3,4]ZX

Ø Medical and Surgical
Y Anatomical Regions, Lower Extremities
H Insertion Definition: Putting in a nonbiological appliance that monitors, assists, performs, or prevents a physiological function but does not physically take the place of a body part

Explanation: None

Body Part Character 4	Approach Character 5	Device Character 6	Qualifier Character 7
Ø Buttock, Right 1 Buttock, Left 5 Inguinal Region, Right Inguinal canal Inguinal triangle 6 Inguinal Region, Left *See 5 Inguinal Region, Right* 7 Femoral Region, Right 8 Femoral Region, Left 9 Lower Extremity, Right B Lower Extremity, Left C Upper Leg, Right D Upper Leg, Left F Knee Region, Right G Knee Region, Left H Lower Leg, Right J Lower Leg, Left K Ankle Region, Right L Ankle Region, Left M Foot, Right N Foot, Left	Ø Open 3 Percutaneous 4 Percutaneous Endoscopic	1 Radioactive Element 3 Infusion Device Y Other Device	Z No Qualifier

DRG Non-OR ØYH[Ø,1,5,6,7,8,9,B,C,D,F,G,H,J,K,L,M,N][Ø,3,4][3,Y]Z

Ø Medical and Surgical
Y Anatomical Regions, Lower Extremities
J Inspection Definition: Visually and/or manually exploring a body part

Explanation: Visual exploration may be performed with or without optical instrumentation. Manual exploration may be performed directly or through intervening body layers.

Body Part Character 4	Approach Character 5	Device Character 6	Qualifier Character 7
Ø Buttock, Right **1** Buttock, Left **5** Inguinal Region, Right Inguinal canal Inguinal triangle **6** Inguinal Region, Left *See 5 Inguinal Region, Right* **7** Femoral Region, Right **8** Femoral Region, Left **9** Lower Extremity, Right **A** Inguinal Region, Bilateral *See 5 Inguinal Region, Right* **B** Lower Extremity, Left **C** Upper Leg, Right **D** Upper Leg, Left **E** Femoral Region, Bilateral **F** Knee Region, Right **G** Knee Region, Left **H** Lower Leg, Right **J** Lower Leg, Left **K** Ankle Region, Right **L** Ankle Region, Left **M** Foot, Right **N** Foot, Left	**Ø** Open **3** Percutaneous **4** Percutaneous Endoscopic **X** External	**Z** No Device	**Z** No Qualifier

DRG Non-OR ØYJ[Ø,1,8,9,B,C,D,E,F,G,H,J,K,L,M,N]ØZZ
Non-OR ØYJ[Ø,1,9,B,C,D,F,G,H,J,K,L,M,N][3,4,X]ZZ
Non-OR ØYJ[5,6,7,8,A,E][3,X]ZZ

Ø Medical and Surgical
Y Anatomical Regions, Lower Extremities
M Reattachment Definition: Putting back in or on all or a portion of a separated body part to its normal location or other suitable location

Explanation: Vascular circulation and nervous pathways may or may not be reestablished

Body Part Character 4	Approach Character 5	Device Character 6	Qualifier Character 7
Ø Buttock, Right **1 Buttock, Left** **2 Hindquarter, Right** **3 Hindquarter, Left** **4 Hindquarter, Bilateral** **5 Inguinal Region, Right** Inguinal canal Inguinal triangle **6 Inguinal Region, Left** *See 5 Inguinal Region, Right* **7 Femoral Region, Right** **8 Femoral Region, Left** **9 Lower Extremity, Right** **B Lower Extremity, Left** **C Upper Leg, Right** **D Upper Leg, Left** **F Knee Region, Right** **G Knee Region, Left** **H Lower Leg, Right** **J Lower Leg, Left** **K Ankle Region, Right** **L Ankle Region, Left** **M Foot, Right** **N Foot, Left** **P 1st Toe, Right** Hallux **Q 1st Toe, Left** *See 1st Toe, Right* **R 2nd Toe, Right** **S 2nd Toe, Left** **T 3rd Toe, Right** **U 3rd Toe, Left** **V 4th Toe, Right** **W 4th Toe, Left** **X 5th Toe, Right** **Y 5th Toe, Left**	**Ø Open**	**Z No Device**	**Z No Qualifier**

Ø Medical and Surgical
Y Anatomical Regions, Lower Extremities
P Removal Definition: Taking out or off a device from a body part

Explanation: If a device is taken out and a similar device put in without cutting or puncturing the skin or mucous membrane, the procedure is coded to the root operation CHANGE. Otherwise, the procedure for taking out the device is coded to the root operation REMOVAL.

Body Part Character 4	Approach Character 5	Device Character 6	Qualifier Character 7
9 Lower Extremity, Right **B Lower Extremity, Left**	**Ø Open** **3 Percutaneous** **4 Percutaneous Endoscopic** **X External**	**Ø Drainage Device** **1 Radioactive Element** **3 Infusion Device** **7 Autologous Tissue Substitute** **J Synthetic Substitute** **K Nonautologous Tissue Substitute** **Y Other Device**	**Z No Qualifier**

Non-OR All body part, approach, device, and qualifier values

Ø Medical and Surgical
Y Anatomical Regions, Lower Extremities
Q Repair Definition: Restoring, to the extent possible, a body part to its normal anatomic structure and function
Explanation: Used only when the method to accomplish the repair is not one of the other root operations

Body Part Character 4	Approach Character 5	Device Character 6	Qualifier Character 7
Ø Buttock, Right 1 Buttock, Left 5 Inguinal Region, Right Inguinal canal Inguinal triangle 6 Inguinal Region, Left *See 5 Inguinal Region, Right* 7 Femoral Region, Right 8 Femoral Region, Left 9 Lower Extremity, Right A Inguinal Region, Bilateral *See 5 Inguinal Region, Right* B Lower Extremity, Left C Upper Leg, Right D Upper Leg, Left E Femoral Region, Bilateral F Knee Region, Right G Knee Region, Left H Lower Leg, Right J Lower Leg, Left K Ankle Region, Right L Ankle Region, Left M Foot, Right N Foot, Left P 1st Toe, Right Hallux Q 1st Toe, Left *See 1st Toe, Right* R 2nd Toe, Right S 2nd Toe, Left T 3rd Toe, Right U 3rd Toe, Left V 4th Toe, Right W 4th Toe, Left X 5th Toe, Right Y 5th Toe, Left	Ø Open 3 Percutaneous 4 Percutaneous Endoscopic X External	Z No Device	Z No Qualifier

Non-OR ØYQ[5,6,7,8,A,E]XZZ

Ø Medical and Surgical
Y Anatomical Regions, Lower Extremities
U Supplement Definition: Putting in or on biological or synthetic material that physically reinforces and/or augments the function of a portion of a body part

Explanation: The biological material is non-living, or is living and from the same individual. The body part may have been previously replaced, and the SUPPLEMENT procedure is performed to physically reinforce and/or augment the function of the replaced body part.

Body Part Character 4	Approach Character 5	Device Character 6	Qualifier Character 7
Ø Buttock, Right **1** Buttock, Left **5** Inguinal Region, Right Inguinal canal Inguinal triangle **6** Inguinal Region, Left *See 5 Inguinal Region, Right* **7** Femoral Region, Right **8** Femoral Region, Left **9** Lower Extremity, Right **A** Inguinal Region, Bilateral *See 5 Inguinal Region, Right* **B** Lower Extremity, Left **C** Upper Leg, Right **D** Upper Leg, Left **E** Femoral Region, Bilateral **F** Knee Region, Right **G** Knee Region, Left **H** Lower Leg, Right **J** Lower Leg, Left **K** Ankle Region, Right **L** Ankle Region, Left **M** Foot, Right **N** Foot, Left **P** 1st Toe, Right Hallux **Q** 1st Toe, Left *See 1st Toe, Right* **R** 2nd Toe, Right **S** 2nd Toe, Left **T** 3rd Toe, Right **U** 3rd Toe, Left **V** 4th Toe, Right **W** 4th Toe, Left **X** 5th Toe, Right **Y** 5th Toe, Left	**Ø** Open **4** Percutaneous Endoscopic	**7** Autologous Tissue Substitute **J** Synthetic Substitute **K** Nonautologous Tissue Substitute	**Z** No Qualifier

Ø Medical and Surgical
Y Anatomical Regions, Lower Extremities
W Revision Definition: Correcting, to the extent possible, a portion of a malfunctioning device or the position of a displaced device

Explanation: Revision can include correcting a malfunctioning or displaced device by taking out or putting in components of the device such as a screw or pin

Body Part Character 4	Approach Character 5	Device Character 6	Qualifier Character 7
9 Lower Extremity, Right **B** Lower Extremity, Left	**Ø** Open **3** Percutaneous **4** Percutaneous Endoscopic **X** External	**Ø** Drainage Device **3** Infusion Device **7** Autologous Tissue Substitute **J** Synthetic Substitute **K** Nonautologous Tissue Substitute **Y** Other Device	**Z** No Qualifier

DRG Non-OR ØYW[9,B][Ø,3,4][Ø,3,7,J,K,Y]Z
Non-OR ØYW[9,B]X[Ø,3,7,J,K,Y]Z

Obstetrics 1Ø2–1ØY

Character Meanings

This Character Meaning table is provided as a guide to assist the user in the identification of character members that may be found in this section of code tables. It **SHOULD NOT** be used to build a PCS code.

Ø: Pregnancy

Operation–Character 3	Body Part–Character 4	Approach–Character 5	Device–Character 6	Qualifier–Character 7
2 Change	Ø Products of Conception	Ø Open	3 Monitoring Electrode	Ø High
9 Drainage	1 Products of Conception, Retained	3 Percutaneous	Y Other Device	1 Low
A Abortion	2 Products of Conception, Ectopic	4 Percutaneous Endoscopic	Z No Device	2 Extraperitoneal
D Extraction		7 Via Natural or Artificial Opening		3 Low Forceps
E Delivery		8 Via Natural or Artificial Opening Endoscopic		4 Mid Forceps
H Insertion		X External		5 High Forceps
J Inspection				6 Vacuum
P Removal				7 Internal Version
Q Repair				8 Other
S Reposition				9 Fetal Blood OR Manual
T Resection				A Fetal Cerebrospinal Fluid
Y Transplantation				B Fetal Fluid, Other
				C Amniotic Fluid, Therapeutic
				D Fluid, Other
				E Nervous System
				F Cardiovascular System
				G Lymphatics & Hemic
				H Eye
				J Ear, Nose & Sinus
				K Respiratory System
				L Mouth & Throat
				M Gastrointestinal System
				N Hepatobiliary & Pancreas
				P Endocrine System
				Q Skin
				R Musculoskeletal System
				S Urinary System
				T Female Reproductive System
				U Amniotic Fluid, Diagnostic
				V Male Reproductive System
				W Laminaria
				X Abortifacient
				Y Other Body System
				Z No Qualifier

AHA Coding Clinic for table 1Ø9

2014, 3Q, 12 Fetoscopic laser photocoagulation and laser microseptostomy for twin-twin transfusion syndrome
2014, 2Q, 9 Pitocin administration to augment labor

AHA Coding Clinic for table 1ØD

2021, 1Q, 52 Removal of ectopic pregnancy via laparotomy
2020, 4Q, 59-60 Extraction of ectopic products of conception
2018, 4Q, 49-51 Revised qualifier values for root operation "extraction" (cesarean delivery)
2018, 2Q, 17 High transverse cesarean section
2016, 1Q, 9 Vaginal delivery assisted by vacuum and low forceps extraction
2014, 4Q, 43 Cesarean delivery assisted by vacuum extraction
2014, 4Q, 43 Vacuum dilation and curettage for blighted ovum

AHA Coding Clinic for table 1ØE

2017, 3Q, 5 Delivery of placenta
2016, 2Q, 34 Assisted vaginal delivery
2014, 4Q, 17 RH (D) alloimmunization (sensitization)
2014, 2Q, 9 Pitocin administration to augment labor

AHA Coding Clinic for table 1ØH

2013, 2Q, 36 Intrauterine pressure monitor

AHA Coding Clinic for table 1ØQ

2021, 2Q, 21 Ex Utero intrapartum treatment procedure
2014, 3Q, 12 Fetoscopic laser photocoagulation and laser microseptostomy for twin-twin transfusion syndrome

AHA Coding Clinic for table 1ØT

2020, 3Q, 47 Removal of ectopic cornual pregnancy
2015, 3Q, 31 Laparoscopic partial salpingectomy for ectopic pregnancy

1 Obstetrics
Ø Pregnancy
2 Change Definition: Taking out or off a device from a body part and putting back an identical or similar device in or on the same body part without cutting or puncturing the skin or a mucous membrane

Explanation: None

Body Part Character 4	Approach Character 5	Device Character 6	Qualifier Character 7
Ø Products of Conception ♀	7 Via Natural or Artificial Opening	3 Monitoring Electrode Y Other Device	Z No Qualifier

Non-OR All body part, approach, device, and qualifier values
♀ All body part, approach, device, and qualifier values

1 Obstetrics
Ø Pregnancy
9 Drainage Definition: Taking or letting out fluids and/or gases from a body part

Explanation: None

Body Part Character 4	Approach Character 5	Device Character 6	Qualifier Character 7
Ø Products of Conception ♀	Ø Open 3 Percutaneous 4 Percutaneous Endoscopic 7 Via Natural or Artificial Opening 8 Via Natural or Artificial Opening Endoscopic	Z No Device	9 Fetal Blood A Fetal Cerebrospinal Fluid B Fetal Fluid, Other C Amniotic Fluid, Therapeutic D Fluid, Other U Amniotic Fluid, Diagnostic

Non-OR All body part, approach, device, and qualifier values
♀ All body part, approach, device, and qualifier values

1 Obstetrics
Ø Pregnancy
A Abortion Definition: Artificially terminating a pregnancy

Explanation: None

Body Part Character 4	Approach Character 5	Device Character 6	Qualifier Character 7
Ø Products of Conception ♀	Ø Open 3 Percutaneous 4 Percutaneous Endoscopic 8 Via Natural or Artificial Opening Endoscopic	Z No Device	Z No Qualifier
Ø Products of Conception ♀	7 Via Natural or Artificial Opening	Z No Device	6 Vacuum W Laminaria X Abortifacient Z No Qualifier

Non-OR 1ØAØ7Z[6,W,X]
♀ All body part, approach, device, and qualifier values

1 Obstetrics
Ø Pregnancy
D Extraction Definition: Pulling or stripping out or off all or a portion of a body part by the use of force

Explanation: None

Body Part Character 4	Approach Character 5	Device Character 6	Qualifier Character 7
Ø Products of Conception QA ♀	Ø Open	Z No Device	Ø High 1 Low 2 Extraperitoneal
Ø Products of Conception QA ♀	7 Via Natural or Artificial Opening	Z No Device	3 Low Forceps 4 Mid Forceps 5 High Forceps 6 Vacuum 7 Internal Version 8 Other
1 Products of Conception, Retained ♀	7 Via Natural or Artificial Opening 8 Via Natural or Artificial Opening Endoscopic	Z No Device	9 Manual Z No Qualifier
2 Products of Conception, Ectopic ♀	Ø Open 4 Percutaneous Endoscopic 7 Via Natural or Artificial Opening 8 Via Natural or Artificial Opening Endoscopic	Z No Device	Z No Qualifier

DRG Non-OR 1ØDØ7Z[3,4,5,6,7,8]
QA 1ØDØØZ[Ø,1,2] except when a corresponding SDX of Z37.Ø-Z37.9 is also reported
QA 1ØDØ7Z[3,4,5,7] except when a corresponding SDX of Z37.Ø-Z37.9 is also reported
♀ All body part, approach, device, and qualifier values

1 Obstetrics
Ø Pregnancy
E Delivery Definition: Assisting the passage of the products of conception from the genital canal
Explanation: None

Body Part Character 4	Approach Character 5	Device Character 6	Qualifier Character 7
Ø Products of Conception QA ♀	X External	Z No Device	Z No Qualifier

DRG Non-OR 1ØEØXZZ
QA 1ØEØXZZ except when a corresponding SDX of Z37.Ø-Z37.9 is also reported
♀ All body part, approach, device, and qualifier values

1 Obstetrics
Ø Pregnancy
H Insertion Definition: Putting in a nonbiological appliance that monitors, assists, performs, or prevents a physiological function but does not physically take the place of a body part
Explanation: None

Body Part Character 4	Approach Character 5	Device Character 6	Qualifier Character 7
Ø Products of Conception ♀	Ø Open 7 Via Natural or Artificial Opening	3 Monitoring Electrode Y Other Device	Z No Qualifier

Non-OR All body part, approach, device, and qualifier values
♀ All body part, approach, device, and qualifier values

1 Obstetrics
Ø Pregnancy
J Inspection Definition: Visually and/or manually exploring a body part
Explanation: Visual exploration may be performed with or without optical instrumentation. Manual exploration may be performed directly or through intervening body layers.

Body Part Character 4	Approach Character 5	Device Character 6	Qualifier Character 7
Ø Products of Conception ♀ 1 Products of Conception, Retained ♀ 2 Products of Conception, Ectopic ♀	Ø Open 3 Percutaneous 4 Percutaneous Endoscopic 7 Via Natural or Artificial Opening 8 Via Natural or Artificial Opening Endoscopic X External	Z No Device	Z No Qualifier

Non-OR All body part, approach, device, and qualifier values
♀ All body part, approach, device, and qualifier values

1 Obstetrics
Ø Pregnancy
P Removal Definition: Taking out or off a device from a body part, region or orifice
Explanation: If a device is taken out and a similar device put in without cutting or puncturing the skin or mucous membrane, the procedure is coded to the root operation CHANGE. Otherwise, the procedure for taking out a device is coded to the root operation REMOVAL.

Body Part Character 4	Approach Character 5	Device Character 6	Qualifier Character 7
Ø Products of Conception ♀	Ø Open 7 Via Natural or Artificial Opening	3 Monitoring Electrode Y Other Device	Z No Qualifier

Non-OR All body part, approach, device, and qualifier values
♀ All body part, approach, device, and qualifier values

1 Obstetrics
Ø Pregnancy
Q Repair Definition: Restoring, to the extent possible, a body part to its normal anatomic structure and function
Explanation: Used only when the method to accomplish the repair is not one of the other root operations

Body Part Character 4	Approach Character 5	Device Character 6	Qualifier Character 7
Ø Products of Conception ♀	Ø Open 3 Percutaneous 4 Percutaneous Endoscopic 7 Via Natural or Artificial Opening 8 Via Natural or Artificial Opening Endoscopic	Y Other Device Z No Device	E Nervous System F Cardiovascular System G Lymphatics and Hemic H Eye J Ear, Nose and Sinus K Respiratory System L Mouth and Throat M Gastrointestinal System N Hepatobiliary and Pancreas P Endocrine System Q Skin R Musculoskeletal System S Urinary System T Female Reproductive System V Male Reproductive System Y Other Body System

Non-OR All body part, approach, device, and qualifier values
♀ All body part, approach, device, and qualifier values

1 Obstetrics
Ø Pregnancy
S Reposition Definition: Moving to its normal location, or other suitable location, all or a portion of a body part

Explanation: The body part is moved to a new location from an abnormal location, or from a normal location where it is not functioning correctly. The body part may or may not be cut out or off to be moved to the new location.

Body Part Character 4	Approach Character 5	Device Character 6	Qualifier Character 7
Ø Products of Conception ♀	7 Via Natural or Artificial Opening X External	Z No Device	Z No Qualifier
2 Products of Conception, Ectopic ♀	Ø Open 3 Percutaneous 4 Percutaneous Endoscopic 7 Via Natural or Artificial Opening 8 Via Natural or Artificial Opening Endoscopic	Z No Device	Z No Qualifier

Non-OR 10SØ[7,X]ZZ ♀ All body part, approach, device, and qualifier values

1 Obstetrics
Ø Pregnancy
T Resection Definition: Cutting out or off, without replacement, all of a body part

Explanation: None

Body Part Character 4	Approach Character 5	Device Character 6	Qualifier Character 7
2 Products of Conception, Ectopic ♀	Ø Open 3 Percutaneous 4 Percutaneous Endoscopic 7 Via Natural or Artificial Opening 8 Via Natural or Artificial Opening Endoscopic	Z No Device	Z No Qualifier

♀ All body part, approach, device, and qualifier values

1 Obstetrics
Ø Pregnancy
Y Transplantation Definition: Putting in or on all or a portion of a living body part taken from another individual or animal to physically take the place and/or function of all or a portion of a similar body part

Explanation: The native body part may or may not be taken out, and the transplanted body part may take over all or a portion of its function

Body Part Character 4	Approach Character 5	Device Character 6	Qualifier Character 7
Ø Products of Conception ♀	3 Percutaneous 4 Percutaneous Endoscopic 7 Via Natural or Artificial Opening	Z No Device	E Nervous System F Cardiovascular System G Lymphatics and Hemic H Eye J Ear, Nose and Sinus K Respiratory System L Mouth and Throat M Gastrointestinal System N Hepatobiliary and Pancreas P Endocrine System Q Skin R Musculoskeletal System S Urinary System T Female Reproductive System V Male Reproductive System Y Other Body System

Non-OR All body part, approach, device, and qualifier values ♀ All body part, approach, device, and qualifier values

Placement 2WØ–2Y5

AHA Coding Clinic for table 2W6
2015, 2Q, 35 Application of tongs to reduce and stabilize cervical fracture
2013, 2Q, 39 Application of cervical tongs for reduction of cervical fracture

AHA Coding Clinic for table 2Y4
2018, 4Q, 38 Control of epistaxis
2017, 4Q, 106 Nasal packing for epistaxis

2 Placement
W Anatomical Regions
Ø Change Definition: Taking out or off a device from a body part and putting back an identical or similar device in or on the same body part without cutting or puncturing the skin or a mucous membrane

Body Region Character 4	Approach Character 5	Device Character 6	Qualifier Character 7
Ø Head 2 Neck 3 Abdominal Wall 4 Chest Wall 5 Back 6 Inguinal Region, Right 7 Inguinal Region, Left 8 Upper Extremity, Right 9 Upper Extremity, Left A Upper Arm, Right B Upper Arm, Left C Lower Arm, Right D Lower Arm, Left E Hand, Right F Hand, Left G Thumb, Right H Thumb, Left J Finger, Right K Finger, Left L Lower Extremity, Right M Lower Extremity, Left N Upper Leg, Right P Upper Leg, Left Q Lower Leg, Right R Lower Leg, Left S Foot, Right T Foot, Left U Toe, Right V Toe, Left	X External	Ø Traction Apparatus 1 Splint 2 Cast 3 Brace 4 Bandage 5 Packing Material 6 Pressure Dressing 7 Intermittent Pressure Device Y Other Device	Z No Qualifier
1 Face	X External	Ø Traction Apparatus 1 Splint 2 Cast 3 Brace 4 Bandage 5 Packing Material 6 Pressure Dressing 7 Intermittent Pressure Device 9 Wire Y Other Device	Z No Qualifier

2 Placement
W Anatomical Regions
1 Compression Definition: Putting pressure on a body region

Body Region Character 4	Approach Character 5	Device Character 6	Qualifier Character 7
Ø Head 1 Face 2 Neck 3 Abdominal Wall 4 Chest Wall 5 Back 6 Inguinal Region, Right 7 Inguinal Region, Left 8 Upper Extremity, Right 9 Upper Extremity, Left A Upper Arm, Right B Upper Arm, Left C Lower Arm, Right D Lower Arm, Left E Hand, Right F Hand, Left G Thumb, Right H Thumb, Left J Finger, Right K Finger, Left L Lower Extremity, Right M Lower Extremity, Left N Upper Leg, Right P Upper Leg, Left Q Lower Leg, Right R Lower Leg, Left S Foot, Right T Foot, Left U Toe, Right V Toe, Left	X External	6 Pressure Dressing 7 Intermittent Pressure Device	Z No Qualifier

2 Placement
W Anatomical Regions
2 Dressing Definition: Putting material on a body region for protection

Body Region Character 4	Approach Character 5	Device Character 6	Qualifier Character 7
Ø Head 1 Face 2 Neck 3 Abdominal Wall 4 Chest Wall 5 Back 6 Inguinal Region, Right 7 Inguinal Region, Left 8 Upper Extremity, Right 9 Upper Extremity, Left A Upper Arm, Right B Upper Arm, Left C Lower Arm, Right D Lower Arm, Left E Hand, Right F Hand, Left G Thumb, Right H Thumb, Left J Finger, Right K Finger, Left L Lower Extremity, Right M Lower Extremity, Left N Upper Leg, Right P Upper Leg, Left Q Lower Leg, Right R Lower Leg, Left S Foot, Right T Foot, Left U Toe, Right V Toe, Left	X External	4 Bandage	Z No Qualifier

2 Placement
W Anatomical Regions
3 Immobilization Definition: Limiting or preventing motion of a body region

Body Region Character 4	Approach Character 5	Device Character 6	Qualifier Character 7
Ø Head 2 Neck 3 Abdominal Wall 4 Chest Wall 5 Back 6 Inguinal Region, Right 7 Inguinal Region, Left 8 Upper Extremity, Right 9 Upper Extremity, Left A Upper Arm, Right B Upper Arm, Left C Lower Arm, Right D Lower Arm, Left E Hand, Right F Hand, Left G Thumb, Right H Thumb, Left J Finger, Right K Finger, Left L Lower Extremity, Right M Lower Extremity, Left N Upper Leg, Right P Upper Leg, Left Q Lower Leg, Right R Lower Leg, Left S Foot, Right T Foot, Left U Toe, Right V Toe, Left	X External	1 Splint 2 Cast 3 Brace Y Other Device	Z No Qualifier
1 Face	X External	1 Splint 2 Cast 3 Brace 9 Wire Y Other Device	Z No Qualifier

2 Placement
W Anatomical Regions
4 Packing Definition: Putting material in a body region or orifice

Body Region Character 4	Approach Character 5	Device Character 6	Qualifier Character 7
Ø Head 1 Face 2 Neck 3 Abdominal Wall 4 Chest Wall 5 Back 6 Inguinal Region, Right 7 Inguinal Region, Left 8 Upper Extremity, Right 9 Upper Extremity, Left A Upper Arm, Right B Upper Arm, Left C Lower Arm, Right D Lower Arm, Left E Hand, Right F Hand, Left G Thumb, Right H Thumb, Left J Finger, Right K Finger, Left L Lower Extremity, Right M Lower Extremity, Left N Upper Leg, Right P Upper Leg, Left Q Lower Leg, Right R Lower Leg, Left S Foot, Right T Foot, Left U Toe, Right V Toe, Left	X External	5 Packing Material	Z No Qualifier

2 Placement
W Anatomical Regions
5 Removal Definition: Taking out or off a device from a body part

Body Region Character 4	Approach Character 5	Device Character 6	Qualifier Character 7
Ø Head **2** Neck **3** Abdominal Wall **4** Chest Wall **5** Back **6** Inguinal Region, Right **7** Inguinal Region, Left **8** Upper Extremity, Right **9** Upper Extremity, Left **A** Upper Arm, Right **B** Upper Arm, Left **C** Lower Arm, Right **D** Lower Arm, Left **E** Hand, Right **F** Hand, Left **G** Thumb, Right **H** Thumb, Left **J** Finger, Right **K** Finger, Left **L** Lower Extremity, Right **M** Lower Extremity, Left **N** Upper Leg, Right **P** Upper Leg, Left **Q** Lower Leg, Right **R** Lower Leg, Left **S** Foot, Right **T** Foot, Left **U** Toe, Right **V** Toe, Left	**X** External	**Ø** Traction Apparatus **1** Splint **2** Cast **3** Brace **4** Bandage **5** Packing Material **6** Pressure Dressing **7** Intermittent Pressure Device **Y** Other Device	**Z** No Qualifier
1 Face	**X** External	**Ø** Traction Apparatus **1** Splint **2** Cast **3** Brace **4** Bandage **5** Packing Material **6** Pressure Dressing **7** Intermittent Pressure Device **9** Wire **Y** Other Device	**Z** No Qualifier

2 Placement
W Anatomical Regions
6 Traction Definition: Exerting a pulling force on a body region in a distal direction

Body Region Character 4	Approach Character 5	Device Character 6	Qualifier Character 7
Ø Head 1 Face 2 Neck 3 Abdominal Wall 4 Chest Wall 5 Back 6 Inguinal Region, Right 7 Inguinal Region, Left 8 Upper Extremity, Right 9 Upper Extremity, Left A Upper Arm, Right B Upper Arm, Left C Lower Arm, Right D Lower Arm, Left E Hand, Right F Hand, Left G Thumb, Right H Thumb, Left J Finger, Right K Finger, Left L Lower Extremity, Right M Lower Extremity, Left N Upper Leg, Right P Upper Leg, Left Q Lower Leg, Right R Lower Leg, Left S Foot, Right T Foot, Left U Toe, Right V Toe, Left	X External	Ø Traction Apparatus Z No Device	Z No Qualifier

2 Placement
Y Anatomical Orifices
Ø Change Definition: Taking out or off a device from a body part and putting back an identical or similar device in or on the same body part without cutting or puncturing the skin or a mucous membrane

Body Region Character 4	Approach Character 5	Device Character 6	Qualifier Character 7
Ø Mouth and Pharynx 1 Nasal 2 Ear 3 Anorectal 4 Female Genital Tract ♀ 5 Urethra	X External	5 Packing Material	Z No Qualifier

♀ 2YØ4X5Z

2 Placement
Y Anatomical Orifices
4 Packing Definition: Putting material in a body region or orifice

Body Region Character 4	Approach Character 5	Device Character 6	Qualifier Character 7
Ø Mouth and Pharynx 1 Nasal 2 Ear 3 Anorectal 4 Female Genital Tract ♀ 5 Urethra	X External	5 Packing Material	Z No Qualifier

♀ 2Y44X5Z

2 Placement
Y Anatomical Orifices
5 Removal Definition: Taking out or off a device from a body part

Body Region Character 4	Approach Character 5	Device Character 6	Qualifier Character 7
Ø Mouth and Pharynx 1 Nasal 2 Ear 3 Anorectal 4 Female Genital Tract ♀ 5 Urethra	X External	5 Packing Material	Z No Qualifier

♀ 2Y54X5Z

Administration 3Ø2–3E1

AHA Coding Clinic for table 3Ø2

2020, 4Q, 60-61	Transfusion stem cell progenitor cells
2019, 4Q, 35	Transfusion of blood products
2019, 4Q, 36	T-cell depleted hematopoietic stem cells for transplantation
2016, 4Q, 113	Bone marrow and stem cell transfusion (Transplantation)

AHA Coding Clinic for table 3EØ

2021, 1Q, 49	Frequently asked questions regarding ICD-1Ø-CM and ICD-1Ø-PCS coding for COVID-19
2020, 4Q, 49-50	Intravascular ultrasound assisted thrombolysis
2020, 4Q, 95	Frequently Asked Questions Regarding ICD-1Ø-PCS Coding for COVID-19
2020, 3Q, 17-21	New procedure codes for introduction or infusion of therapeutics
2019, 4Q, 36-37	Hyperthermic antineoplastic chemotherapy
2018, 3Q, 7	Coronary brachytherapy with angioplasty
2018, 1Q, 8	Placement of bone morphogenetic protein & spinal fusion surgery
2017, 2Q, 14	Infusion of tPA into pleural cavity
2017, 1Q, 37	Injection of glue into enteric fistula tract
2016, 4Q, 113-114	Substances applied to cranial cavity and brain
2016, 3Q, 29	Closure of bilateral alveolar clefts
2016, 1Q, 20	Metatarsophalangeal joint resection arthroplasty
2015, 3Q, 24	Esophagogastroduodenoscopy with epinephrine injection for control of bleeding

AHA Coding Clinic for table 3EØ (Continued)

2015, 3Q, 29	Placement of adhesion barrier
2015, 2Q, 29	Insertion of nasogastric tube for drainage and feeding
2015, 2Q, 31	Thoracoscopic talc pleurodesis
2015, 1Q, 31	Intrathecal chemotherapy
2015, 1Q, 38	Chemoembolization of the hepatic artery
2014, 4Q, 16	Administration of RH (D) immunoglobulin
2014, 4Q, 17	RH (D) alloimmunization (sensitization)
2014, 4Q, 19	Ultrasound accelerated thrombolysis
2014, 4Q, 34	Resection of brain malignancy with implantation of chemotherapeutic wafer
2014, 4Q, 38	Placement of saline and seprafilm solution into abdominal cavity
2014, 3Q, 26	Coil embolization of gastroduodenal artery with chemoembolization of hepatic artery
2014, 2Q, 8	Medical induction of labor with Cervidil tampon insertion
2014, 2Q, 10	Prophylactic Neulasta injection for infection prevention
2013, 4Q, 124	Administration of tPA for stroke treatment prior to transfer
2013, 1Q, 27	Injection of sclerosing agent into an esophageal varix

AHA Coding Clinic for table 3E1

2019, 4Q, 38	Irrigation of joint using irrigating substance
2017, 3Q, 14	Bronchoscopy with suctioning and washings for removal of mucus plug

3 Administration
Ø Circulatory
2 Transfusion Definition: Putting in blood or blood products

Body System/Region Character 4	Approach Character 5	Substance Character 6	Qualifier Character 7
3 Peripheral Vein NC 4 Central Vein NC	3 Percutaneous	A Stem Cells, Embryonic	Z No Qualifier
3 Peripheral Vein 4 Central Vein	3 Percutaneous	C Hematopoietic Stem/Progenitor Cells, Genetically Modified	Ø Autologous
3 Peripheral Vein 4 Central Vein	3 Percutaneous	D Pathogen Reduced Cryoprecipitated Fibrinogen Complex	1 Nonautologous
3 Peripheral Vein NC 4 Central Vein NC	3 Percutaneous	G Bone Marrow X Stem Cells, Cord Blood Y Stem Cells, Hematopoietic	Ø Autologous 2 Allogeneic, Related 3 Allogeneic, Unrelated 4 Allogeneic, Unspecified
3 Peripheral Vein 4 Central Vein	3 Percutaneous	H Whole Blood J Serum Albumin K Frozen Plasma L Fresh Plasma M Plasma Cryoprecipitate N Red Blood Cells P Frozen Red Cells Q White Cells R Platelets S Globulin T Fibrinogen V Antihemophilic Factors W Factor IX	Ø Autologous 1 Nonautologous
3 Peripheral Vein 4 Central Vein	3 Percutaneous	U Stem Cells, T-cell Depleted Hematopoietic	2 Allogeneic, Related 3 Allogeneic, Unrelated 4 Allogeneic, Unspecified
7 Products of Conception, Circulatory ♀	3 Percutaneous 7 Via Natural or Artificial Opening	H Whole Blood J Serum Albumin K Frozen Plasma L Fresh Plasma M Plasma Cryoprecipitate N Red Blood Cells P Frozen Red Cells Q White Cells R Platelets S Globulin T Fibrinogen V Antihemophilic Factors W Factor IX	1 Nonautologous
8 Vein	3 Percutaneous	B 4-Factor Prothrombin Complex Concentrate	1 Nonautologous

DRG Non-OR 3Ø2[3,4]3AZ
DRG Non-OR 3Ø2[3,4]3CØ
DRG Non-OR 3Ø2[3,4]3[G,X,Y][Ø,2,3,4]
DRG Non-OR 3Ø2[3,4]3U[2,3,4]

NC 3Ø2[3,4]3AZ Only when reported with PDx or SDx of C91.ØØ, C92.ØØ, C92.1Ø, C92.11, C92.4Ø, C92.5Ø, C92.6Ø, C92.AØ, C93.ØØ, C94.ØØ, C95.ØØ
NC 3Ø2[3,4]3[G,Y]Ø Only when reported with PDx or SDx of C91.ØØ, C92.ØØ, C92.1Ø, C92.11, C92.4Ø, C92.5Ø, C92.6Ø, C92.AØ, C93.ØØ, C94.ØØ, C95.ØØ
♀ 3Ø27[3,7][H,J,K,L,M,N,P,Q,R,S,T,V,W]1

3 Administration
C Indwelling Device
1 Irrigation Definition: Putting in or on a cleansing substance

Body System/Region Character 4	Approach Character 5	Substance Character 6	Qualifier Character 7
Z None	**X** External	**8** Irrigating Substance	**Z** No Qualifier

3 Administration
E Physiological Systems and Anatomical Regions
Ø Introduction Definition: Putting in or on a therapeutic, diagnostic, nutritional, physiological, or prophylactic substance except blood or blood products

Body System/Region Character 4	Approach Character 5	Substance Character 6	Qualifier Character 7
Ø Skin and Mucous Membranes	**X** External	**Ø** Antineoplastic	**5** Other Antineoplastic **M** Monoclonal Antibody
Ø Skin and Mucous Membranes	**X** External	**2** Anti-infective	**8** Oxazolidinones **9** Other Anti-infective
Ø Skin and Mucous Membranes	**X** External	**3** Anti-inflammatory **4** Serum, Toxoid and Vaccine **B** Anesthetic Agent **K** Other Diagnostic Substance **M** Pigment **N** Analgesics, Hypnotics, Sedatives **T** Destructive Agent	**Z** No Qualifier
Ø Skin and Mucous Membranes	**X** External	**G** Other Therapeutic Substance	**C** Other Substance
1 Subcutaneous Tissue	**Ø** Open	**2** Anti-infective	**A** Anti-Infective Envelope
1 Subcutaneous Tissue	**3** Percutaneous	**Ø** Antineoplastic	**5** Other Antineoplastic **M** Monoclonal Antibody
1 Subcutaneous Tissue	**3** Percutaneous	**2** Anti-infective	**8** Oxazolidinones **9** Other Anti-infective **A** Anti-Infective Envelope
1 Subcutaneous Tissue	**3** Percutaneous	**3** Anti-inflammatory **6** Nutritional Substance **7** Electrolytic and Water Balance Substance **B** Anesthetic Agent **H** Radioactive Substance **K** Other Diagnostic Substance **N** Analgesics, Hypnotics, Sedatives **T** Destructive Agent	**Z** No Qualifier
1 Subcutaneous Tissue	**3** Percutaneous	**4** Serum, Toxoid and Vaccine	**Ø** Influenza Vaccine **Z** No Qualifier
1 Subcutaneous Tissue	**3** Percutaneous	**G** Other Therapeutic Substance	**C** Other Substance
1 Subcutaneous Tissue	**3** Percutaneous	**V** Hormone	**G** Insulin **J** Other Hormone
2 Muscle	**3** Percutaneous	**Ø** Antineoplastic	**5** Other Antineoplastic **M** Monoclonal Antibody
2 Muscle	**3** Percutaneous	**2** Anti-infective	**8** Oxazolidinones **9** Other Anti-infective
2 Muscle	**3** Percutaneous	**3** Anti-inflammatory **6** Nutritional Substance **7** Electrolytic and Water Balance Substance **B** Anesthetic Agent **H** Radioactive Substance **K** Other Diagnostic Substance **N** Analgesics, Hypnotics, Sedatives **T** Destructive Agent	**Z** No Qualifier
2 Muscle	**3** Percutaneous	**4** Serum, Toxoid and Vaccine	**Ø** Influenza Vaccine **Z** No Qualifier
2 Muscle	**3** Percutaneous	**G** Other Therapeutic Substance	**C** Other Substance
3 Peripheral Vein	**Ø** Open	**Ø** Antineoplastic	**2** High-dose Interleukin-2 **3** Low-dose Interleukin-2 **5** Other Antineoplastic **M** Monoclonal Antibody **P** Clofarabine
3 Peripheral Vein	**Ø** Open	**1** Thrombolytic	**6** Recombinant Human- activated Protein C **7** Other Thrombolytic
3 Peripheral Vein	**Ø** Open	**2** Anti-infective	**8** Oxazolidinones **9** Other Anti-infective

DRG Non-OR 3EØ3ØØ2
DRG Non-OR 3EØ3Ø17

3EØ Continued on next page

3EØ Continued

3 Administration
E Physiological Systems and Anatomical Regions
Ø Introduction Definition: Putting in or on a therapeutic, diagnostic, nutritional, physiological, or prophylactic substance except blood or blood products

Body System/Region Character 4	Approach Character 5	Substance Character 6	Qualifier Character 7
3 Peripheral Vein	Ø Open	3 Anti-inflammatory 4 Serum, Toxoid and Vaccine 6 Nutritional Substance 7 Electrolytic and Water Balance Substance F Intracirculatory Anesthetic H Radioactive Substance K Other Diagnostic Substance N Analgesics, Hypnotics, Sedatives P Platelet Inhibitor R Antiarrhythmic T Destructive Agent X Vasopressor	Z No Qualifier
3 Peripheral Vein	Ø Open	G Other Therapeutic Substance	C Other Substance N Blood Brain Barrier Disruption
3 Peripheral Vein	Ø Open	U Pancreatic Islet Cells	Ø Autologous 1 Nonautologous
3 Peripheral Vein	Ø Open	V Hormone	G Insulin H Human B-type Natriuretic Peptide J Other Hormone
3 Peripheral Vein	Ø Open	W Immunotherapeutic	K Immunostimulator L Immunosuppressive
3 Peripheral Vein	3 Percutaneous	Ø Antineoplastic	2 High-dose Interleukin-2 3 Low-dose Interleukin-2 5 Other Antineoplastic M Monoclonal Antibody P Clofarabine
3 Peripheral Vein	3 Percutaneous	1 Thrombolytic	6 Recombinant Human- activated Protein C 7 Other Thrombolytic
3 Peripheral Vein	3 Percutaneous	2 Anti-infective	8 Oxazolidinones 9 Other Anti-infective
3 Peripheral Vein	3 Percutaneous	3 Anti-inflammatory 4 Serum, Toxoid and Vaccine 6 Nutritional Substance 7 Electrolytic and Water Balance Substance F Intracirculatory Anesthetic H Radioactive Substance K Other Diagnostic Substance N Analgesics, Hypnotics, Sedatives P Platelet Inhibitor R Antiarrhythmic T Destructive Agent X Vasopressor	Z No Qualifier
3 Peripheral Vein	3 Percutaneous	G Other Therapeutic Substance	C Other Substance N Blood Brain Barrier Disruption Q Glucarpidase
3 Peripheral Vein	3 Percutaneous	U Pancreatic Islet Cells	Ø Autologous 1 Nonautologous
3 Peripheral Vein	3 Percutaneous	V Hormone	G Insulin H Human B-type Natriuretic Peptide J Other Hormone
3 Peripheral Vein	3 Percutaneous	W Immunotherapeutic	K Immunostimulator L Immunosuppressive
4 Central Vein	Ø Open	Ø Antineoplastic	2 High-dose Interleukin-2 3 Low-dose Interleukin-2 5 Other Antineoplastic M Monoclonal Antibody P Clofarabine
4 Central Vein	Ø Open	1 Thrombolytic	6 Recombinant Human- activated Protein C 7 Other Thrombolytic

Valid OR 3EØ3ØTZ
DRG Non-OR 3EØ3ØU[Ø,1]
DRG Non-OR 3EØ33Ø2
DRG Non-OR 3EØ3317
DRG Non-OR 3EØ33U[Ø,1]
DRG Non-OR 3EØ4ØØ2
DRG Non-OR 3EØ4Ø17

3EØ Continued on next page

Administration

3EØ Continued

3 Administration
E Physiological Systems and Anatomical Regions
Ø Introduction Definition: Putting in or on a therapeutic, diagnostic, nutritional, physiological, or prophylactic substance except blood or blood products

Body System/Region Character 4	Approach Character 5	Substance Character 6	Qualifier Character 7
4 Central Vein	Ø Open	2 Anti-infective	8 Oxazolidinones 9 Other Anti-infective
4 Central Vein	Ø Open	3 Anti-inflammatory 4 Serum, Toxoid and Vaccine 6 Nutritional Substance 7 Electrolytic and Water Balance Substance F Intracirculatory Anesthetic H Radioactive Substance K Other Diagnostic Substance N Analgesics, Hypnotics, Sedatives P Platelet Inhibitor R Antiarrhythmic T Destructive Agent X Vasopressor	Z No Qualifier
4 Central Vein	Ø Open	G Other Therapeutic Substance	C Other Substance N Blood Brain Barrier Disruption
4 Central Vein	Ø Open	V Hormone	G Insulin H Human B-type Natriuretic Peptide J Other Hormone
4 Central Vein	Ø Open	W Immunotherapeutic	K Immunostimulator L Immunosuppressive
4 Central Vein	3 Percutaneous	Ø Antineoplastic	2 High-dose Interleukin-2 3 Low-dose Interleukin-2 5 Other Antineoplastic M Monoclonal Antibody P Clofarabine
4 Central Vein	3 Percutaneous	1 Thrombolytic	6 Recombinant Human- activated Protein C 7 Other Thrombolytic
4 Central Vein	3 Percutaneous	2 Anti-infective	8 Oxazolidinones 9 Other Anti-infective
4 Central Vein	3 Percutaneous	3 Anti-inflammatory 4 Serum, Toxoid and Vaccine 6 Nutritional Substance 7 Electrolytic and Water Balance Substance F Intracirculatory Anesthetic H Radioactive Substance K Other Diagnostic Substance N Analgesics, Hypnotics, Sedatives P Platelet Inhibitor R Antiarrhythmic T Destructive Agent X Vasopressor	Z No Qualifier
4 Central Vein	3 Percutaneous	G Other Therapeutic Substance	C Other Substance N Blood Brain Barrier Disruption Q Glucarpidase
4 Central Vein	3 Percutaneous	V Hormone	G Insulin H Human B-type Natriuretic Peptide J Other Hormone
4 Central Vein	3 Percutaneous	W Immunotherapeutic	K Immunostimulator L Immunosuppressive
5 Peripheral Artery 6 Central Artery	Ø Open 3 Percutaneous	Ø Antineoplastic	2 High-dose Interleukin-2 3 Low-dose Interleukin-2 5 Other Antineoplastic M Monoclonal Antibody P Clofarabine
5 Peripheral Artery 6 Central Artery	Ø Open 3 Percutaneous	1 Thrombolytic	6 Recombinant Human- activated Protein C 7 Other Thrombolytic
5 Peripheral Artery 6 Central Artery	Ø Open 3 Percutaneous	2 Anti-infective	8 Oxazolidinones 9 Other Anti-infective

Valid OR 3EØ4ØTZ
DRG Non-OR 3EØ43Ø2
DRG Non-OR 3EØ4317
DRG Non-OR 3EØ[5,6][Ø,3]Ø2
DRG Non-OR 3EØ[5,6][Ø,3]17

3EØ Continued on next page

3EØ–3EØ

3 Administration
E Physiological Systems and Anatomical Regions
Ø Introduction Definition: Putting in or on a therapeutic, diagnostic, nutritional, physiological, or prophylactic substance except blood or blood products

3EØ Continued

Body System/Region Character 4	Approach Character 5	Substance Character 6	Qualifier Character 7
5 Peripheral Artery 6 Central Artery	Ø Open 3 Percutaneous	3 Anti-inflammatory 4 Serum, Toxoid and Vaccine 6 Nutritional Substance 7 Electrolytic and Water Balance Substance F Intracirculatory Anesthetic H Radioactive Substance K Other Diagnostic Substance N Analgesics, Hypnotics, Sedatives P Platelet Inhibitor R Antiarrhythmic T Destructive Agent X Vasopressor	Z No Qualifier
5 Peripheral Artery 6 Central Artery	Ø Open 3 Percutaneous	G Other Therapeutic Substance	C Other Substance N Blood Brain Barrier Disruption
5 Peripheral Artery 6 Central Artery	Ø Open 3 Percutaneous	V Hormone	G Insulin H Human B-type Natriuretic Peptide J Other Hormone
5 Peripheral Artery 6 Central Artery	Ø Open 3 Percutaneous	W Immunotherapeutic	K Immunostimulator L Immunosuppressive
7 Coronary Artery 8 Heart	Ø Open 3 Percutaneous	1 Thrombolytic	6 Recombinant Human- activated Protein C 7 Other Thrombolytic
7 Coronary Artery 8 Heart	Ø Open 3 Percutaneous	G Other Therapeutic Substance	C Other Substance
7 Coronary Artery 8 Heart	Ø Open 3 Percutaneous	K Other Diagnostic Substance P Platelet Inhibitor	Z No Qualifier
7 Coronary Artery 8 Heart	4 Percutaneous Endoscopic	G Other Therapeutic Substance	C Other Substance
9 Nose	3 Percutaneous 7 Via Natural or Artificial Opening X External	Ø Antineoplastic	5 Other Antineoplastic M Monoclonal Antibody
9 Nose	3 Percutaneous 7 Via Natural or Artificial Opening X External	2 Anti-infective	8 Oxazolidinones 9 Other Anti-infective
9 Nose	3 Percutaneous 7 Via Natural or Artificial Opening X External	3 Anti-inflammatory 4 Serum, Toxoid and Vaccine B Anesthetic Agent H Radioactive Substance K Other Diagnostic Substance N Analgesics, Hypnotics, Sedatives T Destructive Agent	Z No Qualifier
9 Nose	3 Percutaneous 7 Via Natural or Artificial Opening X External	G Other Therapeutic Substance	C Other Substance
A Bone Marrow	3 Percutaneous	Ø Antineoplastic	5 Other Antineoplastic M Monoclonal Antibody
A Bone Marrow	3 Percutaneous	G Other Therapeutic Substance	C Other Substance
B Ear	3 Percutaneous 7 Via Natural or Artificial Opening X External	Ø Antineoplastic	4 Liquid Brachytherapy Radioisotope 5 Other Antineoplastic M Monoclonal Antibody
B Ear	3 Percutaneous 7 Via Natural or Artificial Opening X External	2 Anti-infective	8 Oxazolidinones 9 Other Anti-infective
B Ear	3 Percutaneous 7 Via Natural or Artificial Opening X External	3 Anti-inflammatory B Anesthetic Agent H Radioactive Substance K Other Diagnostic Substance N Analgesics, Hypnotics, Sedatives T Destructive Agent	Z No Qualifier
B Ear	3 Percutaneous 7 Via Natural or Artificial Opening X External	G Other Therapeutic Substance	C Other Substance

DRG Non-OR 3EØ8[Ø,3]17

3EØ Continued on next page

3 Administration
E Physiological Systems and Anatomical Regions
Ø Introduction Definition: Putting in or on a therapeutic, diagnostic, nutritional, physiological, or prophylactic substance except blood or blood products

3EØ Continued

Body System/Region Character 4	Approach Character 5	Substance Character 6	Qualifier Character 7
C Eye	3 Percutaneous 7 Via Natural or Artificial Opening X External	Ø Antineoplastic	4 Liquid Brachytherapy Radioisotope 5 Other Antineoplastic M Monoclonal Antibody
C Eye	3 Percutaneous 7 Via Natural or Artificial Opening X External	2 Anti-infective	8 Oxazolidinones 9 Other Anti-infective
C Eye	3 Percutaneous 7 Via Natural or Artificial Opening X External	3 Anti-inflammatory B Anesthetic Agent H Radioactive Substance K Other Diagnostic Substance M Pigment N Analgesics, Hypnotics, Sedatives T Destructive Agent	Z No Qualifier
C Eye	3 Percutaneous 7 Via Natural or Artificial Opening X External	G Other Therapeutic Substance	C Other Substance
C Eye	3 Percutaneous 7 Via Natural or Artificial Opening X External	S Gas	F Other Gas
D Mouth and Pharynx	3 Percutaneous 7 Via Natural or Artificial Opening X External	Ø Antineoplastic	4 Liquid Brachytherapy Radioisotope 5 Other Antineoplastic M Monoclonal Antibody
D Mouth and Pharynx	3 Percutaneous 7 Via Natural or Artificial Opening X External	2 Anti-infective	8 Oxazolidinones 9 Other Anti-infective
D Mouth and Pharynx	3 Percutaneous 7 Via Natural or Artificial Opening X External	3 Anti-inflammatory 4 Serum, Toxoid and Vaccine 6 Nutritional Substance 7 Electrolytic and Water Balance Substance B Anesthetic Agent H Radioactive Substance K Other Diagnostic Substance N Analgesics, Hypnotics, Sedatives R Antiarrhythmic T Destructive Agent	Z No Qualifier
D Mouth and Pharynx	3 Percutaneous 7 Via Natural or Artificial Opening X External	G Other Therapeutic Substance	C Other Substance
E Products of Conception ♀ G Upper GI H Lower GI K Genitourinary Tract N Male Reproductive ♂	3 Percutaneous 7 Via Natural or Artificial Opening 8 Via Natural or Artificial Opening Endoscopic	Ø Antineoplastic	4 Liquid Brachytherapy Radioisotope 5 Other Antineoplastic M Monoclonal Antibody
E Products of Conception ♀ G Upper GI H Lower GI K Genitourinary Tract N Male Reproductive ♂	3 Percutaneous 7 Via Natural or Artificial Opening 8 Via Natural or Artificial Opening Endoscopic	2 Anti-infective	8 Oxazolidinones 9 Other Anti-infective
E Products of Conception ♀ G Upper GI H Lower GI K Genitourinary Tract N Male Reproductive ♂	3 Percutaneous 7 Via Natural or Artificial Opening 8 Via Natural or Artificial Opening Endoscopic	3 Anti-inflammatory 6 Nutritional Substance 7 Electrolytic and Water Balance Substance B Anesthetic Agent H Radioactive Substance K Other Diagnostic Substance N Analgesics, Hypnotics, Sedatives T Destructive Agent	Z No Qualifier
E Products of Conception ♀ G Upper GI H Lower GI K Genitourinary Tract N Male Reproductive ♂	3 Percutaneous 7 Via Natural or Artificial Opening 8 Via Natural or Artificial Opening Endoscopic	G Other Therapeutic Substance	C Other Substance

♂ All approach, substance, and qualifier values for body system/region (character 4) with this icon
♀ All approach, substance, and qualifier values for body system/region (character 4) with this icon

3EØ Continued on next page

3 Administration
E Physiological Systems and Anatomical Regions
Ø Introduction Definition: Putting in or on a therapeutic, diagnostic, nutritional, physiological, or prophylactic substance except blood or blood products

3EØ Continued

Body System/Region Character 4	Approach Character 5	Substance Character 6	Qualifier Character 7
E Products of Conception ♀ **G** Upper GI **H** Lower GI **K** Genitourinary Tract **N** Male Reproductive ♂	**3** Percutaneous **7** Via Natural or Artificial Opening **8** Via Natural or Artificial Opening Endoscopic	**S** Gas	**F** Other Gas
E Products of Conception ♀ **G** Upper GI **H** Lower GI **K** Genitourinary Tract **N** Male Reproductive ♂	**4** Percutaneous Endoscopic	**G** Other Therapeutic Substance	**C** Other Substance
F Respiratory Tract	**3** Percutaneous **7** Via Natural or Artificial Opening **8** Via Natural or Artificial Opening Endoscopic	**Ø** Antineoplastic	**4** Liquid Brachytherapy Radioisotope **5** Other Antineoplastic **M** Monoclonal Antibody
F Respiratory Tract	**3** Percutaneous **7** Via Natural or Artificial Opening **8** Via Natural or Artificial Opening Endoscopic	**2** Anti-infective	**8** Oxazolidinones **9** Other Anti-infective
F Respiratory Tract	**3** Percutaneous **7** Via Natural or Artificial Opening **8** Via Natural or Artificial Opening Endoscopic	**3** Anti-inflammatory **6** Nutritional Substance **7** Electrolytic and Water Balance Substance **B** Anesthetic Agent **H** Radioactive Substance **K** Other Diagnostic Substance **N** Analgesics, Hypnotics, Sedatives **T** Destructive Agent	**Z** No Qualifier
F Respiratory Tract	**3** Percutaneous **7** Via Natural or Artificial Opening **8** Via Natural or Artificial Opening Endoscopic	**G** Other Therapeutic Substance	**C** Other Substance
F Respiratory Tract	**3** Percutaneous **7** Via Natural or Artificial Opening **8** Via Natural or Artificial Opening Endoscopic	**S** Gas	**D** Nitric Oxide **F** Other Gas
F Respiratory Tract	**4** Percutaneous Endoscopic	**G** Other Therapeutic Substance	**C** Other Substance
J Biliary and Pancreatic Tract	**3** Percutaneous **7** Via Natural or Artificial Opening **8** Via Natural or Artificial Opening Endoscopic	**Ø** Antineoplastic	**4** Liquid Brachytherapy Radioisotope **5** Other Antineoplastic **M** Monoclonal Antibody
J Biliary and Pancreatic Tract	**3** Percutaneous **7** Via Natural or Artificial Opening **8** Via Natural or Artificial Opening Endoscopic	**2** Anti-infective	**8** Oxazolidinones **9** Other Anti-infective
J Biliary and Pancreatic Tract	**3** Percutaneous **7** Via Natural or Artificial Opening **8** Via Natural or Artificial Opening Endoscopic	**3** Anti-inflammatory **6** Nutritional Substance **7** Electrolytic and Water Balance Substance **B** Anesthetic Agent **H** Radioactive Substance **K** Other Diagnostic Substance **N** Analgesics, Hypnotics, Sedatives **T** Destructive Agent	**Z** No Qualifier
J Biliary and Pancreatic Tract	**3** Percutaneous **7** Via Natural or Artificial Opening **8** Via Natural or Artificial Opening Endoscopic	**G** Other Therapeutic Substance	**C** Other Substance
J Biliary and Pancreatic Tract	**3** Percutaneous **7** Via Natural or Artificial Opening **8** Via Natural or Artificial Opening Endoscopic	**S** Gas	**F** Other Gas

♂ All approach, substance, and qualifier values for body system/region (character 4) with this icon
♀ All approach, substance, and qualifier values for body system/region (character 4) with this icon

3EØ Continued on next page

3 Administration ***3EØ Continued***
E Physiological Systems and Anatomical Regions
Ø Introduction Definition: Putting in or on a therapeutic, diagnostic, nutritional, physiological, or prophylactic substance except blood or blood products

Body System/Region Character 4	Approach Character 5	Substance Character 6	Qualifier Character 7
J Biliary and Pancreatic Tract	**3 Percutaneous** **7 Via Natural or Artificial Opening** **8 Via Natural or Artificial Opening Endoscopic**	**U Pancreatic Islet Cells**	**Ø Autologous** **1 Nonautologous**
J Biliary and Pancreatic Tract	**4 Percutaneous Endoscopic**	**G Other Therapeutic Substance**	**C Other Substance**
L Pleural Cavity	**Ø Open**	**5 Adhesion Barrier**	**Z No Qualifier**
L Pleural Cavity	**3 Percutaneous**	**Ø Antineoplastic**	**4 Liquid Brachytherapy Radioisotope** **5 Other Antineoplastic** **M Monoclonal Antibody**
L Pleural Cavity	**3 Percutaneous**	**2 Anti-infective**	**8 Oxazolidinones** **9 Other Anti-infective**
L Pleural Cavity	**3 Percutaneous**	**3 Anti-inflammatory** **5 Adhesion Barrier** **6 Nutritional Substance** **7 Electrolytic and Water Balance Substance** **B Anesthetic Agent** **H Radioactive Substance** **K Other Diagnostic Substance** **N Analgesics, Hypnotics, Sedatives** **T Destructive Agent**	**Z No Qualifier**
L Pleural Cavity	**3 Percutaneous**	**G Other Therapeutic Substance**	**C Other Substance**
L Pleural Cavity	**3 Percutaneous**	**S Gas**	**F Other Gas**
L Pleural Cavity	**4 Percutaneous Endoscopic**	**5 Adhesion Barrier**	**Z No Qualifier**
L Pleural Cavity	**4 Percutaneous Endoscopic**	**G Other Therapeutic Substance**	**C Other Substance**
L Pleural Cavity	**7 Via Natural or Artificial Opening**	**Ø Antineoplastic**	**4 Liquid Brachytherapy Radioisotope** **5 Other Antineoplastic** **M Monoclonal Antibody**
L Pleural Cavity	**7 Via Natural or Artificial Opening**	**S Gas**	**F Other Gas**
M Peritoneal Cavity	**Ø Open**	**5 Adhesion Barrier**	**Z No Qualifier**
M Peritoneal Cavity	**3 Percutaneous**	**Ø Antineoplastic**	**4 Liquid Brachytherapy Radioisotope** **5 Other Antineoplastic** **M Monoclonal Antibody** **Y Hyperthermic**
M Peritoneal Cavity	**3 Percutaneous**	**2 Anti-infective**	**8 Oxazolidinones** **9 Other Anti-infective**
M Peritoneal Cavity	**3 Percutaneous**	**3 Anti-inflammatory** **5 Adhesion Barrier** **6 Nutritional Substance** **7 Electrolytic and Water Balance Substance** **B Anesthetic Agent** **H Radioactive Substance** **K Other Diagnostic Substance** **N Analgesics, Hypnotics, Sedatives** **T Destructive Agent**	**Z No Qualifier**
M Peritoneal Cavity	**3 Percutaneous**	**G Other Therapeutic Substance**	**C Other Substance**
M Peritoneal Cavity	**3 Percutaneous**	**S Gas**	**F Other Gas**
M Peritoneal Cavity	**4 Percutaneous Endoscopic**	**5 Adhesion Barrier**	**Z No Qualifier**
M Peritoneal Cavity	**4 Percutaneous Endoscopic**	**G Other Therapeutic Substance**	**C Other Substance**
M Peritoneal Cavity	**7 Via Natural or Artificial Opening**	**Ø Antineoplastic**	**4 Liquid Brachytherapy Radioisotope** **5 Other Antineoplastic** **M Monoclonal Antibody**
M Peritoneal Cavity	**7 Via Natural or Artificial Opening**	**S Gas**	**F Other Gas**
P Female Reproductive ♀	**Ø Open**	**5 Adhesion Barrier**	**Z No Qualifier**
P Female Reproductive ♀	**3 Percutaneous**	**Ø Antineoplastic**	**4 Liquid Brachytherapy Radioisotope** **5 Other Antineoplastic** **M Monoclonal Antibody**
P Female Reproductive ♀	**3 Percutaneous**	**2 Anti-infective**	**8 Oxazolidinones** **9 Other Anti-infective**

Valid OR 3EØL4GC
DRG Non-OR 3EØJ[3,7,8]U[Ø,1]
♀ All approach, substance, and qualifier values for body system/region (character 4) with this icon

3EØ Continued on next page

3 Administration
E Physiological Systems and Anatomical Regions
Ø Introduction Definition: Putting in or on a therapeutic, diagnostic, nutritional, physiological, or prophylactic substance except blood or blood products

3EØ Continued

Body System/Region Character 4	Approach Character 5	Substance Character 6	Qualifier Character 7
P Female Reproductive ♀	3 Percutaneous	3 Anti-inflammatory 5 Adhesion Barrier 6 Nutritional Substance 7 Electrolytic and Water Balance Substance B Anesthetic Agent H Radioactive Substance K Other Diagnostic Substance L Sperm N Analgesics, Hypnotics, Sedatives T Destructive Agent V Hormone	Z No Qualifier
P Female Reproductive ♀	3 Percutaneous	G Other Therapeutic Substance	C Other Substance
P Female Reproductive ♀	3 Percutaneous	Q Fertilized Ovum	Ø Autologous 1 Nonautologous
P Female Reproductive ♀	3 Percutaneous	S Gas	F Other Gas
P Female Reproductive ♀	4 Percutaneous Endoscopic	5 Adhesion Barrier	Z No Qualifier
P Female Reproductive ♀	4 Percutaneous Endoscopic	G Other Therapeutic Substance	C Other Substance
P Female Reproductive ♀	7 Via Natural or Artificial Opening	Ø Antineoplastic	4 Liquid Brachytherapy Radioisotope 5 Other Antineoplastic M Monoclonal Antibody
P Female Reproductive ♀	7 Via Natural or Artificial Opening	2 Anti-infective	8 Oxazolidinones 9 Other Anti-infective
P Female Reproductive ♀	7 Via Natural or Artificial Opening	3 Anti-inflammatory 6 Nutritional Substance 7 Electrolytic and Water Balance Substance B Anesthetic Agent H Radioactive Substance K Other Diagnostic Substance L Sperm N Analgesics, Hypnotics, Sedatives T Destructive Agent V Hormone	Z No Qualifier
P Female Reproductive ♀	7 Via Natural or Artificial Opening	G Other Therapeutic Substance	C Other Substance
P Female Reproductive ♀	7 Via Natural or Artificial Opening	Q Fertilized Ovum	Ø Autologous 1 Nonautologous
P Female Reproductive ♀	7 Via Natural or Artificial Opening	S Gas	F Other Gas
P Female Reproductive ♀	8 Via Natural or Artificial Opening Endoscopic	Ø Antineoplastic	4 Liquid Brachytherapy Radioisotope 5 Other Antineoplastic M Monoclonal Antibody
P Female Reproductive ♀	8 Via Natural or Artificial Opening Endoscopic	2 Anti-infective	8 Oxazolidinones 9 Other Anit-infection
P Female Reproductive ♀	8 Via Natural or Artificial Opening Endoscopic	3 Anti-inflammatory 6 Nutritional Substance 7 Electrolytic and Water Balance Substance B Anesthetic Agent H Radioactive Substance K Other Diagnostic Substance N Analgesics, Hypnotics, Sedative T Destructive Agent	Z No Qualifier
P Female Reproductive ♀	8 Via Natural or Artificial Opening Endoscopic	G Other Therapeutic Substance	C Other Substance
P Female Reproductive ♀	8 Via Natural or Artificial Opening Endoscopic	S Gas	F Other Gas
Q Cranial Cavity and Brain	Ø Open 3 Percutaneous	Ø Antineoplastic	4 Liquid Brachytherapy Radioisotope 5 Other Antineoplastic M Monoclonal Antibody
Q Cranial Cavity and Brain	Ø Open 3 Percutaneous	2 Anti-infective	8 Oxazolidinones 9 Other Anti-infective

Valid OR 3EØP3Q[Ø,1]
Valid OR 3EØP7Q[Ø,1]
DRG Non-OR 3EØQ[Ø,3]Ø5
♀ All approach, substance, and qualifier values for body system/region (character 4) with this icon

3EØ Continued on next page

Administration

3EØ–3EØ

3 Administration *3EØ Continued*
E Physiological Systems and Anatomical Regions
Ø Introduction Definition: Putting in or on a therapeutic, diagnostic, nutritional, physiological, or prophylactic substance except blood or blood products

Body System/Region Character 4	Approach Character 5	Substance Character 6	Qualifier Character 7
Q Cranial Cavity and Brain	Ø Open 3 Percutaneous	3 Anti-inflammatory 6 Nutritional Substance 7 Electrolytic and Water Balance Substance A Stem Cells, Embryonic B Anesthetic Agent H Radioactive Substance K Other Diagnostic Substance N Analgesics, Hypnotics, Sedatives T Destructive Agent	Z No Qualifier
Q Cranial Cavity and Brain	Ø Open 3 Percutaneous	E Stem Cells, Somatic	Ø Autologous 1 Nonautologous
Q Cranial Cavity and Brain	Ø Open 3 Percutaneous	G Other Therapeutic Substance	C Other Substance
Q Cranial Cavity and Brain	Ø Open 3 Percutaneous	S Gas	F Other Gas
Q Cranial Cavity and Brain	7 Via Natural or Artificial Opening	Ø Antineoplastic	4 Liquid Brachytherapy Radioisotope 5 Other Antineoplastic M Monoclonal Antibody
Q Cranial Cavity and Brain	7 Via Natural or Artificial Opening	S Gas	F Other Gas
R Spinal Canal	Ø Open	A Stem Cells, Embryonic	Z No Qualifier
R Spinal Canal	Ø Open	E Stem Cells, Somatic	Ø Autologous 1 Nonautologous
R Spinal Canal	3 Percutaneous	Ø Antineoplastic	2 High-dose Interleukin-2 3 Low-dose Interleukin-2 4 Liquid Brachytherapy Radioisotope 5 Other Antineoplastic M Monoclonal Antibody
R Spinal Canal	3 Percutaneous	2 Anti-infective	8 Oxazolidinones 9 Other Anti-infective
R Spinal Canal	3 Percutaneous	3 Anti-inflammatory 6 Nutritional Substance 7 Electrolytic and Water Balance Substance A Stem Cells, Embryonic B Anesthetic Agent H Radioactive Substance K Other Diagnostic Substance N Analgesics, Hypnotics, Sedatives T Destructive Agent	Z No Qualifier
R Spinal Canal	3 Percutaneous	E Stem Cells, Somatic	Ø Autologous 1 Nonautologous
R Spinal Canal	3 Percutaneous	G Other Therapeutic Substance	C Other Substance
R Spinal Canal	3 Percutaneous	S Gas	F Other Gas
R Spinal Canal	7 Via Natural or Artificial Opening	S Gas	F Other Gas
S Epidural Space	3 Percutaneous	Ø Antineoplastic	2 High-dose Interleukin-2 3 Low-dose Interleukin-2 4 Liquid Brachytherapy Radioisotope 5 Other Antineoplastic M Monoclonal Antibody
S Epidural Space	3 Percutaneous	2 Anti-infective	8 Oxazolidinones 9 Other Anti-infective
S Epidural Space	3 Percutaneous	3 Anti-inflammatory 6 Nutritional Substance 7 Electrolytic and Water Balance Substance B Anesthetic Agent H Radioactive Substance K Other Diagnostic Substance N Analgesics, Hypnotics, Sedatives T Destructive Agent	Z No Qualifier

DRG Non-OR 3EØQ7Ø5
DRG Non-OR 3EØR3Ø2
DRG Non-OR 3EØS3Ø2

3EØ Continued on next page

3 Administration
E Physiological Systems and Anatomical Regions
Ø Introduction Definition: Putting in or on a therapeutic, diagnostic, nutritional, physiological, or prophylactic substance except blood or blood products

3EØ Continued

Body System/Region Character 4	Approach Character 5	Substance Character 6	Qualifier Character 7
S Epidural Space	3 Percutaneous	G Other Therapeutic Substance	C Other Substance
S Epidural Space	3 Percutaneous	S Gas	F Other Gas
S Epidural Space	7 Via Natural or Artificial Opening	S Gas	F Other Gas
T Peripheral Nerves and Plexi X Cranial Nerves	3 Percutaneous	3 Anti-inflammatory B Anesthetic Agent T Destructive Agent	Z No Qualifier
T Peripheral Nerves and Plexi X Cranial Nerves	3 Percutaneous	G Other Therapeutic Substance	C Other Substance
U Joints	Ø Open	2 Anti-infective	8 Oxazolidinones 9 Other Anti-infective
U Joints	Ø Open	G Other Therapeutic Substance	B Recombinant Bone Morphogenetic Protein
U Joints	3 Percutaneous	Ø Antineoplastic	4 Liquid Brachytherapy Radioisotope 5 Other Antineoplastic M Monoclonal Antibody
U Joints	3 Percutaneous	2 Anti-infective	8 Oxazolidinones 9 Other Anti-infective
U Joints	3 Percutaneous	3 Anti-inflammatory 6 Nutritional Substance 7 Electrolytic and Water Balance Substance B Anesthetic Agent H Radioactive Substance K Other Diagnostic Substance N Analgesics, Hypnotics, Sedatives T Destructive Agent	Z No Qualifier
U Joints	3 Percutaneous	G Other Therapeutic Substance	B Recombinant Bone Morphogenetic Protein C Other Substance
U Joints	3 Percutaneous	S Gas	F Other Gas
U Joints	4 Percutaneous Endoscopic	G Other Therapeutic Substance	C Other Substance
V Bones	Ø Open	G Other Therapeutic Substance	B Recombinant Bone Morphogenetic Protein
V Bones	3 Percutaneous	Ø Antineoplastic	5 Other Antineoplastic M Monoclonal Antibody
V Bones	3 Percutaneous	2 Anti-infective	8 Oxazolidinones 9 Other Anti-infective
V Bones	3 Percutaneous	3 Anti-inflammatory 6 Nutritional Substance 7 Electrolytic and Water Balance Substance B Anesthetic Agent H Radioactive Substance K Other Diagnostic Substance N Analgesics, Hypnotics, Sedatives T Destructive Agent	Z No Qualifier
V Bones	3 Percutaneous	G Other Therapeutic Substance	B Recombinant Bone Morphogenetic Protein C Other Substance
W Lymphatics	3 Percutaneous	Ø Antineoplastic	5 Other Antineoplastic M Monoclonal Antibody
W Lymphatics	3 Percutaneous	2 Anti-infective	8 Oxazolidinones 9 Other Anti-infective
W Lymphatics	3 Percutaneous	3 Anti-inflammatory 6 Nutritional Substance 7 Electrolytic and Water Balance Substance B Anesthetic Agent H Radioactive Substance K Other Diagnostic Substance N Analgesics, Hypnotics, Sedatives T Destructive Agent	Z No Qualifier
W Lymphatics	3 Percutaneous	G Other Therapeutic Substance	C Other Substance

3EØ Continued on next page

3EØ Continued

3 Administration
E Physiological Systems and Anatomical Regions
Ø Introduction Definition: Putting in or on a therapeutic, diagnostic, nutritional, physiological, or prophylactic substance except blood or blood products

Body System/Region Character 4	Approach Character 5	Substance Character 6	Qualifier Character 7
Y Pericardial Cavity	3 Percutaneous	Ø Antineoplastic	4 Liquid Brachytherapy Radioisotope 5 Other Antineoplastic M Monoclonal Antibody
Y Pericardial Cavity	3 Percutaneous	2 Anti-infective	8 Oxazolidinones 9 Other Anti-infective
Y Pericardial Cavity	3 Percutaneous	3 Anti-inflammatory 6 Nutritional Substance 7 Electrolytic and Water Balance Substance B Anesthetic Agent H Radioactive Substance K Other Diagnostic Substance N Analgesics, Hypnotics, Sedatives T Destructive Agent	Z No Qualifier
Y Pericardial Cavity	3 Percutaneous	G Other Therapeutic Substance	C Other Substance
Y Pericardial Cavity	3 Percutaneous	S Gas	F Other Gas
Y Pericardial Cavity	4 Percutaneous Endoscopic	G Other Therapeutic Substance	C Other Substance
Y Pericardial Cavity	7 Via Natural or Artificial Opening	Ø Antineoplastic	4 Liquid Brachytherapy Radioisotope 5 Other Antineoplastic M Monoclonal Antibody
Y Pericardial Cavity	7 Via Natural or Artificial Opening	S Gas	F Other Gas

3 Administration
E Physiological Systems and Anatomical Regions
1 Irrigation Definition: Putting in or on a cleansing substance

Body System/Region Character 4	Approach Character 5	Substance Character 6	Qualifier Character 7
Ø Skin and Mucous Membranes C Eye	3 Percutaneous X External	8 Irrigating Substance	X Diagnostic Z No Qualifier
9 Nose B Ear F Respiratory Tract G Upper GI H Lower GI J Biliary and Pancreatic Tract K Genitourinary Tract N Male Reproductive ♂ P Female Reproductive ♀	3 Percutaneous 7 Via Natural or Artificial Opening 8 Via Natural or Artificial Opening Endoscopic	8 Irrigating Substance	X Diagnostic Z No Qualifier
L Pleural Cavity Q Cranial Cavity and Brain R Spinal Canal S Epidural Space Y Pericardial Cavity	3 Percutaneous	8 Irrigating Substance	X Diagnostic Z No Qualifier
M Peritoneal Cavity	3 Percutaneous	8 Irrigating Substance	X Diagnostic Z No Qualifier
M Peritoneal Cavity	3 Percutaneous	9 Dialysate	Z No Qualifier
M Peritoneal Cavity	4 Percutaneous Endoscopic	8 Irrigating Substance	X Diagnostic Z No Qualifier
U Joints	3 Percutaneous 4 Percutaneous Endoscopic	8 Irrigating Substance	X Diagnostic Z No Qualifier

♂ 3E1N[3,7,8]8[X,Z]
♀ 3E1P[3,7,8]8[X,Z]

Measurement and Monitoring 4AØ–4BØ

AHA Coding Clinic for table 4AØ

2020, 4Q, 62	Measurement of intracranial arterial flow
2020, 4Q, 62	Percutaneous endoscopic measurement of portal venous pressure
2020, 4Q, 63	Intercompartmental pressure measurement
2019, 3Q, 32	Endomyocardial biopsy and right heart catheterization
2018, 1Q, 12	Percutaneous balloon valvuloplasty & cardiac catheterization with ventriculogram
2016, 3Q, 37	Fractional flow reserve
2015, 3Q, 29	Approach value for esophageal electrophysiology study

AHA Coding Clinic for table 4A1

2019, 4Q, 38-39	Intraoperative fluorescence lymphatic mapping using Indocyanine green dye
2016, 4Q, 114	Fluorescence vascular angiography
2016, 2Q, 29	Decompressive craniectomy with cryopreservation and storage of bone flap
2016, 2Q, 33	Monitoring of arterial pressure & pulse
2015, 3Q, 35	Swan Ganz catheterization
2015, 2Q, 14	Intraoperative EMG monitoring via endotracheal tube
2015, 1Q, 26	Intraoperative monitoring using Sentio MMG®
2014, 4Q, 28	Removal and replacement of displaced growing rods

4 Measurement and Monitoring
A Physiological Systems
Ø Measurement Definition: Determining the level of a physiological or physical function at a point in time

Body System Character 4	Approach Character 5	Function/Device Character 6	Qualifier Character 7
Ø Central Nervous	Ø Open	2 Conductivity 4 Electrical Activity B Pressure	Z No Qualifier
Ø Central Nervous	3 Percutaneous 7 Via Natural or Artificial Opening 8 Via Natural or Artificial Opening Endoscopic	4 Electrical Activity	Z No Qualifier
Ø Central Nervous	3 Percutaneous 7 Via Natural or Artificial Opening 8 Via Natural or Artificial Opening Endoscopic	B Pressure K Temperature R Saturation	D Intracranial
Ø Central Nervous	X External	2 Conductivity 4 Electrical Activity	Z No Qualifier
1 Peripheral Nervous	Ø Open 3 Percutaneous 7 Via Natural or Artificial Opening 8 Via Natural or Artificial Opening Endoscopic X External	2 Conductivity	9 Sensory B Motor
1 Peripheral Nervous	Ø Open 3 Percutaneous 7 Via Natural or Artificial Opening 8 Via Natural or Artificial Opening Endoscopic X External	4 Electrical Activity	Z No Qualifier
2 Cardiac	Ø Open 3 Percutaneous 7 Via Natural or Artificial Opening 8 Via Natural or Artificial Opening Endoscopic	4 Electrical Activity 9 Output C Rate F Rhythm H Sound P Action Currents	Z No Qualifier
2 Cardiac	Ø Open 3 Percutaneous 7 Via Natural or Artificial Opening 8 Via Natural or Artificial Opening Endoscopic	N Sampling and Pressure	6 Right Heart 7 Left Heart 8 Bilateral
2 Cardiac	X External	4 Electrical Activity	A Guidance Z No Qualifier
2 Cardiac	X External	9 Output C Rate F Rhythm H Sound P Action Currents	Z No Qualifier
2 Cardiac	X External	M Total Activity	4 Stress
3 Arterial	Ø Open 3 Percutaneous	5 Flow J Pulse	1 Peripheral 3 Pulmonary C Coronary
3 Arterial	Ø Open 3 Percutaneous	B Pressure	1 Peripheral 3 Pulmonary C Coronary F Other Thoracic

DRG Non-OR 4AØ2[3,7,8]FZ
DRG Non-OR 4AØ2[Ø,3,7,8]N[6,7,8]

4AØ Continued on next page

Measurement and Monitoring

4AØ Continued

4 Measurement and Monitoring
A Physiological Systems
Ø Measurement Definition: Determining the level of a physiological or physical function at a point in time

Body System Character 4	Approach Character 5	Function/Device Character 6	Qualifier Character 7
3 Arterial	Ø Open 3 Percutaneous	H Sound R Saturation	1 Peripheral
3 Arterial	X External	5 Flow NT	1 Peripheral D Intracranial
3 Arterial	X External	B Pressure H Sound J Pulse R Saturation	1 Peripheral
4 Venous	Ø Open 3 Percutaneous	5 Flow B Pressure J Pulse	Ø Central 1 Peripheral 2 Portal 3 Pulmonary
4 Venous	Ø Open 3 Percutaneous	R Saturation	1 Peripheral
4 Venous	4 Percutaneous Endoscopic	B Pressure	2 Portal
4 Venous	X External	5 Flow B Pressure J Pulse R Saturation	1 Peripheral
5 Circulatory	X External	L Volume	Z No Qualifier
6 Lymphatic	Ø Open 3 Percutaneous 7 Via Natural or Artificial Opening 8 Via Natural or Artificial Opening Endoscopic	5 Flow B Pressure	Z No Qualifier
7 Visual	X External	Ø Acuity 7 Mobility B Pressure	Z No Qualifier
8 Olfactory	X External	Ø Acuity	Z No Qualifier
9 Respiratory	7 Via Natural or Artificial Opening 8 Via Natural or Artificial Opening Endoscopic X External	1 Capacity 5 Flow C Rate D Resistance L Volume M Total Activity	Z No Qualifier
B Gastrointestinal	7 Via Natural or Artificial Opening 8 Via Natural or Artificial Opening Endoscopic	8 Motility B Pressure G Secretion	Z No Qualifier
C Biliary	3 Percutaneous 4 Percutaneous Endoscopic 7 Via Natural or Artificial Opening 8 Via Natural or Artificial Opening Endoscopic	5 Flow B Pressure	Z No Qualifier
D Urinary	7 Via Natural or Artificial Opening 8 Via Natural or Artificial Opening Endoscopic	3 Contractility 5 Flow B Pressure D Resistance L Volume	Z No Qualifier
F Musculoskeletal	3 Percutaneous	3 Contractility	Z No Qualifier
F Musculoskeletal	3 Percutaneous	B Pressure	E Compartment
F Musculoskeletal	X External	3 Contractility	Z No Qualifier
H Products of Conception, Cardiac ♀	7 Via Natural or Artificial Opening 8 Via Natural or Artificial Opening Endoscopic X External	4 Electrical Activity C Rate F Rhythm H Sound	Z No Qualifier
J Products of Conception, Nervous ♀	7 Via Natural or Artificial Opening 8 Via Natural or Artificial Opening Endoscopic X External	2 Conductivity 4 Electrical Activity B Pressure	Z No Qualifier
Z None	7 Via Natural or Artificial Opening	6 Metabolism K Temperature	Z No Qualifier
Z None	X External	6 Metabolism K Temperature Q Sleep	Z No Qualifier

Valid OR 4AØ6Ø[5,B]Z
Valid OR 4AØC4[5,B]Z
NT 4AØ3X5D for use of ContaCT
♀ 4AØH[7,8,X][4,C,F,H]Z
♀ 4AØJ[7,8,X][2,4,B]Z

4 Measurement and Monitoring
A Physiological Systems
1 Monitoring Definition: Determining the level of a physiological or physical function repetitively over a period of time

Body System Character 4	Approach Character 5	Function/Device Character 6	Qualifier Character 7
Ø Central Nervous	Ø Open	2 Conductivity B Pressure	Z No Qualifier
Ø Central Nervous	Ø Open	4 Electrical Activity	G Intraoperative Z No Qualifier
Ø Central Nervous	3 Percutaneous 7 Via Natural or Artificial Opening 8 Via Natural or Artificial Opening Endoscopic	4 Electrical Activity	G Intraoperative Z No Qualifier
Ø Central Nervous	3 Percutaneous 7 Via Natural or Artificial Opening 8 Via Natural or Artificial Opening Endoscopic	B Pressure K Temperature R Saturation	D Intracranial
Ø Central Nervous	X External	2 Conductivity	Z No Qualifier
Ø Central Nervous	X External	4 Electrical Activity	G Intraoperative Z No Qualifier
1 Peripheral Nervous	Ø Open 3 Percutaneous 7 Via Natural or Artificial Opening 8 Via Natural or Artificial Opening Endoscopic X External	2 Conductivity	9 Sensory B Motor
1 Peripheral Nervous	Ø Open 3 Percutaneous 7 Via Natural or Artificial Opening 8 Via Natural or Artificial Opening Endoscopic X External	4 Electrical Activity	G Intraoperative Z No Qualifier
2 Cardiac	Ø Open 3 Percutaneous 7 Via Natural or Artificial Opening 8 Via Natural or Artificial Opening Endoscopic	4 Electrical Activity 9 Output C Rate F Rhythm H Sound	Z No Qualifier
2 Cardiac	X External	4 Electrical Activity	5 Ambulatory Z No Qualifier
2 Cardiac	X External	9 Output C Rate F Rhythm H Sound	Z No Qualifier
2 Cardiac	X External	M Total Activity	4 Stress
2 Cardiac	X External	S Vascular Perfusion	H Indocyanine Green Dye
3 Arterial	Ø Open 3 Percutaneous	5 Flow B Pressure J Pulse	1 Peripheral 3 Pulmonary C Coronary
3 Arterial	Ø Open 3 Percutaneous	H Sound R Saturation	1 Peripheral
3 Arterial	X External	5 Flow B Pressure H Sound J Pulse R Saturation	1 Peripheral
4 Venous	Ø Open 3 Percutaneous	5 Flow B Pressure J Pulse	Ø Central 1 Peripheral 2 Portal 3 Pulmonary
4 Venous	Ø Open 3 Percutaneous	R Saturation	Ø Central 2 Portal 3 Pulmonary
4 Venous	X External	5 Flow B Pressure J Pulse	1 Peripheral
6 Lymphatic	Ø Open 3 Percutaneous 7 Via Natural or Artificial Opening 8 Via Natural or Artificial Opening Endoscopic	5 Flow	H Indocyanine Green Dye Z No Qualifier

Valid OR 4A16Ø5Z

4A1 Continued on next page

Measurement and Monitoring

4A1 Continued

4 Measurement and Monitoring
A Physiological Systems
1 Monitoring Definition: Determining the level of a physiological or physical function repetitively over a period of time

Body System Character 4	Approach Character 5	Function/Device Character 6	Qualifier Character 7
6 Lymphatic	Ø Open 3 Percutaneous 7 Via Natural or Artificial Opening 8 Via Natural or Artificial Opening Endoscopic	B Pressure	Z No Qualifier
9 Respiratory	7 Via Natural or Artificial Opening X External	1 Capacity 5 Flow C Rate D Resistance L Volume	Z No Qualifier
B Gastrointestinal	7 Via Natural or Artificial Opening 8 Via Natural or Artificial Opening Endoscopic	8 Motility B Pressure G Secretion	Z No Qualifier
B Gastrointestinal	X External	S Vascular Perfusion	H Indocyanine Green Dye
D Urinary	7 Via Natural or Artificial Opening 8 Via Natural or Artificial Opening Endoscopic	3 Contractility 5 Flow B Pressure D Resistance L Volume	Z No Qualifier
G Skin and Breast	X External	S Vascular Perfusion	H Indocyanine Green Dye
H Products of Conception, Cardiac ♀	7 Via Natural or Artificial Opening 8 Via Natural or Artificial Opening Endoscopic X External	4 Electrical Activity C Rate F Rhythm H Sound	Z No Qualifier
J Products of Conception, Nervous ♀	7 Via Natural or Artificial Opening 8 Via Natural or Artificial Opening Endoscopic X External	2 Conductivity 4 Electrical Activity B Pressure	Z No Qualifier
Z None	7 Via Natural or Artificial Opening	K Temperature	Z No Qualifier
Z None	X External	K Temperature Q Sleep	Z No Qualifier

Valid OR 4A16ØBZ
♀ 4A1H[7,8,X][4,C,F,H]Z
♀ 4A1J[7,8,X][2,4,B]Z

4 Measurement and Monitoring
B Physiological Devices
Ø Measurement Definition: Determining the level of a physiological or physical function at a point in time

Body System Character 4	Approach Character 5	Function/Device Character 6	Qualifier Character 7
Ø Central Nervous	X External	V Stimulator	Z No Qualifier
Ø Central Nervous	X External	W Cerebrospinal Fluid Shunt	Ø Wireless Sensor
1 Peripheral Nervous F Musculoskeletal	X External	V Stimulator	Z No Qualifier
2 Cardiac	X External	S Pacemaker T Defibrillator	Z No Qualifier
9 Respiratory	X External	S Pacemaker	Z No Qualifier

Extracorporeal or Systemic Assistance and Performance 5AØ–5A2

AHA Coding Clinic for table 5AØ

2021, 2Q, 12	Repositioning of displaced intra-aortic balloon pump
2020, 4Q, 64-65	Ventilatory assistance by high flow or high velocity nasal cannula devices
2020, 1Q, 10	Intermittent use of continuous positive airway pressure
2018, 2Q, 3-5	Intra-aortic balloon pump
2017, 4Q, 43-44	Insertion of external heart assist devices
2017, 3Q, 18	Intra-aortic balloon pump removal
2017, 1Q, 10-11	External heart assist device
2017, 1Q, 29	Newborn resuscitation using positive pressure ventilation
2017, 1Q, 29	Newborn noninvasive ventilation
2016, 4Q, 137-139	Heart assist device systems
2014, 4Q, 9	Mechanical ventilation
2014, 3Q, 19	Ablation of ventricular tachycardia with Impella® support
2013, 3Q, 18	Heart transplant surgery

AHA Coding Clinic for table 5A1

2019, 4Q, 39-41	Intraoperative extracorporeal membrane oxygenation
2019, 3Q, 19	Insertion of left ventricular catheter
2019, 3Q, 20	Removal and revision of ECMO component
2019, 3Q, 21	Exchange of extracorporeal membrane oxygenation component (oxygenator)
2019, 2Q, 36	Veno-arterial extracorporeal membrane oxygenation via sternotomy
2019, 3Q, 22	Extracorporeal membrane oxygenation and Centrimag™ pump
2019, 3Q, 22	Extracorporeal membrane oxygenation transfers
2018, 4Q, 52-54	Percutaneous extracorporeal membrane oxygenation
2018, 1Q, 13	Mechanical ventilation using patient's equipment
2017, 4Q, 71-73	Hemodialysis and renal replacement therapy
2017, 3Q, 7	Senning procedure (arterial switch)
2017, 1Q, 19	Norwood Sano procedure
2016, 1Q, 27	Aortocoronary bypass graft utilizing Y-graft
2016, 1Q, 28	Extracorporeal liver assist device
2016, 1Q, 29	Duration of hemodialysis
2015, 4Q, 22-24	Congenital heart corrective procedures
2014, 4Q, 3-10	Mechanical ventilation
2014, 4Q, 11-15	Sequencing of mechanical ventilation with other procedures
2014, 3Q, 16	Repair of Tetralogy of Fallot
2014, 3Q, 20	MAZE procedure performed with coronary artery bypass graft
2014, 1Q, 10	Repair of thoracic aortic aneurysm & coronary artery bypass graft
2013, 3Q, 18	Heart transplant surgery

5 Extracorporeal or Systemic Assistance and Performance
A Physiological Systems
Ø Assistance Definition: Taking over a portion of a physiological function by extracorporeal means

Body System Character 4	Duration Character 5	Function Character 6	Qualifier Character 7
2 Cardiac	1 Intermittent 2 Continuous	1 Output	Ø Balloon Pump 5 Pulsatile Compression 6 Other Pump D Impeller Pump
5 Circulatory	1 Intermittent 2 Continuous	2 Oxygenation	1 Hyperbaric C Supersaturated
9 Respiratory	2 Continuous	Ø Filtration	Z No Qualifier
9 Respiratory	3 Less than 24 Consecutive Hours 4 24-96 Consecutive Hours 5 Greater than 96 Consecutive Hours	5 Ventilation	7 Continuous Positive Airway Pressure 8 Intermittent Positive Airway Pressure 9 Continuous Negative Airway Pressure A High Nasal Flow/Velocity B Intermittent Negative Airway Pressure Z No Qualifier

Valid OR 5AØ2[1,2]1[Ø,6,D]

5 Extracorporeal or Systemic Assistance and Performance
A Physiological Systems
1 Performance Definition: Completely taking over a physiological function by extracorporeal means

Body System Character 4	Duration Character 5	Function Character 6	Qualifier Character 7
2 Cardiac	Ø Single	1 Output	2 Manual
2 Cardiac	1 Intermittent	3 Pacing	Z No Qualifier
2 Cardiac	2 Continuous	1 Output	J Automated Z No Qualifier
2 Cardiac	2 Continuous	3 Pacing	Z No Qualifier
5 Circulatory	2 Continuous A Intraoperative	2 Oxygenation	F Membrane, Central G Membrane, Peripheral Veno-arterial H Membrane, Peripheral Veno-venous
9 Respiratory	Ø Single	5 Ventilation	4 Nonmechanical
9 Respiratory	3 Less than 24 Consecutive Hours 4 24-96 Consecutive Hours 5 Greater than 96 Consecutive Hours	5 Ventilation	Z No Qualifier
C Biliary	Ø Single 6 Multiple	Ø Filtration	Z No Qualifier
D Urinary	7 Intermittent, Less than 6 Hours per day 8 Prolonged Intermittent, 6-18 Hours per day 9 Continuous, Greater than 18 Hours per day	Ø Filtration	Z No Qualifier

Valid OR 5A1522F
DRG Non-OR 5A1522[G,H]
DRG Non-OR 5A19[3,4]5Z
DRG Non-OR 5A1955Z Length of stay must be > 4 consecutive days.
DRG Non-OR 5A1D[7,8,9]ØZ

5 Extracorporeal or Systemic Assistance and Performance
A Physiological Systems
2 Restoration Definition: Returning, or attempting to return, a physiological function to its original state by extracorporeal means.

Body System Character 4	Duration Character 5	Function Character 6	Qualifier Character 7
2 Cardiac	Ø Single	4 Rhythm	Z No Qualifier

Extracorporeal or Systemic Therapies 6AØ–6AB

AHA Coding Clinic for table 6A4
2019, 2Q, 17 Cryoamputation of lower leg

AHA Coding Clinic for table 6A7
2014, 4Q, 19 Ultrasound accelerated thrombolysis

AHA Coding Clinic for table 6AB
2016, 4Q, 115 Donor organ perfusion

6 Extracorporeal or Systemic Therapies
A Physiological Systems
Ø Atmospheric Control Definition: Extracorporeal control of atmospheric pressure and composition

Body System Character 4	Duration Character 5	Qualifier Character 6	Qualifier Character 7
Z None	Ø Single 1 Multiple	Z No Qualifier	Z No Qualifier

6 Extracorporeal or Systemic Therapies
A Physiological Systems
1 Decompression Definition: Extracorporeal elimination of undissolved gas from body fluids

Body System Character 4	Duration Character 5	Qualifier Character 6	Qualifier Character 7
5 Circulatory	Ø Single 1 Multiple	Z No Qualifier	Z No Qualifier

6 Extracorporeal or Systemic Therapies
A Physiological Systems
2 Electromagnetic Therapy Definition: Extracorporeal treatment by electromagnetic rays

Body System Character 4	Duration Character 5	Qualifier Character 6	Qualifier Character 7
1 Urinary 2 Central Nervous	Ø Single 1 Multiple	Z No Qualifier	Z No Qualifier

6 Extracorporeal or Systemic Therapies
A Physiological Systems
3 Hyperthermia Definition: Extracorporeal raising of body temperature

Body System Character 4	Duration Character 5	Qualifier Character 6	Qualifier Character 7
Z None	Ø Single 1 Multiple	Z No Qualifier	Z No Qualifier

6 Extracorporeal or Systemic Therapies
A Physiological Systems
4 Hypothermia Definition: Extracorporeal lowering of body temperature

Body System Character 4	Duration Character 5	Qualifier Character 6	Qualifier Character 7
Z None	Ø Single 1 Multiple	Z No Qualifier	Z No Qualifier

6 Extracorporeal or Systemic Therapies
A Physiological Systems
5 Pheresis Definition: Extracorporeal separation of blood products

Body System Character 4	Duration Character 5	Qualifier Character 6	Qualifier Character 7
5 Circulatory	Ø Single 1 Multiple	Z No Qualifier	Ø Erythrocytes 1 Leukocytes 2 Platelets 3 Plasma T Stem Cells, Cord Blood V Stem Cells, Hematopoietic

6 Extracorporeal or Systemic Therapies
A Physiological Systems
6 Phototherapy Definition: Extracorporeal treatment by light rays

Body System Character 4	Duration Character 5	Qualifier Character 6	Qualifier Character 7
Ø Skin 5 Circulatory	Ø Single 1 Multiple	Z No Qualifier	Z No Qualifier

6 Extracorporeal or Systemic Therapies
A Physiological Systems
7 Ultrasound Therapy Definition: Extracorporeal treatment by ultrasound

Body System Character 4	Duration Character 5	Qualifier Character 6	Qualifier Character 7
5 Circulatory	Ø Single 1 Multiple	Z No Qualifier	4 Head and Neck Vessels 5 Heart 6 Peripheral Vessels 7 Other Vessels Z No Qualifier

6 Extracorporeal or Systemic Therapies
A Physiological Systems
8 Ultraviolet Light Therapy Definition: Extracorporeal treatment by ultraviolet light

Body System Character 4	Duration Character 5	Qualifier Character 6	Qualifier Character 7
Ø Skin	Ø Single 1 Multiple	Z No Qualifier	Z No Qualifier

6 Extracorporeal or Systemic Therapies
A Physiological Systems
9 Shock Wave Therapy Definition: Extracorporeal treatment by shock waves

Body System Character 4	Duration Character 5	Qualifier Character 6	Qualifier Character 7
3 Musculoskeletal	Ø Single 1 Multiple	Z No Qualifier	Z No Qualifier

6 Extracorporeal or Systemic Therapies
A Physiological Systems
B Perfusion Definition: Extracorporeal treatment by diffusion of therapeutic fluid

Body System Character 4	Duration Character 5	Qualifier Character 6	Qualifier Character 7
5 Circulatory B Respiratory System F Hepatobiliary System and Pancreas T Urinary System	Ø Single	B Donor Organ	Z No Qualifier

Osteopathic 7WØ

7 Osteopathic
W Anatomical Regions
Ø Treatment Definition: Manual treatment to eliminate or alleviate somatic dysfunction and related disorders

Body Region Character 4	Approach Character 5	Method Character 6	Qualifier Character 7
Ø Head 1 Cervical 2 Thoracic 3 Lumbar 4 Sacrum 5 Pelvis 6 Lower Extremities 7 Upper Extremities 8 Rib Cage 9 Abdomen	X External	Ø Articulatory-Raising 1 Fascial Release 2 General Mobilization 3 High Velocity-Low Amplitude 4 Indirect 5 Low Velocity-High Amplitude 6 Lymphatic Pump 7 Muscle Energy-Isometric 8 Muscle Energy-Isotonic 9 Other Method	Z None

Other Procedures 8CØ–8EØ

AHA Coding Clinic for table 8EØ

2021, 2Q, 19	Electromagnetic stealth guided ventriculoperitoneal shunt insertion with endoscopy
2020, 4Q, 53	Bypass pancreatic duct to stomach
2020, 4Q, 65-66	Near infrared spectroscopy for tissue viability assessment
2020, 4Q, 99	Robotic-assisted prostatectomy with extension of incision for specimen removal
2020, 4Q, 100	Robotic-assisted sigmoid colectomy with extension of incision for specimen removal
2019, 4Q, 41-42	Intraoperative fluorescence guidance
2019, 1Q, 30	Laparoscopic-assisted rectopexy with manual reduction of prolapse
2015, 1Q, 33	Robotic-assisted laparoscopic hysterectomy converted to open procedure
2014, 4Q, 33	Radical prostatectomy

8 Other Procedures
C Indwelling Device
Ø Other Procedures Definition: Methodologies which attempt to remediate or cure a disorder or disease

Body Region Character 4	Approach Character 5	Method Character 6	Qualifier Character 7
1 Nervous System	**X** External	**6** Collection	**J** Cerebrospinal Fluid **L** Other Fluid
2 Circulatory System	**X** External	**6** Collection	**K** Blood **L** Other Fluid

8 Other Procedures
E Physiological Systems and Anatomical Regions
Ø Other Procedures Definition: Methodologies which attempt to remediate or cure a disorder or disease

Body Region Character 4	Approach Character 5	Method Character 6	Qualifier Character 7
1 Nervous System **U** Female Reproductive System ♀	**X** External	**Y** Other Method	**7** Examination
2 Circulatory System	**3** Percutaneous **X** External	**D** Near Infrared Spectroscopy	**Z** No Qualifier
9 Head and Neck Region	**Ø** Open	**C** Robotic Assisted Procedure	**Z** No Qualifier
9 Head and Neck Region	**Ø** Open	**E** Fluorescence Guided Procedure	**M** Aminolevulinic Acid **Z** No Qualifier
9 Head and Neck Region	**3** Percutaneous **4** Percutaneous Endoscopic **7** Via Natural or Artificial Opening **8** Via Natural or Artificial Opening Endoscopic	**C** Robotic Assisted Procedure **E** Fluorescence Guided Procedure	**Z** No Qualifier
9 Head and Neck Region	**X** External	**B** Computer Assisted Procedure	**F** With Fluoroscopy **G** With Computerized Tomography **H** With Magnetic Resonance Imaging **Z** No Qualifier
9 Head and Neck Region	**X** External	**C** Robotic Assisted Procedure	**Z** No Qualifier
9 Head and Neck Region	**X** External	**Y** Other Method	**8** Suture Removal
H Integumentary System and Breast	**3** Percutaneous	**Ø** Acupuncture	**Ø** Anesthesia **Z** No Qualifier
H Integumentary System and Breast ♀	**X** External	**6** Collection	**2** Breast Milk
H Integumentary System and Breast	**X** External	**Y** Other Method	**9** Piercing
K Musculoskeletal System	**X** External	**1** Therapeutic Massage	**Z** No Qualifier
K Musculoskeletal System	**X** External	**Y** Other Method	**7** Examination
V Male Reproductive System ♂	**X** External	**1** Therapeutic Massage	**C** Prostate **D** Rectum
V Male Reproductive System ♂	**X** External	**6** Collection	**3** Sperm
W Trunk Region	**Ø** Open **3** Percutaneous **4** Percutaneous Endoscopic **7** Via Natural or Artificial Opening **8** Via Natural or Artificial Opening Endoscopic	**C** Robotic Assisted Procedure **E** Fluorescence Guided Procedure	**Z** No Qualifier
W Trunk Region	**X** External	**B** Computer Assisted Procedure	**F** With Fluoroscopy **G** With Computerized Tomography **H** With Magnetic Resonance Imaging **Z** No Qualifier
W Trunk Region	**X** External	**C** Robotic Assisted Procedure	**Z** No Qualifier
W Trunk Region	**X** External	**Y** Other Method	**8** Suture Removal
X Upper Extremity **Y** Lower Extremity	**Ø** Open **3** Percutaneous **4** Percutaneous Endoscopic	**C** Robotic Assisted Procedure **E** Fluorescence Guided Procedure	**Z** No Qualifier

♂	8EØVX1C	♀	8EØUXY7
♂	8EØVX63	♀	8EØHX62

8EØ Continued on next page

8 Other Procedures
E Physiological Systems and Anatomical Regions
Ø Other Procedures Definition: Methodologies which attempt to remediate or cure a disorder or disease

8EØ Continued

Body Region Character 4	Approach Character 5	Method Character 6	Qualifier Character 7
X Upper Extremity Y Lower Extremity	X External	B Computer Assisted Procedure	F With Fluoroscopy G With Computerized Tomography H With Magnetic Resonance Imaging Z No Qualifier
X Upper Extremity Y Lower Extremity	X External	C Robotic Assisted Procedure	Z No Qualifier
X Upper Extremity Y Lower Extremity	X External	Y Other Method	8 Suture Removal
Z None	X External	Y Other Method	1 In Vitro Fertilization 4 Yoga Therapy 5 Meditation 6 Isolation

Chiropractic 9WB

9 Chiropractic
W Anatomical Regions
B Manipulation Definition: Manual procedure that involves a directed thrust to move a joint past the physiological range of motion, without exceeding the anatomical limit

Body Region Character 4	Approach Character 5	Method Character 6	Qualifier Character 7
Ø Head 1 Cervical 2 Thoracic 3 Lumbar 4 Sacrum 5 Pelvis 6 Lower Extremities 7 Upper Extremities 8 Rib Cage 9 Abdomen	X External	B Non-Manual C Indirect Visceral D Extra-Articular F Direct Visceral G Long Lever Specific Contact H Short Lever Specific Contact J Long and Short Lever Specific Contact K Mechanically Assisted L Other Method	Z None

Imaging B00–BY4

AHA Coding Clinic for table B21
2018, 1Q, 12 Percutaneous balloon valvuloplasty & cardiac catheterization with ventriculogram
2016, 3Q, 36 Type of contrast medium for angiography (high osmolar, low osmolar, and other)

AHA Coding Clinic for table B41
2015, 3Q, 9 Aborted endovascular stenting of superficial femoral artery

AHA Coding Clinic for table B51
2015, 4Q, 30 Vascular access devices

AHA Coding Clinic for table BF4
2014, 3Q, 15 Drainage of pancreatic pseudocyst
2020, 4Q, 66 Other imaging type

AHA Coding Clinic for table BF5
2020, 4Q, 66 Other imaging type
2020, 4Q, 66-67 Fluorescence imaging of hepatobiliary system

AHA Coding Clinic for table BW5
2020, 4Q, 66 Other imaging type
2020, 4Q, 68 Bacterial autofluorescence detection

B Imaging
0 Central Nervous System
0 Plain Radiography Definition: Planar display of an image developed from the capture of external ionizing radiation on photographic or photoconductive plate

Body Part Character 4	Contrast Character 5	Qualifier Character 6	Qualifier Character 7
B Spinal Cord	0 High Osmolar 1 Low Osmolar Y Other Contrast Z None	Z None	Z None

B Imaging
0 Central Nervous System
1 Fluoroscopy Definition: Single plane or bi-plane real time display of an image developed from the capture of external ionizing radioation on a fluorescent screen. The image may also be stored by either digital or analog means.

Body Part Character 4	Contrast Character 5	Qualifier Character 6	Qualifier Character 7
B Spinal Cord	0 High Osmolar 1 Low Osmolar Y Other Contrast Z None	Z None	Z None

B Imaging
0 Central Nervous System
2 Computerized Tomography (CT Scan) Definition: Computer reformatted digital display of multiplanar images developed from the capture of multiple exposures of external ionizing radiation

Body Part Character 4	Contrast Character 5	Qualifier Character 6	Qualifier Character 7
0 Brain 7 Cisterna 8 Cerebral Ventricle(s) 9 Sella Turcica/Pituitary Gland B Spinal Cord	0 High Osmolar 1 Low Osmolar Y Other Contrast	0 Unenhanced and Enhanced Z None	Z None
0 Brain 7 Cisterna 8 Cerebral Ventricle(s) 9 Sella Turcica/Pituitary Gland B Spinal Cord	Z None	Z None	Z None

B Imaging
0 Central Nervous System
3 Magnetic Resonance Imaging (MRI) Definition: Computer reformatted digital display of multiplanar images developed from the capture of radio-frequency signals emitted by nuclei in a body site excited within a magnetic field

Body Part Character 4	Contrast Character 5	Qualifier Character 6	Qualifier Character 7
0 Brain 9 Sella Turcica/Pituitary Gland B Spinal Cord C Acoustic Nerves	Y Other Contrast	0 Unenhanced and Enhanced Z None	Z None
0 Brain 9 Sella Turcica/Pituitary Gland B Spinal Cord C Acoustic Nerves	Z None	Z None	Z None

B Imaging
Ø Central Nervous System
4 Ultrasonography Definition: Real time display of images of anatomy or flow information developed from the capture of reflected and attenuated high frequency sound waves

Body Part Character 4	Contrast Character 5	Qualifier Character 6	Qualifier Character 7
Ø Brain **B** Spinal Cord	**Z** None	**Z** None	**Z** None

B Imaging
2 Heart
Ø Plain Radiography Definition: Planar display of an image developed from the capture of external ionizing radiation on photographic or photoconductive plate

Body Part Character 4	Contrast Character 5	Qualifier Character 6	Qualifier Character 7
Ø Coronary Artery, Single **1** Coronary Arteries, Multiple **2** Coronary Artery Bypass Graft, Single **3** Coronary Artery Bypass Grafts, Multiple **4** Heart, Right **5** Heart, Left **6** Heart, Right and Left **7** Internal Mammary Bypass Graft, Right **8** Internal Mammary Bypass Graft, Left **F** Bypass Graft, Other	**Ø** High Osmolar **1** Low Osmolar **Y** Other Contrast	**Z** None	**Z** None

DRG Non-OR All body part, contrast, and qualifier values

B Imaging
2 Heart
1 Fluoroscopy Definition: Single plane or bi-plane real time display of an image developed from the capture of external ionizing radioation on a fluorescent screen. The image may also be stored by either digital or analog means.

Body Part Character 4	Contrast Character 5	Qualifier Character 6	Qualifier Character 7
Ø Coronary Artery, Single **1** Coronary Arteries, Multiple **2** Coronary Artery Bypass Graft, Single **3** Coronary Artery Bypass Grafts, Multiple	**Ø** High Osmolar **1** Low Osmolar **Y** Other Contrast	**1** Laser	**Ø** Intraoperative
Ø Coronary Artery, Single **1** Coronary Arteries, Multiple **2** Coronary Artery Bypass Graft, Single **3** Coronary Artery Bypass Grafts, Multiple	**Ø** High Osmolar **1** Low Osmolar **Y** Other Contrast	**Z** None	**Z** None
4 Heart, Right **5** Heart, Left **6** Heart, Right and Left **7** Internal Mammary Bypass Graft, Right **8** Internal Mammary Bypass Graft, Left **F** Bypass Graft, Other	**Ø** High Osmolar **1** Low Osmolar **Y** Other Contrast	**Z** None	**Z** None

DRG Non-OR B21[Ø,1,2,3][Ø,1,Y]ZZ
DRG Non-OR B21[4,5,6,7,8,F][Ø,1,Y]ZZ

B Imaging
2 Heart
2 Computerized Tomography (CT Scan) Definition: Computer reformatted digital display of multiplanar images developed from the capture of multiple exposures of external ionizing radiation

Body Part Character 4	Contrast Character 5	Qualifier Character 6	Qualifier Character 7
1 Coronary Arteries, Multiple **3** Coronary Artery Bypass Grafts, Multiple **6** Heart, Right and Left	**Ø** High Osmolar **1** Low Osmolar **Y** Other Contrast	**Ø** Unenhanced and Enhanced **Z** None	**Z** None
1 Coronary Arteries, Multiple **3** Coronary Artery Bypass Grafts, Multiple **6** Heart, Right and Left	**Z** None	**2** Intravascular Optical Coherence **Z** None	**Z** None

B Imaging
2 Heart
3 Magnetic Resonance Imaging (MRI) Definition: Computer reformatted digital display of multiplanar images developed from the capture of radio-frequency signals emitted by nuclei in a body site excited within a magnetic field

Body Part Character 4	Contrast Character 5	Qualifier Character 6	Qualifier Character 7
1 Coronary Arteries, Multiple 3 Coronary Artery Bypass Grafts, Multiple 6 Heart, Right and Left	Y Other Contrast	Ø Unenhanced and Enhanced Z None	Z None
1 Coronary Arteries, Multiple 3 Coronary Artery Bypass Grafts, Multiple 6 Heart, Right and Left	Z None	Z None	Z None

B Imaging
2 Heart
4 Ultrasonography Definition: Real time display of images of anatomy or flow information developed from the capture of reflected and attenuated high frequency sound waves

Body Part Character 4	Contrast Character 5	Qualifier Character 6	Qualifier Character 7
Ø Coronary Artery, Single 1 Coronary Arteries, Multiple 4 Heart, Right 5 Heart, Left 6 Heart, Right and Left B Heart with Aorta C Pericardium D Pediatric Heart	Y Other Contrast	Z None	Z None
Ø Coronary Artery, Single 1 Coronary Arteries, Multiple 4 Heart, Right 5 Heart, Left 6 Heart, Right and Left B Heart with Aorta C Pericardium D Pediatric Heart	Z None	Z None	3 Intravascular 4 Transesophageal Z None

B Imaging
3 Upper Arteries
Ø Plain Radiography Definition: Planar display of an image developed from the capture of external ionizing radiation on photographic or photoconductive plate

Body Part Character 4	Contrast Character 5	Qualifier Character 6	Qualifier Character 7
Ø Thoracic Aorta 1 Brachiocephalic-Subclavian Artery, Right 2 Subclavian Artery, Left 3 Common Carotid Artery, Right 4 Common Carotid Artery, Left 5 Common Carotid Arteries, Bilateral 6 Internal Carotid Artery, Right 7 Internal Carotid Artery, Left 8 Internal Carotid Arteries, Bilateral 9 External Carotid Artery, Right B External Carotid Artery, Left C External Carotid Arteries, Bilateral D Vertebral Artery, Right F Vertebral Artery, Left G Vertebral Arteries, Bilateral H Upper Extremity Arteries, Right J Upper Extremity Arteries, Left K Upper Extremity Arteries, Bilateral L Intercostal and Bronchial Arteries M Spinal Arteries N Upper Arteries, Other P Thoraco-Abdominal Aorta Q Cervico-Cerebral Arch R Intracranial Arteries S Pulmonary Artery, Right T Pulmonary Artery, Left	Ø High Osmolar 1 Low Osmolar Y Other Contrast Z None	Z None	Z None

B Imaging
3 Upper Arteries
1 Fluoroscopy Definition: Single plane or bi-plane real time display of an image developed from the capture of external ionizing radiation on a fluorescent screen. The image may also be stored by either digital or analog means.

Body Part Character 4	Contrast Character 5	Qualifier Character 6	Qualifier Character 7
Ø Thoracic Aorta 1 Brachiocephalic-Subclavian Artery, Right 2 Subclavian Artery, Left 3 Common Carotid Artery, Right 4 Common Carotid Artery, Left 5 Common Carotid Arteries, Bilateral 6 Internal Carotid Artery, Right 7 Internal Carotid Artery, Left 8 Internal Carotid Arteries, Bilateral 9 External Carotid Artery, Right B External Carotid Artery, Left C External Carotid Arteries, Bilateral D Vertebral Artery, Right F Vertebral Artery, Left G Vertebral Arteries, Bilateral H Upper Extremity Arteries, Right J Upper Extremity Arteries, Left K Upper Extremity Arteries, Bilateral L Intercostal and Bronchial Arteries M Spinal Arteries N Upper Arteries, Other P Thoraco-Abdominal Aorta Q Cervico-Cerebral Arch R Intracranial Arteries S Pulmonary Artery, Right T Pulmonary Artery, Left U Pulmonary Trunk	Ø High Osmolar 1 Low Osmolar Y Other Contrast	1 Laser	Ø Intraoperative
Ø Thoracic Aorta 1 Brachiocephalic-Subclavian Artery, Right 2 Subclavian Artery, Left 3 Common Carotid Artery, Right 4 Common Carotid Artery, Left 5 Common Carotid Arteries, Bilateral 6 Internal Carotid Artery, Right 7 Internal Carotid Artery, Left 8 Internal Carotid Arteries, Bilateral 9 External Carotid Artery, Right B External Carotid Artery, Left C External Carotid Arteries, Bilateral D Vertebral Artery, Right F Vertebral Artery, Left G Vertebral Arteries, Bilateral H Upper Extremity Arteries, Right J Upper Extremity Arteries, Left K Upper Extremity Arteries, Bilateral L Intercostal and Bronchial Arteries M Spinal Arteries N Upper Arteries, Other P Thoraco-Abdominal Aorta Q Cervico-Cerebral Arch R Intracranial Arteries S Pulmonary Artery, Right T Pulmonary Artery, Left U Pulmonary Trunk	Ø High Osmolar 1 Low Osmolar Y Other Contrast	Z None	Z None

B31 Continued on next page

B31 Continued

B Imaging
3 Upper Arteries
1 Fluoroscopy Definition: Single plane or bi-plane real time display of an image developed from the capture of external ionizing radiation on a fluorescent screen. The image may also be stored by either digital or analog means.

Body Part Character 4	Contrast Character 5	Qualifier Character 6	Qualifier Character 7
Ø Thoracic Aorta 1 Brachiocephalic-Subclavian Artery, Right 2 Subclavian Artery, Left 3 Common Carotid Artery, Right 4 Common Carotid Artery, Left 5 Common Carotid Arteries, Bilateral 6 Internal Carotid Artery, Right 7 Internal Carotid Artery, Left 8 Internal Carotid Arteries, Bilateral 9 External Carotid Artery, Right B External Carotid Artery, Left C External Carotid Arteries, Bilateral D Vertebral Artery, Right F Vertebral Artery, Left G Vertebral Arteries, Bilateral H Upper Extremity Arteries, Right J Upper Extremity Arteries, Left K Upper Extremity Arteries, Bilateral L Intercostal and Bronchial Arteries M Spinal Arteries N Upper Arteries, Other P Thoraco-Abdominal Aorta Q Cervico-Cerebral Arch R Intracranial Arteries S Pulmonary Artery, Right T Pulmonary Artery, Left U Pulmonary Trunk	Z None	Z None	Z None

B Imaging
3 Upper Arteries
2 Computerized Tomography (CT Scan) Definition: Computer reformatted digital display of multiplanar images developed from the capture of multiple exposures of external ionizing radiation

Body Part Character 4	Contrast Character 5	Qualifier Character 6	Qualifier Character 7
Ø Thoracic Aorta 5 Common Carotid Arteries, Bilateral 8 Internal Carotid Arteries, Bilateral G Vertebral Arteries, Bilateral R Intracranial Arteries S Pulmonary Artery, Right T Pulmonary Artery, Left	Ø High Osmolar 1 Low Osmolar Y Other Contrast	Z None	Z None
Ø Thoracic Aorta 5 Common Carotid Arteries, Bilateral 8 Internal Carotid Arteries, Bilateral G Vertebral Arteries, Bilateral R Intracranial Arteries S Pulmonary Artery, Right T Pulmonary Artery, Left	Z None	2 Intravascular Optical Coherence Z None	Z None

B Imaging
3 Upper Arteries
3 Magnetic Resonance Imaging (MRI) Definition: Computer reformatted digital display of multiplanar images developed from the capture of radio-frequency signals emitted by nuclei in a body site excited within a magnetic field

Body Part Character 4	Contrast Character 5	Qualifier Character 6	Qualifier Character 7
Ø Thoracic Aorta 5 Common Carotid Arteries, Bilateral 8 Internal Carotid Arteries, Bilateral G Vertebral Arteries, Bilateral H Upper Extremity Arteries, Right J Upper Extremity Arteries, Left K Upper Extremity Arteries, Bilateral M Spinal Arteries Q Cervico-Cerebral Arch R Intracranial Arteries	Y Other Contrast	Ø Unenhanced and Enhanced Z None	Z None
Ø Thoracic Aorta 5 Common Carotid Arteries, Bilateral 8 Internal Carotid Arteries, Bilateral G Vertebral Arteries, Bilateral H Upper Extremity Arteries, Right J Upper Extremity Arteries, Left K Upper Extremity Arteries, Bilateral M Spinal Arteries Q Cervico-Cerebral Arch R Intracranial Arteries	Z None	Z None	Z None

B Imaging
3 Upper Arteries
4 Ultrasonography Definition: Real time display of images of anatomy or flow information developed from the capture of reflected and attenuated high frequency sound waves

Body Part Character 4	Contrast Character 5	Qualifier Character 6	Qualifier Character 7
Ø Thoracic Aorta 1 Brachiocephalic-Subclavian Artery, Right 2 Subclavian Artery, Left 3 Common Carotid Artery, Right 4 Common Carotid Artery, Left 5 Common Carotid Arteries, Bilateral 6 Internal Carotid Artery, Right 7 Internal Carotid Artery, Left 8 Internal Carotid Arteries, Bilateral H Upper Extremity Arteries, Right J Upper Extremity Arteries, Left K Upper Extremity Arteries, Bilateral R Intracranial Arteries S Pulmonary Artery, Right T Pulmonary Artery, Left V Ophthalmic Arteries	Z None	Z None	3 Intravascular Z None

B Imaging
4 Lower Arteries
Ø Plain Radiography Definition: Planar display of an image developed from the capture of external ionizing radiation on photographic or photoconductive plate

Body Part Character 4	Contrast Character 5	Qualifier Character 6	Qualifier Character 7
Ø Abdominal Aorta 2 Hepatic Artery 3 Splenic Arteries 4 Superior Mesenteric Artery 5 Inferior Mesenteric Artery 6 Renal Artery, Right 7 Renal Artery, Left 8 Renal Arteries, Bilateral 9 Lumbar Arteries B Intra-Abdominal Arteries, Other C Pelvic Arteries D Aorta and Bilateral Lower Extremity Arteries F Lower Extremity Arteries, Right G Lower Extremity Arteries, Left J Lower Arteries, Other M Renal Artery Transplant	Ø High Osmolar 1 Low Osmolar Y Other Contrast	Z None	Z None

B Imaging
4 Lower Arteries
1 Fluoroscopy Definition: Single plane or bi-plane real time display of an image developed from the capture of external ionizing radiation on a fluorescent screen. The image may also be stored by either digital or analog means.

Body Part Character 4	Contrast Character 5	Qualifier Character 6	Qualifier Character 7
Ø Abdominal Aorta 2 Hepatic Artery 3 Splenic Arteries 4 Superior Mesenteric Artery 5 Inferior Mesenteric Artery 6 Renal Artery, Right 7 Renal Artery, Left 8 Renal Arteries, Bilateral 9 Lumbar Arteries B Intra-Abdominal Arteries, Other C Pelvic Arteries D Aorta and Bilateral Lower Extremity Arteries F Lower Extremity Arteries, Right G Lower Extremity Arteries, Left J Lower Arteries, Other	Ø High Osmolar 1 Low Osmolar Y Other Contrast	1 Laser	Ø Intraoperative
Ø Abdominal Aorta 2 Hepatic Artery 3 Splenic Arteries 4 Superior Mesenteric Artery 5 Inferior Mesenteric Artery 6 Renal Artery, Right 7 Renal Artery, Left 8 Renal Arteries, Bilateral 9 Lumbar Arteries B Intra-Abdominal Arteries, Other C Pelvic Arteries D Aorta and Bilateral Lower Extremity Arteries F Lower Extremity Arteries, Right G Lower Extremity Arteries, Left J Lower Arteries, Other	Ø High Osmolar 1 Low Osmolar Y Other Contrast	Z None	Z None
Ø Abdominal Aorta 2 Hepatic Artery 3 Splenic Arteries 4 Superior Mesenteric Artery 5 Inferior Mesenteric Artery 6 Renal Artery, Right 7 Renal Artery, Left 8 Renal Arteries, Bilateral 9 Lumbar Arteries B Intra-Abdominal Arteries, Other C Pelvic Arteries D Aorta and Bilateral Lower Extremity Arteries F Lower Extremity Arteries, Right G Lower Extremity Arteries, Left J Lower Arteries, Other	Z None	Z None	Z None

B Imaging
4 Lower Arteries
2 Computerized Tomography (CT Scan) Definition: Computer reformatted digital display of multiplanar images developed from the capture of multiple exposures of external ionizing radiation

Body Part Character 4	Contrast Character 5	Qualifier Character 6	Qualifier Character 7
Ø Abdominal Aorta 1 Celiac Artery 4 Superior Mesenteric Artery 8 Renal Arteries, Bilateral C Pelvic Arteries F Lower Extremity Arteries, Right G Lower Extremity Arteries, Left H Lower Extremity Arteries, Bilateral M Renal Artery Transplant	Ø High Osmolar 1 Low Osmolar Y Other Contrast	Z None	Z None
Ø Abdominal Aorta 1 Celiac Artery 4 Superior Mesenteric Artery 8 Renal Arteries, Bilateral C Pelvic Arteries F Lower Extremity Arteries, Right G Lower Extremity Arteries, Left H Lower Extremity Arteries, Bilateral M Renal Artery Transplant	Z None	2 Intravascular Optical Coherence Z None	Z None

B Imaging
4 Lower Arteries
3 Magnetic Resonance Imaging (MRI) Definition: Computer reformatted digital display of multiplanar images developed from the capture of radio-frequency signals emitted by nuclei in a body site excited within a magnetic field

Body Part Character 4	Contrast Character 5	Qualifier Character 6	Qualifier Character 7
Ø Abdominal Aorta 1 Celiac Artery 4 Superior Mesenteric Artery 8 Renal Arteries, Bilateral C Pelvic Arteries F Lower Extremity Arteries, Right G Lower Extremity Arteries, Left H Lower Extremity Arteries, Bilateral	Y Other Contrast	Ø Unenhanced and Enhanced Z None	Z None
Ø Abdominal Aorta 1 Celiac Artery 4 Superior Mesenteric Artery 8 Renal Arteries, Bilateral C Pelvic Arteries F Lower Extremity Arteries, Right G Lower Extremity Arteries, Left H Lower Extremity Arteries, Bilateral	Z None	Z None	Z None

B Imaging
4 Lower Arteries
4 Ultrasonography Definition: Real time display of images of anatomy or flow information developed from the capture of reflected and attenuated high frequency sound waves

Body Part Character 4	Contrast Character 5	Qualifier Character 6	Qualifier Character 7
Ø Abdominal Aorta 4 Superior Mesenteric Artery 5 Inferior Mesenteric Artery 6 Renal Artery, Right 7 Renal Artery, Left 8 Renal Arteries, Bilateral B Intra-Abdominal Arteries, Other F Lower Extremity Arteries, Right G Lower Extremity Arteries, Left H Lower Extremity Arteries, Bilateral K Celiac and Mesenteric Arteries L Femoral Artery N Penile Arteries	Z None	Z None	3 Intravascular Z None

B Imaging
5 Veins
Ø Plain Radiography Definition: Planar display of an image developed from the capture of external ionizing radiation on photographic or photoconductive plate

Body Part Character 4	Contrast Character 5	Qualifier Character 6	Qualifier Character 7
Ø Epidural Veins 1 Cerebral and Cerebellar Veins 2 Intracranial Sinuses 3 Jugular Veins, Right 4 Jugular Veins, Left 5 Jugular Veins, Bilateral 6 Subclavian Vein, Right 7 Subclavian Vein, Left 8 Superior Vena Cava 9 Inferior Vena Cava B Lower Extremity Veins, Right C Lower Extremity Veins, Left D Lower Extremity Veins, Bilateral F Pelvic (Iliac) Veins, Right G Pelvic (Iliac) Veins, Left H Pelvic (Iliac) Veins, Bilateral J Renal Vein, Right K Renal Vein, Left L Renal Veins, Bilateral M Upper Extremity Veins, Right N Upper Extremity Veins, Left P Upper Extremity Veins, Bilateral Q Pulmonary Vein, Right R Pulmonary Vein, Left S Pulmonary Veins, Bilateral T Portal and Splanchnic Veins V Veins, Other W Dialysis Shunt/Fistula	Ø High Osmolar 1 Low Osmolar Y Other Contrast	Z None	Z None

B Imaging
5 Veins
1 Fluoroscopy Definition: Single plane or bi-plane real time display of an image developed from the capture of external ionizing radioation on a fluorescent screen. The image may also be stored by either digital or analog means.

Body Part Character 4	Contrast Character 5	Qualifier Character 6	Qualifier Character 7
Ø Epidural Veins 1 Cerebral and Cerebellar Veins 2 Intracranial Sinuses 3 Jugular Veins, Right 4 Jugular Veins, Left 5 Jugular Veins, Bilateral 6 Subclavian Vein, Right 7 Subclavian Vein, Left 8 Superior Vena Cava 9 Inferior Vena Cava B Lower Extremity Veins, Right C Lower Extremity Veins, Left D Lower Extremity Veins, Bilateral F Pelvic (Iliac) Veins, Right G Pelvic (Iliac) Veins, Left H Pelvic (Iliac) Veins, Bilateral J Renal Vein, Right K Renal Vein, Left L Renal Veins, Bilateral M Upper Extremity Veins, Right N Upper Extremity Veins, Left P Upper Extremity Veins, Bilateral Q Pulmonary Vein, Right R Pulmonary Vein, Left S Pulmonary Veins, Bilateral T Portal and Splanchnic Veins V Veins, Other W Dialysis Shunt/Fistula	Ø High Osmolar 1 Low Osmolar Y Other Contrast Z None	Z None	A Guidance Z None

B Imaging
5 Veins
2 Computerized Tomography (CT Scan) Definition: Computer reformatted digital display of multiplanar images developed from the capture of multiple exposures of external ionizing radiation

Body Part Character 4	Contrast Character 5	Qualifier Character 6	Qualifier Character 7
2 Intracranial Sinuses 8 Superior Vena Cava 9 Inferior Vena Cava F Pelvic (Iliac) Veins, Right G Pelvic (Iliac) Veins, Left H Pelvic (Iliac) Veins, Bilateral J Renal Vein, Right K Renal Vein, Left L Renal Veins, Bilateral Q Pulmonary Vein, Right R Pulmonary Vein, Left S Pulmonary Veins, Bilateral T Portal and Splanchnic Veins	Ø High Osmolar 1 Low Osmolar Y Other Contrast	Ø Unenhanced and Enhanced Z None	Z None
2 Intracranial Sinuses 8 Superior Vena Cava 9 Inferior Vena Cava F Pelvic (Iliac) Veins, Right G Pelvic (Iliac) Veins, Left H Pelvic (Iliac) Veins, Bilateral J Renal Vein, Right K Renal Vein, Left L Renal Veins, Bilateral Q Pulmonary Vein, Right R Pulmonary Vein, Left S Pulmonary Veins, Bilateral T Portal and Splanchnic Veins	Z None	2 Intravascular Optical Coherence Z None	Z None

B Imaging
5 Veins
3 Magnetic Resonance Imaging (MRI) Definition: Computer reformatted digital display of multiplanar images developed from the capture of radio-frequency signals emitted by nuclei in a body site excited within a magnetic field

Body Part Character 4	Contrast Character 5	Qualifier Character 6	Qualifier Character 7
1 Cerebral and Cerebellar Veins 2 Intracranial Sinuses 5 Jugular Veins, Bilateral 8 Superior Vena Cava 9 Inferior Vena Cava B Lower Extremity Veins, Right C Lower Extremity Veins, Left D Lower Extremity Veins, Bilateral H Pelvic (Iliac) Veins, Bilateral L Renal Veins, Bilateral M Upper Extremity Veins, Right N Upper Extremity Veins, Left P Upper Extremity Veins, Bilateral S Pulmonary Veins, Bilateral T Portal and Splanchnic Veins V Veins, Other	Y Other Contrast	Ø Unenhanced and Enhanced Z None	Z None
1 Cerebral and Cerebellar Veins 2 Intracranial Sinuses 5 Jugular Veins, Bilateral 8 Superior Vena Cava 9 Inferior Vena Cava B Lower Extremity Veins, Right C Lower Extremity Veins, Left D Lower Extremity Veins, Bilateral H Pelvic (Iliac) Veins, Bilateral L Renal Veins, Bilateral M Upper Extremity Veins, Right N Upper Extremity Veins, Left P Upper Extremity Veins, Bilateral S Pulmonary Veins, Bilateral T Portal and Splanchnic Veins V Veins, Other	Z None	Z None	Z None

B Imaging
5 Veins
4 Ultrasonography Definition: Real time display of images of anatomy or flow information developed from the capture of reflected and attenuated high frequency sound waves

Body Part Character 4	Contrast Character 5	Qualifier Character 6	Qualifier Character 7
3 Jugular Veins, Right 4 Jugular Veins, Left 6 Subclavian Vein, Right 7 Subclavian Vein, Left 8 Superior Vena Cava 9 Inferior Vena Cava B Lower Extremity Veins, Right C Lower Extremity Veins, Left D Lower Extremity Veins, Bilateral J Renal Vein, Right K Renal Vein, Left L Renal Veins, Bilateral M Upper Extremity Veins, Right N Upper Extremity Veins, Left P Upper Extremity Veins, Bilateral T Portal and Splanchnic Veins	Z None	Z None	3 Intravascular A Guidance Z None

B Imaging
7 Lymphatic System
Ø Plain Radiography Definition: Planar display of an image developed from the capture of external ionizing radiation on photographic or photoconductive plate

Body Part Character 4	Contrast Character 5	Qualifier Character 6	Qualifier Character 7
Ø Abdominal/Retroperitoneal Lymphatics, Unilateral 1 Abdominal/Retroperitoneal Lymphatics, Bilateral 4 Lymphatics, Head and Neck 5 Upper Extremity Lymphatics, Right 6 Upper Extremity Lymphatics, Left 7 Upper Extremity Lymphatics, Bilateral 8 Lower Extremity Lymphatics, Right 9 Lower Extremity Lymphatics, Left B Lower Extremity Lymphatics, Bilateral C Lymphatics, Pelvic	Ø High Osmolar 1 Low Osmolar Y Other Contrast	Z None	Z None

B Imaging
8 Eye
Ø Plain Radiography Definition: Planar display of an image developed from the capture of external ionizing radiation on photographic or photoconductive plate

Body Part Character 4	Contrast Character 5	Qualifier Character 6	Qualifier Character 7
Ø Lacrimal Duct, Right 1 Lacrimal Duct, Left 2 Lacrimal Ducts, Bilateral	Ø High Osmolar 1 Low Osmolar Y Other Contrast	Z None	Z None
3 Optic Foramina, Right 4 Optic Foramina, Left 5 Eye, Right 6 Eye, Left 7 Eyes, Bilateral	Z None	Z None	Z None

B Imaging
8 Eye
2 Computerized Tomography (CT Scan) Definition: Computer reformatted digital display of multiplanar images developed from the capture of multiple exposures of external ionizing radiation

Body Part Character 4	Contrast Character 5	Qualifier Character 6	Qualifier Character 7
5 Eye, Right 6 Eye, Left 7 Eyes, Bilateral	Ø High Osmolar 1 Low Osmolar Y Other Contrast	Ø Unenhanced and Enhanced Z None	Z None
5 Eye, Right 6 Eye, Left 7 Eyes, Bilateral	Z None	Z None	Z None

B Imaging
8 Eye
3 Magnetic Resonance Imaging (MRI) Definition: Computer reformatted digital display of multiplanar images developed from the capture of radio-frequency signals emitted by nuclei in a body site excited within a magnetic field

Body Part Character 4	Contrast Character 5	Qualifier Character 6	Qualifier Character 7
5 Eye, Right 6 Eye, Left 7 Eyes, Bilateral	Y Other Contrast	Ø Unenhanced and Enhanced Z None	Z None
5 Eye, Right 6 Eye, Left 7 Eyes, Bilateral	Z None	Z None	Z None

B Imaging
8 Eye
4 Ultrasonography Definition: Real time display of images of anatomy or flow information developed from the capture of reflected and attenuated high frequency sound waves

Body Part Character 4	Contrast Character 5	Qualifier Character 6	Qualifier Character 7
5 Eye, Right 6 Eye, Left 7 Eyes, Bilateral	Z None	Z None	Z None

B Imaging
9 Ear, Nose, Mouth and Throat
Ø Plain Radiography Definition: Planar display of an image developed from the capture of external ionizing radiation on photographic or photoconductive plate

Body Part Character 4	Contrast Character 5	Qualifier Character 6	Qualifier Character 7
2 Paranasal Sinuses F Nasopharynx/Oropharynx H Mastoids	Z None	Z None	Z None
4 Parotid Gland, Right 5 Parotid Gland, Left 6 Parotid Glands, Bilateral 7 Submandibular Gland, Right 8 Submandibular Gland, Left 9 Submandibular Glands, Bilateral B Salivary Gland, Right C Salivary Gland, Left D Salivary Glands, Bilateral	Ø High Osmolar 1 Low Osmolar Y Other Contrast	Z None	Z None

B Imaging
9 Ear, Nose, Mouth and Throat
1 Fluoroscopy Definition: Single plane or bi-plane real time display of an image developed from the capture of external ionizing radioation on a fluorescent screen. The image may also be stored by either digital or analog means.

Body Part Character 4	Contrast Character 5	Qualifier Character 6	Qualifier Character 7
G Pharynx and Epiglottis J Larynx	Y Other Contrast Z None	Z None	Z None

B Imaging
9 Ear, Nose, Mouth and Throat
2 Computerized Tomography (CT Scan) Definition: Computer reformatted digital display of multiplanar images developed from the capture of multiple exposures of external ionizing radiation

Body Part Character 4	Contrast Character 5	Qualifier Character 6	Qualifier Character 7
Ø Ear 2 Paranasal Sinuses 6 Parotid Glands, Bilateral 9 Submandibular Glands, Bilateral D Salivary Glands, Bilateral F Nasopharynx/Oropharynx J Larynx	Ø High Osmolar 1 Low Osmolar Y Other Contrast	Ø Unenhanced and Enhanced Z None	Z None
Ø Ear 2 Paranasal Sinuses 6 Parotid Glands, Bilateral 9 Submandibular Glands, Bilateral D Salivary Glands, Bilateral F Nasopharynx/Oropharynx J Larynx	Z None	Z None	Z None

B Imaging
9 Ear, Nose, Mouth and Throat
3 Magnetic Resonance Imaging (MRI) Definition: Computer reformatted digital display of multiplanar images developed from the capture of radio-frequency signals emitted by nuclei in a body site excited within a magnetic field

Body Part Character 4	Contrast Character 5	Qualifier Character 6	Qualifier Character 7
Ø Ear 2 Paranasal Sinuses 6 Parotid Glands, Bilateral 9 Submandibular Glands, Bilateral D Salivary Glands, Bilateral F Nasopharynx/Oropharynx J Larynx	Y Other Contrast	Ø Unenhanced and Enhanced Z None	Z None
Ø Ear 2 Paranasal Sinuses 6 Parotid Glands, Bilateral 9 Submandibular Glands, Bilateral D Salivary Glands, Bilateral F Nasopharynx/Oropharynx J Larynx	Z None	Z None	Z None

B Imaging
B Respiratory System
Ø Plain Radiography Definition: Planar display of an image developed from the capture of external ionizing radiation on photographic or photoconductive plate

Body Part Character 4	Contrast Character 5	Qualifier Character 6	Qualifier Character 7
7 Tracheobronchial Tree, Right 8 Tracheobronchial Tree, Left 9 Tracheobronchial Trees, Bilateral	Y Other Contrast	Z None	Z None
D Upper Airways	Z None	Z None	Z None

B Imaging
B Respiratory System
1 Fluoroscopy Definition: Single plane or bi-plane real time display of an image developed from the capture of external ionizing radioation on a fluorescent screen. The image may also be stored by either digital or analog means.

Body Part Character 4	Contrast Character 5	Qualifier Character 6	Qualifier Character 7
2 Lung, Right 3 Lung, Left 4 Lungs, Bilateral 6 Diaphragm C Mediastinum D Upper Airways	Z None	Z None	Z None
7 Tracheobronchial Tree, Right 8 Tracheobronchial Tree, Left 9 Tracheobronchial Trees, Bilateral	Y Other Contrast	Z None	Z None

B Imaging
B Respiratory System
2 Computerized Tomography (CT Scan) Definition: Computer reformatted digital display of multiplanar images developed from the capture of multiple exposures of external ionizing radiation

Body Part Character 4	Contrast Character 5	Qualifier Character 6	Qualifier Character 7
4 Lungs, Bilateral 7 Tracheobronchial Tree, Right 8 Tracheobronchial Tree, Left 9 Tracheobronchial Trees, Bilateral F Trachea/Airways	Ø High Osmolar 1 Low Osmolar Y Other Contrast	Ø Unenhanced and Enhanced Z None	Z None
4 Lungs, Bilateral 7 Tracheobronchial Tree, Right 8 Tracheobronchial Tree, Left 9 Tracheobronchial Trees, Bilateral F Trachea/Airways	Z None	Z None	Z None

B Imaging
B Respiratory System
3 Magnetic Resonance Imaging (MRI) Definition: Computer reformatted digital display of multiplanar images developed from the capture of radio-frequency signals emitted by nuclei in a body site excited within a magnetic field

Body Part Character 4	Contrast Character 5	Qualifier Character 6	Qualifier Character 7
G Lung Apices	Y Other Contrast	Ø Unenhanced and Enhanced Z None	Z None
G Lung Apices	Z None	Z None	Z None

B Imaging
B Respiratory System
4 Ultrasonography Definition: Real time display of images of anatomy or flow information developed from the capture of reflected and attenuated high frequency sound waves

Body Part Character 4	Contrast Character 5	Qualifier Character 6	Qualifier Character 7
B Pleura C Mediastinum	Z None	Z None	Z None

B Imaging
D Gastrointestinal System
1 Fluoroscopy Definition: Single plane or bi-plane real time display of an image developed from the capture of external ionizing radioation on a fluorescent screen. The image may also be stored by either digital or analog means.

Body Part Character 4	Contrast Character 5	Qualifier Character 6	Qualifier Character 7
1 Esophagus 2 Stomach 3 Small Bowel 4 Colon 5 Upper GI 6 Upper GI and Small Bowel 9 Duodenum B Mouth/Oropharynx	Y Other Contrast Z None	Z None	Z None

B Imaging
D Gastrointestinal System
2 Computerized Tomography (CT Scan) Definition: Computer reformatted digital display of multiplanar images developed from the capture of multiple exposures of external ionizing radiation

Body Part Character 4	Contrast Character 5	Qualifier Character 6	Qualifier Character 7
4 Colon	Ø High Osmolar 1 Low Osmolar Y Other Contrast	Ø Unenhanced and Enhanced Z None	Z None
4 Colon	Z None	Z None	Z None

B Imaging
D Gastrointestinal System
4 Ultrasonography Definition: Real time display of images of anatomy or flow information developed from the capture of reflected and attenuated high frequency sound waves

Body Part Character 4	Contrast Character 5	Qualifier Character 6	Qualifier Character 7
1 Esophagus 2 Stomach 7 Gastrointestinal Tract 8 Appendix 9 Duodenum C Rectum	Z None	Z None	Z None

B Imaging
F Hepatobiliary System and Pancreas
Ø Plain Radiography Definition: Planar display of an image developed from the capture of external ionizing radiation on photographic or photoconductive plate

Body Part Character 4	Contrast Character 5	Qualifier Character 6	Qualifier Character 7
Ø Bile Ducts 3 Gallbladder and Bile Ducts C Hepatobiliary System, All	Ø High Osmolar 1 Low Osmolar Y Other Contrast	Z None	Z None

B Imaging
F Hepatobiliary System and Pancreas
1 Fluoroscopy Definition: Single plane or bi-plane real time display of an image developed from the capture of external ionizing radioation on a fluorescent screen. The image may also be stored by either digital or analog means.

Body Part Character 4	Contrast Character 5	Qualifier Character 6	Qualifier Character 7
Ø Bile Ducts **1** Biliary and Pancreatic Ducts **2** Gallbladder **3** Gallbladder and Bile Ducts **4** Gallbladder, Bile Ducts and Pancreatic Ducts **8** Pancreatic Ducts	**Ø** High Osmolar **1** Low Osmolar **Y** Other Contrast	**Z** None	**Z** None
5 Liver	**Ø** High Osmolar **1** Low Osmolar **Y** Other Contrast	**Z** None	**Z** None
5 Liver	**Z** None	**Z** None	**A** Guidance

B Imaging
F Hepatobiliary System and Pancreas
2 Computerized Tomography (CT Scan) Definition: Computer reformatted digital display of multiplanar images developed from the capture of multiple exposures of external ionizing radiation

Body Part Character 4	Contrast Character 5	Qualifier Character 6	Qualifier Character 7
5 Liver **6** Liver and Spleen **7** Pancreas **C** Hepatobiliary System, All	**Ø** High Osmolar **1** Low Osmolar **Y** Other Contrast	**Ø** Unenhanced and Enhanced **Z** None	**Z** None
5 Liver **6** Liver and Spleen **7** Pancreas **C** Hepatobiliary System, All	**Z** None	**Z** None	**Z** None

B Imaging
F Hepatobiliary System and Pancreas
3 Magnetic Resonance Imaging (MRI) Definition: Computer reformatted digital display of multiplanar images developed from the capture of radio-frequency signals emitted by nuclei in a body site excited within a magnetic field

Body Part Character 4	Contrast Character 5	Qualifier Character 6	Qualifier Character 7
5 Liver **6** Liver and Spleen **7** Pancreas	**Y** Other Contrast	**Ø** Unenhanced and Enhanced **Z** None	**Z** None
5 Liver **6** Liver and Spleen **7** Pancreas	**Z** None	**Z** None	**Z** None

B Imaging
F Hepatobiliary System and Pancreas
4 Ultrasonography Definition: Real time display of images of anatomy or flow information developed from the capture of reflected and attenuated high frequency sound waves

Body Part Character 4	Contrast Character 5	Qualifier Character 6	Qualifier Character 7
Ø Bile Ducts **2** Gallbladder **3** Gallbladder and Bile Ducts **5** Liver **6** Liver and Spleen **7** Pancreas **C** Hepatobiliary System, All	**Z** None	**Z** None	**Z** None

B Imaging
F Hepatobiliary System and Pancreas
5 Other Imaging Definition: Other specified modality for visualizing a body part

Body Part Character 4	Contrast Character 5	Qualifier Character 6	Qualifier Character 7
Ø Bile Ducts **2** Gallbladder **3** Gallbladder and Bile Ducts **5** Liver **6** Liver and Spleen **7** Pancreas **C** Hepatobiliary System, All	**2** Fluorescing Agent	**Ø** Indocyanine Green Dye **Z** None	**Ø** Intraoperative **Z** None

B Imaging
G Endocrine System
2 Computerized Tomography (CT Scan) Definition: Computer reformatted digital display of multiplanar images developed from the capture of multiple exposures of external ionizing radiation

Body Part Character 4	Contrast Character 5	Qualifier Character 6	Qualifier Character 7
2 Adrenal Glands, Bilateral 3 Parathyroid Glands 4 Thyroid Gland	Ø High Osmolar 1 Low Osmolar Y Other Contrast	Ø Unenhanced and Enhanced Z None	Z None
2 Adrenal Glands, Bilateral 3 Parathyroid Glands 4 Thyroid Gland	Z None	Z None	Z None

B Imaging
G Endocrine System
3 Magnetic Resonance Imaging (MRI) Definition: Computer reformatted digital display of multiplanar images developed from the capture of radio-frequency signals emitted by nuclei in a body site excited within a magnetic field

Body Part Character 4	Contrast Character 5	Qualifier Character 6	Qualifier Character 7
2 Adrenal Glands, Bilateral 3 Parathyroid Glands 4 Thyroid Gland	Y Other Contrast	Ø Unenhanced and Enhanced Z None	Z None
2 Adrenal Glands, Bilateral 3 Parathyroid Glands 4 Thyroid Gland	Z None	Z None	Z None

B Imaging
G Endocrine System
4 Ultrasonography Definition: Real time display of images of anatomy or flow information developed from the capture of reflected and attenuated high frequency sound waves

Body Part Character 4	Contrast Character 5	Qualifier Character 6	Qualifier Character 7
Ø Adrenal Gland, Right 1 Adrenal Gland, Left 2 Adrenal Glands, Bilateral 3 Parathyroid Glands 4 Thyroid Gland	Z None	Z None	Z None

B Imaging
H Skin, Subcutaneous Tissue and Breast
Ø Plain Radiography Definition: Planar display of an image developed from the capture of external ionizing radiation on photographic or photoconductive plate

Body Part Character 4	Contrast Character 5	Qualifier Character 6	Qualifier Character 7
Ø Breast, Right 1 Breast, Left 2 Breasts, Bilateral	Z None	Z None	Z None
3 Single Mammary Duct, Right 4 Single Mammary Duct, Left 5 Multiple Mammary Ducts, Right 6 Multiple Mammary Ducts, Left	Ø High Osmolar 1 Low Osmolar Y Other Contrast Z None	Z None	Z None

B Imaging
H Skin, Subcutaneous Tissue and Breast
3 Magnetic Resonance Imaging (MRI) Definition: Computer reformatted digital display of multiplanar images developed from the capture of radio-frequency signals emitted by nuclei in a body site excited within a magnetic field

Body Part Character 4	Contrast Character 5	Qualifier Character 6	Qualifier Character 7
Ø Breast, Right 1 Breast, Left 2 Breasts, Bilateral D Subcutaneous Tissue, Head/Neck F Subcutaneous Tissue, Upper Extremity G Subcutaneous Tissue, Thorax H Subcutaneous Tissue, Abdomen and Pelvis J Subcutaneous Tissue, Lower Extremity	Y Other Contrast	Ø Unenhanced and Enhanced Z None	Z None
Ø Breast, Right 1 Breast, Left 2 Breasts, Bilateral D Subcutaneous Tissue, Head/Neck F Subcutaneous Tissue, Upper Extremity G Subcutaneous Tissue, Thorax H Subcutaneous Tissue, Abdomen and Pelvis J Subcutaneous Tissue, Lower Extremity	Z None	Z None	Z None

B Imaging
H Skin, Subcutaneous Tissue and Breast
4 Ultrasonography Definition: Real time display of images of anatomy or flow information developed from the capture of reflected and attenuated high frequency sound waves

Body Part Character 4	Contrast Character 5	Qualifier Character 6	Qualifier Character 7
Ø Breast, Right 1 Breast, Left 2 Breasts, Bilateral 7 Extremity, Upper 8 Extremity, Lower 9 Abdominal Wall B Chest Wall C Head and Neck	Z None	Z None	Z None

B Imaging
L Connective Tissue
3 Magnetic Resonance Imaging (MRI) Definition: Computer reformatted digital display of multiplanar images developed from the capture of radio-frequency signals emitted by nuclei in a body site excited within a magnetic field

Body Part Character 4	Contrast Character 5	Qualifier Character 6	Qualifier Character 7
Ø Connective Tissue, Upper Extremity 1 Connective Tissue, Lower Extremity 2 Tendons, Upper Extremity 3 Tendons, Lower Extremity	Y Other Contrast	Ø Unenhanced and Enhanced Z None	Z None
Ø Connective Tissue, Upper Extremity 1 Connective Tissue, Lower Extremity 2 Tendons, Upper Extremity 3 Tendons, Lower Extremity	Z None	Z None	Z None

B Imaging
L Connective Tissue
4 Ultrasonography Definition: Real time display of images of anatomy or flow information developed from the capture of reflected and attenuated high frequency sound waves

Body Part Character 4	Contrast Character 5	Qualifier Character 6	Qualifier Character 7
Ø Connective Tissue, Upper Extremity 1 Connective Tissue, Lower Extremity 2 Tendons, Upper Extremity 3 Tendons, Lower Extremity	Z None	Z None	Z None

B Imaging
N Skull and Facial Bones
Ø Plain Radiography Definition: Planar display of an image developed from the capture of external ionizing radiation on photographic or photoconductive plate

Body Part Character 4	Contrast Character 5	Qualifier Character 6	Qualifier Character 7
Ø Skull 1 Orbit, Right 2 Orbit, Left 3 Orbits, Bilateral 4 Nasal Bones 5 Facial Bones 6 Mandible B Zygomatic Arch, Right C Zygomatic Arch, Left D Zygomatic Arches, Bilateral G Tooth, Single H Teeth, Multiple J Teeth, All	Z None	Z None	Z None
7 Temporomandibular Joint, Right 8 Temporomandibular Joint, Left 9 Temporomandibular Joints, Bilateral	Ø High Osmolar 1 Low Osmolar Y Other Contrast Z None	Z None	Z None

B Imaging
N Skull and Facial Bones
1 Fluoroscopy Definition: Single plane or bi-plane real time display of an image developed from the capture of external ionizing radioation on a fluorescent screen. The image may also be stored by either digital or analog means.

Body Part Character 4	Contrast Character 5	Qualifier Character 6	Qualifier Character 7
7 Temporomandibular Joint, Right 8 Temporomandibular Joint, Left 9 Temporomandibular Joints, Bilateral	Ø High Osmolar 1 Low Osmolar Y Other Contrast Z None	Z None	Z None

B Imaging
N Skull and Facial Bones
2 Computerized Tomography (CT Scan) Definition: Computer reformatted digital display of multiplanar images developed from the capture of multiple exposures of external ionizing radiation

Body Part Character 4	Contrast Character 5	Qualifier Character 6	Qualifier Character 7
Ø Skull 3 Orbits, Bilateral 5 Facial Bones 6 Mandible 9 Temporomandibular Joints, Bilateral F Temporal Bones	Ø High Osmolar 1 Low Osmolar Y Other Contrast Z None	Z None	Z None

B Imaging
N Skull and Facial Bones
3 Magnetic Resonance Imaging (MRI) Definition: Computer reformatted digital display of multiplanar images developed from the capture of radio-frequency signals emitted by nuclei in a body site excited within a magnetic field

Body Part Character 4	Contrast Character 5	Qualifier Character 6	Qualifier Character 7
9 Temporomandibular Joints, Bilateral	Y Other Contrast Z None	Z None	Z None

B Imaging
P Non-Axial Upper Bones
Ø Plain Radiography Definition: Planar display of an image developed from the capture of external ionizing radiation on photographic or photoconductive plate

Body Part Character 4	Contrast Character 5	Qualifier Character 6	Qualifier Character 7
Ø Sternoclavicular Joint, Right 1 Sternoclavicular Joint, Left 2 Sternoclavicular Joints, Bilateral 3 Acromioclavicular Joints, Bilateral 4 Clavicle, Right 5 Clavicle, Left 6 Scapula, Right 7 Scapula, Left A Humerus, Right B Humerus, Left E Upper Arm, Right F Upper Arm, Left J Forearm, Right K Forearm, Left N Hand, Right P Hand, Left R Finger(s), Right S Finger(s), Left X Ribs, Right Y Ribs, Left	Z None	Z None	Z None
8 Shoulder, Right 9 Shoulder, Left C Hand/Finger Joint, Right D Hand/Finger Joint, Left G Elbow, Right H Elbow, Left L Wrist, Right M Wrist, Left	Ø High Osmolar 1 Low Osmolar Y Other Contrast Z None	Z None	Z None

B Imaging
P Non-Axial Upper Bones
1 Fluoroscopy Definition: Single plane or bi-plane real time display of an image developed from the capture of external ionizing radioation on a fluorescent screen. The image may also be stored by either digital or analog means.

Body Part Character 4	Contrast Character 5	Qualifier Character 6	Qualifier Character 7
Ø Sternoclavicular Joint, Right 1 Sternoclavicular Joint, Left 2 Sternoclavicular Joints, Bilateral 3 Acromioclavicular Joints, Bilateral 4 Clavicle, Right 5 Clavicle, Left 6 Scapula, Right 7 Scapula, Left A Humerus, Right B Humerus, Left E Upper Arm, Right F Upper Arm, Left J Forearm, Right K Forearm, Left N Hand, Right P Hand, Left R Finger(s), Right S Finger(s), Left X Ribs, Right Y Ribs, Left	Z None	Z None	Z None
8 Shoulder, Right 9 Shoulder, Left L Wrist, Right M Wrist, Left	Ø High Osmolar 1 Low Osmolar Y Other Contrast Z None	Z None	Z None
C Hand/Finger Joint, Right D Hand/Finger Joint, Left G Elbow, Right H Elbow, Left	Ø High Osmolar 1 Low Osmolar Y Other Contrast	Z None	Z None

B Imaging
P Non-Axial Upper Bones
2 Computerized Tomography (CT Scan) Definition: Computer reformatted digital display of multiplanar images developed from the capture of multiple exposures of external ionizing radiation

Body Part Character 4	Contrast Character 5	Qualifier Character 6	Qualifier Character 7
Ø Sternoclavicular Joint, Right **1** Sternoclavicular Joint, Left **W** Thorax	**Ø** High Osmolar **1** Low Osmolar **Y** Other Contrast	**Z** None	**Z** None
2 Sternoclavicular Joints, Bilateral **3** Acromioclavicular Joints, Bilateral **4** Clavicle, Right **5** Clavicle, Left **6** Scapula, Right **7** Scapula, Left **8** Shoulder, Right **9** Shoulder, Left **A** Humerus, Right **B** Humerus, Left **E** Upper Arm, Right **F** Upper Arm, Left **G** Elbow, Right **H** Elbow, Left **J** Forearm, Right **K** Forearm, Left **L** Wrist, Right **M** Wrist, Left **N** Hand, Right **P** Hand, Left **Q** Hands and Wrists, Bilateral **R** Finger(s), Right **S** Finger(s), Left **T** Upper Extremity, Right **U** Upper Extremity, Left **V** Upper Extremities, Bilateral **X** Ribs, Right **Y** Ribs, Left	**Ø** High Osmolar **1** Low Osmolar **Y** Other Contrast **Z** None	**Z** None	**Z** None
C Hand/Finger Joint, Right **D** Hand/Finger Joint, Left	**Z** None	**Z** None	**Z** None

B Imaging
P Non-Axial Upper Bones
3 Magnetic Resonance Imaging (MRI) Definition: Computer reformatted digital display of multiplanar images developed from the capture of radio-frequency signals emitted by nuclei in a body site excited within a magnetic field

Body Part Character 4	Contrast Character 5	Qualifier Character 6	Qualifier Character 7
8 Shoulder, Right **9** Shoulder, Left **C** Hand/Finger Joint, Right **D** Hand/Finger Joint, Left **E** Upper Arm, Right **F** Upper Arm, Left **G** Elbow, Right **H** Elbow, Left **J** Forearm, Right **K** Forearm, Left **L** Wrist, Right **M** Wrist, Left	**Y** Other Contrast	**Ø** Unenhanced and Enhanced **Z** None	**Z** None
8 Shoulder, Right **9** Shoulder, Left **C** Hand/Finger Joint, Right **D** Hand/Finger Joint, Left **E** Upper Arm, Right **F** Upper Arm, Left **G** Elbow, Right **H** Elbow, Left **J** Forearm, Right **K** Forearm, Left **L** Wrist, Right **M** Wrist, Left	**Z** None	**Z** None	**Z** None

B Imaging
P Non-Axial Upper Bones
4 Ultrasonography Definition: Real time display of images of anatomy or flow information developed from the capture of reflected and attenuated high frequency sound waves

Body Part Character 4	Contrast Character 5	Qualifier Character 6	Qualifier Character 7
8 Shoulder, Right **9** Shoulder, Left **G** Elbow, Right **H** Elbow, Left **L** Wrist, Right **M** Wrist, Left **N** Hand, Right **P** Hand, Left	**Z** None	**Z** None	**1** Densitometry **Z** None

B Imaging
Q Non-Axial Lower Bones
Ø Plain Radiography Definition: Planar display of an image developed from the capture of external ionizing radiation on photographic or photoconductive plate

Body Part Character 4	Contrast Character 5	Qualifier Character 6	Qualifier Character 7
Ø Hip, Right **1** Hip, Left	**Ø** High Osmolar **1** Low Osmolar **Y** Other Contrast	**Z** None	**Z** None
Ø Hip, Right **1** Hip, Left	**Z** None	**Z** None	**1** Densitometry **Z** None
3 Femur, Right **4** Femur, Left	**Z** None	**Z** None	**1** Densitometry **Z** None
7 Knee, Right **8** Knee, Left **G** Ankle, Right **H** Ankle, Left	**Ø** High Osmolar **1** Low Osmolar **Y** Other Contrast **Z** None	**Z** None	**Z** None
D Lower Leg, Right **F** Lower Leg, Left **J** Calcaneus, Right **K** Calcaneus, Left **L** Foot, Right **M** Foot, Left **P** Toe(s), Right **Q** Toe(s), Left **V** Patella, Right **W** Patella, Left	**Z** None	**Z** None	**Z** None
X Foot/Toe Joint, Right **Y** Foot/Toe Joint, Left	**Ø** High Osmolar **1** Low Osmolar **Y** Other Contrast	**Z** None	**Z** None

B Imaging
Q Non-Axial Lower Bones
1 Fluoroscopy Definition: Single plane or bi-plane real time display of an image developed from the capture of external ionizing radioation on a fluorescent screen. The image may also be stored by either digital or analog means.

Body Part Character 4	Contrast Character 5	Qualifier Character 6	Qualifier Character 7
Ø Hip, Right **1** Hip, Left **7** Knee, Right **8** Knee, Left **G** Ankle, Right **H** Ankle, Left **X** Foot/Toe Joint, Right **Y** Foot/Toe Joint, Left	**Ø** High Osmolar **1** Low Osmolar **Y** Other Contrast **Z** None	**Z** None	**Z** None
3 Femur, Right **4** Femur, Left **D** Lower Leg, Right **F** Lower Leg, Left **J** Calcaneus, Right **K** Calcaneus, Left **L** Foot, Right **M** Foot, Left **P** Toe(s), Right **Q** Toe(s), Left **V** Patella, Right **W** Patella, Left	**Z** None	**Z** None	**Z** None

B Imaging
Q Non-Axial Lower Bones
2 Computerized Tomography (CT Scan) Definition: Computer reformatted digital display of multiplanar images developed from the capture of multiple exposures of external ionizing radiation

Body Part Character 4	Contrast Character 5	Qualifier Character 6	Qualifier Character 7
Ø Hip, Right **1** Hip, Left **3** Femur, Right **4** Femur, Left **7** Knee, Right **8** Knee, Left **D** Lower Leg, Right **F** Lower Leg, Left **G** Ankle, Right **H** Ankle, Left **J** Calcaneus, Right **K** Calcaneus, Left **L** Foot, Right **M** Foot, Left **P** Toe(s), Right **Q** Toe(s), Left **R** Lower Extremity, Right **S** Lower Extremity, Left **V** Patella, Right **W** Patella, Left **X** Foot/Toe Joint, Right **Y** Foot/Toe Joint, Left	**Ø** High Osmolar **1** Low Osmolar **Y** Other Contrast **Z** None	**Z** None	**Z** None
B Tibia/Fibula, Right **C** Tibia/Fibula, Left	**Ø** High Osmolar **1** Low Osmolar **Y** Other Contrast	**Z** None	**Z** None

B Imaging
Q Non-Axial Lower Bones
3 Magnetic Resonance Imaging (MRI) Definition: Computer reformatted digital display of multiplanar images developed from the capture of radio-frequency signals emitted by nuclei in a body site excited within a magnetic field

Body Part Character 4	Contrast Character 5	Qualifier Character 6	Qualifier Character 7
Ø Hip, Right **1** Hip, Left **3** Femur, Right **4** Femur, Left **7** Knee, Right **8** Knee, Left **D** Lower Leg, Right **F** Lower Leg, Left **G** Ankle, Right **H** Ankle, Left **J** Calcaneus, Right **K** Calcaneus, Left **L** Foot, Right **M** Foot, Left **P** Toe(s), Right **Q** Toe(s), Left **V** Patella, Right **W** Patella, Left	**Y** Other Contrast	**Ø** Unenhanced and Enhanced **Z** None	**Z** None
Ø Hip, Right **1** Hip, Left **3** Femur, Right **4** Femur, Left **7** Knee, Right **8** Knee, Left **D** Lower Leg, Right **F** Lower Leg, Left **G** Ankle, Right **H** Ankle, Left **J** Calcaneus, Right **K** Calcaneus, Left **L** Foot, Right **M** Foot, Left **P** Toe(s), Right **Q** Toe(s), Left **V** Patella, Right **W** Patella, Left	**Z** None	**Z** None	**Z** None

B Imaging
Q Non-Axial Lower Bones
4 Ultrasonography Definition: Real time display of images of anatomy or flow information developed from the capture of reflected and attenuated high frequency sound waves

Body Part Character 4	Contrast Character 5	Qualifier Character 6	Qualifier Character 7
Ø Hip, Right 1 Hip, Left 2 Hips, Bilateral 7 Knee, Right 8 Knee, Left 9 Knees, Bilateral	Z None	Z None	Z None

B Imaging
R Axial Skeleton, Except Skull and Facial Bones
Ø Plain Radiography Definition: Planar display of an image developed from the capture of external ionizing radiation on photographic or photoconductive plate

Body Part Character 4	Contrast Character 5	Qualifier Character 6	Qualifier Character 7
Ø Cervical Spine 7 Thoracic Spine 9 Lumbar Spine G Whole Spine	Z None	Z None	1 Densitometry Z None
1 Cervical Disc(s) 2 Thoracic Disc(s) 3 Lumbar Disc(s) 4 Cervical Facet Joint(s) 5 Thoracic Facet Joint(s) 6 Lumbar Facet Joint(s) D Sacroiliac Joints	Ø High Osmolar 1 Low Osmolar Y Other Contrast Z None	Z None	Z None
8 Thoracolumbar Joint B Lumbosacral Joint C Pelvis F Sacrum and Coccyx H Sternum	Z None	Z None	Z None

B Imaging
R Axial Skeleton, Except Skull and Facial Bones
1 Fluoroscopy Definition: Single plane or bi-plane real time display of an image developed from the capture of external ionizing radioation on a fluorescent screen. The image may also be stored by either digital or analog means.

Body Part Character 4	Contrast Character 5	Qualifier Character 6	Qualifier Character 7
Ø Cervical Spine 1 Cervical Disc(s) 2 Thoracic Disc(s) 3 Lumbar Disc(s) 4 Cervical Facet Joint(s) 5 Thoracic Facet Joint(s) 6 Lumbar Facet Joint(s) 7 Thoracic Spine 8 Thoracolumbar Joint 9 Lumbar Spine B Lumbosacral Joint C Pelvis D Sacroiliac Joints F Sacrum and Coccyx G Whole Spine H Sternum	Ø High Osmolar 1 Low Osmolar Y Other Contrast Z None	Z None	Z None

B Imaging
R Axial Skeleton, Except Skull and Facial Bones
2 Computerized Tomography (CT Scan) Definition: Computer reformatted digital display of multiplanar images developed from the capture of multiple exposures of external ionizing radiation

Body Part Character 4	Contrast Character 5	Qualifier Character 6	Qualifier Character 7
Ø Cervical Spine 7 Thoracic Spine 9 Lumbar Spine C Pelvis D Sacroiliac Joints F Sacrum and Coccyx	Ø High Osmolar 1 Low Osmolar Y Other Contrast Z None	Z None	Z None

B Imaging
R Axial Skeleton, Except Skull and Facial Bones
3 Magnetic Resonance Imaging (MRI) Definition: Computer reformatted digital display of multiplanar images developed from the capture of radio-frequency signals emitted by nuclei in a body site excited within a magnetic field

Body Part Character 4	Contrast Character 5	Qualifier Character 6	Qualifier Character 7
Ø Cervical Spine 1 Cervical Disc(s) 2 Thoracic Disc(s) 3 Lumbar Disc(s) 7 Thoracic Spine 9 Lumbar Spine C Pelvis F Sacrum and Coccyx	Y Other Contrast	Ø Unenhanced and Enhanced Z None	Z None
Ø Cervical Spine 1 Cervical Disc(s) 2 Thoracic Disc(s) 3 Lumbar Disc(s) 7 Thoracic Spine 9 Lumbar Spine C Pelvis F Sacrum and Coccyx	Z None	Z None	Z None

B Imaging
R Axial Skeleton, Except Skull and Facial Bones
4 Ultrasonography Definition: Real time display of images of anatomy or flow information developed from the capture of reflected and attenuated high frequency sound waves

Body Part Character 4	Contrast Character 5	Qualifier Character 6	Qualifier Character 7
Ø Cervical Spine 7 Thoracic Spine 9 Lumbar Spine F Sacrum and Coccyx	Z None	Z None	Z None

B Imaging
T Urinary System
Ø Plain Radiography Definition: Planar display of an image developed from the capture of external ionizing radiation on photographic or photoconductive plate

Body Part Character 4	Contrast Character 5	Qualifier Character 6	Qualifier Character 7
Ø Bladder 1 Kidney, Right 2 Kidney, Left 3 Kidneys, Bilateral 4 Kidneys, Ureters and Bladder 5 Urethra 6 Ureter, Right 7 Ureter, Left 8 Ureters, Bilateral B Bladder and Urethra C Ileal Diversion Loop	Ø High Osmolar 1 Low Osmolar Y Other Contrast Z None	Z None	Z None

B Imaging
T Urinary System
1 Fluoroscopy Definition: Single plane or bi-plane real time display of an image developed from the capture of external ionizing radioation on a fluorescent screen. The image may also be stored by either digital or analog means.

Body Part Character 4	Contrast Character 5	Qualifier Character 6	Qualifier Character 7
Ø Bladder 1 Kidney, Right 2 Kidney, Left 3 Kidneys, Bilateral 4 Kidneys, Ureters and Bladder 5 Urethra 6 Ureter, Right 7 Ureter, Left B Bladder and Urethra C Ileal Diversion Loop D Kidney, Ureter and Bladder, Right F Kidney, Ureter and Bladder, Left G Ileal Loop, Ureters and Kidneys	Ø High Osmolar 1 Low Osmolar Y Other Contrast Z None	Z None	Z None

B Imaging
T Urinary System
2 Computerized Tomography (CT Scan) Definition: Computer reformatted digital display of multiplanar images developed from the capture of multiple exposures of external ionizing radiation

Body Part Character 4	Contrast Character 5	Qualifier Character 6	Qualifier Character 7
Ø Bladder 1 Kidney, Right 2 Kidney, Left 3 Kidneys, Bilateral 9 Kidney Transplant	Ø High Osmolar 1 Low Osmolar Y Other Contrast	Ø Unenhanced and Enhanced Z None	Z None
Ø Bladder 1 Kidney, Right 2 Kidney, Left 3 Kidneys, Bilateral 9 Kidney Transplant	Z None	Z None	Z None

B Imaging
T Urinary System
3 Magnetic Resonance Imaging (MRI) Definition: Computer reformatted digital display of multiplanar images developed from the capture of radio-frequency signals emitted by nuclei in a body site excited within a magnetic field

Body Part Character 4	Contrast Character 5	Qualifier Character 6	Qualifier Character 7
Ø Bladder 1 Kidney, Right 2 Kidney, Left 3 Kidneys, Bilateral 9 Kidney Transplant	Y Other Contrast	Ø Unenhanced and Enhanced Z None	Z None
Ø Bladder 1 Kidney, Right 2 Kidney, Left 3 Kidneys, Bilateral 9 Kidney Transplant	Z None	Z None	Z None

B Imaging
T Urinary System
4 Ultrasonography Definition: Real time display of images of anatomy or flow information developed from the capture of reflected and attenuated high frequency sound waves

Body Part Character 4	Contrast Character 5	Qualifier Character 6	Qualifier Character 7
Ø Bladder 1 Kidney, Right 2 Kidney, Left 3 Kidneys, Bilateral 5 Urethra 6 Ureter, Right 7 Ureter, Left 8 Ureters, Bilateral 9 Kidney Transplant J Kidneys and Bladder	Z None	Z None	Z None

B Imaging
U Female Reproductive System
Ø Plain Radiography Definition: Planar display of an image developed from the capture of external ionizing radiation on photographic or photoconductive plate

Body Part Character 4	Contrast Character 5	Qualifier Character 6	Qualifier Character 7
Ø Fallopian Tube, Right ♀ 1 Fallopian Tube, Left ♀ 2 Fallopian Tubes, Bilateral ♀ 6 Uterus ♀ 8 Uterus and Fallopian Tubes ♀ 9 Vagina ♀	Ø High Osmolar 1 Low Osmolar Y Other Contrast	Z None	Z None

♀ All body part, contrast, and qualifier values

B Imaging
U Female Reproductive System
1 Fluoroscopy Definition: Single plane or bi-plane real time display of an image developed from the capture of external ionizing radioation on a fluorescent screen. The image may also be stored by either digital or analog means.

Body Part Character 4	Contrast Character 5	Qualifier Character 6	Qualifier Character 7
Ø Fallopian Tube, Right ♀ 1 Fallopian Tube, Left ♀ 2 Fallopian Tubes, Bilateral ♀ 6 Uterus ♀ 8 Uterus and Fallopian Tubes ♀ 9 Vagina ♀	Ø High Osmolar 1 Low Osmolar Y Other Contrast Z None	Z None	Z None

♀ All body part, contrast, and qualifier values

B Imaging
U Female Reproductive System
3 Magnetic Resonance Imaging (MRI) Definition: Computer reformatted digital display of multiplanar images developed from the capture of radio-frequency signals emitted by nuclei in a body site excited within a magnetic field

Body Part Character 4	Contrast Character 5	Qualifier Character 6	Qualifier Character 7
3 Ovary, Right ♀ 4 Ovary, Left ♀ 5 Ovaries, Bilateral ♀ 6 Uterus ♀ 9 Vagina ♀ B Pregnant Uterus ♀ C Uterus and Ovaries ♀	Y Other Contrast	Ø Unenhanced and Enhanced Z None	Z None
3 Ovary, Right ♀ 4 Ovary, Left ♀ 5 Ovaries, Bilateral ♀ 6 Uterus ♀ 9 Vagina ♀ B Pregnant Uterus ♀ C Uterus and Ovaries ♀	Z None	Z None	Z None

♀ All body part, contrast, and qualifier values

B Imaging
U Female Reproductive System
4 Ultrasonography Definition: Real time display of images of anatomy or flow information developed from the capture of reflected and attenuated high frequency sound waves

Body Part Character 4	Contrast Character 5	Qualifier Character 6	Qualifier Character 7
Ø Fallopian Tube, Right ♀ 1 Fallopian Tube, Left ♀ 2 Fallopian Tubes, Bilateral ♀ 3 Ovary, Right ♀ 4 Ovary, Left ♀ 5 Ovaries, Bilateral ♀ 6 Uterus ♀ C Uterus and Ovaries ♀	Y Other Contrast Z None	Z None	Z None

♀ All body part, contrast, and qualifier values

B Imaging
V Male Reproductive System
Ø Plain Radiography Definition: Planar display of an image developed from the capture of external ionizing radiation on photographic or photoconductive plate

Body Part Character 4	Contrast Character 5	Qualifier Character 6	Qualifier Character 7
Ø Corpora Cavernosa ♂ 1 Epididymis, Right ♂ 2 Epididymis, Left ♂ 3 Prostate ♂ 5 Testicle, Right ♂ 6 Testicle, Left ♂ 8 Vasa Vasorum ♂	Ø High Osmolar 1 Low Osmolar Y Other Contrast	Z None	Z None

♂ All body part, contrast, and qualifier values

B Imaging
V Male Reproductive System
1 Fluoroscopy Definition: Single plane or bi-plane real time display of an image developed from the capture of external ionizing radioation on a fluorescent screen. The image may also be stored by either digital or analog means.

Body Part Character 4	Contrast Character 5	Qualifier Character 6	Qualifier Character 7
Ø Corpora Cavernosa ♂ 8 Vasa Vasorum ♂	Ø High Osmolar 1 Low Osmolar Y Other Contrast Z None	Z None	Z None

♂ All body part, contrast, and qualifier values

B Imaging
V Male Reproductive System
2 Computerized Tomography (CT Scan) Definition: Computer reformatted digital display of multiplanar images developed from the capture of multiple exposures of external ionizing radiation

Body Part Character 4	Contrast Character 5	Qualifier Character 6	Qualifier Character 7
3 Prostate ♂	Ø High Osmolar 1 Low Osmolar Y Other Contrast	Ø Unenhanced and Enhanced Z None	Z None
3 Prostate ♂	Z None	Z None	Z None

♂ BV23[Ø,Y][Ø,Z]Z
♂ BV231ØZ
♂ BV23ZZZ

B Imaging
V Male Reproductive System
3 Magnetic Resonance Imaging (MRI) Definition: Computer reformatted digital display of multiplanar images developed from the capture of radio-frequency signals emitted by nuclei in a body site excited within a magnetic field

Body Part Character 4	Contrast Character 5	Qualifier Character 6	Qualifier Character 7
Ø Corpora Cavernosa ♂ 3 Prostate ♂ 4 Scrotum ♂ 5 Testicle, Right ♂ 6 Testicle, Left ♂ 7 Testicles, Bilateral ♂	Y Other Contrast	Ø Unenhanced and Enhanced Z None	Z None
Ø Corpora Cavernosa ♂ 3 Prostate ♂ 4 Scrotum ♂ 5 Testicle, Right ♂ 6 Testicle, Left ♂ 7 Testicles, Bilateral ♂	Z None	Z None	Z None

♂ All body part, contrast, and qualifier values

B Imaging
V Male Reproductive System
4 Ultrasonography Definition: Real time display of images of anatomy or flow information developed from the capture of reflected and attenuated high frequency sound waves

Body Part Character 4	Contrast Character 5	Qualifier Character 6	Qualifier Character 7
4 Scrotum ♂ 9 Prostate and Seminal Vesicles ♂ B Penis ♂	Z None	Z None	Z None

♂ All body part, contrast, and qualifier values

B Imaging
W Anatomical Regions
Ø Plain Radiography Definition: Planar display of an image developed from the capture of external ionizing radiation on photographic or photoconductive plate

Body Part Character 4	Contrast Character 5	Qualifier Character 6	Qualifier Character 7
Ø Abdomen 1 Abdomen and Pelvis 3 Chest B Long Bones, All C Lower Extremity J Upper Extremity K Whole Body L Whole Skeleton M Whole Body, Infant	Z None	Z None	Z None

B Imaging
W Anatomical Regions
1 Fluoroscopy Definition: Single plane or bi-plane real time display of an image developed from the capture of external ionizing radioation on a fluorescent screen. The image may also be stored by either digital or analog means.

Body Part Character 4	Contrast Character 5	Qualifier Character 6	Qualifier Character 7
1 Abdomen and Pelvis 9 Head and Neck C Lower Extremity J Upper Extremity	Ø High Osmolar 1 Low Osmolar Y Other Contrast Z None	Z None	Z None

B Imaging
W Anatomical Regions
2 Computerized Tomography (CT Scan) Definition: Computer reformatted digital display of multiplanar images developed from the capture of multiple exposures of external ionizing radiation

Body Part Character 4	Contrast Character 5	Qualifier Character 6	Qualifier Character 7
Ø Abdomen 1 Abdomen and Pelvis 4 Chest and Abdomen 5 Chest, Abdomen and Pelvis 8 Head 9 Head and Neck F Neck G Pelvic Region	Ø High Osmolar 1 Low Osmolar Y Other Contrast	Ø Unenhanced and Enhanced Z None	Z None
Ø Abdomen 1 Abdomen and Pelvis 4 Chest and Abdomen 5 Chest, Abdomen and Pelvis 8 Head 9 Head and Neck F Neck G Pelvic Region	Z None	Z None	Z None

B Imaging
W Anatomical Regions
3 Magnetic Resonance Imaging (MRI) Definition: Computer reformatted digital display of multiplanar images developed from the capture of radio-frequency signals emitted by nuclei in a body site excited within a magnetic field

Body Part Character 4	Contrast Character 5	Qualifier Character 6	Qualifier Character 7
Ø Abdomen 8 Head F Neck G Pelvic Region H Retroperitoneum P Brachial Plexus	Y Other Contrast	Ø Unenhanced and Enhanced Z None	Z None
Ø Abdomen 8 Head F Neck G Pelvic Region H Retroperitoneum P Brachial Plexus	Z None	Z None	Z None
3 Chest	Y Other Contrast	Ø Unenhanced and Enhanced Z None	Z None

B Imaging
W Anatomical Regions
4 Ultrasonography Definition: Real time display of images of anatomy or flow information developed from the capture of reflected and attenuated high frequency sound waves

Body Part Character 4	Contrast Character 5	Qualifier Character 6	Qualifier Character 7
Ø Abdomen 1 Abdomen and Pelvis F Neck G Pelvic Region	Z None	Z None	Z None

B Imaging
W Anatomical Regions
5 Other Imaging Definition: Other specified modality for visualizing a body part

Body Part Character 4	Contrast Character 5	Qualifier Character 6	Qualifier Character 7
2 Trunk 9 Head and Neck C Lower Extremity J Upper Extremity	Z None	1 Bacterial Autofluorescence	Z None

B Imaging
Y Fetus and Obstetrical
3 Magnetic Resonance Imaging (MRI) Definition: Computer reformatted digital display of multiplanar images developed from the capture of radio-frequency signals emitted by nuclei in a body site excited within a magnetic field

Body Part Character 4	Contrast Character 5	Qualifier Character 6	Qualifier Character 7
Ø Fetal Head ♀ 1 Fetal Heart ♀ 2 Fetal Thorax ♀ 3 Fetal Abdomen ♀ 4 Fetal Spine ♀ 5 Fetal Extremities ♀ 6 Whole Fetus ♀	Y Other Contrast	Ø Unenhanced and Enhanced Z None	Z None
Ø Fetal Head ♀ 1 Fetal Heart ♀ 2 Fetal Thorax ♀ 3 Fetal Abdomen ♀ 4 Fetal Spine ♀ 5 Fetal Extremities ♀ 6 Whole Fetus ♀	Z None	Z None	Z None

♀ BY3[Ø,1,2,3,5,6]Y[Ø,Z]Z
♀ BY34YZZ
♀ BY3[Ø,1,2,3,4,5,6]ZZZ

B Imaging
Y Fetus and Obstetrical
4 Ultrasonography Definition: Real time display of images of anatomy or flow information developed from the capture of reflected and attenuated high frequency sound waves

Body Part Character 4	Contrast Character 5	Qualifier Character 6	Qualifier Character 7
7 Fetal Umbilical Cord ♀ 8 Placenta ♀ 9 First Trimester, Single Fetus ♀ B First Trimester, Multiple Gestation ♀ C Second Trimester, Single Fetus ♀ D Second Trimester, Multiple Gestation ♀ F Third Trimester, Single Fetus ♀ G Third Trimester, Multiple Gestation ♀	Z None	Z None	Z None

♀ All body part, contrast, and qualifier values

Nuclear Medicine CØ1–CW7

C Nuclear Medicine
Ø Central Nervous System
1 Planar Nuclear Medicine Imaging Definition: Introduction of radioactive materials into the body for single plane display of images developed from the capture of radioactive emissions

Body Part Character 4	Radionuclide Character 5	Qualifier Character 6	Qualifier Character 7
Ø Brain	1 Technetium 99m (Tc-99m) Y Other Radionuclide	Z None	Z None
5 Cerebrospinal Fluid	D Indium 111 (In-111) Y Other Radionuclide	Z None	Z None
Y Central Nervous System	Y Other Radionuclide	Z None	Z None

C Nuclear Medicine
Ø Central Nervous System
2 Tomographic (Tomo) Nuclear Medicine Imaging Definition: Introduction of radioactive materials into the body for three dimensional display of images developed from the capture of radioactive emissions

Body Part Character 4	Radionuclide Character 5	Qualifier Character 6	Qualifier Character 7
Ø Brain	1 Technetium 99m (Tc-99m) F Iodine 123 (I-123) S Thallium 201 (Tl-201) Y Other Radionuclide	Z None	Z None
5 Cerebrospinal Fluid	D Indium 111 (In-111) Y Other Radionuclide	Z None	Z None
Y Central Nervous System	Y Other Radionuclide	Z None	Z None

C Nuclear Medicine
Ø Central Nervous System
3 Positron Emission Tomographic (PET) Imaging Definition: Introduction of radioactive materials into the body for three dimensional display of images developed from the simultaneous capture, 180 degrees apart, of radioactive emissions

Body Part Character 4	Radionuclide Character 5	Qualifier Character 6	Qualifier Character 7
Ø Brain	B Carbon 11 (C-11) K Fluorine 18 (F-18) M Oxygen 15 (O-15) Y Other Radionuclide	Z None	Z None
Y Central Nervous System	Y Other Radionuclide	Z None	Z None

C Nuclear Medicine
Ø Central Nervous System
5 Nonimaging Nuclear Medicine Probe Definition: Introduction of radioactive materials into the body for the study of distribution and fate of certain substances by the detection of radioactive emissions; or, alternatively, measurement of absorption of radioactive emissions from an external source

Body Part Character 4	Radionuclide Character 5	Qualifier Character 6	Qualifier Character 7
Ø Brain	V Xenon 133 (Xe-133) Y Other Radionuclide	Z None	Z None
Y Central Nervous System	Y Other Radionuclide	Z None	Z None

C Nuclear Medicine
2 Heart
1 Planar Nuclear Medicine Imaging Definition: Introduction of radioactive materials into the body for single plane display of images developed from the capture of radioactive emissions

Body Part Character 4	Radionuclide Character 5	Qualifier Character 6	Qualifier Character 7
6 Heart, Right and Left	1 Technetium 99m (Tc-99m) Y Other Radionuclide	Z None	Z None
G Myocardium	1 Technetium 99m (Tc-99m) D Indium 111 (In-111) S Thallium 201 (Tl-201) Y Other Radionuclide Z None	Z None	Z None
Y Heart	Y Other Radionuclide	Z None	Z None

C Nuclear Medicine
2 Heart
2 Tomographic (Tomo) Nuclear Medicine Imaging Definition: Introduction of radioactive materials into the body for three dimensional display of images developed from the capture of radioactive emissions

Body Part Character 4	Radionuclide Character 5	Qualifier Character 6	Qualifier Character 7
6 Heart, Right and Left	1 Technetium 99m (Tc-99m) Y Other Radionuclide	Z None	Z None
G Myocardium	1 Technetium 99m (Tc-99m) D Indium 111 (In-111) K Fluorine 18 (F-18) S Thallium 201 (Tl-201) Y Other Radionuclide Z None	Z None	Z None
Y Heart	Y Other Radionuclide	Z None	Z None

C Nuclear Medicine
2 Heart
3 Positron Emission Tomographic (PET) Imaging Definition: Introduction of radioactive materials into the body for three dimensional display of images developed from the simultaneous capture, 180 degrees apart, of radioactive emissions

Body Part Character 4	Radionuclide Character 5	Qualifier Character 6	Qualifier Character 7
G Myocardium	K Fluorine 18 (F-18) M Oxygen 15 (O-15) Q Rubidium 82 (Rb-82) R Nitrogen 13 (N-13) Y Other Radionuclide	Z None	Z None
Y Heart	Y Other Radionuclide	Z None	Z None

C Nuclear Medicine
2 Heart
5 Nonimaging Nuclear Medicine Probe Definition: Introduction of radioactive materials into the body for the study of distribution and fate of certain substances by the detection of radioactive emissions; or, alternatively, measurement of absorption of radioactive emissions from an external source

Body Part Character 4	Radionuclide Character 5	Qualifier Character 6	Qualifier Character 7
6 Heart, Right and Left	1 Technetium 99m (Tc-99m) Y Other Radionuclide	Z None	Z None
Y Heart	Y Other Radionuclide	Z None	Z None

C Nuclear Medicine
5 Veins
1 Planar Nuclear Medicine Imaging Definition: Introduction of radioactive materials into the body for single plane display of images developed from the capture of radioactive emissions

Body Part Character 4	Radionuclide Character 5	Qualifier Character 6	Qualifier Character 7
B Lower Extremity Veins, Right C Lower Extremity Veins, Left D Lower Extremity Veins, Bilateral N Upper Extremity Veins, Right P Upper Extremity Veins, Left Q Upper Extremity Veins, Bilateral R Central Veins	1 Technetium 99m (Tc-99m) Y Other Radionuclide	Z None	Z None
Y Veins	Y Other Radionuclide	Z None	Z None

C Nuclear Medicine
7 Lymphatic and Hematologic System
1 Planar Nuclear Medicine Imaging Definition: Introduction of radioactive materials into the body for single plane display of images developed from the capture of radioactive emissions

Body Part Character 4	Radionuclide Character 5	Qualifier Character 6	Qualifier Character 7
Ø Bone Marrow	1 Technetium 99m (Tc-99m) D Indium 111 (In-111) Y Other Radionuclide	Z None	Z None
2 Spleen 5 Lymphatics, Head and Neck D Lymphatics, Pelvic J Lymphatics, Head K Lymphatics, Neck L Lymphatics, Upper Chest M Lymphatics, Trunk N Lymphatics, Upper Extremity P Lymphatics, Lower Extremity	1 Technetium 99m (Tc-99m) Y Other Radionuclide	Z None	Z None
3 Blood	D Indium 111 (In-111) Y Other Radionuclide	Z None	Z None
Y Lymphatic and Hematologic System	Y Other Radionuclide	Z None	Z None

C Nuclear Medicine
7 Lymphatic and Hematologic System
2 Tomographic (Tomo) Nuclear Medicine Imaging Definition: Introduction of radioactive materials into the body for three dimensional display of images developed from the capture of radioactive emissions

Body Part Character 4	Radionuclide Character 5	Qualifier Character 6	Qualifier Character 7
2 Spleen	1 Technetium 99m (Tc-99m) Y Other Radionuclide	Z None	Z None
Y Lymphatic and Hematologic System	Y Other Radionuclide	Z None	Z None

C Nuclear Medicine
7 Lymphatic and Hematologic System
5 Nonimaging Nuclear Medicine Probe Definition: Introduction of radioactive materials into the body for the study of distribution and fate of certain substances by the detection of radioactive emissions; or, alternatively, measurement of absorption of radioactive emissions from an external source

Body Part Character 4	Radionuclide Character 5	Qualifier Character 6	Qualifier Character 7
5 Lymphatics, Head and Neck D Lymphatics, Pelvic J Lymphatics, Head K Lymphatics, Neck L Lymphatics, Upper Chest M Lymphatics, Trunk N Lymphatics, Upper Extremity P Lymphatics, Lower Extremity	1 Technetium 99m (Tc-99m) Y Other Radionuclide	Z None	Z None
Y Lymphatic and Hematologic System	Y Other Radionuclide	Z None	Z None

C Nuclear Medicine
7 Lymphatic and Hematologic System
6 Nonimaging Nuclear Medicine Assay Definition: Introduction of radioactive materials into the body for the study of body fluids and blood elements, by the detection of radioactive emissions

Body Part Character 4	Radionuclide Character 5	Qualifier Character 6	Qualifier Character 7
3 Blood	1 Technetium 99m (Tc-99m) 7 Cobalt 58 (Co-58) C Cobalt 57 (Co-57) D Indium 111 (In-111) H Iodine 125 (I-125) W Chromium (Cr-51) Y Other Radionuclide	Z None	Z None
Y Lymphatic and Hematologic System	Y Other Radionuclide	Z None	Z None

C Nuclear Medicine
8 Eye
1 Planar Nuclear Medicine Imaging Definition: Introduction of radioactive materials into the body for single plane display of images developed from the capture of radioactive emissions

Body Part Character 4	Radionuclide Character 5	Qualifier Character 6	Qualifier Character 7
9 Lacrimal Ducts, Bilateral	1 Technetium 99m (Tc-99m) Y Other Radionuclide	Z None	Z None
Y Eye	Y Other Radionuclide	Z None	Z None

C Nuclear Medicine
9 Ear, Nose, Mouth and Throat
1 Planar Nuclear Medicine Imaging Definition: Introduction of radioactive materials into the body for single plane display of images developed from the capture of radioactive emissions

Body Part Character 4	Radionuclide Character 5	Qualifier Character 6	Qualifier Character 7
B Salivary Glands, Bilateral	1 Technetium 99m (Tc-99m) Y Other Radionuclide	Z None	Z None
Y Ear, Nose, Mouth and Throat	Y Other Radionuclide	Z None	Z None

C Nuclear Medicine
B Respiratory System
1 Planar Nuclear Medicine Imaging Definition: Introduction of radioactive materials into the body for single plane display of images developed from the capture of radioactive emissions

Body Part Character 4	Radionuclide Character 5	Qualifier Character 6	Qualifier Character 7
2 Lungs and Bronchi	1 Technetium 99m (Tc-99m) 9 Krypton (Kr-81m) T Xenon 127 (Xe-127) V Xenon 133 (Xe-133) Y Other Radionuclide	Z None	Z None
Y Respiratory System	Y Other Radionuclide	Z None	Z None

C Nuclear Medicine
B Respiratory System
2 Tomographic (Tomo) Nuclear Medicine Imaging Definition: Introduction of radioactive materials into the body for three dimensional display of images developed from the capture of radioactive emissions

Body Part Character 4	Radionuclide Character 5	Qualifier Character 6	Qualifier Character 7
2 Lungs and Bronchi	1 Technetium 99m (Tc-99m) 9 Krypton (Kr-81m) Y Other Radionuclide	Z None	Z None
Y Respiratory System	Y Other Radionuclide	Z None	Z None

C Nuclear Medicine
B Respiratory System
3 Positron Emission Tomographic (PET) Imaging Definition: Introduction of radioactive materials into the body for three dimensional display of images developed from the simultaneous capture, 180 degrees apart, of radioactive emissions

Body Part Character 4	Radionuclide Character 5	Qualifier Character 6	Qualifier Character 7
2 Lungs and Bronchi	K Fluorine 18 (F-18) Y Other Radionuclide	Z None	Z None
Y Respiratory System	Y Other Radionuclide	Z None	Z None

C Nuclear Medicine
D Gastrointestinal System
1 Planar Nuclear Medicine Imaging Definition: Introduction of radioactive materials into the body for single plane display of images developed from the capture of radioactive emissions

Body Part Character 4	Radionuclide Character 5	Qualifier Character 6	Qualifier Character 7
5 Upper Gastrointestinal Tract 7 Gastrointestinal Tract	1 Technetium 99m (Tc-99m) D Indium 111 (In-111) Y Other Radionuclide	Z None	Z None
Y Digestive System	Y Other Radionuclide	Z None	Z None

C **Nuclear Medicine**
D **Gastrointestinal System**
2 **Tomographic (Tomo) Nuclear Medicine Imaging** Definition: Introduction of radioactive materials into the body for three dimensional display of images developed from the capture of radioactive emissions

Body Part Character 4	Radionuclide Character 5	Qualifier Character 6	Qualifier Character 7
7 Gastrointestinal Tract	1 Technetium 99m (Tc-99m) D Indium 111 (In-111) Y Other Radionuclide	Z None	Z None
Y Digestive System	Y Other Radionuclide	Z None	Z None

C **Nuclear Medicine**
F **Hepatobiliary System and Pancreas**
1 **Planar Nuclear Medicine Imaging** Definition: Introduction of radioactive materials into the body for single plane display of images developed from the capture of radioactive emissions

Body Part Character 4	Radionuclide Character 5	Qualifier Character 6	Qualifier Character 7
4 Gallbladder 5 Liver 6 Liver and Spleen C Hepatobiliary System, All	1 Technetium 99m (Tc-99m) Y Other Radionuclide	Z None	Z None
Y Hepatobiliary System and Pancreas	Y Other Radionuclide	Z None	Z None

C **Nuclear Medicine**
F **Hepatobiliary System and Pancreas**
2 **Tomographic (Tomo) Nuclear Medicine Imaging** Definition: Introduction of radioactive materials into the body for three dimensional display of images developed from the capture of radioactive emissions

Body Part Character 4	Radionuclide Character 5	Qualifier Character 6	Qualifier Character 7
4 Gallbladder 5 Liver 6 Liver and Spleen	1 Technetium 99m (Tc-99m) Y Other Radionuclide	Z None	Z None
Y Hepatobiliary System and Pancreas	Y Other Radionuclide	Z None	Z None

C **Nuclear Medicine**
G **Endocrine System**
1 **Planar Nuclear Medicine Imaging** Definition: Introduction of radioactive materials into the body for single plane display of images developed from the capture of radioactive emissions

Body Part Character 4	Radionuclide Character 5	Qualifier Character 6	Qualifier Character 7
1 Parathyroid Glands	1 Technetium 99m (Tc-99m) S Thallium 201 (Tl-201) Y Other Radionuclide	Z None	Z None
2 Thyroid Gland	1 Technetium 99m (Tc-99m) F Iodine 123 (I-123) G Iodine 131 (I-131) Y Other Radionuclide	Z None	Z None
4 Adrenal Glands, Bilateral	G Iodine 131 (I-131) Y Other Radionuclide	Z None	Z None
Y Endocrine System	Y Other Radionuclide	Z None	Z None

C **Nuclear Medicine**
G **Endocrine System**
2 **Tomographic (Tomo) Nuclear Medicine Imaging** Definition: Introduction of radioactive materials into the body for three dimensional display of images developed from the capture of radioactive emissions

Body Part Character 4	Radionuclide Character 5	Qualifier Character 6	Qualifier Character 7
1 Parathyroid Glands	1 Technetium 99m (Tc-99m) S Thallium 201 (Tl-201) Y Other Radionuclide	Z None	Z None
Y Endocrine System	Y Other Radionuclide	Z None	Z None

C Nuclear Medicine
G Endocrine System
4 Nonimaging Nuclear Medicine Uptake Definition: Introduction of radioactive materials into the body for measurements of organ function, from the detection of radioactive emmissions

Body Part Character 4	Radionuclide Character 5	Qualifier Character 6	Qualifier Character 7
2 Thyroid Gland	1 Technetium 99m (Tc-99m) F Iodine 123 (I-123) G Iodine 131 (I-131) Y Other Radionuclide	Z None	Z None
Y Endocrine System	Y Other Radionuclide	Z None	Z None

C Nuclear Medicine
H Skin, Subcutaneous Tissue and Breast
1 Planar Nuclear Medicine Imaging Definition: Introduction of radioactive materials into the body for single plane display of images developed from the capture of radioactive emissions

Body Part Character 4	Radionuclide Character 5	Qualifier Character 6	Qualifier Character 7
Ø Breast, Right 1 Breast, Left 2 Breasts, Bilateral	1 Technetium 99m (Tc-99m) S Thallium 201 (Tl-201) Y Other Radionuclide	Z None	Z None
Y Skin, Subcutaneous Tissue and Breast	Y Other Radionuclide	Z None	Z None

C Nuclear Medicine
H Skin, Subcutaneous Tissue and Breast
2 Tomographic (Tomo) Nuclear Medicine Imaging Definition: Introduction of radioactive materials into the body for three dimensional display of images developed from the capture of radioactive emissions

Body Part Character 4	Radionuclide Character 5	Qualifier Character 6	Qualifier Character 7
Ø Breast, Right 1 Breast, Left 2 Breasts, Bilateral	1 Technetium 99m (Tc-99m) S Thallium 201 (Tl-201) Y Other Radionuclide	Z None	Z None
Y Skin, Subcutaneous Tissue and Breast	Y Other Radionuclide	Z None	Z None

C Nuclear Medicine
P Musculoskeletal System
1 Planar Nuclear Medicine Imaging Definition: Introduction of radioactive materials into the body for single plane display of images developed from the capture of radioactive emissions

Body Part Character 4	Radionuclide Character 5	Qualifier Character 6	Qualifier Character 7
1 Skull 4 Thorax 5 Spine 6 Pelvis 7 Spine and Pelvis 8 Upper Extremity, Right 9 Upper Extremity, Left B Upper Extremities, Bilateral C Lower Extremity, Right D Lower Extremity, Left F Lower Extremities, Bilateral Z Musculoskeletal System, All	1 Technetium 99m (Tc-99m) Y Other Radionuclide	Z None	Z None
Y Musculoskeletal System, Other	Y Other Radionuclide	Z None	Z None

C Nuclear Medicine
P Musculoskeletal System
2 Tomographic (Tomo) Nuclear Medicine Imaging Definition: Introduction of radioactive materials into the body for three dimensional display of images developed from the capture of radioactive emissions

Body Part Character 4	Radionuclide Character 5	Qualifier Character 6	Qualifier Character 7
1 Skull 2 Cervical Spine 3 Skull and Cervical Spine 4 Thorax 6 Pelvis 7 Spine and Pelvis 8 Upper Extremity, Right 9 Upper Extremity, Left B Upper Extremities, Bilateral C Lower Extremity, Right D Lower Extremity, Left F Lower Extremities, Bilateral G Thoracic Spine H Lumbar Spine J Thoracolumbar Spine	1 Technetium 99m (Tc-99m) Y Other Radionuclide	Z None	Z None
Y Musculoskeletal System, Other	Y Other Radionuclide	Z None	Z None

C Nuclear Medicine
P Musculoskeletal System
5 Nonimaging Nuclear Medicine Probe Definition: Introduction of radioactive materials into the body for the study of distribution and fate of certain substances by the detection of radioactive emissions; or, alternatively, measurement of absorption of radioactive emissions from an external source

Body Part Character 4	Radionuclide Character 5	Qualifier Character 6	Qualifier Character 7
5 Spine N Upper Extremities P Lower Extremities	Z None	Z None	Z None
Y Musculoskeletal System, Other	Y Other Radionuclide	Z None	Z None

C Nuclear Medicine
T Urinary System
1 Planar Nuclear Medicine Imaging Definition: Introduction of radioactive materials into the body for single plane display of images developed from the capture of radioactive emissions

Body Part Character 4	Radionuclide Character 5	Qualifier Character 6	Qualifier Character 7
3 Kidneys, Ureters and Bladder	1 Technetium 99m (Tc-99m) F Iodine 123 (I-123) G Iodine 131 (I-131) Y Other Radionuclide	Z None	Z None
H Bladder and Ureters	1 Technetium 99m (Tc-99m) Y Other Radionuclide	Z None	Z None
Y Urinary System	Y Other Radionuclide	Z None	Z None

C Nuclear Medicine
T Urinary System
2 Tomographic (Tomo) Nuclear Medicine Imaging Definition: Introduction of radioactive materials into the body for three dimensional display of images developed from the capture of radioactive emissions

Body Part Character 4	Radionuclide Character 5	Qualifier Character 6	Qualifier Character 7
3 Kidneys, Ureters and Bladder	1 Technetium 99m (Tc-99m) Y Other Radionuclide	Z None	Z None
Y Urinary System	Y Other Radionuclide	Z None	Z None

C Nuclear Medicine
T Urinary System
6 Nonimaging Nuclear Medicine Assay Definition: Introduction of radioactive materials into the body for the study of body fluids and blood elements, by the detection of radioactive emissions

Body Part Character 4	Radionuclide Character 5	Qualifier Character 6	Qualifier Character 7
3 Kidneys, Ureters and Bladder	1 Technetium 99m (Tc-99m) F Iodine 123 (I-123) G Iodine 131 (I-131) H Iodine 125 (I-125) Y Other Radionuclide	Z None	Z None
Y Urinary System	Y Other Radionuclide	Z None	Z None

C Nuclear Medicine
V Male Reproductive System
1 Planar Nuclear Medicine Imaging Definition: Introduction of radioactive materials into the body for single plane display of images developed from the capture of radioactive emissions

Body Part Character 4	Radionuclide Character 5	Qualifier Character 6	Qualifier Character 7
9 Testicles, Bilateral ♂	**1** Technetium 99m (Tc-99m) **Y** Other Radionuclide	**Z** None	**Z** None
Y Male Reproductive System ♂	**Y** Other Radionuclide	**Z** None	**Z** None

♂ All body part, radionuclide, and qualifier values

C Nuclear Medicine
W Anatomical Regions
1 Planar Nuclear Medicine Imaging Definition: Introduction of radioactive materials into the body for single plane display of images developed from the capture of radioactive emissions

Body Part Character 4	Radionuclide Character 5	Qualifier Character 6	Qualifier Character 7
Ø Abdomen **1** Abdomen and Pelvis **4** Chest and Abdomen **6** Chest and Neck **B** Head and Neck **D** Lower Extremity **J** Pelvic Region **M** Upper Extremity **N** Whole Body	**1** Technetium 99m (Tc-99m) **D** Indium 111 (In-111) **F** Iodine 123 (I-123) **G** Iodine 131 (I-131) **L** Gallium 67 (Ga-67) **S** Thallium 201 (Tl-201) **Y** Other Radionuclide	**Z** None	**Z** None
3 Chest	**1** Technetium 99m (Tc-99m) **D** Indium 111 (In-111) **F** Iodine 123 (I-123) **G** Iodine 131 (I-131) **K** Fluorine 18 (F-18) **L** Gallium 67 (Ga-67) **S** Thallium 201 (Tl-201) **Y** Other Radionuclide	**Z** None	**Z** None
Y Anatomical Regions, Multiple	**Y** Other Radionuclide	**Z** None	**Z** None
Z Anatomical Region, Other	**Z** None	**Z** None	**Z** None

C Nuclear Medicine
W Anatomical Regions
2 Tomographic (Tomo) Nuclear Medicine Imaging Definition: Introduction of radioactive materials into the body for three dimensional display of images developed from the capture of radioactive emissions

Body Part Character 4	Radionuclide Character 5	Qualifier Character 6	Qualifier Character 7
Ø Abdomen **1** Abdomen and Pelvis **3** Chest **4** Chest and Abdomen **6** Chest and Neck **B** Head and Neck **D** Lower Extremity **J** Pelvic Region **M** Upper Extremity	**1** Technetium 99m (Tc-99m) **D** Indium 111 (In-111) **F** Iodine 123 (I-123) **G** Iodine 131 (I-131) **K** Fluorine 18 (F-18) **L** Gallium 67 (Ga-67) **S** Thallium 201 (Tl-201) **Y** Other Radionuclide	**Z** None	**Z** None
Y Anatomical Regions, Multiple	**Y** Other Radionuclide	**Z** None	**Z** None

C Nuclear Medicine
W Anatomical Regions
3 Positron Emission Tomographic (PET) Imaging Definition: Introduction of radioactive materials into the body for three dimensional display of images developed from the simultaneous capture, 180 degrees apart, of radioactive emissions

Body Part Character 4	Radionuclide Character 5	Qualifier Character 6	Qualifier Character 7
N Whole Body	**Y** Other Radionuclide	**Z** None	**Z** None

C Nuclear Medicine
W Anatomical Regions
5 Nonimaging Nuclear Medicine Probe Definition: Introduction of radioactive materials into the body for the study of distribution and fate of certain substances by the detection of radioactive emissions; or, alternatively, measurement of absorption of radioactive emissions from an external source

Body Part Character 4	Radionuclide Character 5	Qualifier Character 6	Qualifier Character 7
Ø Abdomen 1 Abdomen and Pelvis 3 Chest 4 Chest and Abdomen 6 Chest and Neck B Head and Neck D Lower Extremity J Pelvic Region M Upper Extremity	1 Technetium 99m (Tc-99m) D Indium 111 (In-111) Y Other Radionuclide	Z None	Z None

C Nuclear Medicine
W Anatomical Regions
7 Systemic Nuclear Medicine Therapy Definition: Introduction of unsealed radioactive materials into the body for treatment

Body Part Character 4	Radionuclide Character 5	Qualifier Character 6	Qualifier Character 7
Ø Abdomen 3 Chest	N Phosphorus 32 (P-32) Y Other Radionuclide	Z None	Z None
G Thyroid	G Iodine 131 (I-131) Y Other Radionuclide	Z None	Z None
N Whole Body	8 Samarium 153 (Sm-153) G Iodine 131 (I-131) N Phosphorus 32 (P-32) P Strontium 89 (Sr-89) Y Other Radionuclide	Z None	Z None
Y Anatomical Regions, Multiple	Y Other Radionuclide	Z None	Z None

Radiation Therapy DØØ–DWY

AHA Coding Clinic for table DØ1
2020, 4Q, 43-44 Insertion of radioactive element
2020, 4Q, 69-70 Cesium 131 brachytherapy
2019, 4Q, 42-44 Unidirectional source brachytherapy

AHA Coding Clinic for table DØY
2020, 4Q, 70 Intraoperative radiation therapy

AHA Coding Clinic for table D71
2020, 4Q, 43-44 Insertion of radioactive element
2020, 4Q, 69-70 Cesium 131 brachytherapy
2019, 4Q, 42-44 Unidirectional source brachytherapy

AHA Coding Clinic for table D81
2020, 4Q, 43-44 Insertion of radioactive element
2020, 4Q, 69-70 Cesium 131 brachytherapy
2019, 4Q, 42-44 Unidirectional source brachytherapy

AHA Coding Clinic for table D91
2020, 4Q, 43-44 Insertion of radioactive element
2020, 4Q, 69-70 Cesium 131 brachytherapy
2019, 4Q, 42-44 Unidirectional source brachytherapy

AHA Coding Clinic for table DB1
2020, 4Q, 43-44 Insertion of radioactive element
2020, 4Q, 69-70 Cesium 131 brachytherapy
2019, 4Q, 42-44 Unidirectional source brachytherapy

AHA Coding Clinic for table DD1
2020, 4Q, 43-44 Insertion of radioactive element
2020, 4Q, 69-70 Cesium 131 brachytherapy
2019, 4Q, 42-44 Unidirectional source brachytherapy

AHA Coding Clinic for table DF1
2020, 4Q, 43-44 Insertion of radioactive element
2020, 4Q, 69-70 Cesium 131 brachytherapy
2019, 4Q, 42-44 Unidirectional source brachytherapy

AHA Coding Clinic for table DG1
2020, 4Q, 43-44 Insertion of radioactive element
2020, 4Q, 69-70 Cesium 131 brachytherapy
2019, 4Q, 42-44 Unidirectional source brachytherapy

AHA Coding Clinic for table DM1
2020, 4Q, 43-44 Insertion of radioactive element
2020, 4Q, 69-70 Cesium 131 brachytherapy
2019, 4Q, 42-44 Unidirectional source brachytherapy

AHA Coding Clinic for table DT1
2020, 4Q, 43-44 Insertion of radioactive element
2020, 4Q, 69-70 Cesium 131 brachytherapy
2019, 4Q, 42-44 Unidirectional source brachytherapy

AHA Coding Clinic for table DU1
2020, 4Q, 43-44 Insertion of radioactive element
2020, 4Q, 69-70 Cesium 131 brachytherapy
2019, 4Q, 42-44 Unidirectional source brachytherapy
2017, 4Q, 104 Intrauterine brachytherapy & placement of tandems & ovoids

AHA Coding Clinic for table DV1
2020, 4Q, 43-44 Insertion of radioactive element
2020, 4Q, 69-70 Cesium 131 brachytherapy
2019, 4Q, 42-44 Unidirectional source brachytherapy

AHA Coding Clinic for table DW1
2020, 4Q, 43-44 Insertion of radioactive element
2020, 4Q, 69-70 Cesium 131 brachytherapy
2019, 4Q, 42-44 Unidirectional source brachytherapy

AHA Coding Clinic for table DWY
2019, 4Q, 37 Hyperthermic antineoplastic chemotherapy

D Radiation Therapy
Ø Central and Peripheral Nervous System
Ø Beam Radiation

Treatment Site Character 4	Modality Qualifier Character 5	Isotope Character 6	Qualifier Character 7
Ø Brain 1 Brain Stem 6 Spinal Cord 7 Peripheral Nerve	Ø Photons <1 MeV 1 Photons 1 - 10 MeV 2 Photons >10 MeV 4 Heavy Particles (Protons, Ions) 5 Neutrons 6 Neutron Capture	Z None	Z None
Ø Brain 1 Brain Stem 6 Spinal Cord 7 Peripheral Nerve	3 Electrons	Z None	Ø Intraoperative Z None

D Radiation Therapy
Ø Central and Peripheral Nervous System
1 Brachytherapy

Treatment Site Character 4	Modality Qualifier Character 5	Isotope Character 6	Qualifier Character 7
Ø Brain 1 Brain Stem 6 Spinal Cord 7 Peripheral Nerve	9 High Dose Rate (HDR)	7 Cesium 137 (Cs-137) 8 Iridium 192 (Ir-192) 9 Iodine 125 (I-125) B Palladium 103 (Pd-103) C Californium 252 (Cf-252) Y Other Isotope	Z None
Ø Brain 1 Brain Stem 6 Spinal Cord 7 Peripheral Nerve	B Low Dose Rate (LDR)	6 Cesium 131 (Cs-131) 7 Cesium 137 (Cs-137) 8 Iridium 192 (Ir-192) 9 Iodine 125 (I-125) C Californium 252 (Cf-252) Y Other Isotope	Z None
Ø Brain 1 Brain Stem 6 Spinal Cord 7 Peripheral Nerve	B Low Dose Rate (LDR)	B Palladium 103 (Pd-103)	1 Unidirectional Source Z None

Radiation Therapy

D Radiation Therapy
Ø Central and Peripheral Nervous System
2 Stereotactic Radiosurgery

Treatment Site Character 4	Modality Qualifier Character 5	Isotope Character 6	Qualifier Character 7
Ø Brain 1 Brain Stem 6 Spinal Cord 7 Peripheral Nerve	D Stereotactic Other Photon Radiosurgery H Stereotactic Particulate Radiosurgery J Stereotactic Gamma Beam Radiosurgery	Z None	Z None

DRG Non-OR All treatment site, modality, isotope, and qualifier values

D Radiation Therapy
Ø Central and Peripheral Nervous System
Y Other Radiation

Treatment Site Character 4	Modality Qualifier Character 5	Isotope Character 6	Qualifier Character 7
Ø Brain 1 Brain Stem 6 Spinal Cord 7 Peripheral Nerve	7 Contact Radiation 8 Hyperthermia C Intraoperative Radiation Therapy (IORT) F Plaque Radiation K Laser Interstitial Thermal Therapy	Z None	Z None

Valid OR DØY[Ø,1,6,7]KZZ

D Radiation Therapy
7 Lymphatic and Hematologic System
Ø Beam Radiation

Treatment Site Character 4	Modality Qualifier Character 5	Isotope Character 6	Qualifier Character 7
Ø Bone Marrow 1 Thymus 2 Spleen 3 Lymphatics, Neck 4 Lymphatics, Axillary 5 Lymphatics, Thorax 6 Lymphatics, Abdomen 7 Lymphatics, Pelvis 8 Lymphatics, Inguinal	Ø Photons <1 MeV 1 Photons 1- 10 MeV 2 Photons >10 MeV 4 Heavy Particles (Protons, Ions) 5 Neutrons 6 Neutron Capture	Z None	Z None
Ø Bone Marrow 1 Thymus 2 Spleen 3 Lymphatics, Neck 4 Lymphatics, Axillary 5 Lymphatics, Thorax 6 Lymphatics, Abdomen 7 Lymphatics, Pelvis 8 Lymphatics, Inguinal	3 Electrons	Z None	Ø Intraoperative Z None

D Radiation Therapy
7 Lymphatic and Hematologic System
1 Brachytherapy

Treatment Site Character 4	Modality Qualifier Character 5	Isotope Character 6	Qualifier Character 7
Ø Bone Marrow 1 Thymus 2 Spleen 3 Lymphatics, Neck 4 Lymphatics, Axillary 5 Lymphatics, Thorax 6 Lymphatics, Abdomen 7 Lymphatics, Pelvis 8 Lymphatics, Inguinal	9 High Dose Rate (HDR)	7 Cesium 137 (Cs-137) 8 Iridium 192 (Ir-192) 9 Iodine 125 (I-125) B Palladium 103 (Pd-103) C Californium 252 (Cf-252) Y Other Isotope	Z None
Ø Bone Marrow 1 Thymus 2 Spleen 3 Lymphatics, Neck 4 Lymphatics, Axillary 5 Lymphatics, Thorax 6 Lymphatics, Abdomen 7 Lymphatics, Pelvis 8 Lymphatics, Inguinal	B Low Dose Rate (LDR)	6 Cesium 131 (Cs-131) 7 Cesium 137 (Cs-137) 8 Iridium 192 (Ir-192) 9 Iodine 125 (I-125) C Californium 252 (Cf-252) Y Other Isotope	Z None
Ø Bone Marrow 1 Thymus 2 Spleen 3 Lymphatics, Neck 4 Lymphatics, Axillary 5 Lymphatics, Thorax 6 Lymphatics, Abdomen 7 Lymphatics, Pelvis 8 Lymphatics, Inguinal	B Low Dose Rate (LDR)	B Palladium 103 (Pd-103)	1 Unidirectional Source Z None

D Radiation Therapy
7 Lymphatic and Hematologic System
2 Stereotactic Radiosurgery

Treatment Site Character 4	Modality Qualifier Character 5	Isotope Character 6	Qualifier Character 7
Ø Bone Marrow 1 Thymus 2 Spleen 3 Lymphatics, Neck 4 Lymphatics, Axillary 5 Lymphatics, Thorax 6 Lymphatics, Abdomen 7 Lymphatics, Pelvis 8 Lymphatics, Inguinal	D Stereotactic Other Photon Radiosurgery H Stereotactic Particulate Radiosurgery J Stereotactic Gamma Beam Radiosurgery	Z None	Z None

DRG Non-OR All treatment site, modality, isotope, and qualifier values

D Radiation Therapy
7 Lymphatic and Hematologic System
Y Other Radiation

Treatment Site Character 4	Modality Qualifier Character 5	Isotope Character 6	Qualifier Character 7
Ø Bone Marrow 1 Thymus 2 Spleen 3 Lymphatics, Neck 4 Lymphatics, Axillary 5 Lymphatics, Thorax 6 Lymphatics, Abdomen 7 Lymphatics, Pelvis 8 Lymphatics, Inguinal	8 Hyperthermia F Plaque Radiation	Z None	Z None

D Radiation Therapy
8 Eye
Ø Beam Radiation

Treatment Site Character 4	Modality Qualifier Character 5	Isotope Character 6	Qualifier Character 7
Ø Eye	Ø Photons <1 MeV 1 Photons 1- 10 MeV 2 Photons >10 MeV 4 Heavy Particles (Protons, Ions) 5 Neutrons 6 Neutron Capture	Z None	Z None
Ø Eye	3 Electrons	Z None	Ø Intraoperative Z None

D Radiation Therapy
8 Eye
1 Brachytherapy

Treatment Site Character 4	Modality Qualifier Character 5	Isotope Character 6	Qualifier Character 7
Ø Eye	9 High Dose Rate (HDR)	7 Cesium 137 (Cs-137) 8 Iridium 192 (Ir-192) 9 Iodine 125 (I-125) B Palladium 103 (Pd-103) C Californium 252 (Cf-252) Y Other Isotope	Z None
Ø Eye	B Low Dose Rate (LDR)	6 Cesium 131 (Cs-131) 7 Cesium 137 (Cs-137) 8 Iridium 192 (Ir-192) 9 Iodine 125 (I-125) C Californium 252 (Cf-252) Y Other Isotope	Z None
Ø Eye	B Low Dose Rate (LDR)	B Palladium 103 (Pd-103)	1 Unidirectional Source Z None

D Radiation Therapy
8 Eye
2 Stereotactic Radiosurgery

Treatment Site Character 4	Modality Qualifier Character 5	Isotope Character 6	Qualifier Character 7
Ø Eye	D Stereotactic Other Photon Radiosurgery H Stereotactic Particulate Radiosurgery J Stereotactic Gamma Beam Radiosurgery	Z None	Z None

DRG Non-OR All treatment site, modality, isotope, and qualifier values

D Radiation Therapy
8 Eye
Y Other Radiation

Treatment Site Character 4	Modality Qualifier Character 5	Isotope Character 6	Qualifier Character 7
Ø Eye	7 Contact Radiation 8 Hyperthermia F Plaque Radiation	Z None	Z None

D Radiation Therapy
9 Ear, Nose, Mouth and Throat
0 Beam Radiation

Treatment Site Character 4	Modality Qualifier Character 5	Isotope Character 6	Qualifier Character 7
0 Ear 1 Nose 3 Hypopharynx 4 Mouth 5 Tongue 6 Salivary Glands 7 Sinuses 8 Hard Palate 9 Soft Palate B Larynx D Nasopharynx F Oropharynx	0 Photons <1 MeV 1 Photons 1- 10 MeV 2 Photons >10 MeV 4 Heavy Particles (Protons, Ions) 5 Neutrons 6 Neutron Capture	Z None	Z None
0 Ear 1 Nose 3 Hypopharynx 4 Mouth 5 Tongue 6 Salivary Glands 7 Sinuses 8 Hard Palate 9 Soft Palate B Larynx D Nasopharynx F Oropharynx	3 Electrons	Z None	0 Intraoperative Z None

D Radiation Therapy
9 Ear, Nose, Mouth and Throat
1 Brachytherapy

Treatment Site Character 4	Modality Qualifier Character 5	Isotope Character 6	Qualifier Character 7
0 Ear 1 Nose 3 Hypopharynx 4 Mouth 5 Tongue 6 Salivary Glands 7 Sinuses 8 Hard Palate 9 Soft Palate B Larynx D Nasopharynx F Oropharynx	9 High Dose Rate (HDR)	7 Cesium 137 (Cs-137) 8 Iridium 192 (Ir-192) 9 Iodine 125 (I-125) B Palladium 103 (Pd-103) C Californium 252 (Cf-252) Y Other Isotope	Z None
0 Ear 1 Nose 3 Hypopharynx 4 Mouth 5 Tongue 6 Salivary Glands 7 Sinuses 8 Hard Palate 9 Soft Palate B Larynx D Nasopharynx F Oropharynx	B Low Dose Rate (LDR)	6 Cesium 131 (Cs-131) 7 Cesium 137 (Cs-137) 8 Iridium 192 (Ir-192) 9 Iodine 125 (I-125) C Californium 252 (Cf-252) Y Other Isotope	Z None
0 Ear 1 Nose 3 Hypopharynx 4 Mouth 5 Tongue 6 Salivary Glands 7 Sinuses 8 Hard Palate 9 Soft Palate B Larynx D Nasopharynx F Oropharynx	B Low Dose Rate (LDR)	B Palladium 103 (Pd-103)	1 Unidirectional Source Z None

D Radiation Therapy
9 Ear, Nose, Mouth and Throat
2 Stereotactic Radiosurgery

Treatment Site Character 4	Modality Qualifier Character 5	Isotope Character 6	Qualifier Character 7
Ø Ear 1 Nose 4 Mouth 5 Tongue 6 Salivary Glands 7 Sinuses 8 Hard Palate 9 Soft Palate B Larynx C Pharynx D Nasopharynx	D Stereotactic Other Photon Radiosurgery H Stereotactic Particulate Radiosurgery J Stereotactic Gamma Beam Radiosurgery	Z None	Z None

DRG Non-OR All treatment site, modality, isotope, and qualifier values

D Radiation Therapy
9 Ear, Nose, Mouth and Throat
Y Other Radiation

Treatment Site Character 4	Modality Qualifier Character 5	Isotope Character 6	Qualifier Character 7
Ø Ear 1 Nose 5 Tongue 6 Salivary Glands 7 Sinuses 8 Hard Palate 9 Soft Palate	7 Contact Radiation 8 Hyperthermia F Plaque Radiation	Z None	Z None
3 Hypopharynx F Oropharynx	7 Contact Radiation 8 Hyperthermia	Z None	Z None
4 Mouth B Larynx D Nasopharynx	7 Contact Radiation 8 Hyperthermia C Intraoperative Radiation Therapy (IORT) F Plaque Radiation	Z None	Z None
C Pharynx	C Intraoperative Radiation Therapy (IORT) F Plaque Radiation	Z None	Z None

D Radiation Therapy
B Respiratory System
Ø Beam Radiation

Treatment Site Character 4	Modality Qualifier Character 5	Isotope Character 6	Qualifier Character 7
Ø Trachea 1 Bronchus 2 Lung 5 Pleura 6 Mediastinum 7 Chest Wall 8 Diaphragm	Ø Photons <1 MeV 1 Photons 1- 10 MeV 2 Photons >10 MeV 4 Heavy Particles (Protons, Ions) 5 Neutrons 6 Neutron Capture	Z None	Z None
Ø Trachea 1 Bronchus 2 Lung 5 Pleura 6 Mediastinum 7 Chest Wall 8 Diaphragm	3 Electrons	Z None	Ø Intraoperative Z None

D Radiation Therapy
B Respiratory System
1 Brachytherapy

Treatment Site Character 4	Modality Qualifier Character 5	Isotope Character 6	Qualifier Character 7
Ø Trachea 1 Bronchus 2 Lung 5 Pleura 6 Mediastinum 7 Chest Wall 8 Diaphragm	9 High Dose Rate (HDR)	7 Cesium 137 (Cs-137) 8 Iridium 192 (Ir-192) 9 Iodine 125 (I-125) B Palladium 103 (Pd-103) C Californium 252 (Cf-252) Y Other Isotope	Z None
Ø Trachea 1 Bronchus 2 Lung 5 Pleura 6 Mediastinum 7 Chest Wall 8 Diaphragm	B Low Dose Rate (LDR)	6 Cesium 131 (Cs-131) 7 Cesium 137 (Cs-137) 8 Iridium 192 (Ir-192) 9 Iodine 125 (I-125) C Californium 252 (Cf-252) Y Other Isotope	Z None
Ø Trachea 1 Bronchus 2 Lung 5 Pleura 6 Mediastinum 7 Chest Wall 8 Diaphragm	B Low Dose Rate (LDR)	B Palladium 103 (Pd-103)	1 Unidirectional Source Z None

D Radiation Therapy
B Respiratory System
2 Stereotactic Radiosurgery

Treatment Site Character 4	Modality Qualifier Character 5	Isotope Character 6	Qualifier Character 7
Ø Trachea 1 Bronchus 2 Lung 5 Pleura 6 Mediastinum 7 Chest Wall 8 Diaphragm	D Stereotactic Other Photon Radiosurgery H Stereotactic Particulate Radiosurgery J Stereotactic Gamma Beam Radiosurgery	Z None	Z None

DRG Non-OR All treatment site, modality, isotope, and qualifier values

D Radiation Therapy
B Respiratory System
Y Other Radiation

Treatment Site Character 4	Modality Qualifier Character 5	Isotope Character 6	Qualifier Character 7
Ø Trachea 1 Bronchus 2 Lung 5 Pleura 6 Mediastinum 7 Chest Wall 8 Diaphragm	7 Contact Radiation 8 Hyperthermia F Plaque Radiation K Laser Interstitial Thermal Therapy	Z None	Z None

Valid OR DBY[Ø,1,2,5,6,7,8]KZZ

D Radiation Therapy
D Gastrointestinal System
Ø Beam Radiation

Treatment Site Character 4	Modality Qualifier Character 5	Isotope Character 6	Qualifier Character 7
Ø Esophagus 1 Stomach 2 Duodenum 3 Jejunum 4 Ileum 5 Colon 7 Rectum	Ø Photons <1 MeV 1 Photons 1- 10 MeV 2 Photons >10 MeV 4 Heavy Particles (Protons, Ions) 5 Neutrons 6 Neutron Capture	Z None	Z None
Ø Esophagus 1 Stomach 2 Duodenum 3 Jejunum 4 Ileum 5 Colon 7 Rectum	3 Electrons	Z None	Ø Intraoperative Z None

D Radiation Therapy
D Gastrointestinal System
1 Brachytherapy

Treatment Site Character 4	Modality Qualifier Character 5	Isotope Character 6	Qualifier Character 7
Ø Esophagus 1 Stomach 2 Duodenum 3 Jejunum 4 Ileum 5 Colon 7 Rectum	9 High Dose Rate (HDR)	7 Cesium 137 (Cs-137) 8 Iridium 192 (Ir-192) 9 Iodine 125 (I-125) B Palladium 103 (Pd-103) C Californium 252 (Cf-252) Y Other Isotope	Z None
Ø Esophagus 1 Stomach 2 Duodenum 3 Jejunum 4 Ileum 5 Colon 7 Rectum	B Low Dose Rate (LDR)	6 Cesium 131 (Cs-131) 7 Cesium 137 (Cs-137) 8 Iridium 192 (Ir-192) 9 Iodine 125 (I-125) C Californium 252 (Cf-252) Y Other Isotope	Z None
Ø Esophagus 1 Stomach 2 Duodenum 3 Jejunum 4 Ileum 5 Colon 7 Rectum	B Low Dose Rate (LDR)	B Palladium 103 (Pd-103)	1 Unidirectional Source Z None

D Radiation Therapy
D Gastrointestinal System
2 Stereotactic Radiosurgery

Treatment Site Character 4	Modality Qualifier Character 5	Isotope Character 6	Qualifier Character 7
Ø Esophagus 1 Stomach 2 Duodenum 3 Jejunum 4 Ileum 5 Colon 7 Rectum	D Stereotactic Other Photon Radiosurgery H Stereotactic Particulate Radiosurgery J Stereotactic Gamma Beam Radiosurgery	Z None	Z None

DRG Non-OR All treatment site, modality, isotope, and qualifier values

D Radiation therapy
D Gastrointestinal System
Y Other Radiation

Treatment Site Character 4	Modality Qualifier Character 5	Isotope Character 6	Qualifier Character 7
Ø Esophagus	7 Contact Radiation 8 Hyperthermia F Plaque Radiation K Laser Interstitial Thermal Therapy	Z None	Z None
1 Stomach 2 Duodenum 3 Jejunum 4 Ileum 5 Colon 7 Rectum	7 Contact Radiation 8 Hyperthermia C Intraoperative Radiation Therapy (IORT) F Plaque Radiation K Laser Interstitial Thermal Therapy	Z None	Z None
8 Anus	C Intraoperative Radiation Therapy (IORT) F Plaque Radiation K Laser Interstitial Thermal Therapy	Z None	Z None

Valid OR DDYØKZZ
Valid OR DDY[1,2,3,4,5,7]KZZ
Valid OR DDY8KZZ

D Radiation Therapy
F Hepatobiliary System and Pancreas
Ø Beam Radiation

Treatment Site Character 4	Modality Qualifier Character 5	Isotope Character 6	Qualifier Character 7
Ø Liver 1 Gallbladder 2 Bile Ducts 3 Pancreas	Ø Photons <1 MeV 1 Photons 1- 10 MeV 2 Photons >10 MeV 4 Heavy Particles (Protons, Ions) 5 Neutrons 6 Neutron Capture	Z None	Z None
Ø Liver 1 Gallbladder 2 Bile Ducts 3 Pancreas	3 Electrons	Z None	Ø Intraoperative Z None

D Radiation Therapy
F Hepatobiliary System and Pancreas
1 Brachytherapy

Treatment Site Character 4	Modality Qualifier Character 5	Isotope Character 6	Qualifier Character 7
Ø Liver 1 Gallbladder 2 Bile Ducts 3 Pancreas	9 High Dose Rate (HDR)	7 Cesium 137 (Cs-137) 8 Iridium 192 (Ir-192) 9 Iodine 125 (I-125) B Palladium 103 (Pd-103) C Californium 252 (Cf-252) Y Other Isotope	Z None
Ø Liver 1 Gallbladder 2 Bile Ducts 3 Pancreas	B Low Dose Rate (LDR)	6 Cesium 131 (Cs-131) 7 Cesium 137 (Cs-137) 8 Iridium 192 (Ir-192) 9 Iodine 125 (I-125) C Californium 252 (Cf-252) Y Other Isotope	Z None
Ø Liver 1 Gallbladder 2 Bile Ducts 3 Pancreas	B Low Dose Rate (LDR)	B Palladium 103 (Pd-103)	1 Unidirectional Source Z None

D Radiation Therapy
F Hepatobiliary System and Pancreas
2 Stereotactic Radiosurgery

Treatment Site Character 4	Modality Qualifier Character 5	Isotope Character 6	Qualifier Character 7
Ø Liver 1 Gallbladder 2 Bile Ducts 3 Pancreas	D Stereotactic Other Photon Radiosurgery H Stereotactic Particulate Radiosurgery J Stereotactic Gamma Beam Radiosurgery	Z None	Z None

DRG Non-OR All treatment site, modality, isotope, and qualifier values

D Radiation Therapy
F Hepatobiliary System and Pancreas
Y Other Radiation

Treatment Site Character 4	Modality Qualifier Character 5	Isotope Character 6	Qualifier Character 7
Ø Liver 1 Gallbladder 2 Bile Ducts 3 Pancreas	7 Contact Radiation 8 Hyperthermia C Intraoperative Radiation Therapy (IORT) F Plaque Radiation K Laser Interstitial Thermal Therapy	Z None	Z None

Valid OR DFY[Ø,1,2,3]KZZ

D Radiation Therapy
G Endocrine System
Ø Beam Radiation

Treatment Site Character 4	Modality Qualifier Character 5	Isotope Character 6	Qualifier Character 7
Ø Pituitary Gland 1 Pineal Body 2 Adrenal Glands 4 Parathyroid Glands 5 Thyroid	Ø Photons <1 MeV 1 Photons 1- 10 MeV 2 Photons >10 MeV 5 Neutrons 6 Neutron Capture	Z None	Z None
Ø Pituitary Gland 1 Pineal Body 2 Adrenal Glands 4 Parathyroid Glands 5 Thyroid	3 Electrons	Z None	Ø Intraoperative Z None

D Radiation Therapy
G Endocrine System
1 Brachytherapy

Treatment Site Character 4	Modality Qualifier Character 5	Isotope Character 6	Qualifier Character 7
Ø Pituitary Gland 1 Pineal Body 2 Adrenal Glands 4 Parathyroid Glands 5 Thyroid	9 High Dose Rate (HDR)	7 Cesium 137 (Cs-137) 8 Iridium 192 (Ir-192) 9 Iodine 125 (I-125) B Palladium 103 (Pd-103) C Californium 252 (Cf-252) Y Other Isotope	Z None
Ø Pituitary Gland 1 Pineal Body 2 Adrenal Glands 4 Parathyroid Glands 5 Thyroid	B Low Dose Rate (LDR)	6 Cesium 131 (Cs-131) 7 Cesium 137 (Cs-137) 8 Iridium 192 (Ir-192) 9 Iodine 125 (I-125) C Californium 252 (Cf-252) Y Other Isotope	Z None
Ø Pituitary Gland 1 Pineal Body 2 Adrenal Glands 4 Parathyroid Glands 5 Thyroid	B Low Dose Rate (LDR)	B Palladium 103 (Pd-103)	1 Unidirectional Source Z None

D Radiation Therapy
G Endocrine System
2 Stereotactic Radiosurgery

Treatment Site Character 4	Modality Qualifier Character 5	Isotope Character 6	Qualifier Character 7
Ø Pituitary Gland 1 Pineal Body 2 Adrenal Glands 4 Parathyroid Glands 5 Thyroid	D Stereotactic Other Photon Radiosurgery H Stereotactic Particulate Radiosurgery J Stereotactic Gamma Beam Radiosurgery	Z None	Z None

DRG Non-OR All treatment site, modality, isotope, and qualifier values

D Radiation therapy
G Endocrine System
Y Other Radiation

Treatment Site Character 4	Modality Qualifier Character 5	Isotope Character 6	Qualifier Character 7
Ø Pituitary Gland 1 Pineal Body 2 Adrenal Glands 4 Parathyroid Glands 5 Thyroid	7 Contact Radiation 8 Hyperthermia F Plaque Radiation K Laser Interstitial Thermal Therapy	Z None	Z None

Valid OR DGY[Ø,1,2,4,5]KZZ

D Radiation Therapy
H Skin
Ø Beam Radiation

Treatment Site Character 4	Modality Qualifier Character 5	Isotope Character 6	Qualifier Character 7
2 Skin, Face 3 Skin, Neck 4 Skin, Arm 6 Skin, Chest 7 Skin, Back 8 Skin, Abdomen 9 Skin, Buttock B Skin, Leg	Ø Photons <1 MeV 1 Photons 1- 10 MeV 2 Photons >10 MeV 4 Heavy Particles (Protons, Ions) 5 Neutrons 6 Neutron Capture	Z None	Z None
2 Skin, Face 3 Skin, Neck 4 Skin, Arm 6 Skin, Chest 7 Skin, Back 8 Skin, Abdomen 9 Skin, Buttock B Skin, Leg	3 Electrons	Z None	Ø Intraoperative Z None

D Radiation Therapy
H Skin
Y Other Radiation

Treatment Site Character 4	Modality Qualifier Character 5	Isotope Character 6	Qualifier Character 7
2 Skin, Face 3 Skin, Neck 4 Skin, Arm 6 Skin, Chest 7 Skin, Back 8 Skin, Abdomen 9 Skin, Buttock B Skin, Leg	7 Contact Radiation 8 Hyperthermia F Plaque Radiation	Z None	Z None
5 Skin, Hand C Skin, Foot	F Plaque Radiation	Z None	Z None

D Radiation Therapy
M Breast
Ø Beam Radiation

Treatment Site Character 4	Modality Qualifier Character 5	Isotope Character 6	Qualifier Character 7
Ø Breast, Left **1** Breast, Right	**Ø** Photons <1 MeV **1** Photons 1- 10 MeV **2** Photons >10 MeV **4** Heavy Particles (Protons, Ions) **5** Neutrons **6** Neutron Capture	**Z** None	**Z** None
Ø Breast, Left **1** Breast, Right	**3** Electrons	**Z** None	**Ø** Intraoperative **Z** None

D Radiation Therapy
M Breast
1 Brachytherapy

Treatment Site Character 4	Modality Qualifier Character 5	Isotope Character 6	Qualifier Character 7
Ø Breast, Left **1** Breast, Right	**9** High Dose Rate (HDR)	**7** Cesium 137 (Cs-137) **8** Iridium 192 (Ir-192) **9** Iodine 125 (I-125) **B** Palladium 103 (Pd-103) **C** Californium 252 (Cf-252) **Y** Other Isotope	**Z** None
Ø Breast, Left **1** Breast, Right	**B** Low Dose Rate (LDR)	**6** Cesium 131 (Cs-131) **7** Cesium 137 (Cs-137) **8** Iridium 192 (Ir-192) **9** Iodine 125 (I-125) **C** Californium 252 (Cf-252) **Y** Other Isotope	**Z** None
Ø Breast, Left **1** Breast, Right	**B** Low Dose Rate (LDR)	**B** Palladium 103 (Pd-103)	**1** Unidirectional Source **Z** None

D Radiation Therapy
M Breast
2 Stereotactic Radiosurgery

Treatment Site Character 4	Modality Qualifier Character 5	Isotope Character 6	Qualifier Character 7
Ø Breast, Left **1** Breast, Right	**D** Stereotactic Other Photon Radiosurgery **H** Stereotactic Particulate Radiosurgery **J** Stereotactic Gamma Beam Radiosurgery	**Z** None	**Z** None

DRG Non-OR All treatment site, modality, isotope, and qualifier values

D Radiation Therapy
M Breast
Y Other Radiation

Treatment Site Character 4	Modality Qualifier Character 5	Isotope Character 6	Qualifier Character 7
Ø Breast, Left **1** Breast, Right	**7** Contact Radiation **8** Hyperthermia **F** Plaque Radiation **K** Laser Interstitial Thermal Therapy	**Z** None	**Z** None

Valid OR DMY[Ø,1]KZZ

D Radiation Therapy
P Musculoskeletal System
Ø Beam Radiation

Treatment Site Character 4	Modality Qualifier Character 5	Isotope Character 6	Qualifier Character 7
Ø Skull 2 Maxilla 3 Mandible 4 Sternum 5 Rib(s) 6 Humerus 7 Radius/Ulna 8 Pelvic Bones 9 Femur B Tibia/Fibula C Other Bone	Ø Photons <1 MeV 1 Photons 1- 10 MeV 2 Photons >10 MeV 4 Heavy Particles (Protons, Ions) 5 Neutrons 6 Neutron Capture	Z None	Z None
Ø Skull 2 Maxilla 3 Mandible 4 Sternum 5 Rib(s) 6 Humerus 7 Radius/Ulna 8 Pelvic Bones 9 Femur B Tibia/Fibula C Other Bone	3 Electrons	Z None	Ø Intraoperative Z None

D Radiation Therapy
P Musculoskeletal System
Y Other Radiation

Treatment Site Character 4	Modality Qualifier Character 5	Isotope Character 6	Qualifier Character 7
Ø Skull 2 Maxilla 3 Mandible 4 Sternum 5 Rib(s) 6 Humerus 7 Radius/Ulna 8 Pelvic Bones 9 Femur B Tibia/Fibula C Other Bone	7 Contact Radiation 8 Hyperthermia F Plaque Radiation	Z None	Z None

D Radiation Therapy
T Urinary System
Ø Beam Radiation

Treatment Site Character 4	Modality Qualifier Character 5	Isotope Character 6	Qualifier Character 7
Ø Kidney 1 Ureter 2 Bladder 3 Urethra	Ø Photons <1 MeV 1 Photons 1- 10 MeV 2 Photons >10 MeV 4 Heavy Particles (Protons, Ions) 5 Neutrons 6 Neutron Capture	Z None	Z None
Ø Kidney 1 Ureter 2 Bladder 3 Urethra	3 Electrons	Z None	Ø Intraoperative Z None

D Radiation Therapy
T Urinary System
1 Brachytherapy

Treatment Site Character 4	Modality Qualifier Character 5	Isotope Character 6	Qualifier Character 7
Ø Kidney 1 Ureter 2 Bladder 3 Urethra	9 High Dose Rate (HDR)	7 Cesium 137 (Cs-137) 8 Iridium 192 (Ir-192) 9 Iodine 125 (I-125) B Palladium 103 (Pd-103) C Californium 252 (Cf-252) Y Other Isotope	Z None
Ø Kidney 1 Ureter 2 Bladder 3 Urethra	B Low Dose Rate (LDR)	6 Cesium 131 (Cs-131) 7 Cesium 137 (Cs-137) 8 Iridium 192 (Ir-192) 9 Iodine 125 (I-125) C Californium 252 (Cf-252) Y Other Isotope	Z None
Ø Kidney 1 Ureter 2 Bladder 3 Urethra	B Low Dose Rate (LDR)	B Palladium 103 (Pd-103)	1 Unidirectional Source Z None

D Radiation Therapy
T Urinary System
2 Stereotactic Radiosurgery

Treatment Site Character 4	Modality Qualifier Character 5	Isotope Character 6	Qualifier Character 7
Ø Kidney 1 Ureter 2 Bladder 3 Urethra	D Stereotactic Other Photon Radiosurgery H Stereotactic Particulate Radiosurgery J Stereotactic Gamma Beam Radiosurgery	Z None	Z None

DRG Non-OR All treatment site, modality, isotope, and qualifier values

D Radiation Therapy
T Urinary System
Y Other Radiation

Treatment Site Character 4	Modality Qualifier Character 5	Isotope Character 6	Qualifier Character 7
Ø Kidney 1 Ureter 2 Bladder 3 Urethra	7 Contact Radiation 8 Hyperthermia C Intraoperative Radiation Therapy (IORT) F Plaque Radiation	Z None	Z None

D Radiation Therapy
U Female Reproductive System
Ø Beam Radiation

Treatment Site Character 4	Modality Qualifier Character 5	Isotope Character 6	Qualifier Character 7
Ø Ovary ♀ 1 Cervix ♀ 2 Uterus ♀	Ø Photons <1 MeV 1 Photons 1- 10 MeV 2 Photons >10 MeV 4 Heavy Particles (Protons, Ions) 5 Neutrons 6 Neutron Capture	Z None	Z None
Ø Ovary ♀ 1 Cervix ♀ 2 Uterus ♀	3 Electrons	Z None	Ø Intraoperative Z None

♀ All treatment site, modality, isotope, and qualifier values

Radiation Therapy

D Radiation Therapy
U Female Reproductive System
1 Brachytherapy

Treatment Site Character 4	Modality Qualifier Character 5	Isotope Character 6	Qualifier Character 7
Ø Ovary ♀ 1 Cervix ♀ 2 Uterus ♀	9 High Dose Rate (HDR)	7 Cesium 137 (Cs-137) 8 Iridium 192 (Ir-192) 9 Iodine 125 (I-125) B Palladium 103 (Pd-103) C Californium 252 (Cf-252) Y Other Isotope	Z None
Ø Ovary ♀ 1 Cervix ♀ 2 Uterus ♀	B Low Dose Rate (LDR)	6 Cesium 131 (Cs-131) 7 Cesium 137 (Cs-137) 8 Iridium 192 (Ir-192) 9 Iodine 125 (I-125) C Californium 252 (Cf-252) Y Other Isotope	Z None
Ø Ovary ♀ 1 Cervix ♀ 2 Uterus ♀	B Low Dose Rate (LDR)	B Palladium 103 (Pd-103)	1 Unidirectional Source Z None

♀ All treatment site, modality, isotope, and qualifier values

D Radiation Therapy
U Female Reproductive System
2 Stereotactic Radiosurgery

Treatment Site Character 4	Modality Qualifier Character 5	Isotope Character 6	Qualifier Character 7
Ø Ovary ♀ 1 Cervix ♀ 2 Uterus ♀	D Stereotactic Other Photon Radiosurgery H Stereotactic Particulate Radiosurgery J Stereotactic Gamma Beam Radiosurgery	Z None	Z None

DRG Non-OR All treatment site, modality, isotope, and qualifier values
♀ All treatment site, modality, isotope, and qualifier values

D Radiation Therapy
U Female Reproductive System
Y Other Radiation

Treatment Site Character 4	Modality Qualifier Character 5	Isotope Character 6	Qualifier Character 7
Ø Ovary ♀ 1 Cervix ♀ 2 Uterus ♀	7 Contact Radiation 8 Hyperthermia C Intraoperative Radiation Therapy (IORT) F Plaque Radiation	Z None	Z None

♀ All treatment site, modality, isotope, and qualifier values

D Radiation Therapy
V Male Reproductive System
Ø Beam Radiation

Treatment Site Character 4	Modality Qualifier Character 5	Isotope Character 6	Qualifier Character 7
Ø Prostate ♂ 1 Testis ♂	Ø Photons <1 MeV 1 Photons 1- 10 MeV 2 Photons >10 MeV 4 Heavy Particles (Protons, Ions) 5 Neutrons 6 Neutron Capture	Z None	Z None
Ø Prostate ♂ 1 Testis ♂	3 Electrons	Z None	Ø Intraoperative Z None

♂ All treatment site, modality, isotope, and qualifier values

D Radiation Therapy
V Male Reproductive System
1 Brachytherapy

Treatment Site Character 4	Modality Qualifier Character 5	Isotope Character 6	Qualifier Character 7
Ø Prostate ♂ 1 Testis ♂	9 High Dose Rate (HDR)	7 Cesium 137 (Cs-137) 8 Iridium 192 (Ir-192) 9 Iodine 125 (I-125) B Palladium 103 (Pd-103) C Californium 252 (Cf-252) Y Other Isotope	Z None
Ø Prostate ♂ 1 Testis ♂	B Low Dose Rate (LDR)	6 Cesium 131 (Cs-131) 7 Cesium 137 (Cs-137) 8 Iridium 192 (Ir-192) 9 Iodine 125 (I-125) C Californium 252 (Cf-252) Y Other Isotope	Z None
Ø Prostate ♂ 1 Testis ♂	B Low Dose Rate (LDR)	B Palladium 103 (Pd-103)	1 Unidirectional Source Z None

♂ All treatment site, modality, isotope, and qualifier values

D Radiation Therapy
V Male Reproductive System
2 Stereotactic Radiosurgery

Treatment Site Character 4	Modality Qualifier Character 5	Isotope Character 6	Qualifier Character 7
Ø Prostate ♂ 1 Testis ♂	D Stereotactic Other Photon Radiosurgery H Stereotactic Particulate Radiosurgery J Stereotactic Gamma Beam Radiosurgery	Z None	Z None

DRG Non-OR All treatment site, modality, isotope, and qualifier values
♂ All treatment site, modality, isotope, and qualifier values

D Radiation Therapy
V Male Reproductive System
Y Other Radiation

Treatment Site Character 4	Modality Qualifier Character 5	Isotope Character 6	Qualifier Character 7
Ø Prostate ♂	7 Contact Radiation 8 Hyperthermia C Intraoperative Radiation Therapy (IORT) F Plaque Radiation K Laser Interstitial Thermal Therapy	Z None	Z None
1 Testis ♂	7 Contact Radiation 8 Hyperthermia F Plaque Radiation	Z None	Z None

Valid OR DVYØKZZ
♂ All treatment site, modality, isotope, and qualifier values

D Radiation Therapy
W Anatomical Regions
Ø Beam Radiation

Treatment Site Character 4	Modality Qualifier Character 5	Isotope Character 6	Qualifier Character 7
1 Head and Neck 2 Chest 3 Abdomen 4 Hemibody 5 Whole Body 6 Pelvic Region	Ø Photons <1 MeV 1 Photons 1- 10 MeV 2 Photons >10 MeV 4 Heavy Particles (Protons, Ions) 5 Neutrons 6 Neutron Capture	Z None	Z None
1 Head and Neck 2 Chest 3 Abdomen 4 Hemibody 5 Whole Body 6 Pelvic Region	3 Electrons	Z None	Ø Intraoperative Z None

D Radiation Therapy
W Anatomical Regions
1 Brachytherapy

Treatment Site Character 4	Modality Qualifier Character 5	Isotope Character 6	Qualifier Character 7
Ø Cranial Cavity K Upper Back L Lower Back P Gastrointestinal Tract Q Respiratory Tract R Genitourinary Tract X Upper Extremity Y Lower Extremity	B Low Dose Rate (LDR)	B Palladium 103 (Pd-103)	1 Unidirectional Source Z None
1 Head and Neck 2 Chest 3 Abdomen 6 Pelvic Region	9 High Dose Rate (HDR)	7 Cesium 137 (Cs-137) 8 Iridium 192 (Ir-192) 9 Iodine 125 (I-125) B Palladium 103 (Pd-103) C Californium 252 (Cf-252) Y Other Isotope	Z None
1 Head and Neck 2 Chest 3 Abdomen 6 Pelvic Region	B Low Dose Rate (LDR)	6 Cesium 131 (Cs-131) 7 Cesium 137 (Cs-137) 8 Iridium 192 (Ir-192) 9 Iodine 125 (I-125) C Californium 252 (Cf-252) Y Other Isotope	Z None
1 Head and Neck 2 Chest 3 Abdomen 6 Pelvic Region	B Low Dose Rate (LDR)	B Palladium 103 (Pd-103)	1 Unidirectional Source Z None

D Radiation Therapy
W Anatomical Regions
2 Stereotactic Radiosurgery

Treatment Site Character 4	Modality Qualifier Character 5	Isotope Character 6	Qualifier Character 7
1 Head and Neck 2 Chest 3 Abdomen 6 Pelvic Region	D Stereotactic Other Photon Radiosurgery H Stereotactic Particulate Radiosurgery J Stereotactic Gamma Beam Radiosurgery	Z None	Z None

DRG Non-OR All treatment site, modality, isotope, and qualifier values

D Radiation Therapy
W Anatomical Regions
Y Other Radiation

Treatment Site Character 4	Modality Qualifier Character 5	Isotope Character 6	Qualifier Character 7
1 Head and Neck 2 Chest 3 Abdomen 4 Hemibody 6 Pelvic Region	7 Contact Radiation 8 Hyperthermia F Plaque Radiation	Z None	Z None
5 Whole Body	7 Contact Radiation 8 Hyperthermia F Plaque Radiation	Z None	Z None
5 Whole Body	G Isotope Administration	D Iodine 131 (I-131) F Phosphorus 32 (P-32) G Strontium 89 (Sr-89) H Strontium 90 (Sr-90) Y Other Isotope	Z None

Physical Rehabilitation and Diagnostic Audiology FØØ–F15

F Physical Rehabilitation and Diagnostic Audiology
Ø Rehabilitation
Ø Speech Assessment Definition: Measurement of speech and related functions

Body System/Region Character 4	Type Qualifier Character 5	Equipment Character 6	Qualifier Character 7
3 Neurological System - Whole Body	G Communicative/Cognitive Integration Skills	K Audiovisual M Augmentative / Alternative Communication P Computer Y Other Equipment Z None	Z None
Z None	Ø Filtered Speech 3 Staggered Spondaic Word Q Performance Intensity Phonetically Balanced Speech Discrimination R Brief Tone Stimuli S Distorted Speech T Dichotic Stimuli V Temporal Ordering of Stimuli W Masking Patterns	1 Audiometer 2 Sound Field / Booth K Audiovisual Z None	Z None
Z None	1 Speech Threshold 2 Speech/Word Recognition	1 Audiometer 2 Sound Field / Booth 9 Cochlear Implant K Audiovisual Z None	Z None
Z None	4 Sensorineural Acuity Level	1 Audiometer 2 Sound Field / Booth Z None	Z None
Z None	5 Synthetic Sentence Identification	1 Audiometer 2 Sound Field / Booth 9 Cochlear Implant K Audiovisual	Z None
Z None	6 Speech and/or Language Screening 7 Nonspoken Language 8 Receptive/Expressive Language C Aphasia G Communicative/Cognitive Integration Skills L Augmentative/Alternative Communication System	K Audiovisual M Augmentative / Alternative Communication P Computer Y Other Equipment Z None	Z None
Z None	9 Articulation/Phonology	K Audiovisual P Computer Q Speech Analysis Y Other Equipment Z None	Z None
Z None	B Motor Speech	K Audiovisual N Biosensory Feedback P Computer Q Speech Analysis T Aerodynamic Function Y Other Equipment Z None	Z None
Z None	D Fluency	K Audiovisual N Biosensory Feedback P Computer Q Speech Analysis S Voice Analysis T Aerodynamic Function Y Other Equipment Z None	Z None
Z None	F Voice	K Audiovisual N Biosensory Feedback P Computer S Voice Analysis T Aerodynamic Function Y Other Equipment Z None	Z None

DRG Non-OR All body system/region, type qualifier, equipment, and qualifier values

FØØ Continued on next page

Physical Rehabilitation and Diagnostic Audiology

FØØ Continued

F Physical Rehabilitation and Diagnostic Audiology
Ø Rehabilitation
Ø Speech Assessment Definition: Measurement of speech and related functions

Body System/Region Character 4	Type Qualifier Character 5	Equipment Character 6	Qualifier Character 7
Z None	H Bedside Swallowing and Oral Function P Oral Peripheral Mechanism	Y Other Equipment Z None	Z None
Z None	J Instrumental Swallowing and Oral Function	T Aerodynamic Function W Swallowing Y Other Equipment	Z None
Z None	K Orofacial Myofunctional	K Audiovisual P Computer Y Other Equipment Z None	Z None
Z None	M Voice Prosthetic	K Audiovisual P Computer S Voice Analysis V Speech Prosthesis Y Other Equipment Z None	Z None
Z None	N Non-invasive Instrumental Status	N Biosensory Feedback P Computer Q Speech Analysis S Voice Analysis T Aerodynamic Function Y Other Equipment	Z None
Z None	X Other Specified Central Auditory Processing	Z None	Z None

DRG Non-OR All body system/region, type qualifier, equipment, and qualifier values

F Physical Rehabilitation and Diagnostic Audiology
Ø Rehabilitation
1 Motor and/or Nerve Function Assessment Definition: Measurement of motor, nerve, and related functions

Body System/Region Character 4	Type Qualifier Character 5	Equipment Character 6	Qualifier Character 7
Ø Neurological System - Head and Neck 1 Neurological System - Upper Back/ Upper Extremity 2 Neurological System - Lower Back/ Lower Extremity 3 Neurological System - Whole Body	Ø Muscle Performance	E Orthosis F Assistive, Adaptive, Supportive or Protective U Prosthesis Y Other Equipment Z None	Z None
Ø Neurological System - Head and Neck 1 Neurological System - Upper Back/ Upper Extremity 2 Neurological System - Lower Back/ Lower Extremity 3 Neurological System - Whole Body	1 Integumentary Integrity 3 Coordination/Dexterity 4 Motor Function G Reflex Integrity	Z None	Z None
Ø Neurological System - Head and Neck 1 Neurological System - Upper Back/ Upper Extremity 2 Neurological System - Lower Back/ Lower Extremity 3 Neurological System - Whole Body	5 Range of Motion and Joint Integrity 6 Sensory Awareness/Processing/ Integrity	Y Other Equipment Z None	Z None
D Integumentary System - Head and Neck F Integumentary System - Upper Back/ Upper Extremity G Integumentary System - Lower Back/ Lower Extremity H Integumentary System - Whole Body J Musculoskeletal System - Head and Neck K Musculoskeletal System - Upper Back/ Upper Extremity L Musculoskeletal System - Lower Back/ Lower Extremity M Musculoskeletal System - Whole Body	Ø Muscle Performance	E Orthosis F Assistive, Adaptive, Supportive or Protective U Prosthesis Y Other Equipment Z None	Z None

DRG Non-OR All body system/region, type qualifier, equipment, and qualifier values

FØ1 Continued on next page

F Physical Rehabilitation and Diagnostic Audiology
Ø Rehabilitation
1 Motor and/or Nerve Function Assessment Definition: Measurement of motor, nerve, and related functions

FØ1 Continued

Body System/Region Character 4	Type Qualifier Character 5	Equipment Character 6	Qualifier Character 7
D Integumentary System - Head and Neck F Integumentary System - Upper Back/ Upper Extremity G Integumentary System - Lower Back/ Lower Extremity H Integumentary System - Whole Body J Musculoskeletal System - Head and Neck K Musculoskeletal System - Upper Back/ Upper Extremity L Musculoskeletal System - Lower Back/ Lower Extremity M Musculoskeletal System - Whole Body	1 Integumentary Integrity	Z None	Z None
D Integumentary System - Head and Neck F Integumentary System - Upper Back/ Upper Extremity G Integumentary System - Lower Back/ Lower Extremity H Integumentary System - Whole Body J Musculoskeletal System - Head and Neck K Musculoskeletal System - Upper Back/ Upper Extremity L Musculoskeletal System - Lower Back/ Lower Extremity M Musculoskeletal System - Whole Body	5 Range of Motion and Joint Integrity 6 Sensory Awareness/Processing/ Integrity	Y Other Equipment Z None	Z None
N Genitourinary System	Ø Muscle Performance	E Orthosis F Assistive, Adaptive, Supportive or Protective U Prosthesis Y Other Equipment Z None	Z None
Z None	2 Visual Motor Integration	K Audiovisual M Augmentative / Alternative Communication N Biosensory Feedback P Computer Q Speech Analysis S Voice Analysis Y Other Equipment Z None	Z None
Z None	7 Facial Nerve Function	7 Electrophysiologic	Z None
Z None	9 Somatosensory Evoked Potentials	J Somatosensory	Z None
Z None	B Bed Mobility C Transfer F Wheelchair Mobility	E Orthosis F Assistive, Adaptive, Supportive or Protective U Prosthesis Z None	Z None
Z None	D Gait and/or Balance	E Orthosis F Assistive, Adaptive, Supportive or Protective U Prosthesis Y Other Equipment Z None	Z None

DRG Non-OR All body system/region, type qualifier, equipment, and qualifier values

F Physical Rehabilitation and Diagnostic Audiology
Ø Rehabilitation
2 Activities of Daily Living Assessment Definition: Measurement of functional level for activities of daily living

Body System/Region Character 4	Type Qualifier Character 5	Equipment Character 6	Qualifier Character 7
Ø Neurological System - Head and Neck	9 Cranial Nerve Integrity D Neuromotor Development	Y Other Equipment Z None	Z None
1 Neurological System - Upper Back/ Upper Extremity 2 Neurological System - Lower Back/ Lower Extremity 3 Neurological System - Whole Body	D Neuromotor Development	Y Other Equipment Z None	Z None
4 Circulatory System - Head and Neck 5 Circulatory System - Upper Back/ Upper Extremity 6 Circulatory System - Lower Back/ Lower Extremity 8 Respiratory System - Head and Neck 9 Respiratory System - Upper Back/ Upper Extremity B Respiratory System - Lower Back/ Lower Extremity	G Ventilation, Respiration and Circulation	C Mechanical G Aerobic Endurance and Conditioning Y Other Equipment Z None	Z None
7 Circulatory System - Whole Body C Respiratory System - Whole Body	7 Aerobic Capacity and Endurance	E Orthosis G Aerobic Endurance and Conditioning U Prosthesis Y Other Equipment Z None	Z None
7 Circulatory System - Whole Body C Respiratory System - Whole Body	G Ventilation, Respiration and Circulation	C Mechanical G Aerobic Endurance and Conditioning Y Other Equipment Z None	Z None
Z None	Ø Bathing/Showering 1 Dressing 3 Grooming/Personal Hygiene 4 Home Management	E Orthosis F Assistive, Adaptive, Supportive or Protective U Prosthesis Z None	Z None
Z None	2 Feeding/Eating 8 Anthropometric Characteristics F Pain	Y Other Equipment Z None	Z None
Z None	5 Perceptual Processing	K Audiovisual M Augmentative / Alternative Communication N Biosensory Feedback P Computer Q Speech Analysis S Voice Analysis Y Other Equipment Z None	Z None
Z None	6 Psychosocial Skills	Z None	Z None
Z None	B Environmental, Home and Work Barriers C Ergonomics and Body Mechanics	E Orthosis F Assistive, Adaptive, Supportive or Protective U Prosthesis Y Other Equipment Z None	Z None
Z None	H Vocational Activities and Functional Community or Work Reintegration Skills	E Orthosis F Assistive, Adaptive, Supportive or Protective G Aerobic Endurance and Conditioning U Prosthesis Y Other Equipment Z None	Z None

DRG Non-OR All body system/region, type qualifier, equipment, and qualifier values

F Physical Rehabilitation and Diagnostic Audiology
Ø Rehabilitation
6 Speech Treatment Definition: Application of techniques to improve, augment, or compensate for speech and related functional impairment

Body System/Region Character 4	Type Qualifier Character 5	Equipment Character 6	Qualifier Character 7
3 Neurological System - Whole Body	6 Communicative/Cognitive Integration Skills	K Audiovisual M Augmentative / Alternative Communication P Computer Y Other Equipment Z None	Z None
Z None	Ø Nonspoken Language 3 Aphasia 6 Communicative/Cognitive Integration Skills	K Audiovisual M Augmentative / Alternative Communication P Computer Y Other Equipment Z None	Z None
Z None	1 Speech-Language Pathology and Related Disorders Counseling 2 Speech-Language Pathology and Related Disorders Prevention	K Audiovisual Z None	Z None
Z None	4 Articulation/Phonology	K Audiovisual P Computer Q Speech Analysis T Aerodynamic Function Y Other Equipment Z None	Z None
Z None	5 Aural Rehabilitation	K Audiovisual L Assistive Listening M Augmentative / Alternative Communication N Biosensory Feedback P Computer Q Speech Analysis S Voice Analysis Y Other Equipment Z None	Z None
Z None	7 Fluency	4 Electroacoustic Immitance / Acoustic Reflex K Audiovisual N Biosensory Feedback Q Speech Analysis S Voice Analysis T Aerodynamic Function Y Other Equipment Z None	Z None
Z None	8 Motor Speech	K Audiovisual N Biosensory Feedback P Computer Q Speech Analysis S Voice Analysis T Aerodynamic Function Y Other Equipment Z None	Z None
Z None	9 Orofacial Myofunctional	K Audiovisual P Computer Y Other Equipment Z None	Z None
Z None	B Receptive/Expressive Language	K Audiovisual L Assistive Listening M Augmentative / Alternative Communication P Computer Y Other Equipment Z None	Z None

DRG Non-OR All body system/region, type qualifier, equipment, and qualifier values

FØ6 Continued on next page

F Physical Rehabilitation and Diagnostic Audiology
Ø Rehabilitation
6 Speech Treatment Definition: Application of techniques to improve, augment, or compensate for speech and related functional impairment

FØ6 Continued

Body System/Region Character 4	Type Qualifier Character 5	Equipment Character 6	Qualifier Character 7
Z None	C Voice	K Audiovisual N Biosensory Feedback P Computer S Voice Analysis T Aerodynamic Function V Speech Prosthesis Y Other Equipment Z None	Z None
Z None	D Swallowing Dysfunction	M Augmentative / Alternative Communication T Aerodynamic Function V Speech Prosthesis Y Other Equipment Z None	Z None

DRG Non-OR All body system/region, type qualifier, equipment, and qualifier values

F Physical Rehabilitation and Diagnostic Audiology
Ø Rehabilitation
7 Motor Treatment Definition: Exercise or activities to increase or facilitate motor function

Body System/Region Character 4	Type Qualifier Character 5	Equipment Character 6	Qualifier Character 7
Ø Neurological System - Head and Neck 1 Neurological System - Upper Back/ Upper Extremity 2 Neurological System - Lower Back/ Lower Extremity 3 Neurological System - Whole Body D Integumentary System - Head and Neck F Integumentary System - Upper Back/ Upper Extremity G Integumentary System - Lower Back/ Lower Extremity H Integumentary System - Whole Body J Musculoskeletal System - Head and Neck K Musculoskeletal System - Upper Back/ Upper Extremity L Musculoskeletal System - Lower Back/ Lower Extremity M Musculoskeletal System - Whole Body	Ø Range of Motion and Joint Mobility 1 Muscle Performance 2 Coordination/Dexterity 3 Motor Function	E Orthosis F Assistive, Adaptive, Supportive or Protective U Prosthesis Y Other Equipment Z None	Z None
Ø Neurological System - Head and Neck 1 Neurological System - Upper Back/ Upper Extremity 2 Neurological System - Lower Back/ Lower Extremity 3 Neurological System - Whole Body D Integumentary System - Head and Neck F Integumentary System - Upper Back/ Upper Extremity G Integumentary System - Lower Back/ Lower Extremity H Integumentary System - Whole Body J Musculoskeletal System - Head and Neck K Musculoskeletal System - Upper Back/ Upper Extremity L Musculoskeletal System - Lower Back/ Lower Extremity M Musculoskeletal System - Whole Body	6 Therapeutic Exercise	B Physical Agents C Mechanical D Electrotherapeutic E Orthosis F Assistive, Adaptive, Supportive or Protective G Aerobic Endurance and Conditioning H Mechanical or Electromechanical U Prosthesis Y Other Equipment Z None	Z None

DRG Non-OR All body system/region, type qualifier, equipment, and qualifier values

FØ7 Continued on next page

FØ7 Continued

F Physical Rehabilitation and Diagnostic Audiology
Ø Rehabilitation
7 Motor Treatment Definition: Exercise or activities to increase or facilitate motor function

Body System/Region Character 4	Type Qualifier Character 5	Equipment Character 6	Qualifier Character 7
Ø Neurological System - Head and Neck **1** Neurological System - Upper Back/ Upper Extremity **2** Neurological System - Lower Back/ Lower Extremity **3** Neurological System - Whole Body **D** Integumentary System - Head and Neck **F** Integumentary System - Upper Back/ Upper Extremity **G** Integumentary System - Lower Back/ Lower Extremity **H** Integumentary System - Whole Body **J** Musculoskeletal System - Head and Neck **K** Musculoskeletal System - Upper Back/ Upper Extremity **L** Musculoskeletal System - Lower Back/ Lower Extremity **M** Musculoskeletal System - Whole Body	**7** Manual Therapy Techniques	**Z** None	**Z** None
4 Circulatory System - Head and Neck **5** Circulatory System - Upper Back / Upper Extremity **6** Circulatory System - Lower Back / Lower Extremity **7** Circulatory System - Whole Body **8** Respiratory System - Head and Neck **9** Respiratory System - Upper Back / Upper Extremity **B** Respiratory System - Lower Back / Lower Extremity **C** Respiratory System - Whole Body	**6** Therapeutic Exercise	**B** Physical Agents **C** Mechanical **D** Electrotherapeutic **E** Orthosis **F** Assistive, Adaptive, Supportive or Protective **G** Aerobic Endurance and Conditioning **H** Mechanical or Electromechanical **U** Prosthesis **Y** Other Equipment **Z** None	**Z** None
N Genitourinary System	**1** Muscle Performance	**E** Orthosis **F** Assistive, Adaptive, Supportive or Protective **U** Prosthesis **Y** Other Equipment **Z** None	**Z** None
N Genitourinary System	**6** Therapeutic Exercise	**B** Physical Agents **C** Mechanical **D** Electrotherapeutic **E** Orthosis **F** Assistive, Adaptive, Supportive or Protective **G** Aerobic Endurance and Conditioning **H** Mechanical or Electromechanical **U** Prosthesis **Y** Other Equipment **Z** None	**Z** None
Z None	**4** Wheelchair Mobility	**D** Electrotherapeutic **E** Orthosis **F** Assistive, Adaptive, Supportive or Protective **U** Prosthesis **Y** Other Equipment **Z** None	**Z** None
Z None	**5** Bed Mobility	**C** Mechanical **E** Orthosis **F** Assistive, Adaptive, Supportive or Protective **U** Prosthesis **Y** Other Equipment **Z** None	**Z** None
Z None	**8** Transfer Training	**C** Mechanical **D** Electrotherapeutic **E** Orthosis **F** Assistive, Adaptive, Supportive or Protective **U** Prosthesis **Y** Other Equipment **Z** None	**Z** None

DRG Non-OR All body system/region, type qualifier, equipment, and qualifier values

FØ7 Continued on next page

Physical Rehabilitation and Diagnostic Audiology

FØ7 Continued

F Physical Rehabilitation and Diagnostic Audiology
Ø Rehabilitation
7 Motor Treatment Definition: Exercise or activities to increase or facilitate motor function

Body System/Region Character 4	Type Qualifier Character 5	Equipment Character 6	Qualifier Character 7
Z None	9 Gait Training/Functional Ambulation	C Mechanical D Electrotherapeutic E Orthosis F Assistive, Adaptive, Supportive or Protective G Aerobic Endurance and Conditioning U Prosthesis Y Other Equipment Z None	Z None

DRG Non-OR All body system/region, type qualifier, equipment, and qualifier values

F Physical Rehabilitation and Diagnostic Audiology
Ø Rehabilitation
8 Activities of Daily Living Treatment Definition: Exercise or activities to facilitate functional competence for activities of daily living

Body System/Region Character 4	Type Qualifier Character 5	Equipment Character 6	Qualifier Character 7
D Integumentary System - Head and Neck F Integumentary System - Upper Back/ Upper Extremity G Integumentary System - Lower Back/ Lower Extremity H Integumentary System - Whole Body J Musculoskeletal System - Head and Neck K Musculoskeletal System - Upper Back/ Upper Extremity L Musculoskeletal System - Lower Back/ Lower Extremity M Musculoskeletal System - Whole Body	5 Wound Management	B Physical Agents C Mechanical D Electrotherapeutic E Orthosis F Assistive, Adaptive, Supportive or Protective U Prosthesis Y Other Equipment Z None	Z None
Z None	Ø Bathing/Showering Techniques 1 Dressing Techniques 2 Grooming/Personal Hygiene	E Orthosis F Assistive, Adaptive, Supportive or Protective U Prosthesis Y Other Equipment Z None	Z None
Z None	3 Feeding/Eating	C Mechanical D Electrotherapeutic E Orthosis F Assistive, Adaptive, Supportive or Protective U Prosthesis Y Other Equipment Z None	Z None
Z None	4 Home Management	D Electrotherapeutic E Orthosis F Assistive, Adaptive, Supportive or Protective U Prosthesis Y Other Equipment Z None	Z None
Z None	6 Psychosocial Skills	Z None	Z None
Z None	7 Vocational Activities and Functional Community or Work Reintegration Skills	B Physical Agents C Mechanical D Electrotherapeutic E Orthosis F Assistive, Adaptive, Supportive or Protective G Aerobic Endurance and Conditioning U Prosthesis Y Other Equipment Z None	Z None

DRG Non-OR All body system/region, type qualifier, equipment, and qualifier values

F Physical Rehabilitation and Diagnostic Audiology
Ø Rehabilitation
9 Hearing Treatment Definition: Application of techniques to improve, augment, or compensate for hearing and related functional impairment

Body System/Region Character 4	Type Qualifier Character 5	Equipment Character 6	Qualifier Character 7
Z None	Ø Hearing and Related Disorders Counseling 1 Hearing and Related Disorders Prevention	K Audiovisual Z None	Z None
Z None	2 Auditory Processing	K Audiovisual L Assistive Listening P Computer Y Other Equipment Z None	Z None
Z None	3 Cerumen Management	X Cerumen Management Z None	Z None

DRG Non-OR All body system/region, type qualifier, equipment, and qualifier values

F Physical Rehabilitation and Diagnostic Audiology
Ø Rehabilitation
B Cochlear Implant Treatment Definition: Application of techniques to improve the communication abilities of individuals with cochlear implant

Body System/Region Character 4	Type Qualifier Character 5	Equipment Character 6	Qualifier Character 7
Z None	Ø Cochlear Implant Rehabilitation	1 Audiometer 2 Sound Field / Booth 9 Cochlear Implant K Audiovisual P Computer Y Other Equipment	Z None

DRG Non-OR All body system/region, type qualifier, equipment, and qualifier values

F Physical Rehabilitation and Diagnostic Audiology
Ø Rehabilitation
C Vestibular Treatment Definition: Application of techniques to improve, augment, or compensate for vestibular and related functional impairment

Body System/Region Character 4	Type Qualifier Character 5	Equipment Character 6	Qualifier Character 7
3 Neurological System - Whole Body H Integumentary System - Whole Body M Musculoskeletal System - Whole Body	3 Postural Control	E Orthosis F Assistive, Adaptive, Supportive or Protective U Prosthesis Y Other Equipment Z None	Z None
Z None	Ø Vestibular	8 Vestibular / Balance Z None	Z None
Z None	1 Perceptual Processing 2 Visual Motor Integration	K Audiovisual L Assistive Listening N Biosensory Feedback P Computer Q Speech Analysis S Voice Analysis T Aerodynamic Function Y Other Equipment Z None	Z None

DRG Non-OR All body system/region, type qualifier, equipment, and qualifier values

F Physical Rehabilitation and Diagnostic Audiology
Ø Rehabilitation
D Device Fitting Definition: Fitting of a device designed to facilitate or support achievement of a higher level of function

Body System/Region Character 4	Type Qualifier Character 5	Equipment Character 6	Qualifier Character 7
Z None	Ø Tinnitus Masker	5 Hearing Aid Selection / Fitting / Test Z None	Z None
Z None	1 Monaural Hearing Aid 2 Binaural Hearing Aid 5 Assistive Listening Device	1 Audiometer 2 Sound Field / Booth 5 Hearing Aid Selection / Fitting / Test K Audiovisual L Assistive Listening Z None	Z None
Z None	3 Augmentative/Alternative Communication System	M Augmentative / Alternative Communication	Z None
Z None	4 Voice Prosthetic	S Voice Analysis V Speech Prosthesis	Z None
Z None	6 Dynamic Orthosis 7 Static Orthosis 8 Prosthesis 9 Assistive, Adaptive,Supportive or Protective Devices	E Orthosis F Assistive, Adaptive, Supportive or Protective U Prosthesis Z None	Z None

DRG Non-OR FØDZØ[5,Z]Z
DRG Non-OR FØDZ[1, 2,5][1,2,5, K,L,Z]Z
DRG Non-OR FØDZ3MZ
DRG Non-OR FØDZ4[S,V]Z
DRG Non-OR FØDZ[6,7][E,F,U,Z]Z
DRG Non-OR FØDZ8[E,F,U]Z

F Physical Rehabilitation and Diagnostic Audiology
Ø Rehabilitation
F Caregiver Training Definition: Training in activities to support patient's optimal level of function

Body System/Region Character 4	Type Qualifier Character 5	Equipment Character 6	Qualifier Character 7
Z None	Ø Bathing/Showering Technique 1 Dressing 2 Feeding and Eating 3 Grooming/Personal Hygiene 4 Bed Mobility 5 Transfer 6 Wheelchair Mobility 7 Therapeutic Exercise 8 Airway Clearance Techniques 9 Wound Management B Vocational Activities and Functional Community or Work Reintegration Skills C Gait Training/Functional Ambulation D Application, Proper Use and Care of Devices F Application, Proper Use and Care of Orthoses G Application, Proper Use and Care of Prosthesis H Home Management	E Orthosis F Assistive, Adaptive, Supportive or Protective U Prosthesis Z None	Z None
Z None	J Communication Skills	K Audiovisual L Assistive Listening M Augmentative / Alternative Communication P Computer Z None	Z None

DRG Non-OR All body system/region, type qualifier, equipment, and qualifier values

F Physical Rehabilitation and Diagnostic Audiology
1 Diagnostic Audiology
3 Hearing Assessment Definition: Measurement of hearing and related functions

Body System/Region Character 4	Type Qualifier Character 5	Equipment Character 6	Qualifier Character 7
Z None	Ø Hearing Screening	Ø Occupational Hearing 1 Audiometer 2 Sound Field / Booth 3 Tympanometer 8 Vestibular / Balance 9 Cochlear Implant Z None	Z None
Z None	1 Pure Tone Audiometry, Air 2 Pure Tone Audiometry, Air and Bone	Ø Occupational Hearing 1 Audiometer 2 Sound Field / Booth Z None	Z None
Z None	3 Bekesy Audiometry 6 Visual Reinforcement Audiometry 9 Short Increment Sensitivity Index B Stenger C Pure Tone Stenger	1 Audiometer 2 Sound Field / Booth Z None	Z None
Z None	4 Conditioned Play Audiometry 5 Select Picture Audiometry	1 Audiometer 2 Sound Field / Booth K Audiovisual Z None	Z None
Z None	7 Alternate Binaural or Monaural Loudness Balance	1 Audiometer K Audiovisual Z None	Z None
Z None	8 Tone Decay D Tympanometry F Eustachian Tube Function G Acoustic Reflex Patterns H Acoustic Reflex Threshold J Acoustic Reflex Decay	3 Tympanometer 4 Electroacoustic Immitance / Acoustic Reflex Z None	Z None
Z None	K Electrocochleography L Auditory Evoked Potentials	7 Electrophysiologic Z None	Z None
Z None	M Evoked Otoacoustic Emissions, Screening N Evoked Otoacoustic Emissions, Diagnostic	6 Otoacoustic Emission (OAE) Z None	Z None
Z None	P Aural Rehabilitation Status	1 Audiometer 2 Sound Field / Booth 4 Electroacoustic Immitance / Acoustic Reflex 9 Cochlear Implant K Audiovisual L Assistive Listening P Computer Z None	Z None
Z None	Q Auditory Processing	K Audiovisual P Computer Y Other Equipment Z None	Z None

F Physical Rehabilitation and Diagnostic Audiology
1 Diagnostic Audiology
4 Hearing Aid Assessment Definition: Measurement of the appropriateness and/or effectiveness of a hearing device

Body System/Region Character 4	Type Qualifier Character 5	Equipment Character 6	Qualifier Character 7
Z None	Ø Cochlear Implant	1 Audiometer 2 Sound Field / Booth 3 Tympanometer 4 Electroacoustic Immitance / Acoustic Reflex 5 Hearing Aid Selection / Fitting / Test 7 Electrophysiologic 9 Cochlear Implant K Audiovisual L Assistive Listening P Computer Y Other Equipment Z None	Z None
Z None	1 Ear Canal Probe Microphone 6 Binaural Electroacoustic Hearing Aid Check 8 Monaural Electroacoustic Hearing Aid Check	5 Hearing Aid Selection / Fitting / Test Z None	Z None
Z None	2 Monaural Hearing Aid 3 Binaural Hearing Aid	1 Audiometer 2 Sound Field / Booth 3 Tympanometer 4 Electroacoustic Immitance / Acoustic Reflex 5 Hearing Aid Selection / Fitting / Test K Audiovisual L Assistive Listening P Computer Z None	Z None
Z None	4 Assistive Listening System/Device Selection	1 Audiometer 2 Sound Field / Booth 3 Tympanometer 4 Electroacoustic Immitance / Acoustic Reflex K Audiovisual L Assistive Listening Z None	Z None
Z None	5 Sensory Aids	1 Audiometer 2 Sound Field / Booth 3 Tympanometer 4 Electroacoustic Immitance / Acoustic Reflex 5 Hearing Aid Selection / Fitting / Test K Audiovisual L Assistive Listening Z None	Z None
Z None	7 Ear Protector Attentuation	Ø Occupational Hearing Z None	Z None

F Physical Rehabilitation and Diagnostic Audiology
1 Diagnostic Audiology
5 Vestibular Assessment Definition: Measurement of the vestibular system and related functions

Body System/Region Character 4	Type Qualifier Character 5	Equipment Character 6	Qualifier Character 7
Z None	Ø Bithermal, Binaural Caloric Irrigation 1 Bithermal, Monaural Caloric Irrigation 2 Unithermal Binaural Screen 3 Oscillating Tracking 4 Sinusoidal Vertical Axis Rotational 5 Dix-Hallpike Dynamic 6 Computerized Dynamic Posturography	8 Vestibular / Balance Z None	Z None
Z None	7 Tinnitus Masker	5 Hearing Aid Selection / Fitting / Test Z None	Z None

Mental Health GZ1–GZJ

G Mental Health
Z None
1 Psychological Tests Definition: The administration and interpretation of standardized psychological tests and measurement instruments for the assessment of psychological function

Qualifier Character 4	Qualifier Character 5	Qualifier Character 6	Qualifier Character 7
Ø Developmental 1 Personality and Behavioral 2 Intellectual and Psychoeducational 3 Neuropsychological 4 Neurobehavioral and Cognitive Status	Z None	Z None	Z None

G Mental Health
Z None
2 Crisis Intervention Definition: Treatment of a traumatized, acutely disturbed or distressed individual for the purpose of short-term stabilization

Qualifier Character 4	Qualifier Character 5	Qualifier Character 6	Qualifier Character 7
Z None	Z None	Z None	Z None

G Mental Health
Z None
3 Medication Management Definition: Monitoring and adjusting the use of medications for the treatment of a mental health disorder

Qualifier Character 4	Qualifier Character 5	Qualifier Character 6	Qualifier Character 7
Z None	Z None	Z None	Z None

G Mental Health
Z None
5 Individual Psychotherapy Definition: Treatment of an individual with a mental health disorder by behavioral, cognitive, psychoanalytic, psychodynamic or psychophysiological means to improve functioning or well-being

Qualifier Character 4	Qualifier Character 5	Qualifier Character 6	Qualifier Character 7
Ø Interactive 1 Behavioral 2 Cognitive 3 Interpersonal 4 Psychoanalysis 5 Psychodynamic 6 Supportive 8 Cognitive-Behavioral 9 Psychophysiological	Z None	Z None	Z None

G Mental Health
Z None
6 Counseling Definition: The application of psychological methods to treat an individual with normal developmental issues and psychological problems in order to increase function, improve well-being, alleviate distress, maladjustment or resolve crises

Qualifier Character 4	Qualifier Character 5	Qualifier Character 6	Qualifier Character 7
Ø Educational 1 Vocational 3 Other Counseling	Z None	Z None	Z None

G Mental Health
Z None
7 Family Psychotherapy Definition: Treatment that includes one or more family members of an individual with a mental health disorder by behavioral, cognitive, psychoanalytic, psychodynamic or psychophysiological means to improve functioning or well-being

Explanation: Remediation of emotional or behavioral problems presented by one or more family members in cases where psychotherapy with more than one family member is indicated

Qualifier Character 4	Qualifier Character 5	Qualifier Character 6	Qualifier Character 7
2 Other Family Psychotherapy	Z None	Z None	Z None

G Mental Health
Z None
B Electroconvulsive Therapy Definition: The application of controlled electrical voltages to treat a mental health disorder

Qualifier Character 4	Qualifier Character 5	Qualifier Character 6	Qualifier Character 7
Ø Unilateral-Single Seizure 1 Unilateral-Multiple Seizure 2 Bilateral-Single Seizure 3 Bilateral-Multiple Seizure 4 Other Electroconvulsive Therapy	Z None	Z None	Z None

G Mental Health
Z None
C Biofeedback Definition: Provision of information from the monitoring and regulating of physiological processes in conjunction with cognitive-behavioral techniques to improve patient functioning or well-being

Qualifier Character 4	Qualifier Character 5	Qualifier Character 6	Qualifier Character 7
9 Other Biofeedback	Z None	Z None	Z None

G Mental Health
Z None
F Hypnosis Definition: Induction of a state of heightened suggestibility by auditory, visual and tactile techniques to elicit an emotional or behavioral response

Qualifier Character 4	Qualifier Character 5	Qualifier Character 6	Qualifier Character 7
Z None	Z None	Z None	Z None

G Mental Health
Z None
G Narcosynthesis Definition: Administration of intravenous barbiturates in order to release suppressed or repressed thoughts

Qualifier Character 4	Qualifier Character 5	Qualifier Character 6	Qualifier Character 7
Z None	Z None	Z None	Z None

G Mental Health
Z None
H Group Psychotherapy Definition: Treatment of two or more individuals with a mental health disorder by behavioral, cognitive, psychoanalytic, psychodynamic or psychophysiological means to improve functioning or well-being

Qualifier Character 4	Qualifier Character 5	Qualifier Character 6	Qualifier Character 7
Z None	Z None	Z None	Z None

G Mental Health
Z None
J Light Therapy Definition: Application of specialized light treatments to improve functioning or well-being

Qualifier Character 4	Qualifier Character 5	Qualifier Character 6	Qualifier Character 7
Z None	Z None	Z None	Z None

Substance Abuse Treatment HZ2–HZ9

AHA Coding Clinic for table HZ2
2020, 1Q, 21 Inpatient detoxification services

AHA Coding Clinic for table HZ9
2020, 1Q, 21 Inpatient detoxification services

H Substance Abuse Treatment
Z None
2 Detoxification Services Definition: Detoxification from alcohol and/or drugs
Explanation: Not a treatment modality, but helps the patient stabilize physically and psychologically until the body becomes free of drugs and the effects of alcohol

Qualifier Character 4	Qualifier Character 5	Qualifier Character 6	Qualifier Character 7
Z None	Z None	Z None	Z None

H Substance Abuse Treatment
Z None
3 Individual Counseling Definition: The application of psychological methods to treat an individual with addictive behavior
Explanation: Comprised of several different techniques, which apply various strategies to address drug addiction

Qualifier Character 4	Qualifier Character 5	Qualifier Character 6	Qualifier Character 7
Ø Cognitive 1 Behavioral 2 Cognitive-Behavioral 3 12-Step 4 Interpersonal 5 Vocational 6 Psychoeducation 7 Motivational Enhancement 8 Confrontational 9 Continuing Care B Spiritual C Pre/Post-Test Infectious Disease	Z None	Z None	Z None

DRG Non-OR HZ3[Ø,1,2,3,4,5,6,7,8,9,B]ZZZ

H Substance Abuse Treatment
Z None
4 Group Counseling Definition: The application of psychological methods to treat two or more individuals with addictive behavior
Explanation: Provides structured group counseling sessions and healing power through the connection with others

Qualifier Character 4	Qualifier Character 5	Qualifier Character 6	Qualifier Character 7
Ø Cognitive 1 Behavioral 2 Cognitive-Behavioral 3 12-Step 4 Interpersonal 5 Vocational 6 Psychoeducation 7 Motivational Enhancement 8 Confrontational 9 Continuing Care B Spiritual C Pre/Post-Test Infectious Disease	Z None	Z None	Z None

DRG Non-OR HZ4[Ø,1,2,3,4,5,6,7,8,9,B]ZZZ

H Substance Abuse Treatment
Z None
5 Individual Psychotherapy Definition: Treatment of an individual with addictive behavior by behavioral, cognitive, psychoanalytic, psychodynamic or psychophysiological means

Qualifier Character 4	Qualifier Character 5	Qualifier Character 6	Qualifier Character 7
Ø Cognitive 1 Behavioral 2 Cognitive-Behavioral 3 12-Step 4 Interpersonal 5 Interactive 6 Psychoeducation 7 Motivational Enhancement 8 Confrontational 9 Supportive B Psychoanalysis C Psychodynamic D Psychophysiological	Z None	Z None	Z None

DRG Non-OR For all qualifier values

H Substance Abuse Treatment
Z None
6 Family Counseling Definition: The application of psychological methods that includes one or more family members to treat an individual with addictive behavior

Explanation: Provides support and education for family members of addicted individuals. Family member participation is seen as a critical area of substance abuse treatment

Qualifier Character 4	Qualifier Character 5	Qualifier Character 6	Qualifier Character 7
3 Other Family Counseling	Z None	Z None	Z None

H Substance Abuse Treatment
Z None
8 Medication Management Definition: Monitoring or adjusting the use of replacement medications for the treatment of addiction

Qualifier Character 4	Qualifier Character 5	Qualifier Character 6	Qualifier Character 7
Ø Nicotine Replacement 1 Methadone Maintenance 2 Levo-alpha-acetyl-methadol (LAAM) 3 Antabuse 4 Naltrexone 5 Naloxone 6 Clonidine 7 Bupropion 8 Psychiatric Medication 9 Other Replacement Medication	Z None	Z None	Z None

H Substance Abuse Treatment
Z None
9 Pharmacotherapy Definition: The use of replacement medications for the treatment of addiction

Qualifier Character 4	Qualifier Character 5	Qualifier Character 6	Qualifier Character 7
Ø Nicotine Replacement 1 Methadone Maintenance 2 Levo-alpha-acetyl-methadol (LAAM) 3 Antabuse 4 Naltrexone 5 Naloxone 6 Clonidine 7 Bupropion 8 Psychiatric Medication 9 Other Replacement Medication	Z None	Z None	Z None

New Technology X27–XYØ

AHA Coding Clinic for all tables in the New Technology Section
2015, 4Q, 8-11 New Section X codes - New Technology procedures

AHA Coding Clinic for table X27
2019, 4Q, 45-46 Sustained released drug-eluting stent

AHA Coding Clinic for table X2A
2021, 1Q, 16 Placement of Sentinel™ embolic protection device with deployment of single filter
2020, 4Q, 70-71 Cerebral embolic filtration extracorporeal flow reversal circuit
2019, 4Q, 46 Cerebral embolic filtration
2016, 4Q, 115-116 Cerebral embolic filtration

AHA Coding Clinic for table X2C
2016, 4Q, 82-83 Coronary artery, number of arteries
2015, 4Q, 8-14 New Section X codes—New Technology procedures

AHA Coding Clinic for table X2R
2016, 4Q, 116 Aortic valve rapid deployment
2015, 4Q, 8-12 New Section X codes—New Technology procedures

AHA Coding Clinic for table XHR
2016, 4Q, 116 Application of wound matrix

AHA Coding Clinic for table XKØ
2017, 4Q, 74 Intramuscular autologous bone marrow cell therapy

AHA Coding Clinic for table XNS
2017, 4Q, 74-75 Magnetic growth rods
2016, 4Q, 117 Placement of magnetic growth rods

AHA Coding Clinic for table XNU
2020, 4Q, 72 Implantation of vertebral mechanically expandable device

AHA Coding Clinic for table XRG
2017, 4Q, 76 Radiolucent porous interbody fusion device

AHA Coding Clinic for table XT2
2019, 4Q, 46-47 Renal function monitoring

AHA Coding Clinic for table XV5
2018, 4Q, 55 Robotic waterjet ablation

AHA Coding Clinic for table XWØ
2021, 1Q, 49 Frequently asked questions regarding ICD-1Ø-CM and ICD-1Ø-PCS coding for COVID-19
2020, 4Q, 72-76 Introduction of new therapeutic substances
2020, 4Q, 95 Frequently Asked Questions Regarding ICD-1Ø-PCS Coding for COVID-19
2020, 3Q, 17-21 New procedure codes for introduction or infusion of therapeutics
2019, 4Q, 47-50 New therapeutic substances
2018, 4Q, 56 New therapeutic substances
2015, 4Q, 8-15 New Section X codes—New Technology procedures

AHA Coding Clinic for table XW1
2020, 3Q, 17-21 New procedure codes for introduction or infusion of therapeutics

AHA Coding Clinic for table XW2
2020, 4Q, 77-78 Transfusion of chimeric antigen receptor (CAR) T cell immunotherapy

AHA Coding Clinic for table XXE
2020, 4Q, 78-79 Measurement of infection
2020, 4Q, 78-79 Positive blood culture fluorescence hybridization
2020, 4Q, 79 Nucleic acid-base microbial detection
2019, 4Q, 50-51 Whole blood nucleic acid-base microbial detection

AHA Coding Clinic for table XYØ
2017, 4Q, 78 Intraoperative treatment of vascular grafts

X New Technology
2 Cardiovascular System
7 Dilation Definition: Expanding an orifice or the lumen of a tubular body part
Explanation: The orifice can be a natural orifice or an artificially created orifice. Accomplished by stretching a tubular body part using intraluminal pressure or by cutting part of the orifice or wall of the tubular body part.

Body Part Character 4	Approach Character 5	Device/Substance/Technology Character 6	Qualifier Character 7
H Femoral Artery, Right J Femoral Artery, Left K Popliteal Artery, Proximal Right L Popliteal Artery, Proximal Left M Popliteal Artery, Distal Right N Popliteal Artery, Distal Left P Anterior Tibial Artery, Right Q Anterior Tibial Artery, Left R Posterior Tibial Artery, Right S Posterior Tibial Artery, Left T Peroneal Artery, Right U Peroneal Artery, Left	3 Percutaneous	8 Intraluminal Device, Sustained Release Drug-eluting NT 9 Intraluminal Device, Sustained Release Drug-eluting, Two NT B Intraluminal Device, Sustained Release Drug-eluting, Three NT C Intraluminal Device, Sustained Release Drug-eluting, Four or More NT	5 New Technology Group 5

Valid OR All body part, approach, device/substance/technology, and qualifier values
NT X27[H,J,K,L]3[8,9,B,C]5 *See* Appendix H for applicable device trade name

X New Technology
2 Cardiovascular System
A Assistance Definition: Taking over a portion of a physiological function by extracorporeal means
Explanation: None

Body Part Character 4	Approach Character 5	Device/Substance/Technology Character 6	Qualifier Character 7
5 Innominate Artery and Left Common Carotid Artery	3 Percutaneous	1 Cerebral Embolic Filtration, Dual Filter	2 New Technology Group 2
6 Aortic Arch	3 Percutaneous	2 Cerebral Embolic Filtration, Single Deflection Filter	5 New Technology Group 5
H Common Carotid Artery, Right J Common Carotid Artery, Left	3 Percutaneous	3 Cerebral Embolic Filtration, Extracorporeal Flow Reversal Circuit	6 New Technology Group 6

X New Technology
2 Cardiovascular System
C Extirpation Definition: Taking or cutting out solid matter from a body part

Explanation: The solid matter may be an abnormal byproduct of a biological function or a foreign body; it may be imbedded in a body part or in the lumen of a tubular body part. The solid matter may or may not have been previously broken into pieces.

Body Part Character 4	Approach Character 5	Device/Substance/Technology Character 6	Qualifier Character 7
P Abdominal Aorta Q Upper Extremity Vein, Right R Upper Extremity Vein, Left S Lower Extremity Artery, Right T Lower Extremity Artery, Left U Lower Extremity Vein, Right V Lower Extremity Vein, Left Y Great Vessel	3 Percutaneous	T Computer-aided Mechanical Aspiration	7 New Technology Group 7

X New Technology
2 Cardiovascular System
J Inspection Definition: Visually and/or manually exploring a body part

Explanation: None

Body Part Character 4	Approach Character 5	Device/Substance/Technology Character 6	Qualifier Character 7
A Heart	X External	4 Transthoracic Echocardiography, Computer-aided Guidance	7 New Technology Group 7

X New Technology
2 Cardiovascular System
K Bypass Definition: Altering the route of passage of the contents of a tubular body part

Explanation: None

Body Part Character 4	Approach Character 5	Device/Substance/Technology Character 6	Qualifier Character 7
B Radial Artery, Right C Radial Artery, Left	3 Percutaneous	1 Thermal Resistance Energy	7 New Technology Group 7

X New Technology
2 Cardiovascular System
R Replacement Definition: Putting in or on biological or synthetic material that physically takes the place and/or function of all or a portion of a body part

Explanation: The body part may have been taken out or replaced, or may be taken out, physically eradicated, or rendered nonfunctional during the REPLACEMENT procedure. A REMOVAL procedure is coded for taking out the device used in a previous replacement procedure

Body Part Character 4	Approach Character 5	Device/Substance/Technology Character 6	Qualifier Character 7
F Aortic Valve	Ø Open 3 Percutaneous 4 Percutaneous Endoscopic	3 Zooplastic Tissue, Rapid Deployment Technique	2 New Technology Group 2
X Thoracic Aorta, Arch	Ø Open	N Branched Synthetic Substitute with Intraluminal Device	7 New Technology Group 7

Valid OR X2RF[Ø,3,4]32

X New Technology
2 Cardiovascular System
V Restriction Definition: Partially closing an orifice or the lumen of a tubular body part

Explanation: None

Body Part Character 4	Approach Character 5	Device/Substance/Technology Character 6	Qualifier Character 7
7 Coronary Sinus	3 Percutaneous	Q Reduction Device	7 New Technology Group 7
W Thoracic Aorta, Descending	Ø Open	N Branched Synthetic Substitute with Intraluminal Device	7 New Technology Group 7

Valid OR X2V73Q7

X New Technology
D Gastrointestinal System
2 Monitoring Definition: Determining the level of a physiological or physical function repetitively over a period of time

Explanation: None

Body Part Character 4	Approach Character 5	Device/Substance/Technology Character 6	Qualifier Character 7
G Upper GI H Lower GI	4 Percutaneous Endoscopic 8 Via Natural or Artificial Opening Endoscopic	V Oxygen Saturation	7 New Technology Group 7

X New Technology
D Gastrointestinal System
P Irrigation Definition: Putting in or on a cleansing substance
Explanation: None

Body Part Character 4	Approach Character 5	Device/Substance/Technology Character 6	Qualifier Character 7
H Lower GI	8 Via Natural or Artificial Opening Endoscopic	K Intraoperative Single-use Oversleeve	7 New Technology Group 7

X New Technology
F Hepatobiliary System and Pancreas
J Inspection Definition: Visually and/or manually exploring a body part
Explanation: None

Body Part Character 4	Approach Character 5	Device/Substance/Technology Character 6	Qualifier Character 7
B Hepatobiliary Duct D Pancreatic Duct	8 Via Natural or Artificial Opening Endoscopic	A Single-use Duodenoscope	7 New Technology Group 7

X New Technology
H Skin, Subcutaneous Tissue, Fascia and Breast
R Replacement Definition: Putting in or on biological or synthetic material that physically takes the place and/or function of all or a portion of a body part
Explanation: The body part may have been taken out or replaced, or may be taken out, physically eradicated, or rendered nonfunctional during the REPLACEMENT procedure. A REMOVAL procedure is coded for taking out the device used in a previous replacement procedure

Body Part Character 4	Approach Character 5	Device/Substance/Technology Character 6	Qualifier Character 7
P Skin	X External	F Bioengineered Allogeneic Construct	7 New Technology Group 7
P Skin	X External	L Skin Substitute, Porcine Liver Derived	2 New Technology Group 2

Valid OR XHRPXL2

X New Technology
K Muscles, Tendons, Bursae and Ligaments
Ø Introduction Definition: Putting in or on a therapeutic, diagnostic, nutritional, physiological, or prophylactic substance except blood or blood products
Explanation: None

Body Part Character 4	Approach Character 5	Device/Substance/Technology Character 6	Qualifier Character 7
2 Muscle	3 Percutaneous	Ø Concentrated Bone Marrow Aspirate	3 New Technology Group 3

X New Technology
N Bones
S Reposition Definition: Moving to its normal location, or other suitable location, all or a portion of a body part

Explanation: The body part is moved to a new location from an abnormal location, or from a normal location where it is not functioning correctly. The body part may or may not be cut out or off to be moved to the new location.

Body Part Character 4	Approach Character 5	Device/Substance/Technology Character 6	Qualifier Character 7
Ø Lumbar Vertebra	Ø Open	3 Magnetically Controlled Growth Rod(s)	2 New Technology Group 2
Ø Lumbar Vertebra	Ø Open	C Posterior (Dynamic) Distraction Device	7 New Technology Group 7
Ø Lumbar Vertebra	3 Percutaneous	3 Magnetically Controlled Growth Rod(s)	2 New Technology Group 2
Ø Lumbar Vertebra	3 Percutaneous	C Posterior (Dynamic) Distraction Device	7 New Technology Group 7
3 Cervical Vertebra	Ø Open 3 Percutaneous	3 Magnetically Controlled Growth Rod(s)	2 New Technology Group 2
4 Thoracic Vertebra	Ø Open	3 Magnetically Controlled Growth Rod(s)	2 New Technology Group 2
4 Thoracic Vertebra	Ø Open	C Posterior (Dynamic) Distraction Device	7 New Technology Group 7
4 Thoracic Vertebra	3 Percutaneous	3 Magnetically Controlled Growth Rod(s)	2 New Technology Group 2
4 Thoracic Vertebra	3 Percutaneous	C Posterior (Dynamic) Distraction Device	7 New Technology Group 7

Valid OR XNSØØ32
Valid OR XNSØ332
Valid OR XNS3[Ø,3]32
Valid OR XNS4Ø32
Valid OR XNS4332

X New Technology
N Bones
U Supplement Definition: Putting in or on biological or synthetic material that physically reinforces and/or augments the function of a portion of a body part

Explanation: None

Body Part Character 4	Approach Character 5	Device/Substance/Technology Character 6	Qualifier Character 7
Ø Lumbar Vertebra 4 Thoracic Vertebra	3 Percutaneous	5 Synthetic Substitute, Mechanically Expandable (Paired) NT	6 New Technology Group 6

Valid OR XNU[Ø,4]356
NT XNU[Ø,4]356 *See* Appendix H for applicable device trade name

X New Technology
R Joints
G Fusion Definition: Joining together portions of an articular body part rendering the articular body part immobile
Explanation: The body part is joined together by fixation device, bone graft, or other means

Body Part Character 4	Approach Character 5	Device/Substance/Technology Character 6	Qualifier Character 7
Ø Occipital-cervical Joint	Ø Open	9 Interbody Fusion Device, Nanotextured Surface	2 New Technology Group 2
Ø Occipital-cervical Joint	Ø Open	F Interbody Fusion Device, Radiolucent Porous	3 New Technology Group 3
1 Cervical Vertebral Joint	Ø Open	9 Interbody Fusion Device, Nanotextured Surface	2 New Technology Group 2
1 Cervical Vertebral Joint	Ø Open	F Interbody Fusion Device, Radiolucent Porous	3 New Technology Group 3
2 Cervical Vertebral Joints, 2 or more	Ø Open	9 Interbody Fusion Device, Nanotextured Surface	2 New Technology Group 2
2 Cervical Vertebral Joints, 2 or more	Ø Open	F Interbody Fusion Device, Radiolucent Porous	3 New Technology Group 3
4 Cervicothoracic Vertebral Joint	Ø Open	9 Interbody Fusion Device, Nanotextured Surface	2 New Technology Group 2
4 Cervicothoracic Vertebral Joint	Ø Open	F Interbody Fusion Device, Radiolucent Porous	3 New Technology Group 3
6 Thoracic Vertebral Joint	Ø Open	9 Interbody Fusion Device, Nanotextured Surface	2 New Technology Group 2
6 Thoracic Vertebral Joint	Ø Open	F Interbody Fusion Device, Radiolucent Porous	3 New Technology Group 3
7 Thoracic Vertebral Joints, 2 to 7 ⊞	Ø Open	9 Interbody Fusion Device, Nanotextured Surface	2 New Technology Group 2
7 Thoracic Vertebral Joints, 2 to 7 ⊞	Ø Open	F Interbody Fusion Device, Radiolucent Porous	3 New Technology Group 3
8 Thoracic Vertebral Joints, 8 or more	Ø Open	9 Interbody Fusion Device, Nanotextured Surface	2 New Technology Group 2
8 Thoracic Vertebral Joints, 8 or more	Ø Open	F Interbody Fusion Device, Radiolucent Porous	3 New Technology Group 3
A Thoracolumbar Vertebral Joint	Ø Open	9 Interbody Fusion Device, Nanotextured Surface	2 New Technology Group 2
A Thoracolumbar Vertebral Joint	Ø Open	F Interbody Fusion Device, Radiolucent Porous	3 New Technology Group 3
A Thoracolumbar Vertebral Joint	Ø Open 3 Percutaneous 4 Percutaneous Endoscopic	R Interbody Fusion Device, Customizable	7 New Technology Group 7
B Lumbar Vertebral Joint	Ø Open	9 Interbody Fusion Device, Nanotextured Surface	2 New Technology Group 2
B Lumbar Vertebral Joint	Ø Open	F Interbody Fusion Device, Radiolucent Porous	3 New Technology Group 3
B Lumbar Vertebral Joint	Ø Open 3 Percutaneous 4 Percutaneous Endoscopic	R Interbody Fusion Device, Customizable	7 New Technology Group 7
C Lumbar Vertebral Joints, 2 or more ⊞	Ø Open	9 Interbody Fusion Device, Nanotextured Surface	2 New Technology Group 2
C Lumbar Vertebral Joints, 2 or more ⊞	Ø Open	F Interbody Fusion Device, Radiolucent Porous	3 New Technology Group 3
C Lumbar Vertebral Joints, 2 or more	Ø Open 3 Percutaneous 4 Percutaneous Endoscopic	R Interbody Fusion Device, Customizable	7 New Technology Group 7
D Lumbosacral Joint	Ø Open	9 Interbody Fusion Device, Nanotextured Surface	2 New Technology Group 2
D Lumbosacral Joint	Ø Open	F Interbody Fusion Device, Radiolucent Porous	3 New Technology Group 3
D Lumbosacral Joint	Ø Open 3 Percutaneous 4 Percutaneous Endoscopic	R Interbody Fusion Device, Customizable	7 New Technology Group 7

Valid OR All body part, approach, device/substance/technology, and qualifier values
HAC XRG[Ø,1,2,4,6,7,8,A,B,C,D]Ø92 when reported with SDx K68.11 or T81.4Ø–T81.49, T84.6Ø-T84.619, T84.63-T84.7 with 7th character A
HAC XRG[Ø,1,2,4,6,7,8,A,B,C,D]ØF3 when reported with SDx K68.11 or T81.4Ø–T81.49, T84.6Ø-T84.619, T84.63-T84.7 with 7th character A

See Appendix L for Procedure Combinations
⊞ XRG7Ø92
⊞ XRG7ØF3
⊞ XRGCØ92
⊞ XRGCØF3

X New Technology
T Urinary System
2 Monitoring Definition: Determining the level of a physiological or physical function repetitively over a period of time
Explanation: None

Body Part Character 4	Approach Character 5	Device/Substance/Technology Character 6	Qualifier Character 7
5 Kidney	X External	E Fluorescent Pyrazine	5 New Technology Group 5

X New Technology
V Male Reproductive System
5 Destruction Definition: Physical eradication of all or a portion of a body part by the direct use of energy, force, or a destructive agent
Explanation: None of the body part is physically taken out

Body Part Character 4	Approach Character 5	Device/Substance/Technology Character 6	Qualifier Character 7
Ø Prostate	8 Via Natural or Artificial Opening Endoscopic	A Robotic Waterjet Ablation	4 New Technology Group 4

Valid OR All body part, approach, device/substance/technology, and qualifier values

X New Technology
W Anatomical Regions
Ø Introduction Definition: Putting in or on a therapeutic, diagnostic, nutritional, physiological, or prophylactic substance except blood or blood products
Explanation: None

Body Part Character 4	Approach Character 5	Device/Substance/Technology Character 6	Qualifier Character 7
Ø Skin	X External	2 Bromelain-enriched Proteolytic Enzyme	7 New Technology Group 7
1 Subcutaneous Tissue	3 Percutaneous	9 Satralizumab-mwge	7 New Technology Group 7
1 Subcutaneous Tissue	3 Percutaneous	F Other New Technology Therapeutic Substance	5 New Technology Group 5
1 Subcutaneous Tissue	3 Percutaneous	H Other New Technology Monoclonal Antibody K Leronlimab Monoclonal Antibody S COVID-19 Vaccine Dose 1 T COVID-19 Vaccine Dose 2 U COVID-19 Vaccine	6 New Technology Group 6
1 Subcutaneous Tissue	3 Percutaneous	W Caplacizumab NT	5 New Technology Group 5
1 Subcutaneous Tissue	X External	2 Bromelain-enriched Proteolytic Enzyme	7 New Technology Group 7
2 Muscle	3 Percutaneous	S COVID-19 Vaccine Dose 1 T COVID-19 Vaccine Dose 2 U COVID-19 Vaccine	6 New Technology Group 6
3 Peripheral Vein	3 Percutaneous	Ø Brexanolone 2 Nerinitide 3 Durvalumab Antineoplastic NT	6 New Technology Group 6
3 Peripheral Vein	3 Percutaneous	5 Narsoplimab Monoclonal Antibody	7 New Technology Group 7
3 Peripheral Vein	3 Percutaneous	6 Lefamulin Anti-infective NT	6 New Technology Group 6
3 Peripheral Vein	3 Percutaneous	6 Terlipressin	7 New Technology Group 7
3 Peripheral Vein	3 Percutaneous	7 Coagulation Factor Xa, Inactivated NT	2 New Technology Group 2
3 Peripheral Vein	3 Percutaneous	7 Trilaciclib 8 Lurbinectedin	7 New Technology Group 7
3 Peripheral Vein	3 Percutaneous	9 Defibrotide Sodium Anticoagulant	2 New Technology Group 2
3 Peripheral Vein	3 Percutaneous	9 Ceftolozane/Tazobactam Anti-infective NT	6 New Technology Group 6
3 Peripheral Vein	3 Percutaneous	A Bezlotoxumab Monoclonal Antibody	3 New Technology Group 3
3 Peripheral Vein	3 Percutaneous	A Cefiderocol Anti-infective NT	6 New Technology Group 6
3 Peripheral Vein	3 Percutaneous	A Ciltacabtagene Autoleucel	7 New Technology Group 7
3 Peripheral Vein	3 Percutaneous	B Cytarabine and Daunorubicin Liposome Antineoplastic	3 New Technology Group 3
3 Peripheral Vein	3 Percutaneous	B Omadacycline Anti-infective NT	6 New Technology Group 6
3 Peripheral Vein	3 Percutaneous	B Amivantamab Monoclonal Antibody	7 New Technology Group 7
3 Peripheral Vein	3 Percutaneous	C Eculizumab NT	6 New Technology Group 6
3 Peripheral Vein	3 Percutaneous	C Engineered Chimeric Antigen Receptor T-cell Immunotherapy, Autologous	7 New Technology Group 7
3 Peripheral Vein	3 Percutaneous	D Atezolizumab Antineoplastic NT	6 New Technology Group 6
3 Peripheral Vein	3 Percutaneous	E Remdesivir Anti-infective NT	5 New Technology Group 5
3 Peripheral Vein	3 Percutaneous	E Etesevimab Monoclonal Antibody	6 New Technology Group 6
3 Peripheral Vein	3 Percutaneous	F Other New Technology Therapeutic Substance	3 New Technology Group 3
3 Peripheral Vein	3 Percutaneous	F Other New Technology Therapeutic Substance	5 New Technology Group 5
3 Peripheral Vein	3 Percutaneous	F Bamlanivimab Monoclonal Antibody	6 New Technology Group 6
3 Peripheral Vein	3 Percutaneous	G Plazomicin Anti-infective NT	4 New Technology Group 4
3 Peripheral Vein	3 Percutaneous	G Sarilumab	5 New Technology Group 5

DRG Non-OR XWØ33C7 NT XWØ3366 NT XWØ33A6 NT XWØ33D6
NT XWØ13W5 NT XWØ3372 NT XWØ33B6 NT XWØ33E5
NT XWØ3336 NT XWØ3396 NT XWØ33C6 NT XWØ33G4

* For all codes with NT icon *see* Appendix I for registered or trade name of substance

XWØ Continued on next page

XWØ Continued

X New Technology
W Anatomical Regions
Ø Introduction Definition: Putting in or on a therapeutic, diagnostic, nutritional, physiological, or prophylactic substance except blood or blood products

Explanation: None

Body Part Character 4	Approach Character 5	Device/Substance/Technology Character 6	Qualifier Character 7
3 Peripheral Vein	3 Percutaneous	G REGN-COV2 Monoclonal Antibody	6 New Technology Group 6
3 Peripheral Vein	3 Percutaneous	G Engineered Chimeric Antigen Receptor T-cell Immunotherapy, Allogeneic	7 New Technology Group 7
3 Peripheral Vein	3 Percutaneous	H Synthetic Human Angiotensin II	4 New Technology Group 4
3 Peripheral Vein	3 Percutaneous	H Tocilizumab	5 New Technology Group 5
3 Peripheral Vein	3 Percutaneous	H Other New Technology Monoclonal Antibody	6 New Technology Group 6
3 Peripheral Vein	3 Percutaneous	H Axicabtagene Ciloleucel Immunotherapy J Tisagenlecleucel Immunotherapy	7 New Technology Group 7
3 Peripheral Vein	3 Percutaneous	K Fosfomycin Anti-infective	5 New Technology Group 5
3 Peripheral Vein	3 Percutaneous	K Idecabtagene Vicleucel Immunotherapy	7 New Technology Group 7
3 Peripheral Vein	3 Percutaneous	L CD24Fc Immunomodulator	6 New Technology Group 6
3 Peripheral Vein	3 Percutaneous	L Lifileucel Immunotherapy M Brexucabtagene Autoleucel Immunotherapy	7 New Technology Group 7
3 Peripheral Vein	3 Percutaneous	N Meropenem-vaborbactam Anti-infective	5 New Technology Group 5
3 Peripheral Vein	3 Percutaneous	N Lisocabtagene Maraleucel Immunotherapy	7 New Technology Group 7
3 Peripheral Vein	3 Percutaneous	Q Tagraxofusp-erzs Antineoplastic NT S Iobenguane I-131 Antineoplastic NT U Imipenem-cilastatin-relebactam Anti-infective NT W Caplacizumab NT	5 New Technology Group 5
4 Central Vein	3 Percutaneous	Ø Brexanolone 2 Nerinitide 3 Durvalumab Antineoplastic NT	6 New Technology Group 6
4 Central Vein	3 Percutaneous	5 Narsoplimab Monoclonal Antibody	7 New Technology Group 7
4 Central Vein	3 Percutaneous	6 Lefamulin Anti-infective NT	6 New Technology Group 6
4 Central Vein	3 Percutaneous	6 Terlipressin	7 New Technology Group 7
4 Central Vein	3 Percutaneous	7 Coagulation Factor Xa, Inactivated NT	2 New Technology Group 2
4 Central Vein	3 Percutaneous	7 Trilaciclib 8 Lurbinectedin	7 New Technology Group 7
4 Central Vein	3 Percutaneous	9 Defibrotide Sodium Anticoagulant	2 New Technology Group 2
4 Central Vein	3 Percutaneous	9 Ceftolozane/Tazobactam Anti-infective NT	6 New Technology Group 6
4 Central Vein	3 Percutaneous	A Bezlotoxumab Monoclonal Antibody	3 New Technology Group 3
4 Central Vein	3 Percutaneous	A Cefiderocol Anti-infective NT	6 New Technology Group 6
4 Central Vein	3 Percutaneous	A Ciltacabtagene Autoleucel	7 New Technology Group 7
4 Central Vein	3 Percutaneous	B Cytarabine and Daunorubicin Liposome Antineoplastic	3 New Technology Group 3
4 Central Vein	3 Percutaneous	B Omadacycline Anti-infective NT	6 New Technology Group 6
4 Central Vein	3 Percutaneous	B Amivantamab Monoclonal Antibody	7 New Technology Group 7
4 Central Vein	3 Percutaneous	C Eculizumab NT	6 New Technology Group 6
4 Central Vein	3 Percutaneous	C Engineered Chimeric Antigen Receptor T-cell Immunotherapy, Autologous	7 New Technology Group 7
4 Central Vein	3 Percutaneous	D Atezolizumab Antineoplastic NT	6 New Technology Group 6
4 Central Vein	3 Percutaneous	E Remdesivir Anti-infective NT	5 New Technology Group 5
4 Central Vein	3 Percutaneous	E Etesevimab Monoclonal Antibody	6 New Technology Group 6
4 Central Vein	3 Percutaneous	F Other New Technology Therapeutic Substance	3 New Technology Group 3
4 Central Vein	3 Percutaneous	F Other New Technology Therapeutic Substance	5 New Technology Group 5
4 Central Vein	3 Percutaneous	F Bamlanivimab Monoclonal Antibody	6 New Technology Group 6
4 Central Vein	3 Percutaneous	G Plazomicin Anti-infective NT	4 New Technology Group 4

DRG Non-OR XWØ33G7
DRG Non-OR XWØ33[H,J]7
DRG Non-OR XWØ33K7
DRG Non-OR XWØ33[L,M]7
DRG Non-OR XWØ33N7
DRG Non-OR XWØ43C7

NT XWØ33[Q,S,U,W]5
NT XWØ4336
NT XWØ4366
NT XWØ4372
NT XWØ4396
NT XWØ43A6
NT XWØ43B6
NT XWØ43C6
NT XWØ43D6
NT XWØ43E5
NT XWØ43G4

* For all codes with NT icon *see* Appendix I for registered or trade name of substance

XWØ Continued on next page

X New Technology
W Anatomical Regions
Ø Introduction Definition: Putting in or on a therapeutic, diagnostic, nutritional, physiological, or prophylactic substance except blood or blood products
Explanation: None

XWØ Continued

Body Part Character 4	Approach Character 5	Device/Substance/Technology Character 6	Qualifier Character 7
4 Central Vein	3 Percutaneous	G Sarilumab	5 New Technology Group 5
4 Central Vein	3 Percutaneous	G REGN-COV2 Monoclonal Antibody	6 New Technology Group 6
4 Central Vein	3 Percutaneous	G Engineered Chimeric Antigen Receptor T-cell Immunotherapy, Allogeneic	7 New Technology Group 7
4 Central Vein	3 Percutaneous	H Synthetic Human Angiotensin II	4 New Technology Group 4
4 Central Vein	3 Percutaneous	H Tocilizumab	5 New Technology Group 5
4 Central Vein	3 Percutaneous	H Other New Technology Monoclonal Antibody	6 New Technology Group 6
4 Central Vein	3 Percutaneous	H Axicabtagene Ciloleucel Immunotherapy J Tisagenlecleucel Immunotherapy	7 New Technology Group 7
4 Central Vein	3 Percutaneous	K Fosfomycin Anti-infective	5 New Technology Group 5
4 Central Vein	3 Percutaneous	K Idecabtagene Vicleucel Immunotherapy	7 New Technology Group 7
4 Central Vein	3 Percutaneous	L CD24Fc Immunomodulator	6 New Technology Group 6
4 Central Vein	3 Percutaneous	L Lifileucel Immunotherapy M Brexucabtagene Autoleucel Immunotherapy	7 New Technology Group 7
4 Central Vein	3 Percutaneous	N Meropenem-vaborbactam Anti-infective	5 New Technology Group 5
4 Central Vein	3 Percutaneous	N Lisocabtagene Maraleucel Immunotherapy	7 New Technology Group 7
4 Central Vein	3 Percutaneous	Q Tagraxofusp-erzs Antineoplastic NT S Iobenguane I-131 Antineoplastic NT U Imipenem-cilastatin-relebactam Anti-infective NT W Caplacizumab NT	5 New Technology Group 5
9 Nose	7 Via Natural or Artificial Opening	M Esketamine Hydrochloride NT	5 New Technology Group 5
D Mouth and Pharynx	X External	6 Lefamulin Anti-infective NT	6 New Technology Group 6
D Mouth and Pharynx	X External	8 Uridine Triacetate	2 New Technology Group 2
D Mouth and Pharynx	X External	F Other New Technology Therapeutic Substance J Apalutamide Antineoplastic L Erdafitinib Antineoplastic NT	5 New Technology Group 5
D Mouth and Pharynx	X External	M Baricitinib NT	6 New Technology Group 6
D Mouth and Pharynx	X External	R Venetoclax Antineoplastic T Ruxolitinib NT V Gilteritinib Antineoplastic NT	5 New Technology Group 5
G Upper GI H Lower GI	7 Via Natural or Artificial Opening	M Baricitinib NT	6 New Technology Group 6
G Upper GI H Lower GI	8 Via Natural or Artificial Opening Endoscopic	8 Mineral-based Topical Hemostatic Agent NT	6 New Technology Group 6
Q Cranial Cavity and Brain	3 Percutaneous	1 Eladocagene exuparvovec	6 New Technology Group 6
V Bones	Ø Open	P Antibiotic-eluting Bone Void Filler	7 New Technology Group 7

DRG Non-OR XWØ43G7
DRG Non-OR XWØ43[H,J]7
DRG Non-OR XWØ43K7
DRG Non-OR XWØ43[L,M]7
DRG Non-OR XWØ43N7

NT XWØ43[Q,S,U,W]5
NT XWØ97M5
NT XWØDX66
NT XWØDXL5
NT XWØDXM6
NT XWØDX[T,V]5
NT XWØ[G,H]7M6
NT XWØ[G,H]886

* For all codes with NT icon *see* Appendix I for registered or trade name of substance

X New Technology
W Anatomical Regions
1 Transfusion Definition: Putting in blood or blood products
Explanation: None

Body Part Character 4	Approach Character 5	Device/Substance/Technology Character 6	Qualifier Character 7
3 Peripheral Vein	3 Percutaneous	2 Plasma, Convalescent (Nonautologous) NT	5 New Technology Group 5
3 Peripheral Vein	3 Percutaneous	D High-Dose Intravenous Immune Globulin E Hyperimmune Globulin	7 New Technology Group 7
4 Central Vein	3 Percutaneous	2 Plasma, Convalescent (Nonautologous) NT	5 New Technology Group 5
4 Central Vein	3 Percutaneous	D High-Dose Intravenous Immune Globulin E Hyperimmune Globulin	7 New Technology Group 7

NT XW13325
NT XW14325

X New Technology
W Anatomical Regions
H Insertion Definition: Putting in a nonbiological appliance that monitors, assists, performs, or prevents a physiological function but does not physically take the place of a body part
Explanation: None

Body Part Character 4	Approach Character 5	Device/Substance/Technology Character 6	Qualifier Character 7
D Mouth and Pharynx	7 Via Natural or Artificial Opening	Q Neurostimulator Lead	7 New Technology Group 7

X New Technology
X Physiological Systems
E Measurement Definition: Determining the level of a physiological or physical function at a point in time
Explanation: None

Body Part Character 4	Approach Character 5	Device/Substance/Technology Character 6	Qualifier Character 7
Ø Central Nervous	X External	Ø Intracranial Vascular Activity, Computer-aided Assessment	7 New Technology Group 7
3 Arterial	X External	2 Pulmonary Artery Flow, Computer-aided Triage and Notification	7 New Technology Group 7
5 Circulatory	X External	M Infection, Whole Blood Nucleic Acid-base Microbial Detection NT	5 New Technology Group 5
5 Circulatory	X External	N Infection, Positive Blood Culture Fluorescence Hybridization for Organism Identification, Concentration and Susceptibility	6 New Technology Group 6
5 Circulatory	X External	R Infection, Mechanical Initial Specimen Diversion Technique Using Active Negative Pressure T Intracranial Arterial Flow, Whole Blood mRNA V Infection, Serum/Plasma Nanoparticle Fluorescence SARS-CoV-2 Antibody Detection	7 New Technology Group 7
9 Nose	7 Via Natural or Artificial Opening	U Infection, Nasopharyngeal Fluid SARS-CoV-2 Polymerase Chain Reaction	7 New Technology Group 7
B Respiratory	X External	Q Infection, Lower Respiratory Fluid Nucleic Acid-base Microbial Detection	6 New Technology Group 6

NT XXE5XM5 for T2 Bacteria Test Panel

X New Technology
Y Extracorporeal
Ø Introduction Definition: Putting in or on a therapeutic, diagnostic, nutritional, physiological, or prophylactic substance except blood or blood products
Explanation: None

Body Part Character 4	Approach Character 5	Device/Substance/Technology Character 6	Qualifier Character 7
V Vein Graft	X External	8 Endothelial Damage Inhibitor	3 New Technology Group 3
Y Extracorporeal	X External	3 Nafamostat Anticoagulant	7 New Technology Group 7

Appendixes

Appendix A: Components of the Medical and Surgical Approach Definitions

ICD-10-PCS Value	Definition	Access Location	Method	Type of Instrumentation	Example
Open (Ø)	Cutting through the skin or mucous membrane and any other body layers necessary to expose the site of the procedure	Skin or mucous membrane, any other body layers	Cutting	None	Abdominal hysterectomy
Percutaneous (3)	Entry, by puncture or minor incision, of instrumentation through the skin or mucous membrane and any other body layers necessary to reach the site of the procedure	Skin or mucous membrane, any other body layers	Puncture or minor incision	Without visualization	Needle biopsy of liver, Liposuction
Percutaneous endoscopic (4)	Entry, by puncture or minor incision, of instrumentation through the skin or mucous membrane and any other body layers necessary to reach and visualize the site of the procedure	Skin or mucous membrane, any other body layers	Puncture or minor incision	With visualization	Arthroscopy, Laparoscopic cholecystectomy
Via natural or artificial opening (7)	Entry of instrumentation through a natural or artificial external opening to reach the site of the procedure	Natural or artificial external opening	Direct entry	Without visualization	Endotracheal tube insertion, Foley catheter placement
Via natural or artificial opening endoscopic (8)	Entry of instrumentation through a natural or artificial external opening to reach and visualize the site of the procedure	Natural or artificial external opening	Direct entry	With visualization	Sigmoidoscopy, EGD, ERCP
Via natural or artificial opening with percutaneous endoscopic assistance (F)	Entry of instrumentation through a natural or artificial external opening and entry, by puncture or minor incision, of instrumentation through the skin or mucous membrane and any other body layers necessary to aid in the performance of the procedure	Skin or mucous membrane, any other body layers	Direct entry with puncture or minor incision for instrumentation only	With visualization	Laparoscopic-assisted vaginal hysterectomy
External (X)	Procedures performed directly on the skin or mucous membrane and procedures performed indirectly by the application of external force through the skin or mucous membrane	Skin or mucous membrane	Direct or indirect application	None	Closed fracture reduction, Resection of tonsils

Open (Ø)

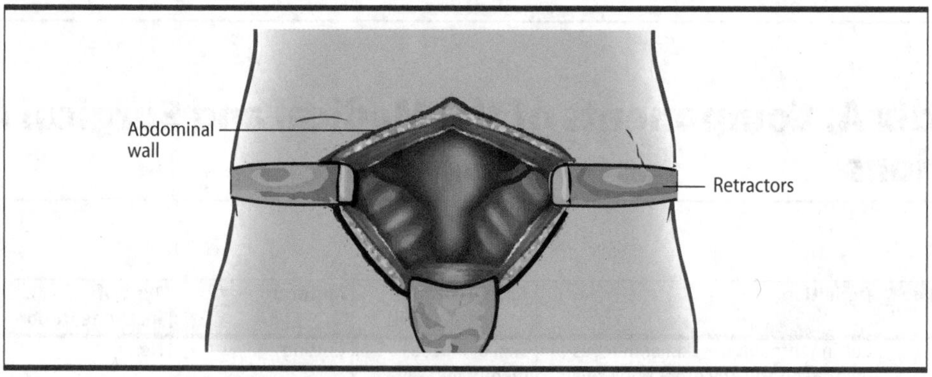

Percutaneous (3)

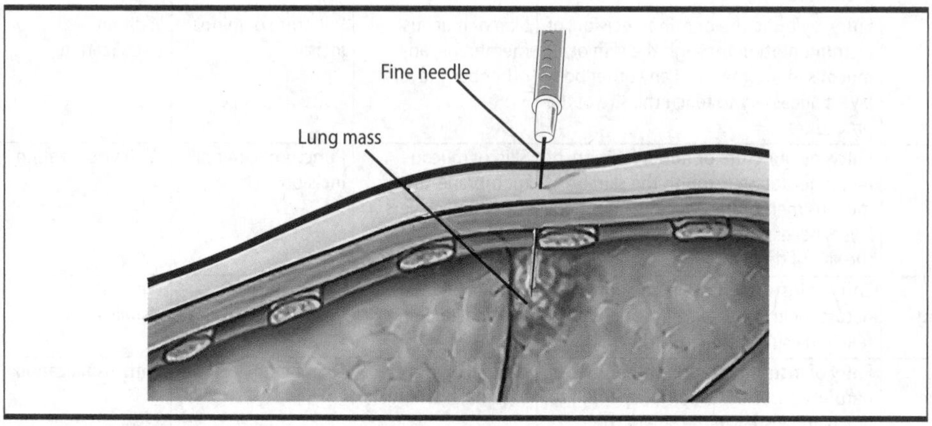

Percutaneous Endoscopic (4)

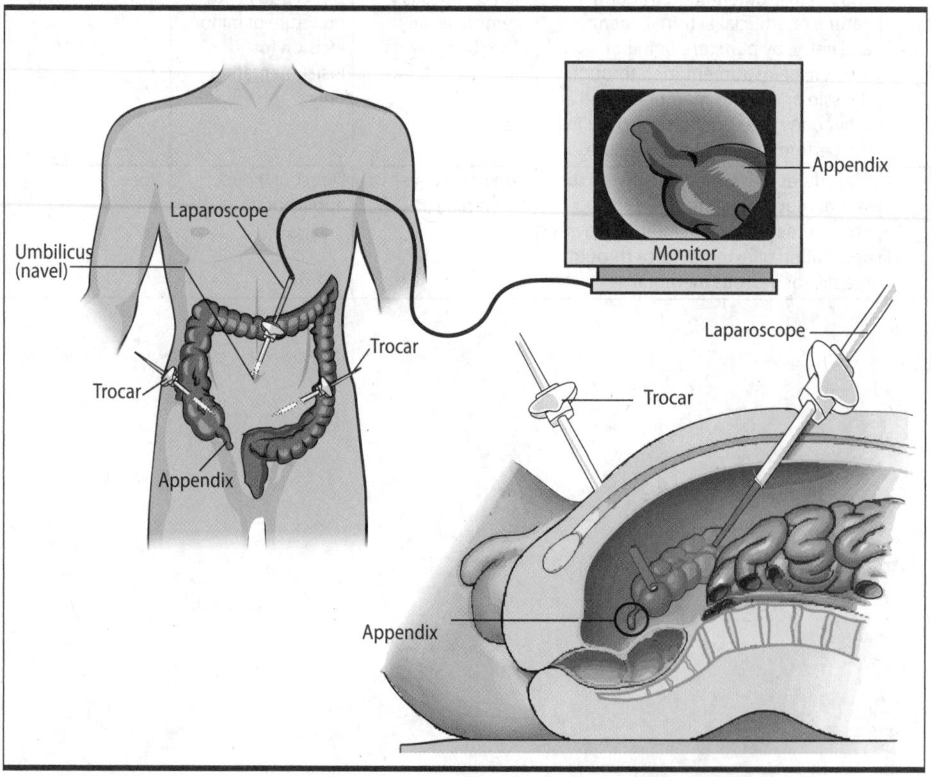

Appendix A: Components of the Medical and Surgical Approach Definitions

Via Natural or Artificial Opening (7)

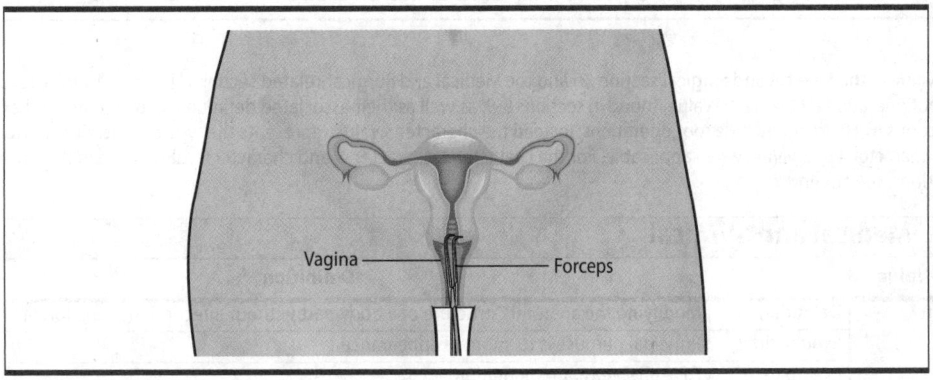

Via Natural or Artificial Opening, Endoscopic (8)

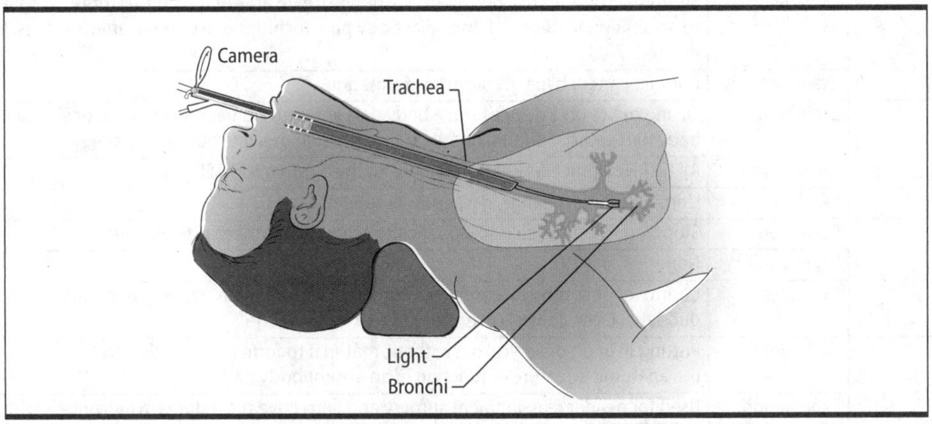

Via Natural or Artificial Opening with Percutaneous Endoscopic Assistance (F)

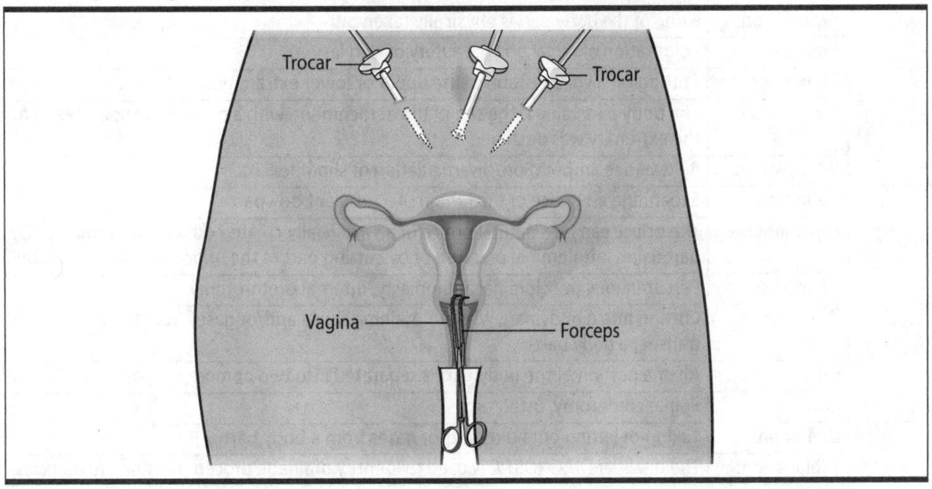

External (X)

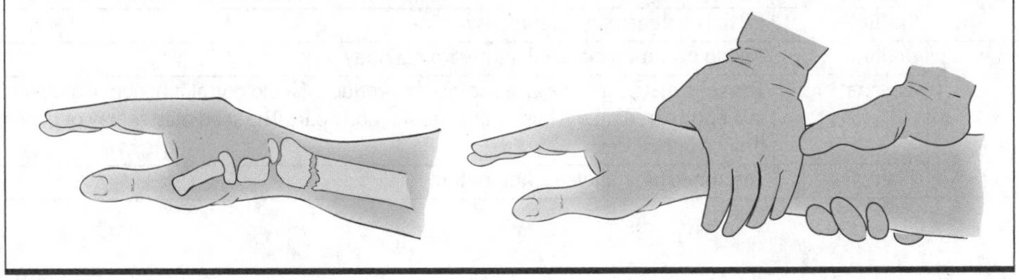

Appendix B: Root Operation Definitions

The character 3 value in the Medical and Surgical section (Ø) and the Medical and Surgical-related sections (1-9) represents the root operation. This resource provides each root operation (character 3) value, found in sections Ø-9, as well as their associated definition, explanation, and examples, where applicable. The Ancillary sections (B-H) do not include root operations; instead the character 3 value represents the type of procedure performed with additional detail provided by the character 4 or 5 value, when applicable. For the character 3, character 4, and character 5 values used in the Ancillary sections of B-H, along with their definitions, see appendix J.

Ø Medical and Surgical

ICD-1Ø-PCS Value		Definition	
Ø	Alteration	Definition:	Modifying the anatomic structure of a body part without affecting the function of the body part
		Explanation:	Principal purpose is to improve appearance
		Examples:	Face lift, breast augmentation
1	Bypass	Definition:	Altering the route of passage of the contents of a tubular body part
		Explanation:	Rerouting contents of a body part to a downstream area of the normal route, to a similar route and body part, or to an abnormal route and dissimilar body part. Includes one or more anastomoses, with or without the use of a device.
		Examples:	Coronary artery bypass, colostomy formation
2	Change	Definition:	Taking out or off a device from a body part and putting back an identical or similar device in or on the same body part without cutting or puncturing the skin or a mucous membrane
		Explanation:	All CHANGE procedures are coded using the approach EXTERNAL
		Example:	Urinary catheter change, gastrostomy tube change
3	Control	Definition:	Stopping, or attempting to stop, postprocedural or other acute bleeding
		Explanation:	None
		Examples:	Control of post-prostatectomy hemorrhage, control of intracranial subdural hemorrhage, control of bleeding duodenal ulcer, control of retroperitoneal hemorrhage
4	Creation	Definition:	Putting in or on biological or synthetic material to form a new body part that to the extent possible replicates the anatomic structure or function of an absent body part
		Explanation:	Used for gender reassignment surgery and corrective procedures in individuals with congenital anomalies
		Examples:	Creation of vagina in a male, creation of right and left atrioventricular valve from common atrioventricular valve
5	Destruction	Definition:	Physical eradication of all or a portion of a body part by the direct use of energy, force, or a destructive agent
		Explanation:	None of the body part is physically taken out
		Examples:	Fulguration of rectal polyp, cautery of skin lesion
6	Detachment	Definition:	Cutting off all or a portion of the upper or lower extremities
		Explanation:	The body part value is the site of the detachment, with a qualifier if applicable to further specify the level where the extremity was detached
		Examples:	Below knee amputation, disarticulation of shoulder
7	Dilation	Definition:	Expanding an orifice or the lumen of a tubular body part
		Explanation:	The orifice can be a natural orifice or an artificially created orifice. Accomplished by stretching a tubular body part using intraluminal pressure or by cutting part of the orifice or wall of the tubular body part.
		Examples:	Percutaneous transluminal angioplasty, internal urethrotomy
8	Division	Definition:	Cutting into a body part, without draining fluids and/or gases from the body part, in order to separate or transect a body part
		Explanation:	All or a portion of the body part is separated into two or more portions
		Examples:	Spinal cordotomy, osteotomy
9	Drainage	Definition:	Taking or letting out fluids and/or gases from a body part
		Explanation:	The qualifier DIAGNOSTIC is used to identify drainage procedures that are biopsies
		Examples:	Thoracentesis, incision and drainage
B	Excision	Definition:	Cutting out or off, without replacement, a portion of a body part
		Explanation:	The qualifier DIAGNOSTIC is used to identify excision procedures that are biopsies
		Examples:	Partial nephrectomy, liver biopsy
C	Extirpation	Definition:	Taking or cutting out solid matter from a body part
		Explanation:	The solid matter may be an abnormal byproduct of a biological function or a foreign body; it may be imbedded in a body part or in the lumen of a tubular body part. The solid matter may or may not have been previously broken into pieces.
		Examples:	Thrombectomy, choledocholithotomy

Continued on next page

Ø Medical and Surgical

Continued from previous page

ICD-1Ø-PCS Value		Definition	
D	Extraction	Definition:	Pulling or stripping out or off all or a portion of a body part by the use of force
		Explanation:	The qualifier DIAGNOSTIC is used to identify extractions that are biopsies
		Examples:	Dilation and curettage, vein stripping
F	Fragmentation	Definition:	Breaking solid matter in a body part into pieces
		Explanation:	Physical force (e.g., manual, ultrasonic) applied directly or indirectly is used to break the solid matter into pieces. The solid matter may be an abnormal byproduct of a biological function or a foreign body. The pieces of solid matter are not taken out.
		Examples:	Extracorporeal shockwave lithotripsy, transurethral lithotripsy
G	Fusion	Definition:	Joining together portions of an articular body part rendering the articular body part immobile
		Explanation:	The body part is joined together by fixation device, bone graft, or other means
		Examples:	Spinal fusion, ankle arthrodesis
H	Insertion	Definition:	Putting in a nonbiological appliance that monitors, assists, performs, or prevents a physiological function but does not physically take the place of a body part
		Explanation:	None
		Examples:	Insertion of radioactive implant, insertion of central venous catheter
J	Inspection	Definition:	Visually and/or manually exploring a body part
		Explanation:	Visual exploration may be performed with or without optical instrumentation. Manual exploration may be performed directly or through intervening body layers.
		Examples:	Diagnostic arthroscopy, exploratory laparotomy
K	Map	Definition:	Locating the route of passage of electrical impulses and/or locating functional areas in a body part
		Explanation:	Applicable only to the cardiac conduction mechanism and the central nervous system
		Examples:	Cardiac mapping, cortical mapping
L	Occlusion	Definition:	Completely closing an orifice or lumen of a tubular body part
		Explanation:	The orifice can be a natural orifice or an artificially created orifice
		Examples:	Fallopian tube ligation, ligation of inferior vena cava
M	Reattachment	Definition:	Putting back in or on all or a portion of a separated body part to its normal location or other suitable location
		Explanation:	Vascular circulation and nervous pathways may or may not be reestablished
		Examples:	Reattachment of hand, reattachment of avulsed kidney
N	Release	Definition:	Freeing a body part from an abnormal physical constraint by cutting or by use of force
		Explanation:	Some of the restraining tissue may be taken out but none of the body part is taken out
		Examples:	Adhesiolysis, carpal tunnel release
P	Removal	Definition:	Taking out or off a device from a body part
		Explanation:	If a device is taken out and a similar device put in without cutting or puncturing the skin or mucous membrane, the procedure is coded to the root operation CHANGE. Otherwise, the procedure for taking out a device is coded to the root operation REMOVAL.
		Examples:	Drainage tube removal, cardiac pacemaker removal
Q	Repair	Definition:	Restoring, to the extent possible, a body part to its normal anatomic structure and function
		Explanation:	Used only when the method to accomplish the repair is not one of the other root operations
		Examples:	Colostomy takedown, suture of laceration
R	Replacement	Definition:	Putting in or on biological or synthetic material that physically takes the place and/or function of all or a portion of a body part
		Explanation:	The body part may have been taken out or replaced, or may be taken out, physically eradicated, or rendered nonfunctional during the REPLACEMENT procedure. A REMOVAL procedure is coded for taking out the device used in a previous replacement procedure.
		Examples:	Total hip replacement, bone graft, free skin graft
S	Reposition	Definition:	Moving to its normal location, or other suitable location, all or a portion of a body part
		Explanation:	The body part is moved to a new location from an abnormal location, or from a normal location where it is not functioning correctly. The body part may or may not be cut out or off to be moved to the new location.
		Examples:	Reposition of undescended testicle, fracture reduction
T	Resection	Definition:	Cutting out or off, without replacement, all of a body part
		Explanation:	None
		Examples:	Total nephrectomy, total lobectomy of lung
V	Restriction	Definition:	Partially closing an orifice or the lumen of a tubular body part
		Explanation:	The orifice can be a natural orifice or an artificially created orifice
		Examples:	Esophagogastric fundoplication, cervical cerclage

Continued on next page

Ø Medical and Surgical

Continued from previous page

ICD-10-PCS Value		Definition	
W	Revision	Definition:	Correcting, to the extent possible, a portion of a malfunctioning device or the position of a displaced device
		Explanation:	Revision can include correcting a malfunctioning or displaced device by taking out or putting in components of the device such as a screw or pin
		Examples:	Adjustment of position of pacemaker lead, recementing of hip prosthesis
U	Supplement	Definition:	Putting in or on biological or synthetic material that physically reinforces and/or augments the function of a portion of a body part
		Explanation:	The biological material is non-living, or is living and from the same individual. The body part may have been previously replaced, and the SUPPLEMENT procedure is performed to physically reinforce and/or augment the function of the replaced body part.
		Examples:	Herniorrhaphy using mesh, mitral valve ring annuloplasty, put a new acetabular liner in a previous hip replacement
X	Transfer	Definition:	Moving, without taking out, all or a portion of a body part to another location to take over the function of all or a portion of a body part
		Explanation:	The body part transferred remains connected to its vascular and nervous supply
		Examples:	Tendon transfer, skin pedicle flap transfer
Y	Transplantation	Definition:	Putting in or on all or a portion of a living body part taken from another individual or animal to physically take the place and/or function of all or a portion of a similar body part
		Explanation:	The native body part may or may not be taken out, and the transplanted body part may take over all or a portion of its function
		Examples:	Kidney transplant, heart transplant

Root Operation Definitions for Other Sections

1 Obstetrics

ICD-10-PCS Value		Definition	
2	Change	Definition:	Taking out or off a device from a body part and putting back an identical or similar device in or on the same body part without cutting or puncturing the skin or a mucous membrane
		Explanation:	None
		Examples:	Replacement of fetal scalp electrode
9	Drainage	Definition:	Taking or letting out fluids and/or gases from a body part
		Explanation:	None
		Examples:	Biopsy of amniotic fluid
A	Abortion	Definition:	Artificially terminating a pregnancy
		Explanation:	None
		Examples:	Transvaginal abortion using vacuum aspiration technique
D	Extraction	Definition:	Pulling or stripping out or off all or a portion of a body part by the use of force
		Explanation:	None
		Examples:	Low-transverse C-section
E	Delivery	Definition:	Assisting the passage of the products of conception from the genital canal
		Explanation:	None
		Examples:	Manually-assisted delivery
H	Insertion	Definition:	Putting in a nonbiological appliance that monitors, assists, performs, or prevents a physiological function but does not physically take the place of a body part
		Explanation:	None
		Examples:	Placement of fetal scalp electrode
J	Inspection	Definition:	Visually and/or manually exploring a body part
		Explanation:	Visual exploration may be performed with or without optical instrumentation. Manual exploration may be performed directly or through intervening body layers.
		Examples:	Bimanual pregnancy exam
P	Removal	Definition:	Taking out or off a device from a body part, region or orifice
		Explanation:	If a device is taken out and a similar device put in without cutting or puncturing the skin or mucous membrane, the procedure is coded to the root operation CHANGE. Otherwise, the procedure for taking out a device is coded to the root operation REMOVAL.
		Examples:	Removal of fetal monitoring electrode

Continued on next page

1 Obstetrics

Continued from previous page

ICD-10-PCS Value			Definition
Q	Repair	Definition:	Restoring, to the extent possible, a body part to its normal anatomic structure and function
		Explanation:	Used only when the method to accomplish the repair is not one of the other root operations
		Examples:	In utero repair of congenital diaphragmatic hernia
S	Reposition	Definition:	Moving to its normal location, or other suitable location, all or a portion of a body part
		Explanation:	The body part is moved to a new location from an abnormal location, or from a normal location where it is not functioning correctly. The body part may or may not be cut out or off to be moved to the new location.
		Examples:	External version of fetus
T	Resection	Definition:	Cutting out or off, without replacement, all of a body part
		Explanation:	None
		Examples:	Total excision of tubal pregnancy
Y	Transplantation	Definition:	Putting in or on all or a portion of a living body part taken from another individual or animal to physically take the place and/or function of all or a portion of a similar body part
		Explanation:	The native body part may or may not be taken out, and the transplanted body part may take over all or a portion of its function
		Examples:	In utero fetal kidney transplant

2 Placement

ICD-10-PCS Value			Definition
Ø	Change	Definition:	Taking out or off a device from a body part and putting back an identical or similar device in or on the same body part without cutting or puncturing the skin or a mucous membrane
		Examples:	Change of vaginal packing
1	Compression	Definition:	Putting pressure on a body region
		Examples:	Placement of pressure dressing on abdominal wall
2	Dressing	Definition:	Putting material on a body region for protection
		Examples:	Application of sterile dressing to head wound
3	Immobilization	Definition:	Limiting or preventing motion of a body region
		Examples:	Placement of splint on left finger
4	Packing	Definition:	Putting material in a body region or orifice
		Examples:	Placement of nasal packing
5	Removal	Definition:	Taking out or off a device from a body part
		Examples:	Removal of stereotactic head frame
6	Traction	Definition:	Exerting a pulling force on a body region in a distal direction
		Examples:	Lumbar traction using motorized split-traction table

3 Administration

ICD-10-PCS Value			Definition
Ø	Introduction	Definition:	Putting in or on a therapeutic, diagnostic, nutritional, physiological, or prophylactic substance except blood or blood products
		Examples:	Nerve block injection to median nerve
1	Irrigation	Definition:	Putting in or on a cleansing substance
		Examples:	Flushing of eye
2	Transfusion	Definition:	Putting in blood or blood products
		Examples:	Transfusion of cell saver red cells into central venous line

4 Measurement and Monitoring

ICD-10-PCS Value			Definition
Ø	Measurement	Definition:	Determining the level of a physiological or physical function at a point in time
		Examples:	External electrocardiogram(EKG), single reading
1	Monitoring	Definition:	Determining the level of a physiological or physical function repetitively over a period of time
		Examples:	Urinary pressure monitoring

5 Extracorporeal or Systemic Assistance and Performance

ICD-10-PCS Value		Definition	
Ø	Assistance	Definition:	Taking over a portion of a physiological function by extracorporeal means
		Examples:	Hyperbaric oxygenation of wound
1	Performance	Definition:	Completely taking over a physiological function by extracorporeal means
		Examples:	Cardiopulmonary bypass in conjunction with CABG
2	Restoration	Definition:	Returning, or attempting to return, a physiological function to its original state by extracorporeal means
		Examples:	Attempted cardiac defibrillation, unsuccessful

6 Extracorporeal or Systemic Therapies

ICD-10-PCS Value		Definition	
Ø	Atmospheric Control	Definition:	Extracorporeal control of atmospheric pressure and composition
		Examples:	Antigen-free air conditioning, series treatment
1	Decompression	Definition:	Extracorporeal elimination of undissolved gas from body fluids
		Examples:	Hyperbaric decompression treatment, single
2	Electromagnetic Therapy	Definition:	Extracorporeal treatment by electromagnetic rays
		Examples:	TMS (transcranial magnetic stimulation), series treatment
3	Hyperthermia	Definition:	Extracorporeal raising of body temperature
		Examples:	None
4	Hypothermia	Definition:	Extracorporeal lowering of body temperature
		Examples:	Whole body hypothermia treatment for temperature imbalances, series
5	Pheresis	Definition:	Extracorporeal separation of blood products
		Examples:	Therapeutic leukopheresis, single treatment
6	Phototherapy	Definition:	Extracorporeal treatment by light rays
		Examples:	Phototherapy of circulatory system, series treatment
7	Ultrasound Therapy	Definition:	Extracorporeal treatment by ultrasound
		Examples:	Therapeutic ultrasound of peripheral vessels, single treatment
8	Ultraviolet Light Therapy	Definition:	Extracorporeal treatment by ultraviolet light
		Examples:	Ultraviolet light phototherapy, series treatment
9	Shock Wave Therapy	Definition:	Extracorporeal treatment by shock waves
		Examples:	Shockwave therapy of plantar fascia, single treatment
B	Perfusion	Definition:	Extracorporeal treatment by diffusion of therapeutic fluid
		Examples:	Perfusion of donor liver while preparing transplant patient

7 Osteopathic

ICD-10-PCS Value		Definition	
Ø	Treatment	Definition:	Manual treatment to eliminate or alleviate somatic dysfunction and related disorders
		Examples:	Fascial release of abdomen, osteopathic treatment

8 Other Procedures

ICD-10-PCS Value		Definition	
Ø	Other Procedures	Definition:	Methodologies which attempt to remediate or cure a disorder or disease
		Examples:	Acupuncture, yoga therapy

9 Chiropractic

ICD-10-PCS Value		Definition	
B	Manipulation	Definition:	Manual procedure that involves a directed thrust to move a joint past the physiological range of motion, without exceeding the anatomical limit
		Examples:	Chiropractic treatment of cervical spine, short lever specific contact

Appendix C: Comparison of Medical and Surgical Root Operations

Note: the character associated with each operation appears in parentheses after its title.

Procedures That Take Out Some or All of a Body Part

Root Operation	Objective of Procedure	Site of Procedure	Example
Destruction (5)	Eradicating without taking out or replacement	Some/all of a body part	Fulguration of endometrium
Detachment (6)	Cutting out/off without replacement	Extremity only, any level	Amputation above elbow
Excision (B)	Cutting out/off without replacement	Some of a body part	Breast lumpectomy
Extraction (D)	Pulling out or off without replacement	Some/all of a body part	Suction D&C
Resection (T)	Cutting out/off without replacement	All of a body part	Total mastectomy

Procedures That Put in/Put Back or Move Some/All of a Body Part

Root Operation	Objective of Procedure	Site of Procedure	Example
Reattachment (M)	Putting back a detached body part	Some/all of a body part	Reattach finger
Reposition (S)	Moving a body part to normal or other suitable location	Some/all of a body part	Move undescended testicle
Transfer (X)	Moving a body part to function for a similar body part	Some/all of a body part	Skin pedicle transfer flap
Transplantation (Y)	Putting in a living body part from a person/animal	Some/all of a body part	Kidney transplant

Procedures That Take Out or Eliminate Solid Matter, Fluids, or Gases From a Body Part

Root Operation	Objective of Procedure	Site of Procedure	Example
Drainage (9)	Taking or letting out	Fluids and/or gases from a body part	Incision and drainage
Extirpation (C)	Taking or cutting out	Solid matter in a body part	Thrombectomy
Fragmentation (F)	Breaking into pieces	Solid matter within a body part	Lithotripsy

Procedures That Involve Only Examination of Body Parts and Regions

Root Operation	Objective of Procedure	Site of Procedure	Example
Inspection (J)	Visual/manual exploration	Some/all of a body part	Diagnostic cystoscopy Exploratory laparoscopy
Map (K)	Locating electrical impulse route/functional areas	Brain/cardiac conduction mechanism	Cardiac mapping

Procedures That Alter the Diameter/Route of a Tubular Body Part

Root Operation	Objective of Procedure	Site of Procedure	Example
Bypass (1)	Altering route of passage of contents	Tubular body part	Coronary artery bypass graft (CABG)
Dilation (7)	Expanding natural or artificially created orifice/lumen	Tubular body part	Percutaneous transluminal coronary angioplasty (PTCA)
Occlusion (L)	Completely closing natural or artificially created orifice/lumen	Tubular body part	Fallopian tube ligation
Restriction (V)	Partially closing natural or artificially created orifice/lumen	Tubular body part	Gastroesophageal fundoplication

Procedures That Always Involve Devices

Root Operation	Objective of Procedure	Site of Procedure	Example
Change (2) DVC	Exchanging device w/out cutting/puncturing	In/on a body part	Gastrostomy tube change
Insertion (H) DVC	Putting in nonbiological device	In/on a body part	Central line insertion
Removal (P) DVC	Taking out device	In/on a body part	Central line removal
Replacement (R) DVC	Putting in device that replaces a body part	Some/all of a body part	Total hip replacement
Revision (W) DVC	Correcting a malfunctioning/displaced device	In/on a body part	Revision of pacemaker
Supplement (U) DVC	Putting in device that reinforces or augments a body part	In/on a body part	Abdominal wall herniorrhaphy using mesh

DVC = Device involved in root operation

Procedures Involving Cutting or Separation Only

Root Operation	Objective of Procedure	Site of Procedure	Example
Division (8)	Cutting into/separating	A body part	Neurotomy
Release (N)	Freeing a body part from constraint	Around a body part	Adhesiolysis

Procedures That Define Other Repairs

Root Operation	Objective of Procedure	Site of Procedure	Example
Control (3)	Stopping/attempting to stop postprocedural or other acute bleeding	Anatomical region or nasal mucosa/soft tissue	Post-prostatectomy bleeding control, control subdural hemorrhage, bleeding ulcer, retroperitoneal hemorrhage
Repair (Q)	Restoring body part to its normal structure/function	Some/all of a body part	Suture laceration

Procedures That Define Other Objectives

Root Operation	Objective of Procedure	Site of Procedure	Example
Alteration (Ø)	Modifying body part for cosmetic purposes without affecting function	Some/all of a body part	Face lift
Creation (4)	Using biological or synthetic material to form a new body part that replicates the anatomic structure or function of a missing body part	Perineum, valve	Sex change/artificial vagina/penis, atrioventricular valve creation
Fusion (G)	Unification or immobilization	Joint or articular body part	Spinal fusion

Appendix D: Body Part Key

Term	ICD-10-PCS Value
Abdominal aortic plexus	Abdominal Sympathetic Nerve
Abdominal esophagus	Esophagus, Lower
Abductor hallucis muscle	Foot Muscle, Right
	Foot Muscle, Left
Accessory cephalic vein	Cephalic Vein, Right
	Cephalic Vein, Left
Accessory obturator nerve	Lumbar Plexus
Accessory phrenic nerve	Phrenic nerve
Accessory spleen	Spleen
Acetabulofemoral joint	Hip Joint, Right
	Hip Joint, Left
Achilles tendon	Lower Leg Tendon, Right
	Lower Leg Tendon, Left
Acromioclavicular ligament	Shoulder Bursa and Ligament, Right
	Shoulder Bursa and Ligament, Left
Acromion (process)	Scapula, Right
	Scapula, Left
Adductor brevis muscle	Upper Leg Muscle, Right
	Upper Leg Muscle, Left
Adductor hallucis muscle	Foot Muscle, Right
	Foot Muscle, Left
Adductor longus muscle	Upper Leg Muscle, Right
	Upper Leg Muscle, Left
Adductor magnus muscle	Upper Leg Muscle, Right
	Upper Leg Muscle, Left
Adenohypophysis	Pituitary Gland
Alar ligament of axis	Head and Neck Bursa and Ligament
Alveolar process of mandible	Mandible, Right
	Mandible, Left
Alveolar process of maxilla	Maxilla
Anal orifice	Anus
Anatomical snuffbox	Lower Arm and Wrist Muscle, Right
	Lower Arm and Wrist Muscle, Left
Angular artery	Face Artery
Angular vein	Face Vein, Right
	Face Vein, Left
Annular ligament	Elbow Bursa and Ligament, Right
	Elbow Bursa and Ligament, Left
Anorectal junction	Rectum
Ansa cervicalis	Cervical Plexus
Antebrachial fascia	Subcutaneous Tissue and Fascia, Right Lower Arm
	Subcutaneous Tissue and Fascia, Left Lower Arm
Anterior (pectoral) lymph node	Lymphatic, Right Axillary
	Lymphatic, Left Axillary
Anterior cerebral artery	Intracranial Artery
Anterior cerebral vein	Intracranial Vein
Anterior choroidal artery	Intracranial Artery
Anterior circumflex humeral artery	Axillary Artery, Right
	Axillary Artery, Left
Anterior communicating artery	Intracranial Artery
Anterior cruciate ligament (ACL)	Knee Bursa and Ligament, Right
	Knee Bursa and Ligament, Left

Term	ICD-10-PCS Value
Anterior crural nerve	Femoral Nerve
Anterior facial vein	Face Vein, Right
	Face Vein, Left
Anterior intercostal artery	Internal Mammary Artery, Right
	Internal Mammary Artery, Left
Anterior interosseous nerve	Median Nerve
Anterior lateral malleolar artery	Anterior Tibial Artery, Right
	Anterior Tibial Artery, Left
Anterior lingual gland	Minor Salivary Gland
Anterior medial malleolar artery	Anterior Tibial Artery, Right
	Anterior Tibial Artery, Left
Anterior spinal artery	Vertebral Artery, Right
	Vertebral Artery, Left
Anterior tibial recurrent artery	Anterior Tibial Artery, Right
	Anterior Tibial Artery, Left
Anterior ulnar recurrent artery	Ulnar Artery, Right
	Ulnar Artery, Left
Anterior vagal trunk	Vagus Nerve
Anterior vertebral muscle	Neck Muscle, Right
	Neck Muscle, Left
Antihelix	External Ear, Right
	External Ear, Left
	External Ear, Bilateral
Antitragus	External Ear, Right
	External Ear, Left
	External Ear, Bilateral
Antrum of Highmore	Maxillary Sinus, Right
	Maxillary Sinus, Left
Aortic annulus	Aortic Valve
Aortic arch	Thoracic Aorta, Ascending/Arch
Aortic intercostal artery	Upper Artery
Apical (subclavicular) lymph node	Lymphatic, Right Axillary
	Lymphatic, Left Axillary
Apneustic center	Pons
Aqueduct of Sylvius	Cerebral Ventricle
Aqueous humour	Anterior Chamber, Right
	Anterior Chamber, Left
Arachnoid mater, intracranial	Cerebral Meninges
Arachnoid mater, spinal	Spinal Meninges
Arcuate artery	Foot Artery, Right
	Foot Artery, Left
Areola	Nipple, Right
	Nipple, Left
Arterial canal (duct)	Pulmonary Artery, Left
Aryepiglottic fold	Larynx
Arytenoid cartilage	Larynx
Arytenoid muscle	Neck Muscle, Right
	Neck Muscle, Left
Ascending aorta	Thoracic Aorta, Ascending/Arch
Ascending palatine artery	Face Artery
Ascending pharyngeal artery	External Carotid Artery, Right
	External Carotid Artery, Left
Atlantoaxial joint	Cervical Vertebral Joint

Term	ICD-10-PCS Value
Atrioventricular node	Conduction Mechanism
Atrium dextrum cordis	Atrium, Right
Atrium pulmonale	Atrium, Left
Auditory tube	Eustachian Tube, Right
	Eustachian Tube, Left
Auerbach's (myenteric)plexus	Abdominal Sympathetic Nerve
Auricle	External Ear, Right
	External Ear, Left
	External Ear, Bilateral
Auricularis muscle	Head Muscle
Axillary fascia	Subcutaneous Tissue and Fascia, Right Upper Arm
	Subcutaneous Tissue and Fascia, Left Upper Arm
Axillary nerve	Brachial Plexus
Bartholin's (greater vestibular) gland	Vestibular Gland
Basal (internal) cerebral vein	Intracranial Vein
Basal nuclei	Basal Ganglia
Base of tongue	Pharynx
Basilar artery	Intracranial Artery
Basis pontis	Pons
Biceps brachii muscle	Upper Arm Muscle, Right
	Upper Arm Muscle, Left
Biceps femoris muscle	Upper Leg Muscle, Right
	Upper Leg Muscle, Left
Bicipital aponeurosis	Subcutaneous Tissue and Fascia, Right Lower Arm
	Subcutaneous Tissue and Fascia, Left Lower Arm
Bicuspid valve	Mitral Valve
Body of femur	Femoral Shaft, Right
	Femoral Shaft, Left
Body of fibula	Fibula, Right
	Fibula, Left
Bony labyrinth	Inner Ear, Right
	Inner Ear, Left
Bony orbit	Orbit, Right
	Orbit, Left
Bony vestibule	Inner Ear, Right
	Inner Ear, Left
Botallo's duct	Pulmonary Artery, Left
Brachial (lateral) lymph node	Lymphatic, Right Axillary
	Lymphatic, Left Axillary
Brachialis muscle	Upper Arm Muscle, Right
	Upper Arm Muscle, Left
Brachiocephalic artery	Innominate Artery
Brachiocephalic trunk	Innominate Artery
Brachiocephalic vein	Innominate Vein, Right
	Innominate Vein, Left
Brachioradialis muscle	Lower Arm and Wrist Muscle, Right
	Lower Arm and Wrist Muscle, Left
Breast procedures, skin only	Skin, Chest
Broad ligament	Uterine Supporting Structure
Bronchial artery	Upper Artery
Bronchus intermedius	Main Bronchus, Right
Buccal gland	Buccal Mucosa

Term	ICD-10-PCS Value
Buccinator lymph node	Lymphatic, Head
Buccinator muscle	Facial Muscle
Bulbospongiosus muscle	Perineum Muscle
Bulbourethral (Cowper's) gland	Urethra
Bundle of His	Conduction Mechanism
Bundle of Kent	Conduction Mechanism
Calcaneocuboid joint	Tarsal Joint, Right
	Tarsal Joint, Left
Calcaneocuboid ligament	Foot Bursa and Ligament, Right
	Foot Bursa and Ligament, Left
Calcaneofibular ligament	Ankle Bursa and Ligament, Right
	Ankle Bursa and Ligament, Left
Calcaneus	Tarsal, Right
	Tarsal, Left
Capitate bone	Carpal, Right
	Carpal, Left
Cardia	Esophagogastric Junction
Cardiac plexus	Thoracic Sympathetic Nerve
Cardioesophageal junction	Esophagogastric Junction
Caroticotympanic artery	Internal Carotid Artery, Right
	Internal Carotid Artery, Left
Carotid glomus	Carotid Body, Right
	Carotid Body, Left
	Carotid Bodies, Bilateral
Carotid sinus	Internal Carotid Artery, Right
	Internal Carotid Artery, Left
Carotid sinus nerve	Glossopharyngeal Nerve
Carpometacarpal ligament	Hand Bursa and Ligament, Right
	Hand Bursa and Ligament, Left
Cauda equina	Lumbar Spinal Cord
Cavernous plexus	Head and Neck Sympathetic Nerve
Celiac ganglion	Abdominal Sympathetic Nerve
Celiac (solar) plexus	Abdominal Sympathetic Nerve
Celiac lymph node	Lymphatic, Aortic
Celiac trunk	Celiac Artery
Central axillary lymph node	Lymphatic, Right Axillary
	Lymphatic, Left Axillary
Cerebral aqueduct (Sylvius)	Cerebral Ventricle
Cerebrum	Brain
Cervical esophagus	Esophagus, Upper
Cervical facet joint	Cervical Vertebral Joint
	Cervical Vertebral Joints, 2 or more
Cervical ganglion	Head and Neck Sympathetic Nerve
Cervical interspinous ligament	Head and Neck Bursa and Ligament
Cervical intertransverse ligament	Head and Neck Bursa and Ligament
Cervical ligamentum flavum	Head and Neck Bursa and Ligament
Cervical lymph node	Lymphatic, Right Neck
	Lymphatic, Left Neck
Cervicothoracic facet joint	Cervicothoracic Vertebral Joint
Choana	Nasopharynx
Chondroglossus muscle	Tongue, Palate, Pharynx Muscle
Chorda tympani	Facial Nerve
Choroid plexus	Cerebral Ventricle
Ciliary body	Eye, Right
	Eye, Left

Term	ICD-10-PCS Value
Ciliary ganglion	Head and Neck Sympathetic Nerve
Circle of Willis	Intracranial Artery
Circumflex illiac artery	Femoral Artery, Right
	Femoral Artery, Left
Claustrum	Basal Ganglia
Coccygeal body	Coccygeal Glomus
Coccygeus muscle	Trunk Muscle, Right
	Trunk Muscle, Left
Cochlea	Inner Ear, Right
	Inner Ear, Left
Cochlear nerve	Acoustic Nerve
Columella	Nasal Mucosa and Soft Tissue
Common digital vein	Foot Vein, Right
	Foot Vein, Left
Common facial vein	Face Vein, Right
	Face Vein, Left
Common fibular nerve	Peroneal Nerve
Common hepatic artery	Hepatic Artery
Common iliac (subaortic) lymph node	Lymphatic, Pelvis
Common interosseous artery	Ulnar Artery, Right
	Ulnar Artery, Left
Common peroneal nerve	Peroneal Nerve
Condyloid process	Mandible, Right
	Mandible, Left
Conus arteriosus	Ventricle, Right
Conus medullaris	Lumbar Spinal Cord
Coracoacromial ligament	Shoulder Bursa and Ligament, Right
	Shoulder Bursa and Ligament, Left
Coracobrachialis muscle	Upper Arm Muscle, Right
	Upper Arm Muscle, Left
Coracoclavicular ligament	Shoulder Bursa and Ligament, Right
	Shoulder Bursa and Ligament, Left
Coracohumeral ligament	Shoulder Bursa and Ligament, Right
	Shoulder Bursa and Ligament, Left
Coracoid process	Scapula, Right
	Scapula, Left
Corniculate cartilage	Larynx
Corpus callosum	Brain
Corpus cavernosum	Penis
Corpus spongiosum	Penis
Corpus striatum	Basal Ganglia
Corrugator supercilii muscle	Facial Muscle
Costocervical trunk	Subclavian Artery, Right
	Subclavian Artery, Left
Costoclavicular ligament	Shoulder Bursa and Ligament, Right
	Shoulder Bursa and Ligament, Left
Costotransverse joint	Thoracic Vertebral Joint
Costotransverse ligament	Rib(s) Bursa and Ligament
Costovertebral joint	Thoracic Vertebral Joint
Costoxiphoid ligament	Sternum Bursa and Ligament
Cowper's (bulbourethral) gland	Urethra
Cremaster muscle	Perineum Muscle
Cribriform plate	Ethmoid Bone, Right
	Ethmoid Bone, Left
Cricoid cartilage	Trachea
Cricothyroid artery	Thyroid Artery, Right
	Thyroid Artery, Left
Cricothyroid muscle	Neck Muscle, Right
	Neck Muscle, Left
Crural fascia	Subcutaneous Tissue and Fascia, Right Upper Leg
	Subcutaneous Tissue and Fascia, Left Upper Leg
Cubital lymph node	Lymphatic, Right Upper Extremity
	Lymphatic, Left Upper Extremity
Cubital nerve	Ulnar Nerve
Cuboid bone	Tarsal, Right
	Tarsal, Left
Cuboideonavicular joint	Tarsal Joint, Right
	Tarsal Joint, Left
Culmen	Cerebellum
Cuneiform cartilage	Larynx
Cuneonavicular joint	Tarsal Joint, Right
	Tarsal Joint, Left
Cuneonavicular ligament	Foot Bursa and Ligament, Right
	Foot Bursa and Ligament, Left
Cutaneous (transverse) cervical nerve	Cervical Plexus
Deep cervical fascia	Subcutaneous Tissue and Fascia, Right Neck
	Subcutaneous Tissue and Fascia, Left Neck
Deep cervical vein	Vertebral Vein, Right
	Vertebral Vein, Left
Deep circumflex iliac artery	External Iliac Artery, Right
	External Iliac Artery, Left
Deep facial vein	Face Vein, Right
	Face Vein, Left
Deep femoral artery	Femoral Artery, Right
	Femoral Artery, Left
Deep femoral (profunda femoris) vein	Femoral Vein, Right
	Femoral Vein, Left
Deep palmar arch	Hand Artery, Right
	Hand Artery, Left
Deep transverse perineal muscle	Perineum Muscle
Deferential artery	Internal Iliac Artery, Right
	Internal Iliac Artery, Left
Deltoid fascia	Subcutaneous Tissue and Fascia, Right Upper Arm
	Subcutaneous Tissue and Fascia, Left Upper Arm
Deltoid ligament	Ankle Bursa and Ligament, Right
	Ankle Bursa and Ligament, Left
Deltoid muscle	Shoulder Muscle, Right
	Shoulder Muscle, Left
Deltopectoral (infraclavicular) lymph node	Lymphatic, Right Upper Extremity
	Lymphatic, Left Upper Extremity
Dens	Cervical Vertebra
Denticulate (dentate) ligament	Spinal Meninges
Depressor anguli oris muscle	Facial Muscle
Depressor labii inferioris muscle	Facial Muscle

Term	ICD-10-PCS Value
Depressor septi nasi muscle	Facial Muscle
Depressor supercilii muscle	Facial Muscle
Dermis	Skin
Descending genicular artery	Femoral Artery, Right
	Femoral Artery, Left
Diaphragma sellae	Dura Mater
Distal humerus	Humeral Shaft, Right
	Humeral Shaft, Left
Distal humerus, involving joint	Elbow Joint, Right
	Elbow Joint, Left
Distal radioulnar joint	Wrist Joint, Right
	Wrist Joint, Left
Dorsal digital nerve	Radial Nerve
Dorsal metacarpal vein	Hand Vein, Right
	Hand Vein, Left
Dorsal metatarsal artery	Foot Artery, Right
	Foot Artery, Left
Dorsal metatarsal vein	Foot Vein, Right
	Foot Vein, Left
Dorsal root ganglion	Cervical Spinal Cord
	Lumbar Spinal Cord
	Spinal Cord
	Thoracic Spinal Cord
Dorsal scapular artery	Subclavian Artery, Right
	Subclavian Artery, Left
Dorsal scapular nerve	Brachial Plexus
Dorsal venous arch	Foot Vein, Right
	Foot Vein, Left
Dorsalis pedis artery	Anterior Tibial Artery, Right
	Anterior Tibial Artery, Left
Duct of Santorini	Pancreatic Duct, Accessory
Duct of Wirsung	Pancreatic Duct
Ductus deferens	Vas Deferens, Right
	Vas Deferens, Left
	Vas Deferens, Bilateral
	Vas Deferens
Duodenal ampulla	Ampulla of Vater
Duodenojejunal flexure	Jejunum
Dura mater, intracranial	Dura Mater
Dura mater, spinal	Spinal Meninges
Dural venous sinus	Intracranial Vein
Earlobe	External Ear, Right
	External Ear, Left
	External Ear, Bilateral
Eighth cranial nerve	Acoustic Nerve
Ejaculatory duct	Vas Deferens, Right
	Vas Deferens, Left
	Vas Deferens, Bilateral
	Vas Deferens
Eleventh cranial nerve	Accessory Nerve
Encephalon	Brain
Ependyma	Cerebral Ventricle
Epidermis	Skin
Epidural space, spinal	Spinal Canal
Epiploic foramen	Peritoneum
Epithalamus	Thalamus
Epitroclear lymph node	Lymphatic, Right Upper Extremity
	Lymphatic, Left Upper Extremity
Erector spinae muscle	Trunk Muscle, Right
	Trunk Muscle, Left
Esophageal artery	Upper Artery
Esophageal plexus	Thoracic Sympathetic Nerve
Ethmoidal air cell	Ethmoid Sinus, Right
	Ethmoid Sinus, Left
Extensor carpi radialis muscle	Lower Arm and Wrist Muscle, Right
	Lower Arm and Wrist Muscle, Left
Extensor carpi ulnaris muscle	Lower Arm and Wrist Muscle, Right
	Lower Arm and Wrist Muscle, Left
Extensor digitorum brevis muscle	Foot Muscle, Right
	Foot Muscle, Left
Extensor digitorum longus muscle	Lower Leg Muscle, Right
	Lower Leg Muscle, Left
Extensor hallucis brevis muscle	Foot Muscle, Right
	Foot Muscle, Left
Extensor hallucis longus muscle	Lower Leg Muscle, Right
	Lower Leg Muscle, Left
External anal sphincter	Anal Sphincter
External auditory meatus	External Auditory Canal, Right
	External Auditory Canal, Left
External maxillary artery	Face Artery
External naris	Nasal Mucosa and Soft Tissue
External oblique aponeurosis	Subcutaneous Tissue and Fascia, Trunk
External oblique muscle	Abdomen Muscle, Right
	Abdomen Muscle, Left
External popliteal nerve	Peroneal Nerve
External pudendal artery	Femoral Artery, Right
	Femoral Artery, Left
External pudenal vein	Saphenous Vein, Right
	Saphenous Vein, Left
External urethral sphincter	Urethra
Extradural space, intracranial	Epidural Space, Intracranial
Extradural space, spinal	Spinal Canal
Facial artery	Face Artery
False vocal cord	Larynx
Falx cerebri	Dura Mater
Fascia lata	Subcutaneous Tissue and Fascia, Right Upper Leg
	Subcutaneous Tissue and Fascia, Left Upper Leg
Femoral head	Upper Femur, Right
	Upper Femur, Left
Femoral lymph node	Lymphatic, Right Lower Extremity
	Lymphatic, Left Lower Extremity
Femoropatellar joint	Knee Joint, Right
	Knee Joint, Left
	Knee Joint, Femoral Surface, Right
	Knee Joint, Femoral Surface, Left
Femorotibial joint	Knee Joint, Right
	Knee Joint, Left
	Knee Joint, Tibial Surface, Right
	Knee Joint, Tibial Surface, Left
Fibular artery	Peroneal Artery, Right
	Peroneal Artery, Left

Term	ICD-10-PCS Value
Fibular sesamoid	Metatarsal, Right
	Metatarsal, Left
Fibularis brevis muscle	Lower Leg Muscle, Right
	Lower Leg Muscle, Left
Fibularis longus muscle	Lower Leg Muscle, Right
	Lower Leg Muscle, Left
Fifth cranial nerve	Trigeminal Nerve
Filum terminale	Spinal Meninges
First cranial nerve	Olfactory Nerve
First intercostal nerve	Brachial Plexus
Flexor carpi radialis muscle	Lower Arm and Wrist Muscle, Right
	Lower Arm and Wrist Muscle, Left
Flexor carpi ulnaris muscle	Lower Arm and Wrist Muscle, Right
	Lower Arm and Wrist Muscle, Left
Flexor digitorum brevis muscle	Foot Muscle, Right
	Foot Muscle, Left
Flexor digitorum longus muscle	Lower Leg Muscle, Right
	Lower Leg Muscle, Left
Flexor hallucis brevis muscle	Foot Muscle, Right
	Foot Muscle, Left
Flexor hallucis longus muscle	Lower Leg Muscle, Right
	Lower Leg Muscle, Left
Flexor pollicis longus muscle	Lower Arm and Wrist Muscle, Right
	Lower Arm and Wrist Muscle, Left
Foramen magnum	Occipital Bone
Foramen of Monro (intraventricular)	Cerebral Ventricle
Foreskin	Prepuce
Fossa of Rosenmuller	Nasopharynx
Fourth cranial nerve	Trochlear Nerve
Fourth ventricle	Cerebral Ventricle
Fovea	Retina, Right
	Retina, Left
Frenulum labii inferioris	Lower Lip
Frenulum labii superioris	Upper Lip
Frenulum linguae	Tongue
Frontal lobe	Cerebral Hemisphere
Frontal vein	Face Vein, Right
	Face Vein, Left
Fundus uteri	Uterus
Galea aponeurotica	Subcutaneous Tissue and Fascia, Scalp
Ganglion impar (ganglion of Walther)	Sacral Sympathetic Nerve
Gasserian ganglion	Trigeminal Nerve
Gastric lymph node	Lymphatic, Aortic
Gastric plexus	Abdominal Sympathetic Nerve
Gastrocnemius muscle	Lower Leg Muscle, Right
	Lower Leg Muscle, Left
Gastrocolic ligament	Omentum
Gastrocolic omentum	Omentum
Gastroduodenal artery	Hepatic Artery
Gastroesophageal (GE) junction	Esophagogastric Junction
Gastrohepatic omentum	Omentum
Gastrophrenic ligament	Omentum
Gastrosplenic ligament	Omentum
Gemellus muscle	Hip Muscle, Right
	Hip Muscle, Left
Geniculate ganglion	Facial Nerve

Term	ICD-10-PCS Value
Geniculate nucleus	Thalamus
Genioglossus muscle	Tongue, Palate, Pharynx Muscle
Genitofemoral nerve	Lumbar Plexus
Glans penis	Prepuce
Glenohumeral joint	Shoulder Joint, Right
	Shoulder Joint, Left
Glenohumeral ligament	Shoulder Bursa and Ligament, Right
	Shoulder Bursa and Ligament, Left
Glenoid fossa (of scapula)	Glenoid Cavity, Right
	Glenoid Cavity, Left
Glenoid ligament (labrum)	Shoulder Joint, Right
	Shoulder Joint, Left
Globus pallidus	Basal Ganglia
Glossoepiglottic fold	Epiglottis
Glottis	Larynx
Gluteal lymph node	Lymphatic, Pelvis
Gluteal vein	Hypogastric Vein, Right
	Hypogastric Vein, Left
Gluteus maximus muscle	Hip Muscle, Right
	Hip Muscle, Left
Gluteus medius muscle	Hip Muscle, Right
	Hip Muscle, Left
Gluteus minimus muscle	Hip Muscle, Right
	Hip Muscle, Left
Gracilis muscle	Upper Leg Muscle, Right
	Upper Leg Muscle, Left
Great auricular nerve	Cervical Plexus
Great cerebral vein	Intracranial Vein
Great(er) saphenous vein	Saphenous Vein, Right
	Saphenous Vein, Left
Greater alar cartilage	Nasal Mucosa and Soft Tissue
Greater occipital nerve	Cervical Nerve
Greater omentum	Omentum
Greater splanchnic nerve	Thoracic Sympathetic Nerve
Greater superficial petrosal nerve	Facial Nerve
Greater trochanter	Upper Femur, Right
	Upper Femur, Left
Greater tuberosity	Humeral Head, Right
	Humeral Head, Left
Greater vestibular (Bartholin's) gland	Vestibular Gland
Greater wing	Sphenoid Bone
Hallux	1st Toe, Right
	1st Toe, Left
Hamate bone	Carpal, Right
	Carpal, Left
Head of fibula	Fibula, Right
	Fibula, Left
Helix	External Ear, Right
	External Ear, Left
	External Ear, Bilateral
Hepatic artery proper	Hepatic Artery
Hepatic flexure	Transverse Colon
Hepatic lymph node	Lymphatic, Aortic
Hepatic plexus	Abdominal Sympathetic Nerve
Hepatic portal vein	Portal Vein
Hepatogastric ligament	Omentum

Term	ICD-10-PCS Value
Hepatopancreatic ampulla	Ampulla of Vater
Humeroradial joint	Elbow Joint, Right
	Elbow Joint, Left
Humeroulnar joint	Elbow Joint, Right
	Elbow Joint, Left
Humerus, distal	Humeral Shaft, Right
	Humeral Shaft, Left
Hyoglossus muscle	Tongue, Palate, Pharynx Muscle
Hyoid artery	Thyroid Artery, Right
	Thyroid Artery, Left
Hypogastric artery	Internal Iliac Artery, Right
	Internal Iliac Artery, Left
Hypopharynx	Pharynx
Hypophysis	Pituitary Gland
Hypothenar muscle	Hand Muscle, Right
	Hand Muscle, Left
Ileal artery	Superior Mesenteric Artery
Ileocolic artery	Superior Mesenteric Artery
Ileocolic vein	Colic Vein
Iliac crest	Pelvic Bone, Right
	Pelvic Bone, Left
Iliac fascia	Subcutaneous Tissue and Fascia, Right Upper Leg
	Subcutaneous Tissue and Fascia, Left Upper Leg
Iliac lymph node	Lymphatic, Pelvis
Iliacus muscle	Hip Muscle, Right
	Hip Muscle, Left
Iliofemoral ligament	Hip Bursa and Ligament, Right
	Hip Bursa and Ligament, Left
Iliohypogastric nerve	Lumbar Plexus
Ilioinguinal nerve	Lumbar Plexus
Iliolumbar artery	Internal Iliac Artery, Right
	Internal Iliac Artery, Left
Iliolumbar ligament	Lower Spine Bursa and Ligament
Iliotibial tract (band)	Subcutaneous Tissue and Fascia, Right Upper Leg
	Subcutaneous Tissue and Fascia, Left Upper Leg
Ilium	Pelvic Bone, Right
	Pelvic Bone, Left
Incus	Auditory Ossicle, Right
	Auditory Ossicle, Left
Inferior cardiac nerve	Thoracic Sympathetic Nerve
Inferior cerebellar vein	Intracranial Vein
Inferior cerebral vein	Intracranial Vein
Inferior epigastric artery	External Iliac Artery, Right
	External Iliac Artery, Left
Inferior epigastric lymph node	Lymphatic, Pelvis
Inferior genicular artery	Popliteal Artery, Right
	Popliteal Artery, Left
Inferior gluteal artery	Internal Iliac Artery, Right
	Internal Iliac Artery, Left
Inferior gluteal nerve	Sacral Plexus
Inferior hypogastric plexus	Abdominal Sympathetic Nerve
Inferior labial artery	Face Artery
Inferior longitudinal muscle	Tongue, Palate, Pharynx Muscle

Term	ICD-10-PCS Value
Inferior mesenteric ganglion	Abdominal Sympathetic Nerve
Inferior mesenteric lymph node	Lymphatic, Mesenteric
Inferior mesenteric plexus	Abdominal Sympathetic Nerve
Inferior oblique muscle	Extraocular Muscle, Right
	Extraocular Muscle, Left
Inferior pancreaticoduodenal artery	Superior Mesenteric Artery
Inferior phrenic artery	Abdominal Aorta
Inferior rectus muscle	Extraocular Muscle, Right
	Extraocular Muscle, Left
Inferior suprarenal artery	Renal Artery, Right
	Renal Artery, Left
Inferior tarsal plate	Lower Eyelid, Right
	Lower Eyelid, Left
Inferior thyroid vein	Innominate Vein, Right
	Innominate Vein, Left
Inferior tibiofibular joint	Ankle Joint, Right
	Ankle Joint, Left
Inferior turbinate	Nasal Turbinate
Inferior ulnar collateral artery	Brachial Artery, Right
	Brachial Artery, Left
Inferior vesical artery	Internal Iliac Artery, Right
	Internal Iliac Artery, Left
Infraauricular lymph node	Lymphatic, Head
Infraclavicular (deltopectoral) lymph node	Lymphatic, Right Upper Extremity
	Lymphatic, Left Upper Extremity
Infrahyoid muscle	Neck Muscle, Right
	Neck Muscle, Left
Infraparotid lymph node	Lymphatic, Head
Infraspinatus fascia	Subcutaneous Tissue and Fascia, Right Upper Arm
	Subcutaneous Tissue and Fascia, Left Upper Arm
Infraspinatus muscle	Shoulder Muscle, Right
	Shoulder Muscle, Left
Infundibulopelvic ligament	Uterine Supporting Structure
Inguinal canal	Inguinal Region, Right
	Inguinal Region, Left
	Inguinal Region, Bilateral
Inguinal triangle	Inguinal Region, Right
	Inguinal Region, Left
	Inguinal Region, Bilateral
Interatrial septum	Atrial Septum
Intercarpal joint	Carpal Joint, Right
	Carpal Joint, Left
Intercarpal ligament	Hand Bursa and Ligament, Right
	Hand Bursa and Ligament, Left
Interclavicular ligament	Shoulder Bursa and Ligament, Right
	Shoulder Bursa and Ligament, Left
Intercostal lymph node	Lymphatic, Thorax
Intercostal muscle	Thorax Muscle, Right
	Thorax Muscle, Left
Intercostal nerve	Thoracic Nerve
Intercostobrachial nerve	Thoracic Nerve
Intercuneiform joint	Tarsal Joint, Right
	Tarsal Joint, Left

Term	ICD-10-PCS Value
Intercuneiform ligament	Foot Bursa and Ligament, Right
	Foot Bursa and Ligament, Left
Intermediate bronchus	Main Bronchus, Right
Intermediate cuneiform bone	Tarsal, Right
	Tarsal, Left
Internal anal sphincter	Anal Sphincter
Internal (basal) cerebral vein	Intracranial Vein
Internal carotid artery, intracranial portion	Intracranial Artery
Internal carotid plexus	Head and Neck Sympathetic Nerve
Internal iliac vein	Hypogastric Vein, Right
	Hypogastric Vein, Left
Internal maxillary artery	External Carotid Artery, Right
	External Carotid Artery, Left
Internal naris	Nasal Mucosa and Soft Tissue
Internal oblique muscle	Abdomen Muscle, Right
	Abdomen Muscle, Left
Internal pudendal artery	Internal Iliac Artery, Right
	Internal Iliac Artery, Left
Internal pudendal vein	Hypogastric Vein, Right
	Hypogastric Vein, Left
Internal thoracic artery	Internal Mammary Artery, Right
	Internal Mammary Artery, Left
	Subclavian Artery, Right
	Subclavian Artery, Left
Internal urethral sphincter	Urethra
Interphalangeal (IP) joint	Finger Phalangeal Joint, Right
	Finger Phalangeal Joint, Left
	Toe Phalangeal Joint, Right
	Toe Phalangeal Joint, Left
Interphalangeal ligament	Foot Bursa and Ligament, Right
	Foot Bursa and Ligament, Left
	Hand Bursa and Ligament, Right
	Hand Bursa and Ligament, Left
Interspinalis muscle	Trunk Muscle, Right
	Trunk Muscle, Left
Interspinous ligament, cervical	Head and Neck Bursa and Ligament
Interspinous ligament, lumbar	Lower Spine Bursa and Ligament
Interspinous ligament, thoracic	Upper Spine Bursa and Ligament
Intertransversarius muscle	Trunk Muscle, Right
	Trunk Muscle, Left
Intertransverse ligament, cervical	Head and Neck Bursa and Ligament
Intertransverse ligament, lumbar	Lower Spine Bursa and Ligament
Intertransverse ligament, thoracic	Upper Spine Bursa and Ligament
Interventricular foramen (Monro)	Cerebral Ventricle
Interventricular septum	Ventricular Septum
Intestinal lymphatic trunk	Cisterna Chyli
Ischiatic nerve	Sciatic Nerve
Ischiocavernosus muscle	Perineum Muscle
Ischiofemoral ligament	Hip Bursa and Ligament, Right
	Hip Bursa and Ligament, Left

Term	ICD-10-PCS Value
Ischium	Pelvic Bone, Right
	Pelvic Bone, Left
Jejunal artery	Superior Mesenteric Artery
Jugular body	Glomus Jugulare
Jugular lymph node	Lymphatic, Right Neck
	Lymphatic, Left Neck
Labia majora	Vulva
Labia minora	Vulva
Labial gland	Upper Lip
	Lower Lip
Lacrimal canaliculus	Lacrimal Duct, Right
	Lacrimal Duct, Left
Lacrimal punctum	Lacrimal Duct, Right
	Lacrimal Duct, Left
Lacrimal sac	Lacrimal Duct, Right
	Lacrimal Duct, Left
Laryngopharynx	Pharynx
Lateral (brachial) lymph node	Lymphatic, Right Axillary
	Lymphatic, Left Axillary
Lateral canthus	Upper Eyelid, Right
	Upper Eyelid, Left
Lateral collateral ligament (LCL)	Knee Bursa and Ligament, Right
	Knee Bursa and Ligament, Left
Lateral condyle of femur	Lower Femur, Right
	Lower Femur, Left
Lateral condyle of tibia	Tibia, Right
	Tibia, Left
Lateral cuneiform bone	Tarsal, Right
	Tarsal, Left
Lateral epicondyle of femur	Lower Femur, Right
	Lower Femur, Left
Lateral epicondyle of humerus	Humeral Shaft, Right
	Humeral Shaft, Left
Lateral femoral cutaneous nerve	Lumbar Plexus
Lateral malleolus	Fibula, Right
	Fibula, Left
Lateral meniscus	Knee Joint, Right
	Knee Joint, Left
Lateral nasal cartilage	Nasal Mucosa and Soft Tissue
Lateral plantar artery	Foot Artery, Right
	Foot Artery, Left
Lateral plantar nerve	Tibial Nerve
Lateral rectus muscle	Extraocular Muscle, Right
	Extraocular Muscle, Left
Lateral sacral artery	Internal Iliac Artery, Right
	Internal Iliac Artery, Left
Lateral sacral vein	Hypogastric Vein, Right
	Hypogastric Vein, Left
Lateral sural cutaneous nerve	Peroneal Nerve
Lateral tarsal artery	Foot Artery, Right
	Foot Artery, Left
Lateral temporo-mandibular ligament	Head and Neck Bursa and Ligament
Lateral thoracic artery	Axillary Artery, Right
	Axillary Artery, Left
Latissimus dorsi muscle	Trunk Muscle, Right
	Trunk Muscle, Left

Term	ICD-10-PCS Value
Least splanchnic nerve	Thoracic Sympathetic Nerve
Left ascending lumbar vein	Hemiazygos Vein
Left atrioventricular valve	Mitral Valve
Left auricular appendix	Atrium, Left
Left colic vein	Colic Vein
Left coronary sulcus	Heart, Left
Left gastric artery	Gastric Artery
Left gastroepiploic artery	Splenic Artery
Left gastroepiploic vein	Splenic Vein
Left inferior phrenic vein	Renal Vein, Left
Left inferior pulmonary vein	Pulmonary Vein, Left
Left jugular trunk	Thoracic Duct
Left lateral ventricle	Cerebral Ventricle
Left ovarian vein	Renal Vein, Left
Left second lumbar vein	Renal Vein, Left
Left subclavian trunk	Thoracic Duct
Left subcostal vein	Hemiazygos Vein
Left superior pulmonary vein	Pulmonary Vein, Left
Left suprarenal vein	Renal Vein, Left
Left testicular vein	Renal Vein, Left
Leptomeninges, intracranial	Cerebral Meninges
Leptomeninges, spinal	Spinal Meninges
Lesser alar cartilage	Nasal Mucosa and Soft Tissue
Lesser occipital nerve	Cervical Plexus
Lesser omentum	Omentum
Lesser saphenous vein	Saphenous Vein, Right
	Saphenous Vein, Left
Lesser splanchnic nerve	Thoracic Sympathetic Nerve
Lesser trochanter	Upper Femur, Right
	Upper Femur, Left
Lesser tuberosity	Humeral Head, Right
	Humeral Head, Left
Lesser wing	Sphenoid Bone
Levator anguli oris muscle	Facial Muscle
Levator ani muscle	Perineum Muscle
Levator labii superioris alaeque nasi muscle	Facial Muscle
Levator labii superioris muscle	Facial Muscle
Levator palpebrae superioris muscle	Upper Eyelid, Right
	Upper Eyelid, Left
Levator scapulae muscle	Neck Muscle, Right
	Neck Muscle, Left
Levator veli palatini muscle	Tongue, Palate, Pharynx Muscle
Levatores costarum muscle	Thorax Muscle, Right
	Thorax Muscle, Left
Ligament of head of fibula	Knee Bursa and Ligament, Right
	Knee Bursa and Ligament, Left
Ligament of the lateral malleolus	Ankle Bursa and Ligament, Right
	Ankle Bursa and Ligament, Left
Ligamentum flavum, cervical	Head and Neck Bursa and Ligament
Ligamentum flavum, lumbar	Lower Spine Bursa and Ligament
Ligamentum flavum, thoracic	Upper Spine Bursa and Ligament

Term	ICD-10-PCS Value
Lingual artery	External Carotid Artery, Right
	External Carotid Artery, Left
Lingual tonsil	Pharynx
Locus ceruleus	Pons
Long thoracic nerve	Brachial Plexus
Lumbar artery	Abdominal Aorta
Lumbar facet joint	Lumbar Vertebral Joint
Lumbar ganglion	Lumbar Sympathetic Nerve
Lumbar lymph node	Lymphatic, Aortic
Lumbar lymphatic trunk	Cisterna Chyli
Lumbar splanchnic nerve	Lumbar Sympathetic Nerve
Lumbosacral facet joint	Lumbosacral Joint
Lumbosacral trunk	Lumbar Nerve
Lunate bone	Carpal, Right
	Carpal, Left
Lunotriquetral ligament	Hand Bursa and Ligament, Right
	Hand Bursa and Ligament, Left
Macula	Retina, Right
	Retina, Left
Malleus	Auditory Ossicle, Right
	Auditory Ossicle, Left
Mammary duct	Breast, Right
	Breast, Left
	Breast, Bilateral
Mammary gland	Breast, Right
	Breast, Left
	Breast, Bilateral
Mammillary body	Hypothalamus
Mandibular nerve	Trigeminal Nerve
Mandibular notch	Mandible, Right
	Mandible, Left
Manubrium	Sternum
Masseter muscle	Head Muscle
Masseteric fascia	Subcutaneous Tissue and Fascia, Face
Mastoid (postauricular) lymph node	Lymphatic, Right Neck
	Lymphatic, Left Neck
Mastoid air cells	Mastoid Sinus, Right
	Mastoid Sinus, Left
Mastoid process	Temporal Bone, Right
	Temporal Bone, Left
Maxillary artery	External Carotid Artery, Right
	External Carotid Artery, Left
Maxillary nerve	Trigeminal Nerve
Medial canthus	Lower Eyelid, Right
	Lower Eyelid, Left
Medial collateral ligament (MCL)	Knee Bursa and Ligament, Right
	Knee Bursa and Ligament, Left
Medial condyle of femur	Lower Femur, Right
	Lower Femur, Left
Medial condyle of tibia	Tibia, Right
	Tibia, Left
Medial cuneiform bone	Tarsal, Right
	Tarsal, Left
Medial epicondyle of femur	Lower Femur, Right
	Lower Femur, Left
Medial epicondyle of humerus	Humeral Shaft, Right
	Humeral Shaft, Left

Term	ICD-10-PCS Value
Medial malleolus	Tibia, Right
	Tibia, Left
Medial meniscus	Knee Joint, Right
	Knee Joint, Left
Medial plantar artery	Foot Artery, Right
	Foot Artery, Left
Medial plantar nerve	Tibial Nerve
Medial popliteal nerve	Tibial Nerve
Medial rectus muscle	Extraocular Muscle, Right
	Extraocular Muscle, Left
Medial sural cutaneous nerve	Tibial Nerve
Median antebrachial vein	Basilic Vein, Right
	Basilic Vein, Left
Median cubital vein	Basilic Vein, Right
	Basilic Vein, Left
Median sacral artery	Abdominal Aorta
Mediastinal cavity	Mediastinum
Mediastinal lymph node	Lymphatic, Thorax
Mediastinal space	Mediastinum
Meissner's (submucous) plexus	Abdominal Sympathetic Nerve
Membranous urethra	Urethra
Mental foramen	Mandible, Right
	Mandible, Left
Mentalis muscle	Facial Muscle
Mesoappendix	Mesentery
Mesocolon	Mesentery
Metacarpal ligament	Hand Bursa and Ligament, Right
	Hand Bursa and Ligament, Left
Metacarpophalangeal ligament	Hand Bursa and Ligament, Right
	Hand Bursa and Ligament, Left
Metatarsal ligament	Foot Bursa and Ligament, Right
	Foot Bursa and Ligament, Left
Metatarsophalangeal ligament	Foot Bursa and Ligament, Right
	Foot Bursa and Ligament, Left
Metatarsophalangeal (MTP) joint	Metatarsal-Phalangeal Joint, Right
	Metatarsal-Phalangeal Joint, Left
Metathalamus	Thalamus
Midcarpal joint	Carpal Joint, Right
	Carpal Joint, Left
Middle cardiac nerve	Thoracic Sympathetic Nerve
Middle cerebral artery	Intracranial Artery
Middle cerebral vein	Intracranial Vein
Middle colic vein	Colic Vein
Middle genicular artery	Popliteal Artery, Right
	Popliteal Artery, Left
Middle hemorrhoidal vein	Hypogastric Vein, Right
	Hypogastric Vein, Left
Middle rectal artery	Internal Iliac Artery, Right
	Internal Iliac Artery, Left
Middle suprarenal artery	Abdominal Aorta
Middle temporal artery	Temporal Artery, Right
	Temporal Artery, Left
Middle turbinate	Nasal Turbinate
Mitral annulus	Mitral Valve
Molar gland	Buccal Mucosa
Musculocutaneous nerve	Brachial Plexus
Musculophrenic artery	Internal Mammary Artery, Right
	Internal Mammary Artery, Left
Musculospiral nerve	Radial Nerve
Myelencephalon	Medulla Oblongata
Myenteric (Auerbach's) plexus	Abdominal Sympathetic Nerve
Myometrium	Uterus
Nail bed	Finger Nail
	Toe Nail
Nail plate	Finger Nail
	Toe Nail
Nasal cavity	Nasal Mucosa and Soft Tissue
Nasal concha	Nasal Turbinate
Nasalis muscle	Facial Muscle
Nasolacrimal duct	Lacrimal Duct, Right
	Lacrimal Duct, Left
Navicular bone	Tarsal, Right
	Tarsal, Left
Neck of femur	Upper Femur, Right
	Upper Femur, Left
Neck of humerus (anatomical) (surgical)	Humeral Head, Right
	Humeral Head, Left
Nerve to the stapedius	Facial Nerve
Neurohypophysis	Pituitary Gland
Ninth cranial nerve	Glossopharyngeal Nerve
Nostril	Nasal Mucosa and Soft Tissue
Obturator artery	Internal Iliac Artery, Right
	Internal Iliac Artery, Left
Obturator lymph node	Lymphatic, Pelvis
Obturator muscle	Hip Muscle, Right
	Hip Muscle, Left
Obturator nerve	Lumbar Plexus
Obturator vein	Hypogastric Vein, Right
	Hypogastric Vein, Left
Obtuse margin	Heart, Left
Occipital artery	External Carotid Artery, Right
	External Carotid Artery, Left
Occipital lobe	Cerebral Hemisphere
Occipital lymph node	Lymphatic, Right Neck
	Lymphatic, Left Neck
Occipitofrontalis muscle	Facial Muscle
Odontoid process	Cervical Vertebra
Olecranon bursa	Elbow Bursa and Ligament, Right
	Elbow Bursa and Ligament, Left
Olecranon process	Ulna, Right
	Ulna, Left
Olfactory bulb	Olfactory Nerve
Ophthalmic artery	Intracranial Artery
Ophthalmic nerve	Trigeminal Nerve
Ophthalmic vein	Intracranial Vein
Optic chiasma	Optic Nerve
Optic disc	Retina, Right
	Retina, Left
Optic foramen	Sphenoid Bone
Orbicularis oculi muscle	Upper Eyelid, Right
	Upper Eyelid, Left
Orbicularis oris muscle	Facial Muscle
Orbital fascia	Subcutaneous Tissue and Fascia, Face

Term	ICD-10-PCS Value
Orbital portion of ethmoid bone	Orbit, Right
	Orbit, Left
Orbital portion of frontal bone	Orbit, Right
	Orbit, Left
Orbital portion of lacrimal bone	Orbit, Right
	Orbit, Left
Orbital portion of maxilla	Orbit, Right
	Orbit, Left
Orbital portion of palatine bone	Orbit, Right
	Orbit, Left
Orbital portion of sphenoid bone	Orbit, Right
	Orbit, Left
Orbital portion of zygomatic bone	Orbit, Right
	Orbit, Left
Oropharynx	Pharynx
Otic ganglion	Head and Neck Sympathetic Nerve
Oval window	Middle Ear, Right
	Middle Ear, Left
Ovarian artery	Abdominal Aorta
Ovarian ligament	Uterine Supporting Structure
Oviduct	Fallopian Tube, Right
	Fallopian Tube, Left
Palatine gland	Buccal Mucosa
Palatine tonsil	Tonsils
Palatine uvula	Uvula
Palatoglossal muscle	Tongue, Palate, Pharynx Muscle
Palatopharyngeal muscle	Tongue, Palate, Pharynx Muscle
Palmar (volar) digital vein	Hand Vein, Right
	Hand Vein, Left
Palmar (volar) metacarpal vein	Hand Vein, Right
	Hand Vein, Left
Palmar cutaneous nerve	Median Nerve
	Radial Nerve
Palmar fascia (aponeurosis)	Subcutaneous Tissue and Fascia, Right Hand
	Subcutaneous Tissue and Fascia, Left Hand
Palmar interosseous muscle	Hand Muscle, Right
	Hand Muscle, Left
Palmar ulnocarpal ligament	Wrist Bursa and Ligament, Right
	Wrist Bursa and Ligament, Left
Palmaris longus muscle	Lower Arm and Wrist Muscle, Right
	Lower Arm and Wrist Muscle, Left
Pancreatic artery	Splenic Artery
Pancreatic plexus	Abdominal Sympathetic Nerve
Pancreatic vein	Splenic Vein
Pancreaticosplenic lymph node	Lymphatic, Aortic
Paraaortic lymph node	Lymphatic, Aortic
Parapharyngeal space	Neck
Pararectal lymph node	Lymphatic, Mesenteric
Parasternal lymph node	Lymphatic, Thorax
Paratracheal lymph node	Lymphatic, Thorax
Paraurethral (Skene's) gland	Vestibular Gland
Parietal lobe	Cerebral Hemisphere
Parotid lymph node	Lymphatic, Head
Parotid plexus	Facial Nerve

Term	ICD-10-PCS Value
Pars flaccida	Tympanic Membrane, Right
	Tympanic Membrane, Left
Patellar ligament	Knee Bursa and Ligament, Right
	Knee Bursa and Ligament, Left
Patellar tendon	Knee Tendon, Right
	Knee Tendon, Left
Patellofemoral joint	Knee Joint, Right
	Knee Joint, Left
	Knee Joint, Femoral Surface, Right
	Knee Joint, Femoral Surface, Left
Pectineus muscle	Upper Leg Muscle, Right
	Upper Leg Muscle, Left
Pectoral (anterior) lymph node	Lymphatic, Right Axillary
	Lymphatic, Left Axillary
Pectoral fascia	Subcutaneous Tissue and Fascia, Chest
Pectoralis major muscle	Thorax Muscle, Right
	Thorax Muscle, Left
Pectoralis minor muscle	Thorax Muscle, Right
	Thorax Muscle, Left
Pelvic splanchnic nerve	Abdominal Sympathetic Nerve
	Sacral Sympathetic Nerve
Penile urethra	Urethra
Pericardiophrenic artery	Internal Mammary Artery, Right
	Internal Mammary Artery, Left
Perimetrium	Uterus
Peroneus brevis muscle	Lower Leg Muscle, Right
	Lower Leg Muscle, Left
Peroneus longus muscle	Lower Leg Muscle, Right
	Lower Leg Muscle, Left
Petrous part of temporal bone	Temporal Bone, Right
	Temporal Bone, Left
Pharyngeal constrictor muscle	Tongue, Palate, Pharynx Muscle
Pharyngeal plexus	Vagus Nerve
Pharyngeal recess	Nasopharynx
Pharyngeal tonsil	Adenoids
Pharyngotympanic tube	Eustachian Tube, Right
	Eustachian Tube, Left
Pia mater, intracranial	Cerebral Meninges
Pia mater, spinal	Spinal Meninges
Pinna	External Ear, Right
	External Ear, Left
	External Ear, Bilateral
Piriform recess (sinus)	Pharynx
Piriformis muscle	Hip Muscle, Right
	Hip Muscle, Left
Pisiform bone	Carpal, Right
	Carpal, Left
Pisohamate ligament	Hand Bursa and Ligament, Right
	Hand Bursa and Ligament, Left
Pisometacarpal ligament	Hand Bursa and Ligament, Right
	Hand Bursa and Ligament, Left
Plantar digital vein	Foot Vein, Right
	Foot Vein, Left
Plantar fascia (aponeurosis)	Subcutaneous Tissue and Fascia, Right Foot
	Subcutaneous Tissue and Fascia, Left Foot

Term	ICD-10-PCS Value
Plantar metatarsal vein	Foot Vein, Right
	Foot Vein, Left
Plantar venous arch	Foot Vein, Right
	Foot Vein, Left
Platysma muscle	Neck Muscle, Right
	Neck Muscle, Left
Plica semilunaris	Conjunctiva, Right
	Conjunctiva, Left
Pneumogastric nerve	Vagus Nerve
Pneumotaxic center	Pons
Pontine tegmentum	Pons
Popliteal ligament	Knee Bursa and Ligament, Right
	Knee Bursa and Ligament, Left
Popliteallymph node	Lymphatic, Left Lower Extremity
	Lymphatic, Right Lower Extremity
Popliteal vein	Femoral Vein, Right
	Femoral Vein, Left
Popliteus muscle	Lower Leg Muscle, Right
	Lower Leg Muscle, Left
Postauricular (mastoid) lymph node	Lymphatic, Right Neck
	Lymphatic, Left Neck
Postcava	Inferior Vena Cava
Posterior (subscapular) lymph node	Lymphatic, Right Axillary
	Lymphatic, Left Axillary
Posterior auricular artery	External Carotid Artery, Right
	External Carotid Artery, Left
Posterior auricular nerve	Facial Nerve
Posterior auricular vein	External Jugular Vein, Right
	External Jugular Vein, Left
Posterior cerebral artery	Intracranial Artery
Posterior chamber	Eye, Right
	Eye, Left
Posterior circumflex humeral artery	Axillary Artery, Right
	Axillary Artery, Left
Posterior communicating artery	Intracranial Artery
Posterior cruciate ligament (PCL)	Knee Bursa and Ligament, Right
	Knee Bursa and Ligament, Left
Posterior facial (retromandibular) vein	Face Vein, Right
	Face Vein, Left
Posterior femoral cutaneous nerve	Sacral Plexus
Posterior inferior cerebellar artery (PICA)	Intracranial Artery
Posterior interosseous nerve	Radial Nerve
Posterior labial nerve	Pudendal Nerve
Posterior scrotal nerve	Pudendal Nerve
Posterior spinal artery	Vertebral Artery, Right
	Vertebral Artery, Left
Posterior tibial recurrent artery	Anterior Tibial Artery, Right
	Anterior Tibial Artery, Left
Posterior ulnar recurrent artery	Ulnar Artery, Right
	Ulnar Artery, Left
Posterior vagal trunk	Vagus Nerve
Preauricular lymph node	Lymphatic, Head
Precava	Superior Vena Cava
Prepatellar bursa	Knee Bursa and Ligament, Right
	Knee Bursa and Ligament, Left

Term	ICD-10-PCS Value
Pretracheal fascia	Subcutaneous Tissue and Fascia, Right Neck
	Subcutaneous Tissue and Fascia, Left Neck
Prevertebral fascia	Subcutaneous Tissue and Fascia, Right Neck
	Subcutaneous Tissue and Fascia, Left Neck
Princeps pollicis artery	Hand Artery, Right
	Hand Artery, Left
Procerus muscle	Facial Muscle
Profunda brachii	Brachial Artery, Right
	Brachial Artery, Left
Profunda femoris (deep femoral) vein	Femoral Vein, Right
	Femoral Vein, Left
Pronator quadratus muscle	Lower Arm and Wrist Muscle, Right
	Lower Arm and Wrist Muscle, Left
Pronator teres muscle	Lower Arm and Wrist Muscle, Right
	Lower Arm and Wrist Muscle, Left
Prostatic urethra	Urethra
Proximal radioulnar joint	Elbow Joint, Right
	Elbow Joint, Left
Psoas muscle	Hip Muscle, Right
	Hip Muscle, Left
Pterygoid muscle	Head Muscle
Pterygoid process	Sphenoid Bone
Pterygopalatine (sphenopalatine) ganglion	Head and Neck Sympathetic Nerve
Pubis	Pelvic Bone, Right
	Pelvic Bone, Left
Pubofemoral ligament	Hip Bursa and Ligament, Right
	Hip Bursa and Ligament, Left
Pudendal nerve	Sacral Plexus
Pulmoaortic canal	Pulmonary Artery, Left
Pulmonary annulus	Pulmonary Valve
Pulmonary plexus	Thoracic Sympathetic Nerve
	Vagus Nerve
Pulmonic valve	Pulmonary Valve
Pulvinar	Thalamus
Pyloric antrum	Stomach, Pylorus
Pyloric canal	Stomach, Pylorus
Pyloric sphincter	Stomach, Pylorus
Pyramidalis muscle	Abdomen Muscle, Right
	Abdomen Muscle, Left
Quadrangular cartilage	Nasal Septum
Quadrate lobe	Liver
Quadratus femoris muscle	Hip Muscle, Right
	Hip Muscle, Left
Quadratus lumborum muscle	Trunk Muscle, Right
	Trunk Muscle, Left
Quadratus plantae muscle	Foot Muscle, Right
	Foot Muscle, Left
Quadriceps (femoris)	Upper Leg Muscle, Right
	Upper Leg Muscle, Left
Radial collateral carpal ligament	Wrist Bursa and Ligament, Right
	Wrist Bursa and Ligament, Left
Radial collateral ligament	Elbow Bursa and Ligament, Right
	Elbow Bursa and Ligament, Left
Radial notch	Ulna, Right
	Ulna, Left

Term	ICD-10-PCS Value
Radial recurrent artery	Radial Artery, Right
	Radial Artery, Left
Radial vein	Brachial Vein, Right
	Brachial Vein, Left
Radialis indicis	Hand Artery, Right
	Hand Artery, Left
Radiocarpal joint	Wrist Joint, Right
	Wrist Joint, Left
Radiocarpal ligament	Wrist Bursa and Ligament, Right
	Wrist Bursa and Ligament, Left
Radioulnar ligament	Wrist Bursa and Ligament, Right
	Wrist Bursa and Ligament, Left
Rectosigmoid junction	Sigmoid Colon
Rectus abdominis muscle	Abdomen Muscle, Right
	Abdomen Muscle, Left
Rectus femoris muscle	Upper Leg Muscle, Right
	Upper Leg Muscle, Left
Recurrent laryngeal nerve	Vagus Nerve
Renal calyx	Kidney, Right
	Kidney, Left
	Kidneys, Bilateral
	Kidney
Renal capsule	Kidney, Right
	Kidney, Left
	Kidneys, Bilateral
	Kidney
Renal cortex	Kidney, Right
	Kidney, Left
	Kidneys, Bilateral
	Kidney
Renal nerve	Abdominal sympathetic Nerve
Renal plexus	Abdominal Sympathetic Nerve
Renal segment	Kidney, Right
	Kidney, Left
	Kidneys, Bilateral
	Kidney
Renal segmental artery	Renal Artery, Right
	Renal Artery, Left
Retroperitoneal cavity	Retroperitoneum
Retroperitoneal lymph node	Lymphatic, Aortic
Retroperitoneal space	Retroperitoneum
Retropharyngeal lymph node	Lymphatic, Right Neck
	Lymphatic, Left Neck
Retropharyngeal space	Neck
Retropubic space	Pelvic Cavity
Rhinopharynx	Nasopharynx
Rhomboid major muscle	Trunk Muscle, Right
	Trunk Muscle, Left
Rhomboid minor muscle	Trunk Muscle, Right
	Trunk Muscle, Left
Right ascending lumbar vein	Azygos Vein
Right atrioventricular valve	Tricuspid Valve
Right auricular appendix	Atrium, Right
Right colic vein	Colic Vein
Right coronary sulcus	Heart, Right
Right gastric artery	Gastric Artery

Term	ICD-10-PCS Value
Right gastroepiploic vein	Superior Mesenteric Vein
Right inferior phrenic vein	Inferior Vena Cava
Right inferior pulmonary vein	Pulmonary Vein, Right
Right jugular trunk	Lymphatic, Right Neck
Right lateral ventricle	Cerebral Ventricle
Right lymphatic duct	Lymphatic, Right Neck
Right ovarian vein	Inferior Vena Cava
Right second lumbar vein	Inferior Vena Cava
Right subclavian trunk	Lymphatic, Right Neck
Right subcostal vein	Azygos Vein
Right superior pulmonary vein	Pulmonary Vein, Right
Right suprarenal vein	Inferior Vena Cava
Right testicular vein	Inferior Vena Cava
Rima glottidis	Larynx
Risorius muscle	Facial Muscle
Round ligament of uterus	Uterine Supporting Structure
Round window	Inner Ear, Right
	Inner Ear, Left
Sacral ganglion	Sacral Sympathetic Nerve
Sacral lymph node	Lymphatic, Pelvis
Sacral splanchnic nerve	Sacral Sympathetic Nerve
Sacrococcygeal ligament	Lower Spine Bursa and Ligament
Sacrococcygeal symphysis	Sacrococcygeal Joint
Sacroiliac ligament	Lower Spine Bursa and Ligament
Sacrospinous ligament	Lower Spine Bursa and Ligament
Sacrotuberous ligament	Lower Spine Bursa and Ligament
Salpingopharyngeus muscle	Tongue, Palate, Pharynx Muscle
Salpinx	Fallopian Tube, Right
	Fallopian Tube, Left
Saphenous nerve	Femoral Nerve
Sartorius muscle	Upper Leg Muscle, Right
	Upper Leg Muscle, Left
Scalene muscle	Neck Muscle, Right
	Neck Muscle, Left
Scaphoid bone	Carpal, Right
	Carpal, Left
Scapholunate ligament	Wrist Bursa and Ligament, Right
	Wrist Bursa and Ligament, Left
Scaphotrapezium ligament	Hand Bursa and Ligament, Right
	Hand Bursa and Ligament, Left
Scarpa's (vestibular) ganglion	Acoustic Nerve
Sebaceous gland	Skin
Second cranial nerve	Optic Nerve
Sella turcica	Sphenoid Bone
Semicircular canal	Inner Ear, Right
	Inner Ear, Left
Semimembranosus muscle	Upper Leg Muscle, Right
	Upper Leg Muscle, Left
Semitendinosus muscle	Upper Leg Muscle, Right
	Upper Leg Muscle, Left
Septal cartilage	Nasal Septum
Serratus anterior muscle	Thorax Muscle, Right
	Thorax Muscle, Left
Serratus posterior muscle	Trunk Muscle, Right
	Trunk Muscle, Left

Term	ICD-10-PCS Value
Seventh cranial nerve	Facial Nerve
Short gastric artery	Splenic Artery
Sigmoid artery	Inferior Mesenteric Artery
Sigmoid flexure	Sigmoid Colon
Sigmoid vein	Inferior Mesenteric Vein
Sinoatrial node	Conduction Mechanism
Sinus venosus	Atrium, Right
Sixth cranial nerve	Abducens Nerve
Skene's (paraurethral) gland	Vestibular Gland
Small saphenous vein	Saphenous Vein, Right
	Saphenous Vein, Left
Solar (celiac) plexus	Abdominal Sympathetic Nerve
Soleus muscle	Lower Leg Muscle, Right
	Lower Leg Muscle, Left
Sphenomandibular ligament	Head and Neck Bursa and Ligament
Sphenopalatine (pterygopalatine) ganglion	Head and Neck Sympathetic Nerve
Spinal nerve, cervical	Cervical Nerve
Spinal nerve, lumbar	Lumbar Nerve
Spinal nerve, sacral	Sacral Nerve
Spinal nerve, thoracic	Thoracic Nerve
Spinous process	Cervical Vertebra
	Lumbar Vertebra
	Thoracic Vertebra
Spiral ganglion	Acoustic Nerve
Splenic flexure	Transverse Colon
Splenic plexus	Abdominal Sympathetic Nerve
Splenius capitis muscle	Head Muscle
Splenius cervicis muscle	Neck Muscle, Right
	Neck Muscle, Left
Stapes	Auditory Ossicle, Right
	Auditory Ossicle, Left
Stellate ganglion	Head and Neck Sympathetic Nerve
Stensen's duct	Parotid Duct, Right
	Parotid Duct, Left
Sternoclavicular ligament	Shoulder Bursa and Ligament, Right
	Shoulder Bursa and Ligament, Left
Sternocleidomastoid artery	Thyroid Artery, Right
	Thyroid Artery, Left
Sternocleidomastoid muscle	Neck Muscle, Right
	Neck Muscle, Left
Sternocostal ligament	Sternum Bursa and Ligament
Styloglossus muscle	Tongue, Palate, Pharynx Muscle
Stylomandibular ligament	Head and Neck Bursa and Ligament
Stylopharyngeus muscle	Tongue, Palate, Pharynx Muscle
Subacromial bursa	Shoulder Bursa and Ligament, Right
	Shoulder Bursa and Ligament, Left
Subaortic (common iliac) lymph node	Lymphatic, Pelvis
Subarachnoid space, spinal	Spinal Canal
Subclavicular (apical) lymph node	Lymphatic, Right Axillary
	Lymphatic, Left Axillary
Subclavius muscle	Thorax Muscle, Right
	Thorax Muscle, Left
Subclavius nerve	Brachial Plexus
Subcostal artery	Upper Artery

Term	ICD-10-PCS Value
Subcostal muscle	Thorax Muscle, Right
	Thorax Muscle, Left
Subcostal nerve	Thoracic Nerve
Subdural space, spinal	Spinal Canal
Submandibular ganglion	Facial Nerve
	Head and Neck Sympathetic Nerve
Submandibular gland	Submaxillary Gland, Right
	Submaxillary Gland, Left
Submandibular lymph node	Lymphatic, Head
Submandibular space	Subcutaneous Tissue and Fascia, Face
Submaxillary ganglion	Head and Neck Sympathetic Nerve
Submaxillary lymph node	Lymphatic, Head
Submental artery	Face Artery
Submental lymph node	Lymphatic, Head
Submucous (Meissner's) plexus	Abdominal Sympathetic Nerve
Suboccipital nerve	Cervical Nerve
Suboccipital venous plexus	Vertebral Vein, Right
	Vertebral Vein, Left
Subparotid lymph node	Lymphatic, Head
Subscapular aponeurosis	Subcutaneous Tissue and Fascia, Right Upper Arm
	Subcutaneous Tissue and Fascia, Left Upper Arm
Subscapular artery	Axillary Artery, Right
	Axillary Artery, Left
Subscapular (posterior) lymph node	Lymphatic, Right Axillary
	Lymphatic, Left Axillary
Subscapularis muscle	Shoulder Muscle, Right
	Shoulder Muscle, Left
Substantia nigra	Basal Ganglia
Subtalar (talocalcaneal) joint	Tarsal Joint, Right
	Tarsal Joint, Left
Subtalar ligament	Foot Bursa and Ligament, Right
	Foot Bursa and Ligament, Left
Subthalamic nucleus	Basal Ganglia
Superficial circumflex iliac vein	Saphenous Vein, Right
	Saphenous Vein, Left
Superficial epigastric artery	Femoral Artery, Right
	Femoral Artery, Left
Superficial epigastric vein	Saphenous Vein, Right
	Saphenous Vein, Left
Superficial palmar arch	Hand Artery, Right
	Hand Artery, Left
Superficial palmar venous arch	Hand Vein, Right
	Hand Vein, Left
Superficial temporal artery	Temporal Artery, Right
	Temporal Artery, Left
Superficial transverse perineal muscle	Perineum Muscle
Superior cardiac nerve	Thoracic Sympathetic Nerve
Superior cerebellar vein	Intracranial Vein
Superior cerebral vein	Intracranial Vein
Superior clunic (cluneal) nerve	Lumbar Nerve
Superior epigastric artery	Internal Mammary Artery, Right
	Internal Mammary Artery, Left

Term	ICD-10-PCS Value
Superior genicular artery	Popliteal Artery, Right
	Popliteal Artery, Left
Superior gluteal artery	Internal Iliac Artery, Right
	Internal Iliac Artery, Left
Superior gluteal nerve	Lumbar Plexus
Superior hypogastric plexus	Abdominal Sympathetic Nerve
Superior labial artery	Face Artery
Superior laryngeal artery	Thyroid Artery, Right
	Thyroid Artery, Left
Superior laryngeal nerve	Vagus Nerve
Superior longitudinal muscle	Tongue, Palate, Pharynx Muscle
Superior mesenteric ganglion	Abdominal Sympathetic Nerve
Superior mesenteric lymph node	Lymphatic, Mesenteric
Superior mesenteric plexus	Abdominal Sympathetic Nerve
Superior oblique muscle	Extraocular Muscle, Right
	Extraocular Muscle, Left
Superior olivary nucleus	Pons
Superior rectal artery	Inferior Mesenteric Artery
Superior rectal vein	Inferior Mesenteric Vein
Superior rectus muscle	Extraocular Muscle, Right
	Extraocular Muscle, Left
Superior tarsal plate	Upper Eyelid, Right
	Upper Eyelid, Left
Superior thoracic artery	Axillary Artery, Right
	Axillary Artery, Left
Superior thyroid artery	External Carotid Artery, Right
	External Carotid Artery, Left
	Thyroid Artery, Right
	Thyroid Artery, Left
Superior turbinate	Nasal Turbinate
Superior ulnar collateral artery	Brachial Artery, Right
	Brachial Artery, Left
Supraclavicular nerve	Cervical Plexus
Supraclavicular (Virchow's) lymph node	Lymphatic, Right Neck
	Lymphatic, Left Neck
Suprahyoid lymph node	Lymphatic, Head
Suprahyoid muscle	Neck Muscle, Right
	Neck Muscle, Left
Suprainguinal lymph node	Lymphatic, Pelvis
Supraorbital vein	Face Vein, Right
	Face Vein, Left
Suprarenal gland	Adrenal Gland, Right
	Adrenal Gland, Left
	Adrenal Glands, Bilateral
	Adrenal Gland
Suprarenal plexus	Abdominal Sympathetic Nerve
Suprascapular nerve	Brachial Plexus
Supraspinatus fascia	Subcutaneous Tissue and Fascia, Right Upper Arm
	Subcutaneous Tissue and Fascia, Left Upper Arm
Supraspinatus muscle	Shoulder Muscle, Right
	Shoulder Muscle, Left
Supraspinous ligament	Upper Spine Bursa and Ligament
	Lower Spine Bursa and Ligament

Term	ICD-10-PCS Value
Suprasternal notch	Sternum
Supratrochlear lymph node	Lymphatic, Right Upper Extremity
	Lymphatic, Left Upper Extremity
Sural artery	Popliteal Artery, Right
	Popliteal Artery, Left
Sweat gland	Skin
Talocalcaneal ligament	Foot Bursa and Ligament, Right
	Foot Bursa and Ligament, Left
Talocalcaneal (subtalar) joint	Tarsal Joint, Right
	Tarsal Joint, Left
Talocalcaneonavicular joint	Tarsal Joint, Right
	Tarsal Joint, Left
Talocalcaneonavicular ligament	Foot Bursa and Ligament, Right
	Foot Bursa and Ligament, Left
Talocrural joint	Ankle Joint, Right
	Ankle Joint, Left
Talofibular ligament	Ankle Bursa and Ligament, Right
	Ankle Bursa and Ligament, Left
Talus bone	Tarsal, Right
	Tarsal, Left
Tarsometatarsal ligament	Foot Bursa and Ligament, Right
	Foot Bursa and Ligament, Left
Temporal lobe	Cerebral Hemisphere
Temporalis muscle	Head Muscle
Temporoparietalis muscle	Head Muscle
Tensor fasciae latae muscle	Hip Muscle, Right
	Hip Muscle, Left
Tensor veli palatini muscle	Tongue, Palate, Pharynx Muscle
Tenth cranial nerve	Vagus Nerve
Tentorium cerebelli	Dura Mater
Teres major muscle	Shoulder Muscle, Right
	Shoulder Muscle, Left
Teres minor muscle	Shoulder Muscle, Right
	Shoulder Muscle, Left
Testicular artery	Abdominal Aorta
Thenar muscle	Hand Muscle, Right
	Hand Muscle, Left
Third cranial nerve	Oculomotor Nerve
Third occipital nerve	Cervical Nerve
Third ventricle	Cerebral Ventricle
Thoracic aortic plexus	Thoracic Sympathetic Nerve
Thoracic esophagus	Esophagus, Middle
Thoracic facet joint	Thoracic Vertebral Joint
Thoracic ganglion	Thoracic Sympathetic Nerve
Thoracoacromial artery	Axillary Artery, Right
	Axillary Artery, Left
Thoracolumbar facet joint	Thoracolumbar Vertebral Joint
Thymus gland	Thymus
Thyroarytenoid muscle	Neck Muscle, Right
	Neck Muscle, Left
Thyrocervical trunk	Thyroid Artery, Right
	Thyroid Artery, Left
Thyroid cartilage	Larynx
Tibial sesamoid	Metatarsal, Right
	Metatarsal, Left
Tibialis anterior muscle	Lower Leg Muscle, Right
	Lower Leg Muscle, Left

Term	ICD-10-PCS Value
Tibialis posterior muscle	Lower Leg Muscle, Right
	Lower Leg Muscle, Left
Tibiofemoral joint	Knee Joint, Right
	Knee Joint, Left
	Knee Joint, Tibial Surface, Right
	Knee Joint, Tibial Surface, Left
Tibioperoneal trunk	Popliteal Artery, Right
	Popliteal Artery, Left
Tongue, base of	Pharynx
Tracheobronchial lymph node	Lymphatic, Thorax
Tragus	External Ear, Right
	External Ear, Left
	External Ear, Bilateral
Transversalis fascia	Subcutaneous Tissue and Fascia, Trunk
Transverse acetabular ligament	Hip Bursa and Ligament, Right
	Hip Bursa and Ligament, Left
Transverse (cutaneous) cervical nerve	Cervical Plexus
Transverse facial artery	Temporal Artery, Right
	Temporal Artery, Left
Transverse foramen	Cervical Vertebra
Transverse humeral ligament	Shoulder Bursa and Ligament, Right
	Shoulder Bursa and Ligament, Left
Transverse ligament of atlas	Head and Neck Bursa and Ligament
Transverse process	Cervical Vertebra
	Thoracic Vertebra
	Lumbar Vertebra
Transverse scapular ligament	Shoulder Bursa and Ligament, Right
	Shoulder Bursa and Ligament, Left
Transverse thoracis muscle	Thorax Muscle, Right
	Thorax Muscle, Left
Transversospinalis muscle	Trunk Muscle, Right
	Trunk Muscle, Left
Transversus abdominis muscle	Abdomen Muscle, Right
	Abdomen Muscle, Left
Trapezium bone	Carpal, Right
	Carpal, Left
Trapezius muscle	Trunk Muscle, Right
	Trunk Muscle, Left
Trapezoid bone	Carpal, Right
	Carpal, Left
Triceps brachii muscle	Upper Arm Muscle, Right
	Upper Arm Muscle, Left
Tricuspid annulus	Tricuspid Valve
Trifacial nerve	Trigeminal Nerve
Trigone of bladder	Bladder
Triquetral bone	Carpal, Right
	Carpal, Left
Trochantericbursa	Hip Bursa and Ligament, Right
	Hip Bursa and Ligament, Left
Twelfth cranial nerve	Hypoglossal Nerve
Tympanic cavity	Middle Ear, Right
	Middle Ear, Left
Tympanic nerve	Glossopharyngeal Nerve
Tympanic part of temoporal bone	Temporal Bone, Right
	Temporal Bone, Left

Term	ICD-10-PCS Value
Ulnar collateral carpal ligament	Wrist Bursa and Ligament, Right
	Wrist Bursa and Ligament, Left
Ulnar collateral ligament	Elbow Bursa and Ligament, Right
	Elbow Bursa and Ligament, Left
Ulnar notch	Radius, Right
	Radius, Left
Ulnar vein	Brachial Vein, Right
	Brachial Vein, Left
Umbilical artery	Internal Iliac Artery, Right
	Internal Iliac Artery, Left
	Lower Artery
Ureteral orifice	Ureter, Right
	Ureter, Left
	Ureters, Bilateral
	Ureter
Ureteropelvic junction (UPJ)	Kidney Pelvis, Right
	Kidney Pelvis, Left
Ureterovesical orifice	Ureter, Right
	Ureter, Left
	Ureters, Bilateral
	Ureter
Uterine artery	Internal Iliac Artery, Right
	Internal Iliac Artery, Left
Uterine cornu	Uterus
Uterine tube	Fallopian Tube, Right
	Fallopian Tube, Left
Uterine vein	Hypogastric Vein, Right
	Hypogastric Vein, Left
Vaginal artery	Internal Iliac Artery, Right
	Internal Iliac Artery, Left
Vaginal vein	Hypogastric Vein, Right
	Hypogastric Vein, Left
Vastus intermedius muscle	Upper Leg Muscle, Right
	Upper Leg Muscle, Left
Vastus lateralis muscle	Upper Leg Muscle, Right
	Upper Leg Muscle, Left
Vastus medialis muscle	Upper Leg Muscle, Right
	Upper Leg Muscle, Left
Ventricular fold	Larynx
Vermiform appendix	Appendix
Vermilion border	Upper Lip
	Lower Lip
Vertebral arch	Cervical Vertebra
	Lumbar Vertebra
	Thoracic Vertebra
Vertebral body	Cervical Vertebra
	Lumbar Vertebra
	Thoracic Vertebra
Vertebral canal	Spinal Canal
Vertebral foramen	Cervical Vertebra
	Lumbar Vertebra
	Thoracic Vertebra
Vertebral lamina	Cervical Vertebra
	Lumbar Vertebra
	Thoracic Vertebra
Vertebral pedicle	Cervical Vertebra
	Lumbar Vertebra
	Thoracic Vertebra

Term	ICD-10-PCS Value
Vesical vein	Hypogastric Vein, Right
	Hypogastric Vein, Left
Vestibular (Scarpa's) ganglion	Acoustic Nerve
Vestibular nerve	Acoustic Nerve
Vestibulocochlear nerve	Acoustic Nerve
Virchow's (supraclavicular) lymph node	Lymphatic, Right Neck
	Lymphatic, Left Neck
Vitreous body	Vitreous, Right
	Vitreous, Left
Vocal fold	Vocal Cord, Right
	Vocal Cord, Left
Volar (palmar) digital vein	Hand Vein, Right
	Hand Vein, Left
Volar (palmar) metacarpal vein	Hand Vein, Right
	Hand Vein, Left
Vomer bone	Nasal Septum
Vomer of nasal septum	Nasal Bone
Xiphoid process	Sternum
Zonule of Zinn	Lens, Right
	Lens, Left
Zygomatic process of frontal bone	Frontal Bone
Zygomatic process of temporal bone	Temporal Bone, Right
	Temporal Bone, Left
Zygomaticus muscle	Facial Muscle

Appendix E: Body Part Definitions

ICD-10-PCS Value	Definition
1st Toe, Left **1st Toe, Right**	**Includes:** Hallux
Abdomen Muscle, Left **Abdomen Muscle, Right**	**Includes:** External oblique muscle Internal oblique muscle Pyramidalis muscle Rectus abdominis muscle Transversus abdominis muscle
Abdominal Aorta	**Includes:** Inferior phrenic artery Lumbar artery Median sacral artery Middle suprarenal artery Ovarian artery Testicular artery
Abdominal Sympathetic Nerve	**Includes:** Abdominal aortic plexus Auerbach's (myenteric) plexus Celiac (solar) plexus Celiac ganglion Gastric plexus Hepatic plexus Inferior hypogastric plexus Inferior mesenteric ganglion Inferior mesenteric plexus Meissner's (submucous) plexus Myenteric (Auerbach's) plexus Pancreatic plexus Pelvic splanchnic nerve Renal nerve Renal plexus Solar (celiac) plexus Splenic plexus Submucous (Meissner's) plexus Superior hypogastric plexus Superior mesenteric ganglion Superior mesenteric plexus Suprarenal plexus
Abducens Nerve	**Includes:** Sixth cranial nerve
Accessory Nerve	**Includes:** Eleventh cranial nerve
Acoustic Nerve	**Includes:** Cochlear nerve Eighth cranial nerve Scarpa's (vestibular) ganglion Spiral ganglion Vestibular (Scarpa's) ganglion Vestibular nerve Vestibulocochlear nerve
Adenoids	**Includes:** Pharyngeal tonsil
Adrenal Gland **Adrenal Gland, Left** **Adrenal Gland, Right** **Adrenal Glands, Bilateral**	**Includes:** Suprarenal gland
Ampulla of Vater	**Includes:** Duodenal ampulla Hepatopancreatic ampulla
Anal Sphincter	**Includes:** External anal sphincter Internal anal sphincter
Ankle Bursa and Ligament, Left **Ankle Bursa and Ligament, Right**	**Includes:** Calcaneofibular ligament Deltoid ligament Ligament of the lateral malleolus Talofibular ligament
Ankle Joint, Left **Ankle Joint, Right**	**Includes:** Inferior tibiofibular joint Talocrural joint
Anterior Chamber, Left **Anterior Chamber, Right**	**Includes:** Aqueous humour
Anterior Tibial Artery, Left **Anterior Tibial Artery, Right**	**Includes:** Anterior lateral malleolar artery Anterior medial malleolar artery Anterior tibial recurrent artery Dorsalis pedis artery Posterior tibial recurrent artery
Anus	**Includes:** Anal orifice
Aortic Valve	**Includes:** Aortic annulus
Appendix	**Includes:** Vermiform appendix
Atrial Septum	**Includes:** Interatrial septum
Atrium, Left	**Includes:** Atrium pulmonale Left auricular appendix
Atrium, Right	**Includes:** Atrium dextrum cordis Right auricular appendix Sinus venosus
Auditory Ossicle, Left **Auditory Ossicle, Right**	**Includes:** Incus Malleus Stapes
Axillary Artery, Left **Axillary Artery, Right**	**Includes:** Anterior circumflex humeral artery Lateral thoracic artery Posterior circumflex humeral artery Subscapular artery Superior thoracic artery Thoracoacromial artery
Azygos Vein	**Includes:** Right ascending lumbar vein Right subcostal vein
Basal Ganglia	**Includes:** Basal nuclei Claustrum Corpus striatum Globus pallidus Substantia nigra Subthalamic nucleus
Basilic Vein, Left **Basilic Vein, Right**	**Includes:** Median antebrachial vein Median cubital vein
Bladder	**Includes:** Trigone of bladder
Brachial Artery, Left **Brachial Artery, Right**	**Includes:** Inferior ulnar collateral artery Profunda brachii Superior ulnar collateral artery

ICD-10-PCS Value	Definition
Brachial Plexus	**Includes:** Axillary nerve Dorsal scapular nerve First intercostal nerve Long thoracic nerve Musculocutaneous nerve Subclavius nerve Suprascapular nerve
Brachial Vein, Left **Brachial Vein, Right**	**Includes:** Radial vein Ulnar vein
Brain	**Includes:** Cerebrum Corpus callosum Encephalon
Breast, Bilateral **Breast, Left** **Breast, Right**	**Includes:** Mammary duct Mammary gland
Buccal Mucosa	**Includes:** Buccal gland Molar gland Palatine gland
Carotid Bodies, Bilateral **Carotid Body, Left** **Carotid Body, Right**	**Includes:** Carotid glomus
Carpal Joint, Left **Carpal Joint, Right**	**Includes:** Intercarpal joint Midcarpal joint
Carpal, Left **Carpal, Right**	**Includes:** Capitate bone Hamate bone Lunate bone Pisiform bone Scaphoid bone Trapezium bone Trapezoid bone Triquetral bone
Celiac Artery	**Includes:** Celiac trunk
Cephalic Vein, Left **Cephalic Vein, Right**	**Includes:** Accessory cephalic vein
Cerebellum	**Includes:** Culmen
Cerebral Hemisphere	**Includes:** Frontal lobe Occipital lobe Parietal lobe Temporal lobe
Cerebral Meninges	**Includes:** Arachnoid mater, intracranial Leptomeninges, intracranial Pia mater, intracranial
Cerebral Ventricle	**Includes:** Aqueduct of Sylvius Cerebral aqueduct (Sylvius) Choroid plexus Ependyma Foramen of Monro (intraventricular) Fourth ventricle Interventricular foramen (Monro) Left lateral ventricle Right lateral ventricle Third ventricle

ICD-10-PCS Value	Definition
Cervical Nerve	**Includes:** Greater occipital nerve Spinal nerve, cervical Suboccipital nerve Third occipital nerve
Cervical Plexus	**Includes:** Ansa cervicalis Cutaneous (transverse) cervical nerve Great auricular nerve Lesser occipital nerve Supraclavicular nerve Transverse (cutaneous) cervical nerve
Cervical Spinal Cord	**Includes:** Dorsal root ganglion
Cervical Vertebra	**Includes:** Dens Odontoid process Spinous process Transverse foramen Transverse process Vertebral arch Vertebral body Vertebral foramen Vertebral lamina Vertebral pedicle
Cervical Vertebral Joint	**Includes:** Atlantoaxial joint Cervical facet joint
Cervical Vertebral Joints, 2 or more	**Includes:** Cervical facet joint
Cervicothoracic Vertebral Joint	**Includes:** Cervicothoracic facet joint
Cisterna Chyli	**Includes:** Intestinal lymphatic trunk Lumbar lymphatic trunk
Coccygeal Glomus	**Includes:** Coccygeal body
Colic Vein	**Includes:** Ileocolic vein Left colic vein Middle colic vein Right colic vein
Conduction Mechanism	**Includes:** Atrioventricular node Bundle of His Bundle of Kent Sinoatrial node
Conjunctiva, Left **Conjunctiva, Right**	**Includes:** Plica semilunaris
Dura Mater	**Includes:** Diaphragma sellae Dura mater, intracranial Falx cerebri Tentorium cerebelli
Elbow Bursa and Ligament, Left **Elbow Bursa and Ligament, Right**	**Includes:** Annular ligament Olecranon bursa Radial collateral ligament Ulnar collateral ligament
Elbow Joint, Left **Elbow Joint, Right**	**Includes:** Distal humerus, involving joint Humeroradial joint Humeroulnar joint Proximal radioulnar joint
Epidural Space, Intracranial	**Includes:** Extradural space, intracranial

ICD-10-PCS Value	Definition
Epiglottis	**Includes:** Glossoepiglottic fold
Esophagogastric Junction	**Includes:** Cardia Cardioesophageal junction Gastroesophageal (GE) junction
Esophagus, Lower	**Includes:** Abdominal esophagus
Esophagus, Middle	**Includes:** Thoracic esophagus
Esophagus, Upper	**Includes:** Cervical esophagus
Ethmoid Bone, Left **Ethmoid Bone, Right**	**Includes:** Cribriform plate
Ethmoid Sinus, Left **Ethmoid Sinus, Right**	**Includes:** Ethmoidal air cell
Eustachian Tube, Left **Eustachian Tube, Right**	**Includes:** Auditory tube Pharyngotympanic tube
External Auditory Canal, Left **External Auditory Canal, Right**	**Includes:** External auditory meatus
External Carotid Artery, Left **External Carotid Artery, Right**	**Includes:** Ascending pharyngeal artery Internal maxillary artery Lingual artery Maxillary artery Occipital artery Posterior auricular artery Superior thyroid artery
External Ear, Bilateral **External Ear, Left** **External Ear, Right**	**Includes:** Antihelix Antitragus Auricle Earlobe Helix Pinna Tragus
External Iliac Artery, Left **External Iliac Artery, Right**	**Includes:** Deep circumflex iliac artery Inferior epigastric artery
External Jugular Vein, Left **External Jugular Vein, Right**	**Includes:** Posterior auricular vein
Extraocular Muscle, Left **Extraocular Muscle, Right**	**Includes:** Inferior oblique muscle Inferior rectus muscle Lateral rectus muscle Medial rectus muscle Superior oblique muscle Superior rectus muscle
Eye, Left **Eye, Right**	**Includes:** Ciliary body Posterior chamber
Face Artery	**Includes:** Angular artery Ascending palatine artery External maxillary artery Facial artery Inferior labial artery Submental artery Superior labial artery

ICD-10-PCS Value	Definition
Face Vein, Left **Face Vein, Right**	**Includes:** Angular vein Anterior facial vein Common facial vein Deep facial vein Frontal vein Posterior facial (retromandibular) vein Supraorbital vein
Facial Muscle	**Includes:** Buccinator muscle Corrugator supercilii muscle Depressor anguli oris muscle Depressor labii inferioris muscle Depressor septi nasi muscle Depressor supercilii muscle Levator anguli oris muscle Levator labii superioris alaeque nasi muscle Levator labii superioris muscle Mentalis muscle Nasalis muscle Occipitofrontalis muscle Orbicularis oris muscle Procerus muscle Risorius muscle Zygomaticus muscle
Facial Nerve	**Includes:** Chorda tympani Geniculate ganglion Greater superficial petrosal nerve Nerve to the stapedius Parotid plexus Posterior auricular nerve Seventh cranial nerve Submandibular ganglion
Fallopian Tube, Left **Fallopian Tube, Right**	**Includes:** Oviduct Salpinx Uterine tube
Femoral Artery, Left **Femoral Artery, Right**	**Includes:** Circumflex iliac artery Deep femoral artery Descending genicular artery External pudendal artery Superficial epigastric artery
Femoral Nerve	**Includes:** Anterior crural nerve Saphenous nerve
Femoral Shaft, Left **Femoral Shaft, Right**	**Includes:** Body of femur
Femoral Vein, Left **Femoral Vein, Right**	**Includes:** Deep femoral (profunda femoris) vein Popliteal vein Profunda femoris (deep femoral) vein
Fibula, Left **Fibula, Right**	**Includes:** Body of fibula Head of fibula Lateral malleolus
Finger Nail	**Includes:** Nail bed Nail plate
Finger Phalangeal Joint, Left **Finger Phalangeal Joint, Right**	**Includes:** Interphalangeal (IP) joint

Appendix E: Body Part Definitions

ICD-10-PCS Value	Definition
Foot Artery, Left **Foot Artery, Right**	**Includes:** Arcuate artery Dorsal metatarsal artery Lateral plantar artery Lateral tarsal artery Medial plantar artery
Foot Bursa and Ligament, Left **Foot Bursa and Ligament, Right**	**Includes:** Calcaneocuboid ligament Cuneonavicular ligament Intercuneiform ligament Interphalangeal ligament Metatarsal ligament Metatarsophalangeal ligament Subtalar ligament Talocalcaneal ligament Talocalcaneonavicular ligament Tarsometatarsal ligament
Foot Muscle, Left **Foot Muscle, Right**	**Includes:** Abductor hallucis muscle Adductor hallucis muscle Extensor digitorum brevis muscle Extensor hallucis brevis muscle Flexor digitorum brevis muscle Flexor hallucis brevis muscle Quadratus plantae muscle
Foot Vein, Left **Foot Vein, Right**	**Includes:** Common digital vein Dorsal metatarsal vein Dorsal venous arch Plantar digital vein Plantar metatarsal vein Plantar venous arch
Frontal Bone	**Includes:** Zygomatic process of frontal bone
Gastric Artery	**Includes:** Left gastric artery Right gastric artery
Glenoid Cavity, Left **Glenoid Cavity, Right**	**Includes:** Glenoid fossa (of scapula)
Glomus Jugulare	**Includes:** Jugular body
Glossopharyngeal Nerve	**Includes:** Carotid sinus nerve Ninth cranial nerve Tympanic nerve
Hand Artery, Left **Hand Artery, Right**	**Includes:** Deep palmar arch Princeps pollicis artery Radialis indicis Superficial palmar arch
Hand Bursa and Ligament, Left **Hand Bursa and Ligament, Right**	**Includes:** Carpometacarpal ligament Intercarpal ligament Interphalangeal ligament Lunotriquetral ligament Metacarpal ligament Metacarpophalangeal ligament Pisohamate ligament Pisometacarpal ligament Scaphotrapezium ligament
Hand Muscle, Left **Hand Muscle, Right**	**Includes:** Hypothenar muscle Palmar interosseous muscle Thenar muscle

ICD-10-PCS Value	Definition
Hand Vein, Left **Hand Vein, Right**	**Includes:** Dorsal metacarpal vein Palmar (volar) digital vein Palmar (volar) metacarpal vein Superficial palmar venous arch Volar (palmar) digital vein Volar (palmar) metacarpal vein
Head and Neck Bursa and Ligament	**Includes:** Alar ligament of axis Cervical interspinous ligament Cervical intertransverse ligament Cervical ligamentum flavum Interspinous ligament, cervical Intertransverse ligament, cervical Lateral temporomandibular ligament Ligamentum flavum, cervical Sphenomandibular ligament Stylomandibular ligament Transverse ligament of atlas
Head and Neck Sympathetic Nerve	**Includes:** Cavernous plexus Cervical ganglion Ciliary ganglion Internal carotid plexus Otic ganglion Pterygopalatine (sphenopalatine) ganglion Sphenopalatine (pterygopalatine) ganglion Stellate ganglion Submandibular ganglion Submaxillary ganglion
Head Muscle	**Includes:** Auricularis muscle Masseter muscle Pterygoid muscle Splenius capitis muscle Temporalis muscle Temporoparietalis muscle
Heart, Left	**Includes:** Left coronary sulcus Obtuse margin
Heart, Right	**Includes:** Right coronary sulcus
Hemiazygos Vein	**Includes:** Left ascending lumbar vein Left subcostal vein
Hepatic Artery	**Includes:** Common hepatic artery Gastroduodenal artery Hepatic artery proper
Hip Bursa and Ligament, Left **Hip Bursa and Ligament, Right**	**Includes:** Iliofemoral ligament Ischiofemoral ligament Pubofemoral ligament Transverse acetabular ligament Trochanteric bursa
Hip Joint, Left **Hip Joint, Right**	**Includes:** Acetabulofemoral joint
Hip Muscle, Left **Hip Muscle, Right**	**Includes:** Gemellus muscle Gluteus maximus muscle Gluteus medius muscle Gluteus minimus muscle Iliacus muscle Obturator muscle Piriformis muscle Psoas muscle Quadratus femoris muscle Tensor fasciae latae muscle

ICD-10-PCS Value	Definition
Humeral Head, Left **Humeral Head, Right**	**Includes:** Greater tuberosity Lesser tuberosity Neck of humerus (anatomical)(surgical)
Humeral Shaft, Left **Humeral Shaft, Right**	**Includes:** Distal humerus Humerus, distal Lateral epicondyle of humerus Medial epicondyle of humerus
Hypogastric Vein, Left **Hypogastric Vein, Right**	**Includes:** Gluteal vein Internal iliac vein Internal pudendal vein Lateral sacral vein Middle hemorrhoidal vein Obturator vein Uterine vein Vaginal vein Vesical vein
Hypoglossal Nerve	**Includes:** Twelfth cranial nerve
Hypothalamus	**Includes:** Mammillary body
Inferior Mesenteric Artery	**Includes:** Sigmoid artery Superior rectal artery
Inferior Mesenteric Vein	**Includes:** Sigmoid vein Superior rectal vein
Inferior Vena Cava	**Includes:** Postcava Right inferior phrenic vein Right ovarian vein Right second lumbar vein Right suprarenal vein Right testicular vein
Inguinal Region, Bilateral **Inguinal Region, Left** **Inguinal Region, Right**	**Includes:** Inguinal canal Inguinal triangle
Inner Ear, Left **Inner Ear, Right**	**Includes:** Bony labyrinth Bony vestibule Cochlea Round window Semicircular canal
Innominate Artery	**Includes:** Brachiocephalic artery Brachiocephalic trunk
Innominate Vein, Left **Innominate Vein, Right**	**Includes:** Brachiocephalic vein Inferior thyroid vein
Internal Carotid Artery, Left **Internal Carotid Artery, Right**	**Includes:** Caroticotympanic artery Carotid sinus

ICD-10-PCS Value	Definition
Internal Iliac Artery, Left **Internal Iliac Artery, Right**	**Includes:** Deferential artery Hypogastric artery Iliolumbar artery Inferior gluteal artery Inferior vesical artery Internal pudendal artery Lateral sacral artery Middle rectal artery Obturator artery Superior gluteal artery Umbilical artery Uterine artery Vaginal artery
Internal Mammary Artery, Left **Internal Mammary Artery, Right**	**Includes:** Anterior intercostal artery Internal thoracic artery Musculophrenic artery Pericardiophrenic artery Superior epigastric artery
Intracranial Artery	**Includes:** Anterior cerebral artery Anterior choroidal artery Anterior communicating artery Basilar artery Circle of Willis Internal carotid artery, intracranial portion Middle cerebral artery Ophthalmic artery Posterior cerebral artery Posterior communicating artery Posterior inferior cerebellar artery (PICA)
Intracranial Vein	**Includes:** Anterior cerebral vein Basal (internal) cerebral vein Dural venous sinus Great cerebral vein Inferior cerebellar vein Inferior cerebral vein Internal (basal) cerebral vein Middle cerebral vein Ophthalmic vein Superior cerebellar vein Superior cerebral vein
Jejunum	**Includes:** Duodenojejunal flexure
Kidney	**Includes:** Renal calyx Renal capsule Renal cortex Renal segment
Kidney Pelvis, Left **Kidney Pelvis, Right**	**Includes:** Ureteropelvic junction (UPJ)
Kidney, Left **Kidney, Right** **Kidneys, Bilateral**	**Includes:** Renal calyx Renal capsule Renal cortex Renal segment
Knee Bursa and Ligament, Left **Knee Bursa and Ligament, Right**	**Includes:** Anterior cruciate ligament (ACL) Lateral collateral ligament (LCL) Ligament of head of fibula Medial collateral ligament (MCL) Patellar ligament Popliteal ligament Posterior cruciate ligament (PCL) Prepatellar bursa

ICD-10-PCS Value	Definition
Knee Joint, Femoral Surface, Left **Knee Joint, Femoral Surface, Right**	**Includes:** Femoropatellar joint Patellofemoral joint
Knee Joint, Left **Knee Joint, Right**	**Includes:** Femoropatellar joint Femorotibial joint Lateral meniscus Medial meniscus Patellofemoral joint Tibiofemoral joint
Knee Joint, Tibial Surface, Left **Knee Joint, Tibial Surface, Right**	**Includes:** Femorotibial joint Tibiofemoral joint
Knee Tendon, Left **Knee Tendon, Right**	**Includes:** Patellar tendon
Lacrimal Duct, Left **Lacrimal Duct, Right**	**Includes:** Lacrimal canaliculus Lacrimal punctum Lacrimal sac Nasolacrimal duct
Larynx	**Includes:** Aryepiglottic fold Arytenoid cartilage Corniculate cartilage Cuneiform cartilage False vocal cord Glottis Rima glottidis Thyroid cartilage Ventricular fold
Lens, Left **Lens, Right**	**Includes:** Zonule of Zinn
Liver	**Includes:** Quadrate lobe
Lower Arm and Wrist Muscle, Left **Lower Arm and Wrist Muscle, Right**	**Includes:** Anatomical snuffbox Brachioradialis muscle Extensor carpi radialis muscle Extensor carpi ulnaris muscle Flexor carpi radialis muscle Flexor carpi ulnaris muscle Flexor pollicis longus muscle Palmaris longus muscle Pronator quadratus muscle Pronator teres muscle
Lower Artery	**Includes:** Umbilical artery
Lower Eyelid, Left **Lower Eyelid, Right**	**Includes:** Inferior tarsal plate Medial canthus
Lower Femur, Left **Lower Femur, Right**	**Includes:** Lateral condyle of femur Lateral epicondyle of femur Medial condyle of femur Medial epicondyle of femur
Lower Leg Muscle, Left **Lower Leg Muscle, Right**	**Includes:** Extensor digitorum longus muscle Extensor hallucis longus muscle Fibularis brevis muscle Fibularis longus muscle Flexor digitorum longus muscle Flexor hallucis longus muscle Gastrocnemius muscle Peroneus brevis muscle Peroneus longus muscle Popliteus muscle Soleus muscle Tibialis anterior muscle Tibialis posterior muscle
Lower Leg Tendon, Left **Lower Leg Tendon, Right**	**Includes:** Achilles tendon
Lower Lip	**Includes:** Frenulum labii inferioris Labial gland Vermilion border
Lower Spine Bursa and Ligament	**Includes:** Iliolumbar ligament Interspinous ligament, lumbar Intertransverse ligament, lumbar Ligamentum flavum, lumbar Sacrococcygeal ligament Sacroiliac ligament Sacrospinous ligament Sacrotuberous ligament Supraspinous ligament
Lumbar Nerve	**Includes:** Lumbosacral trunk Spinal nerve, lumbar Superior clunic (cluneal) nerve
Lumbar Plexus	**Includes:** Accessory obturator nerve Genitofemoral nerve Iliohypogastric nerve Ilioinguinal nerve Lateral femoral cutaneous nerve Obturator nerve Superior gluteal nerve
Lumbar Spinal Cord	**Includes:** Cauda equina Conus medullaris Dorsal root ganglion
Lumbar Sympathetic Nerve	**Includes:** Lumbar ganglion Lumbar splanchnic nerve
Lumbar Vertebra	**Includes:** Spinous process Transverse process Vertebral arch Vertebral body Vertebral foramen Vertebral lamina Vertebral pedicle
Lumbar Vertebral Joint	**Includes:** Lumbar facet joint
Lumbosacral Joint	**Includes:** Lumbosacral facet joint

ICD-10-PCS Value	Definition
Lymphatic, Aortic	**Includes:** Celiac lymph node Gastric lymph node Hepatic lymph node Lumbar lymph node Pancreaticosplenic lymph node Paraaortic lymph node Retroperitoneal lymph node
Lymphatic, Head	**Includes:** Buccinator lymph node Infraauricular lymph node Infraparotid lymph node Parotid lymph node Preauricular lymph node Submandibular lymph node Submaxillary lymph node Submental lymph node Subparotid lymph node Suprahyoid lymph node
Lymphatic, Left Axillary	**Includes:** Anterior (pectoral) lymph node Apical (subclavicular) lymph node Brachial (lateral) lymph node Central axillary lymph node Lateral (brachial) lymph node Pectoral (anterior) lymph node Posterior (subscapular) lymph node Subclavicular (apical) lymph node Subscapular (posterior) lymph node
Lymphatic, Left Lower Extremity	**Includes:** Femoral lymph node Popliteal lymph node
Lymphatic, Left Neck	**Includes:** Cervical lymph node Jugular lymph node Mastoid (postauricular) lymph node Occipital lymph node Postauricular (mastoid) lymph node Retropharyngeal lymph node Supraclavicular (Virchow's) lymph node Virchow's (supraclavicular) lymph node
Lymphatic, Left Upper Extremity	**Includes:** Cubital lymph node Deltopectoral (infraclavicular) lymph node Epitrochlear lymph node Infraclavicular (deltopectoral) lymph node Supratrochlear lymph node
Lymphatic, Mesenteric	**Includes:** Inferior mesenteric lymph node Pararectal lymph node Superior mesenteric lymph node
Lymphatic, Pelvis	**Includes:** Common iliac (subaortic) lymph node Gluteal lymph node Iliac lymph node Inferior epigastric lymph node Obturator lymph node Sacral lymph node Subaortic (common iliac) lymph node Suprainguinal lymph node

ICD-10-PCS Value	Definition
Lymphatic, Right Axillary	**Includes:** Anterior (pectoral) lymph node Apical (subclavicular) lymph node Brachial (lateral) lymph node Central axillary lymph node Lateral (brachial) lymph node Pectoral (anterior) lymph node Posterior (subscapular) lymph node Subclavicular (apical) lymph node Subscapular (posterior) lymph node
Lymphatic, Right Lower Extremity	**Includes:** Femoral lymph node Popliteal lymph node
Lymphatic, Right Neck	**Includes:** Cervical lymph node Jugular lymph node Mastoid (postauricular) lymph node Occipital lymph node Postauricular (mastoid) lymph node Retropharyngeal lymph node Right jugular trunk Right lymphatic duct Right subclavian trunk Supraclavicular (Virchow's) lymph node Virchow's (supraclavicular) lymph node
Lymphatic, Right Upper Extremity	**Includes:** Cubital lymph node Deltopectoral (infraclavicular) lymph node Epitrochlear lymph node Infraclavicular (deltopectoral) lymph node Supratrochlear lymph node
Lymphatic, Thorax	**Includes:** Intercostal lymph node Mediastinal lymph node Parasternal lymph node Paratracheal lymph node Tracheobronchial lymph node
Main Bronchus, Right	**Includes:** Bronchus intermedius Intermediate bronchus
Mandible, Left Mandible, Right	**Includes:** Alveolar process of mandible Condyloid process Mandibular notch Mental foramen
Mastoid Sinus, Left Mastoid Sinus, Right	**Includes:** Mastoid air cells
Metatarsal, Left Metatarsal, Right	**Includes:** Fibular sesamoid Tibial sesamoid
Maxilla	**Includes:** Alveolar process of maxilla
Maxillary Sinus, Left Maxillary Sinus, Right	**Includes:** Antrum of Highmore
Median Nerve	**Includes:** Anterior interosseous nerve Palmar cutaneous nerve
Mediastinum	**Includes:** Mediastinal cavity Mediastinal space
Medulla Oblongata	**Includes:** Myelencephalon
Mesentery	**Includes:** Mesoappendix Mesocolon

ICD-10-PCS Value	Definition
Metatarsal, Right **Metatarsal, Left**	**Includes:** Fibular sesamoid Tibial sesamoid
Metatarsal-Phalangeal Joint, Left **Metatarsal-Phalangeal Joint, Right**	**Includes:** Metatarsophalangeal (MTP) joint
Middle Ear, Left **Middle Ear, Right**	**Includes:** Oval window Tympanic cavity
Minor Salivary Gland	**Includes:** Anterior lingual gland
Mitral Valve	**Includes:** Bicuspid valve Left atrioventricular valve Mitral annulus
Nasal Bone	**Includes:** Vomer of nasal septum
Nasal Mucosa and Soft Tissue	**Includes:** Columella External naris Greater alar cartilage Internal naris Lateral nasal cartilage Lesser alar cartilage Nasal cavity Nostril
Nasal Septum	**Includes:** Quadrangular cartilage Septal cartilage Vomer bone
Nasal Turbinate	**Includes:** Inferior turbinate Middle turbinate Nasal concha Superior turbinate
Nasopharynx	**Includes:** Choana Fossa of Rosenmuller Pharyngeal recess Rhinopharynx
Neck	**Includes:** Parapharyngeal space Retropharyngeal space
Neck Muscle, Left **Neck Muscle, Right**	**Includes:** Anterior vertebral muscle Arytenoid muscle Cricothyroid muscle Infrahyoid muscle Levator scapulae muscle Platysma muscle Scalene muscle Splenius cervicis muscle Sternocleidomastoid muscle Suprahyoid muscle Thyroarytenoid muscle
Nipple, Left **Nipple, Right**	**Includes:** Areola
Occipital Bone	**Includes:** Foramen magnum
Oculomotor Nerve	**Includes:** Third cranial nerve
Olfactory Nerve	**Includes:** First cranial nerve Olfactory bulb

ICD-10-PCS Value	Definition
Omentum	**Includes:** Gastrocolic ligament Gastrocolic omentum Gastrohepatic omentum Gastrophrenic ligament Gastrosplenic ligament Greater Omentum Hepatogastric ligament Lesser Omentum
Optic Nerve	**Includes:** Optic chiasma Second cranial nerve
Orbit, Left **Orbit, Right**	**Includes:** Bony orbit Orbital portion of ethmoid bone Orbital portion of frontal bone Orbital portion of lacrimal bone Orbital portion of maxilla Orbital portion of palatine bone Orbital portion of sphenoid bone Orbital portion of zygomatic bone
Pancreatic Duct	**Includes:** Duct of Wirsung
Pancreatic Duct, Accessory	**Includes:** Duct of Santorini
Parotid Duct, Left **Parotid Duct, Right**	**Includes:** Stensen's duct
Pelvic Bone, Left **Pelvic Bone, Right**	**Includes:** Iliac crest Ilium Ischium Pubis
Pelvic Cavity	**Includes:** Retropubic space
Penis	**Includes:** Corpus cavernosum Corpus spongiosum
Perineum Muscle	**Includes:** Bulbospongiosus muscle Cremaster muscle Deep transverse perineal muscle Ischiocavernosus muscle Levator ani muscle Superficial transverse perineal muscle
Peritoneum	**Includes:** Epiploic foramen
Peroneal Artery, Left **Peroneal Artery, Right**	**Includes:** Fibular artery
Peroneal Nerve	**Includes:** Common fibular nerve Common peroneal nerve External popliteal nerve Lateral sural cutaneous nerve
Pharynx	**Includes:** Base of Tongue Hypopharynx Laryngopharynx Lingual tonsil Oropharynx Piriform recess (sinus) Tongue, base of
Phrenic Nerve	**Includes:** Accessory phrenic nerve
Pituitary Gland	**Includes:** Adenohypophysis Hypophysis Neurohypophysis

ICD-10-PCS Value	Definition
Pons	**Includes:** Apneustic center Basis pontis Locus ceruleus Pneumotaxic center Pontine tegmentum Superior olivary nucleus
Popliteal Artery, Left Popliteal Artery, Right	**Includes:** Inferior genicular artery Middle genicular artery Superior genicular artery Sural artery Tibioperoneal trunk
Portal Vein	**Includes:** Hepatic portal vein
Prepuce	**Includes:** Foreskin Glans penis
Pudendal Nerve	**Includes:** Posterior labial nerve Posterior scrotal nerve
Pulmonary Artery, Left	**Includes:** Arterial canal (duct) Botallo's duct Pulmoaortic canal
Pulmonary Valve	**Includes:** Pulmonary annulus Pulmonic valve
Pulmonary Vein, Left	**Includes:** Left inferior pulmonary vein Left superior pulmonary vein
Pulmonary Vein, Right	**Includes:** Right inferior pulmonary vein Right superior pulmonary vein
Radial Artery, Left Radial Artery, Right	**Includes:** Radial recurrent artery
Radial Nerve	**Includes:** Dorsal digital nerve Musculospiral nerve Palmar cutaneous nerve Posterior interosseous nerve
Radius, Left Radius, Right	**Includes:** Ulnar notch
Rectum	**Includes:** Anorectal junction
Renal Artery, Left Renal Artery, Right	**Includes:** Inferior suprarenal artery Renal segmental artery
Renal Vein, Left	**Includes:** Left inferior phrenic vein Left ovarian vein Left second lumbar vein Left suprarenal vein Left testicular vein
Retina, Left Retina, Right	**Includes:** Fovea Macula Optic disc
Retroperitoneum	**Includes:** Retroperitoneal cavity Retroperitoneal space
Rib(s) Bursa and Ligament	**Includes:** Costotransverse ligament
Sacral Nerve	**Includes:** Spinal nerve, sacral

ICD-10-PCS Value	Definition
Sacral Plexus	**Includes:** Inferior gluteal nerve Posterior femoral cutaneous nerve Pudendal nerve
Sacral Sympathetic Nerve	**Includes:** Ganglion impar (ganglion of Walther) Pelvic splanchnic nerve Sacral ganglion Sacral splanchnic nerve
Sacrococcygeal Joint	**Includes:** Sacrococcygeal symphysis
Saphenous Vein, Left Saphenous Vein, Right	**Includes:** External pudendal vein Great(er) saphenous vein Lesser saphenous vein Small saphenous vein Superficial circumflex iliac vein Superficial epigastric vein
Scapula, Left Scapula, Right	**Includes:** Acromion (process) Coracoid process
Sciatic Nerve	**Includes:** Ischiatic nerve
Shoulder Bursa and Ligament, Left Shoulder Bursa and Ligament, Right	**Includes:** Acromioclavicular ligament Coracoacromial ligament Coracoclavicular ligament Coracohumeral ligament Costoclavicular ligament Glenohumeral ligament Interclavicular ligament Sternoclavicular ligament Subacromial bursa Transverse humeral ligament Transverse scapular ligament
Shoulder Joint, Left Shoulder Joint, Right	**Includes:** Glenohumeral joint Glenoid ligament (labrum)
Shoulder Muscle, Left Shoulder Muscle, Right	**Includes:** Deltoid muscle Infraspinatus muscle Subscapularis muscle Supraspinatus muscle Teres major muscle Teres minor muscle
Sigmoid Colon	**Includes:** Rectosigmoid junction Sigmoid flexure
Skin	**Includes:** Dermis Epidermis Sebaceous gland Sweat gland
Skin, Chest	**Includes:** Breast procedures, skin only
Sphenoid Bone	**Includes:** Greater wing Lesser wing Optic foramen Pterygoid process Sella turcica
Spinal Canal	**Includes:** Epidural space, spinal Extradural space, spinal Subarachnoid space, spinal Subdural space, spinal Vertebral canal

ICD-10-PCS Value	Definition
Spinal Cord	**Includes:** Dorsal root ganglion
Spinal Meninges	**Includes:** Arachnoid mater, spinal Denticulate (dentate) ligament Dura mater, spinal Filum terminale Leptomeninges, spinal Pia mater, spinal
Spleen	**Includes:** Accessory spleen
Splenic Artery	**Includes:** Left gastroepiploic artery Pancreatic artery Short gastric artery
Splenic Vein	**Includes:** Left gastroepiploic vein Pancreatic vein
Sternum	**Includes:** Manubrium Suprasternal notch Xiphoid process
Sternum Bursa and Ligament	**Includes:** Costoxiphoid ligament Sternocostal ligament
Stomach, Pylorus	**Includes:** Pyloric antrum Pyloric canal Pyloric sphincter
Subclavian Artery, Left **Subclavian Artery, Right**	**Includes:** Costocervical trunk Dorsal scapular artery Internal thoracic artery
Subcutaneous Tissue and Fascia, Chest	**Includes:** Pectoral fascia
Subcutaneous Tissue and Fascia, Face	**Includes:** Masseteric fascia Orbital fascia Submandibular space
Subcutaneous Tissue and Fascia, Left Foot	**Includes:** Plantar fascia (aponeurosis)
Subcutaneous Tissue and Fascia, Left Hand	**Includes:** Palmar fascia (aponeurosis)
Subcutaneous Tissue and Fascia, Left Lower Arm	**Includes:** Antebrachial fascia Bicipital aponeurosis
Subcutaneous Tissue and Fascia, Left Neck	**Includes:** Deep cervical fascia Pretracheal fascia Prevertebral fascia
Subcutaneous Tissue and Fascia, Left Upper Arm	**Includes:** Axillary fascia Deltoid fascia Infraspinatus fascia Subscapular aponeurosis Supraspinatus fascia
Subcutaneous Tissue and Fascia, Left Upper Leg	**Includes:** Crural fascia Fascia lata Iliac fascia Iliotibial tract (band)
Subcutaneous Tissue and Fascia, Right Foot	**Includes:** Plantar fascia (aponeurosis)
Subcutaneous Tissue and Fascia, Right Hand	**Includes:** Palmar fascia (aponeurosis)

ICD-10-PCS Value	Definition
Subcutaneous Tissue and Fascia, Right Lower Arm	**Includes:** Antebrachial fascia Bicipital aponeurosis
Subcutaneous Tissue and Fascia, Right Neck	**Includes:** Deep cervical fascia Pretracheal fascia Prevertebral fascia
Subcutaneous Tissue and Fascia, Right Upper Arm	**Includes:** Axillary fascia Deltoid fascia Infraspinatus fascia Subscapular aponeurosis Supraspinatus fascia
Subcutaneous Tissue and Fascia, Right Upper Leg	**Includes:** Crural fascia Fascia lata Iliac fascia Iliotibial tract (band)
Subcutaneous Tissue and Fascia, Scalp	**Includes:** Galea aponeurotica
Subcutaneous Tissue and Fascia, Trunk	**Includes:** External oblique aponeurosis Transversalis fascia
Submaxillary Gland, Left **Submaxillary Gland, Right**	**Includes:** Submandibular gland
Superior Mesenteric Artery	**Includes:** Ileal artery Ileocolic artery Inferior pancreaticoduodenal artery Jejunal artery
Superior Mesenteric Vein	**Includes:** Right gastroepiploic vein
Superior Vena Cava	**Includes:** Precava
Tarsal Joint, Left **Tarsal Joint, Right**	**Includes:** Calcaneocuboid joint Cuboideonavicular joint Cuneonavicular joint Intercuneiform joint Subtalar (talocalcaneal) joint Talocalcaneal (subtalar) joint Talocalcaneonavicular joint
Tarsal, Left **Tarsal, Right**	**Includes:** Calcaneus Cuboid bone Intermediate cuneiform bone Lateral cuneiform bone Medial cuneiform bone Navicular bone Talus bone
Temporal Artery, Left **Temporal Artery, Right**	**Includes:** Middle temporal artery Superficial temporal artery Transverse facial artery
Temporal Bone, Left **Temporal Bone, Right**	**Includes:** Mastoid process Petrous part of temporal bone Tympanic part of temporal bone Zygomatic process of temporal bone
Thalamus	**Includes:** Epithalamus Geniculate nucleus Metathalamus Pulvinar
Thoracic Aorta, Ascending/Arch	**Includes:** Aortic arch Ascending aorta

ICD-10-PCS Value	Definition
Thoracic Duct	**Includes:** Left jugular trunk Left subclavian trunk
Thoracic Nerve	**Includes:** Intercostal nerve Intercostobrachial nerve Spinal nerve, thoracic Subcostal nerve
Thoracic Spinal Cord	**Includes:** Dorsal root ganglion
Thoracic Sympathetic Nerve	**Includes:** Cardiac plexus Esophageal plexus Greater splanchnic nerve Inferior cardiac nerve Least splanchnic nerve Lesser splanchnic nerve Middle cardiac nerve Pulmonary plexus Superior cardiac nerve Thoracic aortic plexus Thoracic ganglion
Thoracic Vertebra	**Includes:** Spinous process Transverse process Vertebral arch Vertebral body Vertebral foramen Vertebral lamina Vertebral pedicle
Thoracic Vertebral Joint	**Includes:** Costotransverse joint Costovertebral joint Thoracic facet joint
Thoracolumbar Vertebral Joint	**Includes:** Thoracolumbar facet joint
Thorax Muscle, Left **Thorax Muscle, Right**	**Includes:** Intercostal muscle Levatores costarum muscle Pectoralis major muscle Pectoralis minor muscle Serratus anterior muscle Subclavius muscle Subcostal muscle Transverse thoracis muscle
Thymus	**Includes:** Thymus gland
Thyroid Artery, Left **Thyroid Artery, Right**	**Includes:** Cricothyroid artery Hyoid artery Sternocleidomastoid artery Superior laryngeal artery Superior thyroid artery Thyrocervical trunk
Tibia, Left **Tibia, Right**	**Includes:** Lateral condyle of tibia Medial condyle of tibia Medial malleolus
Tibial Nerve	**Includes:** Lateral plantar nerve Medial plantar nerve Medial popliteal nerve Medial sural cutaneous nerve
Toe Nail	**Includes:** Nail bed Nail plate

ICD-10-PCS Value	Definition
Toe Phalangeal Joint, Left **Toe Phalangeal Joint, Right**	**Includes:** Interphalangeal (IP) joint
Tongue	**Includes:** Frenulum linguae
Tongue, Palate, Pharynx Muscle	**Includes:** Chondroglossus muscle Genioglossus muscle Hyoglossus muscle Inferior longitudinal muscle Levator veli palatini muscle Palatoglossal muscle Palatopharyngeal muscle Pharyngeal constrictor muscle Salpingopharyngeus muscle Styloglossus muscle Stylopharyngeus muscle Superior longitudinal muscle Tensor veli palatini muscle
Tonsils	**Includes:** Palatine tonsil
Trachea	**Includes:** Cricoid cartilage
Transverse Colon	**Includes:** Hepatic flexure Splenic flexure
Tricuspid Valve	**Includes:** Right atrioventricular valve Tricuspid annulus
Trigeminal Nerve	**Includes:** Fifth cranial nerve Gasserian ganglion Mandibular nerve Maxillary nerve Ophthalmic nerve Trifacial nerve
Trochlear Nerve	**Includes:** Fourth cranial nerve
Trunk Muscle, Left **Trunk Muscle, Right**	**Includes:** Coccygeus muscle Erector spinae muscle Interspinalis muscle Intertransversarius muscle Latissimus dorsi muscle Quadratus lumborum muscle Rhomboid major muscle Rhomboid minor muscle Serratus posterior muscle Transversospinalis muscle Trapezius muscle
Tympanic Membrane, Left **Tympanic Membrane, Right**	**Includes:** Pars flaccida
Ulna, Left **Ulna, Right**	**Includes:** Olecranon process Radial notch
Ulnar Artery, Left **Ulnar Artery, Right**	**Includes:** Anterior ulnar recurrent artery Common interosseous artery Posterior ulnar recurrent artery
Ulnar Nerve	**Includes:** Cubital nerve
Upper Arm Muscle, Left **Upper Arm Muscle, Right**	**Includes:** Biceps brachii muscle Brachialis muscle Coracobrachialis muscle Triceps brachii muscle

ICD-10-PCS Value	Definition
Upper Artery	**Includes:** Aortic intercostal artery Bronchial artery Esophageal artery Subcostal artery
Upper Eyelid, Left **Upper Eyelid, Right**	**Includes:** Lateral canthus Levator palpebrae superioris muscle Orbicularis oculi muscle Superior tarsal plate
Upper Femur, Left **Upper Femur, Right**	**Includes:** Femoral head Greater trochanter Lesser trochanter Neck of femur
Upper Leg Muscle, Left **Upper Leg Muscle, Right**	**Includes:** Adductor brevis muscle Adductor longus muscle Adductor magnus muscle Biceps femoris muscle Gracilis muscle Pectineus muscle Quadriceps (femoris) Rectus femoris muscle Sartorius muscle Semimembranosus muscle Semitendinosus muscle Vastus intermedius muscle Vastus lateralis muscle Vastus medialis muscle
Upper Lip	**Includes:** Frenulum labii superioris Labial gland Vermilion border
Upper Spine Bursa and Ligament	**Includes:** Interspinous ligament, thoracic Intertransverse ligament, thoracic Ligamentum flavum, thoracic Supraspinous ligament
Ureter **Ureter, Left** **Ureter, Right** **Ureters, Bilateral**	**Includes:** Ureteral orifice Ureterovesical orifice
Urethra	**Includes:** Bulbourethral (Cowper's) gland Cowper's (bulbourethral) gland External urethral sphincter Internal urethral sphincter Membranous urethra Penile urethra Prostatic urethra
Uterine Supporting Structure	**Includes:** Broad ligament Infundibulopelvic ligament Ovarian ligament Round ligament of uterus
Uterus	**Includes:** Fundus uteri Myometrium Perimetrium Uterine cornu
Uvula	**Includes:** Palatine uvula

ICD-10-PCS Value	Definition
Vagus Nerve	**Includes:** Anterior vagal trunk Pharyngeal plexus Pneumogastric nerve Posterior vagal trunk Pulmonary plexus Recurrent laryngeal nerve Superior laryngeal nerve Tenth cranial nerve
Vas Deferens **Vas Deferens, Bilateral** **Vas Deferens, Left** **Vas Deferens, Right**	**Includes:** Ductus deferens Ejaculatory duct
Ventricle, Right	**Includes:** Conus arteriosus
Ventricular Septum	**Includes:** Interventricular septum
Vertebral Artery, Left **Vertebral Artery, Right**	**Includes:** Anterior spinal artery Posterior spinal artery
Vertebral Vein, Left **Vertebral Vein, Right**	**Includes:** Deep cervical vein Suboccipital venous plexus
Vestibular Gland	**Includes:** Bartholin's (greater vestibular) gland Greater vestibular (Bartholin's) gland Paraurethral (Skene's) gland Skene's (paraurethral) gland
Vitreous, Left **Vitreous, Right**	**Includes:** Vitreous body
Vocal Cord, Left **Vocal Cord, Right**	**Includes:** Vocal fold
Vulva	**Includes:** Labia majora Labia minora
Wrist Bursa and Ligament, Left **Wrist Bursa and Ligament, Right**	**Includes:** Palmar ulnocarpal ligament Radial collateral carpal ligament Radiocarpal ligament Radioulnar ligament Scapholunate ligament Ulnar collateral carpal ligament
Wrist Joint, Left **Wrist Joint, Right**	**Includes:** Distal radioulnar joint Radiocarpal joint

Appendix F: Device Classification

In most PCS codes, the sixth character of the code classifies the device. The sixth character device value "defines the material or appliance used to accomplish the objective of the procedure that remains in or on the procedure site at the end of the procedure." If the device is the means by which the procedural objective is accomplished, then a specific device value is coded in the sixth character. If no device is used to accomplish the objective of the procedure, the device value No Device is coded in the sixth character. In limited root operations, the classification provides the qualifier values Temporary and Intraoperative, for specific procedures involving clinically significant devices whose purpose is brief use during the procedure or current inpatient stay.

Material that is classified as a PCS device is distinguished from material classified as a PCS substance by its having a specific location. A device is intended to maintain a fixed location at the procedure site where it was put, whereas a substance is intended to disperse or be absorbed in the body. There are circumstances in which a device does not stay where it was put and may need to be "revised" in a subsequent procedure to move the device back to its intended location.

Material classified as a PCS device is also distinguishable by the fact that it is removable. Although it may not be practical to remove some types of devices once they become established at the site, it is physically possible to remove a device for some time after the procedure. A skin graft, for example, once it "takes," may be nearly indistinguishable from the surrounding skin and so is no longer clearly identifiable as a device. Nevertheless, procedures that involve material coded as a device can for the most part be "reversed" by removing the device from the procedure site.

General Device Types

Device Type	Definition	Examples
Grafts	Biological or synthetic material that **takes the place of all or a portion of a body part.**	Full- or partial-thickness skin grafts: • Autologous • Nonautologous • Synthetic • Zooplastic Other tissue grafts: • Bone • Tendon • Vascular
Prosthesis	Biological or synthetic material that **takes the place of all or a portion of a body part.**	Joint prosthesis: • Autologous • Nonautologous • Synthetic
Implants	**Therapeutic** material that is not absorbed by, eliminated by, or incorporated into a body part.	External fixation device Internal fixation device: • Orthopaedic pins • Intramedullary rods Radioactive element implant Mesh
Simple or mechanical appliances	Biological or synthetic material that **assists or prevents a physiological function.**	Drainage device Extraluminal device Endobrachial device Fusion device Intraluminal device (can be temporary) Tracheostomy device IUD
Electronic appliances	Electronic appliances used to **assist, monitor, take the pace of, or prevent a physiological function.**	Cardiac leads Diaphragmatic pacemaker External heart assist system Short-term external heart assist system (Intraoperative) Fetal monitoring Hearing device Monitoring device Neurostimulator
External appliances	Performed without making an incision or a puncture, external appliances are used for the purpose of **protection, immobilization, stretching, compression, or packing.**	Bandage Cast Packing material Pressure dressing Traction apparatus

Transplant/Grafting Tissue Type Terminology

Tissue Type	Terminology
Tissue or organ transferred into a new position in **the body of the same individual**	Autograft Autologous Autoplastic
Having to do with individuals or tissues that have **identical genes**, such as identical twins	Isograft Isologous Syngeneic Syngraft
Tissue or organ taken from **different individuals** of the same species	Allogeneic Allograft Homologous Homograft
Tissue or organ from a **cadaver**	Nonautologous
Tissue or organ from individuals of **different species**	Heterogeneic Heterologous Xenogeneic Xenograft Zooplastic

Appendix G: Device Key and Aggregation Table

This NT symbol next to a device in the Term column identifies that the device has been approved for NTAP (new technology add-on payment). CMS provides incremental payment, in addition to the DRG payment, for technologies that have received an NTAP designation.

Device Key

Term	ICD-10-PCS Value
3f (Aortic) Bioprosthesis valve	Zooplastic Tissue in Heart and Great Vessels
AbioCor® Total Replacement Heart	Synthetic Substitute
Absolute Pro Vascular (OTW) Self-Expanding Stent System	Intraluminal Device
Acculink (RX) Carotid Stent System	Intraluminal Device
Acellular Hydrated Dermis	Nonautologous Tissue Substitute
Acetabular cup	Liner in Lower Joints
Activa PC neurostimulator	Stimulator Generator, Multiple Array for Insertion in Subcutaneous Tissue and Fascia
Activa RC neurostimulator	Stimulator Generator, Multiple Array Rechargeable for Insertion in Subcutaneous Tissue and Fascia
Activa SC neurostimulator	Stimulator Generator, Single Array for Insertion in Subcutaneous Tissue and Fascia
ACUITY™ Steerable Lead	Cardiac Lead, Pacemaker for Insertion in Heart and Great Vessels Cardiac Lead, Defibrillator for Insertion in Heart and Great Vessels
Advisa (MRI)	Pacemaker, Dual Chamber for Insertion in Subcutaneous Tissue and Fascia
AFX® Endovascular AAA System	Intraluminal Device
Alfapump® system	Other Device
AMPLATZER® Muscular VSD Occluder	Synthetic Substitute
AMS 800® Urinary Control System	Artificial Sphincter in Urinary System
AneuRx® AAA Advantage®	Intraluminal Device
Annuloplasty ring	Synthetic Substitute
ApiFix® Minimally Invasive Deformity Correction (MID-C) System (C)	Posterior (Dynamic) Distraction Device in New Technology
Aprevo™	Interbody Fusion Device, Customizable in New Technology
Articulating Spacer (Antibiotic)	Articulating Spacer in Lower Joints
Artificial anal sphincter (AAS)	Artificial Sphincter in Gastrointestinal System
Artificial bowel sphincter (neosphincter)	Artificial Sphincter in Gastrointestinal System
Artificial urinary sphincter (AUS)	Artificial Sphincter in Urinary System
Ascenda Intrathecal Catheter	Infusion Device
Assurant (Cobalt) stent	Intraluminal Device
AtriClip LAA Exclusion System	Extraluminal Device
Attain Ability® Lead	Cardiac Lead, Pacemaker for Insertion in Heart and Great Vessels Cardiac Lead, Defibrillator for Insertion in Heart and Great Vessels
Attain StarFix® (OTW) Lead	Cardiac Lead, Pacemaker for Insertion in Heart and Great Vessels Cardiac Lead, Defibrillator for Insertion in Heart and Great Vessels
Autograft	Autologous Tissue Substitute
Autologous artery graft	Autologous Arterial Tissue in Heart and Great Vessels Autologous Arterial Tissue in Upper Arteries Autologous Arterial Tissue in Lower Arteries Autologous Arterial Tissue in Upper Veins Autologous Arterial Tissue in Lower Veins
Autologous vein graft	Autologous Venous Tissue in Heart and Great Vessels Autologous Venous Tissue in Upper Arteries Autologous Venous Tissue in Lower Arteries Autologous Venous Tissue in Upper Veins Autologous Venous Tissue in Lower Veins
Axial Lumbar Interbody Fusion System	Interbody Fusion Device in Lower Joints
AxiaLIF® System	Interbody Fusion Device in Lower Joints
BAK/C® Interbody Cervical Fusion System	Interbody Fusion Device in Upper Joints
Bard® Composix® (E/X)(LP) mesh	Synthetic Substitute
Bard® Composix® Kugel® patch	Synthetic Substitute
Bard® Dulex™ mesh	Synthetic Substitute
Bard® Ventralex™ hernia patch	Synthetic Substitute
Baroreflex Activation Therapy® (BAT®) NT	Stimulator Lead in Upper Arteries Stimulator Generator in Subcutaneous Tissue and Fascia
Barricaid® Annular Closure Device (ACD)	Synthetic Substitute
Berlin Heart Ventricular Assist Device	Implantable Heart Assist System in Heart and Great Vessels
Bioactive embolization coil(s)	Intraluminal Device, Bioactive in Upper Arteries
Biventricular external heart assist system	Short-term External Heart Assist System in Heart and Great Vessels
Blood glucose monitoring system	Monitoring Device
Bone anchored hearing device	Hearing Device, Bone Conduction for Insertion in Ear, Nose, Sinus Hearing Device, in Head and Facial Bones
Bone bank bone graft	Nonautologous Tissue Substitute
Bone screw (interlocking)(lag)(pedicle)(recessed)	Internal Fixation Device in Head and Facial Bones Internal Fixation Device in Upper Bones Internal Fixation Device in Lower Bones
Bovine pericardial valve	Zooplastic Tissue in Heart and Great Vessels
Bovine pericardium graft	Zooplastic Tissue in Heart and Great Vessels
Brachytherapy seeds	Radioactive Element

Term	ICD-10-PCS Value
BRYAN® Cervical Disc System	Synthetic Substitute
BVS 5000 Ventricular Assist Device	Short-term External Heart Assist System in Heart and Great Vessels
Cardiac contractility modulation lead NT	Cardiac Lead in Heart and Great Vessels
Cardiac event recorder	Monitoring Device
Cardiac resynchronization therapy (CRT) lead	Cardiac Lead, Pacemaker for Insertion in Heart and Great Vessels Cardiac Lead, Defibrillator for Insertion in Heart and Great Vessels
CardioMEMS® pressure sensor	Monitoring Device, Pressure Sensor for Insertion in Heart and Great Vessels
Carmat total artificial heart (TAH)	Biologic with Synthetic Substitute, Autoregulated Electrohydraulic for Replacement in Heart and Great Vessels
Carotid (artery) sinus (baroreceptor) lead	Stimulator Lead in Upper Arteries
Carotid WALLSTENT® Monorail® Endoprosthesis	Intraluminal Device
Centrimag® Blood Pump	Short-term External Heart Assist System in Heart and Great Vessels
Ceramic on ceramic bearing surface	Synthetic Substitute, Ceramic for Replacement in Lower Joints
Cesium-131 Collagen Implant	Radioactive Element, Cesium-131 Collagen Implant for Insertion in Central Nervous System and Cranial Nerves
CivaSheet®	Radioactive Element
Clamp and rod internal fixation system (CRIF)	Internal Fixation Device in Upper Bones Internal Fixation Device in Lower Bones
COALESCE® radiolucent interbody fusion device	Interbody Fusion Device, Radiolucent Porous in New Technology
CoAxia NeuroFlo catheter	Intraluminal Device
Cobalt/chromium head and polyethylene socket	Synthetic Substitute, Metal on Polyethylene for Replacement in Lower Joints
Cobalt/chromium head and socket	Synthetic Substitute, Metal for Replacement in Lower Joints
Cochlear implant (CI), multiple channel (electrode)	Hearing Device, Multiple Channel Cochlear Prosthesis for Insertion in Ear, Nose, Sinus
Cochlear implant (CI), single channel (electrode)	Hearing Device, Single Channel Cochlear Prosthesis for Insertion in Ear, Nose, Sinus
COGNIS® CRT-D	Cardiac Resynchronization Defibrillator Pulse Generator for Insertion in Subcutaneous Tissue and Fascia
COHERE® radiolucent interbody fusion device	Interbody Fusion Device, Radiolucent Porous in New Technology
Colonic Z-Stent®	Intraluminal Device
Complete (SE) stent	Intraluminal Device
Concerto II CRT-D	Cardiac Resynchronization Defibrillator Pulse Generator for Insertion in Subcutaneous Tissue and Fascia
CONSERVE® PLUS Total Resurfacing Hip System	Resurfacing Device in Lower Joints
Consulta CRT-D	Cardiac Resynchronization Defibrillator Pulse Generator for Insertion in Subcutaneous Tissue and Fascia
Consulta CRT-P	Cardiac Resynchronization Pacemaker Pulse Generator for Insertion in Subcutaneous Tissue and Fascia
CONTAK RENEWAL® 3 RF (HE) CRT-D	Cardiac Resynchronization Defibrillator Pulse Generator for Insertion in Subcutaneous Tissue and Fascia
Contegra Pulmonary Valved Conduit	Zooplastic Tissue in Heart and Great Vessels
Continuous Glucose Monitoring (CGM) device	Monitoring Device
Cook Biodesign® Fistula Plug(s)	Nonautologous Tissue Substitute
Cook Biodesign® Hernia Graft(s)	Nonautologous Tissue Substitute
Cook Biodesign® Layered Graft(s)	Nonautologous Tissue Substitute
Cook Zenapro™ Layered Graft(s)	Nonautologous Tissue Substitute
Cook Zenith AAA Endovascular Graft	Intraluminal Device
Cook Zenith® Fenestrated AAA Endovascular Graft	Intraluminal Device, Branched or Fenestrated, One or Two Arteries for Restriction in Lower Arteries Intraluminal Device, Branched or Fenestrated, Three or More Arteries for Restriction in Lower Arteries
CoreValve transcatheter aortic valve	Zooplastic Tissue in Heart and Great Vessels
Cormet Hip Resurfacing System	Resurfacing Device in Lower Joints
CoRoent® XL	Interbody Fusion Device in Lower Joints
Corox (OTW) Bipolar Lead	Cardiac Lead, Pacemaker for Insertion in Heart and Great Vessels Cardiac Lead, Defibrillator for Insertion in Heart and Great Vessels
Cortical strip neurostimulator lead	Neurostimulator Lead in Central Nervous System and Cranial Nerves
Corvia IASD®	Synthetic Substitute
Cultured epidermal cell autograft	Autologous Tissue Substitute
CYPHER® Stent	Intraluminal Device, Drug-eluting in Heart and Great Vessels
Cystostomy tube	Drainage Device
DBS lead	Neurostimulator Lead in Central Nervous System and Cranial Nerves
DeBakey Left Ventricular Assist Device	Implantable Heart Assist System in Heart and Great Vessels
Deep brain neurostimulator lead	Neurostimulator Lead in Central Nervous System and Cranial Nerves
Delta frame external fixator	External Fixation Device, Hybrid for Insertion in Upper Bones External Fixation Device, Hybrid for Reposition in Upper Bones External Fixation Device, Hybrid for Insertion in Lower Bones External Fixation Device, Hybrid for Reposition in Lower Bones
Delta III Reverse shoulder prosthesis	Synthetic Substitute, Reverse Ball and Socket for Replacement in Upper Joints
Diaphragmatic pacemaker generator	Stimulator Generator in Subcutaneous Tissue and Fascia
Direct Lateral Interbody Fusion (DLIF) device	Interbody Fusion Device in Lower Joints
Driver stent (RX) (OTW)	Intraluminal Device
DuraHeart Left Ventricular Assist System	Implantable Heart Assist System in Heart and Great Vessels

Term	ICD-10-PCS Value
Durata® Defibrillation Lead	Cardiac Lead, Defibrillator for Insertion in Heart and Great Vessels
DynaNail®	Internal Fixation Device, Sustained Compression for Fusion in Lower Joints Internal Fixation Device, Sustained Compression for Fusion in Upper Joints
DynaNail Mini®	Internal Fixation Device, Sustained Compression for Fusion in Lower Joints Internal Fixation Device, Sustained Compression for Fusion in Upper Joints
Dynesys® Dynamic Stabilization System	Spinal Stabilization Device, Pedicle-Based for Insertion in Upper Joints Spinal Stabilization Device, Pedicle-Based for Insertion in Lower Joints
E-Luminexx™ (Biliary)(Vascular) Stent	Intraluminal Device
EDWARDS INTUITY Elite valve system	Zooplastic Tissue, Rapid Deployment Technique in New Technology
Electrical bone growth stimulator (EBGS)	Bone Growth Stimulator in Head and Facial Bones Bone Growth Stimulator in Upper Bones Bone Growth Stimulator in Lower Bones
Electrical muscle stimulation (EMS) lead	Stimulator Lead in Muscles
Electronic muscle stimulator lead	Stimulator Lead in Muscles
Eluvia™ Drug-eluting Vascular Stent System NT	Intraluminal Device, Sustained Release Drug-eluting in New Technology Intraluminal Device, Sustained Release Drug-eluting, Two in New Technology Intraluminal Device, Sustained Release Drug-eluting, Three in New Technology Intraluminal Device, Sustained Release Drug-eluting, Four or More in New Technology
Embolization coil(s)	Intraluminal Device
Endeavor® (III)(IV) (Sprint) Zotarolimus-eluting Coronary Stent System	Intraluminal Device, Drug-eluting in Heart and Great Vessels
Endologix AFX® Endovascular AAA System	Intraluminal Device
EndoSure® sensor	Monitoring Device, Pressure Sensor for Insertion in Heart and Great Vessels
ENDOTAK RELIANCE® (G) Defibrillation Lead	Cardiac Lead, Defibrillator for Insertion in Heart and Great Vessels
Endotracheal tube (cuffed)(double-lumen)	Intraluminal Device, Endotracheal Airway in Respiratory System
Endurant® Endovascular Stent Graft	Intraluminal Device
Endurant® II AAA stent graft system	Intraluminal Device
EnRhythm	Pacemaker, Dual Chamber for Insertion in Subcutaneous Tissue and Fascia
Enterra gastric neurostimulator	Stimulator Generator, Multiple Array for Insertion in Subcutaneous Tissue and Fascia
Epic™ Stented Tissue Valve (aortic)	Zooplastic Tissue in Heart and Great Vessels
Epicel® cultured epidermal autograft	Autologous Tissue Substitute
Esophageal obturator airway (EOA)	Intraluminal Device, Airway in Gastrointestinal System
Esteem® implantable hearing system	Hearing Device in Ear, Nose, Sinus
Evera (XT)(S)(DR/VR)	Defibrillator Generator for Insertion in Subcutaneous Tissue and Fascia
Everolimus-eluting coronary stent	Intraluminal Device, Drug-eluting in Heart and Great Vessels
Ex-PRESS™ mini glaucoma shunt	Synthetic Substitute
EXCLUDER® AAA Endoprosthesis	Intraluminal Device Intraluminal Device, Branched or Fenestrated, One or Two Arteries for Restriction in Lower Arteries Intraluminal Device, Branched or Fenestrated, Three or More Arteries for Restriction in Lower Arteries
EXCLUDER® IBE Endoprosthesis	Intraluminal Device, Branched or Fenestrated, One or Two Arteries for Restriction in Lower Arteries
Express® (LD) Premounted Stent System	Intraluminal Device
Express® Biliary SD Monorail® Premounted Stent System	Intraluminal Device
Express® SD Renal Monorail® Premounted Stent System	Intraluminal Device
External fixator	External Fixation Device in Head and Facial Bones External Fixation Device in Upper Bones External Fixation Device in Lower Bones External Fixation Device in Upper Joints External Fixation Device in Lower Joints
EXtreme Lateral Interbody Fusion (XLIF) device	Interbody Fusion Device in Lower Joints
Facet replacement spinal stabilization device	Spinal Stabilization Device, Facet Replacement for Insertion in Upper Joints Spinal Stabilization Device, Facet Replacement for Insertion in Lower Joints
FLAIR® Endovascular Stent Graft	Intraluminal Device
Flexible Composite Mesh	Synthetic Substitute
Flow Diverter embolization device	Intraluminal Device, Flow Diverter for Restriction in Upper Arteries
Foley catheter	Drainage Device
Formula™ Balloon-Expandable Renal Stent System	Intraluminal Device
Freestyle (Stentless) Aortic Root Bioprosthesis	Zooplastic Tissue in Heart and Great Vessels
Fusion screw (compression)(lag)(locking)	Internal Fixation Device in Upper Joints Internal Fixation Device in Lower Joints
GammaTile™	Radioactive Element, Cesium-131 Collagen Implant for Insertion in Central Nervous System and Cranial Nerves
Gastric electrical stimulation (GES) lead	Stimulator Lead in Gastrointestinal System
Gastric pacemaker lead	Stimulator Lead in Gastrointestinal System

Term	ICD-10-PCS Value
GORE EXCLUDER® AAA Endoprosthesis	Intraluminal Device Intraluminal Device, Branched or Fenestrated, One or Two Arteries for Restriction in Lower Arteries Intraluminal Device, Branched or Fenestrated, Three or More Arteries for Restriction in Lower Arteries
GORE EXCLUDER® IBE Endoprosthesis	Intraluminal Device, Branched or Fenestrated, One or Two Arteries for Restriction in Lower Arteries
GORE TAG® Thoracic Endoprosthesis	Intraluminal Device
GORE® DUALMESH®	Synthetic Substitute
Guedel airway	Intraluminal Device, Airway in Mouth and Throat
Hancock Bioprosthesis (aortic)(mitral) valve	Zooplastic Tissue in Heart and Great Vessels
Hancock Bioprosthetic Valved Conduit	Zooplastic Tissue in Heart and Great Vessels
HeartMate 3™ LVAS	Implantable Heart Assist System in Heart and Great Vessels
HeartMate II® Left Ventricular Assist Device (LVAD)	Implantable Heart Assist System in Heart and Great Vessels
HeartMate XVE® Left Ventricular Assist Device (LVAD)	Implantable Heart Assist System in Heart and Great Vessels
Herculink (RX) Elite Renal Stent System	Intraluminal Device
Hip (joint) liner	Liner in Lower Joints
Holter valve ventricular shunt	Synthetic Substitute
IASD® (InterAtrial Shunt Device), Corvia	Synthetic Substitute
Ilizarov external fixator	External Fixation Device, Ring for Insertion in Upper Bones External Fixation Device, Ring for Reposition in Upper Bones External Fixation Device, Ring for Insertion in Lower Bones External Fixation Device, Ring for Reposition in Lower Bones
Ilizarov-Vecklich device	External Fixation Device, Limb Lengthening for Insertion in Upper Bones External Fixation Device, Limb Lengthening for Insertion in Lower Bones
Impella® heart pump	Short-term External Heart Assist System in Heart and Great Vessels
Implantable cardioverter-defibrillator (ICD)	Defibrillator Generator for Insertion in Subcutaneous Tissue and Fascia
Implantable drug infusion pump (anti-spasmodic)(chemotherapy)(pain)	Infusion Device, Pump in Subcutaneous Tissue and Fascia
Implantable glucose monitoring device	Monitoring Device
Implantable hemodynamic monitor (IHM)	Monitoring Device, Hemodynamic for Insertion in Subcutaneous Tissue and Fascia
Implantable hemodynamic monitoring system (IHMS)	Monitoring Device, Hemodynamic for Insertion in Subcutaneous Tissue and Fascia
Implantable Miniature Telescope™ (IMT)	Synthetic Substitute, Intraocular Telescope for Replacement in Eye

Term	ICD-10-PCS Value
Implanted (venous)(access) port	Vascular Access Device, Totally Implantable in Subcutaneous Tissue and Fascia
InDura, intrathecal catheter (1P) (spinal)	Infusion Device
Injection reservoir, port	Vascular Access Device, Totally Implantable in Subcutaneous Tissue and Fascia
Injection reservoir, pump	Infusion Device, Pump in Subcutaneous Tissue and Fascia
InterAtrial Shunt Device IASD®, Corvia	Synthetic Substitute
Interbody fusion (spine) cage	Interbody Fusion Device in Upper Joints Interbody Fusion Device in Lower Joints
Interspinous process spinal stabilization device	Spinal Stabilization Device, Interspinous Process for Insertion in Upper Joints Spinal Stabilization Device, Interspinous Process for Insertion in Lower Joints
InterStim™ Micro Therapy neurostimulator	Stimulator Generator, Single Array Rechargeable for Insertion in Subcutaneous Tissue and Fascia
InterStim® Therapy lead	Neurostimulator Lead in Peripheral Nervous System
InterStim™ II Therapy neurostimulator	Stimulator Generator, Single Array for Insertion in Subcutaneous Tissue and Fascia
Intramedullary (IM) rod (nail)	Internal Fixation Device, Intramedullary in Upper Bones Internal Fixation Device, Intramedullary in Lower Bones
Intramedullary skeletal kinetic distractor (ISKD)	Internal Fixation Device, Intramedullary in Upper Bones Internal Fixation Device, Intramedullary in Lower Bones
Intrauterine Device (IUD)	Contraceptive Device in Female Reproductive System
INTUITY Elite valve system, EDWARDS	Zooplastic Tissue, Rapid Deployment Technique in New Technology
Itrel (3)(4) neurostimulator	Stimulator Generator, Single Array for Insertion in Subcutaneous Tissue and Fascia
Joint fixation plate	Internal Fixation Device in Upper Joints Internal Fixation Device in Lower Joints
Joint liner (insert)	Liner in Lower Joints
Joint spacer (antibiotic)	Spacer in Upper Joints Spacer in Lower Joints
Kappa	Pacemaker, Dual Chamber for Insertion in Subcutaneous Tissue and Fascia
Kirschner wire (K-wire)	Internal Fixation Device in Head and Facial Bones Internal Fixation Device in Upper Bones Internal Fixation Device in Lower Bones Internal Fixation Device in Upper Joints Internal Fixation Device in Lower Joints
Knee (implant) insert	Liner in Lower Joints
Kuntscher nail	Internal Fixation Device, Intramedullary in Upper Bones Internal Fixation Device, Intramedullary in Lower Bones
LAP-BAND® adjustable gastric banding system	Extraluminal Device
LifeStent® (Flexstar)(XL) Vascular Stent System	Intraluminal Device

Term	ICD-10-PCS Value
LIVIAN™ CRT-D	Cardiac Resynchronization Defibrillator Pulse Generator for Insertion in Subcutaneous Tissue and Fascia
Loop recorder, implantable	Monitoring Device
MAGEC® Spinal Bracing and Distraction System	Magnetically Controlled Growth Rod(s) in New Technology
Mark IV Breathing Pacemaker System	Stimulator Generator in Subcutaneous Tissue and Fascia
Maximo II DR (VR)	Defibrillator Generator for Insertion in Subcutaneous Tissue and Fascia
Maximo II DR CRT-D	Cardiac Resynchronization Defibrillator Pulse Generator for Insertion in Subcutaneous Tissue and Fascia
Medtronic Endurant® II AAA stent graft system	Intraluminal Device
Melody® transcatheter pulmonary valve	Zooplastic Tissue in Heart and Great Vessels
Metal on metal bearing surface	Synthetic Substitute, Metal for Replacement in Lower Joints
Micro-Driver stent (RX) (OTW)	Intraluminal Device
MicroMed HeartAssist	Implantable Heart Assist System in Heart and Great Vessels
Micrus CERECYTE microcoil	Intraluminal Device, Bioactive in Upper Arteries
MIRODERM™ Biologic Wound Matrix	Skin Substitute, Porcine Liver Derived in New Technology
MitraClip valve repair system	Synthetic Substitute
Mitroflow® Aortic Pericardial Heart Valve	Zooplastic Tissue in Heart and Great Vessels
Mosaic Bioprosthesis (aortic) (mitral) valve	Zooplastic Tissue in Heart and Great Vessels
MULTI-LINK (VISION)(MINI-VISION)(ULTRA) Coronary Stent System	Intraluminal Device
nanoLOCK™ interbody fusion device	Interbody Fusion Device, Nanotextured Surface in New Technology
Nasopharyngeal airway (NPA)	Intraluminal Device, Airway in Ear, Nose, Sinus
Neovasc Reducer™	Reduction Device in New Technology
Neuromuscular electrical stimulation (NEMS) lead	Stimulator Lead in Muscles
Neurostimulator generator, multiple channel	Stimulator Generator, Multiple Array for Insertion in Subcutaneous Tissue and Fascia
Neurostimulator generator, multiple channel rechargeable	Stimulator Generator, Multiple Array Rechargeable for Insertion in Subcutaneous Tissue and Fascia
Neurostimulator generator, single channel	Stimulator Generator, Single Array for Insertion in Subcutaneous Tissue and Fascia
Neurostimulator generator, single channel rechargeable	Stimulator Generator, Single Array Rechargeable for Insertion in Subcutaneous Tissue and Fascia
Neutralization plate	Internal Fixation Device in Head and Facial Bones Internal Fixation Device in Upper Bones Internal Fixation Device in Lower Bones
Nitinol framed polymer mesh	Synthetic Substitute
Non-tunneled central venous catheter	Infusion Device
Novacor Left Ventricular Assist Device	Implantable Heart Assist System in Heart and Great Vessels
Novation® Ceramic AHS® (Articulation Hip System)	Synthetic Substitute, Ceramic for Replacement in Lower Joints
Omnilink Elite Vascular Balloon Expandable Stent System	Intraluminal Device
Open Pivot Aortic Valve Graft (AVG)	Synthetic Substitute
Open Pivot (mechanical) Valve	Synthetic Substitute
Optimizer™ III implantable pulse generator NT	Contractility Modulation Device for Insertion in Subcutaneous Tissue and Fascia
Oropharyngeal airway (OPA)	Intraluminal Device, Airway in Mouth and Throat
Ovatio™ CRT-D	Cardiac Resynchronization Defibrillator Pulse Generator for Insertion in Subcutaneous Tissue and Fascia
OXINIUM	Synthetic Substitute, Oxidized Zirconium on Polyethylene for Replacement in Lower Joints
Paclitaxel-eluting coronary stent	Intraluminal Device, Drug-eluting in Heart and Great Vessels
Paclitaxel-eluting peripheral stent	Intraluminal Device, Drug-eluting in Upper Arteries Intraluminal Device, Drug-eluting in Lower Arteries
Partially absorbable mesh	Synthetic Substitute
Pedicle-based dynamic stabilization device	Spinal Stabilization Device, Pedicle-Based for Insertion in Upper Joints Spinal Stabilization Device, Pedicle-Based for Insertion in Lower Joints
PERCEPT™ PC neurostimulator	Stimulator Generator, Multiple Array for Insertion in Subcutaneous Tissue and Fascia
Perceval sutureless valve	Zooplastic Tissue, Rapid Deployment Technique in New Technology
Percutaneous endoscopic gastrojejunostomy (PEG/J) tube	Feeding Device in Gastrointestinal System
Percutaneous endoscopic gastrostomy (PEG) tube	Feeding Device in Gastrointestinal System
Percutaneous nephrostomy catheter	Drainage Device
Peripherally inserted central catheter (PICC)	Infusion Device
Pessary ring	Intraluminal Device, Pessary in Female Reproductive System
Phrenic nerve stimulator generator	Stimulator Generator in Subcutaneous Tissue and Fascia
Phrenic nerve stimulator lead	Diaphragmatic Pacemaker Lead in Respiratory System
PHYSIOMESH™ Flexible Composite Mesh	Synthetic Substitute
Pipeline™ (Flex) embolization device	Intraluminal Device, Flow Diverter for Restriction in Upper Arteries
Polyethylene socket	Synthetic Substitute, Polyethylene for Replacement in Lower Joints
Polymethylmethacrylate (PMMA)	Synthetic Substitute
Polypropylene mesh	Synthetic Substitute
Porcine (bioprosthetic) valve	Zooplastic Tissue in Heart and Great Vessels

Term	ICD-10-PCS Value
PRECICE intramedullary limb lengthening system	Internal Fixation Device, Intramedullary Limb Lengthening for Insertion in Upper Bones Internal Fixation Device, Intramedullary Limb Lengthening for Insertion in Lower Bones
PRESTIGE® Cervical Disc	Synthetic Substitute
PrimeAdvanced neurostimulator (SureScan)(MRI Safe)	Stimulator Generator, Multiple Array for Insertion in Subcutaneous Tissue and Fascia
PROCEED™ Ventral Patch	Synthetic Substitute
Prodisc-C	Synthetic Substitute
Prodisc-L	Synthetic Substitute
PROLENE Polypropylene Hernia System (PHS)	Synthetic Substitute
Protecta XT CRT-D	Cardiac Resynchronization Defibrillator Pulse Generator for Insertion in Subcutaneous Tissue and Fascia
Protecta XT DR (XT VR)	Defibrillator Generator for Insertion in Subcutaneous Tissue and Fascia
Protégé® RX Carotid Stent System	Intraluminal Device
Pump reservoir	Infusion Device, Pump in Subcutaneous Tissue and Fascia
REALIZE® Adjustable Gastric Band	Extraluminal Device
Rebound HRD® (Hernia Repair Device)	Synthetic Substitute
Reducer™ System	Reduction Device in New Technology
RestoreAdvanced neurostimulator (SureScan)(MRI Safe)	Stimulator Generator, Multiple Array Rechargeable for Insertion in Subcutaneous Tissue and Fascia
RestoreSensor neurostimulator (SureScan)(MRI Safe)	Stimulator Generator, Multiple Array Rechargeable for Insertion in Subcutaneous Tissue and Fascia
RestoreUltra neurostimulator (SureScan)(MRI Safe)	Stimulator Generator, Multiple Array Rechargeable for Insertion in Subcutaneous Tissue and Fascia
Reveal (LINQ)(DX)(XT)	Monitoring Device
Reverse® Shoulder Prosthesis	Synthetic Substitute, Reverse Ball and Socket for Replacement in Upper Joints
Revo MRI™ SureScan® pacemaker	Pacemaker, Dual Chamber for Insertion in Subcutaneous Tissue and Fascia
Rheos® System device	Stimulator Generator in Subcutaneous Tissue and Fascia
Rheos® System lead	Stimulator Lead in Upper Arteries
RNS System lead	Neurostimulator Lead in Central Nervous System and Cranial Nerves
RNS system neurostimulator generator	Neurostimulator Generator in Head and Facial Bones
S-ICD™ lead	Subcutaneous Defibrillator Lead in Subcutaneous Tissue and Fascia
Sacral nerve modulation (SNM) lead	Stimulator Lead in Urinary System
Sacral neuromodulation lead	Stimulator Lead in Urinary System
SAPIEN transcatheter aortic valve	Zooplastic Tissue in Heart and Great Vessels

Term	ICD-10-PCS Value
SAVAL below-the-knee (BTK) drug-eluting stent system	Intraluminal Device, Sustained Release Drug-eluting in New Technology Intraluminal Device, Sustained Release Drug-eluting, Two in New Technology Intraluminal Device, Sustained Release Drug-eluting, Three in New Technology Intraluminal Device, Sustained Release Drug-eluting, Four or More in New Technology
Secura (DR) (VR)	Defibrillator Generator for Insertion in Subcutaneous Tissue and Fascia
Sheffield hybrid external fixator	External Fixation Device, Hybrid for Insertion in Upper Bones External Fixation Device, Hybrid for Reposition in Upper Bones External Fixation Device, Hybrid for Insertion in Lower Bones External Fixation Device, Hybrid for Reposition in Lower Bones
Sheffield ring external fixator	External Fixation Device, Ring for Insertion in Upper Bones External Fixation Device, Ring for Reposition in Upper Bones External Fixation Device, Ring for Insertion in Lower Bones External Fixation Device, Ring for Reposition in Lower Bones
Single lead pacemaker (atrium)(ventricle)	Pacemaker, Single Chamber for Insertion in Subcutaneous Tissue and Fascia
Single lead rate responsive pacemaker (atrium)(ventricle)	Pacemaker, Single Chamber Rate Responsive for Insertion in Subcutaneous Tissue and Fascia
Sirolimus-eluting coronary stent	Intraluminal Device, Drug-eluting in Heart and Great Vessels
SJM Biocor® Stented Valve System	Zooplastic Tissue in Heart and Great Vessels
Spacer, Articulating (Antibiotic)	Articulating Spacer in Lower Joints
Spacer, Static (Antibiotic)	Spacer in Lower Joints
Spinal cord neurostimulator lead	Neurostimulator Lead in Central Nervous System and Cranial Nerves
Spinal growth rods, magnetically controlled	Magnetically Controlled Growth Rod(s) in New Technology
SpineJack® system NT	Synthetic Substitute, Mechanically Expandable (Paired) in New Technology
Spiration IBV™ Valve System	Intraluminal Device, Endobronchial Valve in Respiratory System
Static Spacer (Antibiotic)	Spacer in Lower Joints
Stent, intraluminal (cardiovascular) (gastrointestinal) (hepatobiliary)(urinary)	Intraluminal Device
Stented tissue valve	Zooplastic Tissue in Heart and Great Vessels
Stratos LV	Cardiac Resynchronization Pacemaker Pulse Generator for Insertion in Subcutaneous Tissue and Fascia
Subcutaneous injection reservoir, port	Vascular Access Device, Totally Implantable in Subcutaneous Tissue and Fascia
Subcutaneous injection reservoir, pump	Infusion Device, Pump in Subcutaneous Tissue and Fascia

Term	ICD-10-PCS Value
Subdermal progesterone implant	Contraceptive Device in Subcutaneous Tissue and Fascia
Surpass Streamline™ Flow Diverter	Intraluminal Device, Flow Diverter for Restriction in Upper Arteries
Sutureless valve, Perceval	Zooplastic Tissue, Rapid Deployment Technique in New Technology
SynCardia (temporary) Total Artificial Heart (TAH)	Synthetic Substitute, Pneumatic for Replacement in Heart and Great Vessels
SynCardia Total Artificial Heart	Synthetic Substitute
Synchra CRT-P	Cardiac Resynchronization Pacemaker Pulse Generator for Insertion in Subcutaneous Tissue and Fascia
SyncroMed Pump	Infusion Device, Pump in Subcutaneous Tissue and Fascia
Talent® Converter	Intraluminal Device
Talent® Occluder	Intraluminal Device
Talent® Stent Graft (abdominal)(thoracic)	Intraluminal Device
TandemHeart® System	Short-term External Heart Assist System in Heart and Great Vessels
TAXUS® Liberté® Paclitaxel-eluting Coronary Stent System	Intraluminal Device, Drug-eluting in Heart and Great Vessels
Therapeutic occlusion coil(s)	Intraluminal Device
Thoracostomy tube	Drainage Device
Thoraflex™ Hybrid device	Branched Synthetic Substitute with Intraluminal Device in New Technology
Thoratec IVAD (Implantable Ventricular Assist Device)	Implantable Heart Assist System in Heart and Great Vessels
Thoratec Paracorporeal Ventricular Assist Device	Short-term External Heart Assist System in Heart and Great Vessels
Tibial insert	Liner in Lower Joints
Tissue bank graft	Nonautologous Tissue Substitute
Tissue expander (inflatable)(injectable)	Tissue Expander in Skin and Breast Tissue Expander in Subcutaneous Tissue and Fascia
Titanium Sternal Fixation System (TSFS)	Internal Fixation Device, Rigid Plate for Insertion in Upper Bones Internal Fixation Device, Rigid Plate for Reposition in Upper Bones
Total artificial (replacement) heart	Synthetic Substitute
Tracheostomy tube	Tracheostomy Device in Respiratory System
Trifecta™ Valve (aortic)	Zooplastic Tissue in Heart and Great Vessels
Tunneled central venous catheter	Vascular Access Device, Tunneled in Subcutaneous Tissue and Fascia
Tunneled spinal (intrathecal) catheter	Infusion Device
Two lead pacemaker	Pacemaker, Dual Chamber for Insertion in Subcutaneous Tissue and Fascia
Ultraflex™ Precision Colonic Stent System	Intraluminal Device
ULTRAPRO Hernia System (UHS)	Synthetic Substitute
ULTRAPRO Partially Absorbable Lightweight Mesh	Synthetic Substitute
ULTRAPRO Plug	Synthetic Substitute
Ultrasonic osteogenic stimulator	Bone Growth Stimulator in Head and Facial Bones Bone Growth Stimulator in Upper Bones Bone Growth Stimulator in Lower Bones
Ultrasound bone healing system	Bone Growth Stimulator in Head and Facial Bones Bone Growth Stimulator in Upper Bones Bone Growth Stimulator in Lower Bones
Uniplanar external fixator	External Fixation Device, Monoplanar for Insertion in Upper Bones External Fixation Device, Monoplanar for Reposition in Upper Bones External Fixation Device, Monoplanar for Insertion in Lower Bones External Fixation Device, Monoplanar for Reposition in Lower Bones
Urinary incontinence stimulator lead	Stimulator Lead in Urinary System
V-Wave Interatrial Shunt System	Synthetic Substitute
Vaginal pessary	Intraluminal Device, Pessary in Female Reproductive System
Valiant Thoracic Stent Graft	Intraluminal Device
Vectra® Vascular Access Graft	Vascular Access Device, Tunneled in Subcutaneous Tissue and Fascia
Ventrio™ Hernia Patch	Synthetic Substitute
Versa	Pacemaker, Dual Chamber for Insertion in Subcutaneous Tissue and Fascia
Virtuoso (II) (DR) (VR)	Defibrillator Generator for Insertion in Subcutaneous Tissue and Fascia
Viva(XT)(S)	Cardiac Resynchronization Defibrillator Pulse Generator for Insertion in Subcutaneous Tissue and Fascia
WALLSTENT® Endoprosthesis	Intraluminal Device
X-STOP® Spacer	Spinal Stabilization Device, Interspinous Process for Insertion in Upper Joints Spinal Stabilization Device, Interspinous Process for Insertion in Lower Joints
Xact Carotid Stent System	Intraluminal Device
Xenograft	Zooplastic Tissue in Heart and Great Vessels
XIENCE Everolimus Eluting Coronary Stent System	Intraluminal Device, Drug-eluting in Heart and Great Vessels
XLIF® System	Interbody Fusion Device in Lower Joints
Zenith® Fenestrated AAA Endovascular Graft	Intraluminal Device, Branched or Fenestrated, One or Two Arteries for Restriction in Lower Arteries Intraluminal Device, Branched or Fenestrated, Three or More Arteries for Restriction in Lower Arteries Intraluminal Device
Zenith Flex® AAA Endovascular Graft	Intraluminal Device
Zenith TX2® TAA Endovascular Graft	Intraluminal Device
Zenith® Renu™ AAA Ancillary Graft	Intraluminal Device
Zilver® PTX® (paclitaxel) Drug-Eluting Peripheral Stent	Intraluminal Device, Drug-eluting in Upper Arteries Intraluminal Device, Drug-eluting in Lower Arteries
Zimmer® NexGen® LPS Mobile Bearing Knee	Synthetic Substitute

Term	ICD-10-PCS Value
Zimmer® NexGen® LPS-Flex Mobile Knee	Synthetic Substitute
Zotarolimus-eluting coronary stent	Intraluminal Device, Drug-eluting in Heart and Great Vessels

Device Aggregation Table

This table crosswalks specific device character value definitions for specific root operations in a specific body system to the more general device character value to be used when the root operation covers a wide range of body parts and the device character represents an entire family of devices.

Specific Device	for Operation	in Body System	General Device
Autologous Arterial Tissue (A)	All applicable	Heart and Great Vessels Lower Arteries Lower Veins Upper Arteries Upper Veins	**7** Autologous Tissue Substitute
Autologous Venous Tissue (9)	All applicable	Heart and Great Vessels Lower Arteries Lower Veins Upper Arteries Upper Veins	**7** Autologous Tissue Substitute
Cardiac Lead, Defibrillator (K)	Insertion	Heart and Great Vessels	**M** Cardiac Lead
Cardiac Lead, Pacemaker (J)	Insertion	Heart and Great Vessels	**M** Cardiac Lead
Cardiac Resynchronization Defibrillator Pulse Generator (9)	Insertion	Subcutaneous Tissue and Fascia	**P** Cardiac Rhythm Related Device
Cardiac Resynchronization Pacemaker Pulse Generator (7)	Insertion	Subcutaneous Tissue and Fascia	**P** Cardiac Rhythm Related Device
Contractility Modulation Device (A)	Insertion	Subcutaneous Tissue and Fascia	**P** Cardiac Rhythm Related Device
Defibrillator Generator (8)	Insertion	Subcutaneous Tissue and Fascia	**P** Cardiac Rhythm Related Device
Epiretinal Visual Prosthesis (5)	All applicable	Eye	**J** Synthetic Substitute
External Fixation Device, Hybrid (D)	Insertion	Lower Bones Upper Bones	**5** External Fixation Device
External Fixation Device, Hybrid (D)	Reposition	Lower Bones Upper Bones	**5** External Fixation Device
External Fixation Device, Limb Lengthening (8)	Insertion	Lower Bones Upper Bones	**5** External Fixation Device
External Fixation Device, Monoplanar (B)	Insertion	Lower Bones Upper Bones	**5** External Fixation Device
External Fixation Device, Monoplanar (B)	Reposition	Lower Bones Upper Bones	**5** External Fixation Device
External Fixation Device, Ring (C)	Insertion	Lower Bones Upper Bones	**5** External Fixation Device
External Fixation Device, Ring (C)	Reposition	Lower Bones Upper Bones	**5** External Fixation Device
Hearing Device, Bone Conduction (4)	Insertion	Ear, Nose, Sinus	**S** Hearing Device
Hearing Device, Multiple Channel Cochlear Prosthesis (6)	Insertion	Ear, Nose, Sinus	**S** Hearing Device
Hearing Device, Single Channel Cochlear Prosthesis (5)	Insertion	Ear, Nose, Sinus	**S** Hearing Device
Internal Fixation Device, Intramedullary (6)	All applicable	Lower Bones Upper Bones	**4** Internal Fixation Device
Internal Fixation Device, Intramedullary Limb Lengthening (7)	Insertion	Lower Bones Upper Bones	**6** Internal Fixation Device, Intramedullary
Internal Fixation Device, Rigid Plate (Ø)	Insertion	Upper Bones	**4** Internal Fixation Device
Internal Fixation Device, Rigid Plate (Ø)	Reposition	Upper Bones	**4** Internal Fixation Device
Intraluminal Device, Airway (B)	All applicable	Ear, Nose, Sinus Gastrointestinal System Mouth and Throat	**D** Intraluminal Device
Intraluminal Device, Bioactive (B)	All applicable	Upper Arteries	**D** Intraluminal Device
Intraluminal Device, Branched or Fenestrated, One or Two Arteries (E)	Restriction	Heart and Great Vessels Lower Arteries	**D** Intraluminal Device

Specific Device	for Operation	in Body System	General Device
Intraluminal Device, Branched or Fenestrated, Three or More Arteries (F)	Restriction	Heart and Great Vessels Lower Arteries	**D** Intraluminal Device
Intraluminal Device, Drug-eluting (4)	All applicable	Heart and Great Vessels Lower Arteries Upper Arteries	**D** Intraluminal Device
Intraluminal Device, Drug-eluting, Four or More (7)	All applicable	Heart and Great Vessels Lower Arteries Upper Arteries	**D** Intraluminal Device
Intraluminal Device, Drug-eluting, Three (6)	All applicable	Heart and Great Vessels Lower Arteries Upper Arteries	**D** Intraluminal Device
Intraluminal Device, Drug-eluting, Two (5)	All applicable	Heart and Great Vessels Lower Arteries Upper Arteries	**D** Intraluminal Device
Intraluminal Device, Endobronchial Valve (G)	All applicable	Respiratory System	**D** Intraluminal Device
Intraluminal Device, Endotracheal Airway (E)	All applicable	Respiratory System	**D** Intraluminal Device
Intraluminal Device, Flow Diverter (H)	Restriction	Upper Arteries	**D** Intraluminal Device
Intraluminal Device, Four or More (G)	All applicable	Heart and Great Vessels Lower Arteries Upper Arteries	**D** Intraluminal Device
Intraluminal Device, Pessary (G)	All applicable	Female Reproductive System	**D** Intraluminal Device
Intraluminal Device, Radioactive (T)	All applicable	Heart and Great Vessels	**D** Intraluminal Device
Intraluminal Device, Three (F)	All applicable	Heart and Great Vessels Lower Arteries Upper Arteries	**D** Intraluminal Device
Intraluminal Device, Two (E)	All applicable	Heart and Great Vessels Lower Arteries Upper Arteries	**D** Intraluminal Device
Monitoring Device, Hemodynamic (Ø)	Insertion	Subcutaneous Tissue and Fascia	**2** Monitoring Device
Monitoring Device, Pressure Sensor (Ø)	Insertion	Heart and Great Vessels	**2** Monitoring Device
Pacemaker, Dual Chamber (6)	Insertion	Subcutaneous Tissue and Fascia	**P** Cardiac Rhythm Related Device
Pacemaker, Single Chamber (4)	Insertion	Subcutaneous Tissue and Fascia	**P** Cardiac Rhythm Related Device
Pacemaker, Single Chamber Rate Responsive (5)	Insertion	Subcutaneous Tissue and Fascia	**P** Cardiac Rhythm Related Device
Spinal Stabilization Device, Facet Replacement (D)	Insertion	Lower Joints Upper Joints	**4** Internal Fixation Device
Spinal Stabilization Device, Interspinous Process (B)	Insertion	Lower Joints Upper Joints	**4** Internal Fixation Device
Spinal Stabilization Device, Pedicle-Based (C)	Insertion	Lower Joints Upper Joints	**4** Internal Fixation Device
Spinal Stabilization Device, Vertebral Body Tether (3)	Reposition	Lower Bones Upper Bones	**4** Internal Fixation Device
Stimulator Generator, Multiple Array (D)	Insertion	Subcutaneous Tissue and Fascia	**M** Stimulator Generator
Stimulator Generator, Multiple Array Rechargeable (E)	Insertion	Subcutaneous Tissue and Fascia	**M** Stimulator Generator
Stimulator Generator, Single Array (B)	Insertion	Subcutaneous Tissue and Fascia	**M** Stimulator Generator
Stimulator Generator, Single Array Rechargeable (C)	Insertion	Subcutaneous Tissue and Fascia	**M** Stimulator Generator
Synthetic Substitute, Ceramic (3)	Replacement	Lower Joints	**J** Synthetic Substitute
Synthetic Substitute, Ceramic on Polyethylene (4)	Replacement	Lower Joints	**J** Synthetic Substitute
Synthetic Substitute, Intraocular Telescope (Ø)	Replacement	Eye	**J** Synthetic Substitute
Synthetic Substitute, Metal (1)	Replacement	Lower Joints	**J** Synthetic Substitute
Synthetic Substitute, Metal on Polyethylene (2)	Replacement	Lower Joints	**J** Synthetic Substitute
Synthetic Substitute, Oxidized Zirconium on Polyethylene (6)	Replacement	Lower Joints	**J** Synthetic Substitute
Synthetic Substitute, Polyethylene (Ø)	Replacement	Lower Joints	**J** Synthetic Substitute
Synthetic Substitute, Reverse Ball and Socket (Ø)	Replacement	Upper Joints	**J** Synthetic Substitute

Appendix H: Device Definitions

This NT symbol next to a device in the Definition column identifies that the device has been approved for NTAP (new technology add-on payment). CMS provides incremental payment, in addition to the DRG payment, for technologies that have received an NTAP designation.

ICD-10-PCS Value	Definition
Articulating Spacer in Lower Joints	**Includes:** Articulating Spacer (Antibiotic) Spacer, Articulating (Antibiotic)
Artificial Sphincter in Gastrointestinal System	**Includes:** Artificial anal sphincter (AAS) Artificial bowel sphincter (neosphincter)
Artificial Sphincter in Urinary System	**Includes:** AMS 800® Urinary Control System Artificial urinary sphincter (AUS)
Autologous Arterial Tissue in Heart and Great Vessels	**Includes:** Autologous artery graft
Autologous Arterial Tissue in Lower Arteries	**Includes:** Autologous artery graft
Autologous Arterial Tissue in Lower Veins	**Includes:** Autologous artery graft
Autologous Arterial Tissue in Upper Arteries	**Includes:** Autologous artery graft
Autologous Arterial Tissue in Upper Veins	**Includes:** Autologous artery graft
Autologous Tissue Substitute	**Includes:** Autograft Cultured epidermal cell autograft Epicel® cultured epidermal autograft
Autologous Venous Tissue in Heart and Great Vessels	**Includes:** Autologous vein graft
Autologous Venous Tissue in Lower Arteries	**Includes:** Autologous vein graft
Autologous Venous Tissue in Lower Veins	**Includes:** Autologous vein graft
Autologous Venous Tissue in Upper Arteries	**Includes:** Autologous vein graft
Autologous Venous Tissue in Upper Veins	**Includes:** Autologous vein graft
Biologic with Synthetic Substitute, Autoregulated Electrohydraulic for Replacement in Heart and Great Vessels	**Includes:** Carmat total artificial heart (TAH)
Bone Growth Stimulator in Head and Facial Bones	**Includes:** Electrical bone growth stimulator (EBGS) Ultrasonic osteogenic stimulator Ultrasound bone healing system
Bone Growth Stimulator in Lower Bones	**Includes:** Electrical bone growth stimulator (EBGS) Ultrasonic osteogenic stimulator Ultrasound bone healing system
Bone Growth Stimulator in Upper Bones	**Includes:** Electrical bone growth stimulator (EBGS) Ultrasonic osteogenic stimulator Ultrasound bone healing system
Branched Synthetic Substitute with Intraluminal Device in New Technology	**Includes:** Thoraflex™ Hybrid device

ICD-10-PCS Value	Definition
Cardiac Lead in Heart and Great Vessels	**Includes:** Cardiac contractility modulation lead NT
Cardiac Lead, Defibrillator for Insertion in Heart and Great Vessels	**Includes:** ACUITY™ Steerable Lead Attain Ability® lead Attain StarFix® (OTW) lead Cardiac resynchronization therapy (CRT) lead Corox (OTW) Bipolar Lead Durata® Defibrillation Lead ENDOTAK RELIANCE® (G) Defibrillation Lead
Cardiac Lead, Pacemaker for Insertion in Heart and Great Vessels	**Includes:** ACUITY™ Steerable Lead Attain Ability® lead Attain StarFix® (OTW) lead Cardiac resynchronization therapy (CRT) lead Corox (OTW) Bipolar Lead
Cardiac Resynchronization Defibrillator Pulse Generator for Insertion in Subcutaneous Tissue and Fascia	**Includes:** COGNIS® CRT-D Concerto II CRT-D Consulta CRT-D CONTAK RENEWA® 3 RF (HE) CRT-D LIVIAN™ CRT-D Maximo II DR CRT-D Ovatio™ CRT-D Protecta XT CRT-D Viva (XT)(S)
Cardiac Resynchronization Pacemaker Pulse Generator for Insertion in Subcutaneous Tissue and Fascia	**Includes:** Consulta CRT-P Stratos LV Synchra CRT-P
Contraceptive Device in Female Reproductive System	**Includes:** Intrauterine device (IUD)
Contraceptive Device in Subcutaneous Tissue and Fascia	**Includes:** Subdermal progesterone implant
Contractility Modulation Device for Insertion in Subcutaneous Tissue and Fascia	**Includes:** Optimizer™ III implantable pulse generator NT
Defibrillator Generator for Insertion in Subcutaneous Tissue and Fascia	**Includes:** Evera (XT)(S)(DR/VR) Implantable cardioverter-defibrillator (ICD) Maximo II DR (VR) Protecta XT DR (XT VR) Secura (DR) (VR) Virtuoso (II) (DR) (VR)
Diaphragmatic Pacemaker Lead in Respiratory System	**Includes:** Phrenic nerve stimulator lead
Drainage Device	**Includes:** Cystostomy tube Foley catheter Percutaneous nephrostomy catheter Thoracostomy tube

ICD-10-PCS Value	Definition
External Fixation Device in Head and Facial Bones	**Includes:** External fixator
External Fixation Device in Lower Bones	**Includes:** External fixator
External Fixation Device in Lower Joints	**Includes:** External fixator
External Fixation Device in Upper Bones	**Includes:** External fixator
External Fixation Device in Upper Joints	**Includes:** External fixator
External Fixation Device, Hybrid for Insertion in Lower Bones	**Includes:** Delta frame external fixator Sheffield hybrid external fixator
External Fixation Device, Hybrid for Insertion in Upper Bones	**Includes:** Delta frame external fixator Sheffield hybrid external fixator
External Fixation Device, Hybrid for Reposition in Lower Bones	**Includes:** Delta frame external fixator Sheffield hybrid external fixator
External Fixation Device, Hybrid for Reposition in Upper Bones	**Includes:** Delta frame external fixator Sheffield hybrid external fixator
External Fixation Device, Limb Lengthening for Insertion in Lower Bones	**Includes:** Ilizarov-Vecklich device
External Fixation Device, Limb Lengthening for Insertion in Upper Bones	**Includes:** Ilizarov-Vecklich device
External Fixation Device, Monoplanar for Insertion in Lower Bones	**Includes:** Uniplanar external fixator
External Fixation Device, Monoplanar for Insertion in Upper Bones	**Includes:** Uniplanar external fixator
External Fixation Device, Monoplanar for Reposition in Lower Bones	**Includes:** Uniplanar external fixator
External Fixation Device, Monoplanar for Reposition in Upper Bones	**Includes:** Uniplanar external fixator
External Fixation Device, Ring for Insertion in Lower Bones	**Includes:** Ilizarov external fixator Sheffield ring external fixator
External Fixation Device, Ring for Insertion in Upper Bones	**Includes:** Ilizarov external fixator Sheffield ring external fixator
External Fixation Device, Ring for Reposition in Lower Bones	**Includes:** Ilizarov external fixator Sheffield ring external fixator
External Fixation Device, Ring for Reposition in Upper Bones	**Includes:** Ilizarov external fixator Sheffield ring external fixator
Extraluminal Device	**Includes:** AtriClip LAA Exclusion System LAP-BAND® adjustable gastric banding system REALIZE® Adjustable Gastric Band
Feeding Device in Gastrointestinal System	**Includes:** Percutaneous endoscopic gastrojejunostomy (PEG/J) tube Percutaneous endoscopic gastrostomy (PEG) tube

ICD-10-PCS Value	Definition
Hearing Device in Ear, Nose, Sinus	**Includes:** Esteem® implantable hearing system
Hearing Device in Head and Facial Bones	**Includes:** Bone anchored hearing device
Hearing Device, Bone Conduction for Insertion in Ear, Nose, Sinus	**Includes:** Bone anchored hearing device
Hearing Device, Multiple Channel Cochlear Prosthesis for Insertion in Ear, Nose, Sinus	**Includes:** Cochlear implant (CI), multiple channel (electrode)
Hearing Device, Single Channel Cochlear Prosthesis for Insertion in Ear, Nose, Sinus	**Includes:** Cochlear implant (CI), single channel (electrode)
Implantable Heart Assist System in Heart and Great Vessels	**Includes:** Berlin Heart Ventricular Assist Device DeBakey Left Ventricular Assist Device DuraHeart Left Ventricular Assist System HeartMate 3™ LVAS HeartMate II® Left Ventricular Assist Device (LVAD) HeartMate XVE® Left Ventricular Assist Device (LVAD) MicroMed HeartAssist Novacor Left Ventricular Assist Device Thoratec IVAD (Implantable Ventricular Assist Device)
Infusion Device	**Includes:** Ascenda Intrathecal Catheter InDura, intrathecal catheter (1P) (spinal) Non-tunneled central venous catheter Peripherally inserted central catheter (PICC) Tunneled spinal (intrathecal) catheter
Infusion Device, Pump in Subcutaneous Tissue and Fascia	**Includes:** Implantable drug infusion pump (anti-spasmodic)(chemotherapy) (pain) Injection reservoir, pump Pump reservoir Subcutaneous injection reservoir, pump SynchroMed pump
Interbody Fusion Device, Customizable in New Technology	**Includes:** aprevo™
Interbody Fusion Device in Lower Joints	**Includes:** Axial Lumbar Interbody Fusion System AxiaLIF® System CoRoent® XL Direct Lateral Interbody Fusion (DLIF) device EXtreme Lateral Interbody Fusion (XLIF) device Interbody fusion (spine) cage XLIF® System
Interbody Fusion Device in Upper Joints	**Includes:** BAK/C® Interbody Cervical Fusion System Interbody fusion (spine) cage
Interbody Fusion Device, Customizable in New Technology	**Includes:** aprevo™
Interbody Fusion Device, Nanotextured Surface in New Technology	**Includes:** nanoLOCK™ interbody fusion device

ICD-10-PCS Value	Definition
Interbody Fusion Device, Radiolucent Porous in New Technology	Includes: COALESCE® radiolucent interbody fusion device COHERE® radiolucent interbody fusion device
Internal Fixation Device in Head and Facial Bones	**Includes:** Bone screw (interlocking)(lag)(pedicle) (recessed) Kirschner wire (K-wire) Neutralization plate
Internal Fixation Device in Lower Bones	**Includes:** Bone screw (interlocking)(lag)(pedicle) (recessed) Clamp and rod internal fixation system (CRIF) Kirschner wire (K-wire) Neutralization plate
Internal Fixation Device in Lower Joints	**Includes:** Fusion screw (compression)(lag)(locking) Joint fixation plate Kirschner wire (K-wire)
Internal Fixation Device in Upper Bones	**Includes:** Bone screw (interlocking)(lag)(pedicle) (recessed) Clamp and rod internal fixation system (CRIF) Kirschner wire (K-wire) Neutralization plate
Internal Fixation Device in Upper Joints	**Includes:** Fusion screw (compression)(lag)(locking) Joint fixation plate Kirschner wire (K-wire)
Internal Fixation Device, Intramedullary in Lower Bones	**Includes:** Intramedullary (IM) rod (nail) Intramedullary skeletal kinetic distractor (ISKD) Kuntscher nail
Internal Fixation Device, Intramedullary in Upper Bones	**Includes:** Intramedullary (IM) rod (nail) Intramedullary skeletal kinetic distractor (ISKD) Kuntscher nail
Internal Fixation Device Intramedullary Limb Lengthening for Insertion in Lower Bones	**Includes:** PRECICE intramedullary limb lengthening system
Internal Fixation Device Intramedullary Limb Lengthening for Insertion in Upper Bones	**Includes:** PRECICE intramedullary limb lengthening system
Internal Fixation Device, Rigid Plate for Insertion in Upper Bones	**Includes:** Titanium Sternal Fixation System (TSFS)
Internal Fixation Device, Rigid Plate for Reposition in Upper Bones	**Includes:** Titanium Sternal Fixation System (TSFS)
Internal Fixation Device, Sustained Compression for Fusion in Lower Joints	**Includes:** DynaNail® DynaNail Mini®
Internal Fixation Device, Sustained Compression for Fusion in Upper Joints	**Includes:** DynaNail® DynaNail Mini®

ICD-10-PCS Value	Definition
Intraluminal Device	**Includes:** Absolute Pro Vascular (OTW) Self-Expanding Stent System Acculink (RX) Carotid Stent System AFX® Endovascular AAA System AneuRx® AAA Advantage® Assurant (Cobalt) stent Carotid WALLSTENT® Monorail® Endoprosthesis CoAxia NeuroFlo catheter Colonic Z-Stent® Complete (SE) stent Cook Zenith AAA Endovascular Graft Driver stent (RX) (OTW) E-Luminexx™ (Biliary)(Vascular) Stent Embolization coil(s) Endologix AFX® Endovascular AAA System Endurant® Endovascular Stent Graft Endurant® II AAA stent graft system EXCLUDER® AAA Endoprosthesis Express® (LD) Premounted Stent System Express® Biliary SD Monorail® Premounted Stent System Express® SD Renal Monorail® Premounted Stent System FLAIR® Endovascular Stent Graft Formula™ Balloon-Expandable Renal Stent System GORE EXCLUDER® AAA Endoprosthesis GORE TAG® Thoracic Endoprosthesis Herculink (RX) Elite Renal Stent System LifeStent® (Flexstar)(XL) Vascular Stent System Medtronic Endurant® II AAA stent graft system Micro-Driver stent (RX) (OTW) MULTI-LINK (VISION)(MINI-VISION)(ULTRA) Coronary Stent System Omnilink Elite Vascular Balloon Expandable Stent System Protege® RX Carotid Stent System Stent, intraluminal (cardiovascular) (gastrointestinal)(hepatobiliary) (urinary) Talent® Converter Talent® Occluder Talent® Stent Graft (abdominal)(thoracic) Therapeutic occlusion coil(s) Ultraflex™ Precision Colonic Stent System Valiant Thoracic Stent Graft WALLSTENT® Endoprosthesis Xact Carotid Stent System Zenith AAA Endovascular Graft Zenith Flex® AAA Endovascular Graft Zenith TX2® TAA Endovascular Graft Zenith® Renu™ AAA Ancillary Graft
Intraluminal Device, Airway in Ear, Nose, Sinus	**Includes:** Nasopharyngeal airway (NPA)
Intraluminal Device, Airway in Gastrointestinal System	**Includes:** Esophageal obturator airway (EOA)
Intraluminal Device, Airway in Mouth and Throat	**Includes:** Guedel airway Oropharyngeal airway (OPA)
Intraluminal Device, Bioactive in Upper Arteries	**Includes:** Bioactive embolization coil(s) Micrus CERECYTE microcoil

ICD-10-PCS Value	Definition
Intraluminal Device, Branched or Fenestrated, One or Two Arteries for Restriction in Lower Arteries	**Includes:** Cook Zenith® Fenestrated AAA Endovascular Graft EXCLUDER® AAA Endoprosthesis EXCLUDER® IBE Endoprosthesis GORE EXCLUDER® AAA Endoprosthesis GORE EXCLUDER®IBE Endoprosthesis Zenith® Fenestrated AAA Endovascular Graft
Intraluminal Device, Branched or Fenestrated, Three or More Arteries for Restriction in Lower Arteries	**Includes:** Cook Zenith® Fenestrated AAA Endovascular Graft EXCLUDER® AAA Endoprosthesis GORE EXCLUDER® AAA Endoprosthesis Zenith® Fenestrated AAA Endovascular Graft
Intraluminal Device, Drug-eluting in Heart and Great Vessels	**Includes:** CYPHER® Stent Endeavor® (III)(IV) (Sprint) Zotarolimus-eluting Coronary Stent System Everolimus-eluting coronary stent Paclitaxel-eluting coronary stent Sirolimus-eluting coronary stent TAXUS® Liberte® Paclitaxel-eluting Coronary Stent System XIENCE Everolimus Eluting Coronary Stent System Zotarolimus-eluting coronary stent
Intraluminal Device, Drug-eluting in Lower Arteries	**Includes:** Paclitaxel-eluting peripheral stent Zilver® PTX® (paclitaxel) Drug-Eluting Peripheral Stent
Intraluminal Device, Drug-eluting in Upper Arteries	**Includes:** Paclitaxel-eluting peripheral stent Zilver® PTX® (paclitaxel) Drug-Eluting Peripheral Stent
Intraluminal Device, Endobronchial Valve in Respiratory System	**Includes:** Spiration IBV™ Valve System
Intraluminal Device, Endotracheal Airway in Respiratory System	**Includes:** Endotracheal tube (cuffed)(double-lumen)
Intraluminal Device, Flow Diverter for Restriction in Upper Arteries	**Includes:** Flow Diverter embolization device Pipeline™ (Flex) embolization device Surpass Streamline™ Flow Diverter
Intraluminal Device, Pessary in Female Reproductive System	**Includes:** Pessary ring Vaginal pessary
Intraluminal Device, Sustained Release Drug-eluting in New Technology	**Includes:** Eluvia™ Drug-eluting Vascular Stent System NT SAVAL below-the-knee (BTK) drug-eluting stent system
Intraluminal Device, Sustained Release Drug-eluting, Four or More in New Technology	**Includes:** Eluvia™ Drug-eluting Vascular Stent System NT SAVAL below-the-knee (BTK) drug-eluting stent system
Intraluminal Device, Sustained Release Drug-eluting, Three in New Technology	**Includes:** Eluvia™ Drug-eluting Vascular Stent System NT SAVAL below-the-knee (BTK) drug-eluting stent system

ICD-10-PCS Value	Definition
Intraluminal Device, Sustained Release Drug-eluting, Two in New Technology	**Includes:** Eluvia™ Drug-eluting Vascular Stent System NT SAVAL below-the-knee (BTK) drug-eluting stent system
Liner in Lower Joints	**Includes:** Acetabular cup Hip (joint) liner Joint liner (insert) Knee (implant) insert Tibial insert
Magnetically Controlled Growth Rod(s) in New Technology	**Includes:** MAGEC® Spinal Bracing and Distraction System Spinal growth rods, magnetically controlled
Monitoring Device	**Includes:** Blood glucose monitoring system Cardiac event recorder Continuous Glucose Monitoring (CGM) device Implantable glucose monitoring device Loop recorder, implantable Reveal (LINQ)(DX)(XT)
Monitoring Device, Hemodynamic for Insertion in Subcutaneous Tissue and Fascia	**Includes:** Implantable hemodynamic monitor (IHM) Implantable hemodynamic monitoring system (IHMS)
Monitoring Device, Pressure Sensor for Insertion in Heart and Great Vessels	**Includes:** CardioMEMS® pressure sensor EndoSure® sensor
Neurostimulator Generator in Head and Facial Bones	**Includes:** RNS system neurostimulator generator
Neurostimulator Lead in Central Nervous System and Cranial Nerves	**Includes:** Cortical strip neurostimulator lead DBS lead Deep brain neurostimulator lead RNS System lead Spinal cord neurostimulator lead
Neurostimulator Lead in Peripheral Nervous System	**Includes:** InterStim® Therapy lead
Nonautologous Tissue Substitute	**Includes:** Acellular Hydrated Dermis Bone bank bone graft Cook Biodesign® Fistula Plug(s) Cook Biodesign® Hernia Graft(s) Cook Biodesign® Layered Graft(s) Cook Zenapro™ Layered Graft(s) Tissue bank graft
Other Device	**Includes:** Alfapump® system
Pacemaker, Dual Chamber for Insertion in Subcutaneous Tissue and Fascia	**Includes:** Advisa (MRI) EnRhythm Kappa Revo MRI™ SureScan® pacemaker Two lead pacemaker Versa
Pacemaker, Single Chamber for Insertion in Subcutaneous Tissue and Fascia	**Includes:** Single lead pacemaker (atrium)(ventricle)

ICD-10-PCS Value	Definition
Pacemaker, Single Chamber Rate Responsive for Insertion in Subcutaneous Tissue and Fascia	**Includes:** Single lead rate responsive pacemaker (atrium)(ventricle)
Posterior (Dynamic) Distraction Device in New Technology	**Includes:** ApiFix® Minimally Invasive Deformity Correction (MID-C) System
Radioactive Element	**Includes:** Brachytherapy seeds CivaSheet®
Radioactive Element, Cesium-131 Collagen Implant for Insertion in Central Nervous System and Cranial Nerves	**Includes:** Cesium-131 Collagen Implant GammaTile™
Reduction Device in New Technology	**Includes:** Neovasc Reducer™ Reducer™ System
Resurfacing Device in Lower Joints	**Includes:** CONSERVE® PLUS Total Resurfacing Hip System Cormet Hip Resurfacing System
Short-term External Heart Assist System in Heart and Great Vessels	**Includes:** Biventricular external heart assist system BVS 5000 Ventricular Assist Device Centrimag® Blood Pump Impella® heart pump TandemHeart® System Thoratec Paracorporeal Ventricular Assist Device
Skin Substitute, Porcine Liver Derived in New Technology	**Includes:** MIRODERM™ Biologic Wound Matrix
Spacer in Lower Joints	**Includes:** Joint spacer (antibiotic) Spacer, Static (Antibiotic) Static Spacer (Antibiotic)
Spacer in Upper Joints	**Includes:** Joint spacer (antibiotic)
Spinal Stabilization Device, Facet Replacement for Insertion in Lower Joints	**Includes:** Facet replacement spinal stabilization device
Spinal Stabilization Device, Facet Replacement for Insertion in Upper Joints	**Includes:** Facet replacement spinal stabilization device
Spinal Stabilization Device, Interspinous Process for Insertion in Lower Joints	**Includes:** Interspinous process spinal stabilization device X-STOP® Spacer
Spinal Stabilization Device, Interspinous Process for Insertion in Upper Joints	**Includes:** Interspinous process spinal stabilization device X-STOP® Spacer
Spinal Stabilization Device, Pedicle- Based for Insertion in Lower Joints	**Includes:** Dynesys® Dynamic Stabilization System Pedicle-based dynamic stabilization device
Spinal Stabilization Device, Pedicle-Based for Insertion in Upper Joints	**Includes:** Dynesys® Dynamic Stabilization System Pedicle-based dynamic stabilization device

ICD-10-PCS Value	Definition
Stimulator Generator in Subcutaneous Tissue and Fascia	**Includes:** Baroreflex Activation Therapy® (BAT®) NT Diaphragmatic pacemaker generator Mark IV Breathing Pacemaker System Phrenic nerve stimulator generator Rheos® System device
Stimulator Generator, Multiple Array for Insertion in Subcutaneous Tissue and Fascia	**Includes:** Activa PC neurostimulator Enterra gastric neurostimulator Neurostimulator generator, multiple channel PERCEPT™ PC neurostimulator PrimeAdvanced neurostimulator (SureScan)(MRI Safe)
Stimulator Generator, Multiple Array Rechargeable for Insertion in Subcutaneous Tissue and Fascia	**Includes:** Activa RC neurostimulator Neurostimulator generator, multiple channel rechargeable RestoreAdvanced neurostimulator (SureScan)(MRI Safe) RestoreSensor neurostimulator (SureScan)(MRI Safe) RestoreUltra neurostimulator (SureScan)(MRI Safe)
Stimulator Generator, Single Array for Insertion in Subcutaneous Tissue and Fascia	**Includes:** Activa SC neurostimulator InterStim™ II Therapy neurostimulator Itrel (3)(4) neurostimulator Neurostimulator generator, single channel
Stimulator Generator, Single Array Rechargeable for Insertion in Subcutaneous Tissue and Fascia	**Includes:** InterStim™ Micro Therapy neurostimulator Neurostimulator generator, single channel rechargeable
Stimulator Lead in Gastrointestinal System	**Includes:** Gastric electrical stimulation (GES) lead Gastric pacemaker lead
Stimulator Lead in Muscles	**Includes:** Electrical muscle stimulation (EMS) lead Electronic muscle stimulator lead Neuromuscular electrical stimulation (NEMS) lead
Stimulator Lead in Upper Arteries	**Includes:** Baroreflex Activation Therapy® (BAT®) NT Carotid (artery) sinus (baroreceptor) lead Rheos® System lead
Stimulator Lead in Urinary System	**Includes:** Sacral nerve modulation (SNM) lead Sacral neuromodulation lead Urinary incontinence stimulator lead
Subcutaneous Defibrillator Lead in Subcutaneous Tissue and Fascia	**Includes:** S-ICD™ lead

ICD-10-PCS Value	Definition
Synthetic Substitute	**Includes:** AbioCor® Total Replacement Heart AMPLATZER® Muscular VSD Occluder Annuloplasty ring Bard® Composix® (E/X) (LP) mesh Bard® Composix® Kugel® patch Bard® Dulex™ mesh Bard® Ventralex™ hernia patch Barricaid® Annular Closure Device (ACD) BRYAN® Cervical Disc System Corvia IASD® Ex-PRESS™ mini glaucoma shunt Flexible Composite Mesh GORE® DUALMESH® Holter valve ventricular shunt IASD® (InterAtrial Shunt Device), Corvia InterAtrial Shunt Device IASD®, Corvia MitraClip valve repair system Nitinol framed polymer mesh Open Pivot (mechanical) valve Open Pivot Aortic Valve Graft (AVG) Partially absorbable mesh PHYSIOMESH™ Flexible Composite Mesh Polymethylmethacrylate (PMMA) Polypropylene mesh PRESTIGE® Cervical Disc PROCEED™ Ventral Patch Prodisc-C Prodisc-L PROLENE Polypropylene Hernia System (PHS) Rebound HRD® (Hernia Repair Device) SynCardia Total Artificial Heart Total artificial (replacement) heart ULTRAPRO Hernia System (UHS) ULTRAPRO Partially Absorbable Lightweight Mesh ULTRAPRO Plug V-Wave Interatrial Shunt System Ventrio™ Hernia Patch Zimmer® NexGen® LPS Mobile Bearing Knee Zimmer® NexGen® LPS-Flex Mobile Knee
Synthetic Substitute, Ceramic for Replacement in Lower Joints	**Includes:** Ceramic on ceramic bearing surface Novation® Ceramic AHS® (Articulation Hip System)
Synthetic Substitute, Intraocular Telescope for Replacement in Eye	**Includes:** Implantable Miniature Telescope™ (IMT)
Synthetic Substitute, Mechanically Expandable (Paired) in New Technology	**Includes:** SpineJack® system NT
Synthetic Substitute, Metal for Replacement in Lower Joints	**Includes:** Cobalt/chromium head and socket Metal on metal bearing surface
Synthetic Substitute, Metal on Polyethylene for Replacement in Lower Joints	**Includes:** Cobalt/chromium head and polyethylene socket
Synthetic Substitute, Oxidized Zirconium on Polyethylene for Replacement in Lower Joints	**Includes:** OXINIUM
Synthetic Substitute, Pneumatic for Replacement in Heart and Great Vessels	**Includes:** SynCardia (temporary) total artificial heart (TAH)
Synthetic Substitute, Polyethylene for Replacement in Lower Joints	**Includes:** Polyethylene socket
Synthetic Substitute, Reverse Ball and Socket for Replacement in Upper Joints	**Includes:** Delta III Reverse shoulder prosthesis Reverse® Shoulder Prosthesis
Tissue Expander in Skin and Breast	**Includes:** Tissue expander (inflatable) (injectable)
Tissue Expander in Subcutaneous Tissue and Fascia	**Includes:** Tissue expander (inflatable) (injectable)
Tracheostomy Device in Respiratory System	**Includes:** Tracheostomy tube
Vascular Access Device, Totally Implantable in Subcutaneous Tissue and Fascia	**Includes:** Implanted (venous)(access) port Injection reservoir, port Subcutaneous injection reservoir, port
Vascular Access Device, Tunneled in Subcutaneous Tissue and Fascia	**Includes:** Tunneled central venous catheter Vectra® Vascular Access Graft
Zooplastic Tissue in Heart and Great Vessels	**Includes:** 3f (Aortic) Bioprosthesis valve Bovine pericardial valve Bovine pericardium graft Contegra Pulmonary Valved Conduit CoreValve transcatheter aortic valve Epic™ Stented Tissue Valve (aortic) Freestyle (Stentless) Aortic Root Bioprosthesis Hancock Bioprosthesis (aortic) (mitral) valve Hancock Bioprosthetic Valved Conduit Melody® transcatheter pulmonary valve Mitroflow® Aortic Pericardial Heart Valve Mosaic Bioprosthesis (aortic) (mitral) valve Porcine (bioprosthetic) valve SAPIEN transcatheter aortic valve SJM Biocor® Stented Valve System Stented tissue valve Trifecta™ Valve (aortic) Xenograft
Zooplastic Tissue, Rapid Deployment Technique in New Technology	**Includes:** EDWARDS INTUITY Elite valve system INTUITY Elite valve system, EDWARDS Perceval sutureless valve Sutureless valve, Perceval

Appendix I: Substance Key/Substance Definitions

Substance Key

This table crosswalks a specific substance, listed by trade name or synonym, to the PCS value that would be used to represent that substance in either the Administration or New Technology section. The ICD-10-PCS value may be located in either the 6th-character Substance column or the 7th-character Qualifier column depending on the section/table to which it is classified. The most specific character is listed in the table.

This NT symbol next to a substance/technology in the Trade Name or Synonym column identifies that the substance/technology has been approved for NTAP (new technology add-on payment). CMS provides incremental payment, in addition to the DRG payment, for technologies that have received an NTAP designation.

Substances denoted by an asterisk (*) in the Trade Name or Synonym column, although not included in the official ICD-1Ø-PCS classification, were added based on information provided in the FY 2Ø22 IPPS proposed rule.

Trade Name or Synonym	ICD-10-PCS Value	PCS Section
ABECMA®	Idecabtagene Vicleucel Immunotherapy (K)	New Technology (X)
ACTEMRA®	Tocilizumab (H)	New Technology (X)
AIGISRx Antibacterial Envelope	Anti-Infective Envelope (A)	Administration (3)
Andexanet Alfa, Factor Xa Inhibitor Reversal Agent	Coagulation Factor Xa, Inactivated (7)	New Technology (X)
Andexxa NT	Coagulation Factor Xa, Inactivated (7)	New Technology (X)
Angiotensin II	Synthetic Human Angiotensin II (H)	New Technology (X)
Antibacterial Envelope (TYRX) (AIGISRx)	Anti-Infective Envelope (A)	Administration (3)
Antimicrobial envelope	Anti-Infective Envelope (A)	Administration (3)
Anti-SARS-CoV-2 hyperimmune globulin	Hyperimmune Globulin (E)	New Technology (X)
AVYCAZ® (ceftazidime-avibactam)	Other Anti-infective (9)	Administration (3)
Axicabtagene Ciloeucel	Axicabtagene Ciloleucel Immunotherapy (H)	New Technology (X)
AZEDRA® NT	Iobenguane I-131 Antineoplastic (S)	New Technology (X)
***Balversa™** NT	Erdafitinib Antineoplastic (L)	New Technology (X)
Blinatumomab	Other Antineoplastic (5)	Administration (3)
BLINCYTO® (blinatumomab)	Other Antineoplastic (5)	Administration (3)
Bone morphogenetic protein 2 (BMP 2)	Recombinant Bone Morphogenetic Protein (B)	Administration (3)
Brexucabtagene Autoleucel	Brexucabtagene Autoleucel Immunotherapy (4)	New Technology (X)
***CABLIVI®** NT	Caplacizumab (W)	New Technology (X)
Casirivimab (REGN1Ø933) and Imdevimab (REGN1Ø987)	REGN-COV2 Monoclonal Antibody (G)	New Technology (X)
CBMA (Concentrated Bone Marrow Aspirate)	Concentrated Bone Marrow Aspirate (Ø)	New Technology (X)
Ceftazidime-avibactam	Other Anti-infective (9)	Administration (3)
CERAMENT® G	Antibiotic-eluting Bone Void Filler (P)	New Technology (X)
cilta-cel	Ciltacabtagene Autoleucel (A)	New Technology (X)
Clolar	Clofarabine (P)	Administration (3)
Coagulation Factor Xa, (Recombinant) Inactivated	Coagulation Factor Xa, Inactivated (7)	New Technology (X)
CONTEPO™	Fosfomycin Anti-infective (K)	New Technology (X)
COSELA™	Trilaciclib (7)	New Technology (X)
CRESEMBA® (isavuconazonium sulfate)	Other Anti-infective (9)	Administration (3)
Defitelio	Defibrotide Sodium Anticoagulant (9)	New Technology (X)
DuraGraft® Endothelial Damage Inhibitor	Endothelial Damage Inhibitor (8)	New Technology (X)
ELZONRIS™ NT	Tagraxofusp-erzs Antineoplastic (Q)	New Technology (X)
ENSPRYNG™	Satralizumab-mwge (9)	New Technology (X)
ERLEADA™	Apalutamide Antineoplastic (J)	New Technology (X)
Factor Xa Inhibitor Reversal Agent, Andexanet Alfa	Coagulation Factor Xa, Inactivated (7)	New Technology (X)
FETROJA® NT	Cefiderocol Anti-infective (A)	New Technology (X)
Fosfomycin injection	Fosfomycin Anti-infective (K)	New Technology (X)
Gammaglobulin	Globulin (S)	Administration (3)
GAMUNEX-C, for COVID-19 treatment	High-Dose Intravenous Immune Globulin (D)	New Technology (X)
GIAPREZA™	Synthetic Human Angiotensin II (H)	New Technology (X)
GS-5734	Remdesivir Anti-infective (E)	New Technology (X)
hdIVIG (high-dose intravenous immunoglobulin), for COVID-19 treatment	High-Dose Intravenous Immune Globulin (D)	New Technology (X)
Hemospray® Endoscopic Hemostat NT	Mineral-based Topical Hemostatic Agent (8)	New Technology (X)
HIG (hyperimmune globulin), for COVID-19 treatment	Hyperimmune Globulin (E)	New Technology (X)

Trade Name or Synonym	ICD-10-PCS Value	PCS Section
High-dose intravenous immunoglobulin (hdIVIG), for COVID-19 treatment	Hyperimmune Globulin (E)	New Technology (X)
hIVIG (hyperimmune intravenous immunoglobulin), for COVID-19 treatment	Hyperimmune Globulin (E)	New Technology (X)
Human angiotensin II, synthetic	Synthetic Human Angiotensin II (H)	New Technology (X)
Hyperimmune globulin	Globulin (S)	Administration (3)
Hyperimmune intravenous immunoglobulin (hIVIG), for COVID-19 treatment	Hyperimmune Globulin (E)	New Technology (X)
Idarucizumab, Pradaxa® (dabigatran) reversal agent	Other Therapeutic Substance (G)	Administration (3)
Idecabtagene Vicleucel	Idecabtagene Vicleucel Immunotherapy (K)	New Technology (X)
Ide-cel	Idecabtagene Vicleucel Immunotherapy (K)	New Technology (X)
IGIV-C, for COVID-19 treatment	Hyperimmune Globulin (E)	New Technology (X)
Imdevimab (REGN10987) and Casirivimab (REGN10933)	REGN-COV2 Monoclonal Antibody (G)	New Technology (X)
IMFINZI® NT	Durvalumab Antineoplastic (3)	New Technology (X)
IMI/REL	Imipenem-cilastatin-relebactam Anti-infective (U)	New Technology (X)
Immunoglobulin	Globulin (S)	Administration (3)
INTERCEPT Blood System for Plasma Pathogen Reduced Cryoprecipitated Fibrinogen Complex	Pathogen Reduced Cryoprecipitated Fibrinogen Complex (D)	Administration (3)
INTERCEPT Fibrinogen Complex	Pathogen Reduced Cryoprecipitated Fibrinogen Complex (D)	Administration (3)
Iobenguane I-131, High Specific Activity (HSA)	Iobenguane I-131 Antineoplastic (S)	New Technology (X)
Isavuconazole (isavuconazonium sulfate)	Other Anti-infective (9)	Administration (3)
Jakafi® NT	Ruxolitinib (T)	New Technology (X)
Kcentra	4-Factor Prothrombin Complex Concentrate (B)	Administration (3)
KEVZARA®	Sarilumab (G)	New Technology (X)
KYMRIAH	Tisagenlecleucel Immunotherapy (J)	New Technology (X)
Lifileucel	Lifileucel Immunotherapy (L)	New Technology (X)
Lisocabtagene Maraleucel	Lisocabtagene Maraleucel Immunotherapy (7)	New Technology (X)
LTX Regional Anticoagulant	Nafamostat Anticoagulant (3)	New Technology (X)
NA-1 (Nerinitide)	Nerinitide (2)	New Technology (X)
Nesiritide	Human B-type Natriuretic Peptide (H)	Administration (3)
NexoBrid™	Bromelain-enriched Proteolytic Enzyme (2)	New Technology (X)
Niyad™	Nafamostat Anticoagulant (3)	New Technology (X)
NUZYRA™ NT	Omadacycline Anti-infective (B)	New Technology (X)
Octagam 10%, for COVID-19 treatment	High-Dose Intravenous Immune Globulin (D)	New Technology (X)
Olumiant® NT	Baricitinib (M)	New Technology (X)
OTL-101	Hematopoietic Stem/Progenitor Cells, Genetically Modified (C)	Administration (3)
OTL-103	Hematopoietic Stem/Progenitor Cells, Genetically Modified (C)	Administration (3)
OTL-200	Hematopoietic Stem/Progenitor Cells, Genetically Modified (C)	Administration (3)
Polyclonal hyperimmune globulin	Globulin (S)	Administration (3)
Praxbind® (idarucizumab), Pradaxa® (dabigatran) reversal agent	Other Therapeutic Substance (G)	Administration (3)
***RECARBRIO™** NT	Imipenem-cilastatin-relebactam Anti-infective (U)	New Technology (X)
rhBMP-2	Recombinant Bone Morphogenetic Protein (B)	Administration (3)
Seprafilm	Adhesion Barrier (5)	Administration (3)
Soliris® NT	Eculizumab (C)	New Technology (X)
SPRAVATO™ NT	Esketamine Hydrochloride (M)	New Technology (X)
STELARA®	Other New Technology Therapeutic Substance (F)	New Technology (X)
StrataGraft®	Bioengineered Allogeneic Construct (F)	New Technology (X)
Tecartus™	Brexucabtagene Autoleucel Immunotherapy (M)	New Technology (X)
TECENTRIQ® NT	Atezolizumab Antineoplastic (D)	New Technology (X)
TERLIVAZ®	Terlipressin (6)	New Technology (X)
Tisagenlecleucel	Tisagenlecleucel Immunotherapy (J)	New Technology (X)
Tissue Plasminogen Activator (tPA)(r- tPA)	Other Thrombolytic (7)	Administration (3)
TYRX Antibacterial Envelope	Anti-Infective Envelope (A)	Administration (3)
Ustekinumab	Other New Technology Therapeutic Substance (F)	New Technology (X)
Vabomere™	Meropenem-vaborbactam Anti-infective (N)	New Technology (X)
Veklury NT	Remdesivir Anti-infective (E)	New Technology (X)
Venclexta®	Ventoclax Antineoplastic (R)	New Technology (X)

Trade Name or Synonym	ICD-10-PCS Value	PCS Section
Vistogard®	Uridine Triacetate (8)	New Technology (X)
Voraxaze	Glucarpidase (Q)	Administration (3)
VYXEOS™	Cytarabine and Daunorubicin Liposome Antineoplastic (B)	New Technology (X)
XENLETA™ NT	Lefamulin Anti-infective (6)	New Technology (X)
XOSPATA® NT	Gilteritinib Antineoplastic (V)	New Technology (X)
***ZEMDRI™** NT	Plazomicin Anti-infective (6)	New Technology (X)
ZEPZELCA™	Lurbinectedin (8)	New Technology (X)
ZERBAXA® NT	Ceftolozane/Tazobactam Anti-infective (9)	New Technology (X)
ZINPLAVA™	Bezlotoxumab Monoclonal Antibody (A)	New Technology (X)
ZULRESSO™	Brexanolone (Ø)	New Technology (X)
Zyvox	Oxazolidinones (8)	Administration (3)

Substance Definitions

This table crosswalks a PCS value, used in the Administration or New Technology section, to a specific substance. The specific substances are listed by trade name or synonym. The ICD-10-PCS value may be located in either the 6th-character Substance column or the 7th-character Qualifier column depending on the section/table to which it is classified.

This NT symbol next to a substance/technology in the Trade Name or Synonym column identifies that the substance/technology has been approved for NTAP (new technology add-on payment). CMS provides incremental payment, in addition to the DRG payment, for technologies that have received an NTAP designation.

Substances denoted by an asterisk (*) in the Trade Name or Synonym column, although not included in the official ICD-1Ø-PCS classification, were added based on information provided in the FY 2Ø22 IPPS proposed rule.

ICD-10-PCS Value	Trade Name or Synonym	PCS Section
4-Factor Prothrombin Complex Concentrate (B)	**Includes:** Kcentra	Administration (3)
Adhesion Barrier (5)	**Includes:** Seprafilm	Administration (3)
Antibiotic-eluting Bone Void Filler (P)	**Includes:** CERAMENT® G	New Technology (X)
Anti-Infective Envelope (A)	**Includes:** AIGISRx Antibacterial Envelope Antimicrobial envelope Antibacterial Envelope (TYRX) (AIGISRx) TYRX Antibacterial Envelope	Administration (3)
Apalutamide Antineoplastic (J)	**Includes:** ERLEADA™	New Technology (X)
Atezolizumab Antineoplastic (D)	**Includes:** TECENTRIQ® NT	New Technology (X)
Axicabtagene Ciloleucel Immunotherapy (H)	**Includes:** Axicabtagene Ciloleucel Yescarta®	New Technology (X)
Baricitinib (M)	**Includes:** Olumiant® NT	New Technology (X)
Bezlotoxumab Monoclonal Antibody (A)	**Includes:** ZINPLAVA™	New Technology (X)
Bioengineered Allogeneic Construct (F)	**Includes:** StrataGraft®	New Technology (X)
Brexanolone (Ø)	**Includes:** ZULRESSO™	New Technology (X)
Brexucabtagene Autoleucel Immunotherapy (M)	**Includes:** Tecartus™	New Technology (X)
Bromelain-enriched Proteolytic Enzyme (2)	**Includes:** NexoBrid™	New Technology (X)
Caplacizumab (W)	**Includes:** *CABLIVI® NT	New Technology (X)
Cefiderocol Anti-infective (A)	**Includes:** FETROJA® NT	New Technology (X)
Ceftolozane/Tazobactam Anti- infective (9)	**Includes:** ZERBAXA® NT	New Technology (X)
Ciltacabtagene Autoleucel (A)	**Includes:** cilta-cel	New Technology (X)
Clofarabine (P)	**Includes:** Clolar	Administration (3)
Coagulation Factor Xa, Inactivated (7)	**Includes:** Andexanet Alfa, Factor Xa Inhibitor Reversal Agent Andexxa NT Coagulation Factor Xa, (Recombinant) Inactivated Factor Xa Inhibitor Reversal Agent, Andexanet Alfa	New Technology (X)
Concentrated Bone Marrow Aspirate (Ø)	**Includes:** CBMA (Concentrated Bone Marrow Aspirate)	New Technology (X)
Cytarabine and Daunorubicin Liposome Antineoplastic (B)	**Includes:** VYXEOS™	New Technology (X)
Defibrotide Sodium Anticoagulant (9)	**Includes:** Defitelio	New Technology (X)
Durvalumab Antineoplastic (3)	**Includes:** IMFINZI® NT	New Technology (X)
Eculizumab (C)	**Includes:** Soliris® NT	New Technology (X)
Endothelial Damage Inhibitor (8)	**Includes:** DuraGraft® Endothelial Damage Inhibitor	New Technology (X)
Erdafitinib Antineoplastic (L)	**Includes:** *Balversa™ NT	New Technology (X)
Esketamine Hydrochloride (M)	**Includes:** SPRAVATO™ NT	New Technology (X)

ICD-10-PCS Value	Trade Name or Synonym	PCS Section
Fosfomycin Anti-infective (K)	**Includes:** CONTEPO™ Fosfomycin injection	New Technology (X)
Gilteritinib Antineoplastic (V)	**Includes:** XOSPATA® NT	New Technology (X)
Globulin (S)	**Includes:** Gammaglobulin Hyperimmune globulin Immunoglobulin Polyclonal hyperimmune globulin	Administration (3)
Glucarpidase (Q)	**Includes:** Voraxaze	Administration (3)
Hematopoietic Stem/Progenitor Cells, Genetically Modified (C)	**Includes:** OTL-101 OTL-103 OTL-200	Administration (3)
High-Dose Intravenous Immune Globulin (D)	**Includes:** GAMUNEX-C, for COVID-19 treatment hdIVIG (high-dose intravenous immunoglobulin), for COVID-19 treatment High-dose intravenous immunoglobulin (hdIVIG), for COVID-19 treatment Octagam 10%, for COVID-19 treatment	New Technology (X)
Human B-type Natriuretic Peptide (H)	**Includes:** Nesiritide	Administration (3)
Hyperimmune Globulin (E)	**Includes:** Anti-SARS-CoV-2 hyperimmune globulin HIG (hyperimmune globulin), for COVID-19 treatment hIVIG (hyperimmune intravenous immunoglobulin), for COVID-19 treatment Hyperimmune intravenous immunoglobulin (hIVIG), for COVID-19 treatment IGIV-C, for COVID-19 treatment	New Technology (X)
Idecabtagene Vicleucel Immunotherapy (K)	**Includes:** ABECMA® Idecabtagene Vicleucel Ide-cel	New Technology (X)
Imipenem-cilastatin-relebactam Anti-infective (U)	**Includes:** IMI/REL *RECARBRIO™ NT	New Technology (X)
Iobenguane I-131 Antineoplastic (S)	**Includes:** AZEDRA® NT Iobenguane I-131, High Specific Activity (HSA)	New Technology (X)
Lefamulin Anti-infective (6)	**Includes:** XENLETA™ NT	New Technology (X)
Lifileucel Immunotherapy (L)	**Includes:** Lifileucel	New Technology (X)
Lisocabtagene Maraleucel Immunotherapy (7)	**Includes:** Lisocabtagene Maraleucel	New Technology (X)
Lurbinectedin (8)	**Includes:** ZEPZELCA™	New Technology (X)
Meropenem-vaborbactam Anti-infective (N)	**Includes:** Vabomere™	New Technology (X)
Mineral-based Topical Hemostatic Agent (8)	**Includes:** Hemospray® Endoscopic Hemostat NT	New Technology (X)
Nafamostat Anticoagulant (3)	**Includes:** LTX Regional Anticoagulant Niyad™	New Technology (X)
Nerinitide (2)	**Includes:** NA-1 (Nerinitide)	New Technology (X)
Omadacycline Anti-infective (B)	**Includes:** NUZYRA™ NT	New Technology (X)
Other Anti-infective (9)	**Includes:** AVYCAZ® (ceftazidime-avibactam) Ceftazidime-avibactam CRESEMBA® (isavuconazonium sulfate) Isavuconazole (isavuconazonium sulfate)	Administration (3)
Other Antineoplastic (5)	**Includes:** Blinatumomab BLINCYTO® (blinatumomab)	Administration (3)
Other New Technology Therapeutic Substance (F)	**Includes:** STELARA® Ustekinumab	New Technology (X)
Other Therapeutic Substance (G)	**Includes:** Idarucizumab, Pradaxa® (dabigatran) reversal agent Praxbind® (idarucizumab), Pradaxa® (dabigatran) reversal agent	Administration (3)
Other Thrombolytic (7)	**Includes:** Tissue Plasminogen Activator (tPA)(r-tPA)	Administration (3)
Oxazolidinones (8)	**Includes:** Zyvox	Administration (3)
Pathogen Reduced Cryoprecipitated Fibrinogen Complex (D)	**Includes:** INTERCEPT Blood System for Plasma Pathogen Reduced Cryoprecipitated Fibrinogen Complex INTERCEPT Fibrinogen Complex	Administration (3)
Plazomicin Anti-infective (G)	**Includes:** *ZEMDRI™ NT	New Technology (X)
Recombinant Bone Morphogenetic Protein (B)	**Includes:** Bone morphogenetic protein 2 (BMP 2) rhBMP-2	Administration (3)
REGN-COV2 Monoclonal Antibody (G)	**Includes:** Casirivimab (REGN10933) and Imdevimab (REGN10987) Imdevimab (REGN10987) and Casirivimab (REGN10933)	New Technology (X)

ICD-10-PCS Value	Trade Name or Synonym		PCS Section
Remdesivir Anti-infective (E)	**Includes:**	GS-5734 Veklury NT	New Technology (X)
Ruxolitinib (T)	**Includes:**	Jakafi® NT	New Technology (X)
Sarilumab (G)	**Includes:**	KEVZARA®	New Technology (X)
Satralizumab-mwge (9)	**Includes:**	ENSPRYNG™	New Technology (X)
Synthetic Human Angiotensin II (H)	**Includes:**	Angiotensin II GIAPREZA™ Human angiotensin II, synthetic	New Technology (X)
Tagraxofusp-erzs Antineoplastic (Q)	**Includes:**	ELZONRIS™ NT	New Technology (X)
Terlipressin (6)	**Includes:**	TERLIVAZ®	New Technology (X)
Tisagenlecleucel Immunotherapy (J)	**Includes:**	KYMRIAH® Tisagenlecleucel	New Technology (X)
Tocilizumab (H)	**Includes:**	ACTEMRA®	New Technology (X)
Trilaciclib (7)	**Includes:**	COSELA™	New Technology (X)
Uridine Triacetate (8)	**Includes:**	Vistogard®	New Technology (X)
Venetoclax Antineoplastic (R)	**Includes:**	Venclexta®	New Technology (X)

Appendix J: Sections B–H Character Definitions

Sections B-H (Imaging through Substance Abuse Treatment) do not include root operations. Instead, the character 3 value represents the type of procedure performed with additional details about that procedure provided by the character 4 or 5 value, when appropriate. This resource provides the specific ICD-10-PCS value and its associated definition for the character 3, character 4, and character 5 values in the ancillary sections of B-H.

Section B–Imaging

ICD-10-PCS Value (Character 3)	Definition
Computerized Tomography (CT Scan) (2)	Computer reformatted digital display of multiplanar images developed from the capture of multiple exposures of external ionizing radiation
Fluoroscopy (1)	Single plane or bi-plane real time display of an image developed from the capture of external ionizing radiation on a fluorescent screen. The image may also be stored by either digital or analog means.
Magnetic Resonance Imaging (MRI) (3)	Computer reformatted digital display of multiplanar images developed from the capture of radiofrequency signals emitted by nuclei in a body site excited within a magnetic field
Other Imaging (5)	Other specified modality for visualizing a body part
Plain Radiography (Ø)	Planar display of an image developed from the capture of external ionizing radiation on photographic or photoconductive plate
Ultrasonography (4)	Real time display of images of anatomy or flow information developed from the capture of reflected and attenuated high frequency sound waves

Section C–Nuclear Medicine

ICD-10-PCS Value (Character 3)	Definition
Nonimaging Nuclear Medicine Assay (6)	Introduction of radioactive materials into the body for the study of body fluids and blood elements, by the detection of radioactive emissions
Nonimaging Nuclear Medicine Probe (5)	Introduction of radioactive materials into the body for the study of distribution and fate of certain substances by the detection of radioactive emissions; or, alternatively, measurement of absorption of radioactive emissions from an external source
Nonimaging Nuclear Medicine Uptake (4)	Introduction of radioactive materials into the body for measurements of organ function, from the detection of radioactive emissions
Planar Nuclear Medicine Imaging (1)	Introduction of radioactive materials into the body for single plane display of images developed from the capture of radioactive emissions
Positron Emission Tomographic (PET) Imaging (3)	Introduction of radioactive materials into the body for three dimensional display of images developed from the simultaneous capture, 18Ø degrees apart, of radioactive emissions
Systemic Nuclear Medicine Therapy (7)	Introduction of unsealed radioactive materials into the body for treatment
Tomographic (Tomo) Nuclear Medicine Imaging (2)	Introduction of radioactive materials into the body for three dimensional display of images developed from the capture of radioactive emissions

Section F–Physical Rehabilitation and Diagnostic Audiology

ICD-10-PCS Value (Character 3)	Definition
Activities of Daily Living Assessment (2)	Measurement of functional level for activities of daily living
Activities of Daily Living Treatment (8)	Exercise or activities to facilitate functional competence for activities of daily living
Caregiver Training (F)	Training in activities to support patient's optimal level of function
Cochlear Implant Treatment (B)	Application of techniques to improve the communication abilities of individuals with cochlear implant
Device Fitting (D)	Fitting of a device designed to facilitate or support achievement of a higher level of function
Hearing Aid Assessment (4)	Measurement of the appropriateness and/or effectiveness of a hearing device
Hearing Assessment (3)	Measurement of hearing and related functions
Hearing Treatment (9)	Application of techniques to improve, augment, or compensate for hearing and related functional impairment
Motor and/or Nerve Function Assessment (1)	Measurement of motor, nerve, and related functions

Continued on next page

Section F–Physical Rehabilitation and Diagnostic Audiology

Continued from previous page

ICD-10-PCS Value (Character 3)	Definition
Motor Treatment (7)	Exercise or activities to increase or facilitate motor function
Speech Assessment (Ø)	Measurement of speech and related functions
Speech Treatment (6)	Application of techniques to improve, augment, or compensate for speech and related functional impairment
Vestibular Assessment (5)	Measurement of the vestibular system and related functions
Vestibular Treatment (C)	Application of techniques to improve, augment, or compensate for vestibular and related functional impairment

Section F–Physical Rehabilitation and Diagnostic Audiology

ICD-10-PCS Value Qualifier (Character 5)	Definition
Acoustic Reflex Decay (J)	Measures reduction in size/strength of acoustic reflex over time Includes/Examples: Includes site of lesion test
Acoustic Reflex Patterns (G)	Defines site of lesion based upon presence/absence of acoustic reflexes with ipsilateral vs. contralateral stimulation
Acoustic Reflex Threshold (H)	Determines minimal intensity that acoustic reflex occurs with ipsilateral and/or contralateral stimulation
Aerobic Capacity and Endurance (7)	Measures autonomic responses to positional changes; perceived exertion, dyspnea or angina during activity; performance during exercise protocols; standard vital signs; and blood gas analysis or oxygen consumption
Alternate Binaural or Monaural Loudness Balance (7)	Determines auditory stimulus parameter that yields the same objective sensation Includes/Examples: Sound intensities that yield same loudness perception
Anthropometric Characteristics (B)	Measures edema, body fat composition, height, weight, length and girth
Aphasia (Assessment) (C)	Measures expressive and receptive speech and language function including reading and writing
Aphasia (Treatment) (3)	Applying techniques to improve, augment, or compensate for receptive/ expressive language impairments
Articulation/Phonology (Assessment) (9)	Measures speech production
Articulation/Phonology (Treatment) (4)	Applying techniques to correct, improve, or compensate for speech productive impairment
Assistive Listening Device (5)	Assists in use of effective and appropriate assistive listening device/system
Assistive Listening System/Device Selection (4)	Measures the effectiveness and appropriateness of assistive listening systems/devices
Assistive, Adaptive, Supportive or Protective Devices (9)	Explanation: Devices to facilitate or support achievement of a higher level of function in wheelchair mobility; bed mobility; transfer or ambulation ability; bath and showering ability; dressing; grooming; personal hygiene; play or leisure
Auditory Evoked Potentials (L)	Measures electric responses produced by the VIIIth cranial nerve and brainstem following auditory stimulation
Auditory Processing (Assessment) (Q)	Evaluates ability to receive and process auditory information and comprehension of spoken language
Auditory Processing (Treatment) (2)	Applying techniques to improve the receiving and processing of auditory information and comprehension of spoken language
Augmentative/Alternative Communication System (Assessment) (L)	Determines the appropriateness of aids, techniques, symbols, and/or strategies to augment or replace speech and enhance communication Includes/Examples: Includes the use of telephones, writing equipment, emergency equipment, and TDD
Augmentative/Alternative Communication System (Treatment) (3)	Includes/Examples: Includes augmentative communication devices and aids
Aural Rehabilitation (5)	Applying techniques to improve the communication abilities associated with hearing loss
Aural Rehabilitation Status (P)	Measures impact of a hearing loss including evaluation of receptive and expressive communication skills
Bathing/Showering (Ø)	Includes/Examples: Includes obtaining and using supplies; soaping, rinsing, and drying body parts; maintaining bathing position; and transferring to and from bathing positions

Continued on next page

Section F–Physical Rehabilitation and Diagnostic Audiology

Continued from previous page

ICD-10-PCS Value Qualifier (Character 5)	Definition
Bathing/Showering Techniques (Ø)	Activities to facilitate obtaining and using supplies, soaping, rinsing and drying body parts, maintaining bathing position, and transferring to and from bathing positions
Bed Mobility (Assessment) (B)	Transitional movement within bed
Bed Mobility (Treatment) (5)	Exercise or activities to facilitate transitional movements within bed
Bedside Swallowing and Oral Function (H)	Includes/Examples: Bedside swallowing includes assessment of sucking, masticating, coughing, and swallowing. Oral function includes assessment of musculature for controlled movements, structures, and functions to determine coordination and phonation.
Bekesy Audiometry (3)	Uses an instrument that provides a choice of discrete or continuously varying pure tones; choice of pulsed or continuous signal
Binaural Electroacoustic Hearing Aid Check (6)	Determines mechanical and electroacoustic function of bilateral hearing aids using hearing aid test box
Binaural Hearing Aid (Assessment) (3)	Measures the candidacy, effectiveness, and appropriateness of a hearing aid Explanation: Measures bilateral fit
Binaural Hearing Aid (Treatment) (2)	Explanation: Assists in achieving maximum understanding and performance
Bithermal, Binaural Caloric Irrigation (Ø)	Measures the rhythmic eye movements stimulated by changing the temperature of the vestibular system
Bithermal, Monaural Caloric Irrigation (1)	Measures the rhythmic eye movements stimulated by changing the temperature of the vestibular system in one ear
Brief Tone Stimuli (R)	Measures specific central auditory process
Cerumen Management (3)	Includes examination of external auditory canal and tympanic membrane and removal of cerumen from external ear canal
Cochlear Implant (Ø)	Measures candidacy for cochlear implant
Cochlear Implant Rehabilitation (Ø)	Applying techniques to improve the communication abilities of individuals with cochlear implant; includes programming the device, providing patients/families with information
Communicative/Cognitive Integration Skills (Assessment) (G)	Measures ability to use higher cortical functions Includes/Examples: Includes orientation, recognition, attention span, initiation and termination of activity, memory, sequencing, categorizing, concept formation, spatial operations, judgment, problem solving, generalization and pragmatic communication
Communicative/Cognitive Integration Skills (Treatment) (6)	Activities to facilitate the use of higher cortical functions Includes/Examples: Includes level of arousal, orientation, recognition, attention span, initiation and termination of activity, memory sequencing, judgment and problem solving, learning and generalization, and pragmatic communication
Computerized Dynamic Posturography (6)	Measures the status of the peripheral and central vestibular system and the sensory/motor component of balance; evaluates the efficacy of vestibular rehabilitation
Conditioned Play Audiometry (4)	Behavioral measures using nonspeech and speech stimuli to obtain frequency-specific and ear-specific information on auditory status from the patient Explanation: Obtains speech reception threshold by having patient point to pictures of spondaic words
Coordination/Dexterity (Assessment) (3)	Measures large and small muscle groups for controlled goal-directed movements Explanation: Dexterity includes object manipulation
Coordination/Dexterity (Treatment) (2)	Exercise or activities to facilitate gross coordination and fine coordination
Cranial Nerve Integrity (9)	Measures cranial nerve sensory and motor functions, including tastes, smell and facial expression
Dichotic Stimuli (T)	Measures specific central auditory process
Distorted Speech (S)	Measures specific central auditory process
Dix-Hallpike Dynamic (5)	Measures nystagmus following Dix-Hallpike maneuver
Dressing (1)	Includes/Examples: Includes selecting clothing and accessories, obtaining clothing from storage, dressing, fastening and adjusting clothing and shoes, and applying and removing personal devices, prosthesis or orthosis
Dressing Techniques (1)	Activities to facilitate selecting clothing and accessories, dressing and undressing, adjusting clothing and shoes, applying and removing devices, prostheses or orthoses
Dynamic Orthosis (6)	Includes/Examples: Includes customized and prefabricated splints, inhibitory casts, spinal and other braces, and protective devices; allows motion through transfer of movement from other body parts or by use of outside forces

Continued on next page

Section F–Physical Rehabilitation and Diagnostic Audiology

Continued from previous page

ICD-10-PCS Value Qualifier (Character 5)	Definition
Ear Canal Probe Microphone (1)	Real ear measures
Ear Protector Attentuation (7)	Measures ear protector fit and effectiveness
Electrocochleography (K)	Measures the VIIIth cranial nerve action potential
Environmental, Home, Work Barriers (B)	Measures current and potential barriers to optimal function, including safety hazards, access problems and home or office design
Ergonomics and Body Mechanics (C)	Ergonomic measurement of job tasks, work hardening or work conditioning needs; functional capacity; and body mechanics
Eustachian Tube Function (F)	Measures eustachian tube function and patency of eustachian tube
Evoked Otoacoustic Emissions, Diagnostic (N)	Measures auditory evoked potentials in a diagnostic format
Evoked Otoacoustic Emissions, Screening (M)	Measures auditory evoked potentials in a screening format
Facial Nerve Function (7)	Measures electrical activity of the VIIth cranial nerve (facial nerve)
Feeding/Eating (Assessment) (2)	Includes/Examples: Includes setting up food, selecting and using utensils and tableware, bringing food or drink to mouth, cleaning face, hands, and clothing, and management of alternative methods of nourishment
Feeding/Eating (Treatment) (3)	Exercise or activities to facilitate setting up food, selecting and using utensils and tableware, bringing food or drink to mouth, cleaning face, hands, and clothing, and management of alternative methods of nourishment
Filtered Speech (Ø)	Uses high or low pass filtered speech stimuli to assess central auditory processing disorders, site of lesion testing
Fluency (Assessment) (D)	Measures speech fluency or stuttering
Fluency (Treatment) (7)	Applying techniques to improve and augment fluent speech
Gait and/or Balance (D)	Measures biomechanical, arthrokinematic and other spatial and temporal characteristics of gait and balance
Gait Training/Functional Ambulation (9)	Exercise or activities to facilitate ambulation on a variety of surfaces and in a variety of environments
Grooming/Personal Hygiene (Assessment) (3)	Includes/Examples: Includes ability to obtain and use supplies in a sequential fashion, general grooming, oral hygiene, toilet hygiene, personal care devices, including care for artificial airways
Grooming/Personal Hygiene (Treatment) (2)	Activities to facilitate obtaining and using supplies in a sequential fashion: general grooming, oral hygiene, toilet hygiene, cleaning body, and personal care devices, including artificial airways
Hearing and Related Disorders Counseling (Ø)	Provides patients/families/caregivers with information, support, referrals to facilitate recovery from a communication disorder Includes/Examples: Includes strategies for psychosocial adjustment to hearing loss for clients and families/caregivers
Hearing and Related Disorders Prevention (1)	Provides patients/families/caregivers with information and support to prevent communication disorders
Hearing Screening (Ø)	Pass/refer measures designed to identify need for further audiologic assessment
Home Management (Assessment) (4)	Obtaining and maintaining personal and household possessions and environment Includes/Examples: Includes clothing care, cleaning, meal preparation and cleanup, shopping, money management, household maintenance, safety procedures, and childcare/parenting
Home Management (Treatment) (4)	Activities to facilitate obtaining and maintaining personal household possessions and environment Includes/Examples: Includes clothing care, cleaning, meal preparation and clean-up, shopping, money management, household maintenance, safety procedures, childcare/parenting
Instrumental Swallowing and Oral Function (J)	Measures swallowing function using instrumental diagnostic procedures Explanation: Methods include videofluoroscopy, ultrasound, manometry, endoscopy
Integumentary Integrity (1)	Includes/Examples: Includes burns, skin conditions, ecchymosis, bleeding, blisters, scar tissue, wounds and other traumas, tissue mobility, turgor and texture
Manual Therapy Techniques (7)	Techniques in which the therapist uses his/her hands to administer skilled movements Includes/Examples: Includes connective tissue massage, joint mobilization and manipulation, manual lymph drainage, manual traction, soft tissue mobilization and manipulation
Masking Patterns (W)	Measures central auditory processing status

Continued on next page

Section F–Physical Rehabilitation and Diagnostic Audiology *Continued from previous page*

ICD-10-PCS Value Qualifier (Character 5)	Definition
Monaural Electroacoustic Hearing Aid Check (8)	Determines mechanical and electroacoustic function of one hearing aid using hearing aid test box
Monaural Hearing Aid (Assessment) (2)	Measures the candidacy, effectiveness, and appropriateness of a hearing aid Explanation: Measures unilateral fit
Monaural Hearing Aid (Treatment) (1)	Explanation: Assists in achieving maximum understanding and performance
Motor Function (Assessment) (4)	Measures the body's functional and versatile movement patterns Includes/Examples: Includes motor assessment scales, analysis of head, trunk and limb movement, and assessment of motor learning
Motor Function (Treatment) (3)	Exercise or activities to facilitate crossing midline, laterality, bilateral integration, praxis, neuromuscular relaxation, inhibition, facilitation, motor function and motor learning
Motor Speech (Assessment) (B)	Measures neurological motor aspects of speech production
Motor Speech (Treatment) (8)	Applying techniques to improve and augment the impaired neurological motor aspects of speech production
Muscle Performance (Assessment) (Ø)	Measures muscle strength, power and endurance using manual testing, dynamometry or computer-assisted electromechanical muscle test; functional muscle strength, power and endurance; muscle pain, tone, or soreness; or pelvic-floor musculature Explanation: Muscle endurance refers to the ability to contract a muscle repeatedly over time
Muscle Performance (Treatment) (1)	Exercise or activities to increase the capacity of a muscle to do work in terms of strength, power, and/or endurance Explanation: Muscle strength is the force exerted to overcome resistance in one maximal effort. Muscle power is work produced per unit of time, or the product of strength and speed. Muscle endurance is the ability to contract a muscle repeatedly over time.
Neuromotor Development (D)	Measures motor development, righting and equilibrium reactions, and reflex and equilibrium reactions
Non-invasive Instrumental Status (N)	Instrumental measures of oral, nasal, vocal, and velopharyngeal functions as they pertain to speech production
Nonspoken Language (Assessment) (7)	Measures nonspoken language (print, sign, symbols) for communication
Nonspoken Language (Treatment) (Ø)	Applying techniques that improve, augment, or compensate spoken communication
Oral Peripheral Mechanism (P)	Structural measures of face, jaw, lips, tongue, teeth, hard and soft palate, pharynx as related to speech production
Orofacial Myofunctional (Assessment) (K)	Measures orofacial myofunctional patterns for speech and related functions
Orofacial Myofunctional (Treatment) (9)	Applying techniques to improve, alter, or augment impaired orofacial myofunctional patterns and related speech production errors
Oscillating Tracking (3)	Measures ability to visually track
Pain (F)	Measures muscle soreness, pain and soreness with joint movement, and pain perception Includes/Examples: Includes questionnaires, graphs, symptom magnification scales or visual analog scales
Perceptual Processing (Assessment) (5)	Measures stereognosis, kinesthesia, body schema, right-left discrimination, form constancy, position in space, visual closure, figure-ground, depth perception, spatial relations and topographical orientation
Perceptual Processing (Treatment) (1)	Exercise and activities to facilitate perceptual processing Explanation: Includes stereognosis, kinesthesia, body schema, right-left discrimination, form constancy, position in space, visual closure, figure-ground, depth perception, spatial relations, and topographical orientation Includes/Examples: Includes stereognosis, kinesthesia, body schema, right-left discrimination, form constancy, position in space, visual closure, figure-ground, depth perception, spatial relations, and topographical orientation
Performance Intensity Phonetically Balanced Speech Discrimination (Q)	Measures word recognition over varying intensity levels
Postural Control (3)	Exercise or activities to increase postural alignment and control
Prosthesis (8)	Explanation: Artificial substitutes for missing body parts that augment performance or function Includes/Examples: Limb prosthesis, ocular prosthesis

Continued on next page

Section F–Physical Rehabilitation and Diagnostic Audiology

Continued from previous page

ICD-10-PCS Value Qualifier (Character 5)	Definition
Psychosocial Skills (Assessment) (6)	The ability to interact in society and to process emotions Includes/Examples: Includes psychological (values, interests, self-concept); social (role performance, social conduct, interpersonal skills, self expression); self-management (coping skills, time management, self-control)
Psychosocial Skills (Treatment) (6)	The ability to interact in society and to process emotions Includes/Examples: Includes psychological (values, interests, self-concept); social (role performance, social conduct, interpersonal skills, self expression); self-management (coping skills, time management, self-control)
Pure Tone Audiometry, Air (1)	Air-conduction pure tone threshold measures with appropriate masking
Pure Tone Audiometry, Air and Bone (2)	Air-conduction and bone-conduction pure tone threshold measures with appropriate masking
Pure Tone Stenger (C)	Measures unilateral nonorganic hearing loss based on simultaneous presentation of pure tones of differing volume
Range of Motion and Joint Integrity (5)	Measures quantity, quality, grade, and classification of joint movement and/or mobility Explanation: Range of Motion is the space, distance or angle through which movement occurs at a joint or series of joints. Joint integrity is the conformance of joints to expected anatomic, biomechanical and kinematic norms.
Range of Motion and Joint Mobility (Ø)	Exercise or activities to increase muscle length and joint mobility
Receptive/Expressive Language (Assessment) (8)	Measures receptive and expressive language
Receptive/Expressive Language (Treatment) (B)	Applying techniques to improve and augment receptive/expressive language
Reflex Integrity (G)	Measures the presence, absence, or exaggeration of developmentally appropriate, pathologic or normal reflexes
Select Picture Audiometry (5)	Establishes hearing threshold levels for speech using pictures
Sensorineural Acuity Level (4)	Measures sensorineural acuity masking presented via bone conduction
Sensory Aids (5)	Determines the appropriateness of a sensory prosthetic device, other than a hearing aid or assistive listening system/device
Sensory Awareness/ Processing/ Integrity (6)	Includes/Examples: Includes light touch, pressure, temperature, pain, sharp/dull, proprioception, vestibular, visual, auditory, gustatory, and olfactory
Short Increment Sensitivity Index (9)	Measures the ear's ability to detect small intensity changes; site of lesion test requiring a behavioral response
Sinusoidal Vertical Axis Rotational (4)	Measures nystagmus following rotation
Somatosensory Evoked Potentials (9)	Measures neural activity from sites throughout the body
Speech/Language Screening (6)	Identifies need for further speech and/or language evaluation
Speech Threshold (1)	Measures minimal intensity needed to repeat spondaic words
Speech-Language Pathology and Related Disorders Counseling (1)	Provides patients/families with information, support, referrals to facilitate recovery from a communication disorder
Speech-Language Pathology and Related Disorders Prevention (2)	Applying techniques to avoid or minimize onset and/or development of a communication disorder
Speech/Word Recognition (2)	Measures ability to repeat/identify single syllable words; scores given as a percentage; includes word recognition/speech discrimination
Staggered Spondaic Word (3)	Measures central auditory processing site of lesion based upon dichotic presentation of spondaic words
Static Orthosis (7)	Includes/Examples: Includes customized and prefabricated splints, inhibitory casts, spinal and other braces, and protective devices; has no moving parts, maintains joint(s) in desired position
Stenger (B)	Measures unilateral nonorganic hearing loss based on simultaneous presentation of signals of differing volume
Swallowing Dysfunction (D)	Activities to improve swallowing function in coordination with respiratory function Includes/Examples: Includes function and coordination of sucking, mastication, coughing, swallowing
Synthetic Sentence Identification (5)	Measures central auditory dysfunction using identification of third order approximations of sentences and competing messages

Continued on next page

Section F–Physical Rehabilitation and Diagnostic Audiology

Continued from previous page

ICD-10-PCS Value Qualifier (Character 5)	Definition
Temporal Ordering of Stimuli (V)	Measures specific central auditory process
Therapeutic Exercise (6)	Exercise or activities to facilitate sensory awareness, sensory processing, sensory integration, balance training, conditioning, reconditioning Includes/Examples: Includes developmental activities, breathing exercises, aerobic endurance activities, aquatic exercises, stretching and ventilatory muscle training
Tinnitus Masker (Assessment) (7)	Determines candidacy for tinnitus masker
Tinnitus Masker (Treatment) (Ø)	Explanation: Used to verify physical fit, acoustic appropriateness, and benefit; assists in achieving maximum benefit
Tone Decay (8)	Measures decrease in hearing sensitivity to a tone; site of lesion test requiring a behavioral response
Transfer (C)	Transitional movement from one surface to another
Transfer Training (8)	Exercise or activities to facilitate movement from one surface to another
Tympanometry (D)	Measures the integrity of the middle ear; measures ease at which sound flows through the tympanic membrane while air pressure against the membrane is varied
Unithermal Binaural Screen (2)	Measures the rhythmic eye movements stimulated by changing the temperature of the vestibular system in both ears using warm water, screening format
Ventilation/Respiration/Circulation (G)	Measures ventilatory muscle strength, power and endurance, pulmonary function and ventilatory mechanics Includes/Examples: Includes ability to clear airway, activities that aggravate or relieve edema, pain, dyspnea or other symptoms, chest wall mobility, cardiopulmonary response to performance of ADL and IAD, cough and sputum, standard vital signs
Vestibular (Ø)	Applying techniques to compensate for balance disorders; includes habituation, exercise therapy, and balance retraining
Visual Motor Integration (Assessment) (2)	Coordinating the interaction of information from the eyes with body movement during activity
Visual Motor Integration (Treatment) (2)	Exercise or activities to facilitate coordinating the interaction of information from eyes with body movement during activity
Visual Reinforcement Audiometry (6)	Behavioral measures using nonspeech and speech stimuli to obtain frequency/ear-specific information on auditory status Includes/Examples: Includes a conditioned response of looking toward a visual reinforcer (e.g., lights, animated toy) every time auditory stimuli are heard
Vocational Activities and Functional Community or Work Reintegration Skills (Assessment) (H)	Measures environmental, home, work (job/school/play) barriers that keep patients from functioning optimally in their environment Includes/Examples: Includes assessment of vocational skills and interests, environment of work (job/school/play), injury potential and injury prevention or reduction, ergonomic stressors, transportation skills, and ability to access and use community resources
Vocational Activities and Functional Community or Work Reintegration Skills (Treatment) (7)	Activities to facilitate vocational exploration, body mechanics training, job acquisition, and environmental or work (job/school/play) task adaptation Includes/Examples: Includes injury prevention and reduction, ergonomic stressor reduction, job coaching and simulation, work hardening and conditioning, driving training, transportation skills, and use of community resources
Voice (Assessment) (F)	Measures vocal structure, function and production
Voice (Treatment) (C)	Applying techniques to improve voice and vocal function
Voice Prosthetic (Assessment) (M)	Determines the appropriateness of voice prosthetic/adaptive device to enhance or facilitate communication
Voice Prosthetic (Treatment) (4)	Includes/Examples: Includes electrolarynx, and other assistive, adaptive, supportive devices
Wheelchair Mobility (Assessment) (F)	Measures fit and functional abilities within wheelchair in a variety of environments
Wheelchair Mobility (Treatment) (4)	Management, maintenance and controlled operation of a wheelchair, scooter or other device, in and on a variety of surfaces and environments
Wound Management (5)	Includes/Examples: Includes non-selective and selective debridement (enzymes, autolysis, sharp debridement), dressings (wound coverings, hydrogel, vacuum-assisted closure), topical agents, etc.

Section G–Mental Health

ICD-10-PCS Value (Character 3)	Definition
Biofeedback (C)	Provision of information from the monitoring and regulating of physiological processes in conjunction with cognitive-behavioral techniques to improve patient functioning or well-being Includes/Examples: Includes EEG, blood pressure, skin temperature or peripheral blood flow, ECG, electrooculogram, EMG, respirometry or capnometry, GSR/EDR, perineometry to monitor/regulate bowel/bladder activity, electrogastrogram to monitor/regulate gastric motility
Counseling (6)	The application of psychological methods to treat an individual with normal developmental issues and psychological problems in order to increase function, improve well-being, alleviate distress, maladjustment or resolve crises
Crisis Intervention (2)	Treatment of a traumatized, acutely disturbed or distressed individual for the purpose of short-term stabilization Includes/Examples: Includes defusing, debriefing, counseling, psychotherapy and/or coordination of care with other providers or agencies
Electroconvulsive Therapy (B)	The application of controlled electrical voltages to treat a mental health disorder Includes/Examples: Includes appropriate sedation and other preparation of the individual
Family Psychotherapy (7)	Treatment that includes one or more family members of an individual with a mental health disorder by behavioral, cognitive, psychoanalytic, psychodynamic or psychophysiological means to improve functioning or well-being Explanation: Remediation of emotional or behavioral problems presented by one or more family members in cases where psychotherapy with more than one family member is indicated
Group Psychotherapy (H)	Treatment of two or more individuals with a mental health disorder by behavioral, cognitive, psychoanalytic, psychodynamic or psychophysiological means to improve functioning or well-being
Hypnosis (F)	Induction of a state of heightened suggestibility by auditory, visual and tactile techniques to elicit an emotional or behavioral response
Individual Psychotherapy (5)	Treatment of an individual with a mental health disorder by behavioral, cognitive, psychoanalytic, psychodynamic or psychophysiological means to improve functioning or well-being
Light Therapy (J)	Application of specialized light treatments to improve functioning or well-being
Medication Management (3)	Monitoring and adjusting the use of medications for the treatment of a mental health disorder
Narcosynthesis (G)	Administration of intravenous barbiturates in order to release suppressed or repressed thoughts
Psychological Tests (1)	The administration and interpretation of standardized psychological tests and measurement instruments for the assessment of psychological function
Behavioral (1)	Primarily to modify behavior Includes/Examples: Includes modeling and role playing, positive reinforcement of target behaviors, response cost, and training of self-management skills
Cognitive (2)	Primarily to correct cognitive distortions and errors
Cognitive-Behavioral (8)	Combining cognitive and behavioral treatment strategies to improve functioning Explanation: Maladaptive responses are examined to determine how cognitions relate to behavior patterns in response to an event. Uses learning principles and information-processing models.
Developmental (Ø)	Age-normed developmental status of cognitive, social and adaptive behavior skills
Intellectual and Psychoeducational (2)	Intellectual abilities, academic achievement and learning capabilities (including behaviors and emotional factors affecting learning)
Interactive (Ø)	Uses primarily physical aids and other forms of non-oral interaction with a patient who is physically, psychologically or developmentally unable to use ordinary language for communication Includes/Examples: Includes the use of toys in symbolic play
Interpersonal (3)	Helps an individual make changes in interpersonal behaviors to reduce psychological dysfunction Includes/Examples: Includes exploratory techniques, encouragement of affective expression, clarification of patient statements, analysis of communication patterns, use of therapy relationship and behavior change techniques
Neurobehavioral and Cognitive Status (4)	Includes neurobehavioral status exam, interview(s), and observation for the clinical assessment of thinking, reasoning and judgment, acquired knowledge, attention, memory, visual spatial abilities, language functions, and planning
Neuropsychological (3)	Thinking, reasoning and judgment, acquired knowledge, attention, memory, visual spatial abilities, language functions, planning
Personality and Behavioral (1)	Mood, emotion, behavior, social functioning, psychopathological conditions, personality traits and characteristics

Continued on next page

Section G–Mental Health

Continued from previous page

ICD-10-PCS Value (Character 3)	Definition
Psychoanalysis (4)	Methods of obtaining a detailed account of past and present mental and emotional experiences to determine the source and eliminate or diminish the undesirable effects of unconscious conflicts Explanation: Accomplished by making the individual aware of their existence, origin, and inappropriate expression in emotions and behavior
Psychodynamic (5)	Exploration of past and present emotional experiences to understand motives and drives using insight-oriented techniques to reduce the undesirable effects of internal conflicts on emotions and behavior Explanation: Techniques include empathetic listening, clarifying self-defeating behavior patterns, and exploring adaptive alternatives
Psychophysiological (9)	Monitoring and alteration of physiological processes to help the individual associate physiological reactions combined with cognitive and behavioral strategies to gain improved control of these processes to help the individual cope more effectively
Supportive (6)	Formation of therapeutic relationship primarily for providing emotional support to prevent further deterioration in functioning during periods of particular stress Explanation: Often used in conjunction with other therapeutic approaches
Vocational (1)	Exploration of vocational interests, aptitudes and required adaptive behavior skills to develop and carry out a plan for achieving a successful vocational placement Includes/Examples: Includes enhancing work related adjustment and/or pursuing viable options in training education or preparation

Section H–Substance Abuse Treatment

ICD-10-PCS Value (Character 3)	Definition
Detoxification Services (2)	Detoxification from alcohol and/or drugs Explanation: Not a treatment modality, but helps the patient stabilize physically and psychologically until the body becomes free of drugs and the effects of alcohol
Family Counseling (6)	The application of psychological methods that includes one or more family members to treat an individual with addictive behavior Explanation: Provides support and education for family members of addicted individuals. Family member participation is seen as a critical area of substance abuse treatment.
Group Counseling (4)	The application of psychological methods to treat two or more individuals with addictive behavior Explanation: Provides structured group counseling sessions and healing power through the connection with others
Individual Counseling (3)	The application of psychological methods to treat an individual with addictive behavior Explanation: Comprised of several different techniques, which apply various strategies to address drug addiction
Individual Psychotherapy (5)	Treatment of an individual with addictive behavior by behavioral, cognitive, psychoanalytic, psychodynamic or psychophysiological means
Medication Management (8)	Monitoring and adjusting the use of replacement medications for the treatment of addiction
Pharmacotherapy (9)	The use of replacement medications for the treatment of addiction

Appendix K: Hospital Acquired Conditions

Hospital acquired conditions (HACs) are conditions considered reasonably preventable through the application of evidence-based guidelines. Although it is the ICD-10-CM diagnosis code that drives a HAC designation, in some cases a specific ICD-10-PCS procedure code must also be present before that diagnosis code can be considered a HAC. This resource provides only those HAC categories that require both an ICD-10-PCS code and an ICD-10-CM diagnosis code. The official descriptions for each code are also provided. To see all 14 HAC categories and their corresponding codes, refer to Optum360's *ICD-10-CM Expert for Hospitals*.

Note: The resource used to compile this list is the proposed, version 39, MS-DRG Grouper software and Definitions Manual files published with the fiscal 2022 IPPS proposed rule. For the final, version 39, MS-DRG Grouper software and Definitions Manual files, refer to the following: https://www.cms.gov/Medicare/Medicare-Fee-for-Service-Payment/AcuteInpatientPPS/MS-DRG-Classifications-and-Software.

HAC 08: Surgical Site Infection of Mediastinitis After Coronary Bypass Graft (CABG) Procedures

Secondary diagnosis not POA:

J98.51 Mediastinitis

J98.59 Other diseases of mediastinum, not elsewhere classified

AND

Any of the following procedures:

0210083 Bypass Coronary Artery, One Artery from Coronary Artery with Zooplastic Tissue, Open Approach

0210088 Bypass Coronary Artery, One Artery from Right Internal Mammary with Zooplastic Tissue, Open Approach

0210089 Bypass Coronary Artery, One Artery from Left Internal Mammary with Zooplastic Tissue, Open Approach

021008C Bypass Coronary Artery, One Artery from Thoracic Artery with Zooplastic Tissue, Open Approach

021008F Bypass Coronary Artery, One Artery from Abdominal Artery with Zooplastic Tissue, Open Approach

021008W Bypass Coronary Artery, One Artery from Aorta with Zooplastic Tissue, Open Approach

0210093 Bypass Coronary Artery, One Artery from Coronary Artery with Autologous Venous Tissue, Open Approach

0210098 Bypass Coronary Artery, One Artery from Right Internal Mammary with Autologous Venous Tissue, Open Approach

0210099 Bypass Coronary Artery, One Artery from Left Internal Mammary with Autologous Venous Tissue, Open Approach

021009C Bypass Coronary Artery, One Artery from Thoracic Artery with Autologous Venous Tissue, Open Approach

021009F Bypass Coronary Artery, One Artery from Abdominal Artery with Autologous Venous Tissue, Open Approach

021009W Bypass Coronary Artery, One Artery from Aorta with Autologous Venous Tissue, Open Approach

02100A3 Bypass Coronary Artery, One Artery from Coronary Artery with Autologous Arterial Tissue, Open Approach

02100A8 Bypass Coronary Artery, One Artery from Right Internal Mammary with Autologous Arterial Tissue, Open Approach

02100A9 Bypass Coronary Artery, One Artery from Left Internal Mammary with Autologous Arterial Tissue, Open Approach

02100AC Bypass Coronary Artery, One Artery from Thoracic Artery with Autologous Arterial Tissue, Open Approach

02100AF Bypass Coronary Artery, One Artery from Abdominal Artery with Autologous Arterial Tissue, Open Approach

02100AW Bypass Coronary Artery, One Artery from Aorta with Autologous Arterial Tissue, Open Approach

02100J3 Bypass Coronary Artery, One Artery from Coronary Artery with Synthetic Substitute, Open Approach

02100J8 Bypass Coronary Artery, One Artery from Right Internal Mammary with Synthetic Substitute, Open Approach

02100J9 Bypass Coronary Artery, One Artery from Left Internal Mammary with Synthetic Substitute, Open Approach

02100JC Bypass Coronary Artery, One Artery from Thoracic Artery with Synthetic Substitute, Open Approach

02100JF Bypass Coronary Artery, One Artery from Abdominal Artery with Synthetic Substitute, Open Approach

02100JW Bypass Coronary Artery, One Artery from Aorta with Synthetic Substitute, Open Approach

02100K3 Bypass Coronary Artery, One Artery from Coronary Artery with Nonautologous Tissue Substitute, Open Approach

02100K8 Bypass Coronary Artery, One Artery from Right Internal Mammary with Nonautologous Tissue Substitute, Open Approach

02100K9 Bypass Coronary Artery, One Artery from Left Internal Mammary with Nonautologous Tissue Substitute, Open Approach

02100KC Bypass Coronary Artery, One Artery from Thoracic Artery with Nonautologous Tissue Substitute, Open Approach

02100KF Bypass Coronary Artery, One Artery from Abdominal Artery with Nonautologous Tissue Substitute, Open Approach

02100KW Bypass Coronary Artery, One Artery from Aorta with Nonautologous Tissue Substitute, Open Approach

02100Z3 Bypass Coronary Artery, One Artery from Coronary Artery, Open Approach

02100Z8 Bypass Coronary Artery, One Artery from Right Internal Mammary, Open Approach

02100Z9 Bypass Coronary Artery, One Artery from Left Internal Mammary, Open Approach

02100ZC Bypass Coronary Artery, One Artery from Thoracic Artery, Open Approach

02100ZF Bypass Coronary Artery, One Artery from Abdominal Artery, Open Approach

0210483 Bypass Coronary Artery, One Artery from Coronary Artery with Zooplastic Tissue, Percutaneous Endoscopic Approach

0210488 Bypass Coronary Artery, One Artery from Right Internal Mammary with Zooplastic Tissue, Percutaneous Endoscopic Approach

0210489 Bypass Coronary Artery, One Artery from Left Internal Mammary with Zooplastic Tissue, Percutaneous Endoscopic Approach

021048C Bypass Coronary Artery, One Artery from Thoracic Artery with Zooplastic Tissue, Percutaneous Endoscopic Approach

021048F Bypass Coronary Artery, One Artery from Abdominal Artery with Zooplastic Tissue, Percutaneous Endoscopic Approach

021048W Bypass Coronary Artery, One Artery from Aorta with Zooplastic Tissue, Percutaneous Endoscopic Approach

0210493 Bypass Coronary Artery, One Artery from Coronary Artery with Autologous Venous Tissue, Percutaneous Endoscopic Approach

0210498 Bypass Coronary Artery, One Artery from Right Internal Mammary with Autologous Venous Tissue, Percutaneous Endoscopic Approach

0210499 Bypass Coronary Artery, One Artery from Left Internal Mammary with Autologous Venous Tissue, Percutaneous Endoscopic Approach

021049C Bypass Coronary Artery, One Artery from Thoracic Artery with Autologous Venous Tissue, Percutaneous Endoscopic Approach

021049F Bypass Coronary Artery, One Artery from Abdominal Artery with Autologous Venous Tissue, Percutaneous Endoscopic Approach

021049W Bypass Coronary Artery, One Artery from Aorta with Autologous Venous Tissue, Percutaneous Endoscopic Approach

02104A3 Bypass Coronary Artery, One Artery from Coronary Artery with Autologous Arterial Tissue, Percutaneous Endoscopic Approach

02104A8 Bypass Coronary Artery, One Artery from Right Internal Mammary with Autologous Arterial Tissue, Percutaneous Endoscopic Approach

02104A9 Bypass Coronary Artery, One Artery from Left Internal Mammary with Autologous Arterial Tissue, Percutaneous Endoscopic Approach

02104AC Bypass Coronary Artery, One Artery from Thoracic Artery with Autologous Arterial Tissue, Percutaneous Endoscopic Approach

02104AF Bypass Coronary Artery, One Artery from Abdominal Artery with Autologous Arterial Tissue, Percutaneous Endoscopic Approach

02104AW Bypass Coronary Artery, One Artery from Aorta with Autologous Arterial Tissue, Percutaneous Endoscopic Approach

02104J3 Bypass Coronary Artery, One Artery from Coronary Artery with Synthetic Substitute, Percutaneous Endoscopic Approach

HAC 08: Surgical Site Infection of Mediastinitis After Coronary Bypass Graft (CABG) Procedures (continued)

Ø2104J8 Bypass Coronary Artery, One Artery from Right Internal Mammary with Synthetic Substitute, Percutaneous Endoscopic Approach
Ø2104J9 Bypass Coronary Artery, One Artery from Left Internal Mammary with Synthetic Substitute, Percutaneous Endoscopic Approach
Ø2104JC Bypass Coronary Artery, One Artery from Thoracic Artery with Synthetic Substitute, Percutaneous Endoscopic Approach
Ø2104JF Bypass Coronary Artery, One Artery from Abdominal Artery with Synthetic Substitute, Percutaneous Endoscopic Approach
Ø2104JW Bypass Coronary Artery, One Artery from Aorta with Synthetic Substitute, Percutaneous Endoscopic Approach
Ø2104K3 Bypass Coronary Artery, One Artery from Coronary Artery with Nonautologous Tissue Substitute, Percutaneous Endoscopic Approach
Ø2104K8 Bypass Coronary Artery, One Artery from Right Internal Mammary with Nonautologous Tissue Substitute, Percutaneous Endoscopic Approach
Ø2104K9 Bypass Coronary Artery, One Artery from Left Internal Mammary with Nonautologous Tissue Substitute, Percutaneous Endoscopic Approach
Ø2104KC Bypass Coronary Artery, One Artery from Thoracic Artery with Nonautologous Tissue Substitute, Percutaneous Endoscopic Approach
Ø2104KF Bypass Coronary Artery, One Artery from Abdominal Artery with Nonautologous Tissue Substitute, Percutaneous Endoscopic Approach
Ø2104KW Bypass Coronary Artery, One Artery from Aorta with Nonautologous Tissue Substitute, Percutaneous Endoscopic Approach
Ø2104Z3 Bypass Coronary Artery, One Artery from Coronary Artery, Percutaneous Endoscopic Approach
Ø2104Z8 Bypass Coronary Artery, One Artery from Right Internal Mammary, Percutaneous Endoscopic Approach
Ø2104Z9 Bypass Coronary Artery, One Artery from Left Internal Mammary, Percutaneous Endoscopic Approach
Ø2104ZC Bypass Coronary Artery, One Artery from Thoracic Artery, Percutaneous Endoscopic Approach
Ø2104ZF Bypass Coronary Artery, One Artery from Abdominal Artery, Percutaneous Endoscopic Approach
Ø211Ø83 Bypass Coronary Artery, Two Arteries from Coronary Artery with Zooplastic Tissue, Open Approach
Ø211Ø88 Bypass Coronary Artery, Two Arteries from Right Internal Mammary with Zooplastic Tissue, Open Approach
Ø211Ø89 Bypass Coronary Artery, Two Arteries from Left Internal Mammary with Zooplastic Tissue, Open Approach
Ø211Ø8C Bypass Coronary Artery, Two Arteries from Thoracic Artery with Zooplastic Tissue, Open Approach
Ø211Ø8F Bypass Coronary Artery, Two Arteries from Abdominal Artery with Zooplastic Tissue, Open Approach
Ø211Ø8W Bypass Coronary Artery, Two Arteries from Aorta with Zooplastic Tissue, Open Approach
Ø211Ø93 Bypass Coronary Artery, Two Arteries from Coronary Artery with Autologous Venous Tissue, Open Approach
Ø211Ø98 Bypass Coronary Artery, Two Arteries from Right Internal Mammary with Autologous Venous Tissue, Open Approach
Ø211Ø99 Bypass Coronary Artery, Two Arteries from Left Internal Mammary with Autologous Venous Tissue, Open Approach
Ø211Ø9C Bypass Coronary Artery, Two Arteries from Thoracic Artery with Autologous Venous Tissue, Open Approach
Ø211Ø9F Bypass Coronary Artery, Two Arteries from Abdominal Artery with Autologous Venous Tissue, Open Approach
Ø211Ø9W Bypass Coronary Artery, Two Arteries from Aorta with Autologous Venous Tissue, Open Approach
Ø211ØA3 Bypass Coronary Artery, Two Arteries from Coronary Artery with Autologous Arterial Tissue, Open Approach
Ø211ØA8 Bypass Coronary Artery, Two Arteries from Right Internal Mammary with Autologous Arterial Tissue, Open Approach
Ø211ØA9 Bypass Coronary Artery, Two Arteries from Left Internal Mammary with Autologous Arterial Tissue, Open Approach
Ø211ØAC Bypass Coronary Artery, Two Arteries from Thoracic Artery with Autologous Arterial Tissue, Open Approach
Ø211ØAF Bypass Coronary Artery, Two Arteries from Abdominal Artery with Autologous Arterial Tissue, Open Approach
Ø211ØAW Bypass Coronary Artery, Two Arteries from Aorta with Autologous Arterial Tissue, Open Approach
Ø211ØJ3 Bypass Coronary Artery, Two Arteries from Coronary Artery with Synthetic Substitute, Open Approach
Ø211ØJ8 Bypass Coronary Artery, Two Arteries from Right Internal Mammary with Synthetic Substitute, Open Approach
Ø211ØJ9 Bypass Coronary Artery, Two Arteries from Left Internal Mammary with Synthetic Substitute, Open Approach
Ø211ØJC Bypass Coronary Artery, Two Arteries from Thoracic Artery with Synthetic Substitute, Open Approach
Ø211ØJF Bypass Coronary Artery, Two Arteries from Abdominal Artery with Synthetic Substitute, Open Approach
Ø211ØJW Bypass Coronary Artery, Two Arteries from Aorta with Synthetic Substitute, Open Approach
Ø211ØK3 Bypass Coronary Artery, Two Arteries from Coronary Artery with Nonautologous Tissue Substitute, Open Approach
Ø211ØK8 Bypass Coronary Artery, Two Arteries from Right Internal Mammary with Nonautologous Tissue Substitute, Open Approach
Ø211ØK9 Bypass Coronary Artery, Two Arteries from Left Internal Mammary with Nonautologous Tissue Substitute, Open Approach
Ø211ØKC Bypass Coronary Artery, Two Arteries from Thoracic Artery with Nonautologous Tissue Substitute, Open Approach
Ø211ØKF Bypass Coronary Artery, Two Arteries from Abdominal Artery with Nonautologous Tissue Substitute, Open Approach
Ø211ØKW Bypass Coronary Artery, Two Arteries from Aorta with Nonautologous Tissue Substitute, Open Approach
Ø211ØZ3 Bypass Coronary Artery, Two Arteries from Coronary Artery, Open Approach
Ø211ØZ8 Bypass Coronary Artery, Two Arteries from Right Internal Mammary, Open Approach
Ø211ØZ9 Bypass Coronary Artery, Two Arteries from Left Internal Mammary, Open Approach
Ø211ØZC Bypass Coronary Artery, Two Arteries from Thoracic Artery, Open Approach
Ø211ØZF Bypass Coronary Artery, Two Arteries from Abdominal Artery, Open Approach
Ø211483 Bypass Coronary Artery, Two Arteries from Coronary Artery with Zooplastic Tissue, Percutaneous Endoscopic Approach
Ø211488 Bypass Coronary Artery, Two Arteries from Right Internal Mammary with Zooplastic Tissue, Percutaneous Endoscopic Approach
Ø211489 Bypass Coronary Artery, Two Arteries from Left Internal Mammary with Zooplastic Tissue, Percutaneous Endoscopic Approach
Ø21148C Bypass Coronary Artery, Two Arteries from Thoracic Artery with Zooplastic Tissue, Percutaneous Endoscopic Approach
Ø21148F Bypass Coronary Artery, Two Arteries from Abdominal Artery with Zooplastic Tissue, Percutaneous Endoscopic Approach
Ø21148W Bypass Coronary Artery, Two Arteries from Aorta with Zooplastic Tissue, Percutaneous Endoscopic Approach
Ø211493 Bypass Coronary Artery, Two Arteries from Coronary Artery with Autologous Venous Tissue, Percutaneous Endoscopic Approach
Ø211498 Bypass Coronary Artery, Two Arteries from Right Internal Mammary with Autologous Venous Tissue, Percutaneous Endoscopic Approach
Ø211499 Bypass Coronary Artery, Two Arteries from Left Internal Mammary with Autologous Venous Tissue, Percutaneous Endoscopic Approach
Ø21149C Bypass Coronary Artery, Two Arteries from Thoracic Artery with Autologous Venous Tissue, Percutaneous Endoscopic Approach
Ø21149F Bypass Coronary Artery, Two Arteries from Abdominal Artery with Autologous Venous Tissue, Percutaneous Endoscopic Approach
Ø21149W Bypass Coronary Artery, Two Arteries from Aorta with Autologous Venous Tissue, Percutaneous Endoscopic Approach
Ø2114A3 Bypass Coronary Artery, Two Arteries from Coronary Artery with Autologous Arterial Tissue, Percutaneous Endoscopic Approach
Ø2114A8 Bypass Coronary Artery, Two Arteries from Right Internal Mammary with Autologous Arterial Tissue, Percutaneous Endoscopic Approach
Ø2114A9 Bypass Coronary Artery, Two Arteries from Left Internal Mammary with Autologous Arterial Tissue, Percutaneous Endoscopic Approach
Ø2114AC Bypass Coronary Artery, Two Arteries from Thoracic Artery with Autologous Arterial Tissue, Percutaneous Endoscopic Approach
Ø2114AF Bypass Coronary Artery, Two Arteries from Abdominal Artery with Autologous Arterial Tissue, Percutaneous Endoscopic Approach

HAC 08: Surgical Site Infection of Mediastinitis After Coronary Bypass Graft (CABG) Procedures (continued)

Ø2114AW Bypass Coronary Artery, Two Arteries from Aorta with Autologous Arterial Tissue, Percutaneous Endoscopic Approach
Ø2114J3 Bypass Coronary Artery, Two Arteries from Coronary Artery with Synthetic Substitute, Percutaneous Endoscopic Approach
Ø2114J8 Bypass Coronary Artery, Two Arteries from Right Internal Mammary with Synthetic Substitute, Percutaneous Endoscopic Approach
Ø2114J9 Bypass Coronary Artery, Two Arteries from Left Internal Mammary with Synthetic Substitute, Percutaneous Endoscopic Approach
Ø2114JC Bypass Coronary Artery, Two Arteries from Thoracic Artery with Synthetic Substitute, Percutaneous Endoscopic Approach
Ø2114JF Bypass Coronary Artery, Two Arteries from Abdominal Artery with Synthetic Substitute, Percutaneous Endoscopic Approach
Ø2114JW Bypass Coronary Artery, Two Arteries from Aorta with Synthetic Substitute, Percutaneous Endoscopic Approach
Ø2114K3 Bypass Coronary Artery, Two Arteries from Coronary Artery with Nonautologous Tissue Substitute, Percutaneous Endoscopic Approach
Ø2114K8 Bypass Coronary Artery, Two Arteries from Right Internal Mammary with Nonautologous Tissue Substitute, Percutaneous Endoscopic Approach
Ø2114K9 Bypass Coronary Artery, Two Arteries from Left Internal Mammary with Nonautologous Tissue Substitute, Percutaneous Endoscopic Approach
Ø2114KC Bypass Coronary Artery, Two Arteries from Thoracic Artery with Nonautologous Tissue Substitute, Percutaneous Endoscopic Approach
Ø2114KF Bypass Coronary Artery, Two Arteries from Abdominal Artery with Nonautologous Tissue Substitute, Percutaneous Endoscopic Approach
Ø2114KW Bypass Coronary Artery, Two Arteries from Aorta with Nonautologous Tissue Substitute, Percutaneous Endoscopic Approach
Ø2114Z3 Bypass Coronary Artery, Two Arteries from Coronary Artery, Percutaneous Endoscopic Approach
Ø2114Z8 Bypass Coronary Artery, Two Arteries from Right Internal Mammary, Percutaneous Endoscopic Approach
Ø2114Z9 Bypass Coronary Artery, Two Arteries from Left Internal Mammary, Percutaneous Endoscopic Approach
Ø2114ZC Bypass Coronary Artery, Two Arteries from Thoracic Artery, Percutaneous Endoscopic Approach
Ø2114ZF Bypass Coronary Artery, Two Arteries from Abdominal Artery, Percutaneous Endoscopic Approach
Ø212Ø83 Bypass Coronary Artery, Three Arteries from Coronary Artery with Zooplastic Tissue, Open Approach
Ø212Ø88 Bypass Coronary Artery, Three Arteries from Right Internal Mammary with Zooplastic Tissue, Open Approach
Ø212Ø89 Bypass Coronary Artery, Three Arteries from Left Internal Mammary with Zooplastic Tissue, Open Approach
Ø212Ø8C Bypass Coronary Artery, Three Arteries from Thoracic Artery with Zooplastic Tissue, Open Approach
Ø212Ø8F Bypass Coronary Artery, Three Arteries from Abdominal Artery with Zooplastic Tissue, Open Approach
Ø212Ø8W Bypass Coronary Artery, Three Arteries from Aorta with Zooplastic Tissue, Open Approach
Ø212Ø93 Bypass Coronary Artery, Three Arteries from Coronary Artery with Autologous Venous Tissue, Open Approach
Ø212Ø98 Bypass Coronary Artery, Three Arteries from Right Internal Mammary with Autologous Venous Tissue, Open Approach
Ø212Ø99 Bypass Coronary Artery, Three Arteries from Left Internal Mammary with Autologous Venous Tissue, Open Approach
Ø212Ø9C Bypass Coronary Artery, Three Arteries from Thoracic Artery with Autologous Venous Tissue, Open Approach
Ø212Ø9F Bypass Coronary Artery, Three Arteries from Abdominal Artery with Autologous Venous Tissue, Open Approach
Ø212Ø9W Bypass Coronary Artery, Three Arteries from Aorta with Autologous Venous Tissue, Open Approach
Ø212ØA3 Bypass Coronary Artery, Three Arteries from Coronary Artery with Autologous Arterial Tissue, Open Approach
Ø212ØA8 Bypass Coronary Artery, Three Arteries from Right Internal Mammary with Autologous Arterial Tissue, Open Approach
Ø212ØA9 Bypass Coronary Artery, Three Arteries from Left Internal Mammary with Autologous Arterial Tissue, Open Approach
Ø212ØAC Bypass Coronary Artery, Three Arteries from Thoracic Artery with Autologous Arterial Tissue, Open Approach
Ø212ØAF Bypass Coronary Artery, Three Arteries from Abdominal Artery with Autologous Arterial Tissue, Open Approach
Ø212ØAW Bypass Coronary Artery, Three Arteries from Aorta with Autologous Arterial Tissue, Open Approach
Ø212ØJ3 Bypass Coronary Artery, Three Arteries from Coronary Artery with Synthetic Substitute, Open Approach
Ø212ØJ8 Bypass Coronary Artery, Three Arteries from Right Internal Mammary with Synthetic Substitute, Open Approach
Ø212ØJ9 Bypass Coronary Artery, Three Arteries from Left Internal Mammary with Synthetic Substitute, Open Approach
Ø212ØJC Bypass Coronary Artery, Three Arteries from Thoracic Artery with Synthetic Substitute, Open Approach
Ø212ØJF Bypass Coronary Artery, Three Arteries from Abdominal Artery with Synthetic Substitute, Open Approach
Ø212ØJW Bypass Coronary Artery, Three Arteries from Aorta with Synthetic Substitute, Open Approach
Ø212ØK3 Bypass Coronary Artery, Three Arteries from Coronary Artery with Nonautologous Tissue Substitute, Open Approach
Ø212ØK8 Bypass Coronary Artery, Three Arteries from Right Internal Mammary with Nonautologous Tissue Substitute, Open Approach
Ø212ØK9 Bypass Coronary Artery, Three Arteries from Left Internal Mammary with Nonautologous Tissue Substitute, Open Approach
Ø212ØKC Bypass Coronary Artery, Three Arteries from Thoracic Artery with Nonautologous Tissue Substitute, Open Approach
Ø212ØKF Bypass Coronary Artery, Three Arteries from Abdominal Artery with Nonautologous Tissue Substitute, Open Approach
Ø212ØKW Bypass Coronary Artery, Three Arteries from Aorta with Nonautologous Tissue Substitute, Open Approach
Ø212ØZ3 Bypass Coronary Artery, Three Arteries from Coronary Artery, Open Approach
Ø212ØZ8 Bypass Coronary Artery, Three Arteries from Right Internal Mammary, Open Approach
Ø212ØZ9 Bypass Coronary Artery, Three Arteries from Left Internal Mammary, Open Approach
Ø212ØZC Bypass Coronary Artery, Three Arteries from Thoracic Artery, Open Approach
Ø212ØZF Bypass Coronary Artery, Three Arteries from Abdominal Artery, Open Approach
Ø212483 Bypass Coronary Artery, Three Arteries from Coronary Artery with Zooplastic Tissue, Percutaneous Endoscopic Approach
Ø212488 Bypass Coronary Artery, Three Arteries from Right Internal Mammary with Zooplastic Tissue, Percutaneous Endoscopic Approach
Ø212489 Bypass Coronary Artery, Three Arteries from Left Internal Mammary with Zooplastic Tissue, Percutaneous Endoscopic Approach
Ø21248C Bypass Coronary Artery, Three Arteries from Thoracic Artery with Zooplastic Tissue, Percutaneous Endoscopic Approach
Ø21248F Bypass Coronary Artery, Three Arteries from Abdominal Artery with Zooplastic Tissue, Percutaneous Endoscopic Approach
Ø21248W Bypass Coronary Artery, Three Arteries from Aorta with Zooplastic Tissue, Percutaneous Endoscopic Approach
Ø212493 Bypass Coronary Artery, Three Arteries from Coronary Artery with Autologous Venous Tissue, Percutaneous Endoscopic Approach
Ø212498 Bypass Coronary Artery, Three Arteries from Right Internal Mammary with Autologous Venous Tissue, Percutaneous Endoscopic Approach
Ø212499 Bypass Coronary Artery, Three Arteries from Left Internal Mammary with Autologous Venous Tissue, Percutaneous Endoscopic Approach
Ø21249C Bypass Coronary Artery, Three Arteries from Thoracic Artery with Autologous Venous Tissue, Percutaneous Endoscopic Approach
Ø21249F Bypass Coronary Artery, Three Arteries from Abdominal Artery with Autologous Venous Tissue, Percutaneous Endoscopic Approach
Ø21249W Bypass Coronary Artery, Three Arteries from Aorta with Autologous Venous Tissue, Percutaneous Endoscopic Approach

HAC 08: Surgical Site Infection of Mediastinitis After Coronary Bypass Graft (CABG) Procedures (continued)

Ø2124A3 Bypass Coronary Artery, Three Arteries from Coronary Artery with Autologous Arterial Tissue, Percutaneous Endoscopic Approach
Ø2124A8 Bypass Coronary Artery, Three Arteries from Right Internal Mammary with Autologous Arterial Tissue, Percutaneous Endoscopic Approach
Ø2124A9 Bypass Coronary Artery, Three Arteries from Left Internal Mammary with Autologous Arterial Tissue, Percutaneous Endoscopic Approach
Ø2124AC Bypass Coronary Artery, Three Arteries from Thoracic Artery with Autologous Arterial Tissue, Percutaneous Endoscopic Approach
Ø2124AF Bypass Coronary Artery, Three Arteries from Abdominal Artery with Autologous Arterial Tissue, Percutaneous Endoscopic Approach
Ø2124AW Bypass Coronary Artery, Three Arteries from Aorta with Autologous Arterial Tissue, Percutaneous Endoscopic Approach
Ø2124J3 Bypass Coronary Artery, Three Arteries from Coronary Artery with Synthetic Substitute, Percutaneous Endoscopic Approach
Ø2124J8 Bypass Coronary Artery, Three Arteries from Right Internal Mammary with Synthetic Substitute, Percutaneous Endoscopic Approach
Ø2124J9 Bypass Coronary Artery, Three Arteries from Left Internal Mammary with Synthetic Substitute, Percutaneous Endoscopic Approach
Ø2124JC Bypass Coronary Artery, Three Arteries from Thoracic Artery with Synthetic Substitute, Percutaneous Endoscopic Approach
Ø2124JF Bypass Coronary Artery, Three Arteries from Abdominal Artery with Synthetic Substitute, Percutaneous Endoscopic Approach
Ø2124JW Bypass Coronary Artery, Three Arteries from Aorta with Synthetic Substitute, Percutaneous Endoscopic Approach
Ø2124K3 Bypass Coronary Artery, Three Arteries from Coronary Artery with Nonautologous Tissue Substitute, Percutaneous Endoscopic Approach
Ø2124K8 Bypass Coronary Artery, Three Arteries from Right Internal Mammary with Nonautologous Tissue Substitute, Percutaneous Endoscopic Approach
Ø2124K9 Bypass Coronary Artery, Three Arteries from Left Internal Mammary with Nonautologous Tissue Substitute, Percutaneous Endoscopic Approach
Ø2124KC Bypass Coronary Artery, Three Arteries from Thoracic Artery with Nonautologous Tissue Substitute, Percutaneous Endoscopic Approach
Ø2124KF Bypass Coronary Artery, Three Arteries from Abdominal Artery with Nonautologous Tissue Substitute, Percutaneous Endoscopic Approach
Ø2124KW Bypass Coronary Artery, Three Arteries from Aorta with Nonautologous Tissue Substitute, Percutaneous Endoscopic Approach
Ø2124Z3 Bypass Coronary Artery, Three Arteries from Coronary Artery, Percutaneous Endoscopic Approach
Ø2124Z8 Bypass Coronary Artery, Three Arteries from Right Internal Mammary, Percutaneous Endoscopic Approach
Ø2124Z9 Bypass Coronary Artery, Three Arteries from Left Internal Mammary, Percutaneous Endoscopic Approach
Ø2124ZC Bypass Coronary Artery, Three Arteries from Thoracic Artery, Percutaneous Endoscopic Approach
Ø2124ZF Bypass Coronary Artery, Three Arteries from Abdominal Artery, Percutaneous Endoscopic Approach
Ø213Ø83 Bypass Coronary Artery, Four or More Arteries from Coronary Artery with Zooplastic Tissue, Open Approach
Ø213Ø88 Bypass Coronary Artery, Four or More Arteries from Right Internal Mammary with Zooplastic Tissue, Open Approach
Ø213Ø89 Bypass Coronary Artery, Four or More Arteries from Left Internal Mammary with Zooplastic Tissue, Open Approach
Ø213Ø8C Bypass Coronary Artery, Four or More Arteries from Thoracic Artery with Zooplastic Tissue, Open Approach
Ø213Ø8F Bypass Coronary Artery, Four or More Arteries from Abdominal Artery with Zooplastic Tissue, Open Approach
Ø213Ø8W Bypass Coronary Artery, Four or More Arteries from Aorta with Zooplastic Tissue, Open Approach
Ø213Ø93 Bypass Coronary Artery, Four or More Arteries from Coronary Artery with Autologous Venous Tissue, Open Approach
Ø213Ø98 Bypass Coronary Artery, Four or More Arteries from Right Internal Mammary with Autologous Venous Tissue, Open Approach
Ø213Ø99 Bypass Coronary Artery, Four or More Arteries from Left Internal Mammary with Autologous Venous Tissue, Open Approach
Ø213Ø9C Bypass Coronary Artery, Four or More Arteries from Thoracic Artery with Autologous Venous Tissue, Open Approach
Ø213Ø9F Bypass Coronary Artery, Four or More Arteries from Abdominal Artery with Autologous Venous Tissue, Open Approach
Ø213Ø9W Bypass Coronary Artery, Four or More Arteries from Aorta with Autologous Venous Tissue, Open Approach
Ø213ØA3 Bypass Coronary Artery, Four or More Arteries from Coronary Artery with Autologous Arterial Tissue, Open Approach
Ø213ØA8 Bypass Coronary Artery, Four or More Arteries from Right Internal Mammary with Autologous Arterial Tissue, Open Approach
Ø213ØA9 Bypass Coronary Artery, Four or More Arteries from Left Internal Mammary with Autologous Arterial Tissue, Open Approach
Ø213ØAC Bypass Coronary Artery, Four or More Arteries from Thoracic Artery with Autologous Arterial Tissue, Open Approach
Ø213ØAF Bypass Coronary Artery, Four or More Arteries from Abdominal Artery with Autologous Arterial Tissue, Open Approach
Ø213ØAW Bypass Coronary Artery, Four or More Arteries from Aorta with Autologous Arterial Tissue, Open Approach
Ø213ØJ3 Bypass Coronary Artery, Four or More Arteries from Coronary Artery with Synthetic Substitute, Open Approach
Ø213ØJ8 Bypass Coronary Artery, Four or More Arteries from Right Internal Mammary with Synthetic Substitute, Open Approach
Ø213ØJ9 Bypass Coronary Artery, Four or More Arteries from Left Internal Mammary with Synthetic Substitute, Open Approach
Ø213ØJC Bypass Coronary Artery, Four or More Arteries from Thoracic Artery with Synthetic Substitute, Open Approach
Ø213ØJF Bypass Coronary Artery, Four or More Arteries from Abdominal Artery with Synthetic Substitute, Open Approach
Ø213ØJW Bypass Coronary Artery, Four or More Arteries from Aorta with Synthetic Substitute, Open Approach
Ø213ØK3 Bypass Coronary Artery, Four or More Arteries from Coronary Artery with Nonautologous Tissue Substitute, Open Approach
Ø213ØK8 Bypass Coronary Artery, Four or More Arteries from Right Internal Mammary with Nonautologous Tissue Substitute, Open Approach
Ø213ØK9 Bypass Coronary Artery, Four or More Arteries from Left Internal Mammary with Nonautologous Tissue Substitute, Open Approach
Ø213ØKC Bypass Coronary Artery, Four or More Arteries from Thoracic Artery with Nonautologous Tissue Substitute, Open Approach
Ø213ØKF Bypass Coronary Artery, Four or More Arteries from Abdominal Artery with Nonautologous Tissue Substitute, Open Approach
Ø213ØKW Bypass Coronary Artery, Four or More Arteries from Aorta with Nonautologous Tissue Substitute, Open Approach
Ø213ØZ3 Bypass Coronary Artery, Four or More Arteries from Coronary Artery, Open Approach
Ø213ØZ8 Bypass Coronary Artery, Four or More Arteries from Right Internal Mammary, Open Approach
Ø213ØZ9 Bypass Coronary Artery, Four or More Arteries from Left Internal Mammary, Open Approach
Ø213ØZC Bypass Coronary Artery, Four or More Arteries from Thoracic Artery, Open Approach
Ø213ØZF Bypass Coronary Artery, Four or More Arteries from Abdominal Artery, Open Approach
Ø213483 Bypass Coronary Artery, Four or More Arteries from Coronary Artery with Zooplastic Tissue, Percutaneous Endoscopic Approach
Ø213488 Bypass Coronary Artery, Four or More Arteries from Right Internal Mammary with Zooplastic Tissue, Percutaneous Endoscopic Approach
Ø213489 Bypass Coronary Artery, Four or More Arteries from Left Internal Mammary with Zooplastic Tissue, Percutaneous Endoscopic Approach
Ø21348C Bypass Coronary Artery, Four or More Arteries from Thoracic Artery with Zooplastic Tissue, Percutaneous Endoscopic Approach

HAC 08: Surgical Site Infection of Mediastinitis After Coronary Bypass Graft (CABG) Procedures (continued)

Ø21348F Bypass Coronary Artery, Four or More Arteries from Abdominal Artery with Zooplastic Tissue, Percutaneous Endoscopic Approach
Ø21348W Bypass Coronary Artery, Four or More Arteries from Aorta with Zooplastic Tissue, Percutaneous Endoscopic Approach
Ø213493 Bypass Coronary Artery, Four or More Arteries from Coronary Artery with Autologous Venous Tissue, Percutaneous Endoscopic Approach
Ø213498 Bypass Coronary Artery, Four or More Arteries from Right Internal Mammary with Autologous Venous Tissue, Percutaneous Endoscopic Approach
Ø213499 Bypass Coronary Artery, Four or More Arteries from Left Internal Mammary with Autologous Venous Tissue, Percutaneous Endoscopic Approach
Ø21349C Bypass Coronary Artery, Four or More Arteries from Thoracic Artery with Autologous Venous Tissue, Percutaneous Endoscopic Approach
Ø21349F Bypass Coronary Artery, Four or More Arteries from Abdominal Artery with Autologous Venous Tissue, Percutaneous Endoscopic Approach
Ø21349W Bypass Coronary Artery, Four or More Arteries from Aorta with Autologous Venous Tissue, Percutaneous Endoscopic Approach
Ø2134A3 Bypass Coronary Artery, Four or More Arteries from Coronary Artery with Autologous Arterial Tissue, Percutaneous Endoscopic Approach
Ø2134A8 Bypass Coronary Artery, Four or More Arteries from Right Internal Mammary with Autologous Arterial Tissue, Percutaneous Endoscopic Approach
Ø2134A9 Bypass Coronary Artery, Four or More Arteries from Left Internal Mammary with Autologous Arterial Tissue, Percutaneous Endoscopic Approach
Ø2134AC Bypass Coronary Artery, Four or More Arteries from Thoracic Artery with Autologous Arterial Tissue, Percutaneous Endoscopic Approach
Ø2134AF Bypass Coronary Artery, Four or More Arteries from Abdominal Artery with Autologous Arterial Tissue, Percutaneous Endoscopic Approach
Ø2134AW Bypass Coronary Artery, Four or More Arteries from Aorta with Autologous Arterial Tissue, Percutaneous Endoscopic Approach
Ø2134J3 Bypass Coronary Artery, Four or More Arteries from Coronary Artery with Synthetic Substitute, Percutaneous Endoscopic Approach
Ø2134J8 Bypass Coronary Artery, Four or More Arteries from Right Internal Mammary with Synthetic Substitute, Percutaneous Endoscopic Approach
Ø2134J9 Bypass Coronary Artery, Four or More Arteries from Left Internal Mammary with Synthetic Substitute, Percutaneous Endoscopic Approach
Ø2134JC Bypass Coronary Artery, Four or More Arteries from Thoracic Artery with Synthetic Substitute, Percutaneous Endoscopic Approach
Ø2134JF Bypass Coronary Artery, Four or More Arteries from Abdominal Artery with Synthetic Substitute, Percutaneous Endoscopic Approach
Ø2134JW Bypass Coronary Artery, Four or More Arteries from Aorta with Synthetic Substitute, Percutaneous Endoscopic Approach
Ø2134K3 Bypass Coronary Artery, Four or More Arteries from Coronary Artery with Nonautologous Tissue Substitute, Percutaneous Endoscopic Approach
Ø2134K8 Bypass Coronary Artery, Four or More Arteries from Right Internal Mammary with Nonautologous Tissue Substitute, Percutaneous Endoscopic Approach
Ø2134K9 Bypass Coronary Artery, Four or More Arteries from Left Internal Mammary with Nonautologous Tissue Substitute, Percutaneous Endoscopic Approach
Ø2134KC Bypass Coronary Artery, Four or More Arteries from Thoracic Artery with Nonautologous Tissue Substitute, Percutaneous Endoscopic Approach
Ø2134KF Bypass Coronary Artery, Four or More Arteries from Abdominal Artery with Nonautologous Tissue Substitute, Percutaneous Endoscopic Approach
Ø2134KW Bypass Coronary Artery, Four or More Arteries from Aorta with Nonautologous Tissue Substitute, Percutaneous Endoscopic Approach
Ø2134Z3 Bypass Coronary Artery, Four or More Arteries from Coronary Artery, Percutaneous Endoscopic Approach
Ø2134Z8 Bypass Coronary Artery, Four or More Arteries from Right Internal Mammary, Percutaneous Endoscopic Approach
Ø2134Z9 Bypass Coronary Artery, Four or More Arteries from Left Internal Mammary, Percutaneous Endoscopic Approach
Ø2134ZC Bypass Coronary Artery, Four or More Arteries from Thoracic Artery, Percutaneous Endoscopic Approach
Ø2134ZF Bypass Coronary Artery, Four or More Arteries from Abdominal Artery, Percutaneous Endoscopic Approach

HAC 10: Deep Vein Thrombosis (DVT) or Pulmonary Embolism (PE) with Total Knee or Hip Replacement

Secondary diagnosis not POA:

I26.Ø2 Saddle embolus of pulmonary artery with acute cor pulmonale
I26.Ø9 Other pulmonary embolism with acute cor pulmonale
I26.92 Saddle embolus of pulmonary artery without acute cor pulmonale
I26.93 Single subsegmental pulmonary embolism without acute cor pulmonale
I26.94 Multiple subsegmental pulmonary emboli without acute cor pulmonale
I26.99 Other pulmonary embolism without acute cor pulmonale
I82.4Ø1 Acute embolism and thrombosis of unspecified deep veins of right lower extremity
I82.4Ø2 Acute embolism and thrombosis of unspecified deep veins of left lower extremity
I82.4Ø3 Acute embolism and thrombosis of unspecified deep veins of lower extremity, bilateral
I82.4Ø9 Acute embolism and thrombosis of unspecified deep veins of unspecified lower extremity
I82.411 Acute embolism and thrombosis of right femoral vein
I82.412 Acute embolism and thrombosis of left femoral vein
I82.413 Acute embolism and thrombosis of femoral vein, bilateral
I82.419 Acute embolism and thrombosis of unspecified femoral vein
I82.421 Acute embolism and thrombosis of right iliac vein
I82.422 Acute embolism and thrombosis of left iliac vein
I82.423 Acute embolism and thrombosis of iliac vein, bilateral
I82.429 Acute embolism and thrombosis of unspecified iliac vein
I82.431 Acute embolism and thrombosis of right popliteal vein
I82.432 Acute embolism and thrombosis of left popliteal vein
I82.433 Acute embolism and thrombosis of popliteal vein, bilateral
I82.439 Acute embolism and thrombosis of unspecified popliteal vein
I82.441 Acute embolism and thrombosis of right tibial vein
I82.442 Acute embolism and thrombosis of left tibial vein
I82.443 Acute embolism and thrombosis of tibial vein, bilateral
I82.449 Acute embolism and thrombosis of unspecified tibial vein
I82.451 Acute embolism and thrombosis of right peroneal vein
I82.452 Acute embolism and thrombosis of left peroneal vein
I82.453 Acute embolism and thrombosis of peroneal vein, bilateral
I82.459 Acute embolism and thrombosis of unspecified peroneal vein
I82.491 Acute embolism and thrombosis of other specified deep vein of right lower extremity
I82.492 Acute embolism and thrombosis of other specified deep vein of left lower extremity
I82.493 Acute embolism and thrombosis of other specified deep vein of lower extremity, bilateral
I82.499 Acute embolism and thrombosis of other specified deep vein of unspecified lower extremity
I82.4Y1 Acute embolism and thrombosis of unspecified deep veins of right proximal lower extremity
I82.4Y2 Acute embolism and thrombosis of unspecified deep veins of left proximal lower extremity
I82.4Y3 Acute embolism and thrombosis of unspecified deep veins of proximal lower extremity, bilateral
I82.4Y9 Acute embolism and thrombosis of unspecified deep veins of unspecified proximal lower extremity
I82.4Z1 Acute embolism and thrombosis of unspecified deep veins of right distal lower extremity
I82.4Z2 Acute embolism and thrombosis of unspecified deep veins of left distal lower extremity
I82.4Z3 Acute embolism and thrombosis of unspecified deep veins of distal lower extremity, bilateral
I82.4Z9 Acute embolism and thrombosis of unspecified deep veins of unspecified distal lower extremity

HAC 10: Deep Vein Thrombosis (DVT) or Pulmonary Embolism (PE) with Total Knee or Hip Replacement (continued)

AND

Any of the following procedures:

ØSR9Ø19 Replacement of Right Hip Joint with Metal Synthetic Substitute, Cemented, Open Approach
ØSR9Ø1A Replacement of Right Hip Joint with Metal Synthetic Substitute, Uncemented, Open Approach
ØSR9Ø1Z Replacement of Right Hip Joint with Metal Synthetic Substitute, Open Approach
ØSR9Ø29 Replacement of Right Hip Joint with Metal on Polyethylene Synthetic Substitute, Cemented, Open Approach
ØSR9Ø2A Replacement of Right Hip Joint with Metal on Polyethylene Synthetic Substitute, Uncemented, Open Approach
ØSR9Ø2Z Replacement of Right Hip Joint with Metal on Polyethylene Synthetic Substitute, Open Approach
ØSR9Ø39 Replacement of Right Hip Joint with Ceramic Synthetic Substitute, Cemented, Open Approach
ØSR9Ø3A Replacement of Right Hip Joint with Ceramic Synthetic Substitute, Uncemented, Open Approach
ØSR9Ø3Z Replacement of Right Hip Joint with Ceramic Synthetic Substitute, Open Approach
ØSR9Ø49 Replacement of Right Hip Joint with Ceramic on Polyethylene Synthetic Substitute, Cemented, Open Approach
ØSR9Ø4A Replacement of Right Hip Joint with Ceramic on Polyethylene Synthetic Substitute, Uncemented, Open Approach
ØSR9Ø4Z Replacement of Right Hip Joint with Ceramic on Polyethylene Synthetic Substitute, Open Approach
ØSR9Ø69 Replacement of Right Hip Joint with Oxidized Zirconium on Polyethylene Synthetic Substitute, Cemented, Open Approach
ØSR9Ø6A Replacement of Right Hip Joint with Oxidized Zirconium on Polyethylene Synthetic Substitute, Uncemented, Open Approach
ØSR9Ø6Z Replacement of Right Hip Joint with Oxidized Zirconium on Polyethylene Synthetic Substitute, Open Approach
ØSR9Ø7Z Replacement of Right Hip Joint with Autologous Tissue Substitute, Open Approach
ØSR9ØEZ Replacement of Right Hip Joint with Articulating Spacer, Open Approach
ØSR9ØJ9 Replacement of Right Hip Joint with Synthetic Substitute, Cemented, Open Approach
ØSR9ØJA Replacement of Right Hip Joint with Synthetic Substitute, Uncemented, Open Approach
ØSR9ØJZ Replacement of Right Hip Joint with Synthetic Substitute, Open Approach
ØSR9ØKZ Replacement of Right Hip Joint with Nonautologous Tissue Substitute, Open Approach
ØSRAØØ9 Replacement of Right Hip Joint, Acetabular Surface with Polyethylene Synthetic Substitute, Cemented, Open Approach
ØSRAØØA Replacement of Right Hip Joint, Acetabular Surface with Polyethylene Synthetic Substitute, Uncemented, Open Approach
ØSRAØØZ Replacement of Right Hip Joint, Acetabular Surface with Polyethylene Synthetic Substitute, Open Approach
ØSRAØ19 Replacement of Right Hip Joint, Acetabular Surface with Metal Synthetic Substitute, Cemented, Open Approach
ØSRAØ1A Replacement of Right Hip Joint, Acetabular Surface with Metal Synthetic Substitute, Uncemented, Open Approach
ØSRAØ1Z Replacement of Right Hip Joint, Acetabular Surface with Metal Synthetic Substitute, Open Approach
ØSRAØ39 Replacement of Right Hip Joint, Acetabular Surface with Ceramic Synthetic Substitute, Cemented, Open Approach
ØSRAØ3A Replacement of Right Hip Joint, Acetabular Surface with Ceramic Synthetic Substitute, Uncemented, Open Approach
ØSRAØ3Z Replacement of Right Hip Joint, Acetabular Surface with Ceramic Synthetic Substitute, Open Approach
ØSRAØ7Z Replacement of Right Hip Joint, Acetabular Surface with Autologous Tissue Substitute, Open Approach
ØSRAØJ9 Replacement of Right Hip Joint, Acetabular Surface with Synthetic Substitute, Cemented, Open Approach
ØSRAØJA Replacement of Right Hip Joint, Acetabular Surface with Synthetic Substitute, Uncemented, Open Approach
ØSRAØJZ Replacement of Right Hip Joint, Acetabular Surface with Synthetic Substitute, Open Approach
ØSRAØKZ Replacement of Right Hip Joint, Acetabular Surface with Nonautologous Tissue Substitute, Open Approach
ØSRBØ19 Replacement of Left Hip Joint with Metal Synthetic Substitute, Cemented, Open Approach
ØSRBØ1A Replacement of Left Hip Joint with Metal Synthetic Substitute, Uncemented, Open Approach
ØSRBØ1Z Replacement of Left Hip Joint with Metal Synthetic Substitute, Open Approach
ØSRBØ29 Replacement of Left Hip Joint with Metal on Polyethylene Synthetic Substitute, Cemented, Open Approach
ØSRBØ2A Replacement of Left Hip Joint with Metal on Polyethylene Synthetic Substitute, Uncemented, Open Approach
ØSRBØ2Z Replacement of Left Hip Joint with Metal on Polyethylene Synthetic Substitute, Open Approach
ØSRBØ39 Replacement of Left Hip Joint with Ceramic Synthetic Substitute, Cemented, Open Approach
ØSRBØ3A Replacement of Left Hip Joint with Ceramic Synthetic Substitute, Uncemented, Open Approach
ØSRBØ3Z Replacement of Left Hip Joint with Ceramic Synthetic Substitute, Open Approach
ØSRBØ49 Replacement of Left Hip Joint with Ceramic on Polyethylene Synthetic Substitute, Cemented, Open Approach
ØSRBØ4A Replacement of Left Hip Joint with Ceramic on Polyethylene Synthetic Substitute, Uncemented, Open Approach
ØSRBØ4Z Replacement of Left Hip Joint with Ceramic on Polyethylene Synthetic Substitute, Open Approach
ØSRBØ69 Replacement of Left Hip Joint with Oxidized Zirconium on Polyethylene Synthetic Substitute, Cemented, Open Approach
ØSRBØ6A Replacement of Left Hip Joint with Oxidized Zirconium on Polyethylene Synthetic Substitute, Uncemented, Open Approach
ØSRBØ6Z Replacement of Left Hip Joint with Oxidized Zirconium on Polyethylene Synthetic Substitute, Open Approach
ØSRBØ7Z Replacement of Left Hip Joint with Autologous Tissue Substitute, Open Approach
ØSRBØEZ Replacement of Left Hip Joint with Articulating Spacer, Open Approach
ØSRBØJ9 Replacement of Left Hip Joint with Synthetic Substitute, Cemented, Open Approach
ØSRBØJA Replacement of Left Hip Joint with Synthetic Substitute, Uncemented, Open Approach
ØSRBØJZ Replacement of Left Hip Joint with Synthetic Substitute, Open Approach
ØSRBØKZ Replacement of Left Hip Joint with Nonautologous Tissue Substitute, Open Approach
ØSRCØ69 Replacement of Right Knee Joint with Oxidized Zirconium on Polyethylene Synthetic Substitute, Cemented, Open Approach
ØSRCØ6A Replacement of Right Knee Joint with Oxidized Zirconium on Polyethylene Synthetic Substitute, Uncemented, Open Approach
ØSRCØ6Z Replacement of Right Knee Joint with Oxidized Zirconium on Polyethylene Synthetic Substitute, Open Approach
ØSRCØ7Z Replacement of Right Knee Joint with Autologous Tissue Substitute, Open Approach
ØSRCØEZ Replacement of Right Knee Joint with Articulating Spacer, Open Approach
ØSRCØJ9 Replacement of Right Knee Joint with Synthetic Substitute, Cemented, Open Approach
ØSRCØJA Replacement of Right Knee Joint with Synthetic Substitute, Uncemented, Open Approach
ØSRCØJZ Replacement of Right Knee Joint with Synthetic Substitute, Open Approach
ØSRCØKZ Replacement of Right Knee Joint with Nonautologous Tissue Substitute, Open Approach
ØSRCØL9 Replacement of Right Knee Joint with Medial Unicondylar Synthetic Substitute, Cemented, Open Approach
ØSRCØLA Replacement of Right Knee Joint with Medial Unicondylar Synthetic Substitute, Uncemented, Open Approach
ØSRCØLZ Replacement of Right Knee Joint with Medial Unicondylar Synthetic Substitute, Open Approach
ØSRCØM9 Replacement of Right Knee Joint with Lateral Unicondylar Synthetic Substitute, Cemented, Open Approach
ØSRCØMA Replacement of Right Knee Joint with Lateral Unicondylar Synthetic Substitute, Uncemented, Open Approach
ØSRCØMZ Replacement of Right Knee Joint with Lateral Unicondylar Synthetic Substitute, Open Approach
ØSRCØN9 Replacement of Right Knee Joint with Patellofemoral Synthetic Substitute, Cemented, Open Approach
ØSRCØNA Replacement of Right Knee Joint with Patellofemoral Synthetic Substitute, Uncemented, Open Approach

HAC 10: Deep Vein Thrombosis (DVT) or Pulmonary Embolism (PE) with Total Knee or Hip Replacement (continued)

ØSRCØNZ Replacement of Right Knee Joint with Patellofemoral Synthetic Substitute, Open Approach
ØSRDØ69 Replacement of Left Knee Joint with Oxidized Zirconium on Polyethylene Synthetic Substitute, Cemented, Open Approach
ØSRDØ6A Replacement of Left Knee Joint with Oxidized Zirconium on Polyethylene Synthetic Substitute, Uncemented, Open Approach
ØSRDØ6Z Replacement of Left Knee Joint with Oxidized Zirconium on Polyethylene Synthetic Substitute, Open Approach
ØSRDØ7Z Replacement of Left Knee Joint with Autologous Tissue Substitute, Open Approach
ØSRDØEZ Replacement of Left Knee Joint with Articulating Spacer, Open Approach
ØSRDØJ9 Replacement of Left Knee Joint with Synthetic Substitute, Cemented, Open Approach
ØSRDØJA Replacement of Left Knee Joint with Synthetic Substitute, Uncemented, Open Approach
ØSRDØJZ Replacement of Left Knee Joint with Synthetic Substitute, Open Approach
ØSRDØKZ Replacement of Left Knee Joint with Nonautologous Tissue Substitute, Open Approach
ØSRDØL9 Replacement of Left Knee Joint with Medial Unicondylar Synthetic Substitute, Cemented, Open Approach
ØSRDØLA Replacement of Left Knee Joint with Medial Unicondylar Synthetic Substitute, Uncemented, Open Approach
ØSRDØLZ Replacement of Left Knee Joint with Medial Unicondylar Synthetic Substitute, Open Approach
ØSRDØM9 Replacement of Left Knee Joint with Lateral Unicondylar Synthetic Substitute, Cemented, Open Approach
ØSRDØMA Replacement of Left Knee Joint with Lateral Unicondylar Synthetic Substitute, Uncemented, Open Approach
ØSRDØMZ Replacement of Left Knee Joint with Lateral Unicondylar Synthetic Substitute, Open Approach
ØSRDØN9 Replacement of Left Knee Joint with Patellofemoral Synthetic Substitute, Cemented, Open Approach
ØSRDØNA Replacement of Left Knee Joint with Patellofemoral Synthetic Substitute, Uncemented, Open Approach
ØSRDØNZ Replacement of Left Knee Joint with Patellofemoral Synthetic Substitute, Open Approach
ØSREØØ9 Replacement of Left Hip Joint, Acetabular Surface with Polyethylene Synthetic Substitute, Cemented, Open Approach
ØSREØØA Replacement of Left Hip Joint, Acetabular Surface with Polyethylene Synthetic Substitute, Uncemented, Open Approach
ØSREØØZ Replacement of Left Hip Joint, Acetabular Surface with Polyethylene Synthetic Substitute, Open Approach
ØSREØ19 Replacement of Left Hip Joint, Acetabular Surface with Metal Synthetic Substitute, Cemented, Open Approach
ØSREØ1A Replacement of Left Hip Joint, Acetabular Surface with Metal Synthetic Substitute, Uncemented, Open Approach
ØSREØ1Z Replacement of Left Hip Joint, Acetabular Surface with Metal Synthetic Substitute, Open Approach
ØSREØ39 Replacement of Left Hip Joint, Acetabular Surface with Ceramic Synthetic Substitute, Cemented, Open Approach
ØSREØ3A Replacement of Left Hip Joint, Acetabular Surface with Ceramic Synthetic Substitute, Uncemented, Open Approach
ØSREØ3Z Replacement of Left Hip Joint, Acetabular Surface with Ceramic Synthetic Substitute, Open Approach
ØSREØ7Z Replacement of Left Hip Joint, Acetabular Surface with Autologous Tissue Substitute, Open Approach
ØSREØJ9 Replacement of Left Hip Joint, Acetabular Surface with Synthetic Substitute, Cemented, Open Approach
ØSREØJA Replacement of Left Hip Joint, Acetabular Surface with Synthetic Substitute, Uncemented, Open Approach
ØSREØJZ Replacement of Left Hip Joint, Acetabular Surface with Synthetic Substitute, Open Approach
ØSREØKZ Replacement of Left Hip Joint, Acetabular Surface with Nonautologous Tissue Substitute, Open Approach
ØSRRØ19 Replacement of Right Hip Joint, Femoral Surface with Metal Synthetic Substitute, Cemented, Open Approach
ØSRRØ1A Replacement of Right Hip Joint, Femoral Surface with Metal Synthetic Substitute, Uncemented, Open Approach
ØSRRØ1Z Replacement of Right Hip Joint, Femoral Surface with Metal Synthetic Substitute, Open Approach
ØSRRØ39 Replacement of Right Hip Joint, Femoral Surface with Ceramic Synthetic Substitute, Cemented, Open Approach
ØSRRØ3A Replacement of Right Hip Joint, Femoral Surface with Ceramic Synthetic Substitute, Uncemented, Open Approach
ØSRRØ3Z Replacement of Right Hip Joint, Femoral Surface with Ceramic Synthetic Substitute, Open Approach
ØSRRØ7Z Replacement of Right Hip Joint, Femoral Surface with Autologous Tissue Substitute, Open Approach
ØSRRØJ9 Replacement of Right Hip Joint, Femoral Surface with Synthetic Substitute, Cemented, Open Approach
ØSRRØJA Replacement of Right Hip Joint, Femoral Surface with Synthetic Substitute, Uncemented, Open Approach
ØSRRØJZ Replacement of Right Hip Joint, Femoral Surface with Synthetic Substitute, Open Approach
ØSRRØKZ Replacement of Right Hip Joint, Femoral Surface with Nonautologous Tissue Substitute, Open Approach
ØSRSØ19 Replacement of Left Hip Joint, Femoral Surface with Metal Synthetic Substitute, Cemented, Open Approach
ØSRSØ1A Replacement of Left Hip Joint, Femoral Surface with Metal Synthetic Substitute, Uncemented, Open Approach
ØSRSØ1Z Replacement of Left Hip Joint, Femoral Surface with Metal Synthetic Substitute, Open Approach
ØSRSØ39 Replacement of Left Hip Joint, Femoral Surface with Ceramic Synthetic Substitute, Cemented, Open Approach
ØSRSØ3A Replacement of Left Hip Joint, Femoral Surface with Ceramic Synthetic Substitute, Uncemented, Open Approach
ØSRSØ3Z Replacement of Left Hip Joint, Femoral Surface with Ceramic Synthetic Substitute, Open Approach
ØSRSØ7Z Replacement of Left Hip Joint, Femoral Surface with Autologous Tissue Substitute, Open Approach
ØSRSØJ9 Replacement of Left Hip Joint, Femoral Surface with Synthetic Substitute, Cemented, Open Approach
ØSRSØJA Replacement of Left Hip Joint, Femoral Surface with Synthetic Substitute, Uncemented, Open Approach
ØSRSØJZ Replacement of Left Hip Joint, Femoral Surface with Synthetic Substitute, Open Approach
ØSRSØKZ Replacement of Left Hip Joint, Femoral Surface with Nonautologous Tissue Substitute, Open Approach
ØSRTØ7Z Replacement of Right Knee Joint, Femoral Surface with Autologous Tissue Substitute, Open Approach
ØSRTØJ9 Replacement of Right Knee Joint, Femoral Surface with Synthetic Substitute, Cemented, Open Approach
ØSRTØJA Replacement of Right Knee Joint, Femoral Surface with Synthetic Substitute, Uncemented, Open Approach
ØSRTØJZ Replacement of Right Knee Joint, Femoral Surface with Synthetic Substitute, Open Approach
ØSRTØKZ Replacement of Right Knee Joint, Femoral Surface with Nonautologous Tissue Substitute, Open Approach
ØSRUØ7Z Replacement of Left Knee Joint, Femoral Surface with Autologous Tissue Substitute, Open Approach
ØSRUØJ9 Replacement of Left Knee Joint, Femoral Surface with Synthetic Substitute, Cemented, Open Approach
ØSRUØJA Replacement of Left Knee Joint, Femoral Surface with Synthetic Substitute, Uncemented, Open Approach
ØSRUØJZ Replacement of Left Knee Joint, Femoral Surface with Synthetic Substitute, Open Approach
ØSRUØKZ Replacement of Left Knee Joint, Femoral Surface with Nonautologous Tissue Substitute, Open Approach
ØSRVØ7Z Replacement of Right Knee Joint, Tibial Surface with Autologous Tissue Substitute, Open Approach
ØSRVØJ9 Replacement of Right Knee Joint, Tibial Surface with Synthetic Substitute, Cemented, Open Approach
ØSRVØJA Replacement of Right Knee Joint, Tibial Surface with Synthetic Substitute, Uncemented, Open Approach
ØSRVØJZ Replacement of Right Knee Joint, Tibial Surface with Synthetic Substitute, Open Approach
ØSRVØKZ Replacement of Right Knee Joint, Tibial Surface with Nonautologous Tissue Substitute, Open Approach
ØSRWØ7Z Replacement of Left Knee Joint, Tibial Surface with Autologous Tissue Substitute, Open Approach
ØSRWØJ9 Replacement of Left Knee Joint, Tibial Surface with Synthetic Substitute, Cemented, Open Approach
ØSRWØJA Replacement of Left Knee Joint, Tibial Surface with Synthetic Substitute, Uncemented, Open Approach
ØSRWØJZ Replacement of Left Knee Joint, Tibial Surface with Synthetic Substitute, Open Approach

HAC 10: Deep Vein Thrombosis (DVT) or Pulmonary Embolism (PE) with Total Knee or Hip Replacement (continued)

ØSRWØKZ Replacement of Left Knee Joint, Tibial Surface with Nonautologous Tissue Substitute, Open Approach
ØSU9ØBZ Supplement Right Hip Joint with Resurfacing Device, Open Approach
ØSUAØBZ Supplement Right Hip Joint, Acetabular Surface with Resurfacing Device, Open Approach
ØSUBØBZ Supplement Left Hip Joint with Resurfacing Device, Open Approach
ØSUEØBZ Supplement Left Hip Joint, Acetabular Surface with Resurfacing Device, Open Approach
ØSURØBZ Supplement Right Hip Joint, Femoral Surface with Resurfacing Device, Open Approach
ØSUSØBZ Supplement Left Hip Joint, Femoral Surface with Resurfacing Device, Open Approach

HAC 11: Surgical Site Infection-Bariatric Surgery

Principal diagnosis of:

E66.Ø1 Morbid (severe) obesity due to excess calories

AND

Secondary diagnosis not POA:

K68.11 Postprocedural retroperitoneal abscess
K95.Ø1 Infection due to gastric band procedure
K95.81 Infection due to other bariatric procedure
T81.4ØXA Infection following a procedure, unspecified, initial encounter
T81.41XA Infection following a procedure, superficial incisional surgical site, initial encounter
T81.42XA Infection following a procedure, deep incisional surgical site, initial encounter
T81.43XA Infection following a procedure, organ and space surgical site, initial encounter
T81.44XA Sepsis following a procedure, initial encounter
T81.49XA Infection following a procedure, other surgical site, initial encounter

AND

Any of the following procedures:

ØD16Ø79 Bypass Stomach to Duodenum with Autologous Tissue Substitute, Open Approach
ØD16Ø7A Bypass Stomach to Jejunum with Autologous Tissue Substitute, Open Approach
ØD16Ø7B Bypass Stomach to Ileum with Autologous Tissue Substitute, Open Approach
ØD16Ø7L Bypass Stomach to Transverse Colon with Autologous Tissue Substitute, Open Approach
ØD16ØJ9 Bypass Stomach to Duodenum with Synthetic Substitute, Open Approach
ØD16ØJA Bypass Stomach to Jejunum with Synthetic Substitute, Open Approach
ØD16ØJB Bypass Stomach to Ileum with Synthetic Substitute, Open Approach
ØD16ØJL Bypass Stomach to Transverse Colon with Synthetic Substitute, Open Approach
ØD16ØK9 Bypass Stomach to Duodenum with Nonautologous Tissue Substitute, Open Approach
ØD16ØKA Bypass Stomach to Jejunum with Nonautologous Tissue Substitute, Open Approach
ØD16ØKB Bypass Stomach to Ileum with Nonautologous Tissue Substitute, Open Approach
ØD16ØKL Bypass Stomach to Transverse Colon with Nonautologous Tissue Substitute, Open Approach
ØD16ØZ9 Bypass Stomach to Duodenum, Open Approach
ØD16ØZA Bypass Stomach to Jejunum, Open Approach
ØD16ØZB Bypass Stomach to Ileum, Open Approach
ØD16ØZL Bypass Stomach to Transverse Colon, Open Approach
ØD16479 Bypass Stomach to Duodenum with Autologous Tissue Substitute, Percutaneous Endoscopic Approach
ØD1647A Bypass Stomach to Jejunum with Autologous Tissue Substitute, Percutaneous Endoscopic Approach
ØD1647B Bypass Stomach to Ileum with Autologous Tissue Substitute, Percutaneous Endoscopic Approach
ØD1647L Bypass Stomach to Transverse Colon with Autologous Tissue Substitute, Percutaneous Endoscopic Approach
ØD164J9 Bypass Stomach to Duodenum with Synthetic Substitute, Percutaneous Endoscopic Approach
ØD164JA Bypass Stomach to Jejunum with Synthetic Substitute, Percutaneous Endoscopic Approach
ØD164JB Bypass Stomach to Ileum with Synthetic Substitute, Percutaneous Endoscopic Approach
ØD164JL Bypass Stomach to Transverse Colon with Synthetic Substitute, Percutaneous Endoscopic Approach
ØD164K9 Bypass Stomach to Duodenum with Nonautologous Tissue Substitute, Percutaneous Endoscopic Approach
ØD164KA Bypass Stomach to Jejunum with Nonautologous Tissue Substitute, Percutaneous Endoscopic Approach
ØD164KB Bypass Stomach to Ileum with Nonautologous Tissue Substitute, Percutaneous Endoscopic Approach
ØD164KL Bypass Stomach to Transverse Colon with Nonautologous Tissue Substitute, Percutaneous Endoscopic Approach
ØD164Z9 Bypass Stomach to Duodenum, Percutaneous Endoscopic Approach
ØD164ZA Bypass Stomach to Jejunum, Percutaneous Endoscopic Approach
ØD164ZB Bypass Stomach to Ileum, Percutaneous Endoscopic Approach
ØD164ZL Bypass Stomach to Transverse Colon, Percutaneous Endoscopic Approach
ØD16879 Bypass Stomach to Duodenum with Autologous Tissue Substitute, Via Natural or Artificial Opening Endoscopic
ØD1687A Bypass Stomach to Jejunum with Autologous Tissue Substitute, Via Natural or Artificial Opening Endoscopic
ØD1687B Bypass Stomach to Ileum with Autologous Tissue Substitute, Via Natural or Artificial Opening Endoscopic
ØD1687L Bypass Stomach to Transverse Colon with Autologous Tissue Substitute, Via Natural or Artificial Opening Endoscopic
ØD168J9 Bypass Stomach to Duodenum with Synthetic Substitute, Via Natural or Artificial Opening Endoscopic
ØD168JA Bypass Stomach to Jejunum with Synthetic Substitute, Via Natural or Artificial Opening Endoscopic
ØD168JB Bypass Stomach to Ileum with Synthetic Substitute, Via Natural or Artificial Opening Endoscopic
ØD168JL Bypass Stomach to Transverse Colon with Synthetic Substitute, Via Natural or Artificial Opening Endoscopic
ØD168K9 Bypass Stomach to Duodenum with Nonautologous Tissue Substitute, Via Natural or Artificial Opening Endoscopic
ØD168KA Bypass Stomach to Jejunum with Nonautologous Tissue Substitute, Via Natural or Artificial Opening Endoscopic
ØD168KB Bypass Stomach to Ileum with Nonautologous Tissue Substitute, Via Natural or Artificial Opening Endoscopic
ØD168KL Bypass Stomach to Transverse Colon with Nonautologous Tissue Substitute, Via Natural or Artificial Opening Endoscopic
ØD168Z9 Bypass Stomach to Duodenum, Via Natural or Artificial Opening Endoscopic
ØD168ZA Bypass Stomach to Jejunum, Via Natural or Artificial Opening Endoscopic
ØD168ZB Bypass Stomach to Ileum, Via Natural or Artificial Opening Endoscopic
ØD168ZL Bypass Stomach to Transverse Colon, Via Natural or Artificial Opening Endoscopic
ØDV64CZ Restriction of Stomach with Extraluminal Device, Percutaneous Endoscopic Approach

HAC 12: Surgical Site Infection-Certain Orthopedic Procedures of the Spine, Shoulder, and Elbow

Secondary diagnosis not POA:

K68.11 Postprocedural retroperitoneal abscess
T81.4ØXA Infection following a procedure, unspecified, initial encounter
T81.41XA Infection following a procedure, superficial incisional surgical site, initial encounter
T81.42XA Infection following a procedure, deep incisional surgical site, initial encounter
T81.43XA Infection following a procedure, organ and space surgical site, initial encounter
T81.44XA Sepsis following a procedure, initial encounter
T81.49XA Infection following a procedure, other surgical site, initial encounter
T84.6ØXA Infection and inflammatory reaction due to internal fixation device of unspecified site, initial encounter
T84.61ØA Infection and inflammatory reaction due to internal fixation device of right humerus, initial encounter
T84.611A Infection and inflammatory reaction due to internal fixation device of left humerus, initial encounter
T84.612A Infection and inflammatory reaction due to internal fixation device of right radius, initial encounter
T84.613A Infection and inflammatory reaction due to internal fixation device of left radius, initial encounter
T84.614A Infection and inflammatory reaction due to internal fixation device of right ulna, initial encounter
T84.615A Infection and inflammatory reaction due to internal fixation device of left ulna, initial encounter
T84.619A Infection and inflammatory reaction due to internal fixation device of unspecified bone of arm, initial encounter
T84.63XA Infection and inflammatory reaction due to internal fixation device of spine, initial encounter
T84.69XA Infection and inflammatory reaction due to internal fixation device of other site, initial encounter

HAC 12: Surgical Site Infection-Certain Orthopedic Procedures of the Spine, Shoulder, and Elbow (continued)

T84.7XXA Infection and inflammatory reaction due to other internal orthopedic prosthetic devices, implants and grafts, initial encounter

AND

Any of the following procedures:

ØRGØØ7Ø Fusion of Occipital-cervical Joint with Autologous Tissue Substitute, Anterior Approach, Anterior Column, Open Approach
ØRGØØ71 Fusion of Occipital-cervical Joint with Autologous Tissue Substitute, Posterior Approach, Posterior Column, Open Approach
ØRGØØ7J Fusion of Occipital-cervical Joint with Autologous Tissue Substitute, Posterior Approach, Anterior Column, Open Approach
ØRGØØAØ Fusion of Occipital-cervical Joint with Interbody Fusion Device, Anterior Approach, Anterior Column, Open Approach
ØRGØØAJ Fusion of Occipital-cervical Joint with Interbody Fusion Device, Posterior Approach, Anterior Column, Open Approach
ØRGØØJØ Fusion of Occipital-cervical Joint with Synthetic Substitute, Anterior Approach, Anterior Column, Open Approach
ØRGØØJ1 Fusion of Occipital-cervical Joint with Synthetic Substitute, Posterior Approach, Posterior Column, Open Approach
ØRGØØJJ Fusion of Occipital-cervical Joint with Synthetic Substitute, Posterior Approach, Anterior Column, Open Approach
ØRGØØKØ Fusion of Occipital-cervical Joint with Nonautologous Tissue Substitute, Anterior Approach, Anterior Column, Open Approach
ØRGØØK1 Fusion of Occipital-cervical Joint with Nonautologous Tissue Substitute, Posterior Approach, Posterior Column, Open Approach
ØRGØØKJ Fusion of Occipital-cervical Joint with Nonautologous Tissue Substitute, Posterior Approach, Anterior Column, Open Approach
ØRGØ37Ø Fusion of Occipital-cervical Joint with Autologous Tissue Substitute, Anterior Approach, Anterior Column, Percutaneous Approach
ØRGØ371 Fusion of Occipital-cervical Joint with Autologous Tissue Substitute, Posterior Approach, Posterior Column, Percutaneous Approach
ØRGØ37J Fusion of Occipital-cervical Joint with Autologous Tissue Substitute, Posterior Approach, Anterior Column, Percutaneous Approach
ØRGØ3AØ Fusion of Occipital-cervical Joint with Interbody Fusion Device, Anterior Approach, Anterior Column, Percutaneous Approach
ØRGØ3AJ Fusion of Occipital-cervical Joint with Interbody Fusion Device, Posterior Approach, Anterior Column, Percutaneous Approach
ØRGØ3JØ Fusion of Occipital-cervical Joint with Synthetic Substitute, Anterior Approach, Anterior Column, Percutaneous Approach
ØRGØ3J1 Fusion of Occipital-cervical Joint with Synthetic Substitute, Posterior Approach, Posterior Column, Percutaneous Approach
ØRGØ3JJ Fusion of Occipital-cervical Joint with Synthetic Substitute, Posterior Approach, Anterior Column, Percutaneous Approach
ØRGØ3KØ Fusion of Occipital-cervical Joint with Nonautologous Tissue Substitute, Anterior Approach, Anterior Column, Percutaneous Approach
ØRGØ3K1 Fusion of Occipital-cervical Joint with Nonautologous Tissue Substitute, Posterior Approach, Posterior Column, Percutaneous Approach
ØRGØ3KJ Fusion of Occipital-cervical Joint with Nonautologous Tissue Substitute, Posterior Approach, Anterior Column, Percutaneous Approach
ØRGØ47Ø Fusion of Occipital-cervical Joint with Autologous Tissue Substitute, Anterior Approach, Anterior Column, Percutaneous Endoscopic Approach
ØRGØ471 Fusion of Occipital-cervical Joint with Autologous Tissue Substitute, Posterior Approach, Posterior Column, Percutaneous Endoscopic Approach
ØRGØ47J Fusion of Occipital-cervical Joint with Autologous Tissue Substitute, Posterior Approach, Anterior Column, Percutaneous Endoscopic Approach
ØRGØ4AØ Fusion of Occipital-cervical Joint with Interbody Fusion Device, Anterior Approach, Anterior Column, Percutaneous Endoscopic Approach
ØRGØ4AJ Fusion of Occipital-cervical Joint with Interbody Fusion Device, Posterior Approach, Anterior Column, Percutaneous Endoscopic Approach
ØRGØ4JØ Fusion of Occipital-cervical Joint with Synthetic Substitute, Anterior Approach, Anterior Column, Percutaneous Endoscopic Approach
ØRGØ4J1 Fusion of Occipital-cervical Joint with Synthetic Substitute, Posterior Approach, Posterior Column, Percutaneous Endoscopic Approach
ØRGØ4JJ Fusion of Occipital-cervical Joint with Synthetic Substitute, Posterior Approach, Anterior Column, Percutaneous Endoscopic Approach
ØRGØ4KØ Fusion of Occipital-cervical Joint with Nonautologous Tissue Substitute, Anterior Approach, Anterior Column, Percutaneous Endoscopic Approach
ØRGØ4K1 Fusion of Occipital-cervical Joint with Nonautologous Tissue Substitute, Posterior Approach, Posterior Column, Percutaneous Endoscopic Approach
ØRGØ4KJ Fusion of Occipital-cervical Joint with Nonautologous Tissue Substitute, Posterior Approach, Anterior Column, Percutaneous Endoscopic Approach
ØRG1Ø7Ø Fusion of Cervical Vertebral Joint with Autologous Tissue Substitute, Anterior Approach, Anterior Column, Open Approach
ØRG1Ø71 Fusion of Cervical Vertebral Joint with Autologous Tissue Substitute, Posterior Approach, Posterior Column, Open Approach
ØRG1Ø7J Fusion of Cervical Vertebral Joint with Autologous Tissue Substitute, Posterior Approach, Anterior Column, Open Approach
ØRG1ØAØ Fusion of Cervical Vertebral Joint with Interbody Fusion Device, Anterior Approach, Anterior Column, Open Approach
ØRG1ØAJ Fusion of Cervical Vertebral Joint with Interbody Fusion Device, Posterior Approach, Anterior Column, Open Approach
ØRG1ØJØ Fusion of Cervical Vertebral Joint with Synthetic Substitute, Anterior Approach, Anterior Column, Open Approach
ØRG1ØJ1 Fusion of Cervical Vertebral Joint with Synthetic Substitute, Posterior Approach, Posterior Column, Open Approach
ØRG1ØJJ Fusion of Cervical Vertebral Joint with Synthetic Substitute, Posterior Approach, Anterior Column, Open Approach
ØRG1ØKØ Fusion of Cervical Vertebral Joint with Nonautologous Tissue Substitute, Anterior Approach, Anterior Column, Open Approach
ØRG1ØK1 Fusion of Cervical Vertebral Joint with Nonautologous Tissue Substitute, Posterior Approach, Posterior Column, Open Approach
ØRG1ØKJ Fusion of Cervical Vertebral Joint with Nonautologous Tissue Substitute, Posterior Approach, Anterior Column, Open Approach
ØRG137Ø Fusion of Cervical Vertebral Joint with Autologous Tissue Substitute, Anterior Approach, Anterior Column, Percutaneous Approach
ØRG1371 Fusion of Cervical Vertebral Joint with Autologous Tissue Substitute, Posterior Approach, Posterior Column, Percutaneous Approach
ØRG137J Fusion of Cervical Vertebral Joint with Autologous Tissue Substitute, Posterior Approach, Anterior Column, Percutaneous Approach
ØRG13AØ Fusion of Cervical Vertebral Joint with Interbody Fusion Device, Anterior Approach, Anterior Column, Percutaneous Approach
ØRG13AJ Fusion of Cervical Vertebral Joint with Interbody Fusion Device, Posterior Approach, Anterior Column, Percutaneous Approach
ØRG13JØ Fusion of Cervical Vertebral Joint with Synthetic Substitute, Anterior Approach, Anterior Column, Percutaneous Approach
ØRG13J1 Fusion of Cervical Vertebral Joint with Synthetic Substitute, Posterior Approach, Posterior Column, Percutaneous Approach
ØRG13JJ Fusion of Cervical Vertebral Joint with Synthetic Substitute, Posterior Approach, Anterior Column, Percutaneous Approach
ØRG13KØ Fusion of Cervical Vertebral Joint with Nonautologous Tissue Substitute, Anterior Approach, Anterior Column, Percutaneous Approach
ØRG13K1 Fusion of Cervical Vertebral Joint with Nonautologous Tissue Substitute, Posterior Approach, Posterior Column, Percutaneous Approach
ØRG13KJ Fusion of Cervical Vertebral Joint with Nonautologous Tissue Substitute, Posterior Approach, Anterior Column, Percutaneous Approach
ØRG147Ø Fusion of Cervical Vertebral Joint with Autologous Tissue Substitute, Anterior Approach, Anterior Column, Percutaneous Endoscopic Approach

HAC 12: Surgical Site Infection-Certain Orthopedic Procedures of the Spine, Shoulder, and Elbow (continued)

ØRG1471 Fusion of Cervical Vertebral Joint with Autologous Tissue Substitute, Posterior Approach, Posterior Column, Percutaneous Endoscopic Approach
ØRG147J Fusion of Cervical Vertebral Joint with Autologous Tissue Substitute, Posterior Approach, Anterior Column, Percutaneous Endoscopic Approach
ØRG14AØ Fusion of Cervical Vertebral Joint with Interbody Fusion Device, Anterior Approach, Anterior Column, Percutaneous Endoscopic Approach
ØRG14AJ Fusion of Cervical Vertebral Joint with Interbody Fusion Device, Posterior Approach, Anterior Column, Percutaneous Endoscopic Approach
ØRG14JØ Fusion of Cervical Vertebral Joint with Synthetic Substitute, Anterior Approach, Anterior Column, Percutaneous Endoscopic Approach
ØRG14J1 Fusion of Cervical Vertebral Joint with Synthetic Substitute, Posterior Approach, Posterior Column, Percutaneous Endoscopic Approach
ØRG14JJ Fusion of Cervical Vertebral Joint with Synthetic Substitute, Posterior Approach, Anterior Column, Percutaneous Endoscopic Approach
ØRG14KØ Fusion of Cervical Vertebral Joint with Nonautologous Tissue Substitute, Anterior Approach, Anterior Column, Percutaneous Endoscopic Approach
ØRG14K1 Fusion of Cervical Vertebral Joint with Nonautologous Tissue Substitute, Posterior Approach, Posterior Column, Percutaneous Endoscopic Approach
ØRG14KJ Fusion of Cervical Vertebral Joint with Nonautologous Tissue Substitute, Posterior Approach, Anterior Column, Percutaneous Endoscopic Approach
ØRG2070 Fusion of 2 or more Cervical Vertebral Joints with Autologous Tissue Substitute, Anterior Approach, Anterior Column, Open Approach
ØRG2071 Fusion of 2 or more Cervical Vertebral Joints with Autologous Tissue Substitute, Posterior Approach, Posterior Column, Open Approach
ØRG207J Fusion of 2 or more Cervical Vertebral Joints with Autologous Tissue Substitute, Posterior Approach, Anterior Column, Open Approach
ØRG20AØ Fusion of 2 or more Cervical Vertebral Joints with Interbody Fusion Device, Anterior Approach, Anterior Column, Open Approach
ØRG20AJ Fusion of 2 or more Cervical Vertebral Joints with Interbody Fusion Device, Posterior Approach, Anterior Column, Open Approach
ØRG20JØ Fusion of 2 or more Cervical Vertebral Joints with Synthetic Substitute, Anterior Approach, Anterior Column, Open Approach
ØRG20J1 Fusion of 2 or more Cervical Vertebral Joints with Synthetic Substitute, Posterior Approach, Posterior Column, Open Approach
ØRG20JJ Fusion of 2 or more Cervical Vertebral Joints with Synthetic Substitute, Posterior Approach, Anterior Column, Open Approach
ØRG20KØ Fusion of 2 or more Cervical Vertebral Joints with Nonautologous Tissue Substitute, Anterior Approach, Anterior Column, Open Approach
ØRG20K1 Fusion of 2 or more Cervical Vertebral Joints with Nonautologous Tissue Substitute, Posterior Approach, Posterior Column, Open Approach
ØRG20KJ Fusion of 2 or more Cervical Vertebral Joints with Nonautologous Tissue Substitute, Posterior Approach, Anterior Column, Open Approach
ØRG2370 Fusion of 2 or more Cervical Vertebral Joints with Autologous Tissue Substitute, Anterior Approach, Anterior Column, Percutaneous Approach
ØRG2371 Fusion of 2 or more Cervical Vertebral Joints with Autologous Tissue Substitute, Posterior Approach, Posterior Column, Percutaneous Approach
ØRG237J Fusion of 2 or more Cervical Vertebral Joints with Autologous Tissue Substitute, Posterior Approach, Anterior Column, Percutaneous Approach
ØRG23AØ Fusion of 2 or more Cervical Vertebral Joints with Interbody Fusion Device, Anterior Approach, Anterior Column, Percutaneous Approach
ØRG23AJ Fusion of 2 or more Cervical Vertebral Joints with Interbody Fusion Device, Posterior Approach, Anterior Column, Percutaneous Approach
ØRG23JØ Fusion of 2 or more Cervical Vertebral Joints with Synthetic Substitute, Anterior Approach, Anterior Column, Percutaneous Approach
ØRG23J1 Fusion of 2 or more Cervical Vertebral Joints with Synthetic Substitute, Posterior Approach, Posterior Column, Percutaneous Approach
ØRG23JJ Fusion of 2 or more Cervical Vertebral Joints with Synthetic Substitute, Posterior Approach, Anterior Column, Percutaneous Approach
ØRG23KØ Fusion of 2 or more Cervical Vertebral Joints with Nonautologous Tissue Substitute, Anterior Approach, Anterior Column, Percutaneous Approach
ØRG23K1 Fusion of 2 or more Cervical Vertebral Joints with Nonautologous Tissue Substitute, Posterior Approach, Posterior Column, Percutaneous Approach
ØRG23KJ Fusion of 2 or more Cervical Vertebral Joints with Nonautologous Tissue Substitute, Posterior Approach, Anterior Column, Percutaneous Approach
ØRG2470 Fusion of 2 or more Cervical Vertebral Joints with Autologous Tissue Substitute, Anterior Approach, Anterior Column, Percutaneous Endoscopic Approach
ØRG2471 Fusion of 2 or more Cervical Vertebral Joints with Autologous Tissue Substitute, Posterior Approach, Posterior Column, Percutaneous Endoscopic Approach
ØRG247J Fusion of 2 or more Cervical Vertebral Joints with Autologous Tissue Substitute, Posterior Approach, Anterior Column, Percutaneous Endoscopic Approach
ØRG24AØ Fusion of 2 or more Cervical Vertebral Joints with Interbody Fusion Device, Anterior Approach, Anterior Column, Percutaneous Endoscopic Approach
ØRG24AJ Fusion of 2 or more Cervical Vertebral Joints with Interbody Fusion Device, Posterior Approach, Anterior Column, Percutaneous Endoscopic Approach
ØRG24JØ Fusion of 2 or more Cervical Vertebral Joints with Synthetic Substitute, Anterior Approach, Anterior Column, Percutaneous Endoscopic Approach
ØRG24J1 Fusion of 2 or more Cervical Vertebral Joints with Synthetic Substitute, Posterior Approach, Posterior Column, Percutaneous Endoscopic Approach
ØRG24JJ Fusion of 2 or more Cervical Vertebral Joints with Synthetic Substitute, Posterior Approach, Anterior Column, Percutaneous Endoscopic Approach
ØRG24KØ Fusion of 2 or more Cervical Vertebral Joints with Nonautologous Tissue Substitute, Anterior Approach, Anterior Column, Percutaneous Endoscopic Approach
ØRG24K1 Fusion of 2 or more Cervical Vertebral Joints with Nonautologous Tissue Substitute, Posterior Approach, Posterior Column, Percutaneous Endoscopic Approach
ØRG24KJ Fusion of 2 or more Cervical Vertebral Joints with Nonautologous Tissue Substitute, Posterior Approach, Anterior Column, Percutaneous Endoscopic Approach
ØRG4070 Fusion of Cervicothoracic Vertebral Joint with Autologous Tissue Substitute, Anterior Approach, Anterior Column, Open Approach
ØRG4071 Fusion of Cervicothoracic Vertebral Joint with Autologous Tissue Substitute, Posterior Approach, Posterior Column, Open Approach
ØRG407J Fusion of Cervicothoracic Vertebral Joint with Autologous Tissue Substitute, Posterior Approach, Anterior Column, Open Approach
ØRG40AØ Fusion of Cervicothoracic Vertebral Joint with Interbody Fusion Device, Anterior Approach, Anterior Column, Open Approach
ØRG40AJ Fusion of Cervicothoracic Vertebral Joint with Interbody Fusion Device, Posterior Approach, Anterior Column, Open Approach
ØRG40JØ Fusion of Cervicothoracic Vertebral Joint with Synthetic Substitute, Anterior Approach, Anterior Column, Open Approach
ØRG40J1 Fusion of Cervicothoracic Vertebral Joint with Synthetic Substitute, Posterior Approach, Posterior Column, Open Approach
ØRG40JJ Fusion of Cervicothoracic Vertebral Joint with Synthetic Substitute, Posterior Approach, Anterior Column, Open Approach
ØRG40KØ Fusion of Cervicothoracic Vertebral Joint with Nonautologous Tissue Substitute, Anterior Approach, Anterior Column, Open Approach
ØRG40K1 Fusion of Cervicothoracic Vertebral Joint with Nonautologous Tissue Substitute, Posterior Approach, Posterior Column, Open Approach
ØRG40KJ Fusion of Cervicothoracic Vertebral Joint with Nonautologous Tissue Substitute, Posterior Approach, Anterior Column, Open Approach
ØRG4370 Fusion of Cervicothoracic Vertebral Joint with Autologous Tissue Substitute, Anterior Approach, Anterior Column, Percutaneous Approach

HAC 12: Surgical Site Infection-Certain Orthopedic Procedures of the Spine, Shoulder, and Elbow (continued)

ØRG4371 Fusion of Cervicothoracic Vertebral Joint with Autologous Tissue Substitute, Posterior Approach, Posterior Column, Percutaneous Approach
ØRG437J Fusion of Cervicothoracic Vertebral Joint with Autologous Tissue Substitute, Posterior Approach, Anterior Column, Percutaneous Approach
ØRG43AØ Fusion of Cervicothoracic Vertebral Joint with Interbody Fusion Device, Anterior Approach, Anterior Column, Percutaneous Approach
ØRG43AJ Fusion of Cervicothoracic Vertebral Joint with Interbody Fusion Device, Posterior Approach, Anterior Column, Percutaneous Approach
ØRG43JØ Fusion of Cervicothoracic Vertebral Joint with Synthetic Substitute, Anterior Approach, Anterior Column, Percutaneous Approach
ØRG43J1 Fusion of Cervicothoracic Vertebral Joint with Synthetic Substitute, Posterior Approach, Posterior Column, Percutaneous Approach
ØRG43JJ Fusion of Cervicothoracic Vertebral Joint with Synthetic Substitute, Posterior Approach, Anterior Column, Percutaneous Approach
ØRG43KØ Fusion of Cervicothoracic Vertebral Joint with Nonautologous Tissue Substitute, Anterior Approach, Anterior Column, Percutaneous Approach
ØRG43K1 Fusion of Cervicothoracic Vertebral Joint with Nonautologous Tissue Substitute, Posterior Approach, Posterior Column, Percutaneous Approach
ØRG43KJ Fusion of Cervicothoracic Vertebral Joint with Nonautologous Tissue Substitute, Posterior Approach, Anterior Column, Percutaneous Approach
ØRG447Ø Fusion of Cervicothoracic Vertebral Joint with Autologous Tissue Substitute, Anterior Approach, Anterior Column, Percutaneous Endoscopic Approach
ØRG4471 Fusion of Cervicothoracic Vertebral Joint with Autologous Tissue Substitute, Posterior Approach, Posterior Column, Percutaneous Endoscopic Approach
ØRG447J Fusion of Cervicothoracic Vertebral Joint with Autologous Tissue Substitute, Posterior Approach, Anterior Column, Percutaneous Endoscopic Approach
ØRG44AØ Fusion of Cervicothoracic Vertebral Joint with Interbody Fusion Device, Anterior Approach, Anterior Column, Percutaneous Endoscopic Approach
ØRG44AJ Fusion of Cervicothoracic Vertebral Joint with Interbody Fusion Device, Posterior Approach, Anterior Column, Percutaneous Endoscopic Approach
ØRG44JØ Fusion of Cervicothoracic Vertebral Joint with Synthetic Substitute, Anterior Approach, Anterior Column, Percutaneous Endoscopic Approach
ØRG44J1 Fusion of Cervicothoracic Vertebral Joint with Synthetic Substitute, Posterior Approach, Posterior Column, Percutaneous Endoscopic Approach
ØRG44JJ Fusion of Cervicothoracic Vertebral Joint with Synthetic Substitute, Posterior Approach, Anterior Column, Percutaneous Endoscopic Approach
ØRG44KØ Fusion of Cervicothoracic Vertebral Joint with Nonautologous Tissue Substitute, Anterior Approach, Anterior Column, Percutaneous Endoscopic Approach
ØRG44K1 Fusion of Cervicothoracic Vertebral Joint with Nonautologous Tissue Substitute, Posterior Approach, Posterior Column, Percutaneous Endoscopic Approach
ØRG44KJ Fusion of Cervicothoracic Vertebral Joint with Nonautologous Tissue Substitute, Posterior Approach, Anterior Column, Percutaneous Endoscopic Approach
ØRG607Ø Fusion of Thoracic Vertebral Joint with Autologous Tissue Substitute, Anterior Approach, Anterior Column, Open Approach
ØRG6Ø71 Fusion of Thoracic Vertebral Joint with Autologous Tissue Substitute, Posterior Approach, Posterior Column, Open Approach
ØRG6Ø7J Fusion of Thoracic Vertebral Joint with Autologous Tissue Substitute, Posterior Approach, Anterior Column, Open Approach
ØRG6ØAØ Fusion of Thoracic Vertebral Joint with Interbody Fusion Device, Anterior Approach, Anterior Column, Open Approach
ØRG6ØAJ Fusion of Thoracic Vertebral Joint with Interbody Fusion Device, Posterior Approach, Anterior Column, Open Approach
ØRG6ØJØ Fusion of Thoracic Vertebral Joint with Synthetic Substitute, Anterior Approach, Anterior Column, Open Approach
ØRG6ØJ1 Fusion of Thoracic Vertebral Joint with Synthetic Substitute, Posterior Approach, Posterior Column, Open Approach
ØRG6ØJJ Fusion of Thoracic Vertebral Joint with Synthetic Substitute, Posterior Approach, Anterior Column, Open Approach
ØRG6ØKØ Fusion of Thoracic Vertebral Joint with Nonautologous Tissue Substitute, Anterior Approach, Anterior Column, Open Approach
ØRG6ØK1 Fusion of Thoracic Vertebral Joint with Nonautologous Tissue Substitute, Posterior Approach, Posterior Column, Open Approach
ØRG6ØKJ Fusion of Thoracic Vertebral Joint with Nonautologous Tissue Substitute, Posterior Approach, Anterior Column, Open Approach
ØRG637Ø Fusion of Thoracic Vertebral Joint with Autologous Tissue Substitute, Anterior Approach, Anterior Column, Percutaneous Approach
ØRG6371 Fusion of Thoracic Vertebral Joint with Autologous Tissue Substitute, Posterior Approach, Posterior Column, Percutaneous Approach
ØRG637J Fusion of Thoracic Vertebral Joint with Autologous Tissue Substitute, Posterior Approach, Anterior Column, Percutaneous Approach
ØRG63AØ Fusion of Thoracic Vertebral Joint with Interbody Fusion Device, Anterior Approach, Anterior Column, Percutaneous Approach
ØRG63AJ Fusion of Thoracic Vertebral Joint with Interbody Fusion Device, Posterior Approach, Anterior Column, Percutaneous Approach
ØRG63JØ Fusion of Thoracic Vertebral Joint with Synthetic Substitute, Anterior Approach, Anterior Column, Percutaneous Approach
ØRG63J1 Fusion of Thoracic Vertebral Joint with Synthetic Substitute, Posterior Approach, Posterior Column, Percutaneous Approach
ØRG63JJ Fusion of Thoracic Vertebral Joint with Synthetic Substitute, Posterior Approach, Anterior Column, Percutaneous Approach
ØRG63KØ Fusion of Thoracic Vertebral Joint with Nonautologous Tissue Substitute, Anterior Approach, Anterior Column, Percutaneous Approach
ØRG63K1 Fusion of Thoracic Vertebral Joint with Nonautologous Tissue Substitute, Posterior Approach, Posterior Column, Percutaneous Approach
ØRG63KJ Fusion of Thoracic Vertebral Joint with Nonautologous Tissue Substitute, Posterior Approach, Anterior Column, Percutaneous Approach
ØRG647Ø Fusion of Thoracic Vertebral Joint with Autologous Tissue Substitute, Anterior Approach, Anterior Column, Percutaneous Endoscopic Approach
ØRG6471 Fusion of Thoracic Vertebral Joint with Autologous Tissue Substitute, Posterior Approach, Posterior Column, Percutaneous Endoscopic Approach
ØRG647J Fusion of Thoracic Vertebral Joint with Autologous Tissue Substitute, Posterior Approach, Anterior Column, Percutaneous Endoscopic Approach
ØRG64AØ Fusion of Thoracic Vertebral Joint with Interbody Fusion Device, Anterior Approach, Anterior Column, Percutaneous Endoscopic Approach
ØRG64AJ Fusion of Thoracic Vertebral Joint with Interbody Fusion Device, Posterior Approach, Anterior Column, Percutaneous Endoscopic Approach
ØRG64JØ Fusion of Thoracic Vertebral Joint with Synthetic Substitute, Anterior Approach, Anterior Column, Percutaneous Endoscopic Approach
ØRG64J1 Fusion of Thoracic Vertebral Joint with Synthetic Substitute, Posterior Approach, Posterior Column, Percutaneous Endoscopic Approach
ØRG64JJ Fusion of Thoracic Vertebral Joint with Synthetic Substitute, Posterior Approach, Anterior Column, Percutaneous Endoscopic Approach
ØRG64KØ Fusion of Thoracic Vertebral Joint with Nonautologous Tissue Substitute, Anterior Approach, Anterior Column, Percutaneous Endoscopic Approach
ØRG64K1 Fusion of Thoracic Vertebral Joint with Nonautologous Tissue Substitute, Posterior Approach, Posterior Column, Percutaneous Endoscopic Approach
ØRG64KJ Fusion of Thoracic Vertebral Joint with Nonautologous Tissue Substitute, Posterior Approach, Anterior Column, Percutaneous Endoscopic Approach
ØRG7Ø7Ø Fusion of 2 to 7 Thoracic Vertebral Joints with Autologous Tissue Substitute, Anterior Approach, Anterior Column, Open Approach
ØRG7Ø71 Fusion of 2 to 7 Thoracic Vertebral Joints with Autologous Tissue Substitute, Posterior Approach, Posterior Column, Open Approach
ØRG7Ø7J Fusion of 2 to 7 Thoracic Vertebral Joints with Autologous Tissue Substitute, Posterior Approach, Anterior Column, Open Approach

HAC 12: Surgical Site Infection-Certain Orthopedic Procedures of the Spine, Shoulder, and Elbow (continued)

ØRG70AØ Fusion of 2 to 7 Thoracic Vertebral Joints with Interbody Fusion Device, Anterior Approach, Anterior Column, Open Approach

ØRG70AJ Fusion of 2 to 7 Thoracic Vertebral Joints with Interbody Fusion Device, Posterior Approach, Anterior Column, Open Approach

ØRG70JØ Fusion of 2 to 7 Thoracic Vertebral Joints with Synthetic Substitute, Anterior Approach, Anterior Column, Open Approach

ØRG70J1 Fusion of 2 to 7 Thoracic Vertebral Joints with Synthetic Substitute, Posterior Approach, Posterior Column, Open Approach

ØRG70JJ Fusion of 2 to 7 Thoracic Vertebral Joints with Synthetic Substitute, Posterior Approach, Anterior Column, Open Approach

ØRG70KØ Fusion of 2 to 7 Thoracic Vertebral Joints with Nonautologous Tissue Substitute, Anterior Approach, Anterior Column, Open Approach

ØRG70K1 Fusion of 2 to 7 Thoracic Vertebral Joints with Nonautologous Tissue Substitute, Posterior Approach, Posterior Column, Open Approach

ØRG70KJ Fusion of 2 to 7 Thoracic Vertebral Joints with Nonautologous Tissue Substitute, Posterior Approach, Anterior Column, Open Approach

ØRG737Ø Fusion of 2 to 7 Thoracic Vertebral Joints with Autologous Tissue Substitute, Anterior Approach, Anterior Column, Percutaneous Approach

ØRG7371 Fusion of 2 to 7 Thoracic Vertebral Joints with Autologous Tissue Substitute, Posterior Approach, Posterior Column, Percutaneous Approach

ØRG737J Fusion of 2 to 7 Thoracic Vertebral Joints with Autologous Tissue Substitute, Posterior Approach, Anterior Column, Percutaneous Approach

ØRG73AØ Fusion of 2 to 7 Thoracic Vertebral Joints with Interbody Fusion Device, Anterior Approach, Anterior Column, Percutaneous Approach

ØRG73AJ Fusion of 2 to 7 Thoracic Vertebral Joints with Interbody Fusion Device, Posterior Approach, Anterior Column, Percutaneous Approach

ØRG73JØ Fusion of 2 to 7 Thoracic Vertebral Joints with Synthetic Substitute, Anterior Approach, Anterior Column, Percutaneous Approach

ØRG73J1 Fusion of 2 to 7 Thoracic Vertebral Joints with Synthetic Substitute, Posterior Approach, Posterior Column, Percutaneous Approach

ØRG73JJ Fusion of 2 to 7 Thoracic Vertebral Joints with Synthetic Substitute, Posterior Approach, Anterior Column, Percutaneous Approach

ØRG73KØ Fusion of 2 to 7 Thoracic Vertebral Joints with Nonautologous Tissue Substitute, Anterior Approach, Anterior Column, Percutaneous Approach

ØRG73K1 Fusion of 2 to 7 Thoracic Vertebral Joints with Nonautologous Tissue Substitute, Posterior Approach, Posterior Column, Percutaneous Approach

ØRG73KJ Fusion of 2 to 7 Thoracic Vertebral Joints with Nonautologous Tissue Substitute, Posterior Approach, Anterior Column, Percutaneous Approach

ØRG747Ø Fusion of 2 to 7 Thoracic Vertebral Joints with Autologous Tissue Substitute, Anterior Approach, Anterior Column, Percutaneous Endoscopic Approach

ØRG7471 Fusion of 2 to 7 Thoracic Vertebral Joints with Autologous Tissue Substitute, Posterior Approach, Posterior Column, Percutaneous Endoscopic Approach

ØRG747J Fusion of 2 to 7 Thoracic Vertebral Joints with Autologous Tissue Substitute, Posterior Approach, Anterior Column, Percutaneous Endoscopic Approach

ØRG74AØ Fusion of 2 to 7 Thoracic Vertebral Joints with Interbody Fusion Device, Anterior Approach, Anterior Column, Percutaneous Endoscopic Approach

ØRG74AJ Fusion of 2 to 7 Thoracic Vertebral Joints with Interbody Fusion Device, Posterior Approach, Anterior Column, Percutaneous Endoscopic Approach

ØRG74JØ Fusion of 2 to 7 Thoracic Vertebral Joints with Synthetic Substitute, Anterior Approach, Anterior Column, Percutaneous Endoscopic Approach

ØRG74J1 Fusion of 2 to 7 Thoracic Vertebral Joints with Synthetic Substitute, Posterior Approach, Posterior Column, Percutaneous Endoscopic Approach

ØRG74JJ Fusion of 2 to 7 Thoracic Vertebral Joints with Synthetic Substitute, Posterior Approach, Anterior Column, Percutaneous Endoscopic Approach

ØRG74KØ Fusion of 2 to 7 Thoracic Vertebral Joints with Nonautologous Tissue Substitute, Anterior Approach, Anterior Column, Percutaneous Endoscopic Approach

ØRG74K1 Fusion of 2 to 7 Thoracic Vertebral Joints with Nonautologous Tissue Substitute, Posterior Approach, Posterior Column, Percutaneous Endoscopic Approach

ØRG74KJ Fusion of 2 to 7 Thoracic Vertebral Joints with Nonautologous Tissue Substitute, Posterior Approach, Anterior Column, Percutaneous Endoscopic Approach

ØRG807Ø Fusion of 8 or More Thoracic Vertebral Joints with Autologous Tissue Substitute, Anterior Approach, Anterior Column, Open Approach

ØRG8071 Fusion of 8 or More Thoracic Vertebral Joints with Autologous Tissue Substitute, Posterior Approach, Posterior Column, Open Approach

ØRG807J Fusion of 8 or More Thoracic Vertebral Joints with Autologous Tissue Substitute, Posterior Approach, Anterior Column, Open Approach

ØRG80AØ Fusion of 8 or More Thoracic Vertebral Joints with Interbody Fusion Device, Anterior Approach, Anterior Column, Open Approach

ØRG80AJ Fusion of 8 or More Thoracic Vertebral Joints with Interbody Fusion Device, Posterior Approach, Anterior Column, Open Approach

ØRG80JØ Fusion of 8 or More Thoracic Vertebral Joints with Synthetic Substitute, Anterior Approach, Anterior Column, Open Approach

ØRG80J1 Fusion of 8 or More Thoracic Vertebral Joints with Synthetic Substitute, Posterior Approach, Posterior Column, Open Approach

ØRG80JJ Fusion of 8 or More Thoracic Vertebral Joints with Synthetic Substitute, Posterior Approach, Anterior Column, Open Approach

ØRG80KØ Fusion of 8 or More Thoracic Vertebral Joints with Nonautologous Tissue Substitute, Anterior Approach, Anterior Column, Open Approach

ØRG80K1 Fusion of 8 or More Thoracic Vertebral Joints with Nonautologous Tissue Substitute, Posterior Approach, Posterior Column, Open Approach

ØRG80KJ Fusion of 8 or More Thoracic Vertebral Joints with Nonautologous Tissue Substitute, Posterior Approach, Anterior Column, Open Approach

ØRG837Ø Fusion of 8 or More Thoracic Vertebral Joints with Autologous Tissue Substitute, Anterior Approach, Anterior Column, Percutaneous Approach

ØRG8371 Fusion of 8 or More Thoracic Vertebral Joints with Autologous Tissue Substitute, Posterior Approach, Posterior Column, Percutaneous Approach

ØRG837J Fusion of 8 or More Thoracic Vertebral Joints with Autologous Tissue Substitute, Posterior Approach, Anterior Column, Percutaneous Approach

ØRG83AØ Fusion of 8 or More Thoracic Vertebral Joints with Interbody Fusion Device, Anterior Approach, Anterior Column, Percutaneous Approach

ØRG83AJ Fusion of 8 or More Thoracic Vertebral Joints with Interbody Fusion Device, Posterior Approach, Anterior Column, Percutaneous Approach

ØRG83JØ Fusion of 8 or More Thoracic Vertebral Joints with Synthetic Substitute, Anterior Approach, Anterior Column, Percutaneous Approach

ØRG83J1 Fusion of 8 or More Thoracic Vertebral Joints with Synthetic Substitute, Posterior Approach, Posterior Column, Percutaneous Approach

ØRG83JJ Fusion of 8 or More Thoracic Vertebral Joints with Synthetic Substitute, Posterior Approach, Anterior Column, Percutaneous Approach

ØRG83KØ Fusion of 8 or More Thoracic Vertebral Joints with Nonautologous Tissue Substitute, Anterior Approach, Anterior Column, Percutaneous Approach

ØRG83K1 Fusion of 8 or More Thoracic Vertebral Joints with Nonautologous Tissue Substitute, Posterior Approach, Posterior Column, Percutaneous Approach

ØRG83KJ Fusion of 8 or More Thoracic Vertebral Joints with Nonautologous Tissue Substitute, Posterior Approach, Anterior Column, Percutaneous Approach

ØRG847Ø Fusion of 8 or More Thoracic Vertebral Joints with Autologous Tissue Substitute, Anterior Approach, Anterior Column, Percutaneous Endoscopic Approach

ØRG8471 Fusion of 8 or More Thoracic Vertebral Joints with Autologous Tissue Substitute, Posterior Approach, Posterior Column, Percutaneous Endoscopic Approach

ØRG847J Fusion of 8 or More Thoracic Vertebral Joints with Autologous Tissue Substitute, Posterior Approach, Anterior Column, Percutaneous Endoscopic Approach

ØRG84AØ Fusion of 8 or More Thoracic Vertebral Joints with Interbody Fusion Device, Anterior Approach, Anterior Column, Percutaneous Endoscopic Approach

HAC 12: Surgical Site Infection-Certain Orthopedic Procedures of the Spine, Shoulder, and Elbow (continued)

ØRG84AJ Fusion of 8 or More Thoracic Vertebral Joints with Interbody Fusion Device, Posterior Approach, Anterior Column, Percutaneous Endoscopic Approach
ØRG84JØ Fusion of 8 or More Thoracic Vertebral Joints with Synthetic Substitute, Anterior Approach, Anterior Column, Percutaneous Endoscopic Approach
ØRG84J1 Fusion of 8 or More Thoracic Vertebral Joints with Synthetic Substitute, Posterior Approach, Posterior Column, Percutaneous Endoscopic Approach
ØRG84JJ Fusion of 8 or More Thoracic Vertebral Joints with Synthetic Substitute, Posterior Approach, Anterior Column, Percutaneous Endoscopic Approach
ØRG84KØ Fusion of 8 or More Thoracic Vertebral Joints with Nonautologous Tissue Substitute, Anterior Approach, Anterior Column, Percutaneous Endoscopic Approach
ØRG84K1 Fusion of 8 or More Thoracic Vertebral Joints with Nonautologous Tissue Substitute, Posterior Approach, Posterior Column, Percutaneous Endoscopic Approach
ØRG84KJ Fusion of 8 or More Thoracic Vertebral Joints with Nonautologous Tissue Substitute, Posterior Approach, Anterior Column, Percutaneous Endoscopic Approach
ØRGAØ7Ø Fusion of Thoracolumbar Vertebral Joint with Autologous Tissue Substitute, Anterior Approach, Anterior Column, Open Approach
ØRGAØ71 Fusion of Thoracolumbar Vertebral Joint with Autologous Tissue Substitute, Posterior Approach, Posterior Column, Open Approach
ØRGAØ7J Fusion of Thoracolumbar Vertebral Joint with Autologous Tissue Substitute, Posterior Approach, Anterior Column, Open Approach
ØRGAØAØ Fusion of Thoracolumbar Vertebral Joint with Interbody Fusion Device, Anterior Approach, Anterior Column, Open Approach
ØRGAØAJ Fusion of Thoracolumbar Vertebral Joint with Interbody Fusion Device, Posterior Approach, Anterior Column, Open Approach
ØRGAØJØ Fusion of Thoracolumbar Vertebral Joint with Synthetic Substitute, Anterior Approach, Anterior Column, Open Approach
ØRGAØJ1 Fusion of Thoracolumbar Vertebral Joint with Synthetic Substitute, Posterior Approach, Posterior Column, Open Approach
ØRGAØJJ Fusion of Thoracolumbar Vertebral Joint with Synthetic Substitute, Posterior Approach, Anterior Column, Open Approach
ØRGAØKØ Fusion of Thoracolumbar Vertebral Joint with Nonautologous Tissue Substitute, Anterior Approach, Anterior Column, Open Approach
ØRGAØK1 Fusion of Thoracolumbar Vertebral Joint with Nonautologous Tissue Substitute, Posterior Approach, Posterior Column, Open Approach
ØRGAØKJ Fusion of Thoracolumbar Vertebral Joint with Nonautologous Tissue Substitute, Posterior Approach, Anterior Column, Open Approach
ØRGA37Ø Fusion of Thoracolumbar Vertebral Joint with Autologous Tissue Substitute, Anterior Approach, Anterior Column, Percutaneous Approach
ØRGA371 Fusion of Thoracolumbar Vertebral Joint with Autologous Tissue Substitute, Posterior Approach, Posterior Column, Percutaneous Approach
ØRGA37J Fusion of Thoracolumbar Vertebral Joint with Autologous Tissue Substitute, Posterior Approach, Anterior Column, Percutaneous Approach
ØRGA3AØ Fusion of Thoracolumbar Vertebral Joint with Interbody Fusion Device, Anterior Approach, Anterior Column, Percutaneous Approach
ØRGA3AJ Fusion of Thoracolumbar Vertebral Joint with Interbody Fusion Device, Posterior Approach, Anterior Column, Percutaneous Approach
ØRGA3JØ Fusion of Thoracolumbar Vertebral Joint with Synthetic Substitute, Anterior Approach, Anterior Column, Percutaneous Approach
ØRGA3J1 Fusion of Thoracolumbar Vertebral Joint with Synthetic Substitute, Posterior Approach, Posterior Column, Percutaneous Approach
ØRGA3JJ Fusion of Thoracolumbar Vertebral Joint with Synthetic Substitute, Posterior Approach, Anterior Column, Percutaneous Approach
ØRGA3KØ Fusion of Thoracolumbar Vertebral Joint with Nonautologous Tissue Substitute, Anterior Approach, Anterior Column, Percutaneous Approach
ØRGA3K1 Fusion of Thoracolumbar Vertebral Joint with Nonautologous Tissue Substitute, Posterior Approach, Posterior Column, Percutaneous Approach
ØRGA3KJ Fusion of Thoracolumbar Vertebral Joint with Nonautologous Tissue Substitute, Posterior Approach, Anterior Column, Percutaneous Approach
ØRGA47Ø Fusion of Thoracolumbar Vertebral Joint with Autologous Tissue Substitute, Anterior Approach, Anterior Column, Percutaneous Endoscopic Approach
ØRGA471 Fusion of Thoracolumbar Vertebral Joint with Autologous Tissue Substitute, Posterior Approach, Posterior Column, Percutaneous Endoscopic Approach
ØRGA47J Fusion of Thoracolumbar Vertebral Joint with Autologous Tissue Substitute, Posterior Approach, Anterior Column, Percutaneous Endoscopic Approach
ØRGA4AØ Fusion of Thoracolumbar Vertebral Joint with Interbody Fusion Device, Anterior Approach, Anterior Column, Percutaneous Endoscopic Approach
ØRGA4AJ Fusion of Thoracolumbar Vertebral Joint with Interbody Fusion Device, Posterior Approach, Anterior Column, Percutaneous Endoscopic Approach
ØRGA4JØ Fusion of Thoracolumbar Vertebral Joint with Synthetic Substitute, Anterior Approach, Anterior Column, Percutaneous Endoscopic Approach
ØRGA4J1 Fusion of Thoracolumbar Vertebral Joint with Synthetic Substitute, Posterior Approach, Posterior Column, Percutaneous Endoscopic Approach
ØRGA4JJ Fusion of Thoracolumbar Vertebral Joint with Synthetic Substitute, Posterior Approach, Anterior Column, Percutaneous Endoscopic Approach
ØRGA4KØ Fusion of Thoracolumbar Vertebral Joint with Nonautologous Tissue Substitute, Anterior Approach, Anterior Column, Percutaneous Endoscopic Approach
ØRGA4K1 Fusion of Thoracolumbar Vertebral Joint with Nonautologous Tissue Substitute, Posterior Approach, Posterior Column, Percutaneous Endoscopic Approach
ØRGA4KJ Fusion of Thoracolumbar Vertebral Joint with Nonautologous Tissue Substitute, Posterior Approach, Anterior Column, Percutaneous Endoscopic Approach
ØRGEØ4Z Fusion of Right Sternoclavicular Joint with Internal Fixation Device, Open Approach
ØRGEØ7Z Fusion of Right Sternoclavicular Joint with Autologous Tissue Substitute, Open Approach
ØRGEØJZ Fusion of Right Sternoclavicular Joint with Synthetic Substitute, Open Approach
ØRGEØKZ Fusion of Right Sternoclavicular Joint with Nonautologous Tissue Substitute, Open Approach
ØRGE34Z Fusion of Right Sternoclavicular Joint with Internal Fixation Device, Percutaneous Approach
ØRGE37Z Fusion of Right Sternoclavicular Joint with Autologous Tissue Substitute, Percutaneous Approach
ØRGE3JZ Fusion of Right Sternoclavicular Joint with Synthetic Substitute, Percutaneous Approach
ØRGE3KZ Fusion of Right Sternoclavicular Joint with Nonautologous Tissue Substitute, Percutaneous Approach
ØRGE44Z Fusion of Right Sternoclavicular Joint with Internal Fixation Device, Percutaneous Endoscopic Approach
ØRGE47Z Fusion of Right Sternoclavicular Joint with Autologous Tissue Substitute, Percutaneous Endoscopic Approach
ØRGE4JZ Fusion of Right Sternoclavicular Joint with Synthetic Substitute, Percutaneous Endoscopic Approach
ØRGE4KZ Fusion of Right Sternoclavicular Joint with Nonautologous Tissue Substitute, Percutaneous Endoscopic Approach
ØRGFØ4Z Fusion of Left Sternoclavicular Joint with Internal Fixation Device, Open Approach
ØRGFØ7Z Fusion of Left Sternoclavicular Joint with Autologous Tissue Substitute, Open Approach
ØRGFØJZ Fusion of Left Sternoclavicular Joint with Synthetic Substitute, Open Approach
ØRGFØKZ Fusion of Left Sternoclavicular Joint with Nonautologous Tissue Substitute, Open Approach
ØRGF34Z Fusion of Left Sternoclavicular Joint with Internal Fixation Device, Percutaneous Approach
ØRGF37Z Fusion of Left Sternoclavicular Joint with Autologous Tissue Substitute, Percutaneous Approach
ØRGF3JZ Fusion of Left Sternoclavicular Joint with Synthetic Substitute, Percutaneous Approach
ØRGF3KZ Fusion of Left Sternoclavicular Joint with Nonautologous Tissue Substitute, Percutaneous Approach
ØRGF44Z Fusion of Left Sternoclavicular Joint with Internal Fixation Device, Percutaneous Endoscopic Approach

HAC 12: Surgical Site Infection-Certain Orthopedic Procedures of the Spine, Shoulder, and Elbow (continued)

ØRGF47Z Fusion of Left Sternoclavicular Joint with Autologous Tissue Substitute, Percutaneous Endoscopic Approach
ØRGF4JZ Fusion of Left Sternoclavicular Joint with Synthetic Substitute, Percutaneous Endoscopic Approach
ØRGF4KZ Fusion of Left Sternoclavicular Joint with Nonautologous Tissue Substitute, Percutaneous Endoscopic Approach
ØRGGØ4Z Fusion of Right Acromioclavicular Joint with Internal Fixation Device, Open Approach
ØRGGØ7Z Fusion of Right Acromioclavicular Joint with Autologous Tissue Substitute, Open Approach
ØRGGØJZ Fusion of Right Acromioclavicular Joint with Synthetic Substitute, Open Approach
ØRGGØKZ Fusion of Right Acromioclavicular Joint with Nonautologous Tissue Substitute, Open Approach
ØRGG34Z Fusion of Right Acromioclavicular Joint with Internal Fixation Device, Percutaneous Approach
ØRGG37Z Fusion of Right Acromioclavicular Joint with Autologous Tissue Substitute, Percutaneous Approach
ØRGG3JZ Fusion of Right Acromioclavicular Joint with Synthetic Substitute, Percutaneous Approach
ØRGG3KZ Fusion of Right Acromioclavicular Joint with Nonautologous Tissue Substitute, Percutaneous Approach
ØRGG44Z Fusion of Right Acromioclavicular Joint with Internal Fixation Device, Percutaneous Endoscopic Approach
ØRGG47Z Fusion of Right Acromioclavicular Joint with Autologous Tissue Substitute, Percutaneous Endoscopic Approach
ØRGG4JZ Fusion of Right Acromioclavicular Joint with Synthetic Substitute, Percutaneous Endoscopic Approach
ØRGG4KZ Fusion of Right Acromioclavicular Joint with Nonautologous Tissue Substitute, Percutaneous Endoscopic Approach
ØRGHØ4Z Fusion of Left Acromioclavicular Joint with Internal Fixation Device, Open Approach
ØRGHØ7Z Fusion of Left Acromioclavicular Joint with Autologous Tissue Substitute, Open Approach
ØRGHØJZ Fusion of Left Acromioclavicular Joint with Synthetic Substitute, Open Approach
ØRGHØKZ Fusion of Left Acromioclavicular Joint with Nonautologous Tissue Substitute, Open Approach
ØRGH34Z Fusion of Left Acromioclavicular Joint with Internal Fixation Device, Percutaneous Approach
ØRGH37Z Fusion of Left Acromioclavicular Joint with Autologous Tissue Substitute, Percutaneous Approach
ØRGH3JZ Fusion of Left Acromioclavicular Joint with Synthetic Substitute, Percutaneous Approach
ØRGH3KZ Fusion of Left Acromioclavicular Joint with Nonautologous Tissue Substitute, Percutaneous Approach
ØRGH44Z Fusion of Left Acromioclavicular Joint with Internal Fixation Device, Percutaneous Endoscopic Approach
ØRGH47Z Fusion of Left Acromioclavicular Joint with Autologous Tissue Substitute, Percutaneous Endoscopic Approach
ØRGH4JZ Fusion of Left Acromioclavicular Joint with Synthetic Substitute, Percutaneous Endoscopic Approach
ØRGH4KZ Fusion of Left Acromioclavicular Joint with Nonautologous Tissue Substitute, Percutaneous Endoscopic Approach
ØRGJØ4Z Fusion of Right Shoulder Joint with Internal Fixation Device, Open Approach
ØRGJØ7Z Fusion of Right Shoulder Joint with Autologous Tissue Substitute, Open Approach
ØRGJØJZ Fusion of Right Shoulder Joint with Synthetic Substitute, Open Approach
ØRGJØKZ Fusion of Right Shoulder Joint with Nonautologous Tissue Substitute, Open Approach
ØRGJ34Z Fusion of Right Shoulder Joint with Internal Fixation Device, Percutaneous Approach
ØRGJ37Z Fusion of Right Shoulder Joint with Autologous Tissue Substitute, Percutaneous Approach
ØRGJ3JZ Fusion of Right Shoulder Joint with Synthetic Substitute, Percutaneous Approach
ØRGJ3KZ Fusion of Right Shoulder Joint with Nonautologous Tissue Substitute, Percutaneous Approach
ØRGJ44Z Fusion of Right Shoulder Joint with Internal Fixation Device, Percutaneous Endoscopic Approach
ØRGJ47Z Fusion of Right Shoulder Joint with Autologous Tissue Substitute, Percutaneous Endoscopic Approach
ØRGJ4JZ Fusion of Right Shoulder Joint with Synthetic Substitute, Percutaneous Endoscopic Approach
ØRGJ4KZ Fusion of Right Shoulder Joint with Nonautologous Tissue Substitute, Percutaneous Endoscopic Approach
ØRGKØ4Z Fusion of Left Shoulder Joint with Internal Fixation Device, Open Approach
ØRGKØ7Z Fusion of Left Shoulder Joint with Autologous Tissue Substitute, Open Approach
ØRGKØJZ Fusion of Left Shoulder Joint with Synthetic Substitute, Open Approach
ØRGKØKZ Fusion of Left Shoulder Joint with Nonautologous Tissue Substitute, Open Approach
ØRGK34Z Fusion of Left Shoulder Joint with Internal Fixation Device, Percutaneous Approach
ØRGK37Z Fusion of Left Shoulder Joint with Autologous Tissue Substitute, Percutaneous Approach
ØRGK3JZ Fusion of Left Shoulder Joint with Synthetic Substitute, Percutaneous Approach
ØRGK3KZ Fusion of Left Shoulder Joint with Nonautologous Tissue Substitute, Percutaneous Approach
ØRGK44Z Fusion of Left Shoulder Joint with Internal Fixation Device, Percutaneous Endoscopic Approach
ØRGK47Z Fusion of Left Shoulder Joint with Autologous Tissue Substitute, Percutaneous Endoscopic Approach
ØRGK4JZ Fusion of Left Shoulder Joint with Synthetic Substitute, Percutaneous Endoscopic Approach
ØRGK4KZ Fusion of Left Shoulder Joint with Nonautologous Tissue Substitute, Percutaneous Endoscopic Approach
ØRGLØ3Z Fusion of Right Elbow Joint with Sustained Compression Internal Fixation Device, Open Approach
ØRGLØ4Z Fusion of Right Elbow Joint with Internal Fixation Device, Open Approach
ØRGLØ5Z Fusion of Right Elbow Joint with External Fixation Device, Open Approach
ØRGLØ7Z Fusion of Right Elbow Joint with Autologous Tissue Substitute, Open Approach
ØRGLØJZ Fusion of Right Elbow Joint with Synthetic Substitute, Open Approach
ØRGLØKZ Fusion of Right Elbow Joint with Nonautologous Tissue Substitute, Open Approach
ØRGL33Z Fusion of Right Elbow Joint with Sustained Compression Internal Fixation Device, Percutaneous Approach
ØRGL34Z Fusion of Right Elbow Joint with Internal Fixation Device, Percutaneous Approach
ØRGL35Z Fusion of Right Elbow Joint with External Fixation Device, Percutaneous Approach
ØRGL37Z Fusion of Right Elbow Joint with Autologous Tissue Substitute, Percutaneous Approach
ØRGL3JZ Fusion of Right Elbow Joint with Synthetic Substitute, Percutaneous Approach
ØRGL3KZ Fusion of Right Elbow Joint with Nonautologous Tissue Substitute, Percutaneous Approach
ØRGL43Z Fusion of Right Elbow Joint with Sustained Compression Internal Fixation Device, Percutaneous Endoscopic Approach
ØRGL44Z Fusion of Right Elbow Joint with Internal Fixation Device, Percutaneous Endoscopic Approach
ØRGL45Z Fusion of Right Elbow Joint with External Fixation Device, Percutaneous Endoscopic Approach
ØRGL47Z Fusion of Right Elbow Joint with Autologous Tissue Substitute, Percutaneous Endoscopic Approach
ØRGL4JZ Fusion of Right Elbow Joint with Synthetic Substitute, Percutaneous Endoscopic Approach
ØRGL4KZ Fusion of Right Elbow Joint with Nonautologous Tissue Substitute, Percutaneous Endoscopic Approach
ØRGMØ3Z Fusion of Left Elbow Joint with Sustained Compression Internal Fixation Device, Open Approach
ØRGMØ4Z Fusion of Left Elbow Joint with Internal Fixation Device, Open Approach
ØRGMØ5Z Fusion of Left Elbow Joint with External Fixation Device, Open Approach
ØRGMØ7Z Fusion of Left Elbow Joint with Autologous Tissue Substitute, Open Approach
ØRGMØJZ Fusion of Left Elbow Joint with Synthetic Substitute, Open Approach
ØRGMØKZ Fusion of Left Elbow Joint with Nonautologous Tissue Substitute, Open Approach
ØRGM33Z Fusion of Left Elbow Joint with Sustained Compression Internal Fixation Device, Percutaneous Approach
ØRGM34Z Fusion of Left Elbow Joint with Internal Fixation Device, Percutaneous Approach
ØRGM35Z Fusion of Left Elbow Joint with External Fixation Device, Percutaneous Approach
ØRGM37Z Fusion of Left Elbow Joint with Autologous Tissue Substitute, Percutaneous Approach
ØRGM3JZ Fusion of Left Elbow Joint with Synthetic Substitute, Percutaneous Approach
ØRGM3KZ Fusion of Left Elbow Joint with Nonautologous Tissue Substitute, Percutaneous Approach
ØRGM43Z Fusion of Left Elbow Joint with Sustained Compression Internal Fixation Device, Percutaneous Endoscopic Approach

HAC 12: Surgical Site Infection-Certain Orthopedic Procedures of the Spine, Shoulder, and Elbow (continued)

ØRGM44Z Fusion of Left Elbow Joint with Internal Fixation Device, Percutaneous Endoscopic Approach
ØRGM45Z Fusion of Left Elbow Joint with External Fixation Device, Percutaneous Endoscopic Approach
ØRGM47Z Fusion of Left Elbow Joint with Autologous Tissue Substitute, Percutaneous Endoscopic Approach
ØRGM4JZ Fusion of Left Elbow Joint with Synthetic Substitute, Percutaneous Endoscopic Approach
ØRGM4KZ Fusion of Left Elbow Joint with Nonautologous Tissue Substitute, Percutaneous Endoscopic Approach
ØRQEØZZ Repair Right Sternoclavicular Joint, Open Approach
ØRQE3ZZ Repair Right Sternoclavicular Joint, Percutaneous Approach
ØRQE4ZZ Repair Right Sternoclavicular Joint, Percutaneous Endoscopic Approach
ØRQEXZZ Repair Right Sternoclavicular Joint, External Approach
ØRQFØZZ Repair Left Sternoclavicular Joint, Open Approach
ØRQF3ZZ Repair Left Sternoclavicular Joint, Percutaneous Approach
ØRQF4ZZ Repair Left Sternoclavicular Joint, Percutaneous Endoscopic Approach
ØRQFXZZ Repair Left Sternoclavicular Joint, External Approach
ØRQGØZZ Repair Right Acromioclavicular Joint, Open Approach
ØRQG3ZZ Repair Right Acromioclavicular Joint, Percutaneous Approach
ØRQG4ZZ Repair Right Acromioclavicular Joint, Percutaneous Endoscopic Approach
ØRQGXZZ Repair Right Acromioclavicular Joint, External Approach
ØRQHØZZ Repair Left Acromioclavicular Joint, Open Approach
ØRQH3ZZ Repair Left Acromioclavicular Joint, Percutaneous Approach
ØRQH4ZZ Repair Left Acromioclavicular Joint, Percutaneous Endoscopic Approach
ØRQHXZZ Repair Left Acromioclavicular Joint, External Approach
ØRQJØZZ Repair Right Shoulder Joint, Open Approach
ØRQJ3ZZ Repair Right Shoulder Joint, Percutaneous Approach
ØRQJ4ZZ Repair Right Shoulder Joint, Percutaneous Endoscopic Approach
ØRQJXZZ Repair Right Shoulder Joint, External Approach
ØRQKØZZ Repair Left Shoulder Joint, Open Approach
ØRQK3ZZ Repair Left Shoulder Joint, Percutaneous Approach
ØRQK4ZZ Repair Left Shoulder Joint, Percutaneous Endoscopic Approach
ØRQKXZZ Repair Left Shoulder Joint, External Approach
ØRQLØZZ Repair Right Elbow Joint, Open Approach
ØRQL3ZZ Repair Right Elbow Joint, Percutaneous Approach
ØRQL4ZZ Repair Right Elbow Joint, Percutaneous Endoscopic Approach
ØRQLXZZ Repair Right Elbow Joint, External Approach
ØRQMØZZ Repair Left Elbow Joint, Open Approach
ØRQM3ZZ Repair Left Elbow Joint, Percutaneous Approach
ØRQM4ZZ Repair Left Elbow Joint, Percutaneous Endoscopic Approach
ØRQMXZZ Repair Left Elbow Joint, External Approach
ØRUEØ7Z Supplement Right Sternoclavicular Joint with Autologous Tissue Substitute, Open Approach
ØRUEØJZ Supplement Right Sternoclavicular Joint with Synthetic Substitute, Open Approach
ØRUEØKZ Supplement Right Sternoclavicular Joint with Nonautologous Tissue Substitute, Open Approach
ØRUE37Z Supplement Right Sternoclavicular Joint with Autologous Tissue Substitute, Percutaneous Approach
ØRUE3JZ Supplement Right Sternoclavicular Joint with Synthetic Substitute, Percutaneous Approach
ØRUE3KZ Supplement Right Sternoclavicular Joint with Nonautologous Tissue Substitute, Percutaneous Approach
ØRUE47Z Supplement Right Sternoclavicular Joint with Autologous Tissue Substitute, Percutaneous Endoscopic Approach
ØRUE4JZ Supplement Right Sternoclavicular Joint with Synthetic Substitute, Percutaneous Endoscopic Approach
ØRUE4KZ Supplement Right Sternoclavicular Joint with Nonautologous Tissue Substitute, Percutaneous Endoscopic Approach
ØRUFØ7Z Supplement Left Sternoclavicular Joint with Autologous Tissue Substitute, Open Approach
ØRUFØJZ Supplement Left Sternoclavicular Joint with Synthetic Substitute, Open Approach
ØRUFØKZ Supplement Left Sternoclavicular Joint with Nonautologous Tissue Substitute, Open Approach
ØRUF37Z Supplement Left Sternoclavicular Joint with Autologous Tissue Substitute, Percutaneous Approach
ØRUF3JZ Supplement Left Sternoclavicular Joint with Synthetic Substitute, Percutaneous Approach
ØRUF3KZ Supplement Left Sternoclavicular Joint with Nonautologous Tissue Substitute, Percutaneous Approach
ØRUF47Z Supplement Left Sternoclavicular Joint with Autologous Tissue Substitute, Percutaneous Endoscopic Approach
ØRUF4JZ Supplement Left Sternoclavicular Joint with Synthetic Substitute, Percutaneous Endoscopic Approach
ØRUF4KZ Supplement Left Sternoclavicular Joint with Nonautologous Tissue Substitute, Percutaneous Endoscopic Approach
ØRUGØ7Z Supplement Right Acromioclavicular Joint with Autologous Tissue Substitute, Open Approach
ØRUGØJZ Supplement Right Acromioclavicular Joint with Synthetic Substitute, Open Approach
ØRUGØKZ Supplement Right Acromioclavicular Joint with Nonautologous Tissue Substitute, Open Approach
ØRUG37Z Supplement Right Acromioclavicular Joint with Autologous Tissue Substitute, Percutaneous Approach
ØRUG3JZ Supplement Right Acromioclavicular Joint with Synthetic Substitute, Percutaneous Approach
ØRUG3KZ Supplement Right Acromioclavicular Joint with Nonautologous Tissue Substitute, Percutaneous Approach
ØRUG47Z Supplement Right Acromioclavicular Joint with Autologous Tissue Substitute, Percutaneous Endoscopic Approach
ØRUG4JZ Supplement Right Acromioclavicular Joint with Synthetic Substitute, Percutaneous Endoscopic Approach
ØRUG4KZ Supplement Right Acromioclavicular Joint with Nonautologous Tissue Substitute, Percutaneous Endoscopic Approach
ØRUHØ7Z Supplement Left Acromioclavicular Joint with Autologous Tissue Substitute, Open Approach
ØRUHØJZ Supplement Left Acromioclavicular Joint with Synthetic Substitute, Open Approach
ØRUHØKZ Supplement Left Acromioclavicular Joint with Nonautologous Tissue Substitute, Open Approach
ØRUH37Z Supplement Left Acromioclavicular Joint with Autologous Tissue Substitute, Percutaneous Approach
ØRUH3JZ Supplement Left Acromioclavicular Joint with Synthetic Substitute, Percutaneous Approach
ØRUH3KZ Supplement Left Acromioclavicular Joint with Nonautologous Tissue Substitute, Percutaneous Approach
ØRUH47Z Supplement Left Acromioclavicular Joint with Autologous Tissue Substitute, Percutaneous Endoscopic Approach
ØRUH4JZ Supplement Left Acromioclavicular Joint with Synthetic Substitute, Percutaneous Endoscopic Approach
ØRUH4KZ Supplement Left Acromioclavicular Joint with Nonautologous Tissue Substitute, Percutaneous Endoscopic Approach
ØRUJØ7Z Supplement Right Shoulder Joint with Autologous Tissue Substitute, Open Approach
ØRUJØJZ Supplement Right Shoulder Joint with Synthetic Substitute, Open Approach
ØRUJØKZ Supplement Right Shoulder Joint with Nonautologous Tissue Substitute, Open Approach
ØRUJ37Z Supplement Right Shoulder Joint with Autologous Tissue Substitute, Percutaneous Approach
ØRUJ3JZ Supplement Right Shoulder Joint with Synthetic Substitute, Percutaneous Approach
ØRUJ3KZ Supplement Right Shoulder Joint with Nonautologous Tissue Substitute, Percutaneous Approach
ØRUJ47Z Supplement Right Shoulder Joint with Autologous Tissue Substitute, Percutaneous Endoscopic Approach
ØRUJ4JZ Supplement Right Shoulder Joint with Synthetic Substitute, Percutaneous Endoscopic Approach
ØRUJ4KZ Supplement Right Shoulder Joint with Nonautologous Tissue Substitute, Percutaneous Endoscopic Approach
ØRUKØ7Z Supplement Left Shoulder Joint with Autologous Tissue Substitute, Open Approach
ØRUKØJZ Supplement Left Shoulder Joint with Synthetic Substitute, Open Approach
ØRUKØKZ Supplement Left Shoulder Joint with Nonautologous Tissue Substitute, Open Approach
ØRUK37Z Supplement Left Shoulder Joint with Autologous Tissue Substitute, Percutaneous Approach
ØRUK3JZ Supplement Left Shoulder Joint with Synthetic Substitute, Percutaneous Approach
ØRUK3KZ Supplement Left Shoulder Joint with Nonautologous Tissue Substitute, Percutaneous Approach

HAC 12: Surgical Site Infection-Certain Orthopedic Procedures of the Spine, Shoulder, and Elbow (continued)

ØRUK47Z Supplement Left Shoulder Joint with Autologous Tissue Substitute, Percutaneous Endoscopic Approach
ØRUK4JZ Supplement Left Shoulder Joint with Synthetic Substitute, Percutaneous Endoscopic Approach
ØRUK4KZ Supplement Left Shoulder Joint with Nonautologous Tissue Substitute, Percutaneous Endoscopic Approach
ØRULØ7Z Supplement Right Elbow Joint with Autologous Tissue Substitute, Open Approach
ØRULØJZ Supplement Right Elbow Joint with Synthetic Substitute, Open Approach
ØRULØKZ Supplement Right Elbow Joint with Nonautologous Tissue Substitute, Open Approach
ØRUL37Z Supplement Right Elbow Joint with Autologous Tissue Substitute, Percutaneous Approach
ØRUL3JZ Supplement Right Elbow Joint with Synthetic Substitute, Percutaneous Approach
ØRUL3KZ Supplement Right Elbow Joint with Nonautologous Tissue Substitute, Percutaneous Approach
ØRUL47Z Supplement Right Elbow Joint with Autologous Tissue Substitute, Percutaneous Endoscopic Approach
ØRUL4JZ Supplement Right Elbow Joint with Synthetic Substitute, Percutaneous Endoscopic Approach
ØRUL4KZ Supplement Right Elbow Joint with Nonautologous Tissue Substitute, Percutaneous Endoscopic Approach
ØRUMØ7Z Supplement Left Elbow Joint with Autologous Tissue Substitute, Open Approach
ØRUMØJZ Supplement Left Elbow Joint with Synthetic Substitute, Open Approach
ØRUMØKZ Supplement Left Elbow Joint with Nonautologous Tissue Substitute, Open Approach
ØRUM37Z Supplement Left Elbow Joint with Autologous Tissue Substitute, Percutaneous Approach
ØRUM3JZ Supplement Left Elbow Joint with Synthetic Substitute, Percutaneous Approach
ØRUM3KZ Supplement Left Elbow Joint with Nonautologous Tissue Substitute, Percutaneous Approach
ØRUM47Z Supplement Left Elbow Joint with Autologous Tissue Substitute, Percutaneous Endoscopic Approach
ØRUM4JZ Supplement Left Elbow Joint with Synthetic Substitute, Percutaneous Endoscopic Approach
ØRUM4KZ Supplement Left Elbow Joint with Nonautologous Tissue Substitute, Percutaneous Endoscopic Approach
ØSGØØ7Ø Fusion of Lumbar Vertebral Joint with Autologous Tissue Substitute, Anterior Approach, Anterior Column, Open Approach
ØSGØØ71 Fusion of Lumbar Vertebral Joint with Autologous Tissue Substitute, Posterior Approach, Posterior Column, Open Approach
ØSGØØ7J Fusion of Lumbar Vertebral Joint with Autologous Tissue Substitute, Posterior Approach, Anterior Column, Open Approach
ØSGØØAØ Fusion of Lumbar Vertebral Joint with Interbody Fusion Device, Anterior Approach, Anterior Column, Open Approach
ØSGØØAJ Fusion of Lumbar Vertebral Joint with Interbody Fusion Device, Posterior Approach, Anterior Column, Open Approach
ØSGØØJØ Fusion of Lumbar Vertebral Joint with Synthetic Substitute, Anterior Approach, Anterior Column, Open Approach
ØSGØØJ1 Fusion of Lumbar Vertebral Joint with Synthetic Substitute, Posterior Approach, Posterior Column, Open Approach
ØSGØØJJ Fusion of Lumbar Vertebral Joint with Synthetic Substitute, Posterior Approach, Anterior Column, Open Approach
ØSGØØKØ Fusion of Lumbar Vertebral Joint with Nonautologous Tissue Substitute, Anterior Approach, Anterior Column, Open Approach
ØSGØØK1 Fusion of Lumbar Vertebral Joint with Nonautologous Tissue Substitute, Posterior Approach, Posterior Column, Open Approach
ØSGØØKJ Fusion of Lumbar Vertebral Joint with Nonautologous Tissue Substitute, Posterior Approach, Anterior Column, Open Approach
ØSGØ37Ø Fusion of Lumbar Vertebral Joint with Autologous Tissue Substitute, Anterior Approach, Anterior Column, Percutaneous Approach
ØSGØ371 Fusion of Lumbar Vertebral Joint with Autologous Tissue Substitute, Posterior Approach, Posterior Column, Percutaneous Approach
ØSGØ37J Fusion of Lumbar Vertebral Joint with Autologous Tissue Substitute, Posterior Approach, Anterior Column, Percutaneous Approach
ØSGØ3AØ Fusion of Lumbar Vertebral Joint with Interbody Fusion Device, Anterior Approach, Anterior Column, Percutaneous Approach
ØSGØ3AJ Fusion of Lumbar Vertebral Joint with Interbody Fusion Device, Posterior Approach, Anterior Column, Percutaneous Approach
ØSGØ3JØ Fusion of Lumbar Vertebral Joint with Synthetic Substitute, Anterior Approach, Anterior Column, Percutaneous Approach
ØSGØ3J1 Fusion of Lumbar Vertebral Joint with Synthetic Substitute, Posterior Approach, Posterior Column, Percutaneous Approach
ØSGØ3JJ Fusion of Lumbar Vertebral Joint with Synthetic Substitute, Posterior Approach, Anterior Column, Percutaneous Approach
ØSGØ3KØ Fusion of Lumbar Vertebral Joint with Nonautologous Tissue Substitute, Anterior Approach, Anterior Column, Percutaneous Approach
ØSGØ3K1 Fusion of Lumbar Vertebral Joint with Nonautologous Tissue Substitute, Posterior Approach, Posterior Column, Percutaneous Approach
ØSGØ3KJ Fusion of Lumbar Vertebral Joint with Nonautologous Tissue Substitute, Posterior Approach, Anterior Column, Percutaneous Approach
ØSGØ47Ø Fusion of Lumbar Vertebral Joint with Autologous Tissue Substitute, Anterior Approach, Anterior Column, Percutaneous Endoscopic Approach
ØSGØ471 Fusion of Lumbar Vertebral Joint with Autologous Tissue Substitute, Posterior Approach, Posterior Column, Percutaneous Endoscopic Approach
ØSGØ47J Fusion of Lumbar Vertebral Joint with Autologous Tissue Substitute, Posterior Approach, Anterior Column, Percutaneous Endoscopic Approach
ØSGØ4AØ Fusion of Lumbar Vertebral Joint with Interbody Fusion Device, Anterior Approach, Anterior Column, Percutaneous Endoscopic Approach
ØSGØ4AJ Fusion of Lumbar Vertebral Joint with Interbody Fusion Device, Posterior Approach, Anterior Column, Percutaneous Endoscopic Approach
ØSGØ4JØ Fusion of Lumbar Vertebral Joint with Synthetic Substitute, Anterior Approach, Anterior Column, Percutaneous Endoscopic Approach
ØSGØ4J1 Fusion of Lumbar Vertebral Joint with Synthetic Substitute, Posterior Approach, Posterior Column, Percutaneous Endoscopic Approach
ØSGØ4JJ Fusion of Lumbar Vertebral Joint with Synthetic Substitute, Posterior Approach, Anterior Column, Percutaneous Endoscopic Approach
ØSGØ4KØ Fusion of Lumbar Vertebral Joint with Nonautologous Tissue Substitute, Anterior Approach, Anterior Column, Percutaneous Endoscopic Approach
ØSGØ4K1 Fusion of Lumbar Vertebral Joint with Nonautologous Tissue Substitute, Posterior Approach, Posterior Column, Percutaneous Endoscopic Approach
ØSGØ4KJ Fusion of Lumbar Vertebral Joint with Nonautologous Tissue Substitute, Posterior Approach, Anterior Column, Percutaneous Endoscopic Approach
ØSG1Ø7Ø Fusion of 2 or More Lumbar Vertebral Joints with Autologous Tissue Substitute, Anterior Approach, Anterior Column, Open Approach
ØSG1Ø71 Fusion of 2 or More Lumbar Vertebral Joints with Autologous Tissue Substitute, Posterior Approach, Posterior Column, Open Approach
ØSG1Ø7J Fusion of 2 or More Lumbar Vertebral Joints with Autologous Tissue Substitute, Posterior Approach, Anterior Column, Open Approach
ØSG1ØAØ Fusion of 2 or More Lumbar Vertebral Joints with Interbody Fusion Device, Anterior Approach, Anterior Column, Open Approach
ØSG1ØAJ Fusion of 2 or More Lumbar Vertebral Joints with Interbody Fusion Device, Posterior Approach, Anterior Column, Open Approach
ØSG1ØJØ Fusion of 2 or More Lumbar Vertebral Joints with Synthetic Substitute, Anterior Approach, Anterior Column, Open Approach
ØSG1ØJ1 Fusion of 2 or More Lumbar Vertebral Joints with Synthetic Substitute, Posterior Approach, Posterior Column, Open Approach
ØSG1ØJJ Fusion of 2 or More Lumbar Vertebral Joints with Synthetic Substitute, Posterior Approach, Anterior Column, Open Approach
ØSG1ØKØ Fusion of 2 or More Lumbar Vertebral Joints with Nonautologous Tissue Substitute, Anterior Approach, Anterior Column, Open Approach

HAC 12: Surgical Site Infection-Certain Orthopedic Procedures of the Spine, Shoulder, and Elbow (continued)

ØSG1ØK1 Fusion of 2 or More Lumbar Vertebral Joints with Nonautologous Tissue Substitute, Posterior Approach, Posterior Column, Open Approach
ØSG1ØKJ Fusion of 2 or More Lumbar Vertebral Joints with Nonautologous Tissue Substitute, Posterior Approach, Anterior Column, Open Approach
ØSG137Ø Fusion of 2 or More Lumbar Vertebral Joints with Autologous Tissue Substitute, Anterior Approach, Anterior Column, Percutaneous Approach
ØSG1371 Fusion of 2 or More Lumbar Vertebral Joints with Autologous Tissue Substitute, Posterior Approach, Posterior Column, Percutaneous Approach
ØSG137J Fusion of 2 or More Lumbar Vertebral Joints with Autologous Tissue Substitute, Posterior Approach, Anterior Column, Percutaneous Approach
ØSG13AØ Fusion of 2 or More Lumbar Vertebral Joints with Interbody Fusion Device, Anterior Approach, Anterior Column, Percutaneous Approach
ØSG13AJ Fusion of 2 or More Lumbar Vertebral Joints with Interbody Fusion Device, Posterior Approach, Anterior Column, Percutaneous Approach
ØSG13JØ Fusion of 2 or More Lumbar Vertebral Joints with Synthetic Substitute, Anterior Approach, Anterior Column, Percutaneous Approach
ØSG13J1 Fusion of 2 or More Lumbar Vertebral Joints with Synthetic Substitute, Posterior Approach, Posterior Column, Percutaneous Approach
ØSG13JJ Fusion of 2 or More Lumbar Vertebral Joints with Synthetic Substitute, Posterior Approach, Anterior Column, Percutaneous Approach
ØSG13KØ Fusion of 2 or More Lumbar Vertebral Joints with Nonautologous Tissue Substitute, Anterior Approach, Anterior Column, Percutaneous Approach
ØSG13K1 Fusion of 2 or More Lumbar Vertebral Joints with Nonautologous Tissue Substitute, Posterior Approach, Posterior Column, Percutaneous Approach
ØSG13KJ Fusion of 2 or More Lumbar Vertebral Joints with Nonautologous Tissue Substitute, Posterior Approach, Anterior Column, Percutaneous Approach
ØSG147Ø Fusion of 2 or More Lumbar Vertebral Joints with Autologous Tissue Substitute, Anterior Approach, Anterior Column, Percutaneous Endoscopic Approach
ØSG1471 Fusion of 2 or More Lumbar Vertebral Joints with Autologous Tissue Substitute, Posterior Approach, Posterior Column, Percutaneous Endoscopic Approach
ØSG147J Fusion of 2 or More Lumbar Vertebral Joints with Autologous Tissue Substitute, Posterior Approach, Anterior Column, Percutaneous Endoscopic Approach
ØSG14AØ Fusion of 2 or More Lumbar Vertebral Joints with Interbody Fusion Device, Anterior Approach, Anterior Column, Percutaneous Endoscopic Approach
ØSG14AJ Fusion of 2 or More Lumbar Vertebral Joints with Interbody Fusion Device, Posterior Approach, Anterior Column, Percutaneous Endoscopic Approach
ØSG14JØ Fusion of 2 or More Lumbar Vertebral Joints with Synthetic Substitute, Anterior Approach, Anterior Column, Percutaneous Endoscopic Approach
ØSG14J1 Fusion of 2 or More Lumbar Vertebral Joints with Synthetic Substitute, Posterior Approach, Posterior Column, Percutaneous Endoscopic Approach
ØSG14JJ Fusion of 2 or More Lumbar Vertebral Joints with Synthetic Substitute, Posterior Approach, Anterior Column, Percutaneous Endoscopic Approach
ØSG14KØ Fusion of 2 or More Lumbar Vertebral Joints with Nonautologous Tissue Substitute, Anterior Approach, Anterior Column, Percutaneous Endoscopic Approach
ØSG14K1 Fusion of 2 or More Lumbar Vertebral Joints with Nonautologous Tissue Substitute, Posterior Approach, Posterior Column, Percutaneous Endoscopic Approach
ØSG14KJ Fusion of 2 or More Lumbar Vertebral Joints with Nonautologous Tissue Substitute, Posterior Approach, Anterior Column, Percutaneous Endoscopic Approach
ØSG307Ø Fusion of Lumbosacral Joint with Autologous Tissue Substitute, Anterior Approach, Anterior Column, Open Approach
ØSG3Ø71 Fusion of Lumbosacral Joint with Autologous Tissue Substitute, Posterior Approach, Posterior Column, Open Approach
ØSG3Ø7J Fusion of Lumbosacral Joint with Autologous Tissue Substitute, Posterior Approach, Anterior Column, Open Approach
ØSG3ØAØ Fusion of Lumbosacral Joint with Interbody Fusion Device, Anterior Approach, Anterior Column, Open Approach
ØSG3ØAJ Fusion of Lumbosacral Joint with Interbody Fusion Device, Posterior Approach, Anterior Column, Open Approach
ØSG3ØJØ Fusion of Lumbosacral Joint with Synthetic Substitute, Anterior Approach, Anterior Column, Open Approach
ØSG3ØJ1 Fusion of Lumbosacral Joint with Synthetic Substitute, Posterior Approach, Posterior Column, Open Approach
ØSG3ØJJ Fusion of Lumbosacral Joint with Synthetic Substitute, Posterior Approach, Anterior Column, Open Approach
ØSG3ØKØ Fusion of Lumbosacral Joint with Nonautologous Tissue Substitute, Anterior Approach, Anterior Column, Open Approach
ØSG3ØK1 Fusion of Lumbosacral Joint with Nonautologous Tissue Substitute, Posterior Approach, Posterior Column, Open Approach
ØSG3ØKJ Fusion of Lumbosacral Joint with Nonautologous Tissue Substitute, Posterior Approach, Anterior Column, Open Approach
ØSG337Ø Fusion of Lumbosacral Joint with Autologous Tissue Substitute, Anterior Approach, Anterior Column, Percutaneous Approach
ØSG3371 Fusion of Lumbosacral Joint with Autologous Tissue Substitute, Posterior Approach, Posterior Column, Percutaneous Approach
ØSG337J Fusion of Lumbosacral Joint with Autologous Tissue Substitute, Posterior Approach, Anterior Column, Percutaneous Approach
ØSG33AØ Fusion of Lumbosacral Joint with Interbody Fusion Device, Anterior Approach, Anterior Column, Percutaneous Approach
ØSG33AJ Fusion of Lumbosacral Joint with Interbody Fusion Device, Posterior Approach, Anterior Column, Percutaneous Approach
ØSG33JØ Fusion of Lumbosacral Joint with Synthetic Substitute, Anterior Approach, Anterior Column, Percutaneous Approach
ØSG33J1 Fusion of Lumbosacral Joint with Synthetic Substitute, Posterior Approach, Posterior Column, Percutaneous Approach
ØSG33JJ Fusion of Lumbosacral Joint with Synthetic Substitute, Posterior Approach, Anterior Column, Percutaneous Approach
ØSG33KØ Fusion of Lumbosacral Joint with Nonautologous Tissue Substitute, Anterior Approach, Anterior Column, Percutaneous Approach
ØSG33K1 Fusion of Lumbosacral Joint with Nonautologous Tissue Substitute, Posterior Approach, Posterior Column, Percutaneous Approach
ØSG33KJ Fusion of Lumbosacral Joint with Nonautologous Tissue Substitute, Posterior Approach, Anterior Column, Percutaneous Approach
ØSG347Ø Fusion of Lumbosacral Joint with Autologous Tissue Substitute, Anterior Approach, Anterior Column, Percutaneous Endoscopic Approach
ØSG3471 Fusion of Lumbosacral Joint with Autologous Tissue Substitute, Posterior Approach, Posterior Column, Percutaneous Endoscopic Approach
ØSG347J Fusion of Lumbosacral Joint with Autologous Tissue Substitute, Posterior Approach, Anterior Column, Percutaneous Endoscopic Approach
ØSG34AØ Fusion of Lumbosacral Joint with Interbody Fusion Device, Anterior Approach, Anterior Column, Percutaneous Endoscopic Approach
ØSG34AJ Fusion of Lumbosacral Joint with Interbody Fusion Device, Posterior Approach, Anterior Column, Percutaneous Endoscopic Approach
ØSG34JØ Fusion of Lumbosacral Joint with Synthetic Substitute, Anterior Approach, Anterior Column, Percutaneous Endoscopic Approach
ØSG34J1 Fusion of Lumbosacral Joint with Synthetic Substitute, Posterior Approach, Posterior Column, Percutaneous Endoscopic Approach
ØSG34JJ Fusion of Lumbosacral Joint with Synthetic Substitute, Posterior Approach, Anterior Column, Percutaneous Endoscopic Approach
ØSG34KØ Fusion of Lumbosacral Joint with Nonautologous Tissue Substitute, Anterior Approach, Anterior Column, Percutaneous Endoscopic Approach
ØSG34K1 Fusion of Lumbosacral Joint with Nonautologous Tissue Substitute, Posterior Approach, Posterior Column, Percutaneous Endoscopic Approach

HAC 12: Surgical Site Infection-Certain Orthopedic Procedures of the Spine, Shoulder, and Elbow (continued)

ØSG34KJ Fusion of Lumbosacral Joint with Nonautologous Tissue Substitute, Posterior Approach, Anterior Column, Percutaneous Endoscopic Approach
ØSG7Ø4Z Fusion of Right Sacroiliac Joint with Internal Fixation Device, Open Approach
ØSG7Ø7Z Fusion of Right Sacroiliac Joint with Autologous Tissue Substitute, Open Approach
ØSG7ØJZ Fusion of Right Sacroiliac Joint with Synthetic Substitute, Open Approach
ØSG7ØKZ Fusion of Right Sacroiliac Joint with Nonautologous Tissue Substitute, Open Approach
ØSG734Z Fusion of Right Sacroiliac Joint with Internal Fixation Device, Percutaneous Approach
ØSG737Z Fusion of Right Sacroiliac Joint with Autologous Tissue Substitute, Percutaneous Approach
ØSG73JZ Fusion of Right Sacroiliac Joint with Synthetic Substitute, Percutaneous Approach
ØSG73KZ Fusion of Right Sacroiliac Joint with Nonautologous Tissue Substitute, Percutaneous Approach
ØSG744Z Fusion of Right Sacroiliac Joint with Internal Fixation Device, Percutaneous Endoscopic Approach
ØSG747Z Fusion of Right Sacroiliac Joint with Autologous Tissue Substitute, Percutaneous Endoscopic Approach
ØSG74JZ Fusion of Right Sacroiliac Joint with Synthetic Substitute, Percutaneous Endoscopic Approach
ØSG74KZ Fusion of Right Sacroiliac Joint with Nonautologous Tissue Substitute, Percutaneous Endoscopic Approach
ØSG8Ø4Z Fusion of Left Sacroiliac Joint with Internal Fixation Device, Open Approach
ØSG8Ø7Z Fusion of Left Sacroiliac Joint with Autologous Tissue Substitute, Open Approach
ØSG8ØJZ Fusion of Left Sacroiliac Joint with Synthetic Substitute, Open Approach
ØSG8ØKZ Fusion of Left Sacroiliac Joint with Nonautologous Tissue Substitute, Open Approach
ØSG834Z Fusion of Left Sacroiliac Joint with Internal Fixation Device, Percutaneous Approach
ØSG837Z Fusion of Left Sacroiliac Joint with Autologous Tissue Substitute, Percutaneous Approach
ØSG83JZ Fusion of Left Sacroiliac Joint with Synthetic Substitute, Percutaneous Approach
ØSG83KZ Fusion of Left Sacroiliac Joint with Nonautologous Tissue Substitute, Percutaneous Approach
ØSG844Z Fusion of Left Sacroiliac Joint with Internal Fixation Device, Percutaneous Endoscopic Approach
ØSG847Z Fusion of Left Sacroiliac Joint with Autologous Tissue Substitute, Percutaneous Endoscopic Approach
ØSG84JZ Fusion of Left Sacroiliac Joint with Synthetic Substitute, Percutaneous Endoscopic Approach
ØSG84KZ Fusion of Left Sacroiliac Joint with Nonautologous Tissue Substitute, Percutaneous Endoscopic Approach
XRGØØ92 Fusion of Occipital-cervical Joint using Nanotextured Surface Interbody Fusion Device, Open Approach, New Technology Group 2
XRGØØF3 Fusion of Occipital-cervical Joint using Radiolucent Porous Interbody Fusion Device, Open Approach, New Technology Group 3
XRG1Ø92 Fusion of Cervical Vertebral Joint using Nanotextured Surface Interbody Fusion Device, Open Approach, New Technology Group 2
XRG1ØF3 Fusion of Cervical Vertebral Joint using Radiolucent Porous Interbody Fusion Device, Open Approach, New Technology Group 3
XRG2Ø92 Fusion of 2 or more Cervical Vertebral Joints using Nanotextured Surface Interbody Fusion Device, Open Approach, New Technology Group 2
XRG2ØF3 Fusion of 2 or more Cervical Vertebral Joints using Radiolucent Porous Interbody Fusion Device, Open Approach, New Technology Group 3
XRG4Ø92 Fusion of Cervicothoracic Vertebral Joint using Nanotextured Surface Interbody Fusion Device, Open Approach, New Technology Group 2
XRG4ØF3 Fusion of Cervicothoracic Vertebral Joint using Radiolucent Porous Interbody Fusion Device, Open Approach, New Technology Group 3
XRG6Ø92 Fusion of Thoracic Vertebral Joint using Nanotextured Surface Interbody Fusion Device, Open Approach, New Technology Group 2
XRG6ØF3 Fusion of Thoracic Vertebral Joint using Radiolucent Porous Interbody Fusion Device, Open Approach, New Technology Group 3
XRG7Ø92 Fusion of 2 to 7 Thoracic Vertebral Joints using Nanotextured Surface Interbody Fusion Device, Open Approach, New Technology Group 2
XRG7ØF3 Fusion of 2 to 7 Thoracic Vertebral Joints using Radiolucent Porous Interbody Fusion Device, Open Approach, New Technology Group 3
XRG8Ø92 Fusion of 8 or more Thoracic Vertebral Joints using Nanotextured Surface Interbody Fusion Device, Open Approach, New Technology Group 2
XRG8ØF3 Fusion of 8 or more Thoracic Vertebral Joints using Radiolucent Porous Interbody Fusion Device, Open Approach, New Technology Group 3
XRGAØ92 Fusion of Thoracolumbar Vertebral Joint using Nanotextured Surface Interbody Fusion Device, Open Approach, New Technology Group 2
XRGAØF3 Fusion of Thoracolumbar Vertebral Joint using Radiolucent Porous Interbody Fusion Device, Open Approach, New Technology Group 3
XRGBØ92 Fusion of Lumbar Vertebral Joint using Nanotextured Surface Interbody Fusion Device, Open Approach, New Technology Group 2
XRGBØF3 Fusion of Lumbar Vertebral Joint using Radiolucent Porous Interbody Fusion Device, Open Approach, New Technology Group 3
XRGCØ92 Fusion of 2 or more Lumbar Vertebral Joints using Nanotextured Surface Interbody Fusion Device, Open Approach, New Technology Group 2
XRGCØF3 Fusion of 2 or more Lumbar Vertebral Joints using Radiolucent Porous Interbody Fusion Device, Open Approach, New Technology Group 3
XRGDØ92 Fusion of Lumbosacral Joint using Nanotextured Surface Interbody Fusion Device, Open Approach, New Technology Group 2
XRGDØF3 Fusion of Lumbosacral Joint using Radiolucent Porous Interbody Fusion Device, Open Approach, New Technology Group 3

HAC 13: Surgical Site Infection (SSI) Following Cardiac Implantable Electronic Device (CIED) Procedures

Secondary diagnosis not POA:
K68.11 Postprocedural retroperitoneal abscess
T81.4ØXA Infection following a procedure, unspecified, initial encounter
T81.41XA Infection following a procedure, superficial incisional surgical site, initial encounter
T81.42XA Infection following a procedure, deep incisional surgical site, initial encounter
T81.43XA Infection following a procedure, organ and space surgical site, initial encounter
T81.44XA Sepsis following a procedure, initial encounter
T81.49XA Infection following a procedure, other surgical site, initial encounter
T82.6XXA Infection and inflammatory reaction due to cardiac valve prosthesis, initial encounter
T82.7XXA Infection and inflammatory reaction due to other internal orthopedic prosthetic devices, implants and grafts, initial encounter

AND

Any of the following procedures:
Ø2H43JZ Insertion of Pacemaker Lead into Coronary Vein, Percutaneous Approach
Ø2H43KZ Insertion of Defibrillator Lead into Coronary Vein, Percutaneous Approach
Ø2H43MZ Insertion of Cardiac Lead into Coronary Vein, Percutaneous Approach
Ø2H63JZ Insertion of Pacemaker Lead into Right Atrium, Percutaneous Approach
Ø2H63MZ Insertion of Cardiac Lead into Right Atrium, Percutaneous Approach
Ø2H73JZ Insertion of Pacemaker Lead into Left Atrium, Percutaneous Approach
Ø2H73MZ Insertion of Cardiac Lead into Left Atrium, Percutaneous Approach
Ø2HK3JZ Insertion of Pacemaker Lead into Right Ventricle, Percutaneous Approach
Ø2HL3JZ Insertion of Pacemaker Lead into Left Ventricle, Percutaneous Approach
Ø2HNØJZ Insertion of Pacemaker Lead into Pericardium, Open Approach
Ø2HNØMZ Insertion of Cardiac Lead into Pericardium, Open Approach
Ø2HN3JZ Insertion of Pacemaker Lead into Pericardium, Percutaneous Approach
Ø2HN3MZ Insertion of Cardiac Lead into Pericardium, Percutaneous Approach
Ø2HN4JZ Insertion of Pacemaker Lead into Pericardium, Percutaneous Endoscopic Approach
Ø2HN4MZ Insertion of Cardiac Lead into Pericardium, Percutaneous Endoscopic Approach
Ø2PAØMZ Removal of Cardiac Lead from Heart, Open Approach
Ø2PA3MZ Removal of Cardiac Lead from Heart, Percutaneous Approach
Ø2PA4MZ Removal of Cardiac Lead from Heart, Percutaneous Endoscopic Approach

HAC 13: Surgical Site Infection (SSI) Following Cardiac Implantable Electronic Device (CIED) Procedures (continued)

Ø2PAXMZ Removal of Cardiac Lead from Heart, External Approach
Ø2WAØMZ Revision of Cardiac Lead in Heart, Open Approach
Ø2WA3MZ Revision of Cardiac Lead in Heart, Percutaneous Approach
Ø2WA4MZ Revision of Cardiac Lead in Heart, Percutaneous Endoscopic Approach
ØJH6Ø4Z Insertion of Pacemaker, Single Chamber into Chest Subcutaneous Tissue and Fascia, Open Approach
ØJH6Ø5Z Insertion of Pacemaker, Single Chamber Rate Responsive into Chest Subcutaneous Tissue and Fascia, Open Approach
ØJH6Ø6Z Insertion of Pacemaker, Dual Chamber into Chest Subcutaneous Tissue and Fascia, Open Approach
ØJH6Ø7Z Insertion of Cardiac Resynchronization Pacemaker Pulse Generator into Chest Subcutaneous Tissue and Fascia, Open Approach
ØJH6Ø8Z Insertion of Defibrillator Generator into Chest Subcutaneous Tissue and Fascia, Open Approach
ØJH6Ø9Z Insertion of Cardiac Resynchronization Defibrillator Pulse Generator into Chest Subcutaneous Tissue and Fascia, Open Approach
ØJH6ØPZ Insertion of Cardiac Rhythm Related Device into Chest Subcutaneous Tissue and Fascia, Open Approach
ØJH634Z Insertion of Pacemaker, Single Chamber into Chest Subcutaneous Tissue and Fascia, Percutaneous Approach
ØJH635Z Insertion of Pacemaker, Single Chamber Rate Responsive into Chest Subcutaneous Tissue and Fascia, Percutaneous Approach
ØJH636Z Insertion of Pacemaker, Dual Chamber into Chest Subcutaneous Tissue and Fascia, Percutaneous Approach
ØJH637Z Insertion of Cardiac Resynchronization Pacemaker Pulse Generator into Chest Subcutaneous Tissue and Fascia, Percutaneous Approach
ØJH638Z Insertion of Defibrillator Generator into Chest Subcutaneous Tissue and Fascia, Percutaneous Approach
ØJH639Z Insertion of Cardiac Resynchronization Defibrillator Pulse Generator into Chest Subcutaneous Tissue and Fascia, Percutaneous Approach
ØJH63PZ Insertion of Cardiac Rhythm Related Device into Chest Subcutaneous Tissue and Fascia, Percutaneous Approach
ØJH8Ø4Z Insertion of Pacemaker, Single Chamber into Abdomen Subcutaneous Tissue and Fascia, Open Approach
ØJH8Ø5Z Insertion of Pacemaker, Single Chamber Rate Responsive into Abdomen Subcutaneous Tissue and Fascia, Open Approach
ØJH8Ø6Z Insertion of Pacemaker, Dual Chamber into Abdomen Subcutaneous Tissue and Fascia, Open Approach
ØJH8Ø7Z Insertion of Cardiac Resynchronization Pacemaker Pulse Generator into Abdomen Subcutaneous Tissue and Fascia, Open Approach
ØJH8Ø8Z Insertion of Defibrillator Generator into Abdomen Subcutaneous Tissue and Fascia, Open Approach
ØJH8Ø9Z Insertion of Cardiac Resynchronization Defibrillator Pulse Generator into Abdomen Subcutaneous Tissue and Fascia, Open Approach
ØJH8ØPZ Insertion of Cardiac Rhythm Related Device into Abdomen Subcutaneous Tissue and Fascia, Open Approach
ØJH834Z Insertion of Pacemaker, Single Chamber into Abdomen Subcutaneous Tissue and Fascia, Percutaneous Approach
ØJH835Z Insertion of Pacemaker, Single Chamber Rate Responsive into Abdomen Subcutaneous Tissue and Fascia, Percutaneous Approach
ØJH836Z Insertion of Pacemaker, Dual Chamber into Abdomen Subcutaneous Tissue and Fascia, Percutaneous Approach
ØJH837Z Insertion of Cardiac Resynchronization Pacemaker Pulse Generator into Abdomen Subcutaneous Tissue and Fascia, Percutaneous Approach
ØJH838Z Insertion of Defibrillator Generator into Abdomen Subcutaneous Tissue and Fascia, Percutaneous Approach
ØJH839Z Insertion of Cardiac Resynchronization Defibrillator Pulse Generator into Abdomen Subcutaneous Tissue and Fascia, Percutaneous Approach
ØJH83PZ Insertion of Cardiac Rhythm Related Device into Abdomen Subcutaneous Tissue and Fascia, Percutaneous Approach
ØJPTØFZ Removal of Subcutaneous Defibrillator Lead from Trunk Subcutaneous Tissue and Fascia, Open Approach
ØJPTØPZ Removal of Cardiac Rhythm Related Device from Trunk Subcutaneous Tissue and Fascia, Open Approach
ØJPT3FZ Removal of Subcutaneous Defibrillator Lead from Trunk Subcutaneous Tissue and Fascia, Percutaneous Approach
ØJPT3PZ Removal of Cardiac Rhythm Related Device from Trunk Subcutaneous Tissue and Fascia, Percutaneous Approach
ØJWTØFZ Revision of Subcutaneous Defibrillator Lead in Trunk Subcutaneous Tissue and Fascia, Open Approach
ØJWTØPZ Revision of Cardiac Rhythm Related Device in Trunk Subcutaneous Tissue and Fascia, Open Approach
ØJWT3FZ Revision of Subcutaneous Defibrillator Lead in Trunk Subcutaneous Tissue and Fascia, Percutaneous Approach
ØJWT3PZ Revision of Cardiac Rhythm Related Device in Trunk Subcutaneous Tissue and Fascia, Percutaneous Approach

HAC 14: Iatrogenic Pneumothorax with Venous Catheterization

Secondary diagnosis not POA:
J95.811 Postprocedural pneumothorax

AND

Any of the following procedures:
Ø2H633Z Insertion of Infusion Device into Right Atrium, Percutaneous Approach
Ø2HK33Z Insertion of Infusion Device into Right Ventricle, Percutaneous Approach
Ø2HS33Z Insertion of Infusion Device into Right Pulmonary Vein, Percutaneous Approach
Ø2HS43Z Insertion of Infusion Device into Right Pulmonary Vein, Percutaneous Endoscopic Approach
Ø2HT33Z Insertion of Infusion Device into Left Pulmonary Vein, Percutaneous Approach
Ø2HT43Z Insertion of Infusion Device into Left Pulmonary Vein, Percutaneous Endoscopic Approach
Ø2HV33Z Insertion of Infusion Device into Superior Vena Cava, Percutaneous Approach
Ø2HV43Z Insertion of Infusion Device into Superior Vena Cava, Percutaneous Endoscopic Approach
Ø5HØ33Z Insertion of Infusion Device into Azygos Vein, Percutaneous Approach
Ø5HØ43Z Insertion of Infusion Device into Azygos Vein, Percutaneous Endoscopic Approach
Ø5H133Z Insertion of Infusion Device into Hemiazygos Vein, Percutaneous Approach
Ø5H143Z Insertion of Infusion Device into Hemiazygos Vein, Percutaneous Endoscopic Approach
Ø5H333Z Insertion of Infusion Device into Right Innominate Vein, Percutaneous Approach
Ø5H343Z Insertion of Infusion Device into Right Innominate Vein, Percutaneous Endoscopic Approach
Ø5H433Z Insertion of Infusion Device into Left Innominate Vein, Percutaneous Approach
Ø5H443Z Insertion of Infusion Device into Left Innominate Vein, Percutaneous Endoscopic Approach
Ø5H533Z Insertion of Infusion Device into Right Subclavian Vein, Percutaneous Approach
Ø5H543Z Insertion of Infusion Device into Right Subclavian Vein, Percutaneous Endoscopic Approach
Ø5H633Z Insertion of Infusion Device into Left Subclavian Vein, Percutaneous Approach
Ø5H643Z Insertion of Infusion Device into Left Subclavian Vein, Percutaneous Endoscopic Approach
Ø5HM33Z Insertion of Infusion Device into Right Internal Jugular Vein, Percutaneous Approach
Ø5HN33Z Insertion of Infusion Device into Left Internal Jugular Vein, Percutaneous Approach
Ø5HP33Z Insertion of Infusion Device into Right External Jugular Vein, Percutaneous Approach
Ø5HQ33Z Insertion of Infusion Device into Left External Jugular Vein, Percutaneous Approach
ØJH63XZ Insertion of Vascular Access Device into Chest Subcutaneous Tissue and Fascia, Percutaneous Approach

Appendix L: Procedure Combination Tables

The tables below were developed to help simplify the relationship between ICD-10-PCS coding and MS-DRG assignment. The Centers for Medicare & Medicaid Services (CMS) has identified in the MS-DRG Definitions Manual certain procedure combinations that must occur in order to assign a specific MS-DRG. There are many factors influencing MS-DRG assignment, including principal and secondary diagnoses, MCC or CC use, sex of the patient, and discharge status. These tables should be used only as a guide. These tables were created based on the proposed, version 39, MS-DRG Grouper software and Definitions Manual files published with the fiscal 2022 IPPS proposed rule. To view the final, version 39, MS-DRG Grouper software and Definitions Manual files, refer to the following: https://www.cms.gov/Medicare/Medicare-Fee-for-Service-Payment/AcuteInpatientPPS/MS-DRG-Classifications-and-Software.

DRG ØØ1-ØØ2 Heart Transplant or Implant of Heart Assist System

Heart Transplant

Replacement of Right and Left Ventricle Ø2RKØJZ and Ø2RLØJZ

Insertion With Removal of Heart Assist System

Type of Heart Assist System	Code as appropriate Insertion by approach	Code also as appropriate Removal of Heart Assist System by approach
Biventricular External	Ø2HA[Ø,3,4]RS	Ø2PA[Ø,3,4]RZ
External	Ø2HA[Ø,4]RZ	Ø2PA[Ø,3,4]RZ

Revision With Removal of Heart Assist System

Type of Heart Assist System	Code as appropriate Revision by approach	Code also as appropriate Removal of Heart Assist System by approach
Implantable	Ø2WA[Ø,3,4]QZ	Ø2PA[Ø,3,4]RZ
External	Ø2WA[Ø,3,4]RZ	Ø2PA[Ø,3,4]RZ

DRG ØØ8 Simultaneous Pancreas/Kidney Transplant

Transplanted Body Part	Code Transplant as appropriate by tissue type			Code also Pancreas Transplant as appropriate by tissue type		
	Allogeneic	Syngeneic	Zooplastic	Allogeneic	Syngeneic	Zooplastic
Kidney, Right	ØTYØØZØ	ØTYØØZ1	ØTYØØZ2	ØFYGØZØ	ØFYGØZ1	ØFYGØZ2
Kidney, Left	ØTY1ØZØ	ØTY1ØZ1	ØTY1ØZ2			

DRG Ø19 Simultaneous Pancreas/Kidney Transplant with Hemodialysis

Transplanted Body Part	Code Transplant as appropriate by tissue type			Code also Pancreas Transplant as appropriate by tissue type			Code also Hemodialysis		
	Allogeneic	Syngeneic	Zooplastic	Allogeneic	Syngeneic	Zooplastic	< 6 Hours	6-18 Hours	> 18 Hours
Kidney, Right	ØTYØØZØ	ØTYØØZ1	ØTYØØZ2	ØFYGØZØ	ØFYGØZ1	ØFYGØZ2	5A1DØ7Z	5A1D8ØZ	5A1D9ØZ
Kidney, Left	ØTY1ØZØ	ØTY1ØZ1	ØTY1ØZ2						

DRG Ø23-Ø27 Craniotomy

Site of Neurostimulator Lead	Code as appropriate Insertion of Lead by approach	Code also as appropriate Insertion of Device by type and subcutaneous site						
		Neuro-stimulator Generator	Stimulator Multiple Array Code as appropriate by approach			Stimulator Multiple Array, Rechargeable Code as appropriate by approach		
		Skull	Chest	Back	Abdomen	Chest	Back	Abdomen
Brain	ØØHØ[Ø,3,4]MZ	ØNHØØNZ	ØJH6[Ø,3]DZ	ØJH7[Ø,3]DZ	ØJH8[Ø,3]DZ	ØJH6[Ø,3]EZ	ØJH7[Ø,3]EZ	ØJH8[Ø,3]EZ
Cerebral Ventricle	ØØH6[Ø,3,4]MZ	ØNHØØNZ	ØJH6[Ø,3]DZ	ØJH7[Ø,3]DZ	ØJH8[Ø,3]DZ	ØJH6[Ø,3]EZ	ØJH7[Ø,3]EZ	ØJH8[Ø,3]EZ

DRG Ø28-Ø3Ø Spinal Procedures

Generator Type	Insertion of Generator by Site			Code also as appropriate Insertion of Neurostimulator Lead by approach	
	Chest	Abdomen	Back	Spinal Canal	Spinal Cord
Single Array	ØJH6[Ø,3]BZ	ØJH8[Ø,3]BZ	ØJH7[Ø,3]BZ	ØØHU[Ø,3,4]MZ	ØØHV[Ø,3,4]MZ
Single Array, Rechargeable	ØJH6[Ø,3]CZ	ØJH8[Ø,3]CZ	ØJH7[Ø,3]CZ	ØØHU[Ø,3,4]MZ	ØØHV[Ø,3,4]MZ
Multiple Array	ØJH6[Ø,3]DZ	ØJH8[Ø,3]DZ	ØJH7[Ø,3]DZ	ØØHU[Ø,3,4]MZ	ØØHV[Ø,3,4]MZ
Multiple Array, Rechargable	ØJH6[Ø,3]EZ	—	ØJH7[Ø,3]EZ	ØØHU[Ø,3,4]MZ	ØØHV[Ø,3,4]MZ
Multiple Array, Rechargable	—	ØJH8[Ø,3]EZ	—	ØØHU[Ø,3,4]MZ	ØØHV[Ø,3,4]MZ

DRG Ø4Ø-Ø42 Peripheral and Cranial Nerve and Other Nervous System Procedures

Insertion of Neurostimulator Lead With Device

Site of Neurostimulator Lead	Code as appropriate Insertion by approach	Code also as appropriate Insertion of Device by type and subcutaneous site					
		Stimulator Single Array Code as appropriate by approach			Stimulator Single Array, Rechargeable Code as appropriate by approach		
		Chest	Back	Abdomen	Chest	Back	Abdomen
Cranial Nerve	ØØHE[Ø,3,4]MZ	ØJH6[Ø,3]BZ	ØJH7[Ø,3]BZ	ØJH8[Ø,3]BZ	ØJH6[Ø,3]CZ	ØJH7[Ø,3]CZ	ØJH8[Ø,3]CZ
Peripheral Nerve	Ø1HY[Ø,3,4]MZ	ØJH6[Ø,3]BZ	ØJH7[Ø,3]BZ	ØJH8[Ø,3]BZ	ØJH6[Ø,3]CZ	ØJH7[Ø,3]CZ	ØJH8[Ø,3]CZ
Stomach	ØDH6[Ø,3,4]MZ	ØJH6[Ø,3]BZ	ØJH7[Ø,3]BZ	ØJH8[Ø,3]BZ	ØJH6[Ø,3]CZ	ØJH7[Ø,3]CZ	ØJH8[Ø,3]CZ
Azygos vein	Ø5HØ[Ø,3,4]MZ	ØJH6[Ø,3]BZ	ØJH7[Ø,S]BZ	ØJH8[Ø,3]BZ	ØJH6[Ø,3]CZ	ØJH7[Ø,S]CZ	ØJH8[Ø,3]CZ
Innominate Vein, Right	Ø5H3[Ø,3,4]MZ	ØJH6[Ø,3]BZ	ØJH7[Ø,S]BZ	ØJH8[Ø,3]BZ	ØJH6[Ø,3]CZ	ØJH7[Ø,S]CZ	ØJH8[Ø,3]CZ
Innominate Vein, Left	Ø5H4[Ø,3,4]MZ	ØJH6[Ø,3]BZ	ØJH7[Ø,S]BZ	ØJH8[Ø,3]BZ	ØJH6[Ø,3]CZ	ØJH7[Ø,S]CZ	ØJH8[Ø,3]CZ
		Stimulator Multiple Array Code as appropriate by approach			Stimulator Multiple Array, Rechargeable Code as appropriate by approach		
		Chest	Back	Abdomen	Chest	Back	Abdomen
Cranial Nerve	ØØHE[Ø,3,4]MZ	ØJH6[Ø,3]DZ	ØJH7[Ø,3]DZ	ØJH8[Ø,3]DZ	ØJH6[Ø,3]EZ	ØJH7[Ø,3]EZ	ØJH8[Ø,3]EZ
Peripheral Nerve	Ø1HY[Ø,3,4]MZ	ØJH6[Ø,3]DZ	ØJH7[Ø,3]DZ	ØJH8[Ø,3]DZ	ØJH6[Ø,3]EZ	ØJH7[Ø,3]EZ	ØJH8[Ø,3]EZ
Stomach	ØDH6[Ø,3,4]MZ	ØJH6[Ø,3]DZ	ØJH7[Ø,3]DZ	ØJH8[Ø,3]DZ	ØJH6[Ø,3]EZ	ØJH7[Ø,3]EZ	ØJH8[Ø,3]EZ
Azygos vein	Ø5HØ[Ø,3,4]MZ	ØJH6[Ø,3]DZ	ØJH7[Ø,S]DZ	ØJH8[Ø,3]DZ	ØJH6[Ø,3]EZ	ØJH7[Ø,S]EZ	ØJH8[Ø,3]EZ
Innominate Vein, Right	Ø5H3[Ø,3,4]MZ	ØJH6[Ø,3]DZ	ØJH7[Ø,S]DZ	ØJH8[Ø,3]DZ	ØJH6[Ø,3]EZ	ØJH7[Ø,S]EZ	ØJH8[Ø,3]EZ
Innominate Vein, Left	Ø5H4[Ø,3,4]MZ	ØJH6[Ø,3]DZ	ØJH7[Ø,S]DZ	ØJH8[Ø,3]DZ	ØJH6[Ø,3]EZ	ØJH7[Ø,S]EZ	ØJH8[Ø,3]EZ

DRG 222-227 Cardiac Defibrillator Implant

Insertion of Generator With Insertion of Lead(s) into Coronary Vein, Atrium or Ventricle

Generator Type	Insertion of Generator by Site		Code also as appropriate Insertion of Leads by site				
			Coronary Vein	Atrium		Ventricle	
	Chest	Abdomen		Right	Left	Right	Left
Defibrillator	ØJH6[Ø,3]8Z	ØJH8[Ø,3]8Z	Ø2H4[Ø,4]KZ	Ø2H6[Ø,3,4]KZ	Ø2H7[Ø,3,4]KZ	Ø2HK[Ø,3,4]KZ	Ø2HL[Ø,3,4]KZ
Cardiac Resynch Defibrillator Pulse Generator	ØJH6[Ø,3]9Z	ØJH8[Ø,3]9Z	Ø2H4[Ø,3,4]KZ or Ø2H43[J,M]Z	Ø2H6[Ø,3,4]KZ	Ø2H7[Ø,3,4]KZ	Ø2HK[Ø,3,4]KZ	Ø2HL[Ø,3,4]KZ
Contractility Modulation Device	ØJH6[Ø,3]AZ	ØJH8[Ø,3]AZ	—	Ø2H6[Ø,3,4]MZ	—	Ø2HK[Ø,3,4]MZ	—

Insertion of Generator with Insertion of Lead(s) into Pericardium or Chest

Generator Type	Insertion of Generator by Site		Code also as appropriate Insertion of Leads by Site and Type			
			Pericardium			Chest
	Chest	Abdomen	Pacemaker	Defibrillator	Cardiac	Subcutaneous
Defibrillator	ØJH6[Ø,3]8Z	ØJH8[Ø,3]8Z	Ø2HN[Ø,3,4]JZ	Ø2HN[Ø,3,4]KZ	Ø2HN[Ø,3,4]MZ	ØJH6[Ø,3]FZ
Cardiac Resynch Defibrillator Pulse Generator	ØJH6[Ø,3]9Z	ØJH8[Ø,3]9Z	Ø2HN[Ø,3,4]JZ	Ø2HN[Ø,3,4]KZ	Ø2HN[Ø,3,4]MZ	ØJH6[Ø,3]FZ

DRG 242-244 Permanent Cardiac Pacemaker Implant

Insertion of Generator and Lead(s) Only

Generator Type	Insertion of Generator by Site		Code also as appropriate Insertion of Leads by site					
	Chest	Abdomen	Coronary Vein	Atrium		Ventricle		Pericardium
				Right	Left	Right	Left	
Single Chamber	ØJH6[Ø,3]4Z	ØJH8[Ø,3]4Z	Ø2H4[Ø,3,4][J,M]Z	Ø2H6[Ø,3,4][J,M]Z	Ø2H7[Ø,3,4][J,M]Z	Ø2HK[Ø,3,4][J,M]Z	Ø2HL[Ø,3,4][J,M]Z	Ø2HN[Ø,3,4][J,M]Z
Single Chamber RR	ØJH6[Ø,3]5Z	ØJH8[Ø,3]5Z	Ø2H4[Ø,3,4][J,M]Z	Ø2H6[Ø,3,4][J,M]Z	Ø2H7[Ø,3,4][J,M]Z	Ø2HK[Ø,3,4][J,M]Z	Ø2HL[Ø,3,4][J,M]Z	Ø2HN[Ø,3,4][J,M]Z
Dual Chamber	ØJH6[Ø,3]6Z	ØJH8[Ø,3]6Z	Ø2H4[Ø,3,4][J,M]Z	Ø2H6[Ø,3,4][J,M]Z	Ø2H7[Ø,3,4][J,M]Z	Ø2HK[Ø,3,4][J,M]Z	Ø2HL[Ø,3,4][J,M]Z	Ø2HN[Ø,3,4][J,M]Z
Cardiac Resynch Pulse Generator	ØJH6[Ø,3]7Z	ØJH8[Ø,3]7Z	Ø2H4[Ø,3,4][J,M]Z	Ø2H6[Ø,3,4][J,M]Z	Ø2H7[Ø,3,4][J,M]Z	Ø2HK[Ø,3,4][J,M]Z	Ø2HL[Ø,3,4][J,M]Z	Ø2HN[Ø,3,4][J,M]Z
Cardiac Rhythm Related	ØJH6[Ø,3]PZ	ØJH8[Ø,3]PZ	Ø2H4[Ø,3,4][J,M]Z	Ø2H6[Ø,3,4][J,M]Z	Ø2H7[Ø,3,4][J,M]Z	Ø2HK[Ø,3,4][J,M]Z	Ø2HL[Ø,3,4][J,M]Z	Ø2HN[Ø,3,4][J,M]Z

DRG 326-328 Stomach, Esophageal and Duodenal Procedures

Site	Resection by Open Approach	Code also as appropriate Resection of Pancreas by Open Approach
Duodenum	ØDT9ØZZ	ØFTGØZZ

DRG 344-346 Minor Small and Large Bowel Procedures

Site	Repair by Open Approach	Code also as appropriate Repair by external approach of Abdominal Wall Stoma
Small Intestine	ØDQ8ØZZ	ØWQFXZ2
Duodenum	ØDQ9ØZZ	ØWQFXZ2
Jejunum	ØDQAØZZ	ØWQFXZ2
Ileum	ØDQBØZZ	ØWQFXZ2
Large Intestine	ØDQEØZZ	ØWQFXZ2
Large Intestine, Right	ØDQFØZZ	ØWQFXZ2
Large Intestine, Left	ØDQGØZZ	ØWQFXZ2
Cecum	ØDQHØZZ	ØWQFXZ2
Ascending Colon	ØDQKØZZ	ØWQFXZ2
Transverse Colon	ØDQLØZZ	ØWQFXZ2
Descending Colon	ØDQMØZZ	ØWQFXZ2
Sigmoid Colon	ØDQNØZZ	ØWQFXZ2

DRG 456-458 Spinal Fusion Except Cervical with Spinal Curvature/Malignancy/ Infection or Extensive Fusions

Fusion of Thoracic and Lumbar Vertebra, Anterior Column

2 to 7 Thoracic Vertebra		Code also 2 or more Lumbar Vertebra	
ØRG[Ø,3,4][7,A,J,K]Ø	XRG7ØF3	ØSG1[Ø,3,4][7,A,J,K]Ø	XRGCØF3

Fusion of Thoracic and Lumbar Vertebra, Posterior Column

2 to 7 Thoracic Vertebra			Code also 2 or more Lumbar Vertebra		
Posterior Approach	Anterior Approach	New Technology	Posterior Approach	Anterior Approach	New Technology
ØRG7[Ø,3,4][7,J,K]1	ØRG7[Ø,3,4][7,A,J,K]J	XRG7Ø92 XRG7ØF3	ØSG1[Ø,3,4][7,J,K]1	ØSG1[Ø,3,4][7,A,J,K]J	XRGCØ92 XRGCØF3

DRG 461-462 Bilateral or Multiple Major Joint Procedures of Lower Extremity

For procedures to qualify as bilateral or multiple joint procedures, at least one replacement code or combination removal and replacement code from two different lower extremity sites from the following table(s) must be reported.

Examples: Left hip and right hip codes (bilateral); left hip and left knee codes (multiple); left hip and right ankle codes (multiple); left knee and right knee codes (bilateral); right hip removal and replacement, with right knee replacement

Hip, RT	Hip, LT	Knee, RT	Knee, LT	Ankle, RT	Ankle, LT
ØSR9Ø19	ØSRBØ19	ØSRCØ69	ØSRDØ69	ØSRFØ7Z	ØSRGØ7Z
ØSR9Ø1A	ØSRBØ1A	ØSRCØ6A	ØSRDØ6A	ØSRFØJ9	ØSRGØJ9
ØSR9Ø1Z	ØSRBØ1Z	ØSRCØ6Z	ØSRDØ6Z	ØSRFØJA	ØSRGØJA
ØSR9Ø29	ØSRBØ29	ØSRCØ7Z	ØSRDØ7Z	ØSRFØJZ	ØSRGØJZ
ØSR9Ø2A	ØSRBØ2A	ØSRCØJ9	ØSRDØJ9	ØSRFØKZ	ØSRGØKZ
ØSR9Ø2Z	ØSRBØ2Z	ØSRCØJA	ØSRDØJA		
ØSR9Ø39	ØSRBØ39	ØSRCØJZ	ØSRDØJZ		
ØSR9Ø3A	ØSRBØ3A	ØSRCØKZ	ØSRDØKZ		
ØSR9Ø3Z	ØSRBØ3Z	ØSRCØL9	ØSRDØL9		
ØSR9Ø49	ØSRBØ49	ØSRCØLA	ØSRDØLA		
ØSR9Ø4A	ØSRBØ4A	ØSRCØLZ	ØSRDØLZ		
ØSR9Ø4Z	ØSRBØ4Z	ØSRCØM9	ØSRDØM9		
ØSR9Ø69	ØSRBØ69	ØSRCØMA	ØSRDØMA		
ØSR9Ø6A	ØSRBØ6A	ØSRCØMZ	ØSRDØMZ		
ØSR9Ø6Z	ØSRBØ6Z	ØSRCØN9	ØSRDØN9		
ØSR9Ø7Z	ØSRBØ7Z	ØSRCØNA	ØSRDØNA		
ØSR9ØJ9	ØSRBØJ9	ØSRCØNZ	ØSRDØNZ		
ØSR9ØJA	ØSRBØJA	ØSRTØ7Z	ØSRUØ7Z		
ØSR9ØJZ	ØSRBØJZ	ØSRTØJ9	ØSRUØJ9		
ØSR9ØKZ	ØSRBØKZ	ØSRTØJA	ØSRUØJA		
ØSRAØØ9	ØSREØØ9	ØSRTØJZ	ØSRUØJZ		
ØSRAØØA	ØSREØØA	ØSRTØKZ	ØSRUØKZ		
ØSRAØØZ	ØSREØØZ	ØSRVØ7Z	ØSRWØ7Z		
ØSRAØ19	ØSREØ19	ØSRVØJ9	ØSRWØJ9		
ØSRAØ1A	ØSREØ1A	ØSRVØJA	ØSRWØJA		
ØSRAØ1Z	ØSREØ1Z	ØSRVØJZ	ØSRWØJZ		
ØSRAØ39	ØSREØ39	ØSRVØKZ	ØSRWØKZ		
ØSRAØ3A	ØSREØ3A	ØSPCØJZ	ØSPDØJZ		
ØSRAØ3Z	ØSREØ3Z				
ØSRAØ7Z	ØSREØ7Z				
ØSRAØJ9	ØSREØJ9				
ØSRAØJA	ØSREØJA				
ØSRAØJZ	ØSREØJZ				
ØSRAØKZ	ØSREØKZ				
ØSRRØ19	ØSRSØ19				
ØSRRØ1A	ØSRSØ1A				
ØSRRØ1Z	ØSRSØ1Z				
ØSRRØ39	ØSRSØ39				
ØSRRØ3A	ØSRSØ3A				
ØSRRØ3Z	ØSRSØ3Z				
ØSRRØ7Z	ØSRSØ7Z				
ØSRRØJ9	ØSRSØJ9				
ØSRRØJA	ØSRSØJA				
ØSRRØJZ	ØSRSØJZ				
ØSRRØKZ	ØSRSØKZ				
ØSU9ØBZ	ØSUBØBZ				
ØSUAØBZ	ØSUEØBZ				
ØSURØBZ	ØSUSØBZ				
ØSP9ØJZ	ØSPBØJZ				

Hip Procedure Combinations

Open Removal of Hip Spacer with Replacement

Removal of Spacer		Code also as appropriate Replacement by Device Type					
		Metal	Metal on Poly	Ceramic	Ceramic on Poly	Oxidized Zirc on Poly	Synth Subst
Hip, RT	ØSP9Ø8Z	ØSR9Ø1[9,A,Z]	ØSR9Ø2[9,A,Z]	ØSR9Ø3[9,A,Z]	ØSR9Ø4[9,A,Z]	ØSR9Ø6[9,A,Z]	ØSR9ØJ[9,A,Z]
Hip, LT	ØSPBØ8Z	ØSRBØ1[9,A,Z]	ØSRBØ2[9,A,Z]	ØSRBØ3[9,A,Z]	ØSRBØ4[9,A,Z]	ØSRBØ6[9,A,Z]	ØSRBØJ[9,A,Z]

Open Removal of Hip Spacer with Replacement

Removal of Spacer		Code also as appropriate Replacement by Device Type						
		Acetabular Surface				Femoral Surface		
		Poly	Metal	Ceramic	Synthetic	Metal	Ceramic	Synth
Hip, RT	ØSP9Ø8Z	ØSRAØØ[9,A,Z]	ØSRAØ1[9,A,Z]	ØSRAØ3[9,A,Z]	ØSRAØJ[9,A,Z]	ØSRRØ1[9,A,Z]	ØSRRØ3[9,A,Z]	ØSRRØJ[9,A,Z]
Hip, LT	ØSPBØ8Z	ØSREØØ[9,A,Z]	ØSREØ1[9,A,Z]	ØSREØ3[9,A,Z]	ØSREØJ[9,A,Z]	ØSRSØ1[9,A,Z]	ØSRSØ3[9,A,Z]	ØSRSØJ[9,A,Z]

Open Removal of Hip Liner with Replacement

Removal of Liner		Code also as appropriate Replacement by Device Type					
		Metal	Metal on Poly	Ceramic	Ceramic on Poly	Oxidized Zirc on Poly	Synth Subst
Hip, RT	ØSP9Ø9Z	ØSR9Ø1[9,A,Z]	ØSR9Ø2[9,A,Z]	ØSR9Ø3[9,A,Z]	ØSR9Ø4[9,A,Z]	ØSR9Ø6[9,A,Z]	ØSR9ØJ[9,A,Z]
Hip, LT	ØSPBØ9Z	ØSRBØ1[9,A,Z]	ØSRBØ2[9,A,Z]	ØSRBØ3[9,A,Z]	ØSRBØ4[9,A,Z]	ØSRBØ6[9,A,Z]	ØSRBØJ[9,A,Z]

Open Removal of Hip Liner with Replacement

Removal of Liner		Code also as appropriate Replacement by Device Type						
		Acetabular Surface				Femoral Surface		
		Poly	Metal	Ceramic	Synthetic	Metal	Ceramic	Synth
Hip, RT	ØSP9Ø9Z	ØSRAØØ[9,A,Z]	ØSRAØ1[9,A,Z]	ØSRAØ3[9,A,Z]	ØSRAØJ[9,A,Z]	ØSRRØ1[9,A,Z]	ØSRRØ3[9,A,Z]	ØSRRØJ[9,A,Z]
Hip, LT	ØSPBØ9Z	ØSREØØ[9,A,Z]	ØSREØ1[9,A,Z]	ØSREØ3[9,A,Z]	ØSREØJ[9,A,Z]	ØSRSØ1[9,A,Z]	ØSRSØ3[9,A,Z]	ØSRSØJ[9,A,Z]

Open Removal of Hip Resurfacing Device with Replacement

Removal of Resurfacing Device		Code also as appropriate Replacement by Device Type					
		Metal	Metal on Poly	Ceramic	Ceramic on Poly	Oxidized Zirc on Poly	Synth Subst
Hip, RT	ØSP9ØBZ	ØSR9Ø1[9,A,Z]	ØSR9Ø2[9,A,Z]	ØSR9Ø3[9,A,Z]	ØSR9Ø4[9,A,Z]	ØSR9Ø6[9,A,Z]	ØSR9ØJ[9,A,Z]
Hip, LT	ØSPBØBZ	ØSRBØ1[9,A,Z]	ØSRBØ2[9,A,Z]	ØSRBØ3[9,A,Z]	ØSRBØ4[9,A,Z]	ØSRBØ6[9,A,Z]	ØSRBØJ[9,A,Z]

Open Removal of Hip Resurfacing Device with Replacement

Removal of Resurfacing Device		Code also as appropriate Replacement by Device Type						
		Acetabular Surface				Femoral Surface		
		Poly	Metal	Ceramic	Synthetic	Metal	Ceramic	Synth
Hip, RT	ØSP9ØBZ	ØSRAØØ[9,A,Z]	ØSRAØ1[9,A,Z]	ØSRAØ3[9,A,Z]	ØSRAØJ[9,A,Z]	ØSRRØ1[9,A,Z]	ØSRRØ3[9,A,Z]	ØSRRØJ[9,A,Z]
Hip, LT	ØSPBØBZ	ØSREØØ[9,A,Z]	ØSREØ1[9,A,Z]	ØSREØ3[9,A,Z]	ØSREØJ[9,A,Z]	ØSRSØ1[9,A,Z]	ØSRSØ3[9,A,Z]	ØSRSØJ[9,A,Z]

Open Removal of Hip Articulating Spacer with Replacement

Removal of Articulating Spacer		Code also as appropriate Replacement by Device Type					
		Metal	Metal on Poly	Ceramic	Ceramic on Poly	Oxidized Zirc on Poly	Synth Subst
Hip, RT	ØSP9ØEZ	ØSR9Ø1[9,A,Z]	ØSR9Ø2[9,A,Z]	ØSR9Ø3[9,A,Z]	ØSR9Ø4[9,A,Z]	ØSR9Ø6[9,A,Z]	ØSR9ØJ[9,A,Z]
Hip, LT	ØSPBØEZ	ØSRBØ1[9,A,Z]	ØSRBØ2[9,A,Z]	ØSRBØ3[9,A,Z]	ØSRBØ4[9,A,Z]	ØSRBØ6[9,A,Z]	ØSRBØJ[9,A,Z]

Open Removal of Hip Articulating Spacer with Replacement

Removal of Articulating Spacer		Code also as appropriate Replacement by Device Type						
		Acetabular Surface				Femoral Surface		
		Poly	Metal	Ceramic	Synthetic	Metal	Ceramic	Synth
Hip, RT	ØSP9ØEZ	ØSRAØØ[9,A,Z]	ØSRAØ1[9,A,Z]	ØSRAØ3[9,A,Z]	ØSRAØJ[9,A,Z]	ØSRRØ1[9,A,Z]	ØSRRØ3[9,A,Z]	ØSRRØJ[9,A,Z]
Hip, LT	ØSPBØEZ	ØSREØØ[9,A,Z]	ØSREØ1[9,A,Z]	ØSREØ3[9,A,Z]	ØSREØJ[9,A,Z]	ØSRSØ1[9,A,Z]	ØSRSØ3[9,A,Z]	ØSRSØJ[9,A,Z]

Open Removal of Hip Synthetic Substitute with Replacement

Removal of Synthetic Substitute		Code also as appropriate Replacement by Device Type					
		Metal	Metal on Poly	Ceramic	Ceramic on Poly	Oxidized Zirc on Poly	Synth Subst
Hip, RT	ØSP[9,A,R]ØJZ	ØSR9Ø1[9,A,Z]	ØSR9Ø2[9,A,Z]	ØSR9Ø3[9,A,Z]	ØSR9Ø4[9,A,Z]	ØSR9Ø6[9,A,Z]	ØSR9ØJ[9,A,Z]
Hip, LT	ØSP[B,E,S]ØJZ	ØSRBØ1[9,A,Z]	ØSRBØ2[9,A,Z]	ØSRBØ3[9,A,Z]	ØSRBØ4[9,A,Z]	ØSRBØ6[9,A,Z]	ØSRBØJ[9,A,Z]

Open Removal of Hip Synthetic Substitute with Replacement

Removal of Synthetic Substitute		Code also as appropriate Replacement by Device Type						
		Acetabular Surface				Femoral Surface		
		Poly	Metal	Ceramic	Synthetic	Metal	Ceramic	Synth
Hip, RT	ØSP[9,A,R]ØJZ	ØSRAØØ[9,A,Z]	ØSRAØ1[9,A,Z]	ØSRAØ3[9,A,Z]	ØSRAØJ[9,A,Z]	ØSRRØ1[9,A,Z]	ØSRRØ3[9,A,Z]	ØSRRØJ[9,A,Z]
Hip, LT	ØSP[B,E,S]ØJZ	ØSREØØ[9,A,Z]	ØSREØ1[9,A,Z]	ØSREØ3[9,A,Z]	ØSREØJ[9,A,Z]	ØSRSØ1[9,A,Z]	ØSRSØ3[9,A,Z]	ØSRSØJ[9,A,Z]

Percutaneous Endoscopic Removal of Hip Spacer with Open Replacement

Removal of Spacer		Code also as appropriate Replacement by Device Type					
		Metal	Metal on Poly	Ceramic	Ceramic on Poly	Oxidized Zirc on Poly	Synth Subst
Hip, RT	ØSP948Z	ØSR9Ø1[9,A,Z]	ØSR9Ø2[9,A,Z]	ØSR9Ø3[9,A,Z]	ØSR9Ø4[9,A,Z]	ØSR9Ø6[9,A,Z]	ØSR9ØJ[9,A,Z]
Hip, LT	ØSPB48Z	ØSRBØ1[9,A,Z]	ØSRBØ2[9,A,Z]	ØSRBØ3[9,A,Z]	ØSRBØ4[9,A,Z]	ØSRBØ6[9,A,Z]	ØSRBØJ[9,A,Z]

Percutaneous Endoscopic Removal of Hip Spacer with Open Replacement

Removal of Spacer		Code also as appropriate Replacement by Device Type						
		Acetabular Surface				Femoral Surface		
		Poly	Metal	Ceramic	Synthetic	Metal	Ceramic	Synth
Hip, RT	ØSP948Z	ØSRAØØ[9,A,Z]	ØSRAØ1[9,A,Z]	ØSRAØ3[9,A,Z]	ØSRAØJ[9,A,Z]	ØSRRØ1[9,A,Z]	ØSRRØ3[9,A,Z]	ØSRRØJ[9,A,Z]
Hip, LT	ØSPB48Z	ØSREØØ[9,A,Z]	ØSREØ1[9,A,Z]	ØSREØ3[9,A,Z]	ØSREØJ[9,A,Z]	ØSRSØ1[9,A,Z]	ØSRSØ3[9,A,Z]	ØSRSØJ[9,A,Z]

Percutaneous Endoscopic Removal of Hip Synthetic Substitute with Open Replacement

Removal of Synthetic Substitute		Code also as appropriate Replacement by Device Type					
		Metal	Metal on Poly	Ceramic	Ceramic on Poly	Oxidized Zirc on Poly	Synth Subst
Hip, RT	ØSP[9,A,R]4JZ	ØSR9Ø1[9,A,Z]	ØSR9Ø2[9,A,Z]	ØSR9Ø3[9,A,Z]	ØSR9Ø4[9,A,Z]	ØSR9Ø6[9,A,Z]	ØSR9ØJ[9,A,Z]
Hip, LT	ØSP[B,E,S]4JZ	ØSRBØ1[9,A,Z]	ØSRBØ2[9,A,Z]	ØSRBØ3[9,A,Z]	ØSRBØ4[9,A,Z]	ØSRBØ6[9,A,Z]	ØSRBØJ[9,A,Z]

Percutaneous Endoscopic Removal of Hip Synthetic Substitute with Open Replacement

Removal of Synthetic Substitute		Code also as appropriate Replacement by Device Type						
		Acetabular Surface				Femoral Surface		
		Poly	Metal	Ceramic	Synthetic	Metal	Ceramic	Synth
Hip, RT	ØSP[9,A,R]4JZ	ØSRAØØ[9,A,Z]	ØSRAØ1[9,A,Z]	ØSRAØ3[9,A,Z]	ØSRAØJ[9,A,Z]	ØSRRØ1[9,A,Z]	ØSRRØ3[9,A,Z]	ØSRRØJ[9,A,Z]
Hip, LT	ØSP[B,E,S]4JZ	ØSREØØ[9,A,Z]	ØSREØ1[9,A,Z]	ØSREØ3[9,A,Z]	ØSREØJ[9,A,Z]	ØSRSØ1[9,A,Z]	ØSRSØ3[9,A,Z]	ØSRSØJ[9,A,Z]

Knee Procedure Combinations

Open Removal of Knee Spacer with Synthetic Substitute Replacement

Removal of Spacer		Code also as appropriate Replacement by Type of Synthetic Substitute				
		Oxidized Zircon on Poly	Synth Subst	Patello-femoral	Femoral Surface	Tibial Surface
Knee, RT	ØSPCØ8Z	ØSRCØ6[9,A,Z]	ØSRCØJ[9,A,Z]	ØSRCØN[9,A,Z]	ØSRTØJ[9,A,Z]	ØSRVØJ[9,A,Z]
Knee, LT	ØSPDØ8Z	ØSRDØ6[9,A,Z]	ØSRDØJ[9,A,Z]	ØSRDØN[9,A,Z]	ØSRUØJ[9,A,Z]	ØSRWØJ[9,A,Z]

Open Removal of Knee Liner with Synthetic Substitute Replacement

Removal of Liner		Code also as appropriate Replacement by Type of Synthetic Substitute						
		Oxidized Zircon on Poly	Synth Subst	Medial Unicondylar	Lateral Unicondylar	Patello-femoral	Femoral Surface	Tibial Surface
Knee, RT	ØSPCØ9Z	ØSRCØ6[9,A,Z]	ØSRCØJ[9,A,Z]	ØSRCØL[9,A,Z]	ØSRCØM[9,A,Z]	ØSRCØN[9,A,Z]	ØSRTØJ[9,A,Z]	ØSRVØJ[9,A,Z]
Knee, LT	ØSPDØ9Z	ØSRDØ6[9,A,Z]	ØSRDØJ[9,A,Z]	ØSRDØL[9,A,Z]	ØSRDØM[9,A,Z]	ØSRDØN[9,A,Z]	ØSRUØJ[9,A,Z]	ØSRWØJ[9,A,Z]

Open Removal of Knee Articulating Spacer with Synthetic Substitute Replacement

Removal of Articulating Spacer		Code also as appropriate Replacement by Type of Synthetic Substitute			
		Oxidized Zircon on Poly	Synth Subst	Femoral Surface	Tibial Surface
Knee, RT	ØSPCØEZ	ØSRCØ6[9,A,Z]	ØSRCØJ[9,A,Z]	ØSRTØJ[9,A,Z]	ØSRVØJ[9,A,Z]
Knee, LT	ØSPØDØEZ	ØSRDØ6[9,A,Z]	ØSRDØJ[9,A,Z]	ØSRUØJ[9,A,Z]	ØSRWØJ[9,A,Z]

Open Removal of Patellar Surface of Knee with Synthetic Substitute Replacement

Removal of Patellar Surface		Code also as appropriate Replacement by Type of Synthetic Substitute				
		Oxidized Zircon on Poly	Synth Subst	Patello-femoral	Femoral Surface	Tibial Surface
Knee, RT	ØSPCØJC	ØSRCØ6[9,A,Z]	ØSRCØJ[9,A,Z]	ØSRCØN[9,A,Z]	ØSRTØJ[9,A,Z]	ØSRVØJ[9,A,Z]
Knee, LT	ØSPDØJC	ØSRDØ6[9,A,Z]	ØSRDØJ[9,A,Z]	ØSRDØN[9,A,Z]	ØSRUØJ[9,A,Z]	ØSRWØJ[9,A,Z]

Open Removal of Knee Synthetic Substitute with Synthetic Substitute Replacement

Removal of Synthetic Substitute		Code also as appropriate Replacement by Type of Synthetic Substitute						
		Oxidized Zircon on Poly	Synth Subst	Medial Unicondylar	Lateral Unicondylar	Patello-femoral	Femoral Surface	Tibial Surface
Knee, RT	ØSPCØJZ	ØSRCØ6[9,A,Z]	ØSRCØJ[9,A,Z]	ØSRCØL[9,A,Z]	ØSRCØM[9,A,Z]	ØSRCØN[9,A,Z]	ØSRTØJ[9,A,Z]	ØSRVØJ[9,A,Z]
Knee, LT	ØSPDØJZ	ØSRDØ6[9,A,Z]	ØSRDØJ[9,A,Z]	ØSRDØL[9,A,Z]	ØSRDØM[9,A,Z]	ØSRDØN[9,A,Z]	ØSRUØJ[9,A,Z]	ØSRWØJ[9,A,Z]

Open Removal of Medial or Lateral Unicondylar Knee with Synthetic Substitute Replacement

Removal of Medial/Lateral Unicondylar Knee		Code also as appropriate Replacement by Type of Synthetic Substitute				
		Oxidized Zircon on Poly	Synth Subst	Medial Unicondylar	Femoral Surface	Tibial Surface
Knee, RT	ØSPCØ[L,M]Z	ØSRCØ6[9,A,Z]	ØSRCØJ[9,A,Z]	ØSRCØL[9,A,Z]	ØSRTØJ[9,A,Z]	ØSRVØJ[9,A,Z]
Knee, LT	ØSPDØ[L,M]Z	ØSRDØ6[9,A,Z]	ØSRDØJ[9,A,Z]	ØSRDØL[9,A,Z]	ØSRUØJ[9,A,Z]	ØSRWØJ[9,A,Z]

Open Removal of Patellofemoral Knee with Synthetic Substitute Replacement

Removal of Patellofemoral Knee		Code also as appropriate Replacement by Type of Synthetic Substitute				
		Oxidized Zircon on Poly	Synth Subst	Medial Unicondylar	Femoral Surface	Tibial Surface
Knee, RT	ØSPCØNZ	ØSRCØ6[9,A,Z]	ØSRCØJ[9,A,Z]	ØSRCØL[9,A,Z]	ØSRTØJ[9,A,Z]	ØSRVØJ[9,A,Z]
Knee, LT	ØSPDØNZ	ØSRDØ6[9,A,Z]	ØSRDØJ[9,A,Z]	ØSRDØL[9,A,Z]	ØSRUØJ[9,A,Z]	ØSRWØJ[9,A,Z]

Open Removal of Femoral/Tibial Surface of Knee with Synthetic Substitute Replacement

Removal of Femoral/Tibial Surface of Knee		Code also as appropriate Replacement by Type of Synthetic Substitute					
		Oxidized Zircon on Poly	Synth Subst	Articulating Spacer	Patello-femoral	Femoral Surface	Tibial Surface
Knee, RT	ØSP[T,V]ØJZ	ØSRCØ6[9,A,Z]	ØSRCØJ[9,A,Z]	ØSRCØEZ	ØSRCØN[9,A,Z]	ØSRTØJ[9,A,Z]	ØSRVØJ[9,A,Z]
Knee, LT	ØSP[U,W]ØJZ	ØSRDØ6[9,A,Z]	ØSRDØJ[9,A,Z]	ØSRDØEZ	ØSRDØN[9,A,Z]	ØSRUØJ[9,A,Z]	ØSRWØJ[9,A,Z]

Percutaneous/Percutaneous Endoscopic Removal of Knee Spacer with Open Synthetic Substitute Replacement

Removal of Spacer		Code also as appropriate Replacement by Type of Synthetic Substitute				
		Oxidized Zircon on Poly	Synth Subst	Patello-femoral	Femoral Surface	Tibial Surface
Knee, RT	ØSPC[3,4]8Z	ØSRCØ6[9,A,Z]	ØSRCØJ[9,A,Z]	ØSRCØN[9,A,Z]	ØSRTØJ[9,A,Z]	ØSRVØJ[9,A,Z]
Knee, LT	ØSPD[3,4]8Z	ØSRDØ6[9,A,Z]	ØSRDØJ[9,A,Z]	ØSRDØN[9,A,Z]	ØSRUØJ[9,A,Z]	ØSRWØJ[9,A,Z]

Percutaneous Endoscopic Removal of Patellar Surface of Knee with Synthetic Substitute Replacement

Removal of Patellar Surface		Code also as appropriate Replacement by Type of Synthetic Substitute				
		Oxidized Zircon on Poly	Synth Subst	Patello-femoral	Femoral Surface	Tibial Surface
Knee, RT	ØSPC4JC	ØSRCØ6[9,A,Z]	ØSRCØJ[9,A,Z]	ØSRCØN[9,A,Z]	ØSRTØJ[9,A,Z]	ØSRVØJ[9,A,Z]
Knee, LT	ØSPD4JC	ØSRDØ6[9,A,Z]	ØSRDØJ[9,A,Z]	ØSRDØN[9,A,Z]	ØSRUØJ[9,A]	ØSRWØJ[9,A,Z]

Percutaneous Endoscopic Removal of Knee Synthetic Substitute with Synthetic Substitute Replacement

Removal of Synthetic Substitute		Code also as appropriate Replacement by Type of Synthetic Substitute						
		Oxidized Zircon on Poly	Synth Subst	Medial Unicondylar	Lateral Unicondylar	Patello-femoral	Femoral Surface	Tibial Surface
Knee, RT	ØSPC4JZ	ØSRCØ6[9,A,Z]	ØSRCØJ[9,A,Z]	ØSRCØL[9,A,Z]	ØSRCØM[9,A,Z]	ØSRCØN[9,A,Z]	ØSRTØJ[9,A,Z]	ØSRVØJ[9,A,Z]
Knee, LT	ØSPD4JZ	ØSRDØ6[9,A,Z]	ØSRDØJ[9,A,Z]	ØSRDØL[9,A,Z]	ØSRDØM[9,A,Z]	ØSRDØN[9,A,Z]	ØSRUØJ[9,A,Z]	ØSRWØJ[9,A,Z]

Percutaneous Endoscopic Removal of Medial or Lateral Unicondylar Knee with Synthetic Substitute Replacement

Removal of Medial/Lateral Unicondylar Knee		Code also as appropriate Replacement by Type of Synthetic Substitute				
		Oxidized Zircon on Poly	Synth Subst	Medial Unicondylar	Femoral Surface	Tibial Surface
Knee, RT	ØSPC4[L,M]Z	ØSRCØ6[9,A,Z]	ØSRCØJ[9,A,Z]	ØSRCØL[9,A,Z]	ØSRTØJ[9,A,Z]	ØSRVØJ[9,A,Z]
Knee, LT	ØSPD4[L,M]Z	ØSRDØ6[9,A,Z]	ØSRDØJ[9,A,Z]	ØSRDØL[9,A,Z]	ØSRUØJ[9,A,Z]	ØSRWØJ[9,A,Z]

Percutaneous Endoscopic Removal of Patellofemoral Knee with Synthetic Substitute Replacement

Removal of Patellofemoral Knee		Code also as appropriate Replacement by Type of Synthetic Substitute				
		Oxidized Zircon on Poly	Synth Subst	Medial Unicondylar	Femoral Surface	Tibial Surface
Knee, RT	ØSPC4NZ	ØSRCØ6[9,A,Z]	ØSRCØJ[9,A,Z]	ØSRCØL[9,A,Z]	ØSRTØJ[9,A,Z]	ØSRVØJ[9,A,Z]
Knee, LT	ØSPD4NZ	ØSRDØ6[9,A,Z]	ØSRDØJ[9,A,Z]	ØSRDØL[9,A,Z]	ØSRUØJ[9,A,Z]	ØSRWØJ[9,A,Z]

Percutaneous Endoscopic Removal of Femoral/Tibial Surface of Knee with Synthetic Substitute Replacement

Removal of Femoral/Tibial Surface of Knee		Code also as appropriate Replacement by Type of Synthetic Substitute					
		Oxidized Zircon on Poly	Synth Subst	Articulating Spacer	Patello-femoral	Femoral Surface	Tibial Surface
Knee, RT	ØSP[T,V]4JZ	ØSRCØ6[9,A,Z]	ØSRCØJ[9,A,Z]	ØSRCØEZ	ØSRCØN[9,A,Z]	ØSRTØJ[9,A,Z]	ØSRVØJ[9,A,Z]
Knee, LT	ØSP[U,W]4JZ	ØSRDØ6[9,A,Z]	ØSRDØJ[9,A,Z]	ØSRDØEZ	ØSRDØN[9,A,Z]	ØSRUØJ[9,A,Z]	ØSRWØJ[9,A,Z]

466-468 Revision of Hip or Knee Replacement

Hip Procedures

Open Removal of Hip Spacer with Replacement

Removal of Spacer		Code also as appropriate Replacement by Device Type						
		Metal	Metal on Poly	Ceramic	Ceramic on Poly	Oxidized Zirc on Poly	Articulating Spacer	Synth Subst
Hip, RT	ØSP9Ø8Z	ØSR9Ø1[9,A,Z]	ØSR9Ø2[9,A,Z]	ØSR9Ø3[9,A,Z]	ØSR9Ø4[9,A,Z]	ØSR9Ø6[9,A,Z]	ØSR9ØEZ	ØSR9ØJ[9,A,Z]
Hip, LT	ØSPBØ8Z	ØSRBØ1[9,A,Z]	ØSRBØ2[9,A,Z]	ØSRBØ3[9,A,Z]	ØSRBØ4[9,A,Z]	ØSRBØ6[9,A,Z]	ØSRBØEZ	ØSRBØJ[9,A,Z]

Open Removal of Hip Spacer with Replacement

Removal of Spacer		Code also as appropriate Replacement by Device Type						
		Acetabular Surface				Femoral Surface		
		Poly	Metal	Ceramic	Synthetic	Metal	Ceramic	Synth
Hip, RT	ØSP9Ø8Z	ØSRAØØ[9,A,Z]	ØSRAØ1[9,A,Z]	ØSRAØ3[9,A,Z]	ØSRAØJ[9,A,Z]	ØSRRØ1[9,A,Z]	ØSRRØ3[9,A,Z]	ØSRRØJ[9,A,Z]
Hip, LT	ØSPBØ8Z	ØSREØØ[9,A,Z]	ØSREØ1[9,A,Z]	ØSREØ3[9,A,Z]	ØSREØJ[9,A,Z]	ØSRSØ1[9,A,Z]	ØSRSØ3[9,A,Z]	ØSRSØJ[9,A,Z]

Open Removal of Hip Spacer with Liner Insertion (supplement)

Removal of Spacer		Code also as appropriate Supplement of Body Part by Site		
		Joint	Acetabular Surface	Femoral Surface
Hip, RT	ØSP9Ø8Z	ØSU9Ø9Z	ØSUAØ9Z	ØSURØ9Z
Hip, LT	ØSPBØ8Z	ØSUBØ9Z	ØSUEØ9Z	ØSUSØ9Z

Open Removal of Hip Liner with Replacement

Removal of Liner		Code also as appropriate Replacement by Device Type						
		Metal	Metal on Poly	Ceramic	Ceramic on Poly	Oxidized Zirc on Poly	Articulating Spacer	Synth Subst
Hip, RT	ØSP9Ø9Z	ØSR9Ø1[9,A,Z]	ØSR9Ø2[9,A,Z]	ØSR9Ø3[9,A,Z]	ØSR9Ø4[9,A,Z]	ØSR9Ø6[9,A,Z]	ØSR9ØEZ	ØSR9ØJ[9,A,Z]
Hip, LT	ØSPBØ9Z	ØSRBØ1[9,A,Z]	ØSRBØ2[9,A,Z]	ØSRBØ3[9,A,Z]	ØSRBØ4[9,A,Z]	ØSRBØ6[9,A,Z]	ØSRBØEZ	ØSRBØJ[9,A,Z]

Open Removal of Hip Liner with Replacement

Removal of Liner		Code also as appropriate Replacement by Device Type						
		Acetabular Surface				Femoral Surface		
		Poly	Metal	Ceramic	Synthetic	Metal	Ceramic	Synth
Hip, RT	ØSP9Ø9Z	ØSRAØØ[9,A,Z]	ØSRAØ1[9,A,Z]	ØSRAØ3[9,A,Z]	ØSRAØJ[9,A,Z]	ØSRRØ1[9,A,Z]	ØSRRØ3[9,A,Z]	ØSRRØJ[9,A,Z]
Hip, LT	ØSPBØ9Z	ØSREØØ[9,A,Z]	ØSREØ1[9,A,Z]	ØSREØ3[9,A,Z]	ØSREØJ[9,A,Z]	ØSRSØ1[9,A,Z]	ØSRSØ3[9,A,Z]	ØSRSØJ[9,A,Z]

Open Removal of Hip Liner with Liner Insertion (supplement)

Removal of Liner		Code also as appropriate Supplement of Body Part by Site		
		Joint	Acetabular Surface	Femoral Surface
Hip, RT	ØSP9Ø9Z	ØSU9Ø9Z	ØSUAØ9Z	ØSURØ9Z
Hip, LT	ØSPBØ9Z	ØSUBØ9Z	ØSUEØ9Z	ØSUSØ9Z

Open Removal of Hip Resurfacing Device with Replacement

Removal of Resurfacing Device		Code also as appropriate Replacement by Device Type						
		Metal	Metal on Poly	Ceramic	Ceramic on Poly	Oxidized Zirc on Poly	Articulating Spacer	Synth Subst
Hip, RT	ØSP9ØBZ	ØSR9Ø1[9,A,Z]	ØSR9Ø2[9,A,Z]	ØSR9Ø3[9,A,Z]	ØSR9Ø4[9,A,Z]	ØSR9Ø6[9,A,Z]	ØSR9ØEZ	ØSR9ØJ[9,A,Z]
Hip, LT	ØSPBØBZ	ØSRBØ1[9,A,Z]	ØSRBØ2[9,A,Z]	ØSRBØ3[9,A,Z]	ØSRBØ4[9,A,Z]	ØSRBØ6[9,A,Z]	ØSRBØEZ	ØSRBØJ[9,A,Z]

Open Removal of Hip Resurfacing Device with Replacement

Removal of Resurfacing Device		Code also as appropriate Replacement by Device Type						
		Acetabular Surface				Femoral Surface		
		Poly	Metal	Ceramic	Synthetic	Metal	Ceramic	Synth
Hip, RT	ØSP9ØBZ	ØSRAØØ[9,A,Z]	ØSRAØ1[9,A,Z]	ØSRAØ3[9,A,Z]	ØSRAØJ[9,A,Z]	ØSRRØ1[9,A,Z]	ØSRRØ3[9,A,Z]	ØSRRØJ[9,A,Z]
Hip, LT	ØSPBØBZ	ØSREØØ[9,A,Z]	ØSREØ1[9,A,Z]	ØSREØ3[9,A,Z]	ØSREØJ[9,A,Z]	ØSRSØ1[9,A,Z]	ØSRSØ3[9,A,Z]	ØSRSØJ[9,A,Z]

Open Removal of Hip Resurfacing Device with Liner Insertion (supplement)

Removal of Resurfacing Device		Code also as appropriate Supplement of Body Part by Site		
		Joint	Acetabular Surface	Femoral Surface
Hip, RT	ØSP9ØBZ	ØSU9Ø9Z	ØSUAØ9Z	ØSURØ9Z
Hip, LT	ØSPBØBZ	ØSUBØ9Z	ØSUEØ9Z	ØSUSØ9Z

Open Removal of Hip Articulating Spacer with Replacement

Removal of Articulating Spacer		Code also as appropriate Replacement by Device Type					
		Metal	Metal on Poly	Ceramic	Ceramic on Poly	Oxidized Zirc on Poly	Synth Subst
Hip, RT	ØSP9ØEZ	ØSR9Ø1[9,A,Z]	ØSR9Ø2[9,A,Z]	ØSR9Ø3[9,A,Z]	ØSR9Ø4[9,A,Z]	ØSR9Ø6[9,A,Z]	ØSR9ØJ[9,A,Z]
Hip, LT	ØSPBØEZ	ØSRBØ1[9,A,Z]	ØSRBØ2[9,A,Z]	ØSRBØ3[9,A,Z]	ØSRBØ4[9,A,Z]	ØSRBØ6[9,A,Z]	ØSRBØJ[9,A,Z]

Open Removal of Hip Articulating Spacer with Replacement

Removal of Articulating Spacer		Code also as appropriate Replacement by Device Type						
		Acetabular Surface				Femoral Surface		
		Poly	Metal	Ceramic	Synthetic	Metal	Ceramic	Synth
Hip, RT	ØSP9ØEZ	ØSRAØØ[9,A,Z]	ØSRAØ1[9,A,Z]	ØSRAØ3[9,A,Z]	ØSRAØJ[9,A,Z]	ØSRRØ1[9,A,Z]	ØSRRØ3[9,A,Z]	ØSRRØJ[9,A,Z]
Hip, LT	ØSPBØEZ	ØSREØØ[9,A,Z]	ØSREØ1[9,A,Z]	ØSREØ3[9,A,Z]	ØSREØJ[9,A,Z]	ØSRSØ1[9,A,Z]	ØSRSØ3[9,A,Z]	ØSRSØJ[9,A,Z]

Open Removal of Hip Articulating Spacer with Liner Insertion (supplement)

Removal of Articulating Spacer		Code also as appropriate Supplement of Body Part by Site		
		Joint	Acetabular Surface	Femoral Surface
Hip, RT	ØSP9ØEZ	ØSU9Ø9Z	ØSUAØ9Z	ØSURØ9Z
Hip, LT	ØSPBØEZ	ØSUBØ9Z	ØSUEØ9Z	ØSUSØ9Z

Open Removal of Hip Synthetic Substitute with Replacement

Removal of Synthetic Substitute		Code also as appropriate Replacement by Device Type						
		Metal	Metal on Poly	Ceramic	Ceramic on Poly	Oxidized Zirc on Poly	Articulating Spacer	Synth Subst
Hip, RT	ØSP[9,A,R]ØJZ	ØSR9Ø1[9,A,Z]	ØSR9Ø2[9,A,Z]	ØSR9Ø3[9,A,Z]	ØSR9Ø4[9,A,Z]	ØSR9Ø6[9,A,Z]	ØSR9ØEZ	ØSR9ØJ[9,A,Z]
Hip, LT	ØSP[B,E,S]ØJZ	ØSRBØ1[9,A,Z]	ØSRBØ2[9,A,Z]	ØSRBØ3[9,A,Z]	ØSRBØ4[9,A,Z]	ØSRBØ6[9,A,Z]	ØSRBØEZ	ØSRBØJ[9,A,Z]

Open Removal of Hip Synthetic Substitute with Replacement

Removal of Synthetic Substitute		Code also as appropriate Replacement by Device Type						
		Acetabular Surface				Femoral Surface		
		Poly	Metal	Ceramic	Synthetic	Metal	Ceramic	Synth
Hip, RT	ØSP[9,A,R]ØJZ	ØSRAØØ[9,A,Z]	ØSRAØ1[9,A,Z]	ØSRAØ3[9,A,Z]	ØSRAØJ[9,A,Z]	ØSRRØ1[9,A,Z]	ØSRRØ3[9,A,Z]	ØSRRØJ[9,A,Z]
Hip, LT	ØSP[B,E,S]ØJZ	ØSREØØ[9,A,Z]	ØSREØ1[9,A,Z]	ØSREØ3[9,A,Z]	ØSREØJ[9,A,Z]	ØSRSØ1[9,A,Z]	ØSRSØ3[9,A,Z]	ØSRSØJ[9,A,Z]

Percutaneous Endoscopic Removal of Hip Spacer with Open Replacement

Removal of Spacer		Code also as appropriate Replacement by Device Type						
		Metal	Metal on Poly	Ceramic	Ceramic on Poly	Oxidized Zirc on Poly	Articulating Spacer	Synth Subst
Hip, RT	ØSP948Z	ØSR9Ø1[9,A,Z]	ØSR9Ø2[9,A,Z]	ØSR9Ø3[9,A,Z]	ØSR9Ø4[9,A,Z]	ØSR9Ø6[9,A,Z]	ØSR9ØEZ	ØSR9ØJ[9,A,Z]
Hip, LT	ØSPB48Z	ØSRBØ1[9,A,Z]	ØSRBØ2[9,A,Z]	ØSRBØ3[9,A,Z]	ØSRBØ4[9,A,Z]	ØSRBØ6[9,A,Z]	ØSRBØEZ	ØSRBØJ[9,A,Z]

Percutaneous Endoscopic Removal of Hip Spacer with Open Replacement

Removal of Spacer		Code also as appropriate Replacement by Device Type						
		Acetabular Surface				Femoral Surface		
		Poly	Metal	Ceramic	Synthetic	Metal	Ceramic	Synth
Hip, RT	ØSP948Z	ØSRAØØ[9,A,Z]	ØSRAØ1[9,A,Z]	ØSRAØ3[9,A,Z]	ØSRAØJ[9,A,Z]	ØSRRØ1[9,A,Z]	ØSRRØ3[9,A,Z]	ØSRRØJ[9,A,Z]
Hip, LT	ØSPB48Z	ØSREØØ[9,A,Z]	ØSREØ1[9,A,Z]	ØSREØ3[9,A,Z]	ØSREØJ[9,A,Z]	ØSRSØ1[9,A,Z]	ØSRSØ3[9,A,Z]	ØSRSØJ[9,A,Z]

Percutaneous Endoscopic Removal of Hip Spacer with Open Liner Insertion (supplement)

Removal of Spacer		Code also as appropriate Supplement of Body Part by Site		
		Joint	Acetabular Surface	Femoral Surface
Hip, RT	ØSP948Z	ØSU9Ø9Z	ØSUAØ9Z	ØSURØ9Z
Hip, LT	ØSPB48Z	ØSUBØ9Z	ØSUEØ9Z	ØSUSØ9Z

Percutaneous Endoscopic Removal of Hip Synthetic Substitute with Open Replacement

Removal of Synthetic Substitute		Code also as appropriate Replacement by Device Type						
		Metal	Metal on Poly	Ceramic	Ceramic on Poly	Oxidized Zirc on Poly	Articulating Spacer	Synth Subst
Hip, RT	ØSP[9,A,R]4JZ	ØSR9Ø1[9,A,Z]	ØSR9Ø2[9,A,Z]	ØSR9Ø3[9,A,Z]	ØSR9Ø4[9,A,Z]	ØSR9Ø6[9,A,Z]	ØSR9ØEZ	ØSR9ØJ[9,A,Z]
Hip, LT	ØSP[B,E,S]4JZ	ØSRBØ1[9,A,Z]	ØSRBØ2[9,A,Z]	ØSRBØ3[9,A,Z]	ØSRBØ4[9,A,Z]	ØSRBØ6[9,A,Z]	ØSRBØEZ	ØSRBØJ[9,A,Z]

Percutaneous Endoscopic Removal of Hip Synthetic Substitute with Open Replacement

Removal of Synthetic Substitute		Code also as appropriate Replacement by Device Type						
		Acetabular Surface				Femoral Surface		
		Poly	Metal	Ceramic	Synthetic	Metal	Ceramic	Synth
Hip, RT	ØSP[9,A,R]4JZ	ØSRAØØ[9,A,Z]	ØSRAØ1[9,A,Z]	ØSRAØ3[9,A,Z]	ØSRAØJ[9,A,Z]	ØSRRØ1[9,A,Z]	ØSRRØ3[9,A,Z]	ØSRRØJ[9,A,Z]
Hip, LT	ØSP[B,E,S]4JZ	ØSREØØ[9,A,Z]	ØSREØ1[9,A,Z]	ØSREØ3[9,A,Z]	ØSREØJ[9,A,Z]	ØSRSØ1[9,A,Z]	ØSRSØ3[9,A,Z]	ØSRSØJ[9,A,Z]

Percutaneous Endoscopic Removal of Hip Synthetic Substitute with Open Liner Insertion (supplement)

Removal of Synthetic Substitute		Code also as appropriate Supplement of Body Part by Site		
		Joint	Acetabular Surface	Femoral Surface
Hip, RT	ØSP[9,A,R]4JZ	ØSU9Ø9Z	ØSUAØ9Z	ØSURØ9Z
Hip, LT	ØSP[B,E,S]4JZ	ØSUBØ9Z	ØSUEØ9Z	ØSUSØ9Z

Knee Procedures

Open Removal of Knee Spacer with Articulating Spacer Replacement

Removal of Spacer		Code also as appropriate Replacement with Articulating Spacer
Knee, RT	ØSPCØ8Z	ØSRCØEZ
Knee, LT	ØSPDØ8Z	ØSRDØEZ

Open Removal of Knee Spacer with Synthetic Substitute Replacement

Removal of Spacer		Code also as appropriate Replacement by Type of Synthetic Substitute				
		Oxidized Zircon on Poly	Synth Subst	Patello-femoral	Femoral Surface	Tibial Surface
Knee, RT	ØSPCØ8Z	ØSRCØ6[9,A,Z]	ØSRCØJ[9,A,Z]	ØSRCØN[9,A,Z]	ØSRTØJ[9,A,Z]	ØSRVØJ[9,A,Z]
Knee, LT	ØSPDØ8Z	ØSRDØ6[9,A,Z]	ØSRDØJ[9,A,Z]	ØSRDØN[9,A,Z]	ØSRUØJ[9,A,Z]	ØSRWØJ[9,A,Z]

Open Removal of Knee Liner with Articulating Spacer Replacement

Removal of Liner		Code also as appropriate Replacement with Articulating Spacer
Knee, RT	ØSPCØ9Z	ØSRCØEZ
Knee, LT	ØSPDØ9Z	ØSRDØEZ

Open Removal of Knee Liner with Synthetic Substitute Replacement

Removal of Liner		Code also as appropriate Replacement by Type of Synthetic Substitute						
		Oxidized Zircon on Poly	Synth Subst	Medial Unicondylar	Lateral Unicondylar	Patello-femoral	Femoral Surface	Tibial Surface
Knee, RT	ØSPCØ9Z	ØSRCØ6[9,A,Z]	ØSRCØJ[9,A,Z]	ØSRCØL[9,A,Z]	ØSRCØM[9,A,Z]	ØSRCØN[9,A,Z]	ØSRTØJ[9,A,Z]	ØSRVØJ[9,A,Z]
Knee, LT	ØSPDØ9Z	ØSRDØ6[9,A,Z]	ØSRDØJ[9,A,Z]	ØSRDØL[9,A,Z]	ØSRDØM[9,A,Z]	ØSRDØN[9,A,Z]	ØSRUØJ[9,A,Z]	ØSRWØJ[9,A,Z]

Open Removal of Knee Articulating Spacer with Synthetic Substitute Replacement

Removal of Articulating Spacer		Code also as appropriate Replacement by Type of Synthetic Substitute			
		Oxidized Zircon on Poly	Synth Subst	Femoral Surface	Tibial Surface
Knee, RT	ØSPCØEZ	ØSRCØ6[9,A,Z]	ØSRCØJ[9,A,Z]	ØSRTØJ[9,A,Z]	ØSRVØJ[9,A,Z]
Knee, LT	ØSPDØEZ	ØSRDØ6[9,A,Z]	ØSRDØJ[9,A,Z]	ØSRUØJ[9,A,Z]	ØSRWØJ[9,A,Z]

Open Removal of Patellar Surface of Knee with Synthetic Substitute Replacement

Removal of Patellar Surface		Code also as appropriate Replacement by Type of Synthetic Substitute				
		Oxidized Zircon on Poly	Synth Subst	Patello-femoral	Femoral Surface	Tibial Surface
Knee, RT	ØSPCØJC	ØSRCØ6[9,A,Z]	ØSRCØJ[9,A,Z]	ØSRCØN[9,A,Z]	ØSRTØJ[9,A,Z]	ØSRVØJ[9,A,Z]
Knee, LT	ØSPDØJC	ØSRDØ6[9,A,Z]	ØSRDØJ[9,A,Z]	ØSRDØN[9,A,Z]	ØSRUØJ[9,A,Z]	ØSRWØJ[9,A,Z]

Open Removal of Patellar Surface of Knee with Articulating Spacer Replacement

Removal of Patellar Surface		Code also as appropriate Replacement with Articulating Spacer
Knee, RT	ØSPCØJC	ØSRCØEZ
Knee, LT	ØSPDØJC	ØSRDØEZ

Open Removal of Knee Synthetic Substitute with Synthetic Substitute Replacement

Removal of Synthetic Substitute		Code also as appropriate Replacement by Type of Synthetic Substitute						
		Oxidized Zircon on Poly	Synth Subst	Medial Unicondylar	Lateral Unicondylar	Patello-femoral	Femoral Surface	Tibial Surface
Knee, RT	ØSPCØJZ	ØSRCØ6[9,A,Z]	ØSRCØJ[9,A,Z]	ØSRCØL[9,A,Z]	ØSRCØM[9,A,Z]	ØSRCØN[9,A,Z]	ØSRTØJ[9,A,Z]	ØSRVØJ[9,A,Z]
Knee, LT	ØSPDØJZ	ØSRDØ6[9,A,Z]	ØSRDØJ[9,A,Z]	ØSRDØL[9,A,Z]	ØSRDØM[9,A,Z]	ØSRDØN[9,A,Z]	ØSRUØJ[9,A,Z]	ØSRWØJ[9,A,Z]

Open Removal of Knee Synthetic Substitute with Articulating Spacer Replacement

Removal of Synthetic Substitute		Code also as appropriate Replacement with Articulating Spacer
Knee, RT	ØSPCØJZ	ØSRCØEZ
Knee, LT	ØSPDØJZ	ØSRDØEZ

Open Removal of Medial or Lateral Unicondylar Knee with Synthetic Substitute Replacement

Removal of Medial/Lateral Unicondylar Knee		Code also as appropriate Replacement by Type of Synthetic Substitute				
		Oxidized Zircon on Poly	Synth Subst	Medial Unicondylar	Femoral Surface	Tibial Surface
Knee, RT	ØSPCØ[L,M]Z	ØSRCØ6[9,A,Z]	ØSRCØJ[9,A,Z]	ØSRCØL[9,A,Z]	ØSRTØJ[9,A,Z]	ØSRVØJ[9,A,Z]
Knee, LT	ØSPDØ[L,M]Z	ØSRDØ6[9,A,Z]	ØSRDØJ[9,A,Z]	ØSRDØL[9,A,Z]	ØSRUØJ[9,A,Z]	ØSRWØJ[9,A,Z]

Open Removal of Patellofemoral Knee with Synthetic Substitute Replacement

Removal of Patellofemoral Knee		Code also as appropriate Replacement by Type of Synthetic Substitute				
		Oxidized Zircon on Poly	Synth Subst	Medial Unicondylar	Femoral Surface	Tibial Surface
Knee, RT	ØSPCØNZ	ØSRCØ6[9,A,Z]	ØSRCØJ[9,A,Z]	ØSRCØL[9,A,Z]	ØSRTØJ[9,A,Z]	ØSRVØJ[9,A,Z]
Knee, LT	ØSPDØNZ	ØSRDØ6[9,A,Z]	ØSRDØJ[9,A,Z]	ØSRDØL[9,A,Z]	ØSRUØJ[9,A,Z]	ØSRWØJ[9,A,Z]

Open Removal of Femoral/Tibial Surface of Knee with Synthetic Substitute Replacement

Removal of Femoral/Tibial Surface of Knee		Code also as appropriate Replacement by Type of Synthetic Substitute					
		Oxidized Zircon on Poly	Synth Subst	Articulating Spacer	Patello-femoral	Femoral Surface	Tibial Surface
Knee, RT	ØSP[T,V]ØJZ	ØSRCØ6[9,A,Z]	ØSRCØJ[9,A,Z]	ØSRCØEZ	ØSRCØN[9,A,Z]	ØSRTØJ[9,A,Z]	ØSRVØJ[9,A,Z]
Knee, LT	ØSP[U,W]ØJZ	ØSRDØ6[9,A,Z]	ØSRDØJ[9,A,Z]	ØSRDØEZ	ØSRDØN[9,A,Z]	ØSRUØJ[9,A,Z]	ØSRWØJ[9,A,Z]

Percutaneous/Percutaneous Endoscopic Removal of Knee Spacer with Open Synthetic Substitute Replacement

Removal of Spacer		Code also as appropriate Replacement by Type of Synthetic Substitute				
		Oxidized Zircon on Poly	Synth Subst	Patello-femoral	Femoral Surface	Tibial Surface
Knee, RT	ØSPC[3,4]8Z	ØSRCØ6[9,A,Z]	ØSRCØJ[9,A,Z]	ØSRCØN[9,A,Z]	ØSRTØJ[9,A,Z]	ØSRVØJ[9,A,Z]
Knee, LT	ØSPD[3,4]8Z	ØSRDØ6[9,A,Z]	ØSRDØJ[9,A,Z]	ØSRDØN[9,A,Z]	ØSRUØJ[9,A,Z]	ØSRWØJ[9,A,Z]

Percutaneous/Percutaneous Endoscopic Removal of Knee Spacer with Open Articulating Spacer Replacement

Removal of Spacer		Code also as appropriate Replacement with Articulating Spacer
Knee, RT	ØSPC[3,4]8Z	ØSRCØEZ
Knee, LT	ØSPD[3,4]8Z	ØSRDØEZ

Percutaneous Endoscopic Removal of Patellar Surface of Knee with Synthetic Substitute Replacement

Removal of Patellar Surface		Code also as appropriate Replacement by Type of Synthetic Substitute				
		Oxidized Zircon on Poly	Synth Subst	Patello-femoral	Femoral Surface	Tibial Surface
Knee, RT	ØSPC4JC	ØSRCØ6[9,A,Z]	ØSRCØJ[9,A,Z]	ØSRCØN[9,A,Z]	ØSRTØJ[9,A,Z]	ØSRVØJ[9,A,Z]
Knee, LT	ØSPD4JC	ØSRDØ6[9,A,Z]	ØSRDØJ[9,A,Z]	ØSRDØN[9,A,Z]	ØSRUØJ[9,A,Z]	ØSRWØJ[9,A,Z]

Percutaneous Endoscopic Removal of Patellar Surface of Knee with Articulating Spacer Replacement

Removal of Patellar Surface		Code also as appropriate Replacement with Articulating Spacer
Knee, RT	ØSPC4JC	ØSRCØEZ
Knee, LT	ØSPD4JC	ØSRDØEZ

Percutaneous Endoscopic Removal of Knee Synthetic Substitute with Synthetic Substitute Replacement

Removal of Synthetic Substitute		Code also as appropriate Replacement by Type of Synthetic Substitute						
		Oxidized Zircon on Poly	Synth Subst	Medial Unicondylar	Lateral Unicondylar	Patello-femoral	Femoral Surface	Tibial Surface
Knee, RT	ØSPC4JZ	ØSRCØ6[9,A,Z]	ØSRCØJ[9,A,Z]	ØSRCØL[9,A,Z]	ØSRCØM[9,A,Z]	ØSRCØN[9,A,Z]	ØSRTØJ[9,A,Z]	ØSRVØJ[9,A,Z]
Knee, LT	ØSPD4JZ	ØSRDØ6[9,A,Z]	ØSRDØJ[9,A,Z]	ØSRDØL[9,A,Z]	ØSRDØM[9,A,Z]	ØSRDØN[9,A,Z]	ØSRUØJ[9,A,Z]	ØSRWØJ[9,A,Z]

Percutaneous Endoscopic Removal of Knee Synthetic Substitute with Articulating Spacer Replacement

Removal of Synthetic Substitute		Code also as appropriate Replacement with Articulating Spacer
Knee, RT	ØSPC4JZ	ØSRCØEZ
Knee, LT	ØSPD4JZ	ØSRDØEZ

Percutaneous Endoscopic Removal of Medial or Lateral Unicondylar Knee with Synthetic Substitute Replacement

Removal of Medial/Lateral Unicondylar Knee		Code also as appropriate Replacement by Type of Synthetic Substitute				
		Oxidized Zircon on Poly	Synth Subst	Medial Unicondylar	Femoral Surface	Tibial Surface
Knee, RT	ØSPC4[L,M]Z	ØSRCØ6[9,A,Z]	ØSRCØJ[9,A,Z]	ØSRCØL[9,A,Z]	ØSRTØJ[9,A,Z]	ØSRVØJ[9,A,Z]
Knee, LT	ØSPD4[L,M]Z	ØSRDØ6[9,A,Z]	ØSRDØJ[9,A,Z]	ØSRDØL[9,A,Z]	ØSRUØJ[9,A,Z]	ØSRWØJ[9,A,Z]

Percutaneous Endoscopic Removal of Patellofemoral Knee with Synthetic Substitute Replacement

Removal of Patellofemoral Knee		Code also as appropriate Replacement by Type of Synthetic Substitute				
		Oxidized Zircon on Poly	Synth Subst	Medial Unicondylar	Femoral Surface	Tibial Surface
Knee, RT	ØSPC4NZ	ØSRCØ6[9,A,Z]	ØSRCØJ[9,A,Z]	ØSRCØL[9,A,Z]	ØSRTØJ[9,A,Z]	ØSRVØJ[9,A,Z]
Knee, LT	ØSPD4NZ	ØSRDØ6[9,A,Z]	ØSRDØJ[9,A,Z]	ØSRDØL[9,A,Z]	ØSRUØJ[9,A,Z]	ØSRWØJ[9,A,Z]

Percutaneous Endoscopic Removal of Femoral/Tibial Surface of Knee with Synthetic Substitute Replacement

Removal of Femoral/Tibial Surface of Knee		Code also as appropriate Replacement by Type of Synthetic Substitute					
		Oxidized Zircon on Poly	Synth Subst	Articulating Spacer	Patello-femoral	Femoral Surface	Tibial Surface
Knee, RT	ØSP[T,V]4JZ	ØSRCØ6[9,A,Z]	ØSRCØJ[9,A,Z]	ØSRCØEZ	ØSRCØN[9,A,Z]	ØSRTØJ[9,A,Z]	ØSRVØJ[9,A,Z]
Knee, LT	ØSP[U,W]4JZ	ØSRDØ6[9,A,Z]	ØSRDØJ[9,A,Z]	ØSRDØEZ	ØSRDØN[9,A,Z]	ØSRUØJ[9,A,Z]	ØSRWØJ[9,A,Z]

DRG 485-489 Knee Procedures

Joint	Removal of Liner by open approach	Code also as appropriate Supplement of Tibial Surface by Site
Knee, RT	ØSPCØ9Z	ØSUVØ9Z
Knee, LT	ØSPDØ9Z	ØSUWØ9Z

DRG 515-517 Other Musculoskeletal System and Connective Tissue Procedures

Site	Reposition of Vertebra by percutaneous approach	Code also as appropriate Supplement With Synthetic Substitute by Percutaneous Approach at site of Repositioned Vertebra
Cervical	ØPS33ZZ	ØPU33JZ
Coccyx	ØQSS3ZZ	ØQUS3JZ
Lumbar	ØQSØ3ZZ	ØQUØ3JZ
Sacrum	ØQS13ZZ	ØQU13JZ
Thoracic	ØPS43ZZ	ØPU43JZ

DRG 518-52Ø Back and Neck Procedures, Except Spinal Fusion, or Disc Devices/Neurostimulators

Generator Type	Insertion of Generator by Site			Code also as appropriate Insertion Neurostimulator Lead by approach and Site	
	Chest	Abdomen	Back	Spinal Canal	Spinal Cord
Single Array	ØJH6[Ø,3]BZ	ØJH8[Ø,3]BZ	ØJH7[Ø,3]BZ	ØØHU[Ø,3,4]MZ	ØØHV[Ø,3,4]MZ
Single Array, Rechargeable	ØJH6[Ø,3]CZ	ØJH8[Ø,3]CZ	ØJH7[Ø,3]CZ	ØØHU[Ø,3,4]MZ	ØØHV[Ø,3,4]MZ
Multiple Array	ØJH6[Ø,3]DZ	ØJH8[Ø,3]DZ	ØJH7[Ø,3]DZ	ØØHU[Ø,3,4]MZ	ØØHV[Ø,3,4]MZ
Multiple Array, Rechargable	ØJH6[Ø,3]EZ	—	ØJH7[Ø,3]EZ	ØØHU[Ø,3,4]MZ	ØØHV[Ø,3,4]MZ
Multiple Array, Rechargable	—	ØJH8[Ø,3]EZ	—	ØØHU[Ø,3,4]MZ	ØØHV[Ø,3,4]MZ

DRG 582-583 Mastectomy for Malignancy

Site	Resection by Open approach	Code also as appropriate Resection of Lymph Nodes by Open approach by site			Code also as appropriate Resection of Thorax Muscle by Open approach	
		Axillary	Internal Mammary	Thorax	Right	Left
Breast, Right	ØHTTØZZ	Ø7T5ØZZ	Ø7T8ØZZ	Ø7T7ØZZ	ØKTHØZZ	—
Breast, Left	ØHTUØZZ	Ø7T6ØZZ	Ø7T9ØZZ	Ø7T7ØZZ	—	ØKTJØZZ
Breast, Bilateral	ØHTVØZZ	Ø7T5ØZZ and Ø7T6ØZZ	Ø7T8ØZZ and Ø7T9ØZZ	Ø7T7ØZZ	ØKTHØZZ	ØKTJØZZ

DRG 584-585 Breast Biopsy, Local Excision and Other Breast Procedures

Resection of Breast With Resection of Lymph Nodes and Thorax Muscle

Site	Resection by Open approach	Code also as appropriate Resection of Lymph Nodes by Open approach by site			Code also as appropriate Resection of Thorax Muscle by Open approach	
		Axillary	Internal Mammary	Thorax	Right	Left
Breast, Right	ØHTTØZZ	Ø7T5ØZZ	Ø7T8ØZZ	Ø7T7ØZZ	ØKTHØZZ	—
Breast, Left	ØHTUØZZ	Ø7T6ØZZ	Ø7T9ØZZ	Ø7T7ØZZ	—	ØKTJØZZ
Breast, Bilateral	ØHTVØZZ	Ø7T5ØZZ and Ø7T6ØZZ	Ø7T8ØZZ and Ø7T9ØZZ	Ø7T7ØZZ	ØKTHØZZ	ØKTJØZZ

Replacement of Breast Tissue

Site	Replacement by Percutaneous approach with Autologous Tissue	Code also as appropriate Extraction of Subcutaneous Tissue by Percutaneous approach					
		Abdomen	Back	Buttock	Chest	Leg, Upper, Right	Leg, Upper, Left
Breast, Right	ØHRT37Z	ØJD83ZZ	ØJD73ZZ	ØJD93ZZ	ØJD63ZZ	ØJDL3ZZ	ØJDM3ZZ
Breast, Left	ØHRU37Z	ØJD83ZZ	ØJD73ZZ	ØJD93ZZ	ØJD63ZZ	ØJDL3ZZ	ØJDM3ZZ
Breast, Bilateral	ØHRV37Z	ØJD83ZZ	ØJD73ZZ	ØJD93ZZ	ØJD63ZZ	ØJDL3ZZ	ØJDM3ZZ

DRG 628-63Ø Other Endocrine, Nutritional and Metabolic Procedures

Hip Procedures

Open Removal of Hip Spacer with Replacement

Removal of Spacer		Code also as appropriate Replacement by Device Type					
		Metal	Metal on Poly	Ceramic	Ceramic on Poly	Oxidized Zirc on Poly	Synthetic Substitute
Hip, RT	ØSP9Ø8Z	ØSR9Ø1[9,A,Z]	ØSR9Ø2[9,A,Z]	ØSR9Ø3[9,A,Z]	ØSR9Ø4[9,A,Z]	ØSR9Ø6[9,A,Z]	ØSR9ØJ[9,A,Z]
Hip, LT	ØSPBØ8Z	ØSRBØ1[9,A,Z]	ØSRBØ2[9,A,Z]	ØSRBØ3[9,A,Z]	ØSRBØ4[9,A,Z]	ØSRBØ6[9,A,Z]	ØSRBØJ[9,A,Z]

Open Removal of Hip Spacer with Replacement

Removal of Spacer		Code also as appropriate Replacement by Device Type						
		Acetabular Surface				Femoral Surface		
		Poly	Metal	Ceramic	Synthetic	Metal	Ceramic	Synthetic
Hip, RT	ØSP9Ø8Z	ØSRAØØ[9,A,Z]	ØSRAØ1[9,A,Z]	ØSRAØ3[9,A,Z]	ØSRAØJ[9,A,Z]	ØSRRØ1[9,A,Z]	ØSRRØ3[9,A,Z]	ØSRRØJ[9,A,Z]
Hip, LT	ØSPBØ8Z	ØSREØØ[9,A,Z]	ØSREØ1[9,A,Z]	ØSREØ3[9,A,Z]	ØSREØJ[9,A,Z]	ØSRSØ1[9,A,Z]	ØSRSØ3[9,A,Z]	ØSRSØJ[9,A,Z]

Open Removal of Hip Spacer with Liner Insertion (supplement)

Removal of Spacer		Code also as appropriate Supplement of Body Part by Site		
		Joint	Acetabular Surface	Femoral Surface
Hip, RT	ØSP9Ø8Z	ØSU9Ø9Z	ØSUAØ9Z	ØSURØ9Z
Hip, LT	ØSPBØ8Z	ØSUBØ9Z	ØSUEØ9Z	ØSUSØ9Z

Open Removal of Hip Liner with Replacement

Removal of Liner		Code also as appropriate Replacement by Device Type					
		Metal	Metal on Poly	Ceramic	Ceramic on Poly	Oxidized Zirc on Poly	Synthetic Substitute
Hip, RT	ØSP9Ø9Z	ØSR9Ø1[9,A,Z]	ØSR9Ø2[9,A,Z]	ØSR9Ø3[9,A,Z]	ØSR9Ø4[9,A,Z]	ØSR9Ø6[9,A,Z]	ØSR9ØJ[9,A,Z]
Hip, LT	ØSPBØ9Z	ØSRBØ1[9,A,Z]	ØSRBØ2[9,A,Z]	ØSRBØ3[9,A,Z]	ØSRBØ4[9,A,Z]	ØSRBØ6[9,A,Z]	ØSRBØJ[9,A,Z]

Open Removal of Hip Liner with Replacement

Removal of Liner		Code also as appropriate Replacement by Device Type						
		Acetabular Surface				Femoral Surface		
		Poly	Metal	Ceramic	Synthetic	Metal	Ceramic	Synthetic
Hip, RT	ØSP9Ø9Z	ØSRAØØ[9,A,Z]	ØSRAØ1[9,A,Z]	ØSRAØ3[9,A,Z]	ØSRAØJ[9,A,Z]	ØSRRØ1[9,A,Z]	ØSRRØ3[9,A,Z]	ØSRRØJ[9,A,Z]
Hip, LT	ØSPBØ9Z	ØSREØØ[9,A,Z]	ØSREØ1[9,A,Z]	ØSREØ3[9,A,Z]	ØSREØJ[9,A,Z]	ØSRSØ1[9,A,Z]	ØSRSØ3[9,A,Z]	ØSRSØJ[9,A,Z]

Open Removal of Hip Liner with Liner Insertion (supplement)

Removal of Liner		Code also as appropriate Supplement of Body Part by Site		
		Joint	Acetabular Surface	Femoral Surface
Hip, RT	ØSP9Ø9Z	ØSU9Ø9Z	ØSUAØ9Z	ØSURØ9Z
Hip, LT	ØSPBØ9Z	ØSUBØ9Z	ØSUEØ9Z	ØSUSØ9Z

Open Removal of Hip Resurfacing Device with Replacement

Removal of Resurfacing Device		Code also as appropriate Replacement by Device Type					
		Metal	Metal on Poly	Ceramic	Ceramic on Poly	Oxidized Zirc on Poly	Synthetic Substitute
Hip, RT	ØSP9ØBZ	ØSR9Ø1[9,A,Z]	ØSR9Ø2[9,A,Z]	ØSR9Ø3[9,A,Z]	ØSR9Ø4[9,A,Z]	ØSR9Ø6[9,A,Z]	ØSR9ØJ[9,A,Z]
Hip, LT	ØSPBØBZ	ØSRBØ1[9,A,Z]	ØSRBØ2[9,A,Z]	ØSRBØ3[9,A,Z]	ØSRBØ4[9,A,Z]	ØSRBØ6[9,A,Z]	ØSRBØJ[9,A,Z]

Open Removal of Hip Resurfacing Device with Replacement

Removal of Resurfacing Device		Code also as appropriate Replacement by Device Type						
		Acetabular Surface				Femoral Surface		
		Poly	Metal	Ceramic	Synthetic	Metal	Ceramic	Synthetic
Hip, RT	ØSP9ØBZ	ØSRAØØ[9,A,Z]	ØSRAØ1[9,A,Z]	ØSRAØ3[9,A,Z]	ØSRAØJ[9,A,Z]	ØSRRØ1[9,A,Z]	ØSRRØ3[9,A,Z]	ØSRRØJ[9,A,Z]
Hip, LT	ØSPBØBZ	ØSREØØ[9,A,Z]	ØSREØ1[9,A,Z]	ØSREØ3[9,A,Z]	ØSREØJ[9,A,Z]	ØSRSØ1[9,A,Z]	ØSRSØ3[9,A,Z]	ØSRSØJ[9,A,Z]

Open Removal of Hip Resurfacing Device with Liner Insertion (supplement)

Removal of Resurfacing Device		Code also as appropriate Supplement of Body Part by Site		
		Joint	Acetabular Surface	Femoral Surface
Hip, RT	ØSP9ØBZ	ØSU9Ø9Z	ØSUAØ9Z	ØSURØ9Z
Hip, LT	ØSPBØBZ	ØSUBØ9Z	ØSUEØ9Z	ØSUSØ9Z

Open Removal of Hip Synthetic Substitute with Replacement

Removal of Synthetic Substitute		Code also as appropriate Replacement by Device Type					
		Metal	Metal on Poly	Ceramic	Ceramic on Poly	Oxidized Zirc on Poly	Synthetic Substitute
Hip, RT	ØSP9ØJZ	ØSR9Ø1[9,A,Z]	ØSR9Ø2[9,A,Z]	ØSR9Ø3[9,A,Z]	ØSR9Ø4[9,A,Z]	ØSR9Ø6[9,A,Z]	ØSR9ØJ[9,A,Z]
Hip, LT	ØSPBØJZ	ØSRBØ1[9,A,Z]	ØSRBØ2[9,A,Z]	ØSRBØ3[9,A,Z]	ØSRBØ4[9,A,Z]	ØSRBØ6[9,A,Z]	ØSRBØJ[9,A,Z]

Open Removal of Hip Synthetic Substitute with Replacement

Removal of Synthetic Substitute		Code also as appropriate Replacement by Device Type						
		Acetabular Surface				Femoral Surface		
		Poly	Metal	Ceramic	Synthetic	Metal	Ceramic	Synthetic
Hip, RT	ØSP9ØJZ	ØSRAØØ[9,A,Z]	ØSRAØ1[9,A,Z]	ØSRAØ3[9,A,Z]	ØSRAØJ[9,A,Z]	ØSRRØ1[9,A,Z]	ØSRRØ3[9,A,Z]	ØSRRØJ[9,A,Z]
Hip, LT	ØSPBØJZ	ØSREØØ[9,A,Z]	ØSREØ1[9,A,Z]	ØSREØ3[9,A,Z]	ØSREØJ[9,A,Z]	ØSRSØ1[9,A,Z]	ØSRSØ3[9,A,Z]	ØSRSØJ[9,A,Z]

Open Removal of Hip Acetabular/Femoral Surface with Replacement

Removal of Acetabular/Femoral Surface		Code also as appropriate Replacement by Device Type					
		Metal	Metal on Poly	Ceramic	Ceramic on Poly	Oxidized Zirc on Poly	Synthetic Substitute
Hip, RT	ØSP[A,R]ØJZ	ØSR9Ø1[9,A,Z]	ØSR9Ø2[9,A,Z]	ØSR9Ø3[9,A,Z]	ØSR9Ø4[9,A,Z]	ØSR9Ø6[9,A,Z]	ØSR9ØJ[9,A,Z]
Hip, LT	ØSP[E,S]ØJZ	ØSRBØ1[9,A,Z]	ØSRBØ2[9,A,Z]	ØSRBØ3[9,A,Z]	ØSRBØ4[9,A,Z]	ØSRBØ6[9,A,Z]	ØSRBØJ[9,A,Z]

Open Removal of Hip Acetabular/Femoral Surface with Replacement

Removal of Acetabular/Femoral Surface		Code also as appropriate Replacement by Device Type						
		Acetabular Surface				Femoral Surface		
		Poly	Metal	Ceramic	Synthetic	Metal	Ceramic	Synthetic
Hip, RT	ØSP[A,R]ØJZ	ØSRAØØ[9,A,Z]	ØSRAØ1[9,A,Z]	ØSRAØ3[9,A,Z]	ØSRAØJ[9,A,Z]	ØSRRØ1[9,A,Z]	ØSRRØ3[9,A,Z]	ØSRRØJ[9,A,Z]
Hip, LT	ØSP[E,S]ØJZ	ØSREØØ[9,A,Z]	ØSREØ1[9,A,Z]	ØSREØ3[9,A,Z]	ØSREØJ[9,A,Z]	ØSRSØ1[9,A,Z]	ØSRSØ3[9,A,Z]	ØSRSØJ[9,A,Z]

Percutaneous Endoscopic Removal of Hip Spacer with Replacement

Removal of Spacer		Code also as appropriate Replacement by Device Type					
		Metal	Metal on Poly	Ceramic	Ceramic on Poly	Oxidized Zirc on Poly	Synthetic Substitute
Hip, RT	ØSP948Z	ØSR9Ø1[9,A,Z]	ØSR9Ø2[9,A,Z]	ØSR9Ø3[9,A,Z]	ØSR9Ø4[9,A,Z]	ØSR9Ø6[9,A,Z]	ØSR9ØJ[9,A,Z]
Hip, LT	ØSPB48Z	ØSRBØ1[9,A,Z]	ØSRBØ2[9,A,Z]	ØSRBØ3[9,A,Z]	ØSRBØ4[9,A,Z]	ØSRBØ6[9,A,Z]	ØSRBØJ[9,A,Z]

Percutaneous Endoscopic Removal of Hip Spacer with Replacement

Removal of Spacer		Code also as appropriate Replacement by Device Type						
		Acetabular Surface				Femoral Surface		
		Poly	Metal	Ceramic	Synthetic	Metal	Ceramic	Synthetic
Hip, RT	ØSP948Z	ØSRAØØ[9,A,Z]	ØSRAØ1[9,A,Z]	ØSRAØ3[9,A,Z]	ØSRAØJ[9,A,Z]	ØSRRØ1[9,A,Z]	ØSRRØ3[9,A,Z]	ØSRRØJ[9,A,Z]
Hip, LT	ØSPB48Z	ØSREØØ[9,A,Z]	ØSREØ1[9,A,Z]	ØSREØ3[9,A,Z]	ØSREØJ[9,A,Z]	ØSRSØ1[9,A,Z]	ØSRSØ3[9,A,Z]	ØSRSØJ[9,A,Z]

Percutaneous Endoscopic Removal of Hip Spacer with Liner Insertion (supplement)

Removal of Spacer		Code also as appropriate Supplement of Body Part by Site		
		Joint	Acetabular Surface	Femoral Surface
Hip, RT	ØSP948Z	ØSU9Ø9Z	ØSUAØ9Z	ØSURØ9Z
Hip, LT	ØSPB48Z	ØSUBØ9Z	ØSUEØ9Z	ØSUSØ9Z

Percutaneous Endoscopic Removal of Hip Synthetic Substitute with Replacement

Removal of Synthetic Substitute		Code also as appropriate Replacement by Device Type					
		Metal	Metal on Poly	Ceramic	Ceramic on Poly	Oxidized Zirc on Poly	Synthetic Substitute
Hip, RT	ØSP94JZ	ØSR9Ø1[9,A,Z]	ØSR9Ø2[9,A,Z]	ØSR9Ø3[9,A,Z]	ØSR9Ø4[9,A,Z]	ØSR9Ø6[9,A,Z]	ØSR9ØJ[9,A,Z]
Hip, LT	ØSPB4JZ	ØSRBØ1[9,A,Z]	ØSRBØ2[9,A,Z]	ØSRBØ3[9,A,Z]	ØSRBØ4[9,A,Z]	ØSRBØ6[9,A,Z]	ØSRBØJ[9,A,Z]

Percutaneous Endoscopic of Hip Synthetic Substitute with Replacement

Removal of Synthetic Substitute		Code also as appropriate Replacement by Device Type						
		Acetabular Surface				Femoral Surface		
		Poly	Metal	Ceramic	Synthetic	Metal	Ceramic	Synthetic
Hip, RT	ØSP94JZ	ØSRAØØ[9,A,Z]	ØSRAØ1[9,A,Z]	ØSRAØ3[9,A,Z]	ØSRAØJ[9,A,Z]	ØSRRØ1[9,A,Z]	ØSRRØ3[9,A,Z]	ØSRRØJ[9,A,Z]
Hip, LT	ØSPB4JZ	ØSREØØ[9,A,Z]	ØSREØ1[9,A,Z]	ØSREØ3[9,A,Z]	ØSREØJ[9,A,Z]	ØSRSØ1[9,A,Z]	ØSRSØ3[9,A,Z]	ØSRSØJ[9,A,Z]

Percutaneous Endoscopic Removal of Hip Synthetic Substitute with Liner Insertion (supplement)

Removal of Synthetic Substitute		Code also as appropriate Supplement of Body Part by Site		
		Joint	Acetabular Surface	Femoral Surface
Hip, RT	ØSP94JZ	ØSU9Ø9Z	ØSUAØ9Z	ØSURØ9Z
Hip, LT	ØSPB4JZ	ØSUBØ9Z	ØSUEØ9Z	ØSUSØ9Z

Percutaneous Endoscopic Removal of Hip Acetabular/Femoral Surface with Replacement

Removal of Acetabular/Femoral Surface		Code also as appropriate Replacement by Device Type					
		Metal	Metal on Poly	Ceramic	Ceramic on Poly	Oxidized Zirc on Poly	Synthetic Substitute
Hip, RT	ØSP[A,R]4JZ	ØSR9Ø1[9,A,Z]	ØSR9Ø2[9,A,Z]	ØSR9Ø3[9,A,Z]	ØSR9Ø4[9,A,Z]	ØSR9Ø6[9,A,Z]	ØSR9ØJ[9,A,Z]
Hip, LT	ØSP[E,S]4JZ	ØSRBØ1[9,A,Z]	ØSRBØ2[9,A,Z]	ØSRBØ3[9,A,Z]	ØSRBØ4[9,A,Z]	ØSRBØ6[9,A,Z]	ØSRBØJ[9,A,Z]

Percutaneous Endoscopic of Hip Acetabular/Femoral Surface with Replacement

Removal of Acetabular/Femoral Surface		Code also as appropriate Replacement by Device Type						
		Acetabular Surface				Femoral Surface		
		Poly	Metal	Ceramic	Synthetic	Metal	Ceramic	Synthetic
Hip, RT	ØSP[A,R]4JZ	ØSRAØØ[9,A,Z]	ØSRAØ1[9,A,Z]	ØSRAØ3[9,A,Z]	ØSRAØJ[9,A,Z]	ØSRRØ1[9,A,Z]	ØSRRØ3[9,A,Z]	ØSRRØJ[9,A,Z]
Hip, LT	ØSP[E,S]4JZ	ØSREØØ[9,A,Z]	ØSREØ1[9,A,Z]	ØSREØ3[9,A,Z]	ØSREØJ[9,A,Z]	ØSRSØ1[9,A,Z]	ØSRSØ3[9,A,Z]	ØSRSØJ[9,A,Z]

Percutaneous Endoscopic Removal of Hip Acetabular/Femoral Surface with Liner Insertion (supplement)

Removal of Acetabular/Femoral Surface		Code also as appropriate Supplement of Body Part by Site		
		Joint	Acetabular Surface	Femoral Surface
Hip, RT	ØSP[A,R]4JZ	ØSU9Ø9Z	ØSUAØ9Z	ØSURØ9Z
Hip, LT	ØSP[E,S]4JZ	ØSUBØ9Z	ØSUEØ9Z	ØSUSØ9Z

Knee Procedures

Open Removal of Knee Liner with Synthetic Substitute Replacement

Removal of Liner		Code also as appropriate Replacement by Type of Synthetic Substitute						
		Oxidized Zircon on Poly	Synthetic Substitute	Medial Unicondylar	Lateral Unicondylar	Patello-femoral	Femoral Surface	Tibial Surface
Knee, RT	ØSPCØ9Z	ØSRCØ6[9,A,Z]	ØSRCØJ[9,A,Z]	ØSRCØL[9,A,Z]	ØSRCØM[9,A,Z]	ØSRCØN[9,A,Z]	ØSRTØJ[9,A,Z]	ØSRVØJ[9,A,Z]
Knee, LT	ØSPDØ9Z	ØSRDØ6[9,A,Z]	ØSRDØJ[9,A,Z]	ØSRDØL[9,A,Z]	ØSRDØM[9,A,Z]	ØSRDØN[9,A,Z]	ØSRUØJ[9,A,Z]	ØSRWØJ[9,A,Z]

Open Removal of Patellar Surface of Knee with Synthetic Substitute Replacement

Removal of Patellar Surface		Code also as appropriate Replacement by Type of Synthetic Substitute	
		Femoral Surface	Tibial Surface
Knee, RT	ØSPCØJC	ØSRTØJ[9,A]	ØSRVØJ[9,A,Z]
Knee, LT	ØSPDØJC	ØSRUØJ[9,A]	ØSRWØJ[9,A,Z]

Open Removal of Knee Synthetic Substitute with Synthetic Substitute Replacement

Removal of Synthetic Substitute		Code also as appropriate Replacement by Type of Synthetic Substitute	
		Femoral Surface	Tibial Surface
Knee, RT	ØSPCØJZ	ØSRTØJ[9,A]	ØSRVØJ[9,A]
Knee, LT	ØSPDØJZ	ØSRUØJ[9,A]	ØSRWØJ[9,A,Z]

Open Removal of Knee Medial/Lateral Unicondylar Device with Synthetic Substitute Replacement

Removal of Medial/Lateral Unicondylar Device		Code also as appropriate Replacement by Type of Synthetic Substitute	
		Femoral Surface	Tibial Surface
Knee, Medial Unicondylar, RT	ØSPCØLZ	ØSRTØJ[9,A]	ØSRVØJ[9,A]
Knee, Medial Unicondylar, LT	ØSPDØLZ	ØSRUØJ[9,A]	ØSRWØJ[9,A,Z]
Knee, Lateral Unicondylar, RT	ØSPCØMZ	ØSRTØJ[9,A]	ØSRVØJ[9,A]
Knee, Lateral Unicondylar, LT	ØSPDØMZ	ØSRUØJ[9,A]	ØSRWØJ[9,A,Z]

Open Removal of Knee Patellofemoral Device with Synthetic Substitute Replacement

Removal of Patellofemoral Device		Code also as appropriate Replacement by Type of Synthetic Substitute	
		Femoral Surface	Tibial Surface
Knee, RT	ØSPCØNZ	ØSRTØJ[9,A]	ØSRVØJ[9,A]
Knee, LT	ØSPDØNZ	ØSRUØJ[9,A]	ØSRWØJ[9,A,Z]

Open Removal of Femoral/Tibial Surface of Knee with Synthetic Substitute Replacement

Removal of Femoral/Tibial Surface		Code also as appropriate Replacement by Type of Synthetic Substitute	
		Femoral Surface	Tibial Surface
Knee, RT	ØSP[T,V]ØJZ	ØSRTØJ[9,A]	ØSRVØJ[9,A]
Knee, LT	ØSP[U,W]ØJZ	ØSRUØJ[9,A]	ØSRWØJ[9,A,Z]

Percutaneous Endoscopic Removal of Patellar Surface of Knee with Synthetic Substitute Replacement

Removal of Patellar Surface		Code also as appropriate Replacement by Type of Synthetic Substitute	
		Femoral Surface	Tibial Surface
Knee, RT	ØSPC4JC	ØSRTØJ[9,A]	ØSRVØJ[9,A]
Knee, LT	ØSPD4JC	ØSRUØJ[9,A]	ØSRWØJ[9,A,Z]

Percutaneous Endoscopic Removal of Knee Synthetic Substitute with Synthetic Substitute Replacement

Removal of Synthetic Substitute		Code also as appropriate Replacement by Type of Synthetic Substitute	
		Femoral Surface	Tibial Surface
Knee, RT	ØSPC4JZ	ØSRTØJ[9,A]	ØSRVØJ[9,A,Z]
Knee, LT	ØSPD4JZ	ØSRUØJ[9,A]	ØSRWØJ[9,A,Z]

Percutaneous Endoscopic Removal of Knee Medial/Lateral Unicondylar Device with Synthetic Substitute Replacement

Removal of Medial/Lateral Unicondylar Device		Code also as appropriate Replacement by Type of Synthetic Substitute	
		Femoral Surface	Tibial Surface
Knee, Medial Unicondylar, RT	ØSPC4LZ	ØSRTØJ[9,A]	ØSRVØJ[9,A]
Knee, Medial Unicondylar, LT	ØSPD4LZ	ØSRUØJ[9,A]	ØSRWØJ[9,A,Z]
Knee, Lateral Unicondylar, RT	ØSPC4MZ	ØSRTØJ[9,A]	ØSRVØJ[9,A]
Knee, Lateral Unicondylar, LT	ØSPD4MZ	ØSRUØJ[9,A]	ØSRWØJ[9,A,Z]

Percutaneous Endoscopic Removal of Knee Patellofemoral Device with Synthetic Substitute Replacement

Removal of Patellofemoral Device		Code also as appropriate Replacement by Type of Synthetic Substitute	
		Femoral Surface	Tibial Surface
Knee, RT	ØSPC4NZ	ØSRTØJ[9,A]	ØSRVØJ[9,A]
Knee, LT	ØSPD4NZ	ØSRUØJ[9,A]	ØSRWØJ[9,A,Z]

Percutaneous Endoscopic Removal of Femoral/Tibial Surface of Knee with Synthetic Substitute Replacement

Removal of Femoral/Tibial Surface		Code also as appropriate Replacement by Type of Synthetic Substitute	
		Femoral Surface	Tibial Surface
Knee, RT	ØSP[T,V]4JZ	ØSRTØJ[9,A]	ØSRVØJ[9,A,Z]
Knee, LT	ØSP[U,W]4JZ	ØSRUØJ[9,A]	ØSRWØJ[9,A,Z]

DRG 662-664 Minor Bladder Procedure

Repair of Bladder	Code also as appropriate Repair of Abdominal Wall	
	with Stoma	without Stoma
ØTQB[Ø,3,4]ZZ	ØWQFXZ2	ØWQFXZZ

DRG 665-667 Prostatectomy

Site	Resection by approach				Code also as appropriate Resection of Seminal Vesicles, Bilateral by approach	
	Open	Percutaneous Endoscopic	Via Natural or Artificial Opening	Via Natural or Artificial Opening Endoscopic	Open	Percutaneous Endoscopic
Prostate	ØVTØØZZ	ØVTØ4ZZ	ØVTØ7ZZ	ØVTØ8ZZ	ØVT3ØZZ	ØVT34ZZ

DRG 7Ø7-7Ø8 Major Male Pelvic Procedures

Site	Resection by approach				Code also as appropriate Resection of Seminal Vesicles, Bilateral by approach	
	Open	Percutaneous Endoscopic	Via Natural or Artificial Opening	Via Natural or Artificial Opening Endoscopic	Open	Percutaneous Endoscopic
Prostate	ØVTØØZZ	ØVTØ4ZZ	ØVTØ7ZZ	ØVTØ8ZZ	ØVT3ØZZ	ØVT34ZZ

DRG 734-735 Pelvic Evisceration, Radical Hysterectomy and Radical Vulvectomy

Pelvic Evisceration

Resection by Site						
Bladder	Cervix	Fallopian Tubes, Bilateral	Ovaries, Bilateral	Urethra	Uterus	Vagina
ØTTBØZZ	ØUTCØZZ	ØUT7ØZZ	ØUT2ØZZ	ØTTDØZZ	ØUT9ØZZ	ØUTGØZZ

Radical Hysterectomy

Approach	Resection by Site		
	Cervix	Uterus	Uterine Support Structure
Vaginal	ØUTC[7,8]ZZ	ØUT9[7,8]ZZ	ØUT4[7,8]ZZ
Abdominal, Endoscopic	ØUTC4ZZ	ØUT9[4,F]ZZ	ØUT44ZZ
Abdominal, Open	ØUTCØZZ	ØUT9ØZZ	ØUT4ØZZ

Radical Vulvectomy

Resection by Site	Code also as appropriate Excision of Inguinal Lymph Nodes by Approach	
Vulva	Right	Left
ØUTM[Ø,X]ZZ	Ø7BH[Ø,4]ZZ	Ø7BJ[Ø,4]ZZ

Non-OR procedure combinations

Note: The following table identifies procedure combinations that are considered Non-OR even though one or more procedures of the combination are considered valid DRG OR procedures

Insertion With Removal of Intraluminal Device

Code as appropriate Insertion of Intraluminal Device into Hepatobiliary Duct	Code also as appropriate Removal of Intraluminal Device by Approach and Site			
	Via Natural or Artificial Opening		External	
	Hepatobiliary Duct	Pancreatic Duct	Hepatobiliary Duct	Pancreatic Duct
ØFHB7DZ	ØFPB[7,8]DZ	ØFPD[7,8]DZ	ØFPBXDZ	ØFPDXDZ

Appendix M: Coding Exercises and Answers

Using the ICD-10-PCS tables construct the code that accurately represents the procedure performed.

Medical Surgical Section

Procedure	Code
1. Excision of malignant melanoma from skin of right ear	
2. Laparoscopy with excision of endometrial implant from left ovary	
3. Percutaneous needle core biopsy of right kidney	
4. EGD with gastric biopsy	
5. Open endarterectomy of left common carotid artery	
6. Excision of basal cell carcinoma of lower lip	
7. Open excision of tail of pancreas	
8. Percutaneous biopsy of right gastrocnemius muscle	
9. Sigmoidoscopy with sigmoid polypectomy	
10. Open excision of lesion from right Achilles tendon	
11. Open resection of cecum	
12. Total excision of pituitary gland, open	
13. Explantation of left failed kidney, open	
14. Open left axillary total lymphadenectomy	
15. Laparoscopic-assisted vaginal hysterectomy	
16. Right total mastectomy, open	
17. Open resection of papillary muscle	
18. Total retropubic prostatectomy, open	
19. Laparoscopic cholecystectomy	
20. Endoscopic bilateral total maxillary sinusectomy	
21. Amputation at right elbow level	
22. Right below-knee amputation, proximal tibia/fibula	
23. Fifth ray carpometacarpal joint amputation, left hand	
24. Right leg and hip amputation through ischium	
25. DIP joint amputation of right thumb	
26. Right wrist joint amputation	
27. Trans-metatarsal amputation of foot at left big toe	
28. Mid-shaft amputation, right humerus	
29. Left fourth toe amputation, mid-proximal phalanx	
30. Right above-knee amputation, distal femur	
31. Cryotherapy of wart on left hand	
32. Percutaneous radiofrequency ablation of right vocal cord lesion	
33. Left heart catheterization with laser destruction of arrhythmogenic focus, A-V node	
34. Cautery of nosebleed	
35. Transurethral endoscopic laser ablation of prostate	
36. Percutaneous cautery of oozing varicose vein, left calf	
37. Laparoscopy with destruction of endometriosis, bilateral ovaries	
38. Laser coagulation of right retinal vessel, percutaneous	
39. Thoracoscopic pleurodesis, left side	
40. Percutaneous insertion of Greenfield IVC filter	
41. Forceps total mouth extraction, upper and lower teeth	

Procedure	Code
42. Removal of left thumbnail	
43. Extraction of right intraocular lens without replacement, percutaneous	
44. Laparoscopy with needle aspiration of ova for in vitro fertilization	
45. Nonexcisional debridement of skin ulcer, right foot	
46. Open stripping of abdominal fascia, right side	
47. Hysteroscopy with D&C, diagnostic	
48. Liposuction for medical purposes, left upper arm	
49. Removal of tattered right ear drum fragments with tweezers	
50. Microincisional phlebectomy of spider veins, right lower leg	
51. Routine Foley catheter placement	
52. Incision and drainage of external anal abscess	
53. Percutaneous drainage of ascites	
54. Laparoscopy with left ovarian cystotomy and drainage	
55. Laparotomy and drain placement for liver abscess, right lobe	
56. Right knee arthrotomy with drain placement	
57. Thoracentesis of left pleural effusion	
58. Phlebotomy of left median cubital vein for polycythemia vera	
59. Percutaneous chest tube placement for right pneumothorax	
60. Endoscopic drainage of left ethmoid sinus	
61. External ventricular CSF drainage catheter placement via burr hole	
62. Removal of foreign body, right cornea	
63. Percutaneous mechanical thrombectomy, left brachial artery	
64. Esophagogastroscopy with removal of bezoar from stomach	
65. Foreign body removal, skin of left thumb	
66. Transurethral cystoscopy with removal of bladder stone	
67. Forceps removal of foreign body in right nostril	
68. Laparoscopy with excision of old suture from mesentery	
69. Incision and removal of right lacrimal duct stone	
70. Nonincisional removal of intraluminal foreign body from vagina	
71. Right common carotid endarterectomy, open	
72. Open excision of retained sliver, subcutaneous tissue of left foot	
73. Extracorporeal shockwave lithotripsy (ESWL), bilateral ureters	
74. Endoscopic retrograde cholangiopancreatography (ERCP) with lithotripsy of common bile duct stone	
75. Thoracotomy with crushing of pericardial calcifications	
76. Transurethral cystoscopy with fragmentation of bladder calculus	
77. Hysteroscopy with intraluminal lithotripsy of left fallopian tube calcification	
78. Division of right foot tendon, percutaneous	

Procedure	Code
79. Left heart catheterization with division of bundle of HIS	
80. Open osteotomy of capitate, left hand	
81. EGD with esophagotomy of esophagogastric junction	
82. Sacral rhizotomy for pain control, percutaneous	
83. Laparotomy with exploration and adhesiolysis of right ureter	
84. Incision of scar contracture, right elbow	
85. Frenulotomy for treatment of tongue-tie syndrome	
86. Right shoulder arthroscopy with coracoacromial ligament release	
87. Mitral valvulotomy for release of fused leaflets, open approach	
88. Percutaneous left Achilles tendon release	
89. Laparoscopy with lysis of peritoneal adhesions	
90. Manual rupture of right shoulder joint adhesions under general anesthesia	
91. Open posterior tarsal tunnel release	
92. Laparoscopy with freeing of left ovary and fallopian tube	
93. Liver transplant with donor matched liver	
94. Orthotopic heart transplant using porcine heart	
95. Right lung transplant, open, using organ donor match	
96. Transplant of large intestine, organ donor match	
97. Left kidney/pancreas organ bank transplant	
98. Replantation of avulsed scalp	
99. Reattachment of severed right ear	
100. Reattachment of traumatic left gastrocnemius avulsion, open	
101. Closed replantation of three avulsed teeth, lower jaw	
102. Reattachment of severed left hand	
103. Right open palmaris longus tendon transfer	
104. Endoscopic radial to median nerve transfer	
105. Fasciocutaneous flap closure of left thigh, open	
106. Transfer left index finger to left thumb position, open	
107. Percutaneous fascia transfer to fill defect, right neck	
108. Trigeminal to facial nerve transfer, percutaneous endoscopic	
109. Endoscopic left leg flexor hallucis longus tendon transfer	
110. Right scalp advancement flap to right temple	
111. Bilateral TRAM pedicle flap reconstruction status post mastectomy, muscle only, open	
112. Skin transfer flap closure of complex open wound, left lower back	
113. Open fracture reduction, right tibia	
114. Laparoscopy with gastropexy for malrotation	
115. Left knee arthroscopy with reposition of anterior cruciate ligament	
116. Open transposition of ulnar nerve	
117. Closed reduction with percutaneous internal fixation of right femoral neck fracture	
118. Trans-vaginal intraluminal cervical cerclage	
119. Cervical cerclage using Shirodkar technique	
120. Thoracotomy with banding of left pulmonary artery using extraluminal device	
121. Restriction of thoracic duct with intraluminal stent, percutaneous	

Procedure	Code
122. Craniotomy with clipping of cerebral aneurysm	
123. Nonincisional, transnasal placement of restrictive stent in right lacrimal duct	
124. Catheter-based temporary restriction of blood flow in abdominal aorta for treatment of cerebral ischemia	
125. Percutaneous ligation of esophageal vein	
126. Percutaneous embolization of left internal carotid-cavernous fistula	
127. Laparoscopy with bilateral occlusion of fallopian tubes using Hulka extraluminal clips	
128. Open suture ligation of failed AV graft, left brachial artery	
129. Percutaneous embolization of vascular supply, intracranial meningioma	
130. Percutaneous embolization of right uterine artery, using coils	
131. Open occlusion of left atrial appendage, using extraluminal pressure clips	
132. Percutaneous suture exclusion of left atrial appendage, via femoral artery access	
133. ERCP with balloon dilation of common bile duct	
134. PTCA of two coronary arteries, LAD with stent placement, RCA with no stent	
135. Cystoscopy with intraluminal dilation of bladder neck stricture	
136. Open dilation of old anastomosis, left femoral artery	
137. Dilation of upper esophageal stricture, direct visualization, with Bougie sound	
138. PTA of right brachial artery stenosis	
139. Transnasal dilation and stent placement in right lacrimal duct	
140. Hysteroscopy with balloon dilation of bilateral fallopian tubes	
141. Tracheoscopy with intraluminal dilation of tracheal stenosis	
142. Cystoscopy with dilation of left ureteral stricture, with stent placement	
143. Open gastric bypass with Roux-en-Y limb to jejunum	
144. Right temporal artery to intracranial artery bypass using Gore-Tex graft, open	
145. Tracheostomy formation with tracheostomy tube placement, percutaneous	
146. PICVA (percutaneous in situ coronary venous arterialization) of single coronary artery	
147. Open left femoral-popliteal artery bypass using cadaver vein graft	
148. Shunting of intrathecal cerebrospinal fluid to peritoneal cavity using synthetic shunt	
149. Colostomy formation, open, transverse colon to abdominal wall	
150. Open urinary diversion, left ureter, using ileal conduit to skin	
151. CABG of LAD using pedicled left internal mammary artery, open off-bypass	
152. Open pleuroperitoneal shunt, right pleural cavity, using synthetic device	
153. Percutaneous placement of ventriculoperitoneal shunt for treatment of hydrocephalus	
154. End-of-life replacement of spinal neurostimulator generator, multiple array, in lower abdomen	
155. Percutaneous insertion of spinal neurostimulator lead, lumbar spinal cord	

Procedure	Code
156. Percutaneous replacement of broken pacemaker lead in left atrium	
157. Open placement of dual chamber pacemaker generator in chest wall	
158. Percutaneous placement of venous central line in right internal jugular, with tip in superior vena cava	
159. Open insertion of multiple channel cochlear implant, left ear	
160. Percutaneous placement of Swan-Ganz catheter in pulmonary trunk	
161. Bronchoscopy with insertion of Low Dose, Pd-103 brachytherapy seeds, right lung	
162. Open insertion of interspinous process device into lumbar vertebral joint	
163. Open placement of bone growth stimulator, left femoral shaft	
164. Cystoscopy with placement of brachytherapy seeds in prostate gland	
165. Percutaneous insertion of Greenfield IVC filter	
166. Full-thickness skin graft to right lower arm, autograft (do not code graft harvest for this exercise)	
167. Excision of necrosed left femoral head with bone bank bone graft to fill the defect, open	
168. Penetrating keratoplasty of right cornea with donor matched cornea, percutaneous approach	
169. Excision of abdominal aorta with Gore-Tex graft replacement, open	
170. Total right knee arthroplasty with insertion of total knee prosthesis	
171. Tenonectomy with graft to right ankle using cadaver graft, open	
172. Mitral valve replacement using porcine valve, open	
173. Percutaneous phacoemulsification of right eye cataract with prosthetic lens insertion	
174. Transcatheter replacement of pulmonary valve using of bovine jugular vein valve	
175. Total left hip replacement using ceramic on ceramic prosthesis, without bone cement	
176. Aortic valve annuloplasty using ring, open	
177. Laparoscopic repair of left inguinal hernia with marlex plug	
178. Autograft nerve graft to right median nerve, percutaneous endoscopic (do not code graft harvest for this exercise)	
179. Exchange of liner in femoral component of previous left hip replacement, open approach	
180. Anterior colporrhaphy with polypropylene mesh reinforcement, open approach	
181. Implantation of CorCap cardiac support device, open approach	
182. Abdominal wall herniorrhaphy, open, using synthetic mesh	
183. Tendon graft to strengthen injured left shoulder using autograft, open (do not code graft harvest for this exercise)	
184. Onlay lamellar keratoplasty of left cornea using autograft, external approach	
185. Resurfacing procedure on right femoral head, open approach	
186. Exchange of drainage tube from right hip joint	
187. Tracheostomy tube exchange	
188. Change chest tube for left pneumothorax	
189. Exchange of cerebral ventriculostomy drainage tube	
190. Foley urinary catheter exchange	
191. Open removal of lumbar sympathetic neurostimulator lead	
192. Nonincisional removal of Swan-Ganz catheter from right pulmonary artery	
193. Laparotomy with removal of pancreatic drain	
194. Extubation, endotracheal tube	
195. Nonincisional PEG tube removal	
196. Transvaginal removal of brachytherapy seeds	
197. Transvaginal removal of extraluminal cervical cerclage	
198. Incision with removal of K-wire fixation, right first metatarsal	
199. Cystoscopy with retrieval of left ureteral stent	
200. Removal of nasogastric drainage tube for decompression	
201. Removal of external fixator, left radial fracture	
202. Trimming and reanastomosis of stenosed femorofemoral synthetic bypass graft, open	
203. Open revision of right hip replacement, with readjustment of prosthesis	
204. Adjustment of position, pacemaker lead in left ventricle, percutaneous	
205. External repositioning of Foley catheter to bladder	
206. Taking out loose screw and putting larger screw in fracture repair plate, left tibia	
207. Revision of totally implantable VAD port placement in chest wall, causing patient discomfort, open	
208. Thoracotomy with exploration of right pleural cavity	
209. Diagnostic laryngoscopy	
210. Exploratory arthrotomy of left knee	
211. Colposcopy with diagnostic hysteroscopy	
212. Digital rectal exam	
213. Diagnostic arthroscopy of right shoulder	
214. Endoscopy of maxillary sinus	
215. Laparotomy with palpation of liver	
216. Transurethral diagnostic cystoscopy	
217. Colonoscopy, discontinued at sigmoid colon	
218. Percutaneous mapping of basal ganglia	
219. Heart catheterization with cardiac mapping	
220. Intraoperative whole brain mapping via craniotomy	
221. Mapping of left cerebral hemisphere, percutaneous endoscopic	
222. Intraoperative cardiac mapping during open heart surgery	
223. Hysteroscopy with cautery of post-hysterectomy oozing and evacuation of clot	
224. Open exploration and ligation of post-op arterial bleeder, left forearm	
225. Control of post-operative retroperitoneal bleeding via laparotomy	
226. Reopening of thoracotomy site with drainage and control of post-op hemopericardium	
227. Arthroscopy with drainage of hemarthrosis at previous operative site, right knee	
228. Radiocarpal fusion of left hand with internal fixation, open	
229. Posterior approach spinal fusion at L1-L3 level with BAK cage interbody fusion device, open	
230. Intercarpal fusion of right hand with bone bank bone graft, open	

Procedure	Code
231. Sacrococcygeal fusion with bone graft from same operative site, open	
232. Interphalangeal fusion of left great toe, percutaneous pin fixation	
233. Suture repair of left radial nerve laceration	
234. Laparotomy with suture repair of blunt force duodenal laceration	
235. Perineoplasty with repair of old obstetric laceration, open	
236. Suture repair of right biceps tendon (upper arm) laceration, open	
237. Closure of abdominal wall stab wound	
238. Cosmetic face lift, open, no other information available	
239. Bilateral breast augmentation with silicone implants, open	
240. Cosmetic rhinoplasty with septal reduction and tip elevation using local tissue graft, open	
241. Abdominoplasty (tummy tuck), open	
242. Liposuction of bilateral thighs	
243. Creation of penis in female patient using tissue bank donor graft	
244. Creation of vagina in male patient using synthetic material	
245. Laparoscopic vertical (sleeve) gastrectomy	
246. Left uterine artery embolization with intraluminal biosphere injection	

Obstetrics

Procedure	Code
1. Abortion by dilation and evacuation following laminaria insertion	
2. Manually assisted spontaneous abortion	
3. Abortion by abortifacient insertion	
4. Bimanual pregnancy examination	
5. Extraperitoneal C-section, low transverse incision	
6. Fetal spinal tap, percutaneous	
7. Fetal kidney transplant, laparoscopic	
8. Open in utero repair of congenital diaphragmatic hernia	
9. Laparoscopy with total excision of tubal pregnancy	
10. Transvaginal removal of fetal monitoring electrode	

Placement

Procedure	Code
1. Placement of packing material, right ear	
2. Mechanical traction of entire left leg	
3. Removal of splint, right shoulder	
4. Placement of neck brace	
5. Change of vaginal packing	
6. Packing of wound, chest wall	
7. Sterile dressing placement to left groin region	
8. Removal of packing material from pharynx	
9. Placement of intermittent pneumatic compression device, covering entire right arm	
10. Exchange of pressure dressing to left thigh	

Administration

Procedure	Code
1. Peritoneal dialysis via indwelling catheter	
2. Transvaginal artificial insemination	
3. Infusion of total parenteral nutrition via central venous catheter	
4. Esophagogastroscopy with Botox injection into esophageal sphincter	
5. Percutaneous irrigation of knee joint	
6. Systemic infusion of recombinant tissue plasminogen activator (r-tPA) via peripheral venous catheter	
7. Transabdominal in vitro fertilization, implantation of donor ovum	
8. Autologous bone marrow transplant via central venous line	
9. Implantation of anti-microbial envelope with cardiac defibrillator placement, open	
10. Sclerotherapy of brachial plexus lesion, alcohol injection	
11. Percutaneous peripheral vein injection, glucarpidase	
12. Introduction of anti-infective envelope into subcutaneous tissue, open	

Measurement and Monitoring

Procedure	Code
1. Cardiac stress test, single measurement	
2. EGD with biliary flow measurement	
3. Right and left heart cardiac catheterization with bilateral sampling and pressure measurements	
4. Temperature monitoring, rectal	
5. Peripheral venous pulse, external, single measurement	
6. Holter monitoring	
7. Respiratory rate, external, single measurement	
8. Fetal heart rate monitoring, transvaginal	
9. Visual mobility test, single measurement	
10. Left ventricular cardiac output monitoring from pulmonary artery wedge (Swan-Ganz) catheter	
11. Olfactory acuity test, single measurement	

Extracorporeal or Systemic Assistance and Performance

Procedure	Code
1. Intermittent mechanical ventilation, 16 hours	
2. Liver dialysis, single encounter	
3. Cardiac countershock with successful conversion to sinus rhythm	
4. IPPB (intermittent positive pressure breathing) for mobilization of secretions, 22 hours	
5. Renal dialysis, 12 hours	
6. IABP (intra-aortic balloon pump) continuous	
7. Intra-operative cardiac pacing, continuous	
8. Intraoperative ECMO (extracorporeal membrane oxygenation), central	
9. Controlled mechanical ventilation (CMV), 45 hours	
10. Pulsatile compression boot with intermittent inflation	

Appendix M: Coding Exercises and Answers

Extracorporeal or Systemic Therapies

Procedure	Code
1. Donor thrombocytapheresis, single encounter	
2. Bili-lite phototherapy, series treatment	
3. Whole body hypothermia, single treatment	
4. Circulatory phototherapy, single encounter	
5. Shock wave therapy of plantar fascia, single treatment	
6. Antigen-free air conditioning, series treatment	
7. TMS (transcranial magnetic stimulation), series treatment	
8. Therapeutic ultrasound of peripheral vessels, single treatment	
9. Plasmapheresis, series treatment	
10. Extracorporeal electromagnetic stimulation (EMS) for urinary incontinence, single treatment	

Osteopathic

Procedure	Code
1. Isotonic muscle energy treatment of right leg	
2. Low velocity-high amplitude osteopathic treatment of head	
3. Lymphatic pump osteopathic treatment of left axilla	
4. Indirect osteopathic treatment of sacrum	
5. Articulatory osteopathic treatment of cervical region	

Other Procedures

Procedure	Code
1. Near infrared spectroscopy of leg vessels	
2. CT computer assisted sinus surgery	
3. Suture removal, abdominal wall	
4. Isolation after infectious disease exposure	
5. Robotic assisted open prostatectomy	
6. In vitro fertilization	

Chiropractic

Procedure	Code
1. Chiropractic treatment of lumbar region using long lever specific contact	
2. Chiropractic manipulation of abdominal region, indirect visceral	
3. Chiropractic extra-articular treatment of hip region	
4. Chiropractic treatment of sacrum using long and short lever specific contact	
5. Mechanically-assisted chiropractic manipulation of head	

Imaging

Procedure	Code
1. Noncontrast CT of abdomen and pelvis	
2. Intravascular ultrasound, left subclavian artery	
3. Fluoroscopic guidance for insertion of central venous catheter in SVC, low osmolar contrast	
4. Chest x-ray, AP/PA and lateral views	
5. Endoluminal ultrasound of gallbladder and bile ducts	
6. MRI of thyroid gland, contrast unspecified	
7. Esophageal videofluoroscopy study with oral barium contrast	
8. Portable x-ray study of right radius/ulna shaft, standard series	
9. Routine fetal ultrasound, second trimester twin gestation	
10. CT scan of bilateral lungs, high osmolar contrast with densitometry	
11. Fluoroscopic guidance for percutaneous transluminal angioplasty (PTA) of left common femoral artery, low osmolar contrast	

Nuclear Medicine

Procedure	Code
1. Tomo scan of right and left heart, unspecified radiopharmaceutical, qualitative gated rest	
2. Technetium pentetate assay of kidneys, ureters, and bladder	
3. Uniplanar scan of spine using technetium oxidronate, with first-pass study	
4. Thallous chloride tomographic scan of bilateral breasts	
5. PET scan of myocardium using rubidium	
6. Gallium citrate scan of head and neck, single plane imaging	
7. Xenon gas nonimaging probe of brain	
8. Upper GI scan, radiopharmaceutical unspecified, for gastric emptying	
9. Carbon 11 PET scan of brain with quantification	
10. Iodinated albumin nuclear medicine assay, blood plasma volume study	

Radiation Therapy

Procedure	Code
1. Plaque radiation of left eye, single port	
2. 8 MeV photon beam radiation to brain	
3. IORT of colon, 3 ports	
4. HDR brachytherapy of prostate using low dose palladium-103, unidirectional source	
5. Electron radiation treatment of right breast, with custom device	
6. Hyperthermia oncology treatment of pelvic region	
7. Contact radiation of tongue	
8. Heavy particle radiation treatment of pancreas, four risk sites	
9. LDR brachytherapy to spinal cord using iodine	
10. Whole body Phosphorus 32 administration with risk to hematopoetic system	

Physical Rehabilitation and Diagnostic Audiology

Procedure	Code
1. Bekesy assessment using audiometer	
2. Individual fitting of left eye prosthesis	
3. Physical therapy for range of motion and mobility, patient right hip, no special equipment	
4. Bedside swallow assessment using assessment kit	
5. Caregiver training in airway clearance techniques	
6. Application of short arm cast in rehabilitation setting	
7. Verbal assessment of patient's pain level	
8. Caregiver training in communication skills using manual communication board	

Procedure	Code
9. Group musculoskeletal balance training exercises, whole body, no special equipment	
10. Individual therapy for auditory processing using tape recorder	

Mental Health

Procedure	Code
1. Cognitive-behavioral psychotherapy, individual	
2. Narcosynthesis	
3. Light therapy	
4. ECT (electroconvulsive therapy), unilateral, multiple seizure	
5. Crisis intervention	
6. Neuropsychological testing	
7. Hypnosis	
8. Developmental testing	
9. Vocational counseling	
10. Family psychotherapy	

Substance Abuse Treatment

Procedure	Code
1. Naltrexone treatment for drug dependency	
2. Substance abuse treatment family counseling	
3. Medication monitoring of patient on methadone maintenance	
4. Individual interpersonal psychotherapy for drug abuse	
5. Patient in for alcohol detoxification treatment	
6. Group motivational counseling	
7. Individual 12-step psychotherapy for substance abuse	
8. Post-test infectious disease counseling for IV drug abuser	
9. Psychodynamic psychotherapy for drug dependent patient	
10. Group cognitive-behavioral counseling for substance abuse	

New Technology

Procedure	Code
1. Infusion of terlipressin via peripheral venous catheter	
2. Transcatheter dilation of left peroneal artery with 2 SAVAL stents	

Answers to Coding Exercises

Medical Surgical Section

Procedure	Code
1. Excision of malignant melanoma from skin of right ear	ØHB2XZZ
2. Laparoscopy with excision of endometrial implant from left ovary	ØUB14ZZ
3. Percutaneous needle core biopsy of right kidney	ØTBØ3ZX
4. EGD with gastric biopsy	ØDB68ZX
5. Open endarterectomy of left common carotid artery	Ø3CJØZZ
6. Excision of basal cell carcinoma of lower lip	ØCB1XZZ
7. Open excision of tail of pancreas	ØFBGØZZ
8. Percutaneous biopsy of right gastrocnemius muscle	ØKBS3ZX
9. Sigmoidoscopy with sigmoid polypectomy	ØDBN8ZZ
10. Open excision of lesion from right Achilles tendon	ØLBNØZZ
11. Open resection of cecum	ØDTHØZZ
12. Total excision of pituitary gland, open	ØGTØØZZ
13. Explantation of left failed kidney, open	ØTT1ØZZ
14. Open left axillary total lymphadenectomy	Ø7T6ØZZ (RESECTION is coded for cutting out a chain of lymph nodes.)
15. Laparoscopic-assisted vaginal hysterectomy	ØUT9FZZ
16. Right total mastectomy, open	ØHTTØZZ
17. Open resection of papillary muscle	Ø2TDØZZ (The papillary muscle refers to the heart and is found in the *Heart and Great Vessels* body system.)
18. Total retropubic prostatectomy, open	ØVTØØZZ
19. Laparoscopic cholecystectomy	ØFT44ZZ
20. Endoscopic bilateral total maxillary sinusectomy	Ø9TQ8ZZ, Ø9TR8ZZ
21. Amputation at right elbow level	ØX6BØZZ
22. Right below-knee amputation, proximal tibia/fibula	ØY6HØZ1 (The qualifier *High* here means the portion of the tib/fib closest to the knee.)
23. Fifth ray carpometacarpal joint amputation, left hand	ØX6KØZ8 (A *complete* ray amputation is through the carpometacarpal joint.)
24. Right leg and hip amputation through ischium	ØY62ØZZ (The *Hindquarter* body part includes amputation along any part of the hip bone.)
25. DIP joint amputation of right thumb	ØX6LØZ3 (The qualifier *low* here means through the distal interphalangeal joint.)
26. Right wrist joint amputation	ØX6JØZØ (Amputation at the wrist joint is actually complete amputation of the hand.)
27. Trans-metatarsal amputation of foot at left big toe	ØY6NØZ9 (A *partial* amputation is through the shaft of the metatarsal bone.)
28. Mid-shaft amputation, right humerus	ØX68ØZ2
29. Left fourth toe amputation, mid-proximal phalanx	ØY6WØZ1 (The qualifier *High* here means anywhere along the proximal phalanx.)
30. Right above-knee amputation, distal femur	ØY6CØZ3
31. Cryotherapy of wart on left hand	ØH5GXZZ
32. Percutaneous radiofrequency ablation of right vocal cord lesion	ØC5T3ZZ
33. Left heart catheterization with laser destruction of arrhythmogenic focus, A-V node	Ø2583ZZ
34. Cautery of nosebleed	Ø93K7ZZ
35. Transurethral endoscopic laser ablation of prostate	ØV5Ø8ZZ
36. Percutaneous cautery of oozing varicose vein, left calf	ØY3J3ZZ
37. Laparoscopy with destruction of endometriosis, bilateral ovaries	ØU524ZZ
38. Laser coagulation of right retinal vessel, percutaneous	Ø85G3ZZ (The *Retinal Vessel* body-part values are in the *Eye* body system.)
39. Thoracoscopic pleurodesis, left side	ØB5P4ZZ
40. Percutaneous insertion of Greenfield IVC filter	Ø6HØ3DZ
41. Forceps total mouth extraction, upper and lower teeth	ØCDWXZ2, ØCDXXZ2
42. Removal of left thumbnail	ØHDQXZZ (No separate body-part value is given for thumbnail, so this is coded to *Fingernail.*)
43. Extraction of right intraocular lens without replacement, percutaneous	Ø8DJ3ZZ
44. Laparoscopy with needle aspiration of ova for in vitro fertilization	ØUDN4ZZ
45. Nonexcisional debridement of skin ulcer, right foot	ØHDMXZZ
46. Open stripping of abdominal fascia, right side	ØJD8ØZZ
47. Hysteroscopy with D&C, diagnostic	ØUDB8ZX
48. Liposuction for medical purposes, left upper arm	ØJDF3ZZ (The *Percutaneous* approach is inherent in the liposuction technique.)
49. Removal of tattered right ear drum fragments with tweezers	Ø9D77ZZ
50. Microincisional phlebectomy of spider veins, right lower leg	Ø6DY3ZZ
51. Routine Foley catheter placement	ØT9B7ØZ
52. Incision and drainage of external anal abscess	ØD9QXZZ
53. Percutaneous drainage of ascites	ØW9G3ZZ (This is drainage of the cavity and not the peritoneal membrane itself.)
54. Laparoscopy with left ovarian cystotomy and drainage	ØU914ZZ
55. Laparotomy and drain placement for liver abscess, right lobe	ØF91ØØZ
56. Right knee arthrotomy with drain placement	ØS9CØØZ
57. Thoracentesis of left pleural effusion	ØW9B3ZZ (This is drainage of the pleural cavity)
58. Phlebotomy of left median cubital vein for polycythemia vera	Ø59C3ZZ (The median cubital vein is a branch of the basilic vein)
59. Percutaneous chest tube placement for right pneumothorax	ØW993ØZ
60. Endoscopic drainage of left ethmoid sinus	Ø99V4ZZ
61. External ventricular CSF drainage catheter placement via burr hole	ØØ963ØZ
62. Removal of foreign body, right cornea	Ø8C8XZZ

Procedure	Code
63. Percutaneous mechanical thrombectomy, left brachial artery	Ø3C83ZZ
64. Esophagogastroscopy with removal of bezoar from stomach	ØDC68ZZ
65. Foreign body removal, skin of left thumb	ØHCGXZZ (There is no specific value for thumb skin, so the procedure is coded to *Hand*.)
66. Transurethral cystoscopy with removal of bladder stone	ØTCB8ZZ
67. Forceps removal of foreign body in right nostril	Ø9CKXZZ (Nostril is coded to the *Nasal muscosa and soft tissue* body-part value.)
68. Laparoscopy with excision of old suture from mesentery	ØDCV4ZZ
69. Incision and removal of right lacrimal duct stone	Ø8CXØZZ
70. Nonincisional removal of intraluminal foreign body from vagina	ØUCG7ZZ (The approach *External* is also a possibility. It is assumed here that since the patient went to the doctor to have the object removed, that it was not in the vaginal orifice.)
71. Right common carotid endarterectomy, open	Ø3CHØZZ
72. Open excision of retained sliver, subcutaneous tissue of left foot	ØJCRØZZ
73. Extracorporeal shockwave lithotripsy (ESWL), bilateral ureters	ØTF6XZZ, ØTF7XZZ (The *Bilateral Ureter* body-part value is not available for the root operation FRAGMENTATION, so the procedures are coded separately.)
74. Endoscopic retrograde cholangiopancreatography (ERCP) with lithotripsy of common bile duct stone	ØFF98ZZ (ERCP is performed through the mouth to the biliary system via the duodenum, so the approach value is *Via Natural or Artificial Opening Endoscopic*.)
75. Thoracotomy with crushing of pericardial calcifications	Ø2FNØZZ
76. Transurethral cystoscopy with fragmentation of bladder calculus	ØTFB8ZZ
77. Hysteroscopy with intraluminal lithotripsy of left fallopian tube calcification	ØUF68ZZ
78. Division of right foot tendon, percutaneous	ØL8V3ZZ
79. Left heart catheterization with division of bundle of HIS	Ø2883ZZ
80. Open osteotomy of capitate, left hand	ØP8NØZZ (The capitate is one of the carpal bones of the hand.)
81. EGD with esophagotomy of esophagogastric junction	ØD948ZZ
82. Sacral rhizotomy for pain control, percutaneous	Ø18R3ZZ
83. Laparotomy with exploration and adhesiolysis of right ureter	ØTN6ØZZ
84. Incision of scar contracture, right elbow	ØHNDXZZ (The skin of the elbow region is coded to *Lower Arm*.)
85. Frenulotomy for treatment of tongue-tie syndrome	ØCN7XZZ (The frenulum is coded to the body-part value *Tongue*.)
86. Right shoulder arthroscopy with coracoacromial ligament release	ØMN14ZZ
87. Mitral valvulotomy for release of fused leaflets, open approach	Ø2NGØZZ
88. Percutaneous left Achilles tendon release	ØLNP3ZZ
89. Laparoscopy with lysis of peritoneal adhesions	ØDNW4ZZ
90. Manual rupture of right shoulder joint adhesions under general anesthesia	ØRNJXZZ
91. Open posterior tarsal tunnel release	Ø1NGØZZ (The nerve released in the posterior tarsal tunnel is the tibial nerve.)
92. Laparoscopy with freeing of left ovary and fallopian tube	ØUN14ZZ, ØUN64ZZ
93. Liver transplant with donor matched liver	ØFYØØZØ
94. Orthotopic heart transplant using porcine heart	Ø2YAØZ2 (The donor heart comes from an animal [pig], so the qualifier value is *Zooplastic*.)
95. Right lung transplant, open, using organ donor match	ØBYKØZØ
96. Transplant of large intestine, organ donor match	ØDYEØZØ
97. Left kidney/pancreas organ bank transplant	ØFYGØZØ, ØTY1ØZØ
98. Replantation of avulsed scalp	ØHMØXZZ
99. Reattachment of severed right ear	Ø9MØXZZ
100. Reattachment of traumatic left gastrocnemius avulsion, open	ØKMTØZZ
101. Closed replantation of three avulsed teeth, lower jaw	ØCMXXZ1
102. Reattachment of severed left hand	ØXMKØZZ
103. Right open palmaris longus tendon transfer	ØLX5ØZZ
104. Endoscopic radial to median nerve transfer	Ø1X64Z5
105. Fasciocutaneous flap closure of left thigh, open	ØJXMØZC (The qualifier identifies the body layers in addition to fascia included in the procedure.)
106. Transfer left index finger to left thumb position, open	ØXXPØZM
107. Percutaneous fascia transfer to fill defect, right neck	ØJX43ZZ
108. Trigeminal to facial nerve transfer, percutaneous endoscopic	ØØXK4ZM
109. Endoscopic left leg flexor hallucis longus tendon transfer	ØLXP4ZZ
110. Right scalp advancement flap to right temple	ØHXØXZZ
111. Bilateral TRAM pedicle flap reconstruction status post mastectomy, muscle only, open	ØKXKØZ6, ØKXLØZ6 (The transverse rectus abdominus muscle (TRAM) flap is coded for each flap developed.)
112. Skin transfer flap closure of complex open wound, left lower back	ØHX6XZZ
113. Open fracture reduction, right tibia	ØQSGØZZ
114. Laparoscopy with gastropexy for malrotation	ØDS64ZZ
115. Left knee arthroscopy with reposition of anterior cruciate ligament	ØMSP4ZZ
116. Open transposition of ulnar nerve	Ø1S4ØZZ
117. Closed reduction with percutaneous internal fixation of right femoral neck fracture	ØQS634Z
118. Trans-vaginal intraluminal cervical cerclage	ØUVC7DZ
119. Cervical cerclage using Shirodkar technique	ØUVC7ZZ
120. Thoracotomy with banding of left pulmonary artery using extraluminal device	Ø2VRØCZ
121. Restriction of thoracic duct with intraluminal stent, percutaneous	Ø7VK3DZ

Procedure	Code
122. Craniotomy with clipping of cerebral aneurysm	Ø3VGØCZ (The clip is placed lengthwise on the outside wall of the widened portion of the vessel.)
123. Nonincisional, transnasal placement of restrictive stent in right lacrimal duct	Ø8VX7DZ
124. Catheter-based temporary restriction of blood flow in abdominal aorta for treatment of cerebral ischemia	Ø4VØ3DJ
125. Percutaneous ligation of esophageal vein	Ø6L33ZZ
126. Percutaneous embolization of left internal carotid-cavernous fistula	Ø3LL3DZ
127. Laparoscopy with bilateral occlusion of fallopian tubes using Hulka extraluminal clips	ØUL74CZ
128. Open suture ligation of failed AV graft, left brachial artery	Ø3L8ØZZ
129. Percutaneous embolization of vascular supply, intracranial meningioma	Ø3LG3DZ
130. Percutaneous embolization of right uterine artery, using coils	Ø4LE3DT
131. Open occlusion of left atrial appendage, using extraluminal pressure clips	Ø2L7ØCK
132. Percutaneous suture exclusion of left atrial appendage, via femoral artery access	Ø2L73ZK
133. ERCP with balloon dilation of common bile duct	ØF798ZZ
134. PTCA of two coronary arteries, LAD with stent placement, RCA with no stent	Ø27Ø3DZ, Ø27Ø3ZZ (A separate procedure is coded for each artery dilated, since the device value differs for each artery.)
135. Cystoscopy with intraluminal dilation of bladder neck stricture	ØT7C8ZZ
136. Open dilation of old anastomosis, left femoral artery	Ø47LØZZ
137. Dilation of upper esophageal stricture, direct visualization, with Bougie sound	ØD717ZZ
138. PTA of right brachial artery stenosis	Ø3773ZZ
139. Transnasal dilation and stent placement in right lacrimal duct	Ø87X7DZ
140. Hysteroscopy with balloon dilation of bilateral fallopian tubes	ØU778ZZ
141. Tracheoscopy with intraluminal dilation of tracheal stenosis	ØB718ZZ
142. Cystoscopy with dilation of left ureteral stricture, with stent placement	ØT778DZ
143. Open gastric bypass with Roux-en-Y limb to jejunum	ØD16ØZA
144. Right temporal artery to intracranial artery bypass using Gore-Tex graft, open	Ø31SØJG
145. Tracheostomy formation with tracheostomy tube placement, percutaneous	ØB113F4
146. PICVA (percutaneous in situ coronary venous arterialization) of single coronary artery	Ø21Ø3D4
147. Open left femoral-popliteal artery bypass using cadaver vein graft	Ø41LØKL
148. Shunting of intrathecal cerebrospinal fluid to peritoneal cavity using synthetic shunt	ØØ16ØJ6
149. Colostomy formation, open, transverse colon to abdominal wall	ØD1LØZ4
150. Open urinary diversion, left ureter, using ileal conduit to skin	ØT17ØZC
151. CABG of LAD using pedicled left internal mammary artery, open off-bypass	Ø21ØØZ9

Procedure	Code
152. Open pleuroperitoneal shunt, right pleural cavity, using synthetic device	ØW19ØJG
153. Percutaneous placement of ventriculoperitoneal shunt for treatment of hydrocephalus	ØØ163J6
154. End-of-life replacement of spinal neurostimulator generator, multiple array, in lower abdomen	ØJH8ØDZ (Taking out of the old generator is coded separately to the root operation *Removal*)
155. Percutaneous insertion of spinal neurostimulator lead, lumbar spinal cord	ØØHV3MZ
156. Percutaneous replacement of broken pacemaker lead in left atrium	Ø2H73JZ (Taking out the broken pacemaker lead is coded separately to the root operation *Removal*.)
157. Open placement of dual chamber pacemaker generator in chest wall	ØJH6Ø6Z
158. Percutaneous placement of venous central line in right internal jugular, with tip in superior vena cava	Ø2HV33Z
159. Open insertion of multiple channel cochlear implant, left ear	Ø9HEØ6Z
160. Percutaneous placement of Swan-Ganz catheter in pulmonary trunk	Ø2HP32Z (The Swan-Ganz catheter is coded to the device value *Monitoring Device* because it monitors pulmonary artery output.)
161. Bronchoscopy with insertion of Low Dose Pd-103 brachytherapy seeds, right lung	ØBHK81Z, DB11BBZ
162. Open insertion of interspinous process device into lumbar vertebral joint	ØSHØØBZ
163. Open placement of bone growth stimulator, left femoral shaft	ØQHYØMZ
164. Cystoscopy with placement of brachytherapy seeds in prostate gland	ØVHØ81Z
165. Percutaneous insertion of Greenfield IVC filter	Ø6HØ3DZ
166. Full-thickness skin graft to right lower arm, autograft (do not code graft harvest for this exercise)	ØHRDX73
167. Excision of necrosed left femoral head with bone bank bone graft to fill the defect, open	ØQR7ØKZ
168. Penetrating keratoplasty of right cornea with donor matched cornea, percutaneous approach	Ø8R83KZ
169. Excision of abdominal aorta with Gore-Tex graft replacement, open	Ø4RØØJZ
170. Total right knee arthroplasty with insertion of total knee prosthesis	ØSRCØJZ
171. Tenonectomy with graft to right ankle using cadaver graft, open	ØLRSØKZ
172. Mitral valve replacement using porcine valve, open	Ø2RGØ8Z
173. Percutaneous phacoemulsification of right eye cataract with prosthetic lens insertion	Ø8RJ3JZ
174. Transcatheter replacement of pulmonary valve using of bovine jugular vein valve	Ø2RH38Z
175. Total left hip replacement using ceramic on ceramic prosthesis, without bone cement	ØSRBØ3A
176. Aortic valve annuloplasty using ring, open	Ø2UFØJZ
177. Laparoscopic repair of left inguinal hernia with marlex plug	ØYU64JZ
178. Autograft nerve graft to right median nerve, percutaneous endoscopic (do not code graft harvest for this exercise)	Ø1U547Z
179. Exchange of liner in femoral component of previous left hip replacement, open approach	ØSUSØ9Z (Taking out of the old liner is coded separately to the root operation *Removal*)

Appendix M: Coding Exercises and Answers

Procedure	Code
180. Anterior colporrhaphy with polypropylene mesh reinforcement, open approach	ØJUCØJZ
181. Implantation of CorCap cardiac support device, open approach	Ø2UAØJZ
182. Abdominal wall herniorrhaphy, open, using synthetic mesh	ØWUFØJZ
183. Tendon graft to strengthen injured left shoulder using autograft, open (do not code graft harvest for this exercise)	ØLU2Ø7Z
184. Onlay lamellar keratoplasty of left cornea using autograft, external approach	Ø8U9X7Z
185. Resurfacing procedure on right femoral head, open approach	ØSURØBZ
186. Exchange of drainage tube from right hip joint	ØS2YXØZ
187. Tracheostomy tube exchange	ØB21XFZ
188. Change chest tube for left pneumothorax	ØW2BXØZ
189. Exchange of cerebral ventriculostomy drainage tube	ØØ2ØXØZ
190. Foley urinary catheter exchange	ØT2BXØZ (This is coded to *Drainage Device* because urine is being drained.)
191. Open removal of lumbar sympathetic neurostimulator lead	Ø1PYØMZ
192. Nonincisional removal of Swan-Ganz catheter from right pulmonary artery	Ø2PYX2Z
193. Laparotomy with removal of pancreatic drain	ØFPGØØZ
194. Extubation, endotracheal tube	ØBP1XDZ
195. Nonincisional PEG tube removal	ØDP6XUZ
196. Transvaginal removal of brachytherapy seeds	ØUPH71Z
197. Transvaginal removal of extraluminal cervical cerclage	ØUPD7CZ
198. Incision with removal of K-wire fixation, right first metatarsal	ØQPNØ4Z
199. Cystoscopy with retrieval of left ureteral stent	ØTP98DZ
200. Removal of nasogastric drainage tube for decompression	ØDP6XØZ
201. Removal of external fixator, left radial fracture	ØPPJX5Z
202. Trimming and reanastomosis of stenosed femorofemoral synthetic bypass graft, open	Ø4WYØJZ
203. Open revision of right hip replacement, with readjustment of prosthesis	ØSW9ØJZ
204. Adjustment of position, pacemaker lead in left ventricle, percutaneous	Ø2WA3MZ
205. External repositioning of Foley catheter to bladder	ØTWBXØZ
206. Taking out loose screw and putting larger screw in fracture repair plate, left tibia	ØQWHØ4Z
207. Revision of totally implantable VAD port placement in chest wall, causing patient discomfort, open	ØJWTØWZ
208. Thoracotomy with exploration of right pleural cavity	ØWJ9ØZZ
209. Diagnostic laryngoscopy	ØCJS8ZZ
210. Exploratory arthrotomy of left knee	ØSJDØZZ
211. Colposcopy with diagnostic hysteroscopy	ØUJD8ZZ
212. Digital rectal exam	ØDJD7ZZ
213. Diagnostic arthroscopy of right shoulder	ØRJJ4ZZ
214. Endoscopy of maxillary sinus	Ø9JY4ZZ
215. Laparotomy with palpation of liver	ØFJØØZZ
216. Transurethral diagnostic cystoscopy	ØTJB8ZZ
217. Colonoscopy, discontinued at sigmoid colon	ØDJD8ZZ
218. Percutaneous mapping of basal ganglia	ØØK83ZZ
219. Heart catheterization with cardiac mapping	Ø2K83ZZ
220. Intraoperative whole brain mapping via craniotomy	ØØKØØZZ

Procedure	Code
221. Mapping of left cerebral hemisphere, percutaneous endoscopic	ØØK74ZZ
222. Intraoperative cardiac mapping during open heart surgery	Ø2K8ØZZ
223. Hysteroscopy with cautery of post-hysterectomy oozing and evacuation of clot	ØW3R8ZZ
224. Open exploration and ligation of post-op arterial bleeder, left forearm	ØX3FØZZ
225. Control of post-operative retroperitoneal bleeding via laparotomy	ØW3HØZZ
226. Reopening of thoracotomy site with drainage and control of post-op hemopericardium	ØW3DØZZ
227. Arthroscopy with drainage of hemarthrosis at previous operative site, right knee	ØY3F4ZZ
228. Radiocarpal fusion of left hand with internal fixation, open	ØRGPØ4Z
229. Posterior approach spinal fusion at L1-L3 level with BAK cage interbody fusion device, open	ØSG1ØAJ
230. Intercarpal fusion of right hand with bone bank bone graft, open	ØRGQØKZ
231. Sacrococcygeal fusion with bone graft from same operative site, open	ØSG5Ø7Z
232. Interphalangeal fusion of left great toe, percutaneous pin fixation	ØSGQ34Z
233. Suture repair of left radial nerve laceration	Ø1Q6ØZZ (The approach value is *Open*, though the surgical exposure may have been created by the wound itself.)
234. Laparotomy with suture repair of blunt force duodenal laceration	ØDQ9ØZZ
235. Perineoplasty with repair of old obstetric laceration, open	ØWQNØZZ
236. Suture repair of right biceps tendon (upper arm) laceration, open	ØLQ3ØZZ
237. Closure of abdominal wall stab wound	ØWQFØZZ
238. Cosmetic face lift, open, no other information available	ØWØ2ØZZ
239. Bilateral breast augmentation with silicone implants, open	ØHØVØJZ
240. Cosmetic rhinoplasty with septal reduction and tip elevation using local tissue graft, open	Ø9ØKØ7Z
241. Abdominoplasty (tummy tuck), open	ØWØFØZZ
242. Liposuction of bilateral thighs	ØJØL3ZZ, ØJØM3ZZ
243. Creation of penis in female patient using tissue bank donor graft	ØW4NØK1
244. Creation of vagina in male patient using synthetic material	ØW4MØJØ
245. Laparoscopic vertical (sleeve) gastrectomy	ØDB64Z3
246. Left uterine artery embolization with intraluminal biosphere injection	Ø4LF3DU

Obstetrics

Procedure	Code
1. Abortion by dilation and evacuation following laminaria insertion	1ØAØ7ZW
2. Manually assisted spontaneous abortion	1ØEØXZZ (Since the pregnancy was not artificially terminated, this is coded to *Delivery* because it captures the procedure objective. The fact that it was an abortion will be identified in the diagnosis code.)
3. Abortion by abortifacient insertion	1ØAØ7ZX

Procedure	Code
4. Bimanual pregnancy examination	1ØJØ7ZZ
5. Extraperitoneal C-section, low transverse incision	1ØDØØZ1
6. Fetal spinal tap, percutaneous	1Ø9Ø3ZA
7. Fetal kidney transplant, laparoscopic	1ØYØ4ZS
8. Open in utero repair of congenital diaphragmatic hernia	1ØQØØZK (Diaphragm is classified to the *Respiratory* body system in the *Medical and Surgical* section.)
9. Laparoscopy with total excision of tubal pregnancy	1ØT24ZZ
10. Transvaginal removal of fetal monitoring electrode	1ØPØ73Z

Placement

Procedure	Code
1. Placement of packing material, right ear	2Y42X5Z
2. Mechanical traction of entire left leg	2W6MXØZ
3. Removal of splint, right shoulder	2W5AX1Z
4. Placement of neck brace	2W32X3Z
5. Change of vaginal packing	2YØ4X5Z
6. Packing of wound, chest wall	2W44X5Z
7. Sterile dressing placement to left groin region	2W27X4Z
8. Removal of packing material from pharynx	2Y5ØX5Z
9. Placement of intermittent pneumatic compression device, covering entire right arm	2W18X7Z
10. Exchange of pressure dressing to left thigh	2WØPX6Z

Administration

Procedure	Code
1. Peritoneal dialysis via indwelling catheter	3E1M39Z
2. Transvaginal artificial insemination	3EØP7LZ
3. Infusion of total parenteral nutrition via central venous catheter	3EØ436Z
4. Esophagogastroscopy with Botox injection into esophageal sphincter	3EØG8GC (Botulinum toxin is a paralyzing agent with temporary effects; it does not sclerose or destroy the nerve.)
5. Percutaneous irrigation of knee joint	3E1U38Z
6. Systemic infusion of recombinant tissue plasminogen activator (r-tPA) via peripheral venous catheter	3EØ3317
7. Transabdominal in vitro fertilization, implantation of donor ovum	3EØP3Q1
8. Autologous bone marrow transplant via central venous line	3Ø243GØ
9. Implantation of anti-microbial envelope with cardiac defibrillator placement, open	3EØ1Ø2A
10. Sclerotherapy of brachial plexus lesion, alcohol injection	3EØT3TZ
11. Percutaneous peripheral vein injection, glucarpidase	3EØ33GQ
12. Introduction of anti-infective envelope into subcutaneous tissue, open	3EØ1Ø2A

Measurement and Monitoring

Procedure	Code
1. Cardiac stress test, single measurement	4AØ2XM4
2. EGD with biliary flow measurement	4AØC85Z
3. Right and left heart cardiac catheterization with bilateral sampling and pressure measurements	4AØ23N8

Procedure	Code
4. Temperature monitoring, rectal	4A1Z7KZ
5. Peripheral venous pulse, external, single measurement	4AØ4XJ1
6. Holter monitoring	4A12X45
7. Respiratory rate, external, single measurement	4AØ9XCZ
8. Fetal heart rate monitoring, transvaginal	4A1H7CZ
9. Visual mobility test, single measurement	4AØ7X7Z
10. Left ventricular cardiac output monitoring from pulmonary artery wedge (Swan-Ganz) catheter	4A1239Z
11. Olfactory acuity test, single measurement	4AØ8XØZ

Extracorporeal or Systemic Assistance and Performance

Procedure	Code
1. Intermittent mechanical ventilation, 16 hours	5A1935Z
2. Liver dialysis, single encounter	5A1CØØZ
3. Cardiac countershock with successful conversion to sinus rhythm	5A22Ø4Z
4. IPPB (intermittent positive pressure breathing) for mobilization of secretions, 22 hours	5AØ9358
5. Renal dialysis, 12 hours	5A1D8ØZ
6. IABP (intra-aortic balloon pump) continuous	5AØ221Ø
7. Intra-operative cardiac pacing, continuous	5A1223Z
8. Intraoperative ECMO (extracorporeal membrane oxygenation), central	5A15A2F
9. Controlled mechanical ventilation (CMV), 45 hours	5A1945Z
10. Pulsatile compression boot with intermittent inflation	5AØ2115 (This is coded to the function value *Cardiac Output*, because the purpose of such compression devices is to return blood to the heart faster.)

Extracorporeal or Systemic Therapies

Procedure	Code
1. Donor thrombocytapheresis, single encounter	6A55ØZ2
2. Bili-lite phototherapy, series treatment	6A6Ø1ZZ
3. Whole body hypothermia, single treatment	6A4ZØZZ
4. Circulatory phototherapy, single encounter	6A65ØZZ
5. Shock wave therapy of plantar fascia, single treatment	6A93ØZZ
6. Antigen-free air conditioning, series treatment	6AØZ1ZZ
7. TMS (transcranial magnetic stimulation), series treatment	6A221ZZ
8. Therapeutic ultrasound of peripheral vessels, single treatment	6A75ØZ6
9. Plasmapheresis, series treatment	6A551Z3
10. Extracorporeal electromagnetic stimulation (EMS) for urinary incontinence, single treatment	6A21ØZZ

Osteopathic

Procedure	Code
1. Isotonic muscle energy treatment of right leg	7WØ6X8Z
2. Low velocity-high amplitude osteopathic treatment of head	7WØØX5Z
3. Lymphatic pump osteopathic treatment of left axilla	7WØ7X6Z
4. Indirect osteopathic treatment of sacrum	7WØ4X4Z
5. Articulatory osteopathic treatment of cervical region	7WØ1XØZ

Other Procedures

Procedure	Code
1. Near infrared spectroscopy of leg vessels	8EØ23DZ
2. CT computer assisted sinus surgery	8EØ9XBG (The primary procedure is coded separately.)
3. Suture removal, abdominal wall	8EØWXY8
4. Isolation after infectious disease exposure	8EØZXY6
5. Robotic assisted open prostatectomy	8EØWØCZ (The primary procedure is coded separately.)
6. In vitro fertilization	8EØZXY1

Chiropractic

Procedure	Code
1. Chiropractic treatment of lumbar region using long lever specific contact	9WB3XGZ
2. Chiropractic manipulation of abdominal region, indirect visceral	9WB9XCZ
3. Chiropractic extra-articular treatment of hip region	9WB6XDZ
4. Chiropractic treatment of sacrum using long and short lever specific contact	9WB4XJZ
5. Mechanically-assisted chiropractic manipulation of head	9WBØXKZ

Imaging

Procedure	Code
1. Noncontrast CT of abdomen and pelvis	BW21ZZZ
2. Intravascular ultrasound, left subclavian artery	B342ZZ3
3. Fluoroscopic guidance for insertion of central venous catheter in SVC, low osmolar contrast	B5181ZA
4. Chest x-ray, AP/PA and lateral views	BWØ3ZZZ
5. Endoluminal ultrasound of gallbladder and bile ducts	BF43ZZZ
6. MRI of thyroid gland, contrast unspecified	BG34YZZ
7. Esophageal videofluoroscopy study with oral barium contrast	BD11YZZ
8. Portable x-ray study of right radius/ulna shaft, standard series	BPØJZZZ
9. Routine fetal ultrasound, second trimester twin gestation	BY4DZZZ
10. CT scan of bilateral lungs, high osmolar contrast with densitometry	BB24ØZZ
11. Fluoroscopic guidance for percutaneous transluminal angioplasty (PTA) of left common femoral artery, low osmolar contrast	B41G1ZZ

Nuclear Medicine

Procedure	Code
1. Tomo scan of right and left heart, unspecified radiopharmaceutical, qualitative gated rest	C226YZZ
2. Technetium pentetate assay of kidneys, ureters, and bladder	CT631ZZ
3. Uniplanar scan of spine using technetium oxidronate, with first-pass study	CP151ZZ
4. Thallous chloride tomographic scan of bilateral breasts	CH22SZZ
5. PET scan of myocardium using rubidium	C23GQZZ
6. Gallium citrate scan of head and neck, single plane imaging	CW1BLZZ
7. Xenon gas nonimaging probe of brain	CØ5ØVZZ
8. Upper GI scan, radiopharmaceutical unspecified, for gastric emptying	CD15YZZ
9. Carbon 11 PET scan of brain with quantification	CØ3ØBZZ
10. Iodinated albumin nuclear medicine assay, blood plasma volume study	C763HZZ

Radiation Therapy

Procedure	Code
1. Plaque radiation of left eye, single port	D8YØFZZ
2. 8 MeV photon beam radiation to brain	DØØ11ZZ
3. IORT of colon, 3 ports	DDY5CZZ
4. HDR brachytherapy of prostate using low dose palladium-103, unidirectional source	DV1ØBB1
5. Electron radiation treatment of right breast, with custom device	DMØ13ZZ
6. Hyperthermia oncology treatment of pelvic region	DWY68ZZ
7. Contact radiation of tongue	D9Y57ZZ
8. Heavy particle radiation treatment of pancreas, four risk sites	DFØ34ZZ
9. LDR brachytherapy to spinal cord using iodine	DØ16B9Z
10. Whole body Phosphorus 32 administration with risk to hematopoetic system	DWY5GFZ

Physical Rehabilitation and Diagnostic Audiology

Procedure	Code
1. Bekesy assessment using audiometer	F13Z31Z
2. Individual fitting of left eye prosthesis	FØDZ8UZ
3. Physical therapy for range of motion and mobility, patient right hip, no special equipment	FØ7LØZZ
4. Bedside swallow assessment using assessment kit	FØØZHYZ
5. Caregiver training in airway clearance techniques	FØFZ8ZZ
6. Application of short arm cast in rehabilitation setting	FØDZ7EZ (Inhibitory cast is listed in the equipment reference table under E, *Orthosis.*)
7. Verbal assessment of patient's pain level	FØ2ZFZZ
8. Caregiver training in communication skills using manual communication board	FØFZJMZ (Manual communication board is listed in the equipment reference table under M, *Augmentative/ Alternative Communication.*)

Procedure	Code
9. Group musculoskeletal balance training exercises, whole body, no special equipment	FØ7M6ZZ (Balance training is included in the motor treatment reference table under *Therapeutic Exercise*.)
10. Individual therapy for auditory processing using tape recorder	FØ9Z2KZ (Tape recorder is listed in the equipment reference table under *Audiovisual Equipment*.)

Mental Health

Procedure	Code
1. Cognitive-behavioral psychotherapy, individual	GZ58ZZZ
2. Narcosynthesis	GZGZZZZ
3. Light therapy	GZJZZZZ
4. ECT (electroconvulsive therapy), unilateral, multiple seizure	GZB1ZZZ
5. Crisis intervention	GZ2ZZZZ
6. Neuropsychological testing	GZ13ZZZ
7. Hypnosis	GZFZZZZ
8. Developmental testing	GZ1ØZZZ
9. Vocational counseling	GZ61ZZZ
10. Family psychotherapy	GZ72ZZZ

Substance Abuse Treatment

Procedure	Code
1. Naltrexone treatment for drug dependency	HZ94ZZZ
2. Substance abuse treatment family counseling	HZ63ZZZ
3. Medication monitoring of patient on methadone maintenance	HZ81ZZZ
4. Individual interpersonal psychotherapy for drug abuse	HZ54ZZZ
5. Patient in for alcohol detoxification treatment	HZ2ZZZZ
6. Group motivational counseling	HZ47ZZZ
7. Individual 12-step psychotherapy for substance abuse	HZ53ZZZ
8. Post-test infectious disease counseling for IV drug abuser	HZ3CZZZ
9. Psychodynamic psychotherapy for drug dependent patient	HZ5CZZZ
10. Group cognitive-behavioral counseling for substance abuse	HZ42ZZZ

New Technology

Procedure	Code
1. Infusion of terlipressin via peripheral venous catheter	XWØ3367
2. Transcatheter dilation of left peroneal artery with 2 SAVAL stents	X27U395